OBSTETRICS — *The history of a book*

In 1913 the W. B. Saunders Company published a memorable book entitled "Principles and Practice of Obstetrics." It was written by Joseph B. DeLee, one of the foremost obstetricians of all times. The book quickly became a necessity for practicing physicians, obstetric specialists and medical students, not only in the United States but also in other countries.

DeLee wrote six more editions of his book. It was my great fortune in 1939 to be asked by both the W. B. Saunders Company and Doctor DeLee to take over its writing. Naturally I was overjoyed with this honor. My first edition was the eighth since 1913 and appeared in 1943. I wrote five more editions, the last one in 1965.

The following principal translations of the book have been made:

DeLee and Greenhill: Principles and Practice of Obstetrics. 8th Edition. Spanish, UTEHA, Mexico City. Published 1945.

DeLee and Greenhill: Principles and Practice of Obstetrics. 9th Edition. Portuguese, Editora Guanabara Koogan, Rio de Janeiro. Published 1949.

DeLee and Greenhill: Principles and Practice of Obstetrics. 9th Edition. Italian, Casa Editrice G. Principato, Milan. Published 1954.

Greenhill: Obstetrics. 11th Edition, 2 volumes. Spanish, UTEHA, Mexico City. Published 1956.

Greenhill: Obstetrics. 12th Edition. Serbo Croat, Medicinska Knjiga, Belgrade. Published 1961.

The present book is entirely new, having been completely rewritten, and contains the combined teaching and practice experiences of Emanuel A. Friedman and myself. We have attempted to maintain the DeLee tradition of excellence in providing a compendium of updated safe obstetric principles and techniques for student and practitioner alike.

J. P. GREENHILL

Biological Principles
and
Modern Practice of
OBSTETRICS

J. P. GREENHILL, M.D.

Senior Attending Obstetrician and Gynecologist, the Michael Reese Hospital; Professor of Gynecology, Emeritus, Cook County Graduate School of Medicine, Chicago

EMANUEL A. FRIEDMAN, M.D., Med. Sc. D.

Professor of Obstetrics and Gynecology, Harvard Medical School; Obstetrician-Gynecologist-in-Chief, Beth Israel Hospital, Boston

W. B. SAUNDERS COMPANY

Philadelphia · London · Toronto

W. B. Saunders Company: West Washington Square
Philadelphia, Pa. 19105

12 Dyott Street
London, WC1A 1DB

833 Oxford Street
Toronto, Ontario M8Z 5T9, Canada

Biological Principles and Modern Practice of Obstetrics   ISBN 0-7216-4257-8

Print No.:   9   8   7   6   5   4   3   2

PREFACE

After exactly sixty years a new name appears as a co-author of the Textbook of Obstetrics first written by the revered and great Joseph B. DeLee who prepared six subsequent editions. It was my great fortune and honor to write six more editions of DeLee's book, the last in 1965. Now it is with the greatest gratification and pride that I welcome Emanuel A. Friedman as co-author of this altogether new text in Obstetrics. He has performed a herculean task and has done by far the major part of writing this edition.

We have deliberately condensed the size of the book considerably, both as regards the text and the number of illustrations, eliminating material that is no longer relevant, reorienting emphasis as needed and adding much that is new. In so doing we hope we have enhanced the quality of the book for teaching students, residents in training, practicing physicians and nurses.

It will be obvious to those who are familiar with previous editions that every page of the book has been entirely rewritten. Hence this is truly a new book. However, in doing this we have again tried to maintain the ideals of Doctor DeLee and brought them up to date.

Both Doctor Friedman and I owe a great debt of gratitude to the officers and staff of the W. B. Saunders Company — especially to John L. Dusseau. Without their assistance and cooperation this book could not have appeared.

We hope this new work will prove as helpful as the previous ones to physicians and medical students throughout the world.

J. P. GREENHILL

CONTENTS

SECTION ONE

PHYSIOLOGY AND CONDUCT OF PREGNANCY

Chapter 1

Introduction

"Whoever she is, I want my mother's body to be a fit factory for the building of my own. I want her mind to be free of oppression and able to want me and to care for me, and to love me as I will one day come to love her. Whatever race I am born to, for the sake of all races, I want my home to be secure enough that no feeling of hopelessness or myth of inferiority will be passed on to me. Whatever schooling is available to me, I want the chance to learn what I will need to learn in order to grow. Under whatever kind of government I am born, I want equal justice under which I will forge my own freedom." In these words, speaking for the fetus, Downs keynoted the first National Congress on the Quality of Life, a recent multidisciplinary conclave devoted to the many serious sociologic, environmental and economic problems which have well-documented adverse effects on pregnancy, the intrauterine milieu and the subsequent growth and development of the infant. This statement hallmarks the recognition and acceptance by society of the critical importance of the intrauterine life that is placed in the care of obstetricians. There can be no doubt whatsoever that the objectives of obstetrics must be to ensure that every child will develop to the fullest measure the potential with which he was endowed at conception.

The origins of the term *obstetrics* are obscure, but it is generally held that it derives from the Latin *obstare*, meaning to stand near or before, or to protect. The Latin feminine noun form *obstetrix* refers to her who stands by or before, that is, the position of the midwife. Use of the word *midwifery* and the phrase *maternity care* is diminishing as they are replaced by *obstetrics*. The term *tocology*, study of the uterus, has not gained wide popularity.

In the narrow academic sense, *obstetrics* is that branch of medicine dealing with reproduction function. Although originally applied specifically to labor and delivery, the term has by usage come to refer to all aspects of the reproductive spectrum, including conception and conception control, pregnancy and its pathology, parturition, lactation and the puerperium. In a much broader sense derived as a consequence of societal emphases on relevance and awareness, obstetrics must deal with the essence of mankind and its survival. While dealing with the epitome of procreation as it relates to sexual instincts and drives, psychological and hormonal influences and the intricacies of embryogenesis, obstetrics must also concern itself with defining and detecting factors which have adverse effects on these processes, aiming to prevent destruction or suboptimal development.

Moreover, this discipline has within its scope considerations relative to the survival of mankind as a whole, not only with reference to factors affecting intrauterine development but also with regard to the global issue of the population crisis which is anticipated by the end of this century if population growth continues to outstrip the availability of consumables while pollution continues to foul the diminishing supplies of usable air and potable water. Thus it becomes imperative that we maximize the quality of life of all conceptuses, attempt to ensure that all are wanted and provide the wherewithal to allow prospective parents the option of conceiving or not. As the number of offspring produced is diminished, it is doubly essential that we optimize outcome for every one conceived.

We are witnessing a decided shift in emphasis toward a critical concern for the surviving infant. This is not at all meant to imply deemphasis of the importance of the mother's health and survival. Nothing could possibly be more important to every physician called upon to deal with pregnant women and obstetric problems. But a healthy mother and a living child are minimal objectives only; we cannot be satisfied with anything short of optimal conditions for the surviving infant. Toward this end we see the development of a new field, *perinatology* or *perinatal medicine*.

Well satisfied with its apparent success in essentially eliminating maternal mortality, obstetrics has turned with enthusiasm to the examination of perinatal mortality and morbidity also. It brings to the attempt the tried tools of statistical analysis, self-criticism and perfection of perinatal care. Perinatal mortality has perhaps declined slightly as a result of initial efforts along these lines, but there remains a solid residue of death and damage, seemingly resistant even to the perfect application of all accepted clinical principles. It is clear that only new approaches will suffice in this regard.

The discipline of obstetrics stands at a turning point in its history. Its accomplishments to date have been prodigious. Indeed, it may be said that what has been done has been the essential task required of it. The appreciation of the fact that fetal and neonatal life are actually a continuum of the same process has resulted in the development of synergistic alliances of individuals whose dissimilar interests, knowledge and expertise can be brought to bear in a cooperative venture for purposes of enhancing comprehensive perinatal care. There is little doubt that the future will require close cooperation between obstetricians, pediatricians, anesthesiologists, biochemists, biophysicists, bioengineers, pathologists, geneticists, statisticians, public health and social workers, as well as specially trained nursing and paramedical personnel.

The most obvious example of the benefits of such cooperative efforts between members of different specialties working toward a common goal is seen in the conquest of Rh isoimmunization (see Chapter 52). By means of the team approach focusing down on this problem, cooperative competence in tangentially interrelated fields was pooled not only to diagnose and treat affected mothers, fetuses and babies but also to uncover underlying pathogenetic mechanisms, to introduce effective therapy and, most recently, essentially to eliminate the problem for future generations by prophylactic measures.

Equally exciting are the newly available techniques for assessing the status of the fetoplacental unit *in utero* in the course of pregnancies complicated by conditions which may affect the fetus adversely (see Chapter 13). The evaluation of such high-risk situations, dealt with at length throughout this book in the various chapters on the specific problems, demands interdisciplinary exchanges between all interested members of the team. Such exchanges not only promote fruitful communication, intellectual stimulation and mutual understanding, but also directly benefit those fetuses at risk.

It is apparent that, in order for obstetrics to fulfill its goal of optimizing fetal outcome, we will ultimately need means for continuously assessing the functional status of the placenta and the well-being of the fetus throughout pregnancy and labor. Moreover, we must be apprised of the diverse and sometimes deleterious effects of drugs ingested by the mother that may endanger the fetus during its intrauterine life (see Chapter 51). Similarly, certain disease states which may have negligible manifestations in the mother, notably certain relatively innocuous viremias (see Chapter 40), may have disastrous effects on the fetus.

The single, pervading objective of obstetrics, as stated earlier, is to minimize maternal risks inherent in pregnancy, while at the same time optimizing fetal outcome to produce a healthy, living infant that will have the capability to attain the full potential he was endowed with at the moment of conception. A physician's management of pregnancy, therefore, has the dual objective of a healthy mother and a healthy baby. However, the fetus is relatively inaccessible before birth. Most of the practical means for diagnosis and treatment must be applied to the mother. The fetus is physiologically dependent on the mother and may be influenced to a considerable extent by treatments administered to her. Nevertheless, the fetus is generally unable to indicate the consequences of such exogenous influences, whether they are subtle or overt. The combination of dependence and inaccessibility, while offering some protection against the hostile outside and intrauterine environment, presents the able practitioner with a challenge to provide both mother and fetus with his full due consideration.

The challenge is difficult to meet because the fetus is obscured by the abdominal and uterine walls and is undergoing phenomenal changes in form and function. As a result the fetus changes its susceptibility to various potentially injurious factors. These changes are especially profound and rapid during the first few weeks following conception. The relationship between fetal vulnerability and the developmental stage is sufficiently well understood that the earliest stages of embryogenesis are the most sensitive (see Chapter 69). However, specific remedial techniques are not yet available and constitute the subject of much ongoing research.

We strive in this book to present standards of good obstetric care that ought to be available and practiced everywhere, even in the absence of sophisticated facilities and programs in perinatal medicine. At the same time, we have indicated those special situations in which perinatology has already made significant inroads toward bridging the gap between theoretically optimal care and that which is currently practiced. There seems to be a salutary trend, particularly in metropolitan areas, to the development of regionalized centers for the intensive care of sick infants. One needs little clairvoyance to visualize a time in the not-too-distant future when selected obstetric patients will be referred, as a matter of course before the baby is born, to regional centers where the intrauterine patient may be studied and treated according to its needs.

The remarkable reduction in maternal and fetal mortality since the turn of this century indicates the great advances that have been made in this discipline. All of our efforts in the first four or five decades were directed toward reduction of maternal deaths in association with childbearing. Today we proudly note that, except for rare instances involving unconscionable neglect or errors in judgment, or occurring in outlying areas where obstetrical care is essentially nonexistent, a maternal death is an unusual and avoidable tragic occurrence. In this new era of obstetrical safety for the mother, our attention is focused more and more on the infant.

Progress has been seen in the 10-fold reduction in neonatal death rates from 1900 to 1970. Although this is substantive and worthy of note, it is certainly not good enough, especially since we are well aware that more than half the infant losses are probably avoidable. This rate of loss of life at birth cannot be equated with death rates in adults. The death of an infant, whose life expectancy is of the order of about 70 years, is not the same as the death of an adult from diseases which strike in the later mature years when natural life expectancy is relatively much shorter. If this difference in terms of relative losses of productive, useful years of life is taken into account, one can begin to understand the real significance of the problem we are faced with and garner an understanding of the importance of this field in perspective.

REFERENCE

Downs, H.: Keynote address. National Congress on the Quality of Life, Chicago, March 22–25, 1972. A.M.A. News, April 3, 1972.

Chapter 2

The Ovum, Ovulation and Conception

OOGENESIS

The adult ovaries are densely fibrous, paired organs situated on the posterior aspect of the broad ligaments (Fig. 1). The ovary is shaped like an unshelled almond and measures 25 to 50 mm. in length, 15 to 30 mm. in width and 7 to 15 mm. in thickness. It normally weighs between 4 and 8 gm. The ovary is suspended to the posterior (dorsocranial) aspect of the broad ligament of the uterus by a transverse fold of peritoneum. At the center of this fold the *mesovarium* contains the vasculature and nerve connections to the ovary. The ovary is attached medially to the uterine cornu by a cylinder of smooth muscle and connective tissue sheathed in a layer of peritoneum, the *utero-ovarian* (or ovarian) *ligament.* Laterally the ovarian artery, veins, lymphatics and nerves course in the free border of the broad ligament, in the

structure called the *infundibulopelvic ligament* (suspensory ligament or plica of the ovary). The ovary itself is covered by a layer of low columnar epithelium, misnamed *germinal epithelium.* The term was applied originally because it was felt that these cells gave rise to ova. This, of course, has been shown to be incorrect but the name remains. Beneath this investiture is a tough *tunica albuginea.* Within the deeper cortical layer are found many oocytes surrounded by a characteristic, highly cellular, reticular connective tissue stroma. Centrally in the hilum are located the ovary's abundant blood supply and lymphatic collecting system as well as numerous fine nerves forming intricate networks.

The primitive gonad, into which the primordial germ cells will ultimately migrate, takes its origin from the urogenital ridge, a longitudinal thickening of the dor-

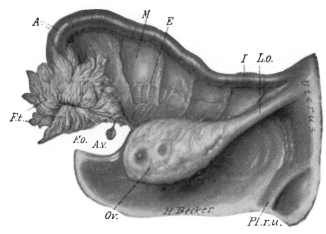

Figure 1 Anatomic configuration of the adult left tube and ovary as seen when observed from above and behind. The uterine tube has been lifted forward and upward to reveal the ovary. *Ov.,* ovary; *A.v.,* appendix vesiculosa; *F.o.,* fimbria ovarica; *F.t.,* fimbriae tubae; *A,* ampulla; *M,* mesosalpinx; *E,* epoophoron; *I,* isthmus; *L.o.,* ligamentum ovarii proprium; *Pl.r.u.,* plica recto-uterina. The infundibulopelvic ligament which contains the ovarian blood vessels and traverses along the upper border of the broad ligament is not shown.

4

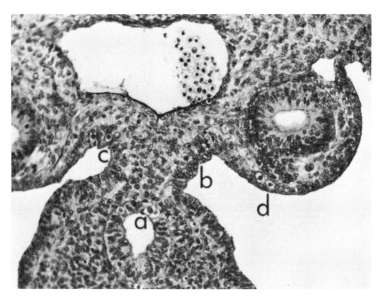

Figure 2 Cross section of an embryo of 28 days age after ovulation, 4.5 mm. crown-rump length, showing primordial germ cells during migration found in either epithelium, mesenchyme, or peritoneum of (*a*) the gut, (*b*) the mesentery, (*c*) the coelomic angle, or (*d*) the urogenital ridge. (Magnification × 200.) (From Witschi, E.: Contrib. Embryol. 32:67, 1948.)

sal coelomic wall (Fig. 2). The ovary is derived from the median aspect of the ridge and is first distinguishable as a thickening of the coelomic epithelium and the mesenchyme beneath it. Gillman was able to detect its existence rather indistinctly by 29 days after ovulation (6.5 mm. crown-rump length), showing it quite clearly set off from the mesonephros by grooved indentations at day 33 (9.5 mm. crown-rump) (Figs. 3 and 4). These grooves continue to deepen to form the mesovarium. The early thickening of the coelomic epithelium into the genital ridge is not homogeneous in that local accumulations of cells move into the mesenchyme as fingerlike sex cords. The intervening epithelium remains to become the covering of the gonad. After about day 34 (10.6 mm. crown-rump length), the primordial germ cells which have remained in the mesenchyme begin to be incorporated into the cords in the outer third of the gonad. They are carried inward as the cords push centrally. By day 37 (15 mm. crown-rump), female differentiation of the embryonic gonad begins. The sex cords become less distinct because they break up into separate clumps of cells destined to form primary ovarian follicles. This lack of distinctness of sex

cords is emphasized by the sparseness of the mesenchyme separating them.

Van Wagenen and Simpson have recently described the embryonic development of the human ovary in still greater detail. They demonstrated two streaks of coelomic mesothelium appearing on the

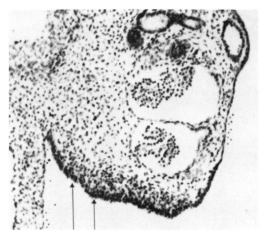

Figure 3 Cross section of the genital ridge of a 6.7 mm. crown-rump embryo of age 31 days showing primordial germ cells in the gonad primordium 4 mm. above the ends of the arrows. They have just become distinguishable because of the thickening of the epithelium and the condensation of the immediately underlying mesenchyme. (From Gillman, J.: Contrib. Embryol. 32:81, 1948.)

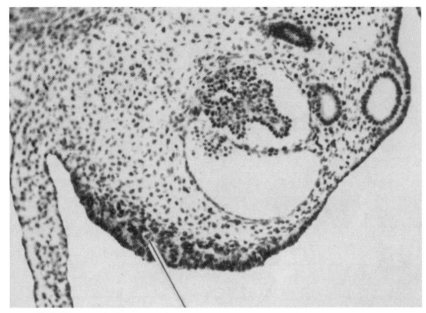

Figure 4 Sex cords forming by means of epithelial proliferation in the genital ridge of an 8.2 mm. crown-rump embryo at age 33 days. One sex cord is shown curving around the primordial germ cells at the end of the arrow. Note the concurrent development of the mesonephros in the dorsolateral aspect of the genital ridge.

posterior wall of the abdomen in the embryo, located on the ventral surface of the wolffian (muellerian) bodies. This thickened mesothelium is seen as early as 28 days following conception (crown-rump length 5.8 mm., menstrual age 42 days). A definite raised genital ridge is recognized in the fetus at 35 days (12 mm. crown-rump length, 49 days menstrual age). Here the surface cells appear to be infiltrating the mesenchyme. Primitive granulosa cells cannot be distinguished from the sex cells. The youngest definitive ovary is obtained from an embryo of ovulation age 40 days (20 mm. crown-rump length). It is composed mostly of cells of uniform size and a few scattered large cells. The ovary is spade shaped at this stage in its development (Fig. 5) with a crenated surface. It increases rapidly in size by mitosis of cells and by cellular enlargement. As it grows and the mesonephros atrophies, the ovary protrudes into the peritoneal cavity, suspended by an increasingly delicate mesovarium. Mesenchymatous tissue from the mesonephric region grows into the gonad, bearing with it blood vessels. Simultaneously, the ovary becomes organized into a structure with a cortex and a medulla.

The connective tissue continues to grow radially from the medulla into the cortex, dividing it into lobules and forming a tunica albuginea. The further development of

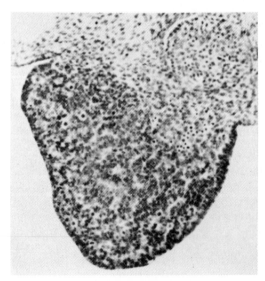

Figure 5 Genital ridge from a 10.6 mm. crown-rump embryo of age 37 days, illustrating primordial germ cells lying between and perhaps within sex cords near the periphery. Here the cords are most widely separated. Centrally, the rete is beginning to form from the tips of the sex cords.

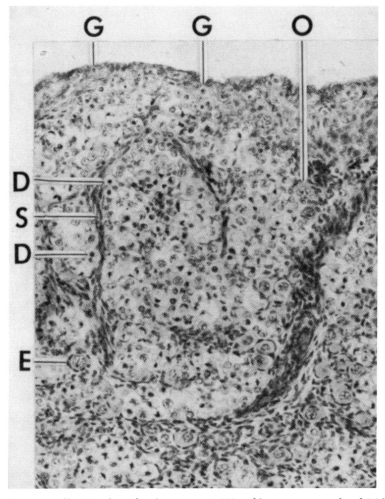

Figure 6   Ovarian germ cells (*G*) enlarged to form oogonia (*O*) and become encapsulated (*E*) by follicle cells or degenerate (*D*) when they come into contact with advancing fetal stroma (*S*) prior to encapsulation. This phenomenon is seen here in a 190 mm. crown-rump embryo of about 22 weeks' menstrual age.

ovarian characteristics involves formation of primary ovarian follicles and fetal ovarian stroma.

Primordial follicles are first formed at the corticomedullary boundary at about the eighteenth week menstrual age (140 mm. crown-rump length) (Fig. 6). The incorporated primordial germ cells arise in the disorganized clumps of cells derived from the sex cords. These enlarged primitive ova or *oogonia* compress the surrounding sex cord cells to form the primitive granulosa or prefollicle cells which encapsulate them. Active mitotic reproduction of oogonia continues until 22 weeks menstrual age (190 mm. crown-

rump length). At this stage of development the total number of germ cells reaches its maximum of about 7 million. Oogonial mitosis rapidly decreases, disappearing entirely from about the thirtieth week menstrual age to term. Thus the ova are nearly all produced during fetal life, although it is conceivable that some are formed during the first year of extrauterine life.

The number of oocytes in a given ovary at birth varies from 422,000 to 575,000 according to Sappy (cited in Häggström). Häggström calculated that the ovaries of a 22-year-old woman contained 420,000 ova. Of these, 1525 had begun to grow beyond the stage of primordial follicles and 141 had developed into graafian follicles. About 1200 follicles of all sizes showed signs of atresia. A total of 67 postovulatory corpora were seen (9 corpora lutea and 58 corpora albicantia). These numbers have been confirmed by both Block and Baker. Nearly all ova will ultimately degenerate through the mechanism of atresia. Perhaps no more than 500 or 0.1 per cent will undergo maturation processes and ovulation and fewer than five or so (0.001 per cent) will ever be fertilized. The maximum number that can take part in ovulation is, of course, based on the duration of reproductive life. Assuming 9 to 13 ovulations annually, one can calculate the number of ovulations possible in a woman whose ovaries can function actively for 30 to 35 years to be between 270 and 455.

Fetal ovarian stroma begins to form after 22 weeks menstrual age by mesenchymal proliferation from the center of the ovary to the periphery. Primitive ova that have not become encapsulated degenerate in the pathway of the advancing stroma. The stroma eventually forms the theca that surrounds ovarian follicles. It is interesting to note that such degeneration of oogonia on contact with proliferating stroma may be followed by a period of renewed proliferation of peripheral coelomic epithelium and germ cells resulting in an invasion similar to that of the sex cords. Zuckerman considers this second proliferation as the primary source of ova for mammals in general. Gillman, on the other hand, considers the first proliferation most important and regards the second as a compensatory phenomenon that is inconstant and variable in the human embryo.

Pinkerton et al. defined the characteristic staining properties of the germ cells and traced their migration into the primitive gonad. They found that migration had been completed by the fourth week following conception and that the number of germ cells had increased to a maximum by the fifteenth week. Thereafter a maturation process occurred in which oogenesis and the development of the surrounding granulosa proceeded apace. Baker found a total of 600,000 ova in serial sections of the human ovary at two months after conception, 7,000,000 at five months, and 2,000,000 at birth. Of those present at birth, one half were already undergoing atresia and by age seven only 300,000 remained. It appears correct that oogenesis ceases at or near birth. Blandau has cinematographically recorded the actual amoeboid locomotion of germ cells in mouse and human embryos.

The germ cells separate from stem cells during early cleavage stages and first become recognizable in embryos at four weeks after conception. They are seen embedded in the dorsal yolk sac epithelium above the allantoic evagination. They migrate during the fifth week of embryonic development to the site of the gonad primordia. They serve as the only source of ova. The ovarian cortex is a specialized strip of peritoneal epithelium that arises as a thickening along the median edge of the mesonephric bodies. The primitive gonad is furnished with follicle cells from the cortex that ultimately become granulosa cells. The cortex is the site of oogenesis and possesses characteristic endocrine potential. The ovarian medulla originates from the medial mesonephric blastema. It gives rise to interstitial cells and contributes to the formation of the follicular theca in advanced stages of oogenesis.

OVULATION

Germ cells develop from primary oocytes into gametes within follicles in the cortex of the ovary (Fig. 7). A *follicle* is composed of an oocyte and the follicular or granulosa cells surrounding it. The resting primordial follicle in the mature ovary is essentially unchanged morphologically when compared with similar structures in the neonatal ovary. Typically, it is located in the periphery of the ovarian cortex. The primary oocyte is about 20μ in diameter. Its cell membrane is not apparent and the cytoplasm is rather pale. The nucleus is large and stains lightly with a nucleolus that is not prominent at first. A single layer of very flattened granulosa cells surrounds the primary oocyte (Fig. 8).

When a follicle begins to develop in the mature ovary, all its elements enlarge and the nucleolus becomes increasingly distinct. The follicle cells become cuboidal

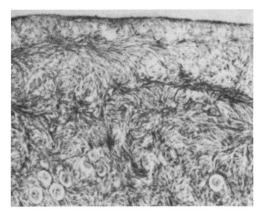

Figure 7 Cortex of an adult human ovary showing germinal epithelium on the outer surface of the dense, fibrous tunica albuginea. There are a few primary follicles in the fibrous tissue of the cortex below the tunica. (Magnification × 110.) (From Witschi, E.: Development of Vertebrates. Philadelphia, W. B. Saunders Company, 1956.)

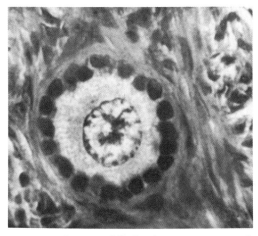

Figure 9 Primary follicle showing oocyte with one layer of cuboidal granulosa cells. (From Shettles, L. B.: Ovum Humanum. New York, Hafner Publishing Company, 1960.)

and the surrounding connective tissue becomes more obvious (Fig. 9). Coincident with enlargement of the primary oocyte, the surrounding granulosa cells proliferate to form multiple layers in an orderly arrangement (Fig. 10).

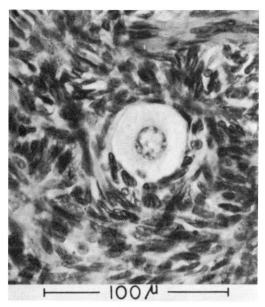

Figure 8 Early stage of a primary follicle in an ovary of a 19-year-old patient. Most of the follicular cells are still flat. The cell membrane of a primary oocyte, as shown here, is unusual to see. (Magnification × 500.)

Growth of the primary oocyte is limited, but the granulosa cells continue to proliferate. A mucoid oolemma or zona pellucida (Braden) begins to develop between the primary oocyte and the surrounding granulosa cells. This membrane is dense and homogeneous, attaining a width of 5μ in the mature follicle (Fig. 11). This membrane is actually perforated by numerous canals through which processes of the oocyte and the granulosa cells extend. This is undoubtedly a mechanism for mediating interchange of vital substances between the oocyte and the granulosa cells.

Thus the immature primary follicle develops into a *vesicular follicle* (graafian follicle) through a mechanism of proliferation of the granulosa cells and accumulation of follicular liquor in the interstitial spaces between the granulosa cells. Although it has long been assumed that the *liquor folliculi* is secreted by the granulosa cells, recent evidence suggests it to be the result of sequestration of ovarian lymph (Short). The fluid spaces fuse to form the *antrum* (Fig. 12). The liquor is clear, viscid, alkaline, albuminoid material containing oil globules and granules. As it continues to accumulate the antrum enlarges and the centrally located primary oocyte comes to lie against the wall of the follicle (Figs. 13 and 14) where it is surrounded by the *cumulus oophorus,* an investing cover-

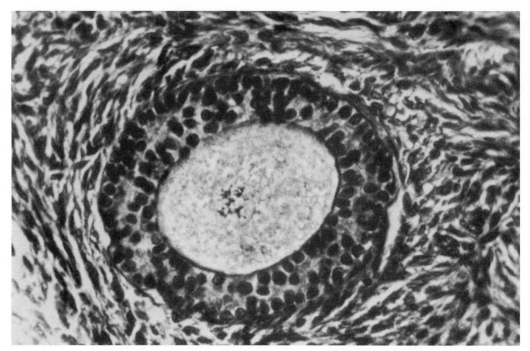

Figure 10   More advanced development of the primary follicle with two or more layers of granulosa cells. (From Shettles, L. B.: Ovum Humanum. New York, Hafner Publishing Company, 1960.)

ing of granulosa cells. Since the liquor accumulates quite rapidly, the granulosa layer becomes relatively thin and the ovum becomes eccentrically displaced to a polar position on the follicular globe. In this location it is embedded in a hillock of granulosa cells, the cumulus oophorus.

The granulosa cells bordering on the ovum become cuboidal in shape and form the *corona radiata*. This name is applied to these granulosa cells because they characteristically remain attached to the ovum after ovulation to form a radiating crown of cells.

The granulosa cells lining the rest of the antrum constitute the *stratum granulosum*. The stratum granulosum is devoid of blood vessels. The follicle rests on a layer of loose, highly vascular connective tissue, the *tunica interna*. This in turn is surrounded by a layer of closely packed fibrous tissue, the *tunica externa*. Both tuni-

cae are derived from the stroma of the ovary and are known collectively as the *theca folliculi* (Fig. 11*f*).

The granulosa cell layers are separated from the theca cells by a prominent basement membrane, called the *membrana propria*. The theca interna is made up of polyhedral cells and the theca externa of fusiform cells. Many fine blood vessels from the ovarian stroma penetrate the thecal layer but do not traverse the membrana propria. As the blood supply of the ovary increases, there is considerable local congestion around the growing follicles.

Vacuoles appear in the cumulus oophorus, loosening the attachment of the ovum and the corona radiata from surrounding granulosa cells. Late in follicular growth, the ovum and its corona radiata may dehisce from the follicular wall to float freely in the antrum. *Ovulation* involves the discharge of this cell mass from

Figure 11   A. Follicle with early formation of oolemma or zona pellucida. (From Shettles, L. B.: Ovum Humanum. New York, Hafner Publishing Co., 1960.) B. Follicle of a slightly later stage at the eighteenth day of the cycle showing *a*, ovum; *b*, oocyte nucleus; *c*, oolemma or zona pellucida; *d*, follicular epithelium with mitochondria; *e*, Call-Exner body or vacuole; *f*, theca folliculi with internal and external layers not yet differentiated; *g*, blood vessels containing erythrocytes; *h*, basement membrane; *i*, mitosis in follicular cell. (Magnification × 345.) Bloom, W., and Fawcett, D. W.: A Textbook of Histology, ed. 9. Philadelphia, W. B. Saunders Company, 1968.)

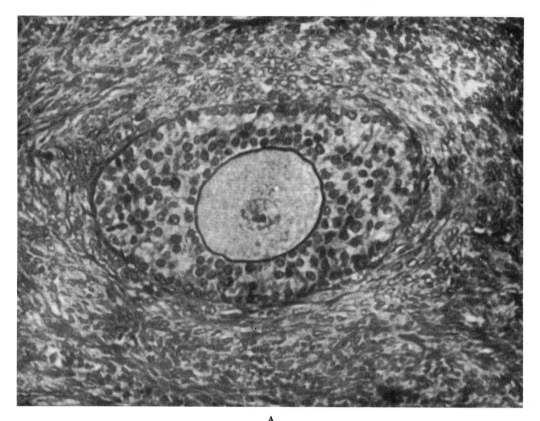

A

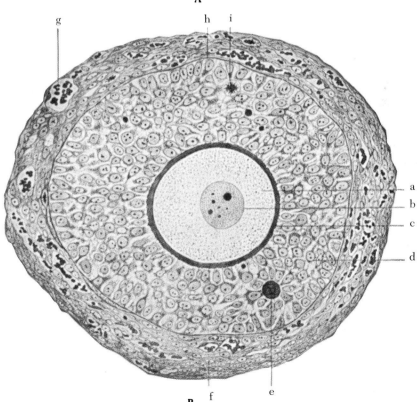

B

Figure 11   See opposite page for legend.

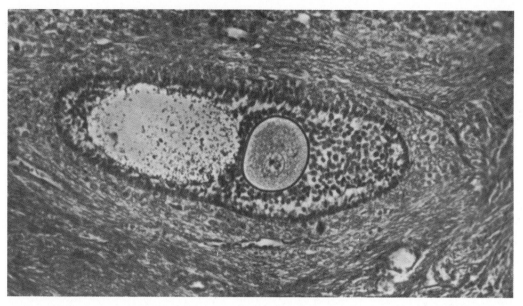

Figure 12   Early vesicular follicle with antrum formation. (From Shettles, L. B.: Ovum Humanum. New York, Hafner Publishing Company, 1960.)

the ovary. At a point nearest to the surface the theca folliculi thickens and its fibers separate. The *stigma* or point of rupture of the follicle becomes necrotic, perhaps as a result of ischemia. Ovulation of the mature vesicular follicle appears to occur following a high peak of luteinizing and follicle stimulating hormone production from the pituitary gland. Although the sequence of events after this peak is rather unclear, certain factors have been suggested. Alteration of vascular flow may occur, producing necrosis at the stigma of the protruding

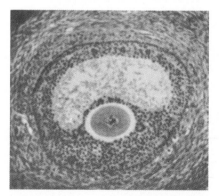

Figure 13   Vesicular follicle with antrum in an intermediate stage of development. (Magnification × 110.) (From Witschi, E.: Development of Vertebrates. Philadelphia, W. B. Saunders Company, 1956.)

follicle. Increased intrafollicular pressure may occur from depolymerization of acid mucopolysaccharides. Local proteolytic enzymatic activity may affect the stigma itself.

The mechanism of ovulation is not well understood. Blandau has shown the process of ovulation in rats to be a slow extrusion rather than an explosive event. Protrusion of the cumulus and follicular contents through the stigma is well demonstrated in the rabbit as well (Fig. 15), where it is apparent that the material remains adherent to the surface to be acted upon subsequently by the ciliary action of the tubal fimbriae. Doyle observed ovulation in women on three occasions by culdoscopy. He found the process to be essentially identical with that in animals, involving gradual opening and oozing out of thin liquor folliculi, followed by viscid liquor and the cumulus containing the ovum.

By the end of the twelfth week of intrauterine life, some oogonia have developed into primary oocytes. At this time they enter a long prophase of the first meiotic division, which results in reduction of the diploid number of chromosomes from 46 (44 autosomes and 2 sex chromosomes) to the haploid number of 23 (22 autosomes

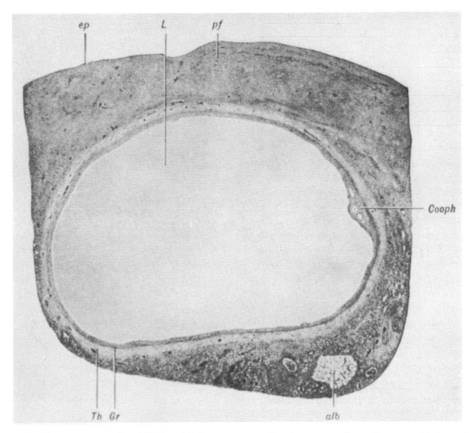

Figure 14　Maturing vesicular follicle with large antrum showing *ep*, surface of ovary with investing germinal epithelium; *L*, follicular liquor; *pf*, primary follicle; *Cooph*, cumulus oophorus with oocyte; *alb*, corpus albicans, the remnant of a previous follicle; *Gr*, granulosa cell layer; *Th*, theca externa and interna. Eighteenth day of cycle, same ovary as Figure 11*B*. (Magnification × 20.) (From Maximow, A. A., and Bloom, W.: A Textbook of Histology. Philadelphia, W. B. Saunders Company, 1957.)

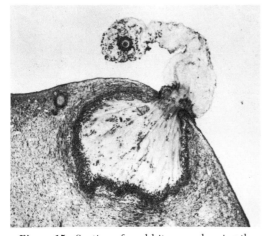 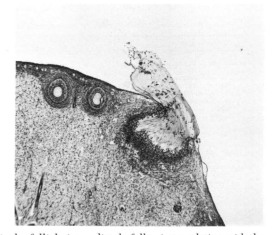

Figure 15　Section of a rabbit ovary showing the vesicular follicle immediately following ovulation with the culumus oophorus and viscid follicular liquor protruding through the stigma and adhering to the surface. (Magnification × 54.) (From Hafez, E. S. E., and Blandau, R. J.: The Mammalian Oviduct. Chicago, University of Chicago Press, 1969.)

and 1 sex chromosome). At birth, the oo-cytes are in the prophase of the first mei-otic division where they remain until the development of the follicles during the reproductive life span that extends from puberty to menopause.

The next maturation division takes place in conjunction with ovulation. Just prior to ovulation the ovum undergoes changes to prepare it for fertilization. A few hours pre-ceding ovulation, the nucleus of the oocyte approaches the surface and undergoes karyokinesis. After resolution of the chro-matin into distinct chromosomes, meiotic division takes place with unequal distribu-tion of the cytoplasm to form a secondary oocyte and the first polar body (Fig. 16). Each of these elements contains the hap-loid number of chromosomes, 23, each in the form of 2 monads. The second matura-tion spindle forms immediately and re-mains at the surface.

Ordinarily, no further development takes place until after ovulation and fertili-zation have occurred. At that time, but prior to union of the male and female pronuclear contributions, another division occurs to reduce the chromosome component of the egg pronucleus to 23 single chromosomes,

each composed of 1 monad. Cytoplasmic division is once again unequal. An *ootid* (the secondary oocyte) and the second polar body are formed. It is the ootid that receives the spermatozoan pronucleus at fertilization. The term *zygote* is used to describe the fertilized egg at any stage prior to cleavage after the male and female pronuclei have joined.

FORMATION OF CORPUS LUTEUM

Liberation of the ovum does not mark the end of the significance of an ovarian follicle. Most of the contained fluid escapes and is accompanied by contraction of the ovarian stroma to reduce the size of its lumen (Fig. 17). Meyer described the morphologic changes in four stages: prolif-eration, vascularization, maturity and re-gression. These are artificial divisions be-cause it is clear that the development of the corpus luteum is a dynamic progres-sion of physiologic and morphologic events.

The most prominent features of the pro-

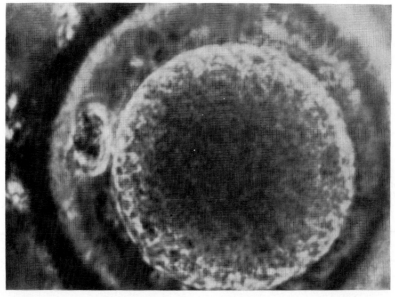

Figure 16   A living human ovum washed from the uterine tube with the zona pellucida completely denuded of cumulus oophorus and corona radiata cells by enzymatic action of tubal mucosa, showing early division into a secondary oocyte with formation of the first polar body. The diameter of the ovum is 100 to 150 μ to the outer surface of the oolemma. (From Shettles, L. B.: Ovum Humanum. New York, Hafner Publishing Company, 1960.)

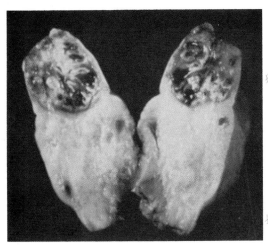

Figure 17 Gross view of a bisected ovary showing the corpus luteum within a few hours after ovulation. Note the collapse of the follicular wall and appearance of hemorrhagic areas. (Life-size.)

liferative stage are vascularity and mitotic activity of the theca. There is an increased storage of lipid material in theca cells and to a lesser extent in granulosa cells. During vascularization the membrana granulosa is invaded by capillaries. At the same time fibroblasts invade the central coagulum that resulted from consolidation of the blood leakage from those vessels injured at the time of rupture of the follicle intermixing with the residue of the follicular contents. A recently ruptured follicle filled with sanguineous coagulated material is called a *corpus hemorrhagicum.*

Using a standard 28 day cycle and assuming ovulation to occur about 14 days prior to menstruation, Corner provided detailed dating of the evolution of a corpus luteum. He noted that, starting with capillary congestion and hemorrhage into the granulosa cell layers on day 1 following ovulation, capillary invasion and progressive luteinization of the granulosa cells from the theca inward occur. By the third day some of the capillaries have penetrated to reach the central cavity and granulosa and theca interna cells have become indistinguishable. Mitoses begin to appear in both layers. Fibroblasts appear in the central cavity by day 4 and the theca cells begin to enlarge. They develop rather large nuclei and vacuolated cytoplasm by day 6. At this time granulosa cells are completely luteinized and densely packed. The fibrin network in the cavity is extensive and fibroblasts begin to line the walls of the cavity. No further mitoses are seen.

Days 6 and 7 mark the peak of cellular activity. Venules appear and fibroblasts enter the central cavity, depositing connective tissue at the margin. Theca cell vacuolation is pronounced during this interval period. Over the next six days vacuolation of the granulosa cells develops to a maximum and this layer begins to shrink, thereby enlarging the central cavity and making the theca more prominent. By day 12 "mulberry cells" appear with many uniform, small vacuoles. These cells indicate that menstruation will occur soon or has already begun. This is followed on the fourteenth day by the appearance of dense, pyknotic nuclei widespread in the granulosa and the theca interna.

Characteristic phospholipin granules develop in the granulosa lutein cells that form the bulk of the *corpus luteum* (yellow body). Its characteristic yellow color is not grossly apparent until enough lutein pigment accumulates in about a week. By the end of the second week after ovulation it has reached a diameter of 10 to 15 mm. and the central coagulum is covered by a thin layer of newly formed connective tissue. The latter in turn is surrounded by a border of lutein cells 1 to 3 mm. thick. During the third week the granulosa lutein cells reach their full size and the structure attains its maximum diameter of 15 to 20 mm. If conception and implantation do not occur, the granulosa cells begin to undergo fatty degeneration, shrink and eventually disappear. Ultimately, nothing remains but connective tissue in a typically silvery white *corpus albicans.* This results through mechanisms of fatty degeneration, phagocytosis and fibrosis.

If pregnancy should occur, the corpus luteum continues to develop. It may grow larger than 25 mm., especially if the stigma sealed promptly following ovulation and the accumulated follicular fluid remained in the cavity. Not only is the overall size greater in pregnancy but also the central cavity is larger, and there is greater vascularity and more connective tissue both in the lutein border and within the central coagulum (Fig. 18). The corpus luteum of

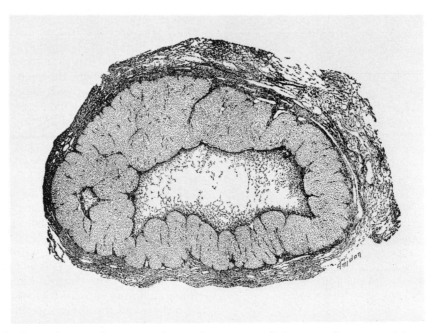

Figure 18 Corpus luteum of pregnancy (corpus luteum verum) showing enlargement of the central cavity and heavily luteinized hyperplastic theca layer.

pregnancy (*corpus luteum verum,* corpus luteum graviditatis) persists for varying intervals of time. Although regression may occur as early as the sixth week following conception, well-developed corpora lutea have been found at term. The characteristic cytologic criterion of the corpus luteum of pregnancy is the finding of calcium or colloid in the luteal cells resembling Call-Exner bodies.

In terms of function, up to the point of follicular rupture, all the changes that the ovary undergoes are directed at delivering mature ova into the peritoneal cavity in preparation for fertilization and, simultaneously, preparing the endometrial lining. Following ovulation, additional changes occur in the ovary in anticipation of fertilization and implantation, to provide for a favorable uterine environment for the development of the conceptus. The chief function of the corpus luteum is the production of progesterone. This hormone is responsible for the uterine changes which precede and accompany implantation of the ovum. Electron microscopic studies of the human corpus luteum (Adams and Hertig) have demonstrated ultrastructural characteristics paralleling progesterone production and physiologic activity of lutein cells.

Although the corpus luteum is essential for the maintenance of pregnancy in various lower animal species, it is probably needed in human pregnancy only for a short period following implantation. There are many instances on record of successful outcome of pregnancy despite early removal or destruction of the corpus luteum. Hall reviewed a series of such cases, demonstrating an abortion rate not significantly greater than that expected in association with other intraabdominal surgery performed during early pregnancy. Only two spontaneous abortions occurred in a group of 14 women who had had corpora lutea removed intentionally by Tulsky and Koff. Thus the corpus luteum functions to produce progesterone for the maintenance of pregnancy. But the human placenta appears to secrete enough progesterone soon after implantation to make the function of the corpus luteum superfluous very early in pregnancy.

Follicular *atresia* is the degenerative process involving most of the ova formed in the ovary and available for oogenesis. Ultimate failure of the ovary to produce ova at the menopause is attributable to the depletion of its supply of follicles. Only a very few will ever be ovulated. All the remainder will be depleted by the process of degeneration and resorption known as atresia. A follicle may undergo this process at any stage of its development short of ovulation. The process is not well understood at all in spite of the fact that atresia is the usual fate of follicles.

Examination of the ovary in the interval prior to ovulation generally reveals the presence of several follicles in various stages of their development. Usually only one will continue its development to become a mature vesicular follicle and ovulate, while all others will undergo some form of intrinsic change to cause them to stop developing and to begin to undergo regressive alterations.

Atretic degeneration of the follicles involves shrinkage of the antrum as it fills with young fibroblasts and ultimately scar formation similar to that of the corpus albicans, albeit smaller and often with a persistent glassy membrane that represents the preexisting basement membrane of the vesicular follicle. Additionally, the follicle in which the oocyte has developed to the point of oolemma formation will present shriveled mucoprotein remnants of this structure in the atretic scar (Fig. 19).

CONCEPTION

The term *conception* refers to the union of the male and female pronuclear elements of procreation from which a new living being develops. It is synonymous with the terms *fecundation, impregnation* and *fertilization*. This puristic definition is obviously incomplete because the moment of fertilization represents only one phase of a long train of processes. Aside from organogenesis of sexual organs, oogenesis and spermatogenesis, the events leading up to conception deal with endocrinologic developmental aspects as well as neurologic and psychologic factors. Physiologic processes begin with instinctive behavior patterns and psychic stimulation that lead to the development of sexual interests. These eventually result in sex play and coitus. With ejaculation of semen into the vagina there follows transport of sperm through the uterus to the uterine tubes where they encounter the recently ovulated ovum. Fertilization takes place in this location and is followed by transport of the fertilized ovum to the uterus for implantation and continued development.

Conception must be distinguished from *copulation* which merely signifies intromission during sexual intercourse or the insertion of the penis into the vagina, and *insemination* which involves discharge of semen. Fertile coitus and fertilization are nearly synchronous primarily because an unfertilized secondary oocyte lives only a few hours following ovulation. Spermatozoa, on the other hand, reach the uterine tube in less than one hour following coitus (Hartman) where they usually live for 24 hours or so. Spermatozoa have been found in the uterine tube and the peritoneum of the female for much longer periods of time, but it is conjectural whether or not they are still capable of fertilizing an ovum. By studying early cleavage stages in human preparations, Rock and Hertig have shown that ova are fertilized within 12 hours after ovulation.

Concerning sexual behavior, sex play and intercourse, the pioneering studies of Dickinson and the more recent detailed investigations of Masters and Johnson have provided much useful information. Although clearly germane to the broad area of reproductive biology, this material falls outside the scope of this book. Moreover, it is quite clear that foreplay, sexual arousal and orgasm are not essential prerequisites to fertilization. The numbers of pregnancies resulting from forcible rape are testimonies to this premise. By the same token, copulation itself is not essential as evidenced by the successes of artificial insemination and pregnancies reported to have resulted from semen deposited on or near the vulva without intromission. The lack of further discussion of this aspect of human sexuality should not be construed by the reader to indicate that we consider it unimportant.

The object of copulation for the purpose of *procreation* is to place the semen in such a location that its living elements, the spermatozoa, may reach the ovum. Once deposited, the spermatozoa must enter the uterus through the cervical canal, pass through the endometrial cavity and reach the ampullar portion of the uterine tube before an ovum can be fertilized. The first barrier is the cervical mucus. Spermatozoa appear within this viscid material almost

Zona pellucida   Loose connective tissue filling follicular antrum

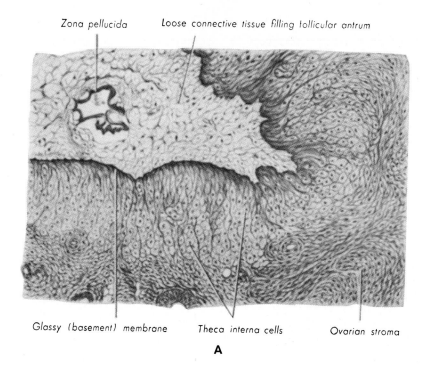

Glassy (basement) membrane   Theca interna cells   Ovarian stroma

A

Invading blood vessels   Ovarian stroma

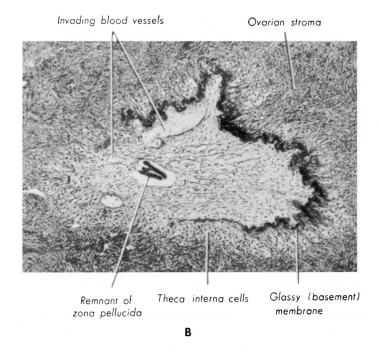

Remnant of   Theca interna cells   Glassy (basement)
zona pellucida   membrane

B

Figure 19 Section of an ovary showing various stages in the development of follicular atresia. *A*, early; *B*, intermediate; *C*, late progression. The ovum and the granulosa cells degenerate early in the course of this process. If the oolemma has been formed about the oocyte, it will persist for long periods of time. The well-developed theca interna disappears, leaving the increasingly prominent glassy basement membrane residua. (From Copenhaver, W. M.: Bailey's Textbook of Histology. Baltimore, Williams and Wilkins Company, 1964.)

Figure 19 continued on opposite page.

Vein

Arteriole

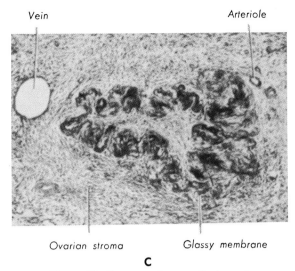

Ovarian stroma

Glassy membrane

C

Figure 19 See opposite page for legend.

immediately after coitus (Sobrero and MacLeod). Harvey has shown that sperm travel at about 27μ per second through cervical mucus. It is likely that the intrinsic motility of the human spermatozoon itself is the mechanism by which it passes into and through the cervical canal. The characteristics of the cervical mucus become very favorable for sperm penetration at the time of ovulation, increasing in amount and altering its electrolyte content and viscosity.

An average ejaculate involves 2 to 5 ml. of semen with sperm count of about 120 to 200 million per milliliter, of which 60 to 90 per cent are morphologically normal. Of this huge number, only one spermatozoon will fertilize the single ootid released at ovulation.

Whereas spermatozoa probably pass through the cervical canal on their own power by means of their flagellae, they appear to ascend through the endometrial cavity by means of uterine contractions (Bickers). Sperm traverse the uterus and reach the uterine tube within a few minutes of coitus. In view of the distances involved, it is clear that transport through the uterus is probably effected chiefly by myometrial contractions and not significantly by the self-propellant activity of the spermatozoa (Sobrero). It is still speculative whether or not prostaglandins, long-chain fatty acid substances found in high concentrations in semen, constitute the agents that initiate uterine contractility under these circumstances.

Although the uterine tube is well supplied with ciliated epithelium which sets up countercurrents in tubal fluid, propulsive transport within the lumen of the tube is probably mediated principally by peristaltic contractions of the muscles in the tubal walls. It is likely that only a few thousand of the original hundreds of millions of spermatozoa that were present in the ejaculate ever enter the uterine tube and many fewer reach the immediate vicinity of the ovum (Austin and Bishop). The chief sites of reduction in sperm number are the cervix, the uterotubal junction and the isthmus of the tube. All other spermatozoa are disposed of in four recognizable ways: passage to the exterior, passage into the peritoneal cavity, phagocytosis by leukocytes and passage into the epithelial lining cells of the endometrial and endosalpingial mucosa. The potential immunologic significance of such phagocytosis in terms of the formation of antisperm antibodies is a matter of considerable theoretical and practical interest (Tyler and Bishop). It is likely that sensitization to spermatozoa may be naturally acquired and affect fertility adversely. Autogenous antibodies are found in both men and women (Franklin and Dukes).

In order for the mature spermatozoon to become capable of fertilizing an ovum it must undergo a process called *capacitation*. The nature of the capacitation phenomenon remains obscure. The duration of this process is variable among mammalian species, ranging from two to six hours.

Chang has shown that it will not take place in rabbits following oophorectomy, during pseudopregnancy or after progesterone administration. Capacitation probably involves detachment of the acrosome from the spermatozoon (Austin and Bishop). Zaneveld et al. discovered an enzyme similar to trypsin in the acrosomes of capacitated rabbit sperm. They also found an inhibitor of this enzyme both in the acrosomes and in seminal fluid. It is theorized that capacitation may involve destruction or deactivation of the inhibitor to permit the trypsinlike enzyme to act on the digestion of the zona pellucida of the ovum thereby enhancing penetration by the spermatozoon. Chang's observation that capacitation is reversible when capaced sperm are resuspended in diluted seminal fluid suggests that the capacitation process may be regarded as a two-stage phenomenon (Austin). This concept appears to be confirmed by the findings of Zaneveld et al.

Transport of the ovum from the vesicular follicle at the time of ovulation to the site of fertilization is undoubtedly the result of ciliary action by tubal mucosa. Direct observations in living animals (Westman; Blandau) have shown that the ovum does not traverse any great distance within the peritoneal cavity. Gross muscular movements of the uterine tube bring the fimbriated end into very close relationship with the ovulating follicle. Although this mechanism has not been directly observed in man, it seems likely to exist. A suction-like mechanism has been postulated, but Clewe and Mastroianni, by placing a ligature around the junction of the fimbria and the ampulla of the tube in the rabbit, showed that ovum transport into the abdominal ostium of the tube was unimpeded. Since it is hard to conceive how any negative pressure could be transmitted through a nonrigid tube, it is generally agreed that ovum transport occurs primarily by ciliary action. Once the ovum has entered the abdominal ostium of the uterine tube, it passes very rapidly to the site of fertilization (Greenwald), which in most mammals is in the ampulla of the tube.

Subsequent migration following fertilization is delayed. For example, the delay is 36 hours in the rabbit before transport to the uterus begins. Transmigration across the tubal isthmus takes about an additional 24 hours so that the rabbit egg enters the uterus about 62 hours after ovulation, in the form of a blastocyst. The human egg, on the other hand, probably passes into the endometrial cavity as a morula about three or three and one-half days after ovulation, which is about average for many mammalian species. The rate of ovum transport through the tube is influenced by ovarian hormones in a complex manner (Austin).

Generally, an ovum enters the uterine tube on the same side as the ovary from which it arose. Exceptions have been noted in nature, however. In some animals with bicornuate uteri, one may observe all embryos in one horn while all corpora lutea from which these ova arose are located in the ovary of the opposite side. This phenomenon is known as *migration of the ovum.* It may also occur in women. External migration of an ovum that escapes from one ovary, traverses the pelvic cavity and enters the tube on the opposite side is not uncommon. Speert et al. have demonstrated that it occurs about once in 10 times as judged by the site of the corpus luteum in tubal pregnancies. Whether it also occurs under other circumstances cannot be determined. When one considers the normal anatomic juxtaposition of both tubes and ovaries on the posterior aspect of a normally anteflexed uterus, this occurrence is not unexpected. Internal migration, that is transmigration of an ovum from the ovary through the ipsilateral uterine tube across the fundus of the endometrial cavity to gain access to the opposite tube, is a theoretical possibility that has yet to be substantiated.

FORMATION OF ZYGOTE

Even the "momentary" event of fertilization may be traced through a number of sequential steps, including contact of the spermatozoa with the ovum, penetration of any residual granulosa cell layers surrounding it, penetration of the zona pellucida, fusion of a spermatid with the ovum, activation of the secondary oocyte with formation of the second polar body and the mature ootid, formation of the male and female pronuclei and finally pairing of the full complement of chromosomes preparatory to cell division.

In order for fertilization to occur it is necessary for spermatozoa to come into contact with the ovum. Chemotaxis, a term denoting attraction of the sperm to the egg, may exist but the evidence in support of this contention is unsubstantiated (Austin). Random collision may be sufficient to explain such contact. The corona radiata of granulosa cells attached to the ovum at the time of ovulation is shed in the course of several hours during transit into the tubal ampulla. It is likely that spermatozoa contact a denuded egg (Fig. 20).

Sperm penetration has been reviewed in detail by Austin and Walton. They found that the eggs of many mammals leave the ovary still surrounded by the cumulus oophorus, a cellular layer with a rich intercellular matrix of hyaluronic acid and protein. Granulosa cells nearest the egg are rather firmly attached to the zona pellucida. In some animals, including man, the cumulus breaks down either at ovulation or very soon thereafter so that the spermatozoon penetrates the denuded oolemma. In other animals, particularly the rodents, the cumulus persists through most of the fertile life of the egg and the fertilizing spermatozoon must penetrate granulosa cell layers to reach the egg.

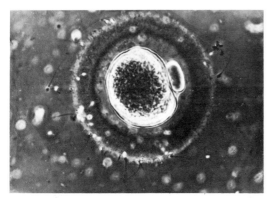

Figure 20 Fertilization of a human ovum *in vitro* showing the denuded ovum surrounded by spermatozoa arranged radially around the zona pellucida. The first polar body lies within the perivitelline space. (From Shettles, L. B.: Ovum Humanum. New York, Hafner Publishing Company, 1960.)

It has been maintained that the enzyme hyaluronidase, carried by the spermatozoon, plays a role in permitting the spermatozoon to penetrate the cumulus. Blandau, however, emphasized that the rat spermatozoon penetrates the granulosa layers faster than would be consistent with depolymerization of the matrix ahead of the sperm.

The zona pellucida is probably penetrated by a mechanism involving an agent associated with the acrosome of the spermatozoon. The canals, which have been demonstrated on electronmicroscopic examination and through which pass the protoplasmic processes of both the corona radiata cells and the oocytes, are probably not involved. The microvilli are undoubtedly instrumental in effecting active transport of metabolites. The passage of the spermatid through the zona pellucida is believed to occur after it loses its acrosome. The sperm makes its way through the membrane with the aid of an active agent or enzyme associated with the acrosome (Austin and Bishop). The sperm then promptly becomes attached to the surface of the vitellus into which it is absorbed after a short delay. Passage through the oolemma appears to occur in an oblique rather than a radial direction, negating the likelihood that the aforementioned microcanals in the zona pellucida serve as pathways.

Immediately after the first spermatid penetrates the oolemma, a reaction spreads throughout this investing layer that prevents any other spermatozoon from penetrating (Austin). Austin and Braden postulate that the zona reaction is probably evoked by contact of the sperm head with the vitelline surface, as a result of which the vitellus releases some substance that passes across the perivitelline space and causes an alteration in the properties of the zona. The rate of this reaction is apparently rather rapid because penetration of ova by more than one sperm is exceedingly rare. In mice and rats it is rather slow, taking at least 10 minutes for completion.

The penetrating spermatid was once considered to enter the vitellus by a process similar to that of phagocytosis. Recent electronmicroscopy studies, how-

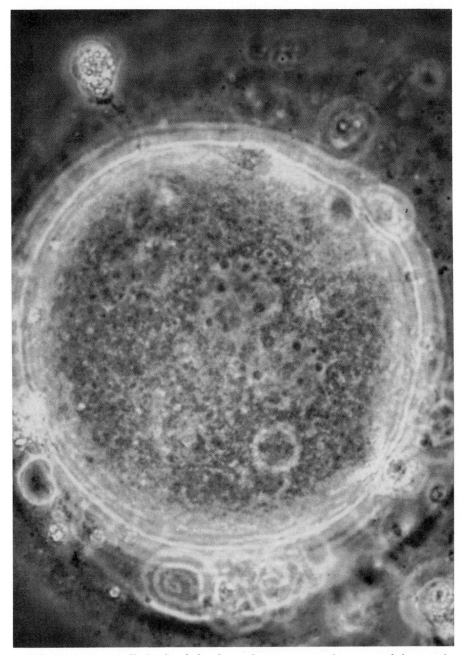

Figure 21 The youngest naturally fertilized, developing human ovum so far recovered shown in living state by phase microscopy. The vitellus is 103 μ diameter in the fresh state. Male and female pronuclei are seen within the cytoplasm of the zygote, both surrounded by nuclear membranes, just prior to coalescence. (From Noyes, R. W., et al.: Science *147*:744, 1965.)

ever, suggest that penetration occurs by fusion. Szollosi and Ris have shown that true fusion occurs upon fertilization in the rat. The sperm plasma membrane becomes continuous with that of the egg and is left behind on the egg surface as the sperm passes deeper into the vitellus. Thus the male pronuclear material lies directly within egg cytoplasm.

Attachment of the sperm to the vitellus stimulates activation of the ovum to resume its second maturation division. At this point, unequal distribution of the cytoplasm occurs and the second polar body is cast off, leaving the female haploid components of chromosomes or pronuclear material within the vitellus. This marks the beginning of embryogenesis. Pronuclear formation occurs and is followed by syngamy and mitosis. Both male and female pronuclear material acquires nuclear membranes (Fig. 21). There is concurrent growth of pronuclei and coalescence of nucleolar material. The pronuclei condense to about half their maximum size but with increased DNA concentration as the nucleoli disappear. The nuclear membranes then also disappear and condensing chromosomes become visible. Those from the separate pronuclei move together to form the metaphase plate, preparatory to the first cell cleavage (Austin). The zygote thus formed represents the beginning of a new life.

REFERENCES

Adams, E. C., and Hertig, A. T.: Studies on the human corpus luteum. I. Observations on the ultrastructure of development and regression of the luteal cells during the menstrual cycle. J. Cell. Biol. *41*:696, 1969.

Adams, E. C., and Hertig, A. T.: Studies on the human corpus luteum. II. Observations on the ultrastructure of luteal cells during pregnancy. J. Cell. Biol. *41*:716, 1969.

Austin, C. R.: Fertilization and transport of the ovum. *In* Hartman, C. G., ed.: Mechanisms Concerned with Conception. New York, The Macmillan Company, 1963.

Austin, C. R., and Bishop, M. W. H.: Some features of the acrosome and perforatorium in mammalian spermatozoa. Proc. Roy. Soc. London (B) *149*:234, 1958.

Austin, C. R., and Bishop, M. W. H.: Role of the rodent acrosome and perforatorium in fertilization. Proc. Roy. Soc. London (B) *149*:241, 1958.

Austin, C. R., and Braden, A. W. H.: Early reactions of the rodent egg to spermatozoon penetration. J. Exp. Biol. *33*:358, 1956.

Austin, C. R., and Walton, A.: Fertilization. *In* Parkes, A. S., ed.: Marshall's Physiology of Reproduction, Vol. 1, Part 2. London, Longmans, Green, 1959.

Baker, T. G.: A quantitative and cytological study of germ cells in human ovaries. Proc. Roy. Soc. (B) *158*:417, 1963.

Bickers, W.: Sperm migration and uterine contractions. Fertil. Steril. *11*:286, 1960.

Blandau, R. J.: Ovulation in the living albino rat. Fertil. Steril. *6*:391, 1955.

Blandau, R. J.: Gamete transport: Comparative aspects. *In* Hafez, E. S. E., and Blandau, R. J., eds.: The Mammalian Oviduct: Comparative Biology and Methodology. Chicago, University of Chicago Press, 1969.

Blandau, R. J., and Money, W. L.: Observations on the rate of transport of spermatozoa in the female genital tract of the rat. Anat. Rec. *90*:255, 1944.

Block, E.: A quantitative morphological investigation of the follicular system in newborn female infants. Acta Anat. *17*:201, 1953.

Braden, A. W. H.: Distribution of sperms in the genital tract of the female rabbit after coitus. Austral. J. Exp. Biol. Med. Sci. *6*:693, 1953.

Chang, M. C.: Development of fertilizing capacity of rabbit spermatozoa in the uterus. Nature *175*:1036, 1955.

Clewe, T. H., and Mastroianni, L., Jr.: Mechanism of ovum pickup. I. Functional capacity of rabbit oviducts ligated near the fimbria. Fertil. Steril. *9*:13, 1958.

Corner, G. W., Jr.: The histological dating of the human corpus luteum of menstruation. Amer. J. Anat. *98*:377, 1956.

Dickinson, R. L.: Human Sex Anatomy. Baltimore, Williams and Wilkins Company, 1933.

Doyle, J. B.: Exploratory culdotomy for observation of tubo-ovarian physiology at ovulation time. Fertil. Steril. *2*:475, 1951.

Franklin, R. R., and Dukes, C. D.: Antispermatozoal antibody and unexplained infertility. Amer. J. Obstet. Gynec. *89*:6, 1964.

Gillman, J.: The development of the gonads in man, with a consideration of the role of fetal endocrines and the histogenesis of ovarian tumors. Contrib. Embryol. *32*:81, 1948.

Greenwald, G. S.: Tubal transport of ova in the rabbit. Anat. Rec. *133*:386, 1959.

Hafez, E. S. E., and Blandau, R. J.: The Mammalian Oviduct: Comparative Biology and Methodology. Chicago, University of Chicago Press, 1969.

Häggström, P.: Zahlenmässige Analyse der Ovarian eines 22-jährigen gesunden Weibes. Upsala Läkaref. Föhr. *26*:1, 1921.

Hall, R. E.: Removal of the corpus luteum in early pregnancy: A review of the literature and report of 2 cases. Bull. Sloane Hosp. *1*:49, 1955.

Hartman, C. G.: How do sperms get into the uterus? Fertil. Steril. *8*:403, 1957.

Harvey, C.: An experimental study of the penetration of human cervical mucus by spermatozoa. J. Obstet. Gynaec. Brit. Emp. *41*:480, 1954.

Harvey, C.: The speed of human spermatozoa and the effect on it of various diluents, with some preliminary observations on clinical material. J. Reprod. Fertil. *1*:84, 1960.

Masters, W. H., and Johnson, V. E.: Human Sexual Response. Boston, Little, Brown and Company, 1966.

Meyer, R.: Über Corpus luteum-Bildung beim Menschen. Arch. Gynäk. *93*:354, 1911.

Noyes, R. W., Dickmann, Z., Clewe, T. H., and Bonney, W. A.: Pronuclear ovum from a patient using an intrauterine device. Science 147:744, 1965.

Pinkerton, J. H. M., McKay, D. G., Adams, E. C., and Hertig, A. T.: Development of the human ovary: Study using histochemical technics. Obstet. Gynec. 18:152, 1961.

Rock, J., and Hertig, A. T.: Information regarding the time of human ovulation derived from a study of 3 unfertilized and 11 fertilized ova. Amer. J. Obstet. Gynec. 47:343, 1944.

Shettles, L. B.: Ovum Humanum: Growth, Maturation, Nourishment, Fertilization and Early Development. New York, Hafner Publishing Company, 1960.

Short, R. V.: Steroid concentrations in the follicular fluid of mares at various stages of the reproductive cycle. J. Endocr. 22:153, 1961.

Sobrero, A. J.: Sperm migration in the female genital tract. In Hartman, C. G., ed.: Mechanisms Concerned with Conception. New York, The Macmillan Company, 1963.

Sobrero, A. J., and MacLeod, J.: The immediate postcoital test. Fertil. Steril. 13:184, 1962.

Speert, H., Nash, W., and Kaplan, A. L.: Tubal pregnancy: Some observations on external migration of the ovum and compensating hypertrophy of the residual ovary. Obstet. Gynec. 7:322, 1956.

Szollosi, D. G., and Ris, H.: Observations of sperm penetration in the rat. J. Biophys. Biochem. Cytol. 10:275, 1961.

Tulsky, A. S., and Koff, A. K.: Some observations on the role of the corpus luteum in early human pregnancy. Fertil. Steril. 8:118, 1957.

Tyler, A., and Bishop, D. W.: Immunological phenomena. In Hartman, C. G., ed.: Mechanisms Concerned with Conception. New York, The Macmillan Company, 1963.

Van Wagenen, G., and Simpson, M. E.: Embryology of the Ovary and Testis *Homo Sapiens* and *Macaca Mulatta*. New Haven, Yale University Press, 1965.

Westman, A.: Beiträge zur Kenntnis des Mechanismus des Eitransportes bei Kaninchen. München Med. Wschr. 73:1793, 1926.

Westman, A.: Investigations into the transport of the ovum. In Engle, E. T., ed.: Proceedings Conference Studies on Testes and Ovary, Eggs and Sperm. Springfield, Ill., Charles C Thomas, 1952.

Witschi, E.: Migration of the germ cells of human embryos from the yolk sac to the primitive gonadal folds. Contrib. Embryol. 32:67, 1948.

Zaneveld, L. J. D., Srivastava, P. N., and Williams, W. L.: Relationship of a trypsin-like enzyme in rabbit spermatozoa to capacitation. J. Reprod. Fertil. 20:337, 1969.

Zuckerman, S.: Origin and development of oocytes in foetal and mature mammals. Mem. Soc. Endocr. 7:63, 1960.

Chapter 3

Implantation and Placentation

Formation of the *zygote* at fertilization by the union of the male and female pronuclei sets into motion a train of events that results in the implantation of the embryo into the uterine wall. When the spermatozoon has penetrated the zona pellucida, the maturation process of the oocyte is concluded. The mature ootid is formed by an unequal cytoplasmic division which also produces the second polar body. At the same time the sperm head fuses with the ovum cytoplasm. By the process of syngamy the male and female chromosomal components of the pronuclei move together to form the metaphase plate in preparation for the first cleavage by mitotic division (Austin).

The zygote is now prepared for *segmentation* or *cleavage* of its nuclear and cytoplasmic substance. This is a very dramatic event when observed microscopically (Fig. 22). The chromosome pairs formed by syngamy arrange themselves on the equatorial plate of the spindle. Rapid anaphase separation of the daughter chromosomes occurs with the appearance of the cleavage furrow as the two daughter cells form with full species chromosome complement and equal cytoplasmic distribution. The achromatic fibers of the spindle which has formed in the segmentation nucleus appear to dissolve centrally as the chromosomes are separated toward the spindle centrosomes. The process of karyokinesis is completed by division of the cytoplasm to form two blastomeres of equal size, each with a full complement of chromosomes, half paternal and half maternal in origin.

Each daughter cell thus formed divides

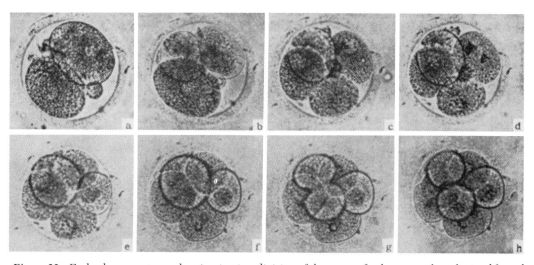

Figure 22 Early cleavage stages showing *in vitro* division of the ovum of a rhesus monkey obtained from the uterine tube and grown in plasma. *a,* two-cell stage at 29½ hours after ovulation; *b,* three-cell at 36 hours; *c* and *d,* four-cell at 37½ hours; *e* and *f,* five-cell at 48½ hours; *g,* six-cell at 49 hours; and *h,* eight-cell at 50 hours. (Magnification × 300.) (From Lewis, W. H., and Hartman, C. G.: Contrib. Embryol. 24:187, 1933.)

again into two. In due course by geometric progression a mass of cells results. This mass resembles a mulberry in shape and is called a *morula*. Multiplication of the blastomeres takes place inside the zona pellucida during the course of transit of the ovum through the uterine tube into the endometrial cavity. Ova have been recovered from the uterine cavity with as few as 12 blastomeres. Since transit time through the tube is approximately three days in duration, one can gather some idea of the rate at which cleavage takes place. In the monkey (Lewis and Hartman), ova were recovered with two blastomeres at about 30 hours following ovulation, four blastomeres at 38 hours, and eight blastomeres at 50 hours.

The process continues to evolve with the development of a *blastula* or blastocyst. It is formed by the gradual accumulation of interstitial fluid between the blastomeres of the morula, ultimately forming a central cavity, the blastocele. The cells of the blastodermic vesicle thus arrange themselves peripherally with a more compact conglomerate mass of cells occupying one pole. This latter mass represents the

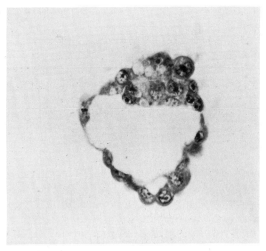

Figure 24 Human blastocyst about five days old that was found free in the uterine cavity on the twenty-seventh day of the menstrual cycle. It measured 153 μ by 115 μ before fixation. The oolemma has disappeared. There are eight larger cells in the inner cell mass and 99 prospective trophoblasts. (Magnification × 600.) (From Hertig, A. T., and Rock, J.: Amer. J. Obstet. Gynec. 47:149, 1944.)

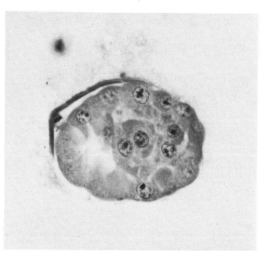

Figure 23 Section of a morula washed from the human uterus on the seventh day of the menstrual cycle showing irregular segmented cavity on the right. There are five larger blastomeres which are presumably embryo-forming and 53 trophoblast-producing cells. The zona pellucida is still intact around the spherical morula which measures 150 μ in the fresh state or about the size of the mature human egg before fertilization. Estimated age—fourth or beginning fifth day. (Magnification × 600.) (From Hertig, A. T., and Rock, J.: Amer. J. Obstet. Gynec. 47:149, 1944.)

progenitor of the embryo itself. The zona pellucida may persist during the early development of the blastula (Fig. 23). In the earliest stages, it is possible to recognize an outer layer of cells that will become the trophoblastic investment and an inner embryo-forming clump of cells. As the blastodermic vesicle continues to develop, the zona pellucida vanishes and the thin trophoblastic layer of cells enclosing the blastocele becomes more apparent (Fig. 24). It is at this stage in its development, approximately seven days following ovulation, that the human blastocyst embeds into the endometrium.

OVUM TRANSPORT

Transmigration of the ovum after extrusion from the vesicular follicle at the time of ovulation to the site of fertilization in the ampulla has been discussed earlier (Chapter 2). In contrast to the rapid transport from ovary to ampulla, subsequent travel of the zygote is relatively slow. In the rabbit, long delays of the order of 36 hours occur before transport to the uterus begins, and an additional 24 hours is required for transit through the isthmus to the uterus (Greenwald). The rabbit ovum enters the uterus in the form of a blastocyst about 62 hours following ovulation. The human ovum traverses the uterine tube in about three days after ovulation and enters the endometrial cavity as a morula. This is about average for many mammalian species.

The rate of ovum transport through the tube is probably under the influence of ovarian hormones (Austin), estrogens apparently augmenting peristaltic activity and progesterone inhibiting it. The true nature of the propulsive mechanism, however, is not well understood, particularly when one considers the need to explain paradoxical transport of spermatozoa in one direction and ova in the other within the uterine tube.

The remaining portion of ovum transport in the human occurs over the next four days, terminating with implantation. There are no studies concerning transit of the human ovum within the endometrial cavity. Animal studies suggest that the egg is propelled to its destination by a mechanism of uterine muscular action and that preconditioning of the muscle by progesterone is necessary. It seems reasonable to assume that a similar mechanism is operant in the human as evidenced by the fact that implantation occurs most often in specific areas on the uterine wall. The most favored site is near the midline about midway between the fundus and the internal os of the cervix, more commonly on the posterior wall.

IMPLANTATION

The process of implantation involves loss of the zona pellucida, adherence of the blastodermic vesicle to the endometrial surface and erosion of the epithelium so that the blastula burrows beneath the endometrial surface. The ovum orients itself by an unknown mechanism so that the pole containing the embryo-forming inner cell mass contacts the endometrial surface first. This situation holds for humans and many other mammals.

Hertig and Rock presented material showing that the youngest observed implanted fertilized human ovum (Fig. 25) appeared as a superficial structure with a central embryonic mass and peripheral blastocele at seven and one-half days following ovulation. It measured about 300μ, which is only about twice the size of the mature ovum. Histological section of this early embryo (Fig. 26) showed rather shallow anchoring with trophoblastic cells and projection of the thin collapsed outer wall of the blastocele into the lumen of the endometrial cavity.

An even earlier stage of implantation of the monkey ovum was shown by Heuser and Streeter (Fig. 27). The very beginning of penetration is occurring with minimal disturbance of the endothelial lining cells. The point of adherence is clearly demonstrated to be closely juxtaposed to the site of the inner cell mass pole. The abembryonic pole of the blastocyst wall projects well into the lumen. The situation in the monkey is substantively different from that in man and the higher apes because implantation tends to be superficial rather than interstitial. The monkey blastocyst embeds itself onto the endometrium and remains essentially an intracavitary structure within the uterus during gestation.

In the human, on the other hand, the blastocyst buries itself in the endometrium, thereby no longer occupying the uterine cavity as such. It does, however, in reality, effect the obliteration of the lumen after about the third month. The human blastocyst penetrates the mucosa by a process of ingrowth until the point of its entrance is covered over by the growth of maternal endometrial cells. The blastocyst expands within the mucosa laterally.

Implantation occurs on an endometrium that has not yet fully developed into decidua. Secretory changes have occurred under the influence of progestational hormonal stimulus from the developing corpus luteum. The endometrium may range in development from about the eighteenth to the twenty-third day of the menstrual cycle.

The biophysical mechanism of implantation of the human ovum is unknown because there is a critical gap in observations of human specimens between those

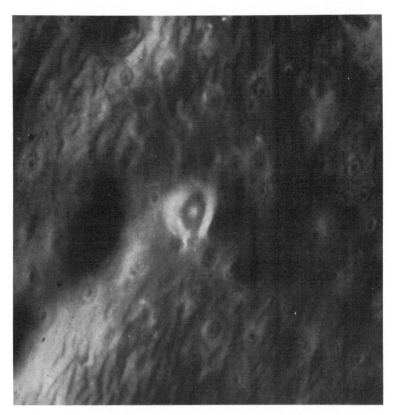

Figure 25 Gross view of earliest normal implantated human fertilized ovum 7½ days from ovulation. Specimen photographed under fluid. Mouths of endometrial glands are evident as tiny dark spots surrounded by concentric rings. The superficially implanted ovum contains a central embryonic mass surrounded by a darker ring of the chorionic cavity and a peripheral opaque outer ring representing the trophoblast seen on edge. (Magnification × 35.) (From Hertig, A. T., and Rock, J.: Contrib. Embryol. *31*:65, 1945.)

free-floating blastocysts in the transport stage and the ova already deeply implanted in the endometrial stroma. Observations in lower primates, particularly the rhesus monkey, tentatively fill this informational hiatus. Böving outlined the steps in the sequence of events in primate implantation based on such composite data. Beginning with a transport stage, the ovum is subjected to phenomena of adhesion, penetration and migration from the uterine lumen through the endometrial lining epithelium to lodge in the stroma. Trophoblastic proliferation ensues while the surface endometrium heals over. It is probable that the zona pellucida is shed during the transport stage before adhesion takes place.

The chemical and mechanical interrelationships involved in this progressive integration of ovum and endometrium have been studied in the rabbit in considerable

detail (Böving). Although this information is probably not applicable to the human, it provides much insight into this complex process. Adhesion of the rabbit ovum to the endometrial lining appears to involve a progesterone-dependent increase of endometrial carbonic anhydrase that accelerates carbon dioxide removal by way of accessible maternal blood vessels, thereby causing a rise of pH in the vicinity of these vessels. The resulting alkalinity renders sticky the *gloiolemma,* the outer layer of mucus and cellular debris condensed or deposited on the rabbit ovum during its transit through the uterine cavity. Whether or not the loosely aggregated layer of mucus and debris that has been observed surrounding human ova acts in a similar manner to effect adhesion is not known. In the rabbit, but not in most other mammals, there is also an inner *mucolemma* deposited on the ovum by the tubal epithelium

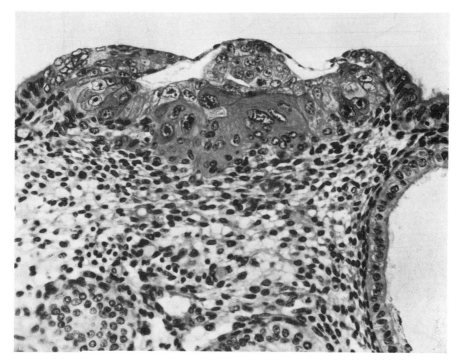

Figure 26 Histological section of the ovum shown in Figure 25 well attached by its trophoblast at the embryonic pole. It is so shallowly implanted at this stage that almost half of it is exposed to the lumen showing characteristics of the blastocyst wall at the abembryonic pole. The primitive character of the trophoblast is evident, with large, dark, multinucleated masses representing primitive syncytiotrophoblast and relatively small, light, discrete cells representing the primitive cytotrophoblast. The embryonic rudiment is the globular mass in the center of the flattened chorionic cavity. It shows primitive endoderm above and ectoderm below. The primordium of the amniotic sac is the tiny cleft between the ectoderm and the trophoblast. (Magnification × 300.)

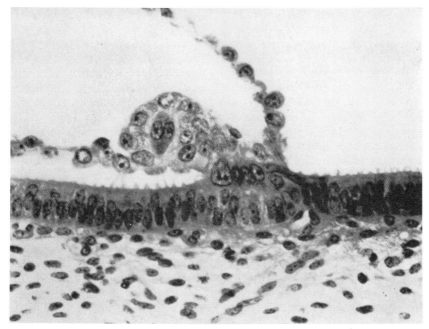

Figure 27 Ovum of the rhesus monkey in the earliest stage of attachment thus far recovered. It exhibits beginning penetration or fusion with disturbance of epithelial cells over a capillary. (Magnification × 200.) (From Heuser, C. H., and Streeter, G. L.: Contrib. Embryol. 29:15, 1941.)

under progesterone influence, and it is probably also altered by alkalinity to favor adhesion.

The innermost layer investing the blastula is the oolemma or zona pellucida, which is common to all mammals. Its removal has been considered indispensable for implantation of the eggs of certain species (Dickmann and Noyes). The simplistic concept that the oolemma serves merely as a barrier that must be removed before implantation can occur is now doubted on the basis of Böving's findings in the rabbit.

Trophoblastic invasion of the endometrium has been attributed to the inherently aggressive nature of these cells as well as a predisposition on the part of the underlying epithelium to invasion. Teleologically, purposeful exploration for nutritional need by the trophoblast and provision of such nutriments by the endometrium have also been proffered as explanations. None of these is entirely satisfactory. The fact that invasion begins at epivascular locations in the rabbit, in sites comparable to those at which adhesion takes place, suggested to Böving that a comparable mechanism existed, namely, that invasion is a consequence of removal of carbon dioxide with subsequent focal alkalinization. Lysis of the lemmas exposes trophoblastic knobs to direct contact with the epithelium, and epivascular alkalinity causes adherence. This is followed by loss of cohesion by endometrial lining cells in the vicinity. Simultaneously, the trophoblastic knobs grow or are pushed through the epithelium by undefined forces. It is believed that the trophoblast does not experience the same cellular dissociation as the endometrial lining cells because it is syncytial rather than cellular. This is speculative. Similarly, the mechanism by which the blastocyst migrates from the endometrial lumen through the epithelium and into the stroma is ill defined.

As the implantation process proceeds, the collapsed blastocyst becomes lodged in the stroma. The trophoblastic outer layer proliferates and invades the stroma. It differentiates a peripheral syncytial layer. The blastocele reexpands and the endometrial lining heals over completely so that the blastocyst is entirely engulfed in the endometrium. The trophoblast at the invading pole increases rapidly and spreads in an undermining fashion into the stroma. Most of the proliferation is accomplished by the central cytotrophoblast. The more peripheral syncytiotrophoblast is considered to be phagocytic and it does not appear to reproduce itself.

The solid trophoblastic elements continue to spread through the stroma at the site of implantation and to envelop maternal blood vessels. *Lacunae* appear in the trophoblast (Fig. 28) by about the ninth day after ovulation (two days after implantation). These vacuolated spaces represent the framework for the maternal circulation of the placenta. It is conceivable that they arise in the endometrial stroma from preexisting engulfed maternal vessels which have lost their endothelial lining. More likely, they form as empty spaces *de novo*. When continuity is established between the lacunae and maternal vessels, the maternal component of the placental circulation is established with maternal blood flowing through spaces that are lined by trophoblast.

DECIDUA FORMATION

The endometrial lining of the uterus consists of a simple columnar epithelium and an underlying stroma (Fig. 29). The epithelium includes ciliated and mucus-secreting cells arranged to form tubular glands that penetrate the stroma and may even enter the underlying muscularis. Under cyclic stimulation of the ovarian hormones, the endometrium undergoes periodic morphologic changes. These are sufficiently characteristic to permit accurate histological dating of the endometrium with reference to the menstrual cycle (Fig. 30).

The typical 28-day cycle is conventionally considered to begin with the onset of menstrual bleeding. The bleeding phase is inconstant in duration but generally lasts about three days. It is associated with debridement of the surface endometrium so that only the glands of the *basalis* remain (Fig. 31).

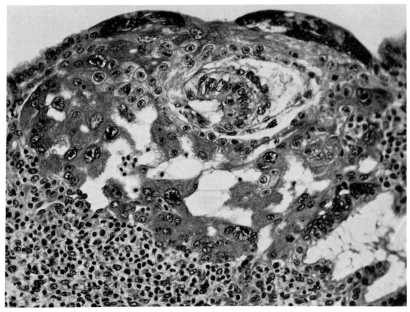

Figure 28 A slightly more advanced early human conceptus nine days after ovulation with blastocele still collapsed but exhibiting much more trophoblastic proliferation and lacunar development within the trophoblast. A maternal vessel is enveloped by trophoblast and shows continuity with the lacunae. No decidual reaction is seen in the stroma, and villi have not yet appeared. (Magnification × 300.) (From Hertig, A. T., et al.: Amer. J. Anat. 98:435, 1956.)

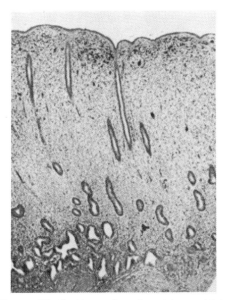

Figure 29 Section of endometrium obtained during the proliferative phase of the menstrual cycle, 11 days after the onset of menstruation. (Magnification × 10.) (Culbertson Collection No. 251, courtesy of G. W. Bartelmez.)

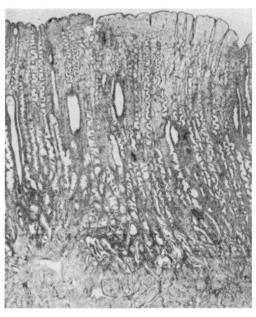

Figure 30 Endometrium of the secretory phase at the twentieth day of the menstrual cycle showing typical saw-toothed convolutions of the endometrial glands. Clear distinction can be made between the zona compacta, zona spongiosa, and zona basalis. (Magnification × 10.) (From Novak, E. R., and Woodruff, J. D.: Novak's Gynecologic and Obstetric Pathology. Philadelphia, W. B. Saunders Company, 1967.)

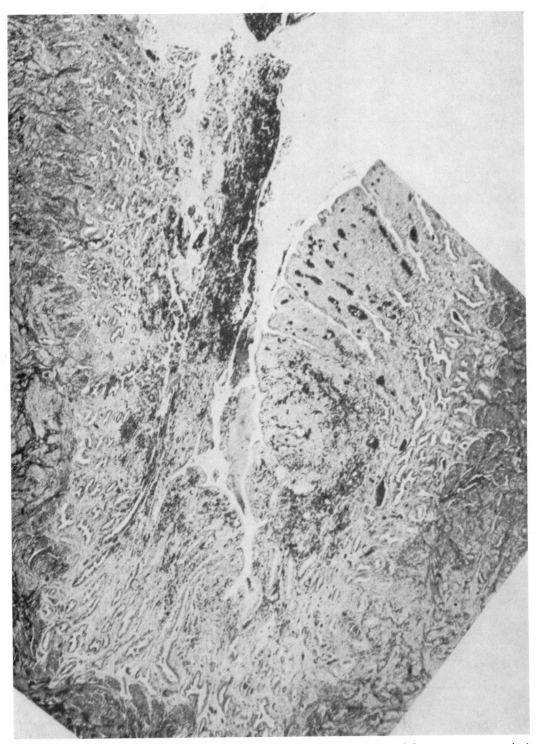

Figure 31 Endometrium on the first day of menstruation showing a spectrum of changes in a counterclock-wise direction. Right, prehemorrhagic congestion with blood appearing as dark sequestrations. Bottom, extravasation is seen. Left, there is clear-cut desquamation. (Magnification × 30.) (From Bartelmez, G. W.: Contrib. Embryol. *24*:141, 1933.)

Endometrium is functionally divisible into three zones: The deepest layer resting on the myometrium, the *basalis,* is composed of the base of undifferentiated endometrial glands incapable of responding to progesterone stimulus with secretory activity. The basalis provides the wherewithal for endometrial regeneration after menstrual sloughing in response to estrogenic stimulus. The superficial or functional zone of the endometrium is divisible into two readily distinguishable strata: *compacta* and *spongiosa.* Both respond to progesterone, but the outer compacta undergoes deciduoid changes as well.

At the conclusion of the menstrual phase, under the stimulating influence of estrogens being produced by a developing group of primordial follicles, the *follicular* or *proliferative* phase begins. It lasts from about the fourth to the fourteenth day after the onset of menstruation. Characteristically, the endometrium develops from a rather thin lining with low cuboidal epithelium and straight, nonconvoluted glands with no evidence of secretory activity. The stroma is compact and appears nonvascular. During the proliferative phase the epithelial cells undergo growth activity as evidenced by mitoses. The surface epithelium becomes taller and columnar and the glands become progressively hypertrophic with steadily increasing numbers of convolutions.

Following ovulation, *secretory* activity begins with the appearance of subnuclear vacuoles containing glycogen granules. At first the cell nuclei are pushed toward the gland lumen by these vacuoles. Later, as the glycogen is secreted into the gland lumen, the cell nuclei return to their original basal position. Concurrently, the stroma becomes abundant and is hyperemic. Late in the secretory phase, the mucosa tends to be thick, measuring 3 to 8 mm., and is usually pale and edematous. The glands are quite tall and tortuous. These secretory changes are brought about under the influence of progesterone.

The superficial layer of the endometrium during the late secretory phase shows abundant stroma between glands (Fig. 32). The stromal cells appear to be hypertrophied, showing abundant perinuclear cytoplasm. This *pseudodecidual reaction* is characterized by a compact layer of epithelioid cells in the stroma near the uterine lumen. The deeper stroma tends to remain somewhat edematous and less cellular.

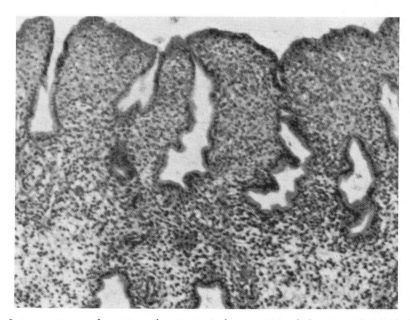

Figure 32 Late secretory endometrium showing typical progestational changes with pseudodecidual reaction characterized by compact layer of epithelioid cells in the stroma near the uterine lumen. The deeper stroma remains somewhat edematous. Infiltration by polymorphonuclear leukocytes has begun. (Magnification × 100.) (From Noyes, R. W., et al.: Fertil. Steril. *1*:3, 1950.)

If conception should not occur, leukopedesis will take place with widespread infiltration by polymorphonuclear leukocytes and round cells. This occurs in response to acute withdrawal of supporting hormones. It is followed by the tissue degeneration and the desquamation of *menstruation.* The basalis layer takes no part in the functional cycle of menstruation so that only the compacta and the spongiosa are sloughed.

When conception takes place, the hypertrophic and secretory changes of the progestational phase are exaggerated. The endometrial glands become even more tortuous and scalloped. The epithelium secretes actively. Stromal cells enlarge and the cytoplasmic content of the cells increases. These polygonal *decidual cells* arrange themselves in a mosaic pattern throughout the superficial stratum compacta where the glands are sparse. In the deeper stratum spongiosum, on the other hand, glandular hypertrophy abounds to form the typical lacy pattern of the decidua of early pregnancy (Fig. 33). Decidual cells are 40 to 50μ in diameter with clear vesicular cytoplasm. They are tightly

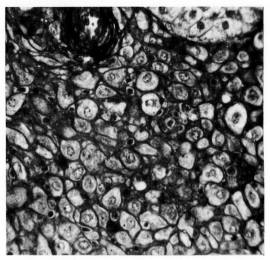

Figure 34   High-power view of the zona compacta of the decidua vera at five weeks' gestational age showing large glycogen-laden decidual cells. Among them are found various types of wandering cells. A deeply stained arteriole and the edge of a gland are seen near the top. (Magnification × 380.)

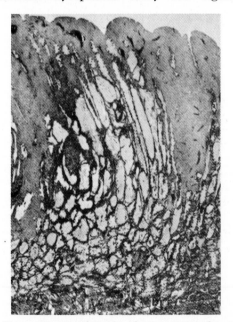

Figure 33   Decidua of early pregnancy showing clearly defined superficial zona compacta contrasting sharply with the lacy network of the zona spongiosa. (Magnification × 10.) (From Novak, E. R., and Woodruff, J. D.: Novak's Gynecologic and Obstetric Pathology. Philadelphia, W. B. Saunders Company, 1967.)

pressed together with little intercellular space. They contain abundant fluid and glycogen (Fig. 34).

It is of interest to note that the decidual changes in stromal cells just described may occur in tissues other than the endometrium. They have been found in the uterine tubes and in ectopic foci of endometrium. They can be produced experimentally in animals by traumatizing the endometrium after appropriate conditioning with progesterone.

Following implantation (see above), trophoblastic proliferation spreads beneath the endometrial mucosa for a considerable distance. As a result the overlying layer of mucous membrane covering the ovum becomes the *decidua capsularis.* The portion on which the ovum rests is termed the *decidua basalis.* The remaining uterine lining is called the *decidua vera* (Fig. 35).

The changes which take place in the various parts of the endometrium during pregnancy vary considerably. The most pronounced changes take place in the decidua basalis. Essentially all trophoblastic development concentrates here. Widespread decidual reaction is seen in the stroma, especially in the superficial third. Glands and blood vessels are mechanically compressed by the growing con-

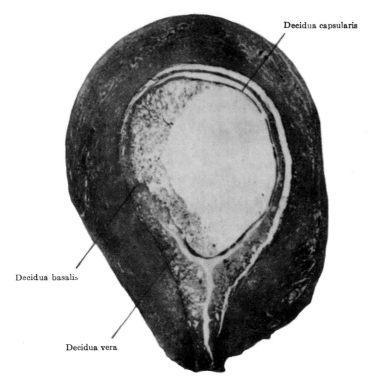

Decidua capsularis

Decidua basalis

Decidua vera

Figure 35 Gross section of the gravid uterus at six weeks showing the three deciduas. The decidua vera has developed in the lower uterine segment. The embryo does not appear in this section. (Magnification × 2.)

ceptus so that vertically oriented glands and blood vessels become distorted and assume oblique or horizontal courses.

By means of mechanical compression and trophoblastic erosion, the decidua basalis is progressively reduced in thickness until it is only a few millimeters in diameter. The glands of the decidua basalis degenerate early in this area of rapid trophoblastic invasion. They are compressed into a low, lamellous layer of spongy tissue. This is the site of the future placenta and the stratum in which separation of the placenta will take place post partum.

The decidua capsularis is that portion of the decidua vera which is stretched over the ovum. It tends to be thick at the equatorial portion and thin at the outer pole, the point at which the ovum buried itself into the mucosa. Trophoblastic invasion occurs in this layer in a manner similar to

that of the decidua basalis. However, because the decidua capsularis provides an unfavorable site, such growth tends to be abortive. Early villi form but soon atrophy because they encounter such little nutritive support. As the embryo continues to grow, moreover, the decidua capsularis atrophies extensively. By the time the conceptus occupies the entire uterine lumen, this layer is thin and fibrous. It fuses with the decidua vera on the opposite wall of the uterus.

The remaining endometrial lining, the decidua vera, continues to develop and thicken until the beginning of the third month, reaching 1 cm. in diameter. It forms smooth, thick folds or *rugae* on the surface. As pregnancy continues, it thins out until at term it is no more than 1 mm. in thickness.

The decidual reaction begins in the

perivascular stroma and spreads widely, sometimes extending deeply into the stroma separating muscle bundles in the myometrium. It is most conspicuous in the superficial third of the endometrium where it may even appear to compress the glands and to constrict their openings into the uterine cavity.

The glandular epithelium shows accentuated secretory activity and hypertrophy of the lining cells with typical corkscrew configuration of the glands. Much inspissated secretion appears within the gland lumina. By the time the conceptus completely occupies the uterine cavity at about the eighth to tenth week of gestation, regression of the decidua vera begins. Mechanical compression results in atrophy of all the tissue elements so that the glands virtually disappear and the decidual cells become smaller.

PLACENTATION

After the blastocyst has implanted in the uterine mucosa by burrowing through the epithelium into the stroma, the trophoblast that arises from the wall of the blastocyst differentiates into two layers. The outer layer, the *syncytiotrophoblast*, is in contact with maternal tissue. It forms a syncytial strip of protoplasm without cell margins and contains many large, oval nuclei. The inner cellular layer of trophoblast, the *cytotrophoblast* or *Langhans' layer*, is composed of cuboidal, mononucleated cells. About day 9 after ovulation, a third layer appears, intervening between the other two, consisting of the *mesoblast*, the connective tissue layer derived from the trophoblast.

Growth of the trophoblast is accomplished by proliferation of Langhans' cells. As it grows, it piles up into fingerlike processes called *chorionic villi*. These project into the surrounding decidual stroma pushing their outer covering of syncytium ahead of them (Fig. 36). The villi subdivide quickly and become increasingly complex, interlacing and anastomosing. Advancing tips of the villi erode the surrounding endometrium, destroying stroma and glands and opening the maternal capillaries.

Blood under low pressure escapes from the capillaries and gains entrance to the trophoblastic lacunae (see above) by way of cytotrophoblastic columns. The lacunar channels gradually become confluent until a single multilocular canalization has formed by the third or fourth week of development. With deeper penetration of trophoblast into the endometrium, the tips of the spiral arterioles are entered so that the head of pressure of maternal blood in the lacunae increases.

After the formation of a unified pool of maternal blood by coalescence of the lacunae, most villi will grow into the pool instead of into the decidua. Villi retaining attachment to the decidua are called anchoring villi (Fig. 36). In time, the maternal blood pool becomes so crowded with villi that its identity is obscured, meriting the commonly used descriptive term *intervillous space* (Figs. 37 and 38).

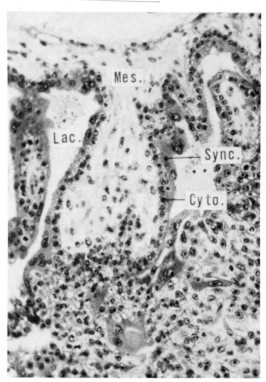

Figure 36 Portion of the wall of an implanted conceptus at approximately 16 days after ovulation. The chorionic cavity lies at the top of the field, the endometrial stroma below. Cytotrophoblast and syncytiotrophoblast are readily distinguished as well as the mesoblast that forms both the core of the villus and the inner wall of the chorion. The lacunae contain a few maternal erythrocytes. (From Heuser, C. H., et al.: Contrib. Embryol. *31*:85, 1945.)

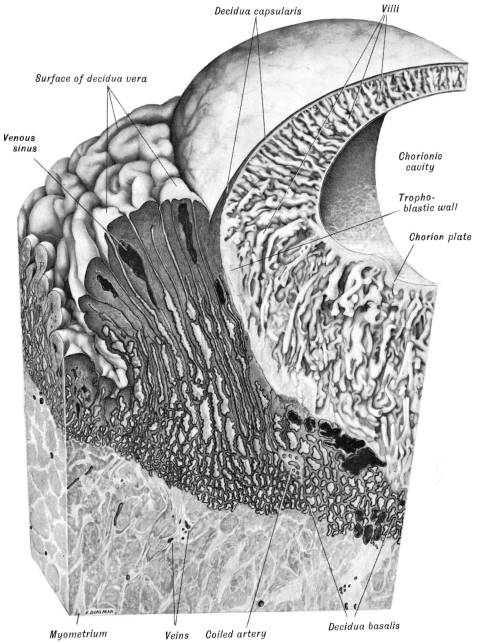

Decidua capsularis

Villi

Surface of decidua vera

Venous sinus

Chorionic cavity

Tropho-blastic wall

Chorion plate

E. DOHLMAN

Myometrium   Veins   Coiled artery

Decidua basalis

Figure 37   Margin of the implantation site of a four-week pregnancy with ovum enclosed in maternal decidua. The superficial chorion with its short villi is attached to the decidua capsularis which protrudes into the uterine lumen. Long villi adjacent to the decidua basalis have many secondary and a few tertiary branches and are anchored to the decidua by a wall of cytotrophoblast. The decidua vera shows its characteristic (1) superficial zona compacta with decidual reaction, (2) zona spongiosa of dilated and sacculated glands in a lacy network, and (3) zona basalis with narrow glands that may be entirely absent. In the implantation site the zona compacta has been obliterated by the developing ovum. (Magnification × 17.) (Courtesy of G. W. Bartelmez, from Bloom, W., and Fawcett, D. W.: A Textbook of Histology, ed. 9. W. B. Saunders Company, 1968.)

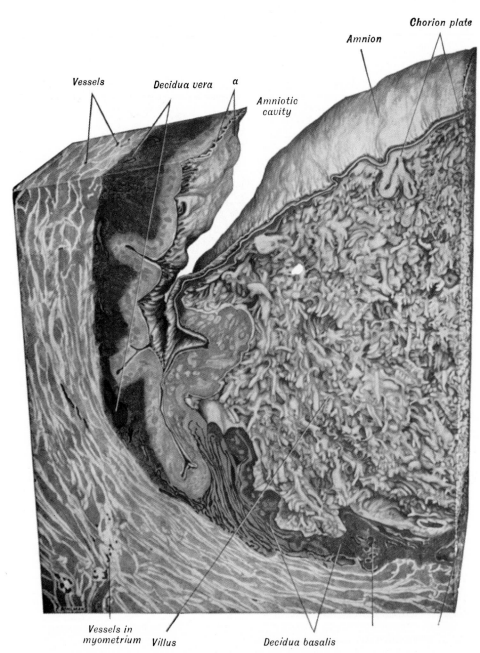

Figure 38   Margin of the placenta of a 16-week pregnancy showing fusion of the connective tissue of amnion and chorion (*a*) obliterating the exocoelom. Fusion of the decidua capsularis and chorion laeve has occurred with regression of the stretched decidua vera, filling the uterine cavity completely to the internal cervical os. Placental villi have grown and branched profusely, increasing the placental volume. The end of each villous trunk remains attached to the decidua basalis while the small twigs float freely in the blood contained in the intervillous space. (Magnification × 7.5.) (Courtesy of G. W. Bartelmez, from Maximow, A. A., and Bloom, W.: Textbook of Histology. Philadelphia, W. B. Saunders Company, 1957.)

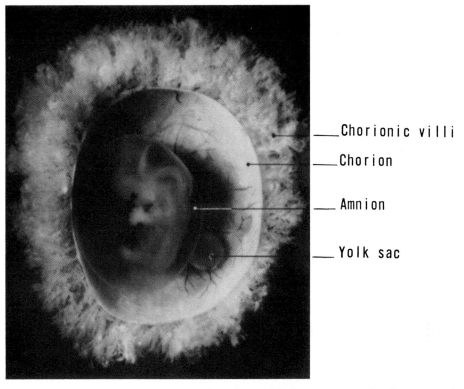

___Chorionic villi

___Chorion

___ Amnion

___ Yolk sac

Figure 39 Human embryo at ovulation age 55 days obtained by hysterectomy. The chorionic sac has been opened but the amnion remains intact. The amnion does not yet completely fill the chorionic sac. The villi at the abembryonic pole, destined to be chorion laeve, already show diminished size when compared with villi at the site of embryonic attachment, the chorion frondosum. (Magnification × 1½.) (Carnegie specimen No. 8537A. From Ramsey, E. M.: Amer. J. Obstet. Gynec. *84*:1649, 1962.)

As the ovum grows, the villi increase in number and complexity. They branch again and again, forming long tufts, and soon the surface of the chorion is covered by a thick brush of villi (Fig. 39). Those villi that grow in the direction of the capsularis find scant nourishment and hence soon atrophy and disappear. The process is started in the fourth week and ends by the ninth. The atrophied chorion is called the *chorion laeve.* If villi persist in the capsularis, a vestigial capsularis placenta may be formed.

The basalis is richly supplied with blood in an almost cavernous structure. Here the villi take on luxuriant growth. This is the site of the future placenta or *chorion frondosum.* As the chorionic sac increases in size, it completely fills the uterine cavity and the chorion laeve fuses with the decidua vera (Fig. 40). The *chorion* thus formed is the first and outermost of the two fetal membranes that enclose the embryo.

The inner membrane or *amnion* is derived from the trophoblastic mesoblast within the cavity of the blastocyst. When the inner cell mass has developed into an elongated plate of epithelial cells, the *ectodermal disk,* a small clear space becomes recognizable between the disk and the wall of the blastocyst. This represents the earliest formation of the amniotic cavity with the ectodermal disk as its floor and the mesoblast as the amnion (Fig. 41).

The mesoblast between the amnion and the trophoblastic wall condenses to form an attachment between the developing embryo and the wall of the chorionic sac. This is the *body stalk* destined to become the umbilical cord (Fig. 42). The major vessels contained in it are the umbilical arteries and vein.

Development of the *amnion* can be traced in Figures 41 and 42. At first overlying the embryonic rudiment, the amniotic sac comes to surround it in the manner in-

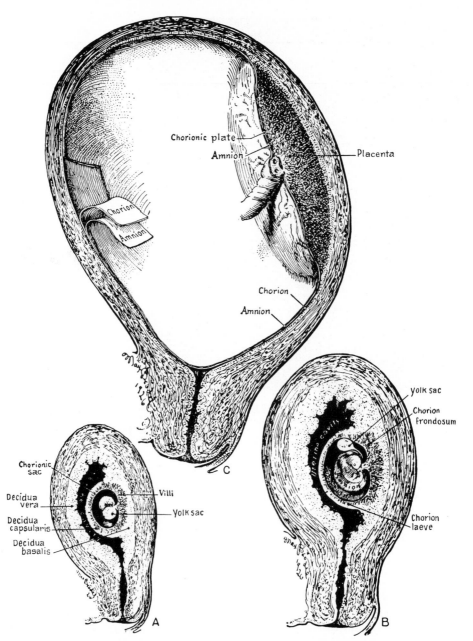

Figure 40 Cross sections of the gravid uterus showing three stages in the formation of placenta and membranes. *A*, At four weeks, the chorionic sac is uniformly covered with villi, but those on the abembryonic side projecting into the uterine cavity are beginning to thin. *B*, At six weeks, the villi have largely disappeared from the capsularis (chorion laeve), leaving only the basal villi to form the placenta (chorion frondosum). *C*, At five months, amnion and chorion have fused together and have become adherent to the opposite wall, thereby obliterating the uterine cavity. (From Williams, J. W.: Amer. J. Obstet. Gynec. *13*:1, 1927.)

dicated by the arrows in Figure 42. Its growing margins are finally merged into the body stalk. The embryo floats within the fluid that accumulates in the amniotic cavity. Early in the third month, the fluid-filled amniotic sac entirely fills the chorionic cavity and its wall fuses with the inner surface of the chorionic membrane (Fig. 43).

The mechanism by which the vestigial *yolk sac* forms is unclear. As the embryonic rudiment develops, the original

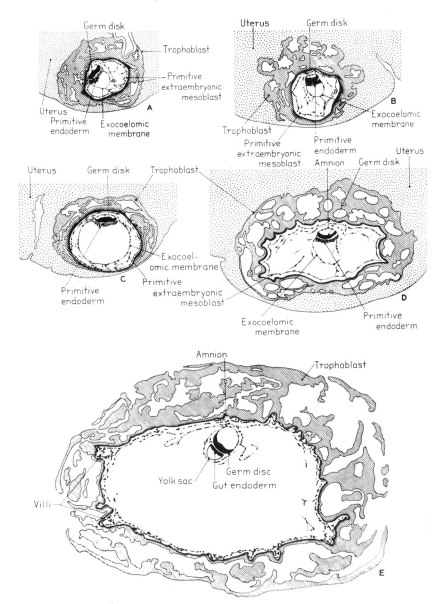

Figure 41 Development of the amnion, yolk sac, primitive mesoblast, trophoblast and villi in early embryos shown diagrammatically. Lacunae are represented by white spaces interspersed in the diagonally shaded trophoblast. The ages of the embryos shown are: *A*, 11 days (Hertig-Rock, Carnegie No. 7699); *B*, 11 days (Miller-Streeter, Carnegie No. 4900); *C*, 12 days (Hertig-Rock, Carnegie No. 7700); *D*, 12 days (Werner-Stieve); and *E*, about 13 days (Edwards-Jones-Brewer). (Magnification × 30.) (From the Carnegie Contributions to Embryology.)

single-layered ectodermal disk differentiates into a two-layered plate, endodermal cells appearing beneath the ectoderm on the side toward the center of the blastocele. The endoderm forms the roof of the yolk sac in the same way that the ectodermal disk forms the floor of the amnion. The rest of the yolk sac wall consists of mesoblast. The yolk sac in primates is never functional and does not grow larger than 1

to 1.5 cm. in diameter. The fluid within the yolk sac soon disappears and the sac atrophies during the fourth month. It persists as a barely recognizable fibrous strand within the umbilical cord.

The *allantois* is also vestigial in man. It originates as an outpocketing of the yolk sac, communicating both with the yolk sac and with the hindgut of the embryo (Fig. 42). Like the yolk sac, the allantois persists

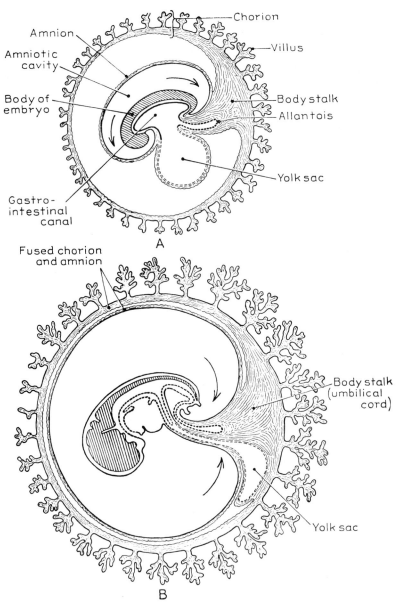

Figure 42 Further development of the amniotic cavity, yolk sac, allantois, and umbilical cord illustrated diagrammatically. Note the gradual distention of the amnion to surround the growing embryo and invest the umbilical cord together with its vestigial remnants of yolk sac and allantois. (From Corner, G. W., 1944.)

as a fibrous remnant embedded in the umbilical cord.

The microscopic structure of the *chorionic villus* (Fig. 44) presents a mesoblastic core and a trophoblastic covering in which syncytium forms the outer layer and Langhans' cells lie just beneath it. Fetal blood vessels are found in the mesoblast and large macrophages or Hofbauer cells are distributed through it.

Smooth muscle fibers have been demonstrated in the wall of the chorion and within the mesoblastic core of the villi (Krantz and Parker). Such muscle is said to occur in discontinuous sheets apparently independent of the muscle in the walls of blood vessels, though often blending with it. The role of the smooth muscle in the placenta is unclear. It may affect volume and flow of blood through the intervillous

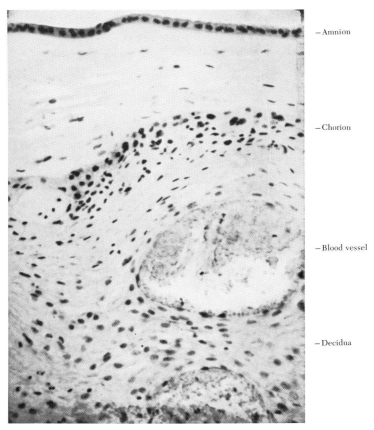

— Amnion

— Chorion

— Blood vessel

— Decidua

Figure 43   Decidua vera at term showing fused amnion and chorion in immediate juxtaposition to vascular decidua. (Magnification × 325.)

space, augmenting circulation by assisting the pulsations of the villi. Whether smooth muscle is present in sufficient quantity to exert an effect on placental circulation is moot. Nerves have not been demonstrated to date either in the chorionic plate or in the villi.

Although there is a basic villus structure, the relative proportions of constituents and their positions vary in different regions of the placenta and according to the stage of pregnancy. Each trunk together with its subdivisions constitutes a *fetal cotyledon,* which numbers 200 rather consistently in the mature placenta (Crawford). The term fetal cotyledon refers specifically to that portion of the placenta related to the ramifications of a single mainstem villus as contrasted with the maternal cotyledon, which refers to that portion of the placenta lying between two complete septa running between decidua and chorion.

Continued growth of the placenta is interstitial and is accomplished not by an increase in the number of cotyledons nor by expansion of the surface attachment to the endometrium but rather by continuous growth of new trophoblastic sprouts into the intervillous space. They are the sites for metabolic transfer of vital substances and wastes. These terminal units are richly supplied with capillaries embedded in a scanty connective tissue matrix. Increasingly larger branches have greater amounts of connective tissue core and carry larger units of the fetal vascular system. In the main trunks are found the major branches of the umbilical vessels surrounded by mature connective tissue sheaths beneath the trophoblastic investiture. Very few terminal units arise directly from the villus trunks. As a result, the region just beneath the chorionic plate, the *subchorial lake,* contains very few villi (Fig. 45).

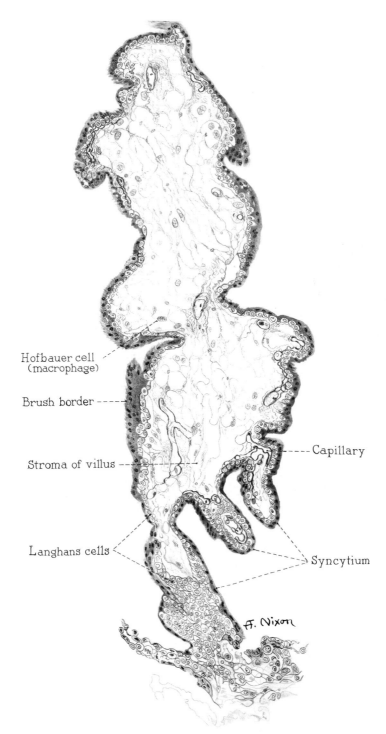

Hofbauer cell
  (macrophage)

Brush border

Stroma of villus

Capillary

Langhans cells

Syncytium

Figure 44   Section of a chorionic villus of a normal 10-week pregnancy showing both morphologic forms of trophoblasts, the dark superficial syncytiotrophoblast and the pale glycogen-laden Langhans' cells of the cytotrophoblast. (Magnification × 170.) (H487, University of Chicago.)

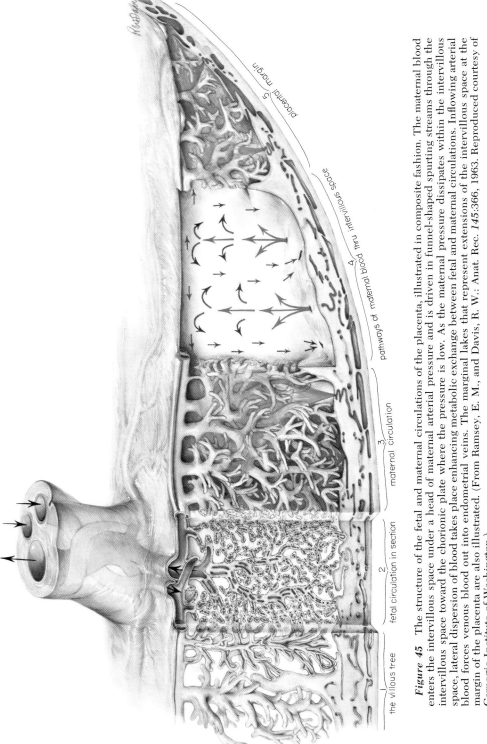

Figure 45 The structure of the fetal and maternal circulations of the placenta, illustrated in composite fashion. The maternal blood enters the intervillous space under a head of maternal arterial pressure and is driven in funnel-shaped spurting streams through the intervillous space toward the chorionic plate where the pressure is low. As the maternal pressure dissipates within the intervillous space, lateral dispersion of blood takes place enhancing metabolic exchange between fetal and maternal circulations. Inflowing arterial blood forces venous blood out into endometrial veins. The marginal lakes that represent extensions of the intervillous space at the margin of the placenta are also illustrated. (From Ramsey, E. M., and Davis, R. W.: Anat. Rec. *145:*366, 1963. Reproduced courtesy of Carnegie Institute of Washington.)

Labels in figure:
1 the villous tree
2 fetal circulation in section
3 maternal circulation
4 pathways of maternal blood thru intervillous space
5 placental margin

Variations in villus structure as correlated with the stage of pregnancy relate primarily to the terminal villi. At the end of the first trimester, for example, capillaries are centrally located in the villus and the stroma is loosely arranged. There is continuity of the Langhans' layer beneath the syncytium characteristically (Fig. 46A). Toward the end of the second trimester, only isolated Langhans' cells are seen, whereas the syncytial layer is still complete. The stroma is more compact and appears to be more cellular. Capillaries lie close to the trophoblastic covering. Often no stroma is seen between the capillary endothelium and the trophoblast. It is probably of some physiologic significance in that this arrangement reduces the amount of tissue that must be traversed by substances passing between the maternal and the fetal blood streams (Fig. 46B).

Evidence of "placental aging" includes deposition of fibrin on the surface of many villi (Fig. 46C). The fibrin may appear in scattered foci or in occasional solid sheets. In normal pregnancies near term, up to eight per cent of the villi may be involved with fibrin deposits. Thickening of the basement membrane may also occur, both of the trophoblast and of the capillary endothelium. A small proportion of villi may also show focal ischemia with secondary degeneration and hyalinization. It is necessary to point out that these features are normal occurrences, but may be considered pathologic where they are abnormally accentuated.

Details of the maternal circulation within the placenta are now available as a result of Ramsey's work. She has shown that both arterial supplying trunks and venous drainage channels are distributed indiscriminately throughout the maternal surface of the placenta. Quite early in embryonic development, the emerging spiral arterioles of the endometrium mature to supply a rich capillary network to the surface stratum. At the same time, the venules draining this network form a grid of vertical and horizontal channels. Prominent venous lakes are formed where the two systems intersect. The spiral arteries continue to grow and become increasingly coiled. They are diverted to oblique directions by increasing compression from the growing conceptus. The coils become looser and wider at midpregnancy when stretching by the uterine contents is most marked. At the same time, the inert thin-walled veins respond by passive dilatation and stretching.

Radioangiographic studies (Ramsey et al.; Freese) have shown that between 50 and 75 arteries communicate with the in-

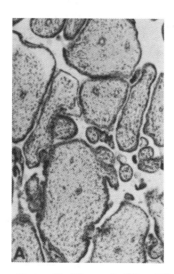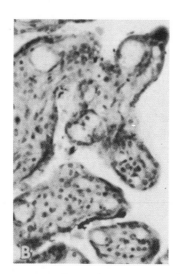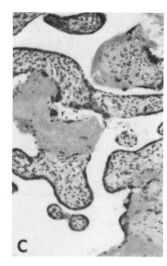

Figure 46 Placental villi at different gestational ages showing varying distances between fetal vessels within villous stroma and maternal intervillous space blood, as well as the amount and types of trophoblast composing the covering layer, and the presence or absence of fibrin. *A*, 12 weeks (Carnegie No. 7957, × 35); *B*, 22 weeks (Carnegie No. 8993, × 140); *C*, 23 weeks (Carnegie No. 9640, × 60.) (From Ramsey, E. M., 1955, 1958, 1962.)

tervillous space of the placenta. The number appears to increase up to about 12 weeks of gestational age and remains constant for the remainder of pregnancy (Crawford). The number of communicating veins, on the other hand, is progressively reduced with advancing pregnancy, especially under the influence of external compression. The persisting venous channels become increasingly distended as a result. The number of uteroplacental veins is very inconstant. Brosens and Dickson estimated this number at 120 spiral arteries in the human placenta at term.

A physiologic concept of the mechanism of circulation in the hemochorial placenta has been formulated by Ramsey. It considers that arterial blood enters by way of the spiral endometrial arterioles through the basal plate under a head of maternal blood pressure so that it spurts toward the chorionic plate before lateral dispersion occurs (Fig. 45). The blood in the intervillous space is drained toward the venous orifices in the basal plate. Mixing and slowing of the circulation takes place within the complex labyrinth of the intervillous space, thus aiding diffusion.

There appear to be no set channels for maternal circulation. Circulation is mediated by maternal blood pressure and restricted by myometrial contractions. Strong uterine contractions may effectively cut off arterial flow into the intervillous space. Similarly, venous outflow is curtailed by myometrial activity. Freese has shown that each placental cotyledon is supplied by one spiral artery which preferentially supplies blood to the *intracotyledonary space.* This concept was confirmed by Reynolds et al. who demonstrated highest pressure readings in the intervillous space located nearest the central cavity of the cotyledon and gradually diminishing pressures toward the subchorial lake.

Much controversy centers on the existence of the "marginal sinus" (Spanner). The vulnerability of the placental margin in terms of separation or rupture makes the vascular relationships in this area important. Although it is likely that no true marginal sinus exists as a separate entity, marginal portions of the intervillous space are present. They merge gradually with the subchorial lake above and with the rest of the intervillous space centrally. Such *marginal lakes* tend to occupy subordinate roles in both placental circulation and function. However, they are important in terms of trauma that may disrupt them. Moreover, distinction should be made between the marginal lakes of the placenta and the maternal venous sinuses located in the decidua lying at the margin of the placenta. The potential effects of rupture of these two types of vasculature are quite different. Whereas disruption of the marginal lake will interfere with placental circulation, rupture of the maternal venous sinus will only affect uterine circulation (Figs. 47 and 48).

THE MATURE PLACENTA

At term the placenta is a cakelike organ and weighs about 500 gm. The weight relationship between the placenta and the fetus is approximately 1:6. Grossly, placentas vary in weight, size, thickness, form and consistency. The placentas of syphilitic and erythroblastotic babies are heavier than those of normal infants of the same size, with the placentofetal ratio reduced to 1:3. Placentas affected by disorders associated with maternal hypertensive or renal diseases, on the other hand, tend to be relatively small with a placentofetal ratio exceeding 1:9. The placenta after delivery may appear small and thick or large and thin, the usual thickness being 1.5 to 2 cm., and the breadth 15 to 18 cm. It is generally discoid in shape, but may assume any shape depending on its growth on the uterine wall (Figs. 49 and 50).

The placenta may be spread over a large area in the form of a *placenta membranacea.* There may also exist accessory lobes, called *placenta succenturiata* (Fig. 51), connected to the main body of the placenta by an artery and vein. This entity carries great clinical significance because of the risks inherent in retention of one of the succenturiate lobes. If there are no blood vessels interconnecting the lobe, it is called a *placenta spuria.*

The shape of the placenta depends to a

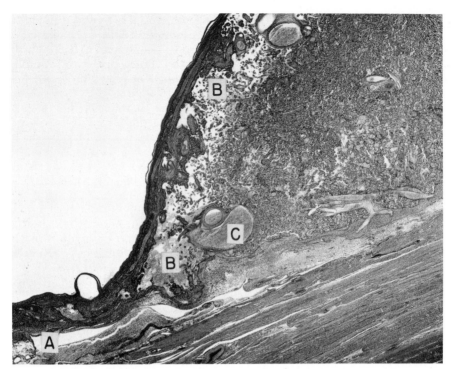

Figure 47   Placental margin of a 28-week pregnancy *in situ* in the uterus at a point where there is no dilatation of the peripheral intervillous space to designate as a marginal lake. A maternal vein (A) forms part of the subplacental wreath. The subchorial lake (B) dips down toward the junction of the decidua and trophoblast. At (C) a villus stalk contains dilated fetal vessels. (Magnification × 8.) (Carnegie No. 9158. From Ramsey, E. M.: Amer. J. Anat. 98:159, 1956.)

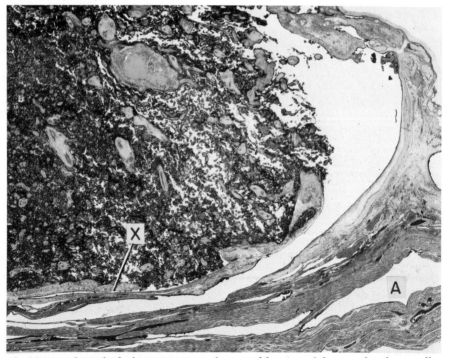

Figure 48   Margin of attached placenta at term showing dilatation of the peripheral intervillous space to form a marginal lake which empties into a wide venous channel leading to a slender vein whose oblique course drains indirectly via an orifice in the trophoblastic plate (X). Maternal veins forming the subplacental wreath are also shown (A). (Magnification × 10.) (Carnegie No. 9033.)

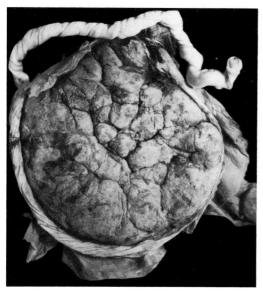 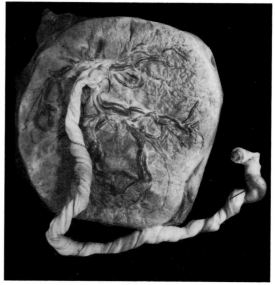

Fig. 49   *Fig. 50*

Figure 49   Gross view of the maternal surface of a full-term placenta showing cotyledonous structure. Chorion laeve and amnion form the membranes which are still attached peripherally.

Figure 50   Gross view of the fetal surface of the placenta shown in Figure 49. The umbilical cord is eccentrically implanted. The amnion has been removed to show the fetal vessels in their typical pattern of distribution.

considerable extent on its implantation site. When the ovum is attached centrally to the anterior or the posterior wall of the uterus, the placenta tends to be round or oval. If embedded near one of the lateral angles, a *bilobate* or *trilobate* placenta may result, ostensibly because the decidua, being thin at this point, offers poor nourishment to villi which then grow eccentrically. Division into lobes may also result from pathologic deposition of fibrin within the placenta.

In the condition known as *placenta circumvallata*, a wedge of decidua overlaps the margin of the placenta, inserting itself between the substance of the placenta and the membranes covering its fetal surface. The circumvallate placenta is not uncommon, various surveys reporting an incidence of 2 to 18 per cent. It presents the picture of a raised white ring around the periphery of the fetal surface of the placenta. A closely allied variant is *placenta marginata* in which a similar overlapping decidual ring is covered by fibrin and debris rather than by fetal membranes.

Some placentas are soft and vascular. Others are harder and more fibrous. The tissue of the organ is dark red, soft and friable, interwoven with tough fibrous tissue

and blood vessels. The maternal surface that has been stripped away from the uterine wall is covered with variably sized tags and sheets of decidua basalis. These are thin, grayish, translucent and slightly roughened membranes which cannot be peeled off readily but tear away from the underlying soft pulp of the placenta. They are attached by anchoring villi and consist of the more superficial and denser portion of the basalis as well as the compacta and the spongiosa.

Examination of the edge of the placenta shows the zone in which the fetal membranes are reflected down onto the surface of the decidua vera (Fig. 47). At the rim of the placenta and extending somewhat under the amnion one often finds a piling up of chorionic ectoderm and decidua to form the *closing ring of Winkler-Waldeyer*. This tucked-in edge is generally no more than a few millimeters in thickness. The maternal component of the ring bears the name *decidua subchorialis*. If the fetal membranes are peeled back in this area so that the interior of the placenta is exposed, components of the *marginal lakes* may be encountered, sometimes with conspicuous drainage channels. This dilatation of the lateral aspect of the intervillous space can

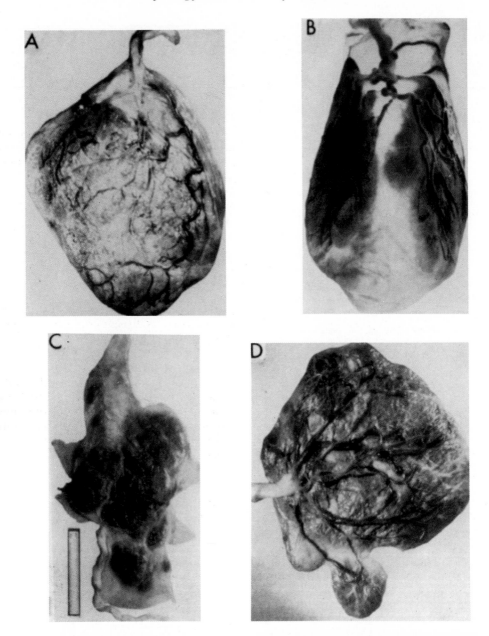

Figure 51 Term placentas showing common variations in shape and in insertion of the umbilical cord. *A, Battledore placenta* with velementous insertion of the umbilical vessels. *B, Bipartite placenta* with two distinct lobes of approximately equal size such as is commonly seen in lower primates, with concurrent velementous insertion of the vessels. *C, Placenta membranacea* with many small succenturiate lobes. *D, Placenta succenturiata* with small accessory lobe interconnected with the main body of placenta by an artery and a vein. (From Potter, E. L.: Pathology of the Fetus and the Infant, ed. 2. Chicago, Year Book Medical Publishers, Inc., 1961.)

sometimes be followed all around the circumference of the placenta, but it is not always continuous and may appear as a succession of chambers.

The maternal surface of the placenta is divided by decidual septa into numerous lobes called *maternal cotyledons* (Fig. 49).

Placental septa (Fig. 45) were once thought to be of trophoblastic origin, but recent sex chromatin studies have established that they originate from maternal tissues. At term most septa are delicate and fenestrated, permitting passage of intervillous blood through and around them.

Others are broad, substantial walls incorporated at one end with the chorion. These structures compartment the placenta into maternal cotyledons. If the cotyledons are pushed aside, the septum is split and the venous sinuses which drain into the intervillous space are disclosed.

Occasionally, a cotyledon will be sessile on the surface of the placenta and may inadvertently be left in the uterus at the time of delivery. Even careful examination of the delivered placenta may fail to reveal the absence of such a retained cotyledon. Hemorrhage or infection may result as a consequence.

The fetal surface of the placenta is covered by a thin glistening amnion through which the placental arteries and veins can be seen coming from the cord and branching in all directions. The smallest twigs discernible disappear into the substance of the placenta. None enter more than about 7 mm. from the edge. The fetal surface is uneven, gray or reddish in appearance, and sometimes dotted with white or yellow areas of fibrous tissue, called *white infarcts*. The amnion may be stripped away from the chorion on the fetal surface of the placenta except at the insertion of the cord where it is attached firmly to Wharton's jelly, which is particularly abundant here. The chorion is the outer, thicker, cloudy and somewhat opaque layer that is easily torn. On the fetal surface, the chorion tends to be inseparably attached to the villus trunks that spring from it. Shreds of endometrial tissue cling to the peripheral portion of the chorion after it has separated from the decidua vera at parturition.

THE UMBILICAL CORD

The umbilical cord is generally inserted near the middle of the fetal surface of the placenta. It may, however, insert at any location. If it inserts at the edge (marginal insertion), the result is a *battledore* placenta (Fig. 51). If the insertion is more distal so that the umbilical vessels course between the amnion and the chorion before reaching the placenta, the condition is known as *velamentous insertion*. Small epithelial amniotic growths or caruncles are occasionally found near the insertion of the cord. Inconstant remnants of the yolk sac duct (vitelline duct) and the remains of the allantois are occasionally encountered. The cord is covered by amnion but not by chorion.

It usually contains two umbilical arteries and one umbilical vein surrounded by Wharton's jelly. Rarely there may be two veins. The appearance of one artery only is abnormal and reflects the possibility of anomalous development. A single umbilical artery is encountered in 1.3 to 1.5 per cent of infants with a frequency of congenital abnormalities, including congenital heart disease and hypospadias, of the order of 25 per cent (Little; Benirschke and Bourne).

The pressure within the blood vessels of the cord during pregnancy distends them. They collapse at delivery after the cord is cut (Fig. 52). Twisting of the normal umbilical cord results from rotatory movements imparted to the fetus by the asymmetric contractions of the uterus. Pathologic torsion or twisting, even to the

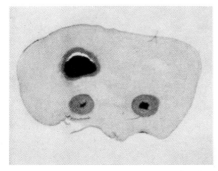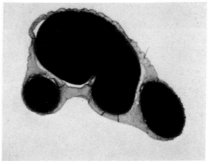

Figure 52 Cross sections of the human umbilical cord of term infants showing characteristic configuration of two arteries and one vein encased in Wharton's jelly. *Left*, Blood vessels are collapsed as seen in conventional preparations obtained after the cord has been cut and the vessels allowed to drain. *Right*, Blood vessels in the same cord distended by blood flowing through it. Note the displacement of Wharton's jelly by the distended vessels. (From Reynolds, S. R. M.: Anat. Rec. *113*:365, 1952.)

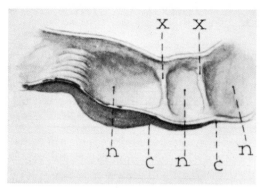

Figure 53 Longitudinal section of a segment of umbilical artery showing the folds of Hoboken (*x*), corresponding constrictions on the outer arterial surface (*c*) and dilatations or *noduli Hobokenii* (*n*). The folds of Hoboken cannot be considered true valves because they are incapable of obstructing backflow. (From Spivack, M.: Anat. Rec. 66:127, 1936.)

point of amputation, appears to be a consequence of fetal death, rather than a cause (Edmonds). Rotational movement of the fetus within the uterus apparently continues even after fetal death.

The amnion with its pavement epithelium is sharply delineated from the skin of the fetus where it juxtaposes at the umbilicus. It is of interest to note that the umbilical arteries are unique in that they possess folds which were described as valves by Hoboken in 1669. More recent investigations have shown that they cannot be regarded functionally or anatomically as valves (Spivack). They are actually

protrusions into the lumen of the arterial wall and include all its layers. They usually occupy a part or all of the circumference of the vessel wall. Histologically, they present thickenings of the media which may or may not be defined on the outer surface by a groove or furrow. Investigation shows them to be incapable of obstructing the backflow of blood as true valves do. Another peculiarity of the umbilical arteries is the presence of gross dilatations on their outer surfaces, known as *gemmulae* or *noduli Hobokenii* (Fig. 53). The umbilical vein possesses semilunar folds which consist of one layer of musculature, the bundles of which assume various directions.

The umbilical arteries are supplied with well-developed muscular coats and are capable of strong contractions. On cross section, their lumina may be narrowed to a slit. The contour of the lumen may be starlike, triangular, or sickle shaped. The capability of the arteries to narrow their lumina to almost complete closure is ascribed to the double spiral course of the muscular fibers in their walls.

Umbilical arteries do not possess an internal elastic lamina in contrast to other arteries of the same caliber, although they do contain elastic tissue within the substance of the media. Elastica appears in tissue sections as specks, clumps or fine wavy fibrils (Fig. 54). In the vein the internal

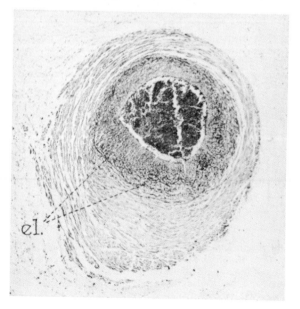

Figure 54 Section of an umbilical artery to illustrate distribution of the elastic tissue (*el.*) within the outer portion of the tunica media of the vessel wall. The elastica appears in the form of fine wavy transverse fibrils. (Magnification × 47, Orcein stain.) (From Spivack, M.: Anat. Rec. 85:85, 1943.)

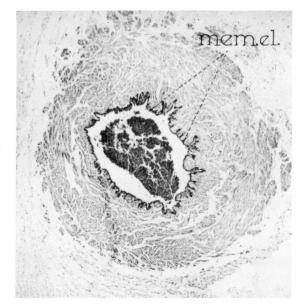

Figure 55 Microscopic section of an umbilical vein showing distinctive location of the well-developed and sharply outlined internal elastic membrane (*mem. el.*) bordering on the vessel lumen. (Magnification × 47, Orcein stain.) (From Spivack, M.: Anat. Rec. 85:85, 1943.)

elastic lamina is well defined as a sharply outlined wavy structure beneath the intima (Fig. 55). Ordinarily the contracted artery with its slitlike lumen is easily differentiated from the wide vein even with routine stains, but in some specimens the differential diagnosis would be difficult if the internal elastic lamina were not present. The umbilical arteries and vein do not possess vasa vasorum. Spivack could find no nerve fibers in any portion of the umbilical cord, but did encounter nonmedullated nerves in the abdominal portions of the umbilical arteries, presenting microscopic evidence for innervation of umbilical vasculature.

REFERENCES

Austin, C. R.: The Mammalian Egg. Springfield, Ill., Charles C Thomas, 1951.

Bartelmez, G. W.: Histological studies on the menstruating mucous membrane of the human uterus. Contrib. Embryol. 24:141, 1933.

Benirschke, K., and Bourne, G. L.: The incidence and prognostic implication of congenital absence of one umbilical artery. Amer. J. Obstet. Gynec. 79:251, 1960.

Bloom, W., and Fawcett, D. W.: A Textbook of Histology, ed. 9. Philadelphia, W. B. Saunders Company, 1968.

Böving, B. G.: Implantation Mechanisms. *In* Hartman, C. G., ed.: Mechanisms Concerned with Conception. New York, The Macmillan Company, 1963.

Brosens, I., and Dickson, H. G.: The anatomy of the maternal side of the placenta. J. Obstet. Gynaec. Brit. Comm. 73:357, 1966.

Crawford, J. M.: Foetal placental circulation: III. Anatomy of cotyledons. J. Obstet. Gynaec. Brit. Emp. 63:542, 1956.

Dickmann, Z., and Noyes, R. W.: The zona pellucida at the time of implantation. Fertil. Steril. 12:310, 1961.

Edmonds, H. W.: The spiral twist of the normal umbilical cord in twins and in singletons. Amer. J. Obstet. Gynec. 67:102, 1954.

Freese, U. E.: The uteroplacental vascular relationship in man. Amer. J. Obstet. Gynec. 101:8, 1968.

Greenwald, G. S.: Tubal transport of ova in the rabbit. Anat. Rec. 133:386, 1959.

Hertig, A. T., and Rock, J.: On the development of the early human ovum with special reference to the trophoblast of the previllous stage: A description of 7 normal and 5 pathological human ova. Amer. J. Obstet. Gynec. 47:149, 1944.

Hertig, A. T., and Rock, J.: Two human ova of previllous stage, having development age of about seven and nine days respectively. Contrib. Embryol. 31:65, 1945.

Hertig, A. T., Rock, J., and Adams, E. C.: A description of 34 human ova within the first 17 days of development. Amer. J. Anat. 98:435, 1956.

Heuser, C. H., and Streeter, G. L.: Development of the macaque embryo. Contrib. Embryol. 29:15, 1941.

Heuser, C. H., Rock, J., and Hertig, A. T.: Two human embryos showing early stages of definitive yolk sac. Contrib. Embryol. 31:85, 1945.

Krantz, K. E., and Parker, J. C.: Contractile properties of the smooth muscle in the human placenta. Clin. Obstet. Gynec. 6:26, 1963.

Lewis, W. H., and Hartman, C. G.: Early cleavage stages of the egg of the monkey, Macaca (Pithecus) rhesus. Contrib. Embryol. 24:187, 1933.

Little, W. A.: Aplasia of the umbilical artery. Bull. Sloane Hosp. 4:127, 1958.

Novak, E. R., and Woodruff, J. D.: Novak's Gynecologic and Obstetric Pathology, ed. 6. Philadelphia, W. B. Saunders Company, 1967.

Noyes, R. W., Hertig, A. T., and Rock, J.: Dating the endometrial biopsy. Fertil. Steril. 1:3, 1950.

Potter, E. L.: Pathology of the Fetus and the Infant, ed. 2. Chicago, Year Book Medical Publishers, Inc., 1961.

Ramsey, E. M.: Vascular patterns in the endometrium and placenta. Angiology 6:321, 1955.

Ramsey, E. M.: Circulation in maternal placenta of rhesus monkey and man, with observations on marginal lakes. Amer. J. Anat. 98:159, 1956.

Ramsey, E. M.: Circulation in the intervillous space of the primate placenta. Amer. J. Obstet. Gynec. 84:1649, 1962.

Ramsey, E. M., and Davis, R. W.: A composite drawing of the placenta to show its structure and circulation. Anat. Rec. 145:366, 1963.

Ramsey, E. M., Corner, G. W., Jr., and Donner, M. W.: Serial and cineradioangiographic visualization of maternal circulation in the primate (hemochorial) placenta. Amer. J. Obstet. Gynec. 86:213, 1963.

Reynolds, S. R. M.: The proportion of Wharton's jelly in relation to distention of the umbilical arteries and vein, with observations on the folds of Hoboken. Anat. Rec. 113:365, 1952.

Reynolds, S. R. M., Freese, U. E., Bieniarz, J., Caldeyro-Barcia, R., Mendez-Bauer, C., and Escarcena, L.: Multiple simultaneous intervillous space pressures recorded in several regions of the hemochorial placenta in relation to functional anatomy of the fetal cotyledon. Amer. J. Obstet. Gynec. 102:1128, 1968.

Spanner, R.: Mutterlicher und kindlicher Kreislauf der menschlichen Plazenta und seine Strombahnen. Z. Anat. Entwicklungsgesch. 105:163, 1935.

Spivack, M.: On the anatomy of the so-called "valves" of the umbilical vessels, with special reference to the "valvulae Hobokenii." Anat. Rec. 66:127, 1936.

Spivack, M.: On the presence or absence of nerves in the umbilical blood vessels of man and guinea pig. Anat. Rec. 85:85, 1943.

Williams, J. W.: Placenta circumvallata. Amer. J. Obstet. Gynec. 13:1, 1927.

Chapter 4

Functional Roles of the Placenta

The placenta is a remarkable organ that takes form, develops into a large complex structure, engages in intricate biologic processes and becomes senescent in a nine-month period. During this time it serves as a means for interchange of many substances between the fetal and maternal bloodstreams maintaining fetal homeostasis. It has many activities which are in part comparable to those of the gastrointestinal, respiratory, circulatory and renal systems of the adult. It is also apparently an active biochemical laboratory in which endocrine substances and enzymes are produced. The placenta, therefore, is an organ of synthesis, degradation and transfer of substances between mother and fetus. These functions of the placenta involve not only regulation of the activities of the reproductive organs throughout the period in which the offspring is dependent on the mother but also maintenance of other organs, such as the adrenals and mammary glands, not directly concerned with the initiation, continuation and termination of pregnancy.

One may subdivide the recognized functions of the placenta into three major categories: (1) those concerned with preparation for parturition and the puerperium, (2) those dealing with the maintenance of pregnancy, and (3) those dealing primarily with fetal support. We will deal in greater detail with the preparatory aspects in our discussions on myometrial function (see Chapter 15). Suffice it to say for now that, under the influence of hormonal substances elaborated by the placenta, the myometrium undergoes hypertrophy and increased production of adenosinetriphosphate, actin and myosin content, and simultaneously there is preparation of accessory organs, such as the breast, for puerperal function. Pregnancy is maintained by independent regulation of the hormonal environment, inhibition of uterine contractility, prevention of the expulsion of the conceptus, interference with mechanisms of heterograft rejection and suppression of cyclic pituitary-ovarian function. For fetal support, there is maintenance of fetal homeostasis, support of oxygenation, nutrition and growth, as well as pathways for waste disposal, while at the same time the fetus is provided with a "barrier" against certain agents and organisms. This chapter will deal separately with these several functions, except for those dealing with preparation of the myometrium and the mammary gland.

HORMONE REGULATION

The concept of the placenta acting as an endocrine organ arose in the first decade of this century partly out of the general interest in ductless glands, and partly out of the endeavor to ascertain how the maternal economy adapted itself to pregnancy. It was also necessary to solve the question of how uterine contents could come to alter the mother's metabolism. The changes induced in the maternal organism by the products of conception are multiple and varied, and even today are not yet fully characterized. It is certainly interesting to realize that the endocrine function of the placenta was completely unknown as recently as 50 years ago. The discovery in 1927 of large amounts of estrogens and gonadotropin in the urine and blood of pregnant women led knowledgeable people to wonder whether the placenta is a gland of internal secretion. This can now be answered unequivocally. Nevertheless, several questions are still unanswered in detail. These include the number and kinds of hormones produced by the placenta, their quantities and the secretory activity of the placenta in different species. Although the specific hormones involved may vary widely from species to species, it is generally agreed that the primary endocrine function of the placenta is concerned with the maintenance of pregnancy.

Two broad categories of hormones are involved: protein *gonadotropins* capable of prolonging the function of the corpus luteum beyond its usual duration of action, and *steroids* capable of reproducing many of the general metabolic effects characteristic of the pregnant state. One of the recurring themes in the story of the evolution of the reproductive process has been the ingenious and diverse endocrine functions assumed by the human placenta. These have been exceeded only by the activities ascribed to this organ which have never been fully confirmed and remain the object of continued research efforts.

From the extensive literature on the subject, it can be stated with reasonable certainty that the hormones of the human placenta include at least chorionic gonadotropin, estrogens and progesterone. Estrogens and progesterone are not peculiar to pregnancy, to the human being or to the placenta. Human chorionic gonadotropin, on the other hand, is an apparently unique substance, but has counterparts in malignant trophoblastic tissue of both sexes. It should be apparent from this that the problems of placental hormone production reflect only one facet of the much larger area of endocrinology. Moreover, hormonal control of pregnancy is not yet completely defined. Rapid advances in our knowledge of the chemistry and biology of the hormones produced by the placenta have made available for discussion and edification many areas of accomplishment. These include the isolation of chemically pure hormones, actual biosynthesis of polypeptide hormones, the evaluation of the relationships between structure and biological activity, the definition of species specificities and the use of immunologic techniques for bioassays.

Chorionic Gonadotropin

There appears to be ample evidence that the placenta is a source of chorionic gonadotropin. There is some question as to what its true function in pregnancy is. Comparative data with lower animals indicate that it has a luteotropic function for maintaining the corpus luteum of pregnancy, but there is no prima facie evidence to support this. The nature and significance of the effects of chorionic gonadotropin on fetal adrenals and gonads have been the subject of intense interest, but whether such effects have biological relevance is difficult to determine. Similarly, the question of gonadotropic influence on the syncytiotrophoblastic elaboration of steroids also remains unanswered. Fluorescent antibody studies have determined that the human chorionic gonadotropin is exclusively located in the syncytium (Thiede and Choate). Whether this actually does represent its site of origin or merely indicates a rapid transfer-storage phenomenon is undetermined at this juncture.

The maternal pituitary as a possible source of gonadotropic substances in pregnancy has been effectively demonstrated. Excretion of urinary gonadotropin was maintained at normal levels in a patient following hypophysectomy for breast cancer (Little et al.). Direct evidence that the cytotrophoblast synthesizes chorionic gonadotropin has been shown utilizing cultures of placental tissue (Gey et al.; Jones et al.).

Human chorionic gonadotropin is a glycoprotein with a molecular weight between 30,000 and 100,000, depending on the method of isolation. It is different structurally from pituitary gonadotropins because the carbohydrate portion of the molecule contains hexosamine and galactose. It is secreted in pregnancy soon after implantation occurs and reaches peak levels between the second and third month. It has been obtained from human pregnancy urine, serum and placental tissue. It has also been produced by trophoblastic cells in tissue culture and by implantation into the anterior chamber of the eye (Stewart). Normally, chorionic gonadotropin is secreted directly into the maternal blood and can be detected as early as eight days after conception. Very little is found in fetal blood (see below). The molecular size of the hormone is such that it approaches the limits of filtration by the renal glomerulus. Its concentration in the urine approximates that in the plasma. The rate of secretion of chorionic gonadotropin parallels cytotrophoblastic activity. Thus, maximum levels occur around 50 to 70 days after conception, coinciding with the greatest concentration of cytotrophoblastic cells.

Blood and Urine Levels. By international agreement under the auspices of the League of Nations Committee for Biological Standards, one international unit of chorionic gonadotropin is the amount of activity equivalent to that in 0.1 mg. of a prepared standard. On this basis, serum concentrations follow a distinctive pattern in pregnancy, rising from base levels between 3 and 30 I.U. per ml. up until about the fortieth day after onset of menstruation (about 26 days after conception) to reach a peak value of about 600 I.U. per ml. between the fiftieth and seventieth day of pregnancy (Fig. 56). Thereafter, the titer begins to fall rapidly, reaching low levels of 5 to 35 I.U. per ml. by the ninetieth day, at which level it persists until delivery. Within 48 hours following expulsion of the placenta, the hormone disappears from the circulating blood.

The urinary excretion levels of the hormone reflect its serum concentrations. Early levels of the order of 5000 I.U. per 24 hours rise rapidly to peak levels of up to 500,000 I.U. per 24 hours between the fiftieth and seventieth day of pregnancy and fall to persistent levels of about 8000 I.U. per 24 hours until delivery. Chorionic gonadotropin can no longer be detected in the urine about three or four days after parturition.

Chorionic gonadotropin is present in fetal blood and tissues in very low concentrations. The ratio of concentrations in maternal and fetal tissues varies from 10:1 to 20:1 (Bruner). The negligible amounts of this hormone in the fetus may reflect its large molecular size and relative inability to cross the placental membrane (see below).

Pregnancy Tests. The presence of chorionic gonadotropin in the urine has formed the basis for the various biological and immunochemical tests for pregnancy. Until the recent availability of a reasonably accurate immunologic pregnancy test, simple qualitative estimations of the hormone were performed by testing its biological effects on ovaries of rodents or on the gonads of amphibia (Hon). The various tests usually become positive within two weeks after the first missed menstrual period. The large amounts of chorionic gonadotropin produced in early pregnancy explain the high accuracy of these tests, ranging from 95 to 98 per cent.

Technical problems associated with unfavorable environment and inappropriate preparation of animals have been largely eliminated with the introduction of newer immunologic testing methods. The biological tests for pregnancy, therefore, are rapidly being replaced, although there is still wide utilization of (1) the time-honored Aschheim-Zondek test, which utilizes immature female mice to demonstrate formation of hemorrhagic follicles or corpora lutea in the ovaries, (2) the Friedman test which utilizes mature, unstimulated, nonpregnant female rabbits for the same purpose, (3) the rat ovarian hyperemia test (Berman), using immature rats and producing characteristic reddened appearance of the ovaries, and (4) the Galli Mainini test, using various toad or frog species to produce sperm ejaculation.

Rapid and simple immunologic assays are based on the availability of antisera against chorionic gonadotropin (Loraine and Bell). Using highly refined (but not yet completely purified) chorionic gonadotropin, antisera can be prepared by provoking antibody response in animals. Some cross-reaction with luteinizing hormone occurs. The latex slide test is a very rapid method for determining the presence of detectable amounts of chorionic gonadotropin by the *immunologic agglutination* of a latex particle. It requires only a few minutes to perform and is not subject to the vagaries of bioassay techniques. *Hemagglutination inhibition* is another form of immunoassay which is very effective, although it requires a somewhat longer time to complete. Tanned erythrocytes that have been

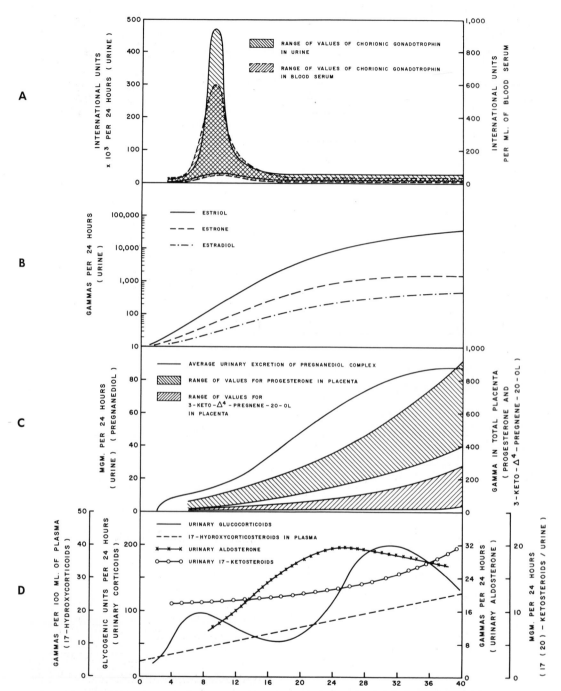

Figure 56 Graphic representation of the progressive changes in hormone levels during normal pregnancy.
A, Chorionic gonadotropin levels in blood and urine (Albert and Berkson, 1951). *B*, Estradiol, estrone and
estriol urinary excretion (Brown, 1956). *C*, Urinary pregnanediol (Davis and Fugo, 1947), and placental progesterone and its precursor, 3-keto-Δ⁴-pregnene-20-ol (Zander, 1958). *D*, Urinary glucocorticoids (Venning,
1948), plasma 17-hydroxycorticoids (Gemzell, 1953), urinary aldosterone (Venning and Dyrenfurth, 1956) and
17-ketosteroids (Plotz et al.: Diabetes 8:14, 1959.)

coated with antigen to chorionic gonadotropin are readily agglutinated by the antibody in gonadotropin antiserum. The antigen contained in urine from a pregnant woman will react with and neutralize the antiserum, preventing the hemagglutination that would be expected to occur when the coated sensitized red cells are added. More recent development of radioimmunoassay techniques holds promise of more accurate and reliably specific determinations.

Function. The precise function of chorionic gonadotropin is unknown. It undoubtedly is concerned with transformation of the corpus luteum of the menstrual cycle into the corpus luteum of pregnancy. This is believed by some to maintain pregnancy until the placental steroid production is sufficient to replace the ovarian secretions. What the duration of this need is cannot be determined precisely, but in humans it is likely not to exceed two to six weeks following conception. It is possible, moreover, that chorionic gonadotropin may also serve in some fashion to regulate steroid synthesis.

Based on the aforementioned biological tests, we have seen that administration of human chorionic gonadotropin to intact, immature mice produces ovulation and the formation of corpora lutea. In the immature hypophysectomized rodent, however, it increases the weight of the ovaries and induces hypertrophy of interstitial ovarian tissue. In the adult hypophysectomized rat, it induces the release of estrogens from corpora lutea already present as determined by keratinization of the vaginal mucosa (Moricard). Administration of large doses of highly purified gonadotropin to normal healthy women during the secretory phase of the menstrual cycle produced a state of pseudopregnancy, demonstrated by the formation of decidua, prolonged excretion of pregnanediol and the presence of well-formed and apparently active corpora lutea (Bradbury et al.).

This clear-cut demonstration of luteotropic activity suggests that chorionic gonadotropin has a major role in ovarian function in pregnancy. The question of its value as an ovulatory hormone remains unanswered. Nevertheless, the analogy between the functional role of chorionic gonadotropin and pituitary gonadotropin is apparent, particularly with regard to its ability to maintain the corpus luteum and prevent it from degenerating, thereby ensuring continued steroid production (see below) and the maintenance of the endometrium for nidation and placentation.

Abnormal Levels. The levels of chorionic gonadotropin may be of clinical significance. Aside from their obvious use in the diagnosis of pregnancy, early pregnancy failures may be indicated by following urine or serum levels. Falling levels of chorionic gonadotropin have been demonstrated in association with pathologic development of the embryo in advance of abortion. At the other extreme, very high levels may be found in conjunction with multiple pregnancies, hydatidiform mole and choriocarcinoma. Elevations in chorionic gonadotropin levels in association with preeclampsia and diabetes (Page) have not been substantiated. Use of serial assays of blood levels and urinary excretion to provide an index of placental function may, under ideal laboratory circumstances, prove valuable but has thus far not gained wide popularity. Rapidly falling human chorionic gonadotropin production may precede clinical evidence of pregnancy failure, but this is not always the case. The value of serial determinations in following treatment efficacy of hydatidiform mole or choriocarcinoma has been well established.

Human Placental Lactogen

A new protein hormone from the placenta was isolated by Josimovich in 1962. Because it has been determined to have actions similar to growth hormone, as well as luteotropic and lactogenic effects, the term *chorionic somato-mammotropin* is currently applied to it. It has a molecular weight between 30,000 and 38,000. It is similar in component amino acid composition to human growth hormone (Sherwood). It is found in high concentrations in the placenta from about the middle of the third week of pregnancy to term. Its concentration in pregnancy serum and urine rises steadily throughout pregnancy. Post partum it disappears from the circulation within 24 hours. Even after hypophysectomy, it persists during pregnancy. Hydatidiform moles and choriocarcinomas (in males also) produce this hormone. It has been shown to be produced in tissue culture placenta, localized by immunofluorescence to the syncytium (Sciarra et al.).

Although suggested as a possible measure of placental function (Spellacy et al.), its ability to detect failing function appears to be limited. It is conceivable that information obtained by serial determinations of placental lactogen can be interpreted meaningfully when used in conjunction with other data, such as estriol excretion, for the evaluation of pregnancies at risk.

The full array of functions ascribable to placental lactogen has not been elucidated. Its actions in experimental animals are well defined, but these verified effects do not necessarily mean that such are its functions in pregnancy. For example, milk production is stimulated in the rabbit, but human placental lactogen has been cleared from the body after delivery well before lactation can begin. Its role in this regard is unknown. Similarly, it is luteotropic in rats, but its luteotropic effects in man are as yet uncertain. It may be instrumental in helping to maintain the corpus luteum of pregnancy. Its synergistic action with human growth hormone has been reported in the rat insofar as its effect in stimulating bone growth is concerned. Alone it has somatotrophic activity in stimulating glucose utilization and protein

synthesis. These have not been confirmed in humans, but there is much speculation as to how fetal growth and development may be influenced by this important hormone.

Estrogens

There is clear evidence that pregnancy is associated with great production of nonprotein phenanthrene steroids (containing a cyclopentenophenanthrene ring nucleus). The biosynthetic pathway (Fig. 57) for their production is undoubtedly very much the same as that which occurs in ovary, adrenal and testis. The evidence for estrogen production by the human placenta includes actual isolation of free steroids from the placenta in relatively high concentrations and recovery from pregnancy urine and blood. Metabolites occur in increasing amounts in the urine as pregnancy progresses, and decrease to nonpregnancy levels soon after delivery. Estrogens are present during pregnancy even after oophorectomy, as well as in pregnant patients with Addison's disease or following hypophysectomy.

Many *in vitro* studies have indicated that the enzymes necessary for estrogen biosynthesis are present in placental tissue. The production of estrogens from placental tissue implanted into the anterior chamber of the eye has also been reported (Stewart). The biosynthesis of estrogens has been detailed in an elaborate series of

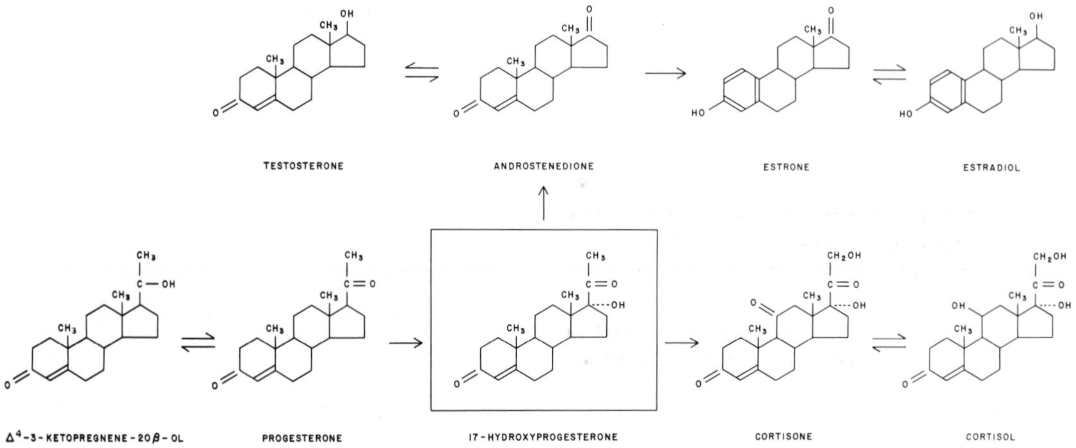

Figure 57 A series of probable hormone interconversions in the placenta involving formation of estrogens and corticosteroids.

steps with ovarian follicular tissue, but several of these important steps have also been established with the human placenta. These include the conversion of pregnenolone to progesterone and of progesterone to 17-hydroxyprogesterone. Although the conversion of 17-hydroxyprogesterone to androgens has thus far only been described in the ovary, conversion of androgens to estrogens has been well documented in the human placenta. Indeed, it appears to be a rather active process, apparently localized to the microsomal fraction, quantitatively producing about 1 mg. of estrone per hour from testosterone *in vitro*. If testosterone is not in fact the normal precursor of estrogens, one may expect the actual precursor to be structurally very similar.

Blood and Urine Levels. Maternal blood in late pregnancy contains 1.5 to 4.6 μg. per 100 ml. estrone, 0.7 to 1.4 μg. per 100 ml. estradiol and 5.2 to 8.0 μg. per 100 ml. estriol (Roy and Brown). Brown has estimated that daily production of estrogen rises from about 1 mg. during the tenth week of gestation to 100 mg. in 24 hours near term (Fig. 56). By contrast, very small amounts of estrogens are produced during the menstrual cycle, varying from 0.08 to 0.34 mg. per 24 hours, with the total amount not exceeding 4.8 mg. during a 30-day cycle.

It is generally agreed that estrogen production during the first five weeks of pregnancy occurs predominantly in the corpus luteum. Considerable quantities of estrogens are found in the corpus luteum during this period and very little thereafter. Surgical extirpation of the ovaries prior to the sixth week of pregnancy is associated with decrease in urinary excretion of estrogens. It remains unchanged, however, when surgery is performed beyond this time in pregnancy. By the seventh week, the estrogen levels in urine rise sharply (Brown), suggesting establishment of the placenta as the major source. Wislocki and Bennett showed histochemical evidence that the syncytiotrophoblast is the probable site of estrogen production.

Only relatively small amounts of estrogens in the placenta are conjugated. The principal estrogens are present as free steroids. Concentrations of the estrogens in the placenta vary with the duration of pregnancy and with the methods used for determination. Urinary excretion rises slowly until about the seventh week of pregnancy when rapid increases occur. They follow a smooth exponential curve which flattens somewhat toward the end of pregnancy. At term both estradiol and estrone levels are about a hundred times greater than those which have been recorded during the luteal phase of the menstrual cycle (0.33 to 0.9 and 0.93 to 2.1 mg. per 24 hours, respectively). Estriol levels, on the other hand, are about a thousand times higher during this time (21 to 41 mg. per 24 hours). Values in late pregnancy and at the onset of labor are similar, supporting the assumption that there is no correlation between estrogen excretion and onset of labor. Following delivery there is a rapid decrease in the urinary estrogen levels. Almost all estrogens in the urine during pregnancy are conjugated, chiefly as glucosiduronates and sulfates.

There has been special interest generated in excretion of estriol. Formation of estriol in the maternal organism is still a matter of doubt. Even though the placenta contains high concentrations of estriol, it has been very difficult to demonstrate the conversion of estradiol to estriol within this tissue (Ryan). The problem is further complicated by the fetus entering into the picture. It appears that the fetus may be the source of estriol. Its estriol concentrations are much higher than that of both estrone and estradiol, and the ratio is even higher than for the mother. Furthermore, the estradiol in the fetus does not appear to be in equilibrium with the general maternal pool, and the fetus appears to metabolize estrogens in a manner different from the mother. The concentration of estriol is five to six times higher in the fetal circulation than in maternal blood (Aitken et al.). Since the isolated placenta elaborates very little if any estriol, it has seemed likely that the production of estriol in such large quantities at term requires the combined efforts of a placenta and a healthy fetus. Use of this fact has been made as a measure of placentofetal function (Greene and Touchstone). Estriol excretion as an index of fetal well-being is an important and useful test (see Chapter 13).

Function. Estrogens are of paramount importance in the physiology of reproduction. They have wide and diverse effects in reproductive function. In the immediate preovulatory phase, they are responsible for the increase in amount of cervical mucus of low viscosity, favoring migration, motility and ascent of spermatozoa. Estrogens stimulate motility of the uterine tubes, bringing the fimbriated end of the tube into intimate contact with the ovarian surface in the region of the mature graafian follicle at the time of ovulation. The expelled ovum is captured by the tube and propelled into the tubal lumen by peristaltic movements which are also under the influence of estrogenic hormones. Estrogens, moreover, cause proliferation of the endometrium and exert a remarkable effect on its vascularity by promoting rapid growth of the spiral arterioles. In conjunction with progesterone, estrogens prepare the endometrium for successful implantation of the fertilized ovum. After implantation, estrogens are primarily responsible for the growth of the myometrium. The muscle cells hypertrophy and concentrations of actomyosin and adenosinetriphosphate increase in the cells. Ductile proliferation of the breasts accompanies estrogen stimulation and lobular-alveolar growth is induced when estrogens act in concert with progesterone.

On a biochemical level, estrogens act on the microsomes. Talalay et al. demonstrated that 17β-estradiol acts as a hydrogen carrier or coenzyme between diphosphopyridine nucleotide (DPN) and triphosphopyridine nucleotide (TPN) in the presence of certain hydroxysteroid dehydrogenases. Villee postulated that the effect of estrogens in promoting growth and increasing functional capacities of the endometrium, myometrium and other estrogen-dependent tissues is mediated by the presence in these tissues of an estrogen-stimulable transhydrogenase. The activity of this enzyme, when increased by estrogens, leads to enhancement in the supply of energy-rich phosphate. This in turn leads to an increase in the rate of synthesis of proteins, fats and nucleic acids. The site of action seems to lie in the Krebs cycle between citrate and α-ketoglutarate.

Recent evidence (Jenson and Jacobson) suggests that the estradiol stimulates uterine growth without undergoing metabolic transformation and that estrone exerts its hormone action on the uterine muscle after first being converted to estradiol. Estrogens are bound to plasma proteins, chiefly albumin, and undergo conjugation with glucuronic acid in the liver, so that the principal form found in urine in pregnancy is estriol glucuronide.

Progesterone

Progesterone appears to be essential for reproduction in all higher forms of animal life. The effects of progesterone on the endometrium, secondary sexual organs and the central nervous system are important preparatory steps for ovulation, fertilization and implantation. Its role after pregnancy has been established involves maintenance of an optimally suitable maternal environment including its actions on myometrial contractility and perhaps an intimate control of the genesis of labor, the mechanism of which is not yet fully understood. Its inhibitory effects on the myometrium during pregnancy and the whole unanswered question of the onset of labor are involved here.

The evidence for placental formation of progesterone includes its isolation from human placentas at all periods of gestation, and from peripheral, uterine and umbilical venous and arterial blood samples. The effluent blood in umbilical and uterine veins contains higher levels of progesterone than the affluent peripheral blood. Similarly, the level in the umbilical vein is higher than in the umbilical artery. Recovery from urine of pregnanediol, a progesterone metabolite, in increasing amounts with progressive pregnancy and its disappearance after delivery are additional evidence. The presence of pregnanediol in the urine has in the past been utilized as a prognostic sign of placental viability with varying, though as yet unsubstantiated, degrees of reliability.

The conversion of cholesterol and pregnenolone to progesterone by placental tissue *in vitro* has been reported. In addition, progesterone can be converted to 17-hydroxyprogesterone in the placenta, and its metabolite in turn, pregnanetriol, has been recovered from pregnancy urine in increasing amounts as pregnancy progresses. It appears that the placenta in late pregnancy produces large amounts of progesterone daily. Both the ovary, that is, the corpus luteum, and the adrenals secrete progesterone, but their contributions seem to be insignificant, since neither oophorectomy nor adrenalectomy materially affects the amount of pregnanediol excreted in pregnancy.

Progesterone is cleared from the bloodstream in a matter of minutes and is rapidly metabolized and conjugated as the glucosiduronate. The turnover time has been calculated to be 3.3 minutes, a rapid replacement rate. Pregnanediol rises in the urine soon after ovulation and continues in pregnancy up to about 32 weeks, when a plateau is reached. The methods for measuring pregnanediol have recently undergone a significant refinement to improve the specificity and accuracy. Studies have indicated that the original values obtained were too high. The average newly reported methods give levels of 40 mg. pregnanediol per 24 hours after the thirty-second week of pregnancy. The original Venning method reported values as high as 80 mg. It is probable that substances other than pregnanediol were being measured by those techniques. Using isotope-dilution techniques, Pearlman estimated the rate of endogenous progesterone production during the last trimester to be about 250 mg. daily.

The corpus luteum appears to be an important source of progesterone in early pregnancy. This certainly applies to most lower animals. However, in humans the gland can be removed relatively early, perhaps after the sixth week, without interrupting the pregnancy (Tulsky and Koff). This suggests that the placenta is capable of taking over production of essential ovarian hormones rather early in pregnancy. With increasing progesterone production by the placenta, there is a sharp rise in pregnanediol excretion into the urine. One of the key pieces of evidence supporting the role of the placenta as the major source of progesterone during pregnancy is the demonstration that human placental tissue is capable of converting certain hormone precursors, including cholesterol and Δ^5-pregnenolone, into progesterone.

Blood and Urine Levels. Progesterone itself is not excreted into the urine directly. Venning and Browne determined that the hormone is metabolized to pregnanediol, which is excreted in turn in large and increasing amounts in the form of its water-soluble glucosiduronate throughout pregnancy. Excretion remains at a level compatible with the corpus luteum phase of the normal menstrual cycle for the first six to eight weeks of pregnancy, ranging between 6 and 15 mg. per 24 hours. Thereafter, excretion increases steadily and peaks late in pregnancy, reaching as high as 80 mg. per 24 hours, depending on the methods used (Fig. 56).

In contrast to the large amounts of progesterone metabolites excreted in the urine, the progesterone concentration in blood plasma is very low. Zander found levels of 0.039 to 0.268 μg. per ml. in plasma during the fourth to ninth months of gestation. Consistently, values in retroplacental blood are much higher. Concentrations in placental tissue are higher during the second and third months than later in pregnancy, but the total content in the placenta rises considerably with advancing pregnancy. Barnes et al. found concentrations of progesterone varying from 0.05 to 0.63 μg. per gram of wet tissue in the myometrium of gravid term uteri. These values exceed the plasma values encountered by these investigators, lending support to the concept that diffusion of progesterone into the underlying myometrium may be a significant event. The relationship of this finding to theoretical consideration of the existence of a "progesterone block" and its relationship to onset of labor will be discussed in detail in Chapter 14.

Using tracer techniques, Bloch demonstrated the conversion of cholesterol to pregnanediol in human pregnancy. This observation suggested that cholesterol is a precursor of progesterone, since pregnanediol is its principal metabolite. In ensuing years the principal pathway of progesterone synthesis has been established from acetate to cholesterol to pregnenolone to progesterone (Fig. 58).

Function. The physiologic effects of

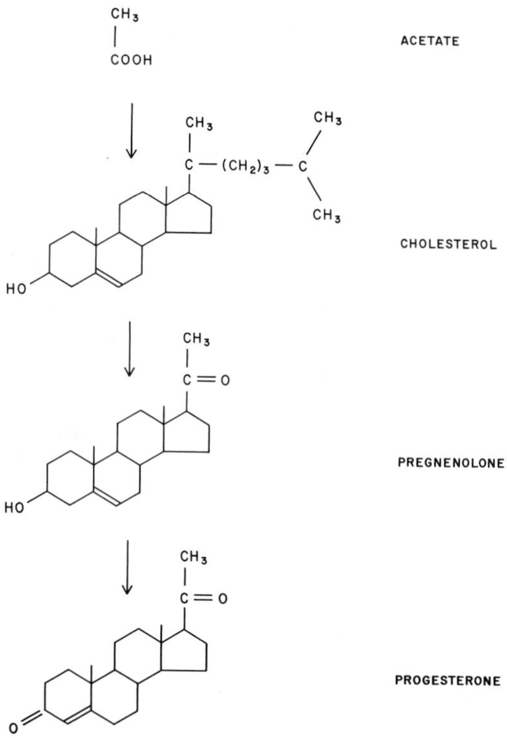

Figure 58 The pathway of the biosynthesis of progesterone from acetate via cholesterol and pregnenolone.

progesterone are demonstrable in the presence of estrogens. Progesterone is partially responsible for the controlled transport of the fertilized ovum to the uterine cavity and for the preparation of the endometrium so that adequate nutrition will be available for the newly implanted conceptus. It accentuates the effect of estrogens on the vascular bed of the endometrium by inducing further growth and coiling of the spiral arterioles, thus increasing the blood supply to the endometrium. Likewise, progesterone is responsible for deciduation in the late secretory phase of the menstrual cycle and in early pregnancy.

The effect of progesterone on uterine motility is still a matter of controversy, but it is currently believed that it acts to inhibit any effect on the biochemical processes involving estrogen and its stimulatory effects on the synthesis of actomyosin and ATP. The growth of the mammary glands during pregnancy is under the influence of both estrogens and proges-

terone. Estrogens stimulate proliferation of the duct system and the growth and pigmentation of the nipples and areolae, while progesterone influences the lobule-alveolar development. Progesterone's effect on the breasts can be elicited only when they have previously been subjected to estrogenic stimulation.

Progesterone produces a rise in basal body temperature during the luteal phase of the cycle (Fig. 59). When pregnancy occurs, the temperature remains elevated. Despite the fact that progesterone secretion by the placenta increases throughout pregnancy, the resultant temperature elevation returns toward normal by about the hundredth day of pregnancy. The mechanism of this thermogenic dissociation is unknown.

Androgens

Reports based on bioassay techniques using placental extracts suggest that the placenta contains androgenic substances. This is not unexpected in view of the current theories of estrogen formation by way of androgens. Specific C-19 steroids, such as testosterone and dehydroepiandrosterone, have not yet been identified in placental tissue. Salhanick et al., however, have reported the presence of androstenedione.

Actually, very little is known about the secretion of androgens in normal pregnancy. There is no change in their urinary excretion as determined by bioassay or by 17-ketosteroid determination. Androsterone and etiocholanolone, the major metabolites of androgenic precursors, are excreted in normal amounts during early pregnancy, although a distinct tendency toward decreased excretion of both compounds during late pregnancy (Fig. 60) has been consistently reported. Similarly, blood levels of dehydroisoandrosterone decrease in late pregnancy (Migeon et al.).

These urinary steroids are believed to originate from precursors elaborated by the maternal adrenal cortex and possibly by the fetal adrenals as well. The significance of these observations is not understood. No evidence exists that the placenta is a major source of androgens in human

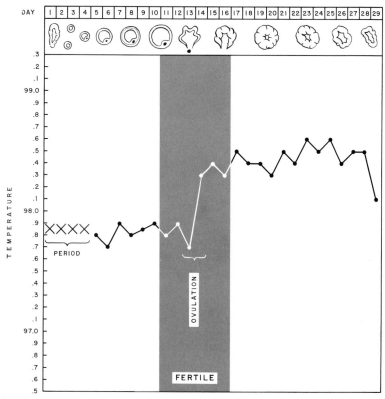

Figure 59 Graphic sequential change in basal body temperature during the course of a menstrual cycle, showing typical systemic thermogenic response to increased progesterone production by the corpus luteum. Progression of the graafian follicle to ovulation, formation of the corpus luteum and its subsequent degeneration are shown pictorially across the top. Precise timing of ovulation is unclear, but the probable fertile period is shown in the shaded area.

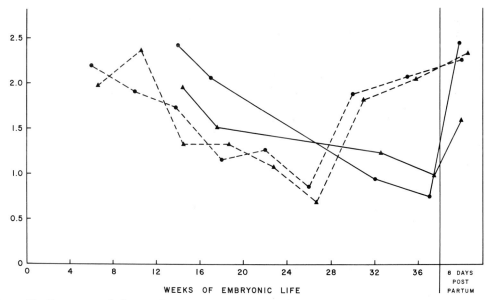

Figure 60 Progressive decline in the urinary excretion of androsterone and etiocholanolone over the course of pregnancy in normal and diabetic women. Solid lines normal, broken lines diabetics; circles androsterone, triangles etiocholanolone. (From Plotz, E. J., et al.: Diabetes 8:14, 1959.)

pregnancy, but androstenedione, an important androgen, has been isolated from both human corpora lutea and the placenta.

Transient hirsutism observed during pregnancy is suggestive of a biological effect. It is possible that theca interna cells which undergo striking hyperplasia during pregnancy may be the source of androgenic hormones causing hirsutism.

Adrenal Cortical Hormones

There is a large body of literature suggesting that certain aspects of adrenal function are increased during pregnancy. The fact that blood concentrations of 17-hydroxycorticosterone increase progressively during human pregnancy suggested that this might be of placental origin. However, it is now generally agreed that this is observed only in patients with intact adrenal glands. Pregnant women with Addison's disease do not show comparable increases. Furthermore, the increased amounts of hormones in the plasma appear to be due to an increased quantity of a specific protein, transcortin, which binds the corticoids. This is believed to be due to an estrogen-induced effect.

It is widely stated that maternal adrenal glands are hyperactive during pregnancy to meet increased demands for adrenal cortical hormones imposed on the maternal organism by gestational changes. Proof of this contention is wanting. Adrenal glands of patients who died suddenly during normal pregnancy, for example, were essentially normal (Whiteley and Stoner).

It has been suggested that the increase in plasma-free 17-hydroxycorticosteroids observed in late pregnancy may be the result of a slow rate of metabolism and destruction, as well as an increased rate of production of adrenal cortical hormones. This assumption is based on the fact that there are no clinical signs of hypercorticalism in human pregnancy despite the high plasma levels of cortical steroids. Moreover, it is likely that increased estrogen production by the placenta plays a role in decreasing the rate of diffusion of cortisol from the bloodstream into body tissues (Christy et al.).

Aldosterone excretion is increased in pregnancy, but does not occur in subjects with adrenal cortical insufficiency. This suggests that the hormone is not elaborated by placental tissue. There is much interest in aldosterone because of its possible action on the electrolyte and water balance problems in pregnancy. There is a progressive increase in the urinary excretion of aldosterone during normal pregnancy followed by a rapid decrease after delivery. Most of it is excreted in conjugated form.

Determinations for total 17-ketosteroids are essentially the same as for nonpregnant women. Excretion of androsterone, etiocholanolone, and dehydroisoandrosterone decreases during the last trimester of pregnancy. It is during this time that hormone production by the placenta should be at its greatest. The observation by Plotz and Davis that administration of large amounts of progesterone in early pregnancy produced a similar decrease in the excretion of androsterone and etiocholanolone supported the concept that the hormone activity of the placenta alters the functional state of the adrenal cortex.

Whether or not the placenta is directly involved in production of adrenal cortical hormones is not entirely clear. The observation by Jailer and Knowlton that pregnant women with Addison's disease excrete 17-ketosteroids and corticoids in almost the same amounts as healthy pregnant women allows one to assume that the placenta is capable of deriving appropriate precursors. *In vitro* studies, however, have failed to demonstrate cortisol production by the placenta.

Placental tissue has the ability to concentrate many hormones from the blood, including ACTH, growth hormone and cortisone. The fact that extracts of placental tissue contain these hormones in quantities higher than those found in maternal plasma is not substantive evidence that they are elaborated by the placenta. The fact that cortisol, cortisone and aldosterone have been found in human placental tissue does not support the conclusion that these hormones are necessarily being produced by the placenta. Their presence may represent simple storage in this organ due to the special ability of the placenta to concentrate hormones.

Moreover, subsequent observations in patients with Addison's disease have not proved to be uniform and it is now apparent that patients with natural adrenal insufficiency or adrenal insufficiency following bilateral adrenalectomy or hypophysectomy produce no significant amounts of adrenal cortical steroids. Similarly, the high serum levels of corticoids noted in pregnancy turned out to be merely reflections of a prolonged half-life and decreased metabolism. The same picture could be mimicked by estrogen administration.

Most placental extraction studies that have indicated elevated adrenal cortical steroids in the placenta have not taken into account the amounts of trapped blood or the ability of the placenta to concentrate adrenal steroids. Thus far direct *in vitro* studies attempting to demonstrate corticoid production have been negative. There is, therefore, little conclusive evidence as yet that the placenta makes any adrenal cortical steroids, but in view of the wide spectrum of activity of other endocrine organs, it would not be surprising if it did.

Studies of aldosterone production in normal pregnant women and those with adrenal insufficiency have shown no evidence for its production by the placenta, even though aldosterone excretion does increase with advancing gestation. The antagonism of its renal effects by progesterone correlates well with this rise.

Prostaglandins

Although prostaglandins have been found in many tissues, the role of the placenta in their production is not determined at all. Nevertheless, they are probably somehow intimately related to the reproductive process. These long-chain fatty acids (20 carbons and a cyclopentane ring) were first found in seminal fluid. Recent evidence indicates they have important actions on myometrial function, particularly as regards induction of abortion or labor (Speroff and Ramwell). Luteolytic effects on the corpus luteum have also been documented in sheep and rhesus monkeys. It is conceivable that naturally occurring prostaglandins or synthetic congeners may someday prove to be of considerable pharmacologic value in this discipline. Their specific roles, however, are not entirely clear today.

The rapidly growing clinical interest in prostaglandins for obstetric use had its impetus in the reports of Karim et al. showing that prostaglandins $F_{2\alpha}$ and E_2 could effectively and with apparent safety initiate labor at term or abort early pregnancy when given intravenously. Others have confirmed these observations in controlled clinical investigations (Anderson et al.; Beazley and Gillespie). Oral administration of these agents, especially prostaglandin-E_2, was also found useful (Karim; Karim and Sharma). Intravaginal, intraamniotic, extraovular and intramyometrial use is now being tested for purposes of producing therapeutic abortion. Side effects are encountered, however, including troublesome diarrhea, nausea and vomiting, as well as some uterine hypertonus. There is much clinical research currently in progress to determine effectiveness, optimal dosage regimen and route, tolerance, safety and constraints. Undoubtedly, these agents will soon become available for wide clinical usage.

Allograft Rejection

Inasmuch as the placenta is a heterologous transplant bearing some of the genetic characteristics of the father, one may conjecture as to why the placenta is not regularly rejected by its recipient host, the mother. The immunochemical aspect of this tumor-host relationship is obscure and warrants serious attention, particularly in this day when organ transplants are realities. Theoretically, the placenta should be rejected by the host within two to three weeks after implantation, in a manner analogous to that which occurs in the rejection of other allografts. The fact that the placenta does not obey such immunologic laws has given rise to much speculation and experimentation in recent years.

Several theories have been advanced to explain this phenomenon: (1) It is speculated that hormonal changes of pregnancy may induce a transient state of tolerance. This has been demonstrated to be incorrect on the basis of the fact that pregnant women are no more tolerant in their ability to accept skin grafts or other heterografts than nonpregnant women. (2) It is further felt that fetal tissues may produce large quantities of histamine that in turn will prevent the vascular ischemia that is associated with graft rejection. It is possible that this factor may play an important role in implantation and early invasion of the trophoblast, but it could not explain the prolonged maternal tolerance to the foreign parasite. (3) The concept that the uterus, like the cheek pouch of the hamster, is a favored location incapable of rejecting homografts has been shown by Simmons not to be the case because normal rejection occurs when other tissues, such as parathyroid, are implanted there. (4) The only explanation that appears to be correct at this time is that the trophoblast may not contain or is unable to express tissue antigens.

Although the placenta as a whole does contain histogenetic antigens, it is possible that there may be some inherent factor within or surrounding the trophoblast that prevents the expected rejection. If indeed the syncytium that is interposed between fetal and maternal tissues is unique in not stimulating tissue response in the host, it is conceivable that it would be recognized by the host as her own tissue and the expected rejection would not take place.

It has been postulated that a special coating surrounds the trophoblast in the form of sialomucin (Currie and Bagshawe) to prevent recognition by the host of the antigens present in the placenta. This hypothesis is rather attractive in that it can explain the lack of immunologic rejection phenomena in the normally developing conceptus on a physicochemical basis. Whether or not this mechanism (or its breakdown) is involved in spontaneous abortions is as yet undetermined.

FETAL SUPPORT MECHANISMS

Little is known about the nutrition of the mammalian embryo prior to the development of the placenta. It is probable that the implanted ovum obtains its nourishment from the surrounding fluids in much the same manner as other cells do. Cell membranes exert an intricate control over exchange of intracellular materials with those in the environment, and it may be suspected that all of the complex transport functions eventually to be undertaken by the placenta may find their primitive counterparts at the cell level.

As the cell continues to divide and the embryo enlarges, the inner core of cells becomes separated from the source of nutrition. The development of a fetal circulation (see Chapter 6) provides for the distribution of essential nutrients throughout the fetus, and the development of the placenta provides a site for the intimate juxtaposition of maternal and fetal circulations and the efficient exchange of materials between them.

The tissue through which these materials must pass in exchanging between mother and fetus has been called the placental barrier, or more correctly the *placental membrane.* This term emphasizes the role of the placenta as an organ for the controlled transfer of materials, instead of one that merely obstructs the transfer of certain materials. The nutritional lifeline of the fetus is actually interrupted by a succession of membranes. For example, the intestinal mucosa first dictates the absorption of food substances into the maternal bloodstream, and the glomerular and tubal membranes of the kidney are effective in maintaining a constant composition of the blood. Progressing toward the fetus, we find the placenta and the fetal membranes, and within the fetus other specialized membranes such as the blood-brain barrier, leading finally to the cell membrane itself. There are also identifiable membranes within the cell, but little is as yet known of their function.

It appears that the common function of all these membranes is to control the rate of transfer of materials. The control is often very specific. Materials differing only slightly in structure may have widely different rates of transfer. In some instances, the transfer rate in one direction is favored over that in the other, producing a gradient in levels of the substances on either side of the membranes. The transfer of some ma-

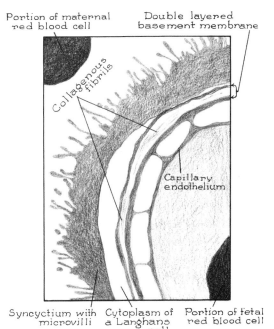

Portion of maternal red blood cell

Double layered basement membrane

Collagenous fibrils

Capillary endothelium

Syncyctium with microvilli   Cytoplasm of a Langhans cell   Portion of fetal red blood cell

Figure 61 The placental "membrane" represented by the tissue intervening between maternal and fetal circulations in a terminal villus of a placenta at term. Drawn from an electronmicroscopic photograph published by Wislocki and Dempsey. (Magnification × 15,000.)

cells, the cytotrophoblasts, which variably persist and may proliferate under abnormal circumstances. These cells appear to function primarily as a source of vital hormones necessary for the maintenance of pregnancy. Underneath the trophoblast there is a double layer of supporting connective tissue, and below this lie the walls of the fetal capillaries, marking the location of the fetal circulation.

In a single placenta, the villi themselves laid end to end extend for perhaps 30 miles and the surface exposed to the maternal bloodstream would be approximately 160 square feet.

When the pregnant woman near term is supine, the pressure of maternal blood in the intervillous space is 7 to 10 mm. Hg, while that in the fetal capillaries exceeds 20 mm. Hg. When the woman sits or stands, however, the pressure in the intervillous space rises to more than 30 mm. Hg, whereas that in the fetal capillaries probably remains constant. Thus, the direction of pressure gradient shifts with reference to maternal posture and undoubtedly is a factor in altering transfer rates. The rate of maternal blood flow through the placenta is of the order of 500 ml. per minute and the rate of fetal blood flow is about 400 ml. per minute. The placental membrane is nourished primarily by the maternal blood, so that occasional occlusion of fetal vessels or even death of the fetus does not necessarily lead to placental degeneration until secondary events occur on the maternal side.

The placenta is, of course, subject to a variety of insults, such as true infarction when the maternal arterial supply is shut off. Under these circumstances, tissue death results. These events occur so frequently in minor degrees that they have been termed normal. It is well to remember, however, that this type of pathologic condition may be undesirable and may indeed be detrimental to both the fetus and its host.

With reference to the placenta as an organ of transfer, not too long ago the placenta was looked upon naively as a simple semipermeable filter. Under this misconception, it was popular to inquire as to which substances would cross the placenta to affect the fetus. Today it can be

terials is so slow that a barrier may be considered to exist, though this is often merely a relative term.

In order to understand this function with regard to the placenta we must be aware of the nature of the placental membrane (Fig. 61). In the human placenta at term, the maternal blood in the intervillous space is directly in contact with the fetal syncytium, a layer of cells which normally clothes all the chorionic villi. The surface of these cells contains a brushlike border, which in reality can be seen on electronmicroscopy to consist of many microvilli, streaming fingers of protoplasm capable of engulfing macromolecules or even whole droplets of plasma and quite possibly transferring them to the fetal capillaries intact by the process of phagocytosis or pinocytosis.

The syncytium is the functional layer of the placental membrane and is responsible for the active enzymatic transfer of selected foodstuffs. It is also the origin of the placental steroid hormones. Beneath the syncytium are found other specialized determined that essentially every substance which exists in the maternal or fetal blood can and does cross the placenta unless it is destroyed or altered, or somehow physiologically inactivated during the passage. Thus, the crucial question is not whether the substance will cross the placenta, but whether it will cross in sufficient quantities per unit of time to have nutritional or physiologic or toxicologic significance.

The distribution of materials across the placenta is very complex (Table 1). We know that many substances, including protein, lipids, fat-soluble vitamins and most hormones occur in higher concentrations in the maternal plasma than in the fetus. On the other hand, water-soluble vitamins, phosphorus compounds, amino acids and certain nitrogenous metabolites are more concentrated on the fetal side. This type of partition cannot be entirely explained on purely physicochemical principles (see below). Page used a classification of substances that was very useful in simplifying the complicated patterns of placental transfer according to the relative importance of the material to the fetal economy. His groups included (1) substances concerned with biochemical homeostasis, (2) substances concerned with fetal nutrition, (3) substances concerned with modifications of growth or the maintenance of pregnancy, and (4) substances of immunologic importance.

Under materials concerned with *biochemical homeostasis* are included those which deal with the immediate maintenance of life, such as water, oxygen, carbon dioxide, as well as electrolytes, urea and certain simple amines. The predominant mechanism of transfer of these substances is by *simple diffusion*. The rates of exchange are apparently exceedingly rapid.

It has been found that water crosses the placental membrane faster than any other known substance with a rate of exchange approximating 180 ml. per second. Most of this water is free but some consists of the water of hydration associated with other molecules. Despite the simplicity of water, the factors which determine its net exchange, that is, factors favoring hydration or dehydration of the fetus, are totally obscure. There are, of course, other routes by which water may reach or leave the fetus. Fetal lungs and kidneys probably contribute water to the amniotic fluid, and the umbilical cord may also be a medium of exchange. Furthermore, the normal fetus appears to drink about one-quarter of its own amniotic fluid every day (see Chapter 5).

Carbon dioxide is highly soluble in the placental membrane and hence probably traverses it with great ease. Oxygen, on the other hand, diffuses with some difficulty and therefore requires a considerable gradient of oxygen pressure on either side of the membrane. Maintenance of this gradient is facilitated by the existence of a unique fetal hemoglobin which takes up and gives off its oxygen at more favorable lower pressures of oxygen (see Chapter 6).

Sodium and potassium cross the placenta very rapidly, albeit at rates slower than water. Flexner et al. showed peak transfer rates of sodium from mother to fetus of the order of 1 mg. per second at about one month prior to term. The rapid transfer of electrolytes by diffusion in either direction appears to protect the fetus against potentially fatal disturbances in osmolarity and acid-base balance.

Some simple compounds, such as histamine, serotonin, angiotensin and epinephrine, are small enough to permit rapid diffusion. However, these may never reach the fetus in active amounts because enzymatic deamination occurs within the placental membrane. This results in unequal

TABLE 1   THE RELATIVE DISTRIBUTION OF SELECTED MATERIALS IN FETAL AND MATERNAL PLASMA

Higher in Fetal Plasma	About Equal	Higher in Maternal Plasma
Amino acids	Sodium	Total proteins
Nonprotein nitrogen	Chloride	Globulins
Creatinine	Creatine	Fibrinogen
Total phosphorus	Urea	Total lipids
Inorganic phosphorus	Uric acid	Phospholipids
Fructose	Magnesium	Fatty acids
Lactate		Glucose
Serum iron		Cholesterol
Calcium		Vitamins A and E
Thiamine chloride		
Pyridoxine		
Riboflavin		
Ascorbic acid		

distribution across the membrane because the diffusible compound is apparently destroyed by the membrane itself.

Among substances concerned primarily with *fetal nutrition*, there are glucose, amino acids and vitamins. These materials seem to be capable of diffusion, but in addition there appears to exist a mechanism of active transport or *facilitated diffusion*, involving enzymatic carrier systems. As an example, the amino acid histidine, one of the essential building blocks for the synthesis of fetal proteins, exists in two forms, the dextro and the levo forms, which are optical isomers or mirror images. In life, only the l-form is used by the fetus for protein synthesis. Experiments performed on pregnant women at term have shown that when the placenta is presented with equimolar concentrations of d- and l-histidine, the l-form is transported to the fetus 12 times faster than the d-form.

A biological membrane cannot distinguish between two isomers with respect to physical diffusion. Therefore, it must be presumed that carrier molecules exist which recognize only the natural form. This rapid transport system requires energy because the fetal plasma normally contains a higher level of histidine than the maternal plasma, so that the transfer occurs against the so-called concentration gradient (Page et al.).

With regard to fetal requirements, considerable progress in the field of nutrition has been made concerning the minimum and optimal amounts of various nutrients required for the growth and the well-being of the human subject. The application of this approach to the fetus would permit the interpretation of placental function in terms of its ability to fulfill nutritional requirements.

Some indication of minimal requirements for growth has been gathered from elemental studies of the composition of fetuses. It has been shown that the fetus does not simply increase in size during its development, but changes substantially in composition. The factors controlling these changes probably exist within the fetus, but it is possible that changes in placental function during gestation also contribute. A major shortcoming in studying the progressive changes in fetal composition is

that these data merely describe minimal requirements as represented by fetal retention of substances and give very little indication of total metabolic needs.

In only a very few instances does our knowledge permit us to attempt to interpret placental function in terms of actual fetal requirements. For these substances information is incompletely available on the nature of materials pertinent to the fetus, the methods of transfer and the qualitative estimates of the rates of transfer.

For example, there is little doubt that the major precursors for fetal protein are the amino acids circulating in the maternal plasma. Radioisotope tracer experiments in animals have demonstrated that amino acids injected into the mother are transferred rapidly and efficiently across the placenta and are readily incorporated into fetal protein. The transfer of amino acids appears to be dependent on a placental mechanism which maintains the fetal level higher than the maternal. It has been suggested that the elevated amino acid level may facilitate the prompt synthesis of protein essential to a rapidly growing organism. Significantly, we have already indicated the lines of evidence that show that transfer of amino acids is dependent on an active placental mechanism. There is also competition among amino acids for transfer. Saturation of the transport mechanism has been demonstrated.

Application of the knowledge concerning the metabolic transfer of amino acids provides an interesting explanation of the experience with two congenital metabolic diseases, namely, phenylketonuria and maple syrup urine disease, in both of which there are disturbances in amino acid metabolism. In both instances, the infants are born normal, although the anomaly must have existed throughout the intrauterine life of the fetus. Shortly after birth, abnormal metabolites are detected in the urine and symptoms begin to appear. These can be reversed by lowering the intake of the offending amino acids. A logical explanation of the absence of symptoms and pathology at birth is that elevation of the blood level of an amino acid in the fetus is followed automatically by a reduction in placental transfer. Thus in phenylketonuria, where there is difficulty in metabolizing phenylalanine, we may expect an elevation in plasma phenylalanine level. This will suppress further transfer of phenylalanine from the mother so that the fetal plasma level never reaches toxic concentrations *in utero*.

With regard to substances of *immunologic importance* it has been definitely shown that macromolecules, such as the plasma proteins and even intact red blood cells, may traverse the human placenta in either direction. The quantities involved, however, are so small that they could hardly be considered to have any nutritional significance. But we do know that they have some rather important immunologic implications. In the case of proteins, the process of *pinocytosis* or *phagocytosis* may be an important mechanism. In animals, antibodies reach the fetus by way of the amniotic fluid, whereas other proteins are found to cross the placenta directly. This has been shown by labeling with radioactive isotopes.

Most of our facts about human subjects are limited to demonstrable antigens and antibodies. Cellular transfer presumably involves minute breaks in the placental barrier. Whether this occurs to a slight extent in all placentas or only in some is unknown. The escape of fetal red blood cells into the maternal circulation is the probable basis of isoimmunization and is now felt to be a substantiated cause of the Rh factor disease, erythroblastosis fetalis.

As intimated earlier, the direction of cellular transfer may depend on such factors as whether the mother is erect or supine. In rare instances, placental leakage may be sufficient to cause profound anemia or even death of the fetus. Such occurrences may result from major pathologic breaks in the placental membrane allowing free interchange between maternal and fetal circulations.

The *rates of exchange* of specific substances are determined by several factors. We have already alluded to the physiologic significance of the substances to be transferred according to the classification detailed above. Relative rates of transfer and the mechanisms of transport may be governed by *physicochemical laws*. Rates of diffusion of simple substances, for example, are a function of a number of well-defined factors, among which are included: (1) the fetomaternal concentration gradient (recognizing that facilitated diffusion commonly occurs against such a gradient), (2) the surface available for transfer, (3) the thickness of the intervening tissue membrane, (4) the degree of ionization of the substances to be transferred, (5) their lipoid solubility, and (6) molecular size.

Undissociated or nonionized forms are recognized to penetrate rapidly across cell membranes and to achieve equilibrium quickly. Moreover, substances with high fat solubility are transferred readily. As to molecular size, the placental membrane is virtually impermeable to substances with molecular weight over 1000 insofar as the simple diffusion mechanism is concerned.

As to permeability of the membrane, it may be altered, impaired or interfered with by various phenomena, including (1) pathologic states (for example, preeclampsia, erythroblastosis, diabetes mellitus), (2) change in maternal and fetal blood flow resulting from uterine contractions, maternal positional or postural changes, anesthesia or umbilical cord compression, (3) maternal asphyxia, (4) hypotension, (5) dehydration, and (6) maternal hemorrhage.

The placenta alters its architecture during the course of pregnancy by increasing the surface area which the villi present to the maternal blood and simultaneously thinning the intervening tissues between the two circulations. This results in an apparent increase in the transfer capabilities during pregnancy. Simultaneously, Langhans' cells largely disappear from the villus, and the capillaries within the villi undergo proliferation and thinning of their walls.

REFERENCES

Aitken, E. H., Preedy, J. R. K., Eton, B., and Short, R. V.: Estrogen and progesterone levels in foetal and maternal plasma at parturition. Lancet 2:1096, 1958.

Albert, A., and Berkson, J.: A clinical bioassay for chorionic gonadotropin. J. Clin. Endocr. *11*:805, 1951.

Anderson, G. G., Hobbins, J. C., and Speroff, L.: Intravenous prostaglandins E₂ and F₂α for the induction of term labor. Amer. J. Obstet. Gynec. *112*:382, 1972.

Aschheim, S., and Zondek, B.: Hypophysenvorderlappenhormon und Ovarialhormon im Harn von Schwangeren. Klin. Wschr. *6*:1322, 1927.

Barnes, A. C., Kumar, D., and Goodno, J. A.: Studies in human myometrium during pregnancy: V. Myometrial tissue progesterone analyses by gas-liquid phase chromatography. Amer. J. Obstet. Gynec. *84*:1207, 1962.

Beazley, J. M., and Gillespie, A.: Double-blind trial of prostaglandin E₂ and oxytocin in induction of labour. Lancet *1*:152, 1971.

Berman, R. L.: Rat hyperemia pregnancy tests: Review, evaluation, comments and interpretation. Fertil. Steril. *7*:276, 1956.

Bloch, K.: The biological conversion of cholesterol to pregnanediol. J. Biol. Chem. *157*:661, 1945.

Bradbury, J. T., Brown, W. E., and Gray, L. A.: Maintenance of the corpus luteum and physiologic actions of progesterone. *In* Pincus, G., ed.: Recent Progress in Hormone Research, Vol. 5. New York, Academic Press, 1950.

Brown, J. B.: Urinary excretion of oestrogens during pregnancy, lactation, and the re-establishment of menstruation. Lancet *1*:704, 1956.

Bruner, J. A.: Distribution of chorionic gonadotropin in mother and fetus at various stages of pregnancy. J. Clin. Endocr. *11*:360, 1951.

Christy, N. P., Wallace, E. Z., Gordon, W. E. L., and Jailer, J. W.: On the rate of hydrocortisone clearance from plasma in pregnant women and in patients with Laennec's cirrhosis. J. Clin. Invest. *36*:299, 1959.

Currie, G. A., and Bagshawe, K. D.: The masking of antigens on trophoblast and cancer cells. Lancet *1*:708, 1967.

Davis, M. E., and Fugo, N. W.: Effects of various sex hormones on the excretion of pregnanediol early in pregnancy. Proc. Soc. Exp. Biol. Med. *65*:283, 1947.

Flexner, L. B., Cowie, D. B., Hellman, L. M., Wilde, W. S., and Vosburgh, G. J.: The permeability of the human placenta to sodium in normal and abnormal pregnancies and the supply of sodium to the human fetus as determined with radioactive sodium. Amer. J. Obstet. Gynec. *55*:469, 1948.

Friedman, M. H., and Lapham, M. E.: A simple rapid method for the laboratory diagnosis of early pregnancies. Amer. J. Obstet. Gynec. *21*:405, 1931.

Galli Mainini, C.: Pregnancy test using male toad. J. Clin. Endocr. *7*:653, 1947.

Gemzell, C. A.: Blood levels of 17-hydroxycorticosteroids in normal pregnancy. J. Clin. Endocr. *13*:898, 1953.

Gey, G. O., Seegar, G. E., and Hellman, L. M.: The production of a gonadotrophic substance (prolan) by placental cells in tissue culture. Science *88*:306, 1938.

Greene, J. W., Jr., and Touchstone, J. C.: Urinary estriol as an index of placental function: A study of 279 cases. Amer. J. Obstet. Gynec. *85*:1, 1963.

Hon, E. H.: A Manual of Pregnancy Testing. Boston, Little, Brown & Company, 1961.

Jailer, J. W., and Knowlton, A. I.: Simulated adrenocortical activity during pregnancy in an Addisonian patient. J. Clin. Invest. *29*:1430, 1950.

Jensen, E. V., and Jacobson, H. I.: Basic guides to the mechanism of estrogen action. *In* Pincus, G., ed.: Recent Progress in Hormone Research, Vol. 18. New York, Academic Press, 1962, p. 387.

Jones, G. E. S., Gey, G. O., and Gey, M. K.: Hormone production by placental cells maintained in continuous culture. Bull. Johns Hopkins Hosp. *72*:26, 1943.

Josimovich, J. B., and MacLaren, J. A.: Presence in the human placental and term serum of a highly lactogenic substance immunologically related to pituitary growth hormone. Endocrin. *71*:209, 1962.

Karim, S. M. M.: Action of prostaglandin in the pregnant woman. Ann. N.Y. Acad. Sci. *180*:483, 1971.

Karim, S. M. M.: Prostaglandins as abortifacients. New Eng. J. Med. *285*:1534, 1971.

Karim, S. M. M., and Sharma, S. D.: Oral administration of prostaglandins E₂ and F₂α for the induction of labour. Brit. Med. J. *1*:260, 1971.

Karim, S. M. M., Trussell, R. R., Hillier, K., and Patel, R. C.: Induction of labour with prostaglandin F₂α. J. Obstet. Gynaec. Brit. Comm. *76*:769, 1969.

Little, B., Smith, O. W., Jessiman, A. G., Selenkow, H. A., Van't Hoff, W., Eglin, J. M., and Moore, F. D.: Hypophysectomy during pregnancy in a patient with cancer of the breast. J. Clin. Endocr. *18*:425, 1958.

Loraine, J. A., and Bell, E. T.: Hormone Assays and Their Clinical Application, ed. 2. Baltimore, Williams and Wilkins, 1966.

Migeon, C. J., Keller, A. R., and Holmstrom, E. G.: Dehydroisoandrosterone, androsterone and 17-hydroxycorticosteroid levels in maternal and cord plasma in cases of vaginal delivery. Bull. Johns Hopkins Hosp. *97*:415, 1955.

Moricard, R.: Effects of chorionic and equine gonadotrophins on hypophysectomized immature rats. Ciba Found. Colloq. Endocr. *5*:33, 1953.

Page, E. W.: Placental dysfunction in eclamptogenic toxemias. Obstet. Gynec. Survey *3*:615, 1948.

Page, E. W.: Transfer of materials across the human placenta. Amer. J. Obstet. Gynec. *74*:705, 1957.

Page, E. W., Glendening, M. B., Margolis, A., and Harper, H. A.: Transfer of d- and l-histidine across the human placenta. Amer. J. Obstet. Gynec. *73*:589, 1957.

Pearlman, W. H.: 16-³H-progesterone metabolism in advanced pregnancy and in oophorectomized-hysterectomized women. Biochem. J. *67*:1, 1957.

Plotz, E. J., and Davis, M. E.: Distribution of radioactivity in human maternal and fetal tissue following administration of C¹⁴-4-progesterone. Proc. Soc. Exp. Biol. Med. *95*:92, 1957.

Plotz, E. J., Davis, M. E., and Ricketts, H. T.: Endocrine studies in pregnant diabetic women. Diabetes *8*:14, 1959.

Roy, E., and Brown, J. B.: Cited by Loraine, J. A.: Ciba Found. Colloq. Endocr. *11*:335, 1957.

Ryan, K. J.: Metabolism of C-16-oxygenated steroids by the human placenta. The formation of estriol. J. Biol. Chem. *234*:2006, 1959.

Salhanick, H. A., Kipnis, D. M., and Vande Wiele, R.

L.: Metabolic Effects of Gonadal Hormones and Contraceptive Steroids. New York, Plenum Press, 1969.

Sciarra, J. J., Kaplan, S. L., and Grumbach, M. M.: Localization of anti-human growth hormone serum within the human placenta: Evidence for a human chorionic "growth hormone-prolactin." Nature 199:1005, 1963.

Sherwood, L. M.: Similarities in the chemical structure of human placental lactogen and pituitary growth hormone. Proc. Nat. Acad. Sci. 58:2307, 1967.

Simmons, R. L.: Histoincompatibility and the survival of the fetus: Current controversies. Transplant. Proc. 1:47, 1969.

Spellacy, W. N., Cohen, W. D., and Carlson, K. L.: Human placental lactogen levels as a measure of placental function. Amer. J. Obstet. Gynec. 97:560, 1967.

Speroff, L., and Ramwell, P. W.: Prostaglandins in reproductive physiology. Amer. J. Obstet. Gynec. 107:1111, 1970.

Stewart, H. L., Jr.: Hormone secretion by human placenta grown in the eyes of rabbits. Amer. J. Obstet. Gynec. 61:990, 1951.

Talalay, P., Hurlock, B., and Williams-Ashman, H. G.: On a coenzymatic function of estradiol-17-beta. Proc. Nat. Acad. Sci. 44:862, 1958.

Thiede, H. A., and Choate, J. W.: Chorionic gonado-

tropin localization in the human placenta by immunofluorescent staining: II. Demonstration of HCG in the trophoblast and amnion epithelium of immature and mature placentas. Obstet. Gynec. 22:433, 1963.

Tulsky, A. S., and Koff, A. K.: Some observations on the role of the corpus luteum in early human pregnancy. Fertil. Steril. 8:118, 1957.

Venning, E. H.: Adrenal function in pregnancy. Endocrinology 39:203, 1946.

Venning, E., and Brown, J. S. L.: Urinary excretion of sodium pregnanediol glucuronidate in the menstrual cycle (an excretion product of progesterone). Amer. J. Physiol. 119:417, 1937.

Venning, E. H., and Dyrenfurth, I.: Aldosterone excretion in pregnancy. J. Clin. Endocr. 16:426, 1956.

Villee, D. B.: Development of endocrine function in the human placenta and fetus. New Eng. J. Med. 281:473, 533, 1969.

Whiteley, H. J., and Stoner, H. B.: The effect of pregnancy on the human adrenal cortex. J. Endocr. 14:325, 1957.

Wislocki, G. B., and Bennett, H. S.: The histology and cytology of the human and monkey placenta with special reference to the trophoblast. Amer. J. Anat. 73:335, 1943.

Zander, J.: Progesteron in menschlichem Blut und Geweben: I. Progesteron im peripheren venösen Blut der Frau. Klin. Wschr. 33:697, 1955.

Chapter 5
Amniotic Fluid

ORIGIN OF AMNIOTIC FLUID

Early in embryologic development, soon after the formation of the amniotic cavity (Chapter 3), a certain amount of clear fluid collects. Throughout its intrauterine life, the fetus is surrounded by this fluid. Its exact origin is not fully understood. In the early months, amniotic fluid is isotonic with maternal serum and its composition approximates that of other protein-poor fluids which are in osmotic equilibrium with blood plasma. This suggests that amniotic fluid originates during this interval as a dialysate in equilibrium with maternal and fetal body fluids.

Later it becomes hypotonic and at term its freezing point and specific gravity are considerably lower than the freezing point and the specific gravity of maternal serum. According to Makepeace et al., the osmolar concentration of amniotic fluid, based on freezing point depression, decreases from 292 to 270 milliosmols per liter during pregnancy, whereas maternal serum concentration is of the order of 296 milliosmols per liter.

The presence of urea and uric acid in the amniotic fluid in late pregnancy indicates that the amniotic fluid becomes more and more diluted by hypotonic fluids, perhaps fetal urine, as pregnancy advances. In this regard, fetal urine was found to have a relatively low osmolar concentration of about 85 milliosmols per liter, suggesting that the hypotonicity of amniotic fluid in late pregnancy was the result of dilution by fetal urine.

The contention that amniotic fluid originates principally as a result of fetal micturition is, however, largely circumstantial. The arguments against this mechanism (Plentl and Gray) are pertinent. For example, the condition of excessive accumulation of amniotic fluid, *hydramnios*, can be found in association with dead fetuses as well as with living fetuses who cannot produce urine, including those with congenital closure of the genitourinary tract or agenesis of the kidneys. Moreover, methylene blue dye, even when given to the mother over long periods of time, cannot be detected in amniotic fluid but is found invariably in fetal urine at birth (Holtermann). On the other hand, *oligohydramnios* may be associated with absent fetal urinary production.

In fact, notwithstanding the wealth of research data in this area, the actual channels of origin and fate of amniotic fluid still remain largely conjectural. The dynamic equilibrium of the amniotic sac compartment and the rapid turnover of its contents, first demonstrated by Vosburgh et al., have been quantitatively detailed in Plentl's laboratory (Hutchinson et al.). Although transcompartmental fluxes have thus been elucidated, this information has done little to define actual anatomic pathways except perhaps by way of inference.

Fetal urine as a partial source is an ancient Hippocratic theorem. It has support in logical implications derived from the clinical observation of oligohydramnios appearing in association with fetal renal agenesis (Bardram; Potter). Further suggestive verification comes from the findings of increased urea and creatinine content and diminishing osmolarity of amniotic fluid with progressive gestational age (Battaglia et al.). This is presumably the result of contributions to the compartment by fetal micturition. Since turnover rate of amniotic fluid is much greater, by a

20-fold factor, than can possibly be attributed to renal sources alone (Alexander et al.; McCance and Widdowson), it is quite reasonable to suggest that other and perhaps more important pathways coexist. These must also be presumed to be active prior to the time when the fetal kidneys begin to excrete actively.

There is some evidence that a major supply of amniotic fluid arrives by way of the chorioamniotic membrane. This is an attractive hypothesis, but quite unproven. Early in pregnancy, the amnion possesses secretory epithelial elements capable of rapid transudation (Danforth and Hull). As pregnancy advances, surface microvilli appear, together with complex intercellular canaliculae (Bourne and Lacy). Fairly rapid osmotic transfer across fresh term amnion has been demonstrated *in vitro* (Scoggin). Furthermore, metabolic activity of chorion, documented to be of the same magnitude as that of intraplacental chorion (Friedman and Sachtleben), makes it likely that transport does take place here and can occur not only by simple diffusion but by carrier or facilitated mechanisms as well (see Chapter 4). This latter is not in vogue to support water transport, but is undoubtedly important insofar as the possible mechanisms by which other substances appear in and are cleared from amniotic fluid.

The surface interface exposed between maternal vascular space and amniotic fluid space is inadequate (even assuming it all to be functional in terms of water exchange) to account for a large measure of amniotic fluid production. Water exchange at term across the normal maternal-fetal interface is about 3600 ml. per hour, as compared with maternal-amnion transfer of 400 ml. per hour. The relative surface areas involved are quite different: placental villus surface area is estimated to be 7 to 12 square meters, whereas maternal-amnion surface area is about 0.2 square meter. The 50:1 relationship in surface area far exceeds the 9:1 ratio of transfer rates.

Additional support for a channel from mother to amniotic fluid, bypassing the fetus, comes from the appearance of certain maternal proteins in amniotic fluid not found in the fetus at all (Ruoslahti et al.)

and from the rapid changes of observed protein patterns as well (Wirtschafter and Williams). Clinically, the maintenance of amniotic fluid volume well beyond the time of fetal death provides another piece of confirmatory evidence to bolster the concept that direct pathways must exist between maternal and amniotic fluid compartments. Moreover, the occasional observation of excessive amniotic fluid, hydramnios, in coassociation with dead fetuses is also supportive.

Transfer across fetal skin perhaps occurs, but probably not beyond midpregnancy to any great extent. This contention is supported by the electronmicroscopic findings of surface microvilli in early embryonic life (Lind et al.). Fetal lung as a speculative location for origin and clearance of amniotic fluid is reasonable on theoretical grounds but investigative data are not completely substantiating. Potter reported coassociation of hypoplasia of lungs and renal agenesis, both in turn related somehow to the appearance of oligohydramnios. Reynolds showed production in the fetal lamb of significant amounts of tracheal fluid similar in composition to amniotic fluid. Alveolar fluid is, of course, quite different in make-up, more nearly resembling serum from which it is derived (Bates; Setnikar et al.; Snyder). Diaphragmatic movements observed to occur *in utero* (Potter and Davis) are unlikely to produce much "respiratory" excursion of fluid in the tracheobronchial tree in either direction, but may aid in mixing amniotic and alveolar fluids at their imaginary interface.

Movement of water across the umbilical cord has been postulated. Embryologically, the lining cells of the umbilical cord are derived from the same fetal ectodermal anlage as amnion and on that basis alone might be expected to have similar properties. The close proximity between intraluminal blood in the umbilical vessels within the cord and the surface of the cord in the living fetus has been demonstrated clearly (see Chapter 3). Rapid transfer has been demonstrated *in vitro* by perfusing the cord (Plentl). More meaningful was the finding of unexpectedly high levels of tracer injected into the amniotic fluid within Wharton's jelly (Hutchinson et al.).

For the sake of completeness, mention should be made of other conjectured sources of amniotic fluid, such as fetal salivary, buccal and mammary glands. Evidence for these pathways is entirely lacking at this time.

FATE OF AMNIOTIC FLUID

Fetal deglutition *in utero* has been thoroughly documented by many investigators utilizing different experimental approaches. The amount that the fetus is capable of swallowing has been quantitated with erythrocytes labeled with isotopic chromium injected into the amniotic sac (Pritchard). At term, the fetus is capable of swallowing as much as 450 ml. of amniotic fluid daily. It is of interest to note that this is approximately the volume the newborn infant is generally capable of ingesting by either bottle or breast feeding.

Absorption of amniotic fluid contents by way of the fetal gastrointestinal tract and disposal through the placental membrane to maternal circulation are well accepted and documented. Whether or not fetal swallowing regulates amniotic fluid volume, however, is not established, although this attractive theory is held by many.

Radiopaque dyes injected into the amniotic fluid are concentrated rapidly in the fetal gastrointestinal tract as a result of deglutition. This phenomenon has proved quite useful in radiographic localization of the fetal peritoneal cavity for purposes of administering blood to fetuses affected by erythroblastosis fetalis (see Chapter 52). The volume of amniotic fluid that can possibly be absorbed by way of the gastrointestinal tract is only a small fraction of the total turnover of amniotic fluid (see below). Therefore, other relevant pathways must exist.

The fetal lung has also been suggested as a site for the removal of amniotic fluid (Macaffee). The observation of lanugo in fetal alveoli is supportive of this contention. Fetal respiratory movements have been observed *in utero* and radiopaque material injected into the amniotic sac has been demonstrated within the lungs of im-

mature fetuses (Davis and Potter). However, the material appeared in the lungs only after long intervals of exposure, concentrating significantly after 18 hours. This suggested that this pathway for clearance of amniotic fluid at best can handle only a very small fraction of the total amount exchanged. Intrauterine fetal respirations have been documented (Snyder and Rosenfeld). There is much debate whether or not intrauterine respiratory activity is necessary for the preparation of the respiratory system for extrauterine function. Nevertheless, insofar as its role in amniotic fluid exchange is concerned, it appears to be negligible.

Transudation of amniotic fluid directly to the mother by way of decidua and placenta is another possible pathway (Szendi). Similarly, the chorioamniotic membranes may serve the same role. Appearance of dyes that have been injected into the amniotic sac within the cytoplasm of amniotic cells may be considered as evidence that absorption occurs by this route. Fetal skin and umbilical cord have already been discussed as possible pathways (see above).

DYNAMICS OF EXCHANGE

The origin, fate and regulation of amniotic fluid and its components in various stages of pregnancy have received much recent attention. The contents of the amniotic sac were considered to be essentially a stagnant pool until the landmark finding by Flexner and Gellhorn, using radioisotope injections in guinea pigs, that water content of the amniotic fluid at all stages of pregnancy is completely replaced at the rather surprisingly rapid rate of about once hourly. This was confirmed in the human by Vosburgh et al. using heavy water (deuterium oxide) and radioactive sodium (Na^{24}) as tracer substances. They determined that amniotic fluid is completely replaced on the average of once every 2.9 hours.

Moreover, it was apparent that water turnover was much more rapid than that of sodium. In the guinea pig, sodium replacement occurred about 50 times slower than water; in the human, about five times slower. Thus, sodium was replaced in the human amniotic sac every 14.5 hours. By actual measurement, Plentl and Hutchinson, also using deuterium oxide, found that the amount of water leaving the amniotic fluid per hour was the same as the transfer rate in the opposite direction from mother to amniotic fluid at 26 mols or about 500 ml. per hour. Identical exchange rates were encountered in patients with oligohydramnios and hydramnios as well (Hutchinson et al.).

Additional investigations have demonstrated that the role of the fetus is appreciable. Direct measurements of water transferred to and from the monkey fetus have indicated that at least 25 per cent and perhaps considerably more of this exchange takes place through the intermedium of the fetus itself (Plentl et al.).

By regarding the system as if it could be represented as three separate compartments, namely, amniotic fluid, maternal and fetal circulations, respectively, Plentl utilized double isotope tracer techniques to measure overall exchange of water between the compartments. A summarization of some of the data derived is shown in Figure 62. Appearance and disappearance rates could be calculated for each of the compartments and calculations made of exchange rates between them.

Although these data do not provide information concerning the actual anatomic pathways for exchange, they do offer useful data on rates of exchange and net circulation. Since neither fetal blood nor amniotic fluid volumes change appreciably during the experimental intervals, it can be assumed that the total gain or loss in any direction is zero. Although the three-compartment exchange system appears simplistic, one must appreciate that, if each compartment exchanges with the other two, there will result six possible transfer rates. These are shown in Figure 62 and indicate that water circulates bidirectionally. Moreover, the sums of the transfer rates in one direction are not equal to those in the opposite direction, suggesting that there exists a net circulation of the order of 500 to 600 ml. per hour from mother to fetus to amniotic fluid and back to mother again.

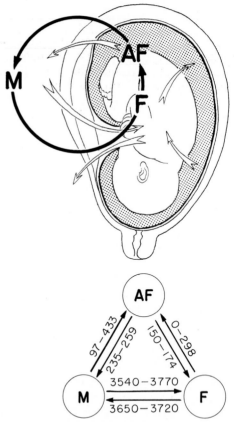

Figure 62 Schematic representation of the three-compartment system of water exchange between mother (*M*), fetus (*F*) and amniotic fluid (*AF*) in normal pregnancy as studied by double-isotope technique. The upper pictorial portion suggests possible anatomic pathways for transfer of water between the several compartments. The lower diagram shows the direction and magnitude of the measured transfer expressed in milliliters of water per hour. The heavy arrows in the upper part of the figure designate the net transfer or "circulation" between the compartments when the differences in bidirectional flow are taken into account. (From Hutchinson, D. L., et al.: J. Clin. Invest. 38:971, 1959.)

Investigations of transfer rates of electrolytes show that these ions are exchanged at their own unique rates. If amniotic fluid were an ultrafiltrate, one would expect all its components, including water, sodium and potassium, to appear and to be removed simultaneously and with equal rates. The 500 ml. of water that leaves the amniotic fluid per hour should be expected to carry with it about 68 mEq. of sodium and 1.9 mEq. of potassium. Since only about one-fifth of these latter amounts are actually transferred, one is led to the assumption that each element exchanges by its own specific independent mechanism. Thus, the amniotic fluid cannot be considered to be a transudate or dialysate of maternal plasma, but rather is in dynamic equilibrium with the maternal system. Verification of this concept exists for the distinctive exchange rates of other substances, including urea, bicarbonate and lactic acid (Friedman et al.; Hutchinson et al.).

Plentl studied normal pregnant women at term and determined that there was an average exchange of 26 mols of water per hour or the equivalent of 468 ml. This may be expressed in terms of clearance rates as indicating that half of the water in the amniotic fluid is exchanged with maternal water every 95 minutes (Fig. 63). This last figure is the disappearance constant or half-value time. Comparable data for hydramnios average 285 minutes and for oligohydramnios 24 minutes (Hutchinson et al.). These figures, although obviously disparate, should not be misinterpreted to indicate that exchange rates for these conditions are also different. It is quite clear that the disappearance constant increases proportionately with increasing volume.

When the true exchange rates are calculated, they are found to be entirely comparable without regard for the actual amount of amniotic fluid present.

Observations were sufficiently consistent to allow the conclusion that the quantity of water transferred in and out of the amniotic sac is constant and independent of the volume of fluid. The accumulation of large amounts of amniotic fluid to form hydramnios, therefore, is not necessarily due to faster or slower exchange rate or to a gross defect in the manner of its removal. Its cause must be searched for in a disturbance of other and probably much more subtle mechanisms. An imbalance in transfer rates is more likely the source of the pathologic process. The existence of the large volume of fluid is merely a reflection of the underlying disorder.

The assumption that the exchange rates in opposite directions are equal is probably justifiable within the constraints of the experimental approach. It is conceivable, for example, that a very small difference of only a few milliliters per hour may result in a slow, but definite increase in volume and ultimately produce the clinical syndrome of hydramnios. Much more precise

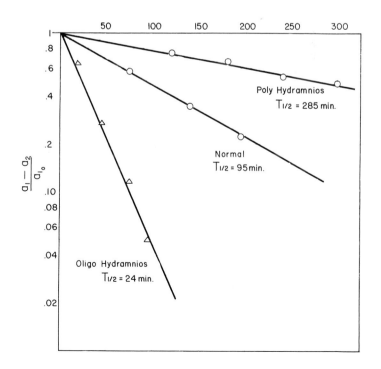

Figure 63 Disappearance constants for the clearance of heavy water (deuterium oxide) injected into amniotic fluid, demonstrated as a linear function of the semilogarithmic plot of the proportion of the tracer element against time. The biological half-life is shown at that point on the decay curve where it crosses 0.5 (50 per cent of the original) concentration. The differences between normal and abnormal patients are based on volume rather than clearance rates. (From Hutchinson, D. L., et al.: Surg. Gynec. Obstet. *100*:391, 1955.)

techniques for studying transfer mechanisms would be required to detect such infinitesimal differences.

VOLUME

The volume of amniotic fluid in early pregnancy has been studied by Monie who found volumes of 8, 20, 45 and 80 ml., respectively, at 6, 8, 10 and 12 weeks after conception. These data have more recently been confirmed by Gillibrand who showed orderly increases in volume throughout pregnancy in coassociation with diminishing osmolality. The volume appears to reach a maximum of between 1000 and 1500 ml. early in the third trimester and to diminish somewhat from this peak as term approaches. It is generally accepted that amniotic fluid volume diminishes more acutely beyond term in prolonged pregnancies. Wide variations in amniotic fluid volume have been reported (Fuchs). The limits of normal have been set rather arbitrarily at between 300 and 2000 ml.

With regard to the condition known as *hydramnios*, in which the volume of amniotic fluid is abnormally great based on clinical impression, it is possible that excessive formation can occur under a variety of circumstances. Some of the sounder theories implicate the fetal circulation and the placenta as causative factors. Stasis in the placental bed, for example, particularly venous stasis in the cotyledons, is said to be a relatively constant finding in hydramnios. Correlation has been reported with various disorders including occlusion of the umbilical vein. Placental infarctions, large placentas and circumvallate placentas are significant coassociated findings which point to the possibility that circulatory defects in the placenta may be etiologic. Maternal diseases which are characteristically coassociated with placental abnormalities, including preeclampsia, diabetes and Rh isoimmunization, have all been implicated as well. The clinical implications of this disorder are discussed in Chapter 54.

A cause and effect relationship has been fairly firmly established between congenital anomalies and hydramnios. There is an average incidence of 26 per cent congenitally abnormal babies which can be expected once hydramnios is diagnosed clinically. Conversely, hydramnios is found in about 50 per cent of pregnancies that terminate in the birth of a congenitally abnormal baby.

The nature of the relationship, however, is far from clear. Anomalies that interfere with fetal swallowing or are associated with obstruction of the upper gastrointestinal tract (duodenal atresias and tracheoesophageal fistulas) are not uncommonly associated with hydramnios, suggesting that interference with deglutition may cause slow accumulation of amniotic fluid volume over the course of time in pregnancy. Although this has not been clearly verified experimentally (see above), it is an attractive hypothesis. The failure of any mechanism designed for the removal of amniotic fluid would theoretically lead to its gradual accumulation. Therefore, obstruction of the gastrointestinal tract, failure of the swallowing mechanism or obstruction of the respiratory passages may indeed be factors of significance.

Anencephalus is often associated with hydramnios also. It has been attributed to increased secretion by the choroid plexus. Proliferation of the highly vascular, thin-walled choroid tissue is commonly seen at the base of the skull in anencephalic infants. Failure of absorption from the lungs may also account for this phenomenon because the lungs are also invariably hypoplastic in anencephalic fetuses.

If these are the pathways for removal of fluid, then many questions still remain unanswered. Hydramnios associated with other varieties of congenital disorders could not be accounted for on these bases. The occurrence of hydramnios in association with essentially normal fetuses would require other explanations. We have already indicated that studies in which tracer elements were used to indicate the total amount of water entering and leaving the amniotic fluid showed that the rates of exchange were the same for patients with and without hydramnios. This exchange of water, however, is of such a large magnitude that a small and perhaps undetectable difference in the exchange rates could bring about the clinical syndrome of hydramnios without its being measurable by our currently available techniques.

CONSTITUENTS

The amniotic fluid at term is pale and clear. It has a slightly alkaline reaction and specific gravity of 1.008. It is composed of more than 98 per cent water. The remainder consists of small quantities of inorganic salts and organic materials. There is also cellular debris sloughed from the surface of the fetus, including sebaceous material from the sweat glands, epithelial cells from its skin, and lanugo.

The detailed composition of amniotic fluid has been reviewed recently by Bonsnes. Protein content averages about 2.6 gm. per liter and is mostly albumin. Its concentration is about one-twentieth that of the serum. Electrophoretically and immunochemically, the protein make-up seems to be about the same as in serum, although two proteins distinctive to amniotic fluid have been reported (Lambotte and Salmon). Amino acid content is also similar to serum. Urea, creatinine and uric acid levels are higher in amniotic fluid, increasing as pregnancy progresses. The implication of this finding with regard to possible contributions by fetal urine has been discussed (see above). Glucose is consistently less concentrated, whereas lactic acid appears in large amounts. Amniotic fluid also contains lipid substances, half in the form of fatty acids.

Electrolytic content is similar to that of extracellular fluid, containing mostly sodium, chloride and bicarbonate ions and small amounts of potassium, magnesium, calcium and phosphate. There is a rapid fall in sodium level with advancing pregnancy beyond 32 to 36 weeks, paralleling the fall in osmolarity.

Some of the constituents of the amniotic fluid are useful indicators of health or disease states. The constituents of the amniotic fluid have been explored extensively for potential value in antenatal diagnosis. Assessments of constituents range from determination of fetal age and sex to detection of inborn errors of metabolism. The greatest potential usefulness involves those tests which help to determine whether the risk of allowing the fetus to remain in its hostile environment is greater or less than the risk inherent in delivery.

Amniotic fluid creatinine, for example, has been tentatively correlated with fetal maturity, as has the per cent of fetal cells which stain orange with Nile blue sulfate, reflecting functional development of fetal sebaceous glands. Its content of bilirubin and bilirubin breakdown products has been determined to be quite useful in evaluating the presence and severity of Rh isoimmunization (see Chapter 52). The presence of lecithin and sphingomyelin has been shown to be useful in evaluating fetal maturity (see Chapter 13). Sequential increase in lecithin correlates with functional maturity of the lungs *in utero*. The ratio of lecithin to sphingomyelin is especially pertinent in this regard.

Study of the epithelial cells within the amniotic fluid for chromatin bodies has been utilized for the purpose of determining the sex of the fetus in instances where sex-linked hereditary disorders can be diagnosed. Culture of amniotic fluid cells is also useful for purposes of chromosome analysis. Tissue culture of these cells can determine the presence or absence of certain hereditable metabolic disorders (see Chapter 13). Biochemical studies of tissue cultures are useful as a means for detecting inborn errors of metabolism *in utero*. Histochemical studies may also offer aid in diagnosing other hereditary disorders.

Many aspects of prenatal diagnosis can be provided by analyzing amniotic fluid for content of steroids, proteins, amino acids and some enzymes. Other investigations are under way along similar lines in an effort to provide diagnostic measures for determining the status of the fetus. Whereas until recent years the amniotic sac was sacrosanct, the ready availability of amniotic fluid for study has opened new and exciting vistas in this discipline.

FUNCTION

From the teleological point of view, the amniotic fluid appears to furnish much protection to the fetus. It ensures a constant pressure and temperature during pregnancy and apparently diminishes the risks of injury to the fetus from outside sources. It allows the fetus to move quite freely and at the same time saves the maternal tissues from much of the direct impact of fetal movements. In labor, especially in its early aspects, the amniotic fluid receives the pressures from uterine contractions directly. Hydrodynamically, the uterine contents are acted upon as a unit. In this way the fluid causes equal distribution of the forces of the uterine contractions. The fetus itself is thus protected for a long period of time during its sojourn *in utero*.

The amniotic fluid provides a liquid environment in which the fetus can grow freely, thereby avoiding the potentially compressing effects of the muscular walls which surround it. Formation of amniotic bands, which have been known to deform fetal limbs and in rare instances to amputate them, has occurred in association with oligohydramnios. Serving as an insulator, the amniotic fluid also protects the fetus against temperature changes.

The hydrostatic action of the fluid when contained within its membranes appears to aid in the dilatation of the maternal soft parts in labor and perhaps to lessen the possibility of injury to the mother. Proof of this contention is wanting. There are other equally unproved purposes ascribed to amniotic fluid, such as its lubricant action after the membranes rupture and its ostensible ability to flush away potentially infectious materials that may have entered during labor. In this regard, however, amniotic fluid is antibacterial to a limited extent.

The role of the amniotic fluid in supplying nutritional substances to the fetus is probably small. Although the fetus swallows substantial amounts of amniotic fluid, its nutritional value is negligible. For example, protein content is quite low as indicated earlier in this chapter, in a range similar to that of interstitial fluid; glucose levels also tend to be quite low, in the range of 40 mg. per 100 ml. The caloric intake represented by the daily ingestion of 450 ml. of this amount of nutritive material cannot be considered to be significant.

REFERENCES

Alexander, D. P., Nixon, D. A., Widdas, W. F., and Wohlzagan, F. S.: Renal function in the sheep fetus. J. Physiol. *140*:14, 1958.

Bardram, E.: Congenital kidney malformations and oligohydramnios. Acta Obstet. Gynec. Scand. *10*:134, 1930.

Bates, H. R.: Comparison of pharyngeal and amniotic fluids in the guinea pig fetus. Amer. J. Obstet. Gynec. 85:484, 1963.

Battaglia, F. C., Prystowsky, H., Smisson, C., Hellegers, A. E., and Bruns, P.: Fetal blood studies: XVI. On the changes in total osmotic pressure and sodium and potassium concentrations of amniotic fluid during the course of gestation. Surg. Gynec. Obstet. *109*:509, 1959.

Bonsnes, R. W.: Composition of amniotic fluid. Clin. Obstet. Gynec. 9:440, 1966.

Bourne, G. L., and Lacy, D.: Ultrastructure of human amnion and its possible relation to the circulation of amniotic fluid. Nature *186*:952, 1960.

Danforth, D. N., and Hull, R. W.: The microscopic anatomy of the fetal membranes with particular reference to the detailed structure of the amnion. Amer. J. Obstet. Gynec. 75:536, 1958.

Davis, M. E., and Potter, E. L.: Intrauterine respiration of the human fetus. J.A.M.A. *131*:1194, 1946.

Flexner, L. B., and Gellhorn, A.: Comparative physi-ology of placental transfer. Amer. J. Obstet. Gynec. *43*:965, 1942.

Friedman, E. A., and Sachtleben, M. R.: Placental oxygen consumption in vitro: I. Baseline studies. Amer. J. Obstet. Gynec. 79:1058, 1960.

Friedman, E. A., Gray, M. J., Grynfogel, M., Hutchinson, D. L., Kelly, W. T., and Plentl, A. A.: Distribution and metabolism of C^{14}-labeled lactic acid and bicarbonate in pregnant primates. J. Clin. Invest. 39:227, 1960.

Fuchs, F.: Volume of amniotic fluid at various stages of pregnancy. Clin. Obstet. Gynec. 9:449, 1966.

Gillibrand, P. N.: Changes in amniotic fluid volume with advancing pregnancy. J. Obstet. Gynaec. Brit. Comm. 76:527, 1969.

Holtermann, C.: Einiges über den Methylenblau-übergang aus dem mutterliehen Organism auf die Frucht. Zbl. Gynäk. 48:2536, 1924.

Hutchinson, D. L., Hunter, C. B., Neslen, E. D., and Plentl, A. A.: Exchange of water and electrolytes in mechanism of amniotic fluid formation and the relationship to hydramnios. Surg. Gynec. Obstet. *100*:391, 1955.

Hutchinson, D. L., Kelly, W. T., Friedman, E. A., and Plentl, A. A.: Distribution and metabolism of carbon-labeled urea in pregnant primates. J. Clin. Invest. 41:1748, 1962.

Hutchinson, D. L., Gray, M. J., Plentl, A. A., Alvarez, H., Caldeyro-Barcia, R., Kaplan, B., and Lind, J.: The role of the fetus in the water exchange of the amniotic fluid of normal and hydramniotic patients. J. Clin. Invest. 38:971, 1959.

Lambotte, R., and Salmon, J.: Étude immunoelectrophoretique du liquide amniotique humain. C. R. Soc. Biol. 156:530, 1962.

Lind, T., Parkin, F. M., and Cheyne, G. A.: Biochemical and cytological changes in liquor amnii with advancing gestation. J. Obstet. Gynaec. Brit. Comm. 76:673, 1969.

Macaffee, C. H. G.: Hydramnios. J. Obstet. Gynaec. Brit. Emp. 57:171, 1950.

Makepeace, A. W., Fremont-Smith, F., Dailey, M. E., and Carroll, M. P.: Nature of amniotic fluid. Surg. Gynec. Obstet. 53:635, 1931.

McCance, R. A., and Widdowson, E. M.: Renal function before birth. Proc. Roy. Soc. 141:488, 1953.

Monie, I. W.: The volume of the amniotic fluid in the early months of pregnancy. Amer. J. Obstet. Gynec. 66:616, 1953.

Plentl, A. A.: The dynamics of the amniotic fluid. Ann. N.Y. Acad. Sci. 75:746, 1959.

Plentl, A. A.: Transfer of water across the perfused umbilical cord. Proc. Soc. Exp. Biol. Med. 107:622, 1961.

Plentl, A. A., and Gray, M. J.: Physiology of the amniotic fluid and the management of hydramnios. Surg. Clin. N. Amer. 37:405, 1957.

Plentl, A. A., and Hutchinson, D. L.: Determination of deuterium exchange rates between maternal circulation and amniotic fluid. Proc. Soc. Exp. Biol. Med. 82:681, 1953.

Plentl, A. A., Gray, M. J., and Neslen, E. D.: Estimation of water transfer from amniotic fluid to fetus. Proc. Soc. Exp. Biol. Med. 92:463, 1956.

Potter, E. L.: Pathology of the Fetus and Infant, ed. 2. Chicago, Year Book Medical Publishers, Inc., 1961.

Potter, E. L., and Davis, M. E.: Intrauterine respiration of human fetus. J.A.M.A. 131:1194, 1946.

Pritchard, J. A.: Deglutition by normal and anencephalic fetuses. Obstet. Gynec. 25:289, 1965.

Pritchard, J. A.: Fetal swallowing and amniotic fluid volume. Obstet. Gynec. 28:606, 1966.

Reynolds, S. R. M.: A source of amniotic fluid in the lamb: The nasopharyngeal and buccal cavities. Nature 172:307, 1953.

Ruoslahti, E., Tallberg, T., and Seppälä, M.: Origin of proteins in amniotic fluid. Nature 212:841, 1966.

Scoggin, W. A.: Exchange and net flow across the human amniochorionic membrane in vitro. Trans. Rochester Trophoblast Conf. 3:108, 1965.

Setnikar, I., Agostone, E., and Taglietti, A.: The fetal lung, a source of amniotic fluid. Proc. Soc. Exp. Biol. Med. 101:842, 1959.

Snyder, F. F.: The rate of entry of amniotic fluid into the pulmonary alveoli during fetal respiration. Amer. J. Obstet. Gynec. 41:224, 1941.

Snyder, F. F., and Rosenfeld, M.: Intra-uterine respiratory movement of the human fetus. J.A.M.A. 108:1946, 1937.

Szendi, B.: Experimentelle Untersuchungen beim Menschen über den Austausch und die intrauterine Rolle des Fruchtwasser. Arch. Gynäk. 170:205, 1940.

Vosburgh, G. J., Flexner, L. F., Cowie, D. B., Hellman, L. M., Procter, N. K., and Wilde, W. S.: Rate of renewal in women of the water and sodium of the amniotic fluid as determined by tracer techniques. Amer. J. Obstet. Gynec. 56:1156, 1948.

Wirtschafter, Z. T., and Williams, D. W.: Dynamics of the amniotic fluid as measured by changes in protein patterns. Amer. J. Obstet. Gynec. 74:309, 1957.

Chapter 6

Fetal and Neonatal Physiology

CIRCULATORY SYSTEM

The yolk sac has only slight nutritive properties. It acquires a store of nutriment from the mother and is involved in hematopoiesis (see below). It constitutes the earliest *vitelline* source of nutrition for the growing embryo. A vitelline circulation develops so that blood flows along the vitelline duct to and from the yolk sac, offering a pathway for exchange of substances with the limited supply within the yolk sac. This circulation is prominent for the first four weeks and then disappears.

As the chorionic villi and the umbilical vessels on the body stalk develop, the fetus is provided with a new and more direct mechanism for nourishment. The capillary system of the umbilical arteries and vein rapidly invades the growing villi, and the intimate osmotic relationship between maternal and fetal blood is soon established. The separate and parallel vitelline and umbilical circulations are shown in Figure 64. The fetal blood now passes from the primitive heart through the primitive aorta and the umbilical arteries to the capillaries lining the periphery of the ovum and dipping into chorionic villi. Blood that has been oxygenated in the placenta and provided with nutritive substances and water for the fetus (see Chapter 4) is collected by the branches of the umbilical vein. Usually, only a single large vein persists in the umbilical cord carrying blood to the fetus. It enters at the umbilicus and ascends behind the parietal peritoneum of the liver. The vein divides within the liver substance into several branches that enter the liver directly. Others anastomose with the portal vein, while one large branch, the *ductus ven-*

osus Arantii, enters the vena cava directly. This pathway is detailed in Figure 65.

Oxygenated blood is then carried into the inferior vena cava where it enters the right atrium, mixing with less oxygenated blood that has reached the superior vena cava from the head and the upper limbs. Blood from the right atrium enters the left atrium by way of the open *foramen ovale* and the right ventricle by way of the mitral valve. From the right ventricle, blood enters the fetal pulmonary circulation, the majority being shunted through the *ductus arteriosus* into the aorta. The blood that has entered the left atrium by way of the foramen ovale is ejected into the left ventricle and out of the aorta to supply the head region of the fetus with maximally oxygenated blood. The blood that travels by way of the aorta along the arch mixes with the deoxygenated blood entering via the ductus arteriosus. This blood travels down the descending aorta and the hypogastric arteries to reach the umbilical arteries and returns to the placenta for oxygenation once again.

After birth (Fig. 66), changes take place in the ductus arteriosus, the ductus venosus, the foramen ovale, the hypogastric arteries and the umbilical cord. Immediately after delivery, the baby begins to breathe and the pulmonary circulation begins to function. The result is that a much larger amount of blood is pumped into the pulmonary arteries by the right ventricle and a smaller amount as a consequence passes through the ductus arteriosus. After the ductus arteriosus becomes obliterated, it is known as the *ligamentum arteriosum*. The umbilical vein no longer has any function once the umbilical cord has been ligated so that less

84

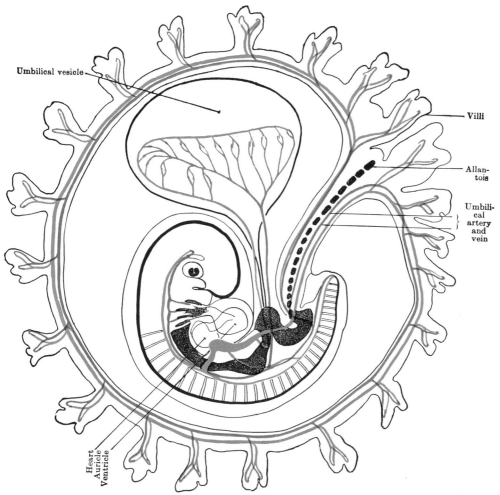

Umbilical vesicle

Villi

Allan-
tois

Umbili-
cal
artery
and
vein

Heart
Auricle
Ventricle

Figure 64 Schematic representation of the vitelline and chorionic circulations of the fetus shown to illustrate the primitive pathway for interchange between the early embryo and its yolk sac (umbilical vesical) and the later and more efficient circulatory exchange pathways via the umbilical vessels to the developing placenta.

blood gains access to the right atrium from the inferior vena cava. This results in a lowered pressure in the right atrium and an increased pressure in the left side of the heart. As a consequence of these changes, the foramen ovale closes. The distal ends of the hypogastric arteries, which in fetal life constituted the origins for the umbilical arteries, cease to function after the pulmonary circulation is established and the umbilical vessels are occluded. The portions of the distal ends that atrophy and become obliterated are known as the *hypogastric ligaments* or obliterated umbilical arteries. The ductus venosus also becomes occluded and is known as the

ligamentum venosum. The obliterated umbilical veins become the *ligamentum teres.*

Angiocardiographic studies in human fetuses have supported the view that mixing of the oxygenated blood from the inferior vena cava and deoxygenated blood from the superior vena cava probably does not take place in the right atrium, but rather that the jetstream of each is such as to minimize admixture (Lind and Wegelius). Blood entering the right atrium appears to be separated into two streams, the larger of which passes through the foramen ovale into the left atrium. Blood from the superior vena cava, on the other hand, passes to

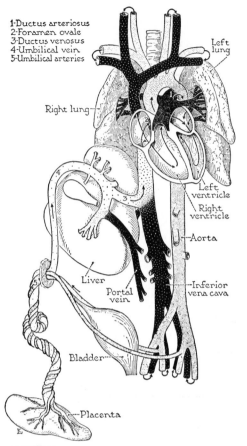

1-Ductus arteriosus
2-Foramen ovale
3-Ductus venosus
4-Umbilical vein
5-Umbilical arteries

Left lung

Right lung

Left ventricle

Right ventricle

Aorta

Liver

Portal vein

Inferior vena cava

Bladder

Placenta

Figure 65 Cardiovascular system of the fetus showing the course of blood flow from the placenta through the umbilical vein (4), ductus venosus (3) into the inferior vena cava and the right atrium, where it crosses through the foramen ovale (2) to course through the left atrium and ventricle to reach the aorta and supply the fetal head with highly oxygenated blood. Returning blood from the superior vena cava enters the right atrium and courses through the right ventricle to the pulmonary artery where it is shunted via the ductus arteriosus (1) into the descending aorta for return to the placenta by way of the umbilical arteries (5). (Courtesy of W. F. Windle.)

the pulmonary artery by way of the right atrium and ventricle. Here an extracardiac shunt through the ductus arteriosus directs most of the pulmonary arterial circulation into the descending aorta with only a small portion actually entering the pulmonary circulation.

Permanent anatomic closure of the ductus arteriosus takes place several weeks after birth. Functional closing, which requires only acute constriction of the vessel wall by fibers which are present

at birth, takes place much earlier. Irreversible closure has been accomplished by the second month after birth.

Based on studies in the sheep, more than half (55 per cent) of the combined outflow from the ventricles flows to the placenta. Of the remaining 45 per cent, only about 10 per cent perfuses the fetal lungs. When respirations begin and the lungs expand, there is a marked fall in pulmonary vascular resistance. Resistance appears to decrease as a direct result of rising oxygen tension and falling carbon dioxide tension, the effect apparently mediated directly on the blood vessels themselves. During the first few hours of life the pressure within the left atrium falls to levels that are lower than those in the normal adult. Small pressure differences between right and left atria probably result in persistence of the shunt through the foramen ovale from right to left for extended periods of time. The transition from fetal to adult circulations with closure of the foramen ovale and ductus arteriosus occurs slowly, usually during the first day of life. As the pulmonary vascular resistance declines, blood flowing through the ductus arteriosus reverses its direction so that flow occurs from left to right until such time as the ductus arteriosus closes functionally. Constriction occurs in response to increased arterial oxygen tension. The fetal pattern of circulation may be reestablished as a result of hypoxia with reopening of the ductus arteriosus in conjunction with increased pulmonary vascular resistance.

Functional closure of the ductus arteriosus is not an immediate phenomenon in normal infants. Blood may flow through it in either direction depending on whether the pulmonary or the systemic pressure is temporarily higher. Regardless of whether the ductus remains temporarily open or not, the neonatal circulation functions so effectively that there is usually uniform distribution throughout the arterial circulation of blood with oxygen saturation in excess of 92 per cent well within an hour after birth. Normal resting pulse rate in the newborn is 110 to 140 per minute. Blood volume is approximately 85 ml. per kg. body weight. Cardiac output is 500 to 600 ml. per minute. In proportion to

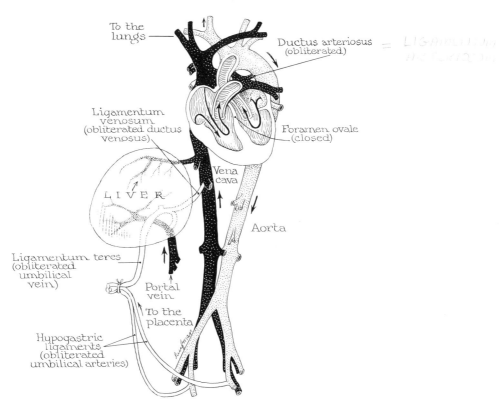

To the lungs

Ductus arteriosus (obliterated)

Ligamentum venosum (obliterated ductus venosus)

Foramen ovale (closed)

Vena cava

LIVER

Aorta

Ligamentum teres (obliterated umbilical vein)

Portal vein

To the placenta

Hypogastric ligaments (obliterated umbilical arteries)

Figure 66 Circulatory system of the newborn infant illustrating the changes which occur after ligation of the umbilical cord. The occluded remnants of the umbilical vein (ligamentum teres), ductus venosus (ligamentum venosum), foramen ovale, ductus arteriosus, and umbilical arteries (hypogastric ligaments) are illustrated. The circulatory pathways are essentially identical with that of the adult.

its body weight, fetal cardiac output is somewhat more than twice that for the normal adult. In view of the fact that this output is achieved at a pulse rate of twice the adult, the cardiac stroke volume must be roughly proportional by weight to that of the adult.

Relative to body weight, the newborn heart is rather large. Similarly, it appears to occupy a sizable portion of the thoracic shadow on x-ray examination. There is a transient increase and subsequent decrease in cardiac volume during the first hour after birth. The standard of 50 per cent thoracic diameter as an upper limit of normal cardiac diameter is probably not valid unless its absolute maximum measurement is greater than 5.7 cm. in a term infant. It is of special significance if enlargement persists or progresses.

Cardiac murmurs, other than those that indicate temporary flow through the

ductus arteriosus, are heard in approximately one to two per cent of all newborn infants. Less than one in 10 of these persists as evidence of organic heart disease, suggesting that most are merely functional. By the same token, it is recognized that murmurs of organic valvulopathy may not necessarily be heard with regularity at birth.

With onset of respirations at the time of birth, a negative intrathoracic pressure occurs. This appears to be instrumental in expanding the pulmonary capillary bed. With rapid fall in pulmonary resistance, blood is diverted into the pulmonary tree and the right atrial pressure falls. The pressure gradient thus established between the two cardiac atria results in closure of the foramen ovale. Establishment of pulmonary circulation causes increasing blood return from the pulmonary veins to further increase pressure in the left atrium, ensuring permanent functional closure of the foramen ovale. As a consequence, blood entering the aorta rapidly becomes fully saturated with oxygen.

Closure of the ductus arteriosus cannot be so readily explained. It appears to occur over the course of several hours and to be related to expansion of the pulmonary circulation and increased oxygen saturation. The mechanism by which the ductus arteriosus closes is not clarified. Assali et al. affected flow through the ductus by altering the pO_2 of the blood. With increased oxygenation, ductus flow was reduced. The effect appeared to be mediated directly on the ductus wall.

RESPIRATORY SYSTEM

Respiratory movements of the fetal diaphragm *in utero* have been observed from the second trimester to term. This coordinated muscular activity is apparently capable of moving amniotic fluid into and out of the alveoli as early as the fourteenth week of pregnancy. The possible role of this activity in the formation or clearance of amniotic fluid has already been discussed (see Chapter 5). Whether or not this pathway is significant is undecided. Nonetheless, the observations indicate that intrauterine respiratory excursions may be useful in the development of pulmonary parenchyma and circulation as well as the musculature necessary to provide appropriate ventilation during extrauterine life.

Embryologic development of the lung begins early with outpocketing of the primitive gut around the twenty-fourth day. Alveoli lined by cuboidal epithelium are recognizable by the sixteenth week. Capillary vessels are seen in the alveolar interstices shortly thereafter. The fluid within the alveoli is closely analogous in composition to that of the plasma, albeit somewhat more acidic and containing larger amounts of chloride. Reabsorption occurs quite rapidly with the onset of respirations. The mature lung contains surface-active substances, lipoprotein in nature, that appear to be essential to reduce surface tension and to aid expansion of the lung at the time of the first breath.

Dilatation of the alveoli at birth is attributable to the development of negative intrathoracic pressure which in turn permits inspiration of air. At the first breath, surface tension within the tracheobronchial tree and the alveoli offers considerable resistance to expansion. Donald showed that the newborn fetus was capable of developing a momentary intrathoracic negative pressure of the order of 40 cm. of water. This is clearly in excess of that which is required to establish normal respiration.

The thorax is compressed during its passage through the birth canal, conceivably aiding in eliminating some of the tracheobronchial fluid. Such compression is likely to be effective in helping to rid the fetus of the more viscid mucus in the upper tract. At birth, thoracic recoil combines with diaphragmatic movements to transmit a large negative pressure to the lung substance. Venous and lymphatic channels are opened and both blood and lymph flow augmented. Lung fluid within the alveoli is resorbed rapidly. The phospholipid-protein complex that constitutes *surfactant,* the essential substance that reduces surface tension significantly, comes to line the alveolar surfaces and aid in the expansion of the alveoli for gaseous exchange. Surfactant appears to be quite essential for appropriate expansion of the alveoli and commencement of respiratory function both initially at the crucial moment of separation of the fetus from its placental attachment to the mother and subsequently during neonatal life when resorption atelectases may be a serious problem leading to respiratory distress.

Under circumstances where increased lung parenchymal elasticity prevents expansion, respiratory embarrassment may result. This may be brought about as a result of immature development, hypoplasia or obstruction. The appearance of lipoprotein in the amniotic fluid, especially lecithin, is a reflection of maturation of the pulmonary system. Lecithin is the major component of the surface-active layer lining the pulmonary alveoli. As the alveoli mature and become more stable, lecithin biosynthesis occurs. Because the finding of significant amounts of lecithin in the amniotic fluid is nearly a constant occurrence in pregnancies near term, it has been used effectively as a measure of fetal maturity as well as a means for predicting whether or not the fetus is at risk for developing respiratory distress after birth (Gluck et al.; Gluck and Kulovich). This is discussed more extensively in Chapter 68, but briefly, surface activity describes a phenomenon of the normal lung by which the surface tension of the air-alveolar lining interface is lowered with expiration. If there were no surface activity, the wall tension would rise as the alveolar radius becomes smaller during expiration and the alveolus would collapse. Surface activity, therefore, ensures that the lung will not collapse and that a residual volume will be maintained during expiration. In the absence of surface activity, atelectasis will result and the characteristic respiratory distress syndrome will develop (see Chapter 68).

The first inspiration is usually followed by a cry in infants delivered of mothers who have not been heavily sedated or anesthetized. The infant expires forcibly against a partially closed glottis. This creates a high positive intrathoracic pressure to about 40 cm. of water which aids expansion further. The newborn breathes at a rate of 30 to 40 per minute at term. The tidal volume is about 20 ml. and minute volume about 600 ml.

Regulation of the respiratory pattern in the newborn infant is unclear. The infant's breathing begins so promptly after birth as to suggest that it is a reflex response to sensory stimuli of exposure. Its smoothly integrated rhythmicity verifies that central mechanisms are intact and have developed to a high degree of function during pregnancy. Under less favorable circumstances, namely those associated with anesthesia or narcosis, breathing appears to begin as a result of chemical responses that are secondary to the sudden withdrawal of maternal oxygenation via the placenta. Here it is likely that chemoreceptors are responding to low oxygen tension to stimulate the central respiratory center. Respirations produce increased ventilatory volume, rising blood oxygen tension and falling carbon dioxide.

This mechanism produces disintegrated, irregular and gasping respirations of a primitive nature. As a consequence, the respiratory pattern under these circumstances is cyclic and may persist for days or weeks after birth. Characteristically, ventilatory excursions are slow and shallow, rising crescendo fashion to a maximum and then falling again. This pattern is particularly seen in premature infants. Although they tend not to be cyanotic or dyspneic, and their arterial blood is well saturated with oxygen, increasing the oxygen in their inspired air will usually result in a change from periodic to regular respiration.

THE HEMATOPOIETIC SYSTEM

Hematopoietic centers which contain formed blood elements are encountered in the early yolk sac. As embryogenesis progresses, blood formation sites appear in various areas, including those destined to become the splenic, renal and hepatic systems. Ultimately, of course, this function comes to be the exclusive province of the bone marrow. The yolk sac persists in its hematopoietic function from about day 14 to two and one-half months of gestational age. The liver in turn takes on its major role in this regard from about six weeks to the end of pregnancy. Its peak function in red cell formation occurs about the third month. Beyond the fourth month, the bone marrow becomes increasingly prominent as the primary site for the production of formed blood elements (Brown).

The red cells formed in the yolk sac are largely megaloblasts; those formed in the liver include megaloblasts as well as megalocytes and macrocytes; normocytes begin to appear when the bone marrow assumes its function in hematopoiesis. Thus, early red cells are all nucleated. As pregnancy progresses, the relative incidence of nucleated erythrocytes falls until comparatively few are seen at term (about 5 to 10 nucleated red cells per 100 white cells). Characteristically at birth, the newborn infant's blood demonstrates both erthyrocytosis and macrocytosis. The red cell count is higher than that in the adult, with values up to 6 million per cubic millimeter recorded commonly. At the same time, the hematocrit at term may be in the 60 per cent range. All blood values rapidly return to normal within the first few weeks of extrauterine life.

The life span of the megaloblasts formed in the yolk sac is quite short (Kleihauer et al.), averaging eight weeks as compared with 120 days in the adult. Even at term the life span of the red cell is shorter than in the adult (Pearson). It is undoubtedly the combination of foreshortened survival time and diminished marrow production that results in the rapid return of the neonatal blood picture to the adult pattern. Although hemolysis is postulated and supported by the common occurrence of neonatal hyperbilirubinemia and jaundice, it is likely that these latter findings arise more from the diminished capability of the liver to clear the bloodstream of the breakdown products of hemoglobin degeneration. The polycythemic state of the fetus at term and of the newborn has been explained as a response to a chronic state of relative intrauterine hypoxia (Barcroft). It is analogous to the response seen during acclimatization to low oxygen pressures at high altitudes.

The hemoglobin that is synthesized in the various hematopoietic sites during the course of pregnancy tends to vary somewhat. In the mesoblastic period, the yolk sac sites produce mostly primitive embryonic hemoglobin of the Gower varieties (containing four or two epsilon-peptide chains per molecule of globin). The yolk sac is also capable of elaborating the so-called fetal hemoglobin with alpha and gamma chains. All other sites in the developing fetus synthesize both fetal (F) and adult (A) hemoglobins, the latter in increasing relative amounts. Adult hemoglobin, in contrast to the other forms, contains two alpha-peptide chains and either two beta chains (hemoglobin A_1) or two delta chains (hemoglobin A_2). Hemoglobin A_2 makes its appearance in the term fetus and increases in relative concentration during extrauterine life.

There is a substantive difference in oxygen affinity of the fetal red blood cells which contain hemoglobin F and those containing mostly hemoglobin A. Oxygen dissociation curves characteristically demonstrate that at a given oxygen tension and blood pH, erythrocytes containing hemoglobin F are capable of binding substantially more oxygen than those containing

hemoglobin A (Fig. 67). This concept has been seriously challenged recently (Kirschbaum et al.). It has been shown (Allen et al.) that solutions of human fetal and adult hemoglobins have identical oxygen dissociation curves. If there are differences, they may exist in other features of fetal blood corpuscles, such as carbonic anhydrase activity (Nechtman and Huisman), rather than in special properties of the hemoglobin molecule (Dawes). At term the ratio of fetal to adult hemoglobin is usually 3:1. Moreover, erythrocytes at birth are about 20 per cent larger than in the adult and contain correspondingly more hemoglobin.

During the first two weeks of extrauterine life, a small decrease in red cell count occurs in association with a rather marked decline in the hemoglobin concentration and hematocrit, the latter falling to 45 per cent by the tenth day. The marrow stops forming macrocytes and begins

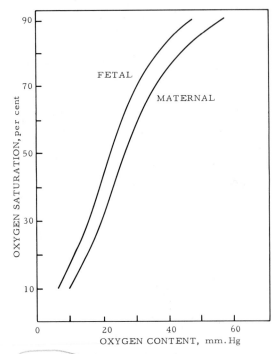

Figure 67 Oxygen dissociation curves of blood obtained from infants at birth as compared with pregnant and nonpregnant women, indicating the shift of the adult maternal curve to the right and the infant curve to the left. The apparently greater affinity of fetal blood to become saturated with oxygen at relatively lower oxygen tensions than maternal blood favors oxygen transport across the placenta to the fetus. (From Darling, R. C., et al.: J. Clin. Invest. 20:739, 1941.)

to elaborate smaller cells containing less hemoglobin at a much slower rate. This process continues throughout the first year. It is probable that there is little if any active or increased destruction of red cells, but rather a sharp reduction in erythropoiesis. There appears to be no change in the fragility of red cells, nor any lowering of osmotic or mechanical resistance during this interval.

Substantial polymorphonuclear leucocytosis may occur with white cell counts as high as 45,000 per cubic millimeter at birth, although most often they range around 20,000. Lower white counts are generally encountered in premature infants. In general, the leucocytosis rapidly disappears. Alternatively or simultaneously, there may be a progressive increase in the relative numbers of lymphocytes so that, at seven days of age, the white count may be halved and the picture be one of a lymphocytosis. Both the relative and absolute numbers of monocytes may increase. Relevance of this occurrence to immunologic response to bacterial invasion is discussed below.

Hemoglobin F differs in several significant ways from adult hemoglobin. It has a useful characteristic in that it is quite resistant to denaturation by alkaline agents. This serves as the basis for identifying it and estimating its concentration in blood. There is a clear-cut correlation between the relative contents of fetal and adult hemoglobin in fetal blood with advancing gestational age. There is a three to four per cent decrease in hemoglobin F during gestation. This rate of decline persists after birth as well. The synthesis of hemoglobin F appears to be favored over the production of adult hemoglobin under the stimulus of low oxygen tensions and low glucose concentrations (Allen and Jandl).

GASTROINTESTINAL SYSTEM

The well-developed swallowing function that the fetus is capable of expressing from relatively early in its embryonic life has already been discussed in reference to the fate of the amniotic fluid (see Chapter 5). By the fourth month of intrauterine life, the gastrointestinal system is sufficiently well developed to permit the fetus to swallow amniotic fluid in large amounts as indicated by radiopaque material injected into the amniotic sac (Davis and Potter). This material is propelled along the bowel so that visualization of the entire tract is possible by x-ray. Moreover, absorption occurs from the gastric and intestinal mucosa.

Confirmatory evidence of intrauterine swallowing consists of the findings of lanugo, desquamated epithelial cells and vernix caseosa in the initial fecal content passed after birth, the *meconium*. The dark green color of the meconium is due to its content of bilirubin breakdown products. Meconium may be passed *per anum* by the fetus under certain conditions. Although characteristically the result of intense hypoxia with coassociated peristaltic bowel hyperactivity and relaxation of the anal sphincter, meconium staining of the amniotic fluid may also be seen in other circumstances as well. For example, intrauterine forces are such as to favor evacuation of the fetal bowel during labor in breech presentations. Likewise, some pharmacologic agents capable of stimulating peristaltic rushes in the adult are sometimes equally effective when absorbed by the fetus via the placenta.

Quantitatively, the fetus swallows approximately 450 ml. of amniotic fluid daily (Pritchard). Although this amount is negligible insofar as the turnover of amniotic fluid is concerned (see Chapter 5), it is approximately equal to the amount which the newborn infant will ingest under normal circumstances by either breast or bottle feeding. Whether or not the act of swallowing is essential for the morphologic maturation of the gastrointestinal tract and the development of its ultimate role in providing for neonatal nutrition cannot be determined definitively. Neither consideration seems likely in view of the fact that fetuses that are unable to swallow actively because of neurologic or developmental disorders or whose gastrointestinal tract is obstructed by anatomic anomalies tend to have otherwise well-developed and apparently normally functional gastrointestinal systems.

As indicated earlier, liver function, particularly as regards its hematopoietic role, is apparent by the fourth month of intrauterine life. Carbohydrate metabolism can be demonstrated in the fetus by the sixteenth week. Glycogen stores in the liver are relatively small in midpregnancy. At term, glycogen concentrations increase markedly so that levels in excess of those in the adult liver are seen at birth. The stores are rapidly consumed following delivery. Other substances, including fats and fat-soluble vitamins A and D, are also stored in the liver during late pregnancy.

The immaturity of liver function during gestation and in the neonatal period is evident in the relative inability of the liver to clear blood breakdown products from the circulation. The placenta (and maternal liver) performs this function almost exclusively during pregnancy. Nevertheless, a small amount of bilirubin is conjugated by the fetal liver and finds its way into the intestinal tract via the biliary tree where it is oxidized to biliverdin. It is this pigmented breakdown product that is responsible for the green discoloration of the meconium. The rapid clearance of unconjugated bilirubin by the placenta is well established. Under conditions of rapid blood hemolysis, this mechanism may not be ample. The resultant hyperbilirubinemia may be further reflected in high levels of this substance and its related breakdown pigments in the amniotic fluid. Such a condition is erythroblastosis fetalis, and the appearance of bilirubin and related pigment in the amniotic fluid has been used effectively for its detection and evaluation (see Chapter 52).

This aspect of immaturity of enzymatic function within the liver results from a deficiency of the enzyme glucuronyl transferase which persists into the neonatal period for a variable interval. It is particularly poorly developed in premature infants, resulting in an almost total inability of the fetus to conjugate bilirubin and thereby effect clearance of hemoglobin breakdown products via the liver. Concurrent deficiencies in essential transport proteins that are believed responsible for intracellular transport of bilirubin by way of hepatic cells to the bile canaliculi for excretion into the bowel are probably also present under these circumstances. The so-called physiologic jaundice of the new-

born is undoubtedly the result of such deficiencies of liver function. Glucuronyl transferase activity can be increased pharmacologically by enzyme induction agents, including phenobarbital and alcohol. The potential usefulness of this mechanism in therapeusis has not as yet been fully explored.

RENAL SYSTEM

The glomerular nephrons develop within the renal cortex from about the eighth week of fetal life, increasing steadily throughout pregnancy in number and maturity. The numbers increase from 350,000 at 20 weeks to 820,000 at term (Osathanondh and Potter).

The fetal kidney is functional by the third month of intrauterine life as evidenced by the presence of urine in the fetal bladder. The contribution of fetal urine to the make-up of amniotic fluid has been discussed earlier (see Chapter 5). The urine produced by the fetal kidneys is quite hypotonic. Its electrolyte content is small as might be expected in view of the fact that the placenta performs the major excretory function for the fetus. The newborn bladder may contain up to 44 ml. of urine (Tausch). Urine production in newborn premature infants has been reported to average 0.05 to 0.09 ml. per minute (Vernier and Smith). A diuretic response to water loading is not encountered in newborn infants under three days of age; beyond five or six days of age, full term and premature infants respond almost exactly like adults to water loading. A similar lack of immediate responsiveness to antidiuretic hormone has also been observed in the first week of extrauterine life.

Studies by Assali et al. in sheep have shown that the blood supply to the fetal kidneys is relatively small, based on rather high vascular resistance within the renal arterial system. Although the data are not necessarily comparable with the human, Alexander et al. found plasma clearances in fetal sheep to be essentially the same for urea, fructose and creatinine, decreasing from 2.4 ml. per min. per kg. body weight in early pregnancy to 0.4 at term. These data and the results of other comparable studies have demonstrated that renal clearances in the fetus are very low when compared with the adult.

The renal circulatory pattern described by Assali et al. may be explained by the relatively low vascular resistance within the placenta which preferentially receives in excess of 65 per cent of the fetal cardiac output. By contrast, the kidneys operate at a high vascular resistance and resultant reduced flow. When the cord is ligated, redistribution of flow occurs with appropriate increase in renal blood flow during the neonatal period. However, renal circulation and glomerular filtration remain below adult levels.

RETICULOENDOTHELIAL SYSTEM

Evidence of the beginning development of immunologic function in the human fetus is seen by the eighth week of intrauterine life with the appearance of lymphocytes in and around the epithelium of the third and fourth branchial arches. This is the anlage for the future thymus. The numbers of lymphocytes increase rapidly during fetal life in the peripheral blood as well as in widely scattered lymphoid follicles, reaching maximum absolute numbers at birth (Smith). Splenic development lags somewhat behind. At birth, the spleen consists mostly of red pulp. Primary follicles containing lymphoid cells appear subsequently and by the second month of neonatal life they are increasing rapidly in number and size. Infectious diseases in early extrauterine life accelerate their development.

There is considerable evidence that the fetus is capable of elaborating immunologic substances. It was once believed that the fetus is not competent to do so; this tenet is incorrect. Humoral antibodies are produced by the lymphoid cells in the form of immunoglobulin molecules consisting of symmetric pairs of polypeptide units. These exist as a single molecule in gamma-G or as linked polymers in gamma-A and gamma-M immunoglobulins. The gamma-G varieties are the most prevalent in the adult circulation. They are found in very small amounts during late fetal life, being synthesized in large amounts after the second month of extrauterine life.

Most of the gamma-G globulin in the fetus is derived from the mother by way of the placenta.

Studies in sheep and monkeys have revealed a pattern of stepwise appearance of immunologic competence to a spectrum of antigens from early embryonic life. Intrauterine infections of the human fetus have verified the existence of comparable potential response to infections such as syphilis, toxoplasmosis and cytomegalovirus. These result in the development of germinal centers, plasmacytosis, secondary follicle formation and synthesis of gamma-M antibody. Similarly, gamma-M immunoglobulin has appeared following cytomegalovirus infections. Antibody response function thus appears to exist in the human fetus as early as the fifth month of gestation.

Maternal gamma-G globulins readily cross the placenta from the third month of gestation to term. The heavy chains of gamma-M and gamma-A immunoglobulins prevent their transfer in measurable amounts. Gamma-A globulins first appear in the serum during the second month of life, but are present in secretions shortly after birth. The gamma-A varieties are the chief secretory immunoglobulins present on the surfaces of the gastrointestinal and respiratory tracts, appearing in salivary, pancreatic and genitourinary secretions. These immunoglobulins appear to be synthesized early and rapidly. Gamma-G production falls swiftly after birth to low levels between six weeks and three months of age. Gamma-M levels rise rapidly during early neonatal life in response to interaction with the bacterial flora of the intestinal tract.

The role of the immunoglobulins in combating neonatal sepsis is undoubtedly very important. This probably applies most pertinently to the gamma-M immunoglobulins which are nearly 1000 times more effective in destroying enteric bacteria than the gamma-G variety. The vulnerability of the newborn to such infections is great since it is protected only by gamma-G immunoglobulins of maternal origin. In addition, protection is offered by the surface immunoglobulins of the gamma-A class. Some newborn infants may not be fully equipped to withstand bacterial challenges and will acquire sepsis.

The passive protection afforded by the mother's gamma-G immunoglobulins which have been transferred across the placenta may be effective to a limited degree. Among these are antibodies against diphtheria and tetanus, as well as antiviral globulins against measles, smallpox, vaccinia, poliomyelitis, Coxsackie virus and herpes simplex. It is generally agreed that, if the maternal antibody concentrations are high, the infant will probably be protected against the specific disease entity for an interval of six months or longer. Shorter lived or quantitatively reduced resistance is expected for circulating antibodies against strains of pneumococci, influenza bacilli, streptococci, staphylococci, and the H antigens of typhoid bacillus. Some antibacterial resistance to dysentery bacilli may occur in the newborn infant, but essentially none exists against *Escherichia*

coli as compared to the usual level of maternal resistance. Transmission of antibodies against pertussis can be demonstrated, but the level of protection afforded is usually small.

Antibodies appear in the maternal colostrum. Although no passive immunity can be expected from absorption of this ingested material by way of the intestinal tract of the newborn infant, it is possible that the gamma-A immunoglobulin present in the colostrum may aid in protecting the infant against enterobacilli by its unique efficiency to function on surfaces. Rh isoimmunization, resulting in erythroblastosis fetalis, is an example of the potentially harmful effects of gamma-G immunoglobulin crossing the placenta from the mother to the fetus, where it causes destruction of the fetal erythrocytes (see Chapter 52).

REFERENCES

Alexander, D. P., Nixon, D. A., Widdas, W. F., and Wohlzogen, F. X. Renal function in the sheep foetus. J. Physiol. *140*:14, 1958.

Allen, D. W., and Jandl, J. H.: Factors influencing relative rates of synthesis of adult and fetal hemoglobin in vitro. J. Clin. Invest. *39*:1107, 1960.

Allen, D. W., Wyman, J., and Smith, C. A.: The oxygen equilibrium of fetal and adult human hemoglobin. J. Biol. Chem. *203*:81, 1953.

Assali, N. S., Bekey, G. A., and Morrison, L. W.: Fetal and neonatal circulation. In Assali, N. S., ed.: Biology of Gestation, Vol. 2. New York, Academic Press, 1968.

Barcroft, J.: Researches on Prenatal Life. Springfield, Ill., Charles C Thomas, 1948.

Brown, A. K.: Bilirubin metabolism in the developing liver. In Assali, N. S., ed.: Biology of Gestation, Vol. 2. New York, Academic Press, 1968.

Darling, R. C., Smith, C. A., Asmussen, E., and Cohen, F. M.: Some properties of human fetal and maternal blood. J. Clin. Invest. *20*:739, 1941.

Davis, M. E., and Potter, E. L.: Intrauterine respirations of the human fetus. J.A.M.A. *131*:1194, 1946.

Dawes, G. S.: Foetal and Neonatal Physiology: A Comparative Study of the Changes at Birth. Chicago, Year Book Medical Publishers, Inc., 1968.

Donald, I.: Atelectasis neonatorum. J. Obstet. Gynaec. Brit. Emp. *61*:725, 1954.

Gluck, L., and Kulovich, M. V.: Measuring the functional maturation of the fetus with the lecithin-sphingomyelin ratio. In Greenhill, J. P., ed.: The Year Book of Obstetrics and Gynecology. Chicago, Year Book Medical Publishers, Inc., 1972.

Gluck, L., Kulovich, M. V., Borer, R. C., Jr., Brenner, P. H., Anderson, G. G., and Spellacy, W. N.: Diagnosis of the respiratory distress syndrome by amniocentesis. Amer. J. Obstet. Gynec. *109*:440, 1971.

Kirschbaum, T. H., DeHaven, J. C., Shapiro, N., and

Assali, N. S.: Oxyhemoglobin dissociation characteristics of human and sheep maternal and fetal blood. Amer. J. Obstet. Gynec. *96*:741, 1966.

Kleihauer, E., Tang, D., and Betke, K.: Die intrazelluläre Verteilung von embryonalem Hämoglobin in roten Blutzellen menschlicher Embryonen: Ein Beitrag zur Ontogenese menschlicher Hämoglobine. Acta Haemat. *38*:264, 1967.

Lind, J., and Wegelius, C.: Angiocardiographic studies on the human foetal circulation: Preliminary report. Pediatrics *4*:391, 1949.

Lind, J., and Wegelius, C.: Human fetal circulation: Changes in the cardiovascular system at birth and disturbances in the post-natal closure of the foramen ovale and ductus arteriosus. Cold Spring Harbor Symp. Quant. Biol. *19*:109, 1954.

Nechtman, C. M., and Huisman, T. H. J.: Comparative studies of oxygen equilibria of human adult and cord blood red cell hemolysates and suspensions. Clin. Chim. Acta *10*:165, 1964.

Osathanondh, V., and Potter, E. L.: Development of human kidney as shown by microdissection: IV. Development of tubular portions of nephrons. Arch. Path. *82*:391, 1966.

Pearson, H. A.: Recent advances in hematology. J. Pediat. *69*:466, 1966.

Pritchard, J. A.: Deglutition by normal and anencephalic fetuses. Obstet. Gynec. *25*:289, 1965.

Rudolph, A. M., and Heymann, M. A.: The fetal circulation. Ann. Rev. Med. *19*:195, 1968.

Smith, R. T.: Fetal and neonatal immunological function. In Assali, N. S., ed.: Biology of Gestation, Vol. 2. New York, Academic Press, 1968.

Tausch, M.: Der Fetalharn. Arch. Gynäk. *162*:217, 1936.

Vernier, R. L., and Smith, F. G., Jr.: Fetal and neonatal kidney. In Assali, N. S., ed.: Biology of Gestation, Vol. 2. New York, Academic Press, 1968.

Chapter 7

Effects of Pregnancy on the Maternal Organism

THE UTERUS

Pronounced alterations occur in the uterus during pregnancy. The normal uterus of a nulligravida is a pear-shaped organ 7 to 9 cm. long, 4 cm. thick and 6 cm. wide, weighing 40 to 60 gm. In a multipara the uterus is 8 to 10 cm. long, 5 to 6 cm. thick and 6 to 7 cm. wide, weighing 50 to 80 gm. It consists largely of unstriated muscle, covered in part by the peritoneum, moored to the pelvis by eight ligaments, and attached to the pelvic floor through the vagina.

The wall of the uterus, about 8 mm. average in thickness before pregnancy, grows to about 25 mm. by the fourth month. After this the decidua capsularis lies on and fuses with the decidua vera. By the end of pregnancy the uterine wall has decreased to 4 to 10 mm. in thickness. The uterus at full term weighs about 675 gm. (1.5 lbs.) (Fig. 68). The muscular fibers of the nongravid uterus are spindle shaped, about 50μ long. Those of the full-term gravid uterus are much larger (200 to 600μ) and present fine longitudinal fibrillations (Figs. 69 and 70).

The fibroelastic tissue of the uterus is of great importance in view of the functions of the organ and its accommodation to distention during gestation. The corpus has much less elastic tissue than the cervix. Elastic fibers are most numerous in the outer layers of the uterus and around the vessels.

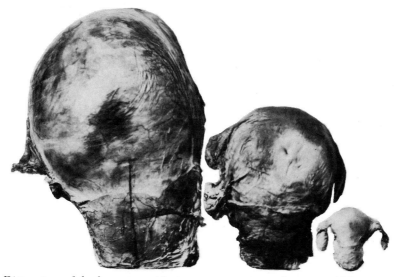

Figure 68 Dimensions of the human gravid uterus at term prior to the onset of labor (left), relative to that of the uterus immediately following delivery (center) and in the nonpregnant state (right). (One-fifth natural size.) (From Knaus, H. H.: Geburtsh. u. Gynäk. *129*:122, 1948.)

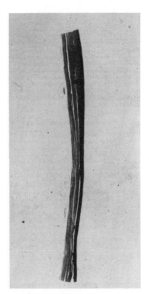

Figure 69　Cross section of the uterine wall just prior to the onset of labor showing how markedly thinned and stretched it is. (Natural size.) (From Knaus, H. H.: Geburtsh. u. Gynäk. *129*:122, 1948.)

The arrangement of the muscular fibers is rather complex. There is an intertwining of muscular elements from frankly circular fibers in the lowest part of the uterus, to obliquely spiral fibers over the fundus to frankly longitudinal outer fibers. The latter find their principal origin in the longitudinal musculature of the tubes and continue downward over the entire length of the corpus. The uterine tubes and the ligaments, that is, the round, ovarian and uterosacral ligaments, provide the chief foci for attachment of the radiating and obliquely spiral fibers. The fibrous tissues of the cervix provide the primary insertion for the longitudinal fibers. Thus, the upper half of the uterus and the fundus contain a preponderance of muscular elements; their origin is mainly in the uterine tubes. Goerttler points out that in the entire body there is no other organ in which such complete harmony exists between morphologic and functional activities. A comparable organ is perhaps the heart.

The uterine musculature follows a distinct plan during pregnancy. The peculiar structure is based on the "spiral course" of the muscular fibers and is directed in the uterine wall from outward toward the inside of the uterus. The action of these muscles is the same on both sides of the uterus. The muscles cross each other (Fig. 71). The function of the uterus, particularly during pregnancy and labor, is based on this peculiar anatomic arrangement. Although it is not altered during gestation, characteristic shiftings of the muscle fibers take place and are easily demonstrable anatomically. The result of these changes is to allow an ever-increasing space to develop inside the uterine cavity (Fig. 72) to accommodate the growing conceptus.

Normally, the cervix possesses a much smaller complement of muscle fibers than the corpus uteri, its bulk being composed largely of fibrous connective tissues. Nevertheless, those muscle fibers present in the cervix are arranged in a relatively simpler pattern than those of the corpus. At the isthmus the circular layers are prominent, especially at the insertion of the retractor fibers in the rear, that is, at the site of insertion of the uterosacral ligaments. The plicae palmatae are made up of longitudinal fibers. Externally, the cervix shows a layer of longitudinal and oblique fibers which spread out into the bladder through the vesicouterine ligaments and into the bases of the broad ligaments. The

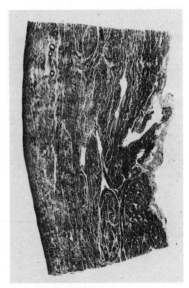

Figure 70　Section of comparable area in the uterine wall as shown in Figure 69, but obtained immediately following delivery. (Natural size.) (From Knaus, H. H.: Geburtsh. u. Gynäk. *129*:122, 1948.)

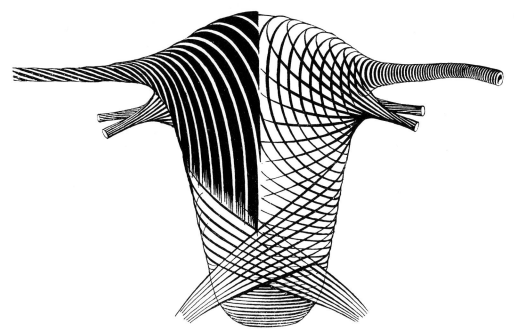

Figure 71 Highly schematized representation of the complex interlacing of the myometrial fibers, showing external longitudinal bands and internal circular arrangement. (From Bumm, E.: Grundriss zum Studium der Geburtshülfe, ed. 13. Wiesbaden, J. F. Bergmann, 1921.)

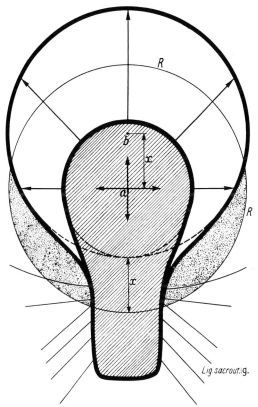

Figure 72 Diagrammatic presentation of the progressive changes in uterine shape in the course of normal pregnancy. The nongravid uterus is shown in the cross-hatched area. The conceptus begins its growth at the midpoint (*a*) of the corpus uteri, expanding radially in the direction of the arrows. The uterus should be expected to grow in response to this circumferential growth by expanding concentrically to the circle *R*; instead, growth of the uterus progresses cranially as the isthmus stretches upward. The center of the ovum comes to lie at point *b*, seemingly having moved from point *a* by the distance *x*. The gravid uterus, shown heavily outlined, has grown in all dimensions to accommodate the enlarging conceptus, having been "unfolded" and displaced upward. (From Goerttler: Morphol. Jahrbuch 65:45, 1930.)

portio vaginalis presents an inner submucous and circular layer, an outer longitudinal layer (both derived from the vagina) and a middle, vascular and inconspicuous layer derived from the similar layer of the corpus which is intermingled with the ligaments entering the cervix.

The cervix, even in a newborn baby, shows a tendency to form two lips, an anterior and a posterior. The fibromuscular bulk of tissue at the sides of the cervix is thinner. The uterus of a woman who has never conceived may sometimes appear to have bilateral lacerations. During pregnancy shallow lateral grooves are palpable. During labor tears usually occur at these sites of functional and anatomic weakness.

Blood Supply of the Uterus

The blood vessels undergo hypertrophy and probably hyperplasia during pregnancy. The arterial supply of the uterus is derived mainly from three paired trunks: (1) the uterine artery, a branch of the hypogastric, (2) the ovarian artery, a branch of the aorta, and (3) the funicular artery, a branch of the vesical which passes up the round ligament and joins the ovarian artery at the fundus. The tortuous uterine artery approaches the uterus from the lateral aspect at the level of the cervix. It extends several large branches which go down to the vagina. The main trunk ascends in the broad ligament close to the side of the uterus. At the level of the internal os it gives off numerous branches which cross into and through the substance of the uterus. These branches anastomose with the branches of the other side. The main trunk extends branches over its entire pathway alongside the uterus and anastomoses with the ovarian artery. The ovarian artery enters the broad ligament within the infundibulopelvic ligament, sends branches to the uterine tube and a main supply to the ovary, continuing to the lateral aspect of the uterine cornu. Here it joins the ascending branch of the uterine artery. All uterine vessels are extensively convoluted and anastomose frequently.

The veins in general follow the same course as the arteries. They penetrate all the layers of the uterus, especially the middle, anastomose freely and empty into the plexuses at the sides of the uterus in the broad ligaments. The ovarian veins empty into the renal vein on the left or the vena cava on the right. The veins of the broad ligaments empty into the hypogastric vein and then into the common iliac. The uterine veins have no valves.

Microscopically, both arteries and veins in the uterine wall are different from vessels elsewhere in the body. They lose their outer coats and lie on the muscular bundles, with only an intima or at most with some tunica media. These form large blood spaces called sinuses.

From comparative measurements of the diameter of the ovarian vascular pedicle in nonpregnant and pregnant women, Hodgkinson estimated that the capacity of these veins is increased more than 60 times by the thirty-sixth week of pregnancy. The ability of the veins to dilate is an important, unique function of the ovarian and pelvic veins. Anatomically, these veins are particularly suited for such a function because they lack supportive fascial sheaths, such as are found in the veins of the legs and arms. It appears likely that changes in systemic venous pressure are neutralized through this function. The pampiniform plexuses of the broad ligaments possibly weaken the potentially deleterious influences of sudden high central pressure, such as occur from acute straining efforts. They may also minimize the effects of local vascular occlusion.

Microscopic study suggests that hypertrophy of the smooth muscle fibers within the vessel walls takes place. This permits an active physiologic effort on the part of the vein wall to compensate for the increased workload imposed by pregnancy. The magnitude of the alterations in workload for the ovarian veins is unparalleled in human vein physiology. It appears likely that blood flow in the pelvic venous system is great. The term "blood depot" is considered anatomically descriptive of the quantitatively large volume of blood required to fill the pelvic system of veins. Physiologically, however, the term is ill chosen, as it implies stagnation of blood. For the same reason the descriptive anatomic simile "arteriovenous fistula" is not considered to describe adequately the physiologic activity of the placenta. Despite this, all evidence supports the contention that the placenta functions as a most efficient organ for the exchange of substances and for metabolism.

Measurements of uterine blood flow, oxygen consumption and uterine vascular resistance in normal pregnancy and in the prepartum and postpartum periods were made by Assali et al. During the last month of pregnancy the uterine blood flow averages 15 ml. per 100 gm. of uterine weight per minute and falls to 9 ml. within the first 24 hours after delivery; oxygen consumption averages 1.9 ml. per 100 gm. per minute and falls to 1 ml. per 100 gm. per minute; vascular resistance averages 6 mm. and rises to 9 mm. of Hg per 100 gm. per minute in the postpartum period. The gravid uterus extracts much more oxygen per unit of blood flow than does the brain. The fetus is probably directly responsible for this large oxygen consumption. In addition, the placenta also consumes significant amounts of oxygen as an actively metabolizing organ (Friedman and Sachtleben), perhaps at times even in competition with the fetus.

Lymph Vessels of the Uterus

These enlarge and multiply during pregnancy, so that the full-term organ is honeycombed by them. They begin as large spaces under the endometrium and the serosa, following the course of the muscular bundles and blood vessels. They anastomose freely under the serosa, and empty into the collecting afferent trunks of the broad ligaments. The lymph vessels of the corpus and the isthmus drain primarily by way of the subovarian lymphatic plexus in the broad ligament and thence via the large afferent channels in the infundibulopelvic ligament along the psoas muscle retroperitoneally to terminate in nodes located in juxtaposition to the aorta and the inferior vena cava at the level of the renal vascular pedicles or the lower pole of the kidneys.

Those of the cervix drain into the interiliac and common iliac lymph nodes. Lymphatics of the round ligaments empty into the upper set of deep femoral glands. Those of the lowermost part of the vagina and of the vulva reach the deep and superficial femoral glands, and through these to the glands around the external iliac arteries (Plentl and Friedman). The lymphatic system plays an important role in puerperal infection.

Nerve Supply of the Uterus

The uterus is innervated by both the sympathetic and the cerebrospinal systems. Motor fibers are derived from the sympathetic system passing down from the aortic plexus. They are reinforced by fibers from the solar, renal and genital ganglia. A large plexus of sympathetic motor fibers is formed above the promontory of the sacrum near the bifurcation of the aorta; it is called the *hypogastric plexus* (Fig. 73). From here the fibers pass on either side of the rectum through the hypogastric nerves to the sides of the uterus. Cerebrospinal fibers arising from the pneumogastric, phrenic and splanchnic nerves follow the same course. The uterus is also innervated from the lumbosacral autonomic system via the pelvic nerves (second, third and fourth sacrals) to the uterovaginal plexus.

Sensory fibers arise from the spinal cord through the sacral nerves. They are also distributed via the great cervical or *Frankenhäuser ganglion* which is a triangular mass of ganglionic cells and nerve fibers lying behind and at the side of the cervix and upper part of the vagina. Because the sensory fibers arise from the spinal cord in this way, labor is painless in paraplegic women. Uterine pain is obtunded after anesthetizing them by intrathecal injection. Sensory receptors have not been identified within the uterus except in the cervix, where various Paccinian-type structures have been found.

It is well established that the completely denervated uterus, both *in vivo* and *in vitro*, can respond in a perfectly normal manner, exhibiting rhythmic contractility and even the evolution of labor progression. This is seen, for example, in paraplegic women after transverse section of the spinal cord or in women who have had

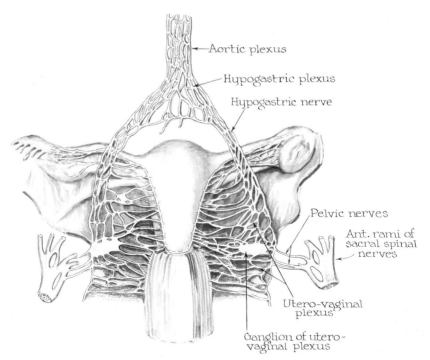

Figure 73 Innervation of the pelvic organs showing the formation of the large presacral hypogastric plexus and the distribution of nerves in the broad ligament. (From Dahl, W.: Z. Geburtsh. Gynäk. 78:539, 1916.)

presacral neurectomy (removal of the superior hypogastric plexus) for dysmenorrhea. These observations raise questions concerning the interrelationships between nervous and hormonal influences on uterine activity (See Chapter 15).

Joseph summarized current concepts of uterine innervation: (1) There is an efferent nerve supply of the uterus which influences muscle, blood vessels and endometrium, including glands (the last is dubious because nerves to the glands have not been demonstrated). (2) There is an afferent nerve supply of the uterus. (3) Anatomic studies show that different parts of the uterus have different nerve supplies. (4) It is misleading to draw conclusions about the nervous system of the human uterus and its functions from animal experiments. There are considerable differences between the reactions of different animal species to the same experiment. Moreover, within species, reactions are not necessarily the same in pregnancy as in the nonpregnant state. Nixon emphasizes that the cervix uteri in early pregnancy has a contractility independent of the corpus.

Changes in Uterine Size and Shape

The uterus grows extensively during pregnancy, accommodating its capacity to the needs of the growing conceptus. There is a limit to its growth. This growth is related to the degree and the shape of the enlarging conceptus. There comes a time in normal pregnancy when the size of the fetus becomes too large for its environment. During the initial period of uterine enlargement the conceptus is spheroidal. During the subsequent period of uterine stretching it becomes elongated and cylindrical in shape. The uterus behaves physically just like a hollow, elastic membrane. Attention centers on the nature of the process of conversion from a spheroid to a cylinder. In the rabbit this takes place over a period of a few hours. Thus, the uterus is at first subjected to increasing tension until a critical condition develops. Then suddenly, by changing shape, the resistance to the continued growth of the conceptus, imposed on it by the spheroidal membrane which surrounds it on all sides, is reduced. The conceptus is then restricted in the cylindric form by the confining action of the tissues of the uterus along its length.

The growth of the conceptus during the early period of greatest uterine growth is subjected to increasing tension all around, whereas during rapid fetal growth and uterine stretching the resistance is reduced to a minimum. This conversion of the uterus from one shape to another at a given time marks a physiologic change of some moment in uterine accommodation (Reynolds). The duration of uterine stretching depends on and is proportional to the rapid growth of the fetus. Gillespie studied uterine enlargement in gravid women by x-ray and weighed their emptied uteri at various stages of gestation. From a review of necropsy studies he found that the uterus at the onset of pregnancy is pear shaped and that by the middle of the pregnancy it assumes a spherical outline. Beyond the twentieth week it begins to elongate rapidly and becomes cylindroid for the last 20 weeks of pregnancy. The rate of elongation decreases somewhat at the thirty-second week; at this time there is some increase in the anteroposterior measurements.

During the elongation the maximal transverse measurement of the fundus also increases and continues to increase until term. This increase is most rapid up to the last month of pregnancy, when the rate of growth decreases somewhat.

For the first 20 weeks of pregnancy, there is a rapid increase in uterine weight (Fig. 74). This is taken as presumptive evidence of actual myometrial growth, as opposed to mere stretching. As evidence of this is the observation that myometrial thickness is maintained during this time. During the last 20 weeks the uterus (exclusive of its contents) ceases to increase in weight and the myometrium becomes progressively thinner (Fig. 75). Concomitantly, fetal weight gain is rapidly accelerated after the twentieth week.

At term, uteri are of various shapes — ovoid, elliptic, cordate and asymmetric. Developmental anomalies are occasionally encountered, based on incomplete fusion or development of the muellerian ducts during embryogenesis.

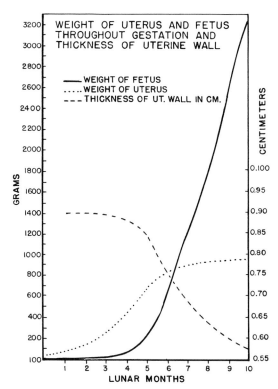

Figure 74 Fetal weight as related to weight and thickness of the uterus during the course of pregnancy. Uterine mass reaches a plateau at about 20 weeks of pregnancy at a time when the uterine wall is becoming progressively thinner and the fetal weight is increasing rapidly. (From Gillespie, E. C.: Amer. J. Obstet. Gynec. 59:949, 1950.)

The fundus may present a shallow groove (Fig. 76), an *arcuate uterus*. Sometimes one horn is developed more than the other (Fig. 77).

Changes in Uterine Consistency and Position

Soon after implantation of the ovum the shape of the uterus begins to change. Usually, the part of the uterus that contains the ovum is thicker and softer and a groove is sometimes encountered there between this portion and the rest of the corpus. Knaus demonstrated that the portion of the uterine wall which lies immediately against the ovum is subject to the influence of a double growth stimulus and actu-

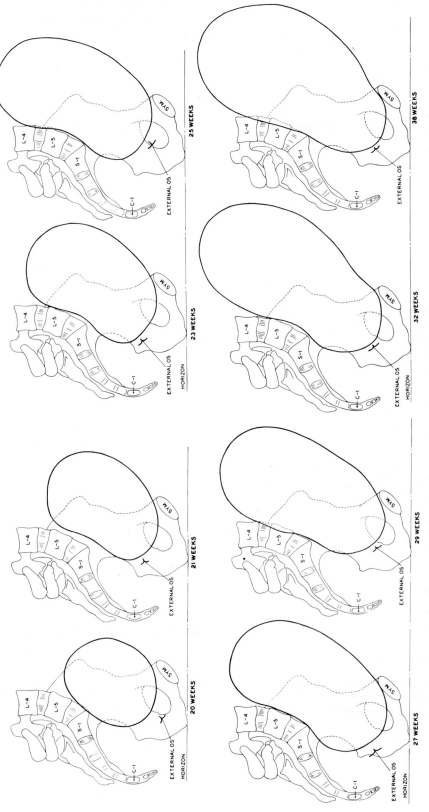

Figure 75   Sequential enlargement of the gravid uterus from the twentieth week of pregnancy to term. Diagrams drawn from actual lateral x-ray views illustrating change from globular to elongated ovoid up to the thirty-second week, followed by a slight progressive increase in anteroposterior diameter. (From Gillespie, E. C.: Amer. J. Obstet. Gynec. 59:949, 1950.)

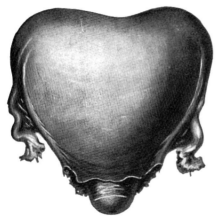

Figure 76 Characteristic appearance of an arcuate uterus with overall heart shape and midline fundal indentation.

ally grows more than those parts of the muscular organ that are unoccupied.

The cervix softens, especially in its supravaginal portion. The acquired compressibility of the isthmus between cervix and corpus is known as *Hegar's sign* of pregnancy, in which the two parts of the uterus appear to be structurally disassociated. The never-pregnant uterus is shaped like a flattened pear, with a capacity of 2 ml. or less; the uterus at full term resembles an immense gourd with a capacity of 4000 to 5000 ml.

The uterus at term, in 80 per cent of women, deviates to the right and twists on

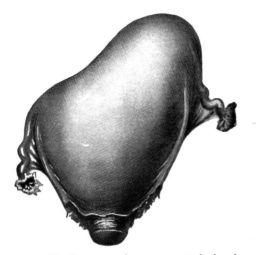

Figure 77 Uterus with asymmetrical development, possibly representing hypoplastic left horn of a bicornuate uterus.

itself from left to right, so that the left adnexa may be located anteriorly near the midline. The round ligament is more prominent on the left side. For cesarean section it is necessary to return the uterus to its midline position before the incision is made.

For the first two months of pregnancy the uterus does not extend above the pelvic brim. As it enlarges it becomes anteverted and anteflexed and lies on the bladder. The corpus is readily felt through the anterior vaginal fornix. The cervix is directed forward (Fig. 78). As the fetus develops the uterus progressively fills the lower abdomen and in time lies against the anterior wall. The intestines, the cecum and the appendix, if mobile, are forced upward and outward. The uterus at term reaches to about the level of the second lumbar vertebra.

The axis of the uterus varies in its relation to that of the pelvic inlet. In primigravidas in an erect position the two axes are usually perpendicular (Fig. 79). In multigravidas the lax abdominal wall allows the uterus to fall forward. If the rectus abdominis muscles are widely separated, a condition called *diastasis recti,* the corpus may protrude through the herniation between them. The *pendulous abdomen* (Fig. 80) that results is characteristic. In the supine position the uterine axis sinks back so that the corpus lies upon the vertebral column (Fig. 81). In late pregnancy pressure of the gravid uterus on the inferior vena cava in the supine position may cause significant changes in venous return to the heart, resulting in the *supine hypotension syndrome.*

Conclusions as to the duration of pregnancy based on the height of the fundus above the pubis are not entirely reliable. Bartholomew's "rule of fourths" (Fig. 82) is a simple and helpful guide. The top or *fundus* of the uterus grows approximately one-fourth of the distance from the symphysis pubis to the umbilicus each month, reaching the level of the umbilicus at about the fifth month. The fundus then rises one-fourth of the way to the ensiform process each month until the ninth, after which it sinks to the level it occupied at eight months. Methods of determining the duration of pregnancy by uterine height

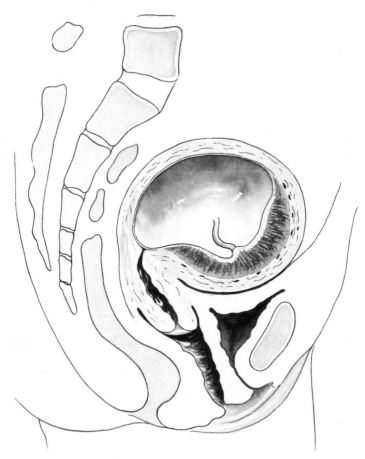

Figure 78 Sharply anteflexed gravid uterus at the end of the third month of pregnancy illustrating how the corpus may compress the bladder as it enlarges out of the pelvis and becomes an abdominal organ.

(see Chapter 8) cannot be considered accurate because the location of the umbilicus is inconstant and the thickness of the abdominal wall varies, as does the amount of amniotic fluid and the size of the fetus. Multiple pregnancy compounds the problem additionally. Nevertheless, attempts should be made to estimate its duration. At times the estimates will be fairly accurate. Serial examinations during the course of pregnancy are also useful in assessing normal progressive development of the conceptus.

Lightening

Two to three weeks before labor in primigravidas the uterus sinks downward and forward. This is called "settling" or "dropping" in lay terms; the technical term is *lightening*. It occurs in about 65 per cent of pregnancies; it is due to the gradual sinking of the fetal head into the true pelvis (a process called *engagement*); it is usual in primigravidas with normal pelves and is sometimes seen in multigravidas with well-preserved abdominal muscles. It appears to be caused by the elongation or ballooning out of the lower uterine segment. It is associated with a distinctive reduction in the height of the uterine fundus. It signifies incorporation of the lower uterine segment (see below) into the wall of the uterus. Lightening usually occurs gradually, but it may be a sudden event.

When the uterus sinks, intestines and stomach are less compressed, the epigas-

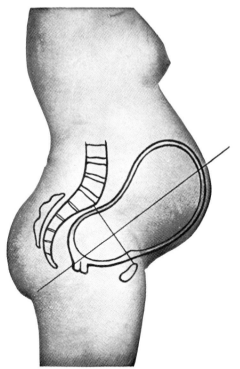

Figure 79 Diagrammatic relationship of the main longitudinal axis of the gravid uterus near term to the axis of the plane of the pelvic inlet as seen in the primigravida when she is standing erect. Note the perpendicularity.

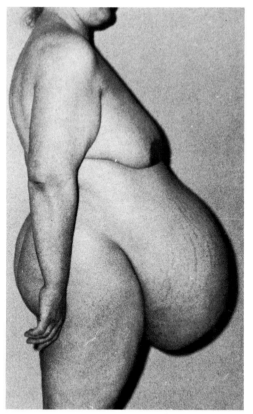

Figure 80 Extreme relaxation of the anterior abdominal wall with diastasis recti allowing forward herniation of the gravid uterus. (Courtesy of K. Kaiser.)

trium is freer, and the diaphragm approximates its usual level. Clothes fit better. However, the fetal head presses against the bladder and the rectum, producing symptoms; walking becomes more difficult, and some women complain of pain in the pelvis.

The Cervix

The cervix consists chiefly of fibrous tissue. Its canal is lined by typical convoluted endocervical glands consisting of large columnar cells containing clear mucus material. The exocervix is uniformly lined by orderly squamous epithelium under normal circumstances. The glandular structures have been shown to consist not of racemose tubular glands but of a system of complicated clefts and tunnels (Fluhmann). It has been conjectured that this arrangement may allow the mucosa to stretch out like an accordion during dilatation and recede after delivery, leaving the cervix without damage. The endocervical epithelium responds to the hormonal stimulus of pregnancy with an intense proliferation. Not uncommonly, the endocervical mucosa may descend onto the portio vaginalis to give the appearance of a so-called circumoral erosion at the external os.

The *cervix uteri* is the lower portion of the uterus and extends from the fibromuscular junction at the anatomic internal os to the vaginal reflection. The *corpus uteri* is the upper part and includes the *fundus,* which strictly speaking refers to the innermost aspect of this hollow organ (analogous to the *fundus oculi*), namely that region lying above the lateral points where the tubes enter the uterine wall. In common usage, the term *uterine fundus* refers to the top of the corpus. The existence of an *isthmus uteri* as a distinct area located

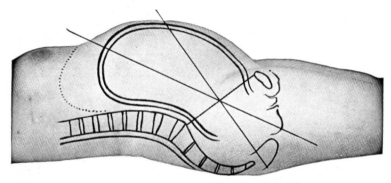

Figure 81   Relationship of the uterine axis to the axis of the pelvic inlet of the same patient shown in Figure 79 when she is lying supine. The uterus falls back on the vertebral column so that its longitudinal axis is no longer perpendicular to the plane of the inlet.

between the corpus and the cervix was maintained by Aschoff, but it has been shown conclusively (Danforth; Danforth and Chapman) that it is more correct to consider it as merely the lower attenuated portion of the corpus (see below).

The fibromuscular junction is said to form an irregular ring that has a sphincteric action. Although anatomic studies have failed to demonstrate a true sphincter, the presence of interlacing muscle fibers that run in transverse and oblique directions may be capable of producing a sphincteric effect when they contract. X-ray evidence exists to support this concept (Asplund; Youssef). It is probably under hormonal control, so that the junction is relatively relaxed under the influence of estrogen and tightly contracted in the luteal phase of the cycle and during pregnancy. The hypothetical role of the sphincter in the maintenance of pregnancy is obvious. Its failure may be reflected in habitual abortion during the second trimester of pregnancy, a condition called *incompetent cervix.*

The cervix in the nonpregnant woman is cylindric in shape but tapering at the lower end. According to the point at which the vaginal mucosa is reflected from the cervix, it is divided into an upper part, the *portio supravaginalis,* and a lower part, the *portio vaginalis,* which are approximately of equal length. The vaginal *fornices* (singular, *fornix*) are formed at the vault of the vagina where the vaginal mucosa is reflected off the cervix. They are designated anterior, posterior or lateral fornix according to their location relative

to the cervix. The supravaginal portion of cervix is in close apposition to the bladder in front. Posteriorly, it is covered by peritoneum that extends onto the posterior vaginal wall and is reflected over the rectum.

The canal of the cervix measures 2.5 to 3 cm. in length and is fusiform, flattened from front to back and slightly dilated in its

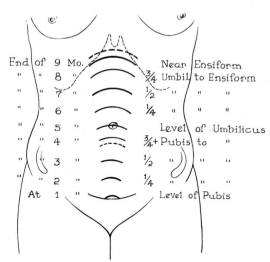

Figure 82   The relative level of the fundus of the gravid uterus during each successive month of pregnancy according to Bartholomew's "rule of fourths." Beginning with the uterus at the level of the pubis at the end of the first month of pregnancy, it is expected to grow one quarter of the way to the umbilicus each month until the fifth month (with slight positive variation from the dotted line at the end of the fourth month) and one-fourth of the remaining distance to the ensiform process (with slight negative variation in the last month) with each succeeding month.

middle third. The average transverse diameter at its widest point is 7 mm.; sagittally, it is about 4 mm. It is continuous with the uterine cavity above at the *internal os.* The *external os* is the opening in the portio vaginalis that connects the cervical canal with the vagina. In the never-pregnant uterus it is usually nearly circular, but there may be many variations in women who have borne children and have had lacerations. Most commonly, the parous cervix is "fish-mouthed" in appearance, forming a transverse slit.

Changes in the cervix begin very early in pregnancy. There is a definite increase in the number of blood and lymph vessels, which also dilate and lengthen. The connective tissue stroma becomes edematous, the cells increase in number and size and young growing cells make their appearance. These stromal alterations are most prominent in the first three months. They are associated with changes in consistency, form and position of the cervix. Softening becomes noticeable within a few weeks. It is very apparent by the fourth and fifth months. During the first three months the cervix is directed downward and backward, but as the uterus enlarges and rises in the abdomen it assumes a more vertical direction.

The increased vascularity and edema of the stroma result in enlargement of the cervix after about the third month. It is more pronounced radially than in length. This change in the volume is due mostly to proliferation of the epithelial structures. As term approaches, the cervix undergoes additional softening. *Effacement* occurs with progressive shortening of the canal as the lower segment unfolds (see below). This process tends to occur earlier in primigravidas then in multiparas. In women who are having their first baby, effacement may actually be complete prior to the onset of labor. Complete effacement exists when the cervix is so thinned that its wall is flush with the lower segment. In effect the depth of the canal equals the thickness of the cervical wall at this time.

The thinning or effacement occurs from above downward, and once labor begins, thinning continues until the cervix is only a few millimeters to 1 cm. thick. The cervix eventually forms the distal 4 to 6 cm. of the uterine canal. The internal os can no longer be identified as a distinct ridge or ring at this stage of development.

Dilatation of the cervix occurs before and during the first stage of labor. It may begin before effacement is complete. The external os eventually reaches a maximal expansion of about 10 cm. Maximal or *full dilatation* is achieved when the cervix is retracted about the fetal presenting part. Since the cervix will dilate no more than is necessary to permit the presenting part to pass, the degree of full cervical dilatation depends on the size of the presenting fetal diameters. The smaller the fetus, the smaller the dimension of the cervical diameter at full dilatation. The larger the fetus or the more unfavorable the presenting diameters, the more the cervix will be required to dilate before it will allow the fetus to descend. The role of the cervix is passive during labor. It merely opens up to allow the passage of the fetus.

The epithelial lining of the portio and of the cervical canal reflects the intense hormonal stimulation of pregnancy. The endocervical columnar cells secrete actively. They are tall and their nuclei are elevated above the base. Marked proliferation takes place and this layer tends to become stratified and to form small cellular projections. This condition has been given various names, including squamous metaplasia and epidermidalization. It is frequently present at all levels of the canal. The endocervical columnar cells undergo intensive growth in pregnancy so that the mucosa progressively increases in thickness. In the nonpregnant state the depth of the mucosa varies from 1.2 to 3.5 mm. in the fixed specimen, but at term it reaches 3 to 6 mm. Irregularities in size, shape and staining quality of the basal cells may occasionally be seen, together with numerous mitotic figures, epithelial buds extending into the underlying stroma, multiple nucleoli and coarsely granular chromatin clumps of the nuclei (Danforth). These changes are important because they must be distinguished from *carcinoma in situ.* The distinction is not difficult to make for knowledgeable pathologists.

The cervical mucus is modified from its characteristics in the nonpregnant state. It becomes thick, viscous and opaque. It forms a *mucous plug* that fills the cervical canal and provides a mechanical antibacterial barrier to the uterine cavity. Cervical smears obtained by spreading a small amount of mucus on a glass slide and allowing it to dry provide interesting information. Dried smears will form a microscopic pattern of arborization, called *ferning,* around the time of ovulation from about the seventh to the eighteenth days of the menstrual cycle. In pregnancy, the pattern is replaced by a cellular or beadlike picture. In normal pregnancy, one sees an abundance of leukocytes, cervical epithelial cells and vaginal cells. Under normal conditions a fernlike pattern is usually absent. The absence of ferning is considered evidence of the predominant influence of progesterone. This picture is characteristic of the postovulatory phase of the menstrual cycle, continues during early pregnancy and persists until a few days before labor. Fernlike smears, which result from an estrogenic effect, can be obtained in approximately 10 per cent of patients during the first 14 weeks of gestation. This finding suggests the possibility of a progesterone deficiency. About half of the patients with such smears will abort (Zondek et al.; Ullery and Shabanah). The appearance of ferning later in gestation apparently does not have the same adverse prognosis. A favorable interpretation is given when the smears show large amounts of mucoid material and abundant exfoliation in addition to a minor degree of the fernlike pattern.

The connective tissue stroma of the cervix undergoes a fundamental transformation that enables it to stretch so that the cervical canal will reach adequate dilatation to permit the fetus to deliver (Danforth et al.; Harkness and Harkness). The collagen fibers prior to labor appear small, edematous and loosened; after delivery, they become smaller and highly branched, giving the impression that there is a dissociation of these fibrils. A diminution of the content of hydroxyproline also suggests a decrease in the concentration of collagen. It has been conjectured that a dissociation and not a dissolution of the fibrils results in the softening and dilatability of the cervix. The fundamental changes appear to involve the ground substances that bind the fibers together rather than the collagen itself.

The Lower Uterine Segment

The inferior boundary of the lower uterine segment is located at the fibromuscular junction of the principally fibrous cervix with the muscular corpus. Its superior border is less obvious. No point of junction between upper and lower segments can be distinguished up to the fifth month of pregnancy. The lower uterine segment does not develop into a definitive, clearly evident structure until later. The lower uterine segment may be defined functionally as that portion of the uterine musculature which must undergo circumferential dilatation to allow the fetus to pass through. This differentiation may begin either in early labor or in the uterine adjustments which immediately precede labor (Fig. 83). Thinning is a necessary accompaniment to this circumferential dilatation of the lower pole of the uterus in response to contractions of the thick, strongly muscular upper segment of the gravid uterus. Longitudinal shortening of the lower uterine segment, with consequent dilatation and thinning, proceeds

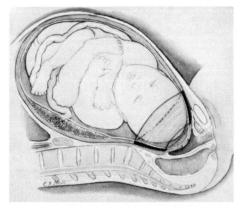

Figure 83 Cut-away view of the lower uterine segment, shown as a shaded truncated cone. It is well ballooned out to accommodate the presenting fetal head, a situation that is characteristic for the nullipara at term and in early labor. (From Danforth and Ivy.)

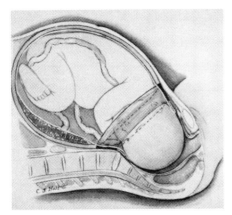

Figure 84 Further development of the lower uterine segment beyond that shown in Figure 83, during the course of active labor, illustrating its shortening and thinning as a result of circumferential dilatation of the cervix and lower segment with subsequent retraction of the cervix to about the level of the pelvic inlet. (From Danforth and Ivy.)

gradually and progressively from above downward until the cervix itself is involved. Circumferential dilatation of the cervix ensues in active labor (see Chapter 15). When the cervix is fully dilated, the cervical lips are at about the level of the pelvic inlet (Fig. 84).

Ivy summarized the evidence pertaining to the growth and unfolding or inclusion of the uterine isthmus into the general uterine cavity to form the lower uterine segment as follows: (1) Histologically, the uterine isthmus increases from two to three times in length during the first three months of pregnancy and then unfolds and is included in the general uterine cavity. (2) The muscular fasciculi of the isthmus in pregnancy assume a more longitudinal or steeper course, but the architecture of the remainder of cervix and corpus is not significantly modified. (3) The mucosa of the lower segment differs histologically from that of the upper segment. (4) The changes in the shape of the uterus in pregnancy (see above) are compatible with and suggest the occurrence of some event between the third and fourth month which contributes to elongation of the cavity. (5) Muscular fasciculi of the isthmus and of the corpus both increase equally in longitudinal length. An isthmus only 1 cm. in length in the nongravid state may hypertrophy until it is 7 to 10 cm. at term.

Borell and Fernström, through iliac arteriography and hysterography, found that the width of the isthmus increases under the influence of estrogen and decreases under the influence of progesterone. Therefore, the isthmus can be regarded as an entity which differs from the corpus and cervix uteri in respect to function.

Danforth found the nongravid cervix to be composed predominantly of fibrous connective tissue with about 15 per cent smooth muscle. The uterine tissue superior to the cervix is composed predominantly of smooth muscle. The transition from fibrous to muscular tissue is usually abrupt. If the change is gradual its transition may extend over 5 to 10 mm. The superior border of the isthmus uteri (the anatomic internal os of Aschoff) cannot be precisely delineated. In 45 per cent of women neither can its lower border (the histologic internal os) be distinguished.

Early in pregnancy the cervix does not change significantly. In the third month the isthmus elongates (Fig. 85). This is a hypertrophic response to pregnancy similar to that occurring elsewhere in the muscularis. Before elongation occurs, the conceptus is confined to the portion of the uterus superior to the isthmic canal. With continuing enlargement of the conceptus, the musculature of the isthmus unfolds to accommodate it so that this musculature makes up a part of the wall of the ovular chamber. The unfolding is limited inferiorly by the fibrous cervix. When the isthmus is unfolded it is not possible to distinguish the isthmic segment from the remainder of the corpus.

From the anatomic and functional points of view the isthmus forms a unit with the remainder of the uterine musculature. Therefore, the concept of the isthmus uteri as a separate, distinct entity is probably inappropriate. The uterus should be considered as being composed of two major parts, the corpus and the cervix, according to whether the fundamental structure is chiefly muscular or chiefly fibrous. The isthmus is merely a part of the corpus (just as the fundus is part of the corpus). Specifically, it is that part of the corpus which lies between the fibromuscular junction of the cervix with the corpus and the plane of the inferior level of the uterine cavity.

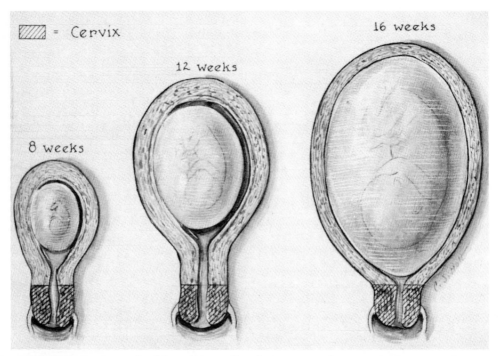

Figure 85 Differential growth of the uterine wall and consequent change in its shape in early pregnancy shown diagrammatically. Compare with Figure 72. The cervix is cross-hatched to represent its passive fibrous nature as contrasted with the muscularity of the remainder of the uterine wall. The uterine configuration at eight weeks is similar to that of the nonpregnant uterus. At 12 weeks muscular hyperplasia is seen throughout, together with comparable thickening and elongation of the isthmic segment. At 16 weeks, the conceptus occupies all of the available space and has begun to unfold a part of the lower uterine segment, thereby elongating the cavity. Unfolding is effectively stopped inferiorly at the level where the fibrous tissue of the cervix begins. (From Danforth, D. N.: Amer. J. Obstet. Gynec. 53:541, 1947.)

THE UTERINE LIGAMENTS

The *round ligaments* are fibromuscular structures arising from both uterine cornua, passing anterolaterally within a peritoneal investiture, exiting from the pelvis in the inguinal canal and anchoring in the upper labium majus. The muscular elements of the round ligaments are continuous with the uterine muscle and hypertrophy with it. Late in pregnancy these ligaments may be 1 to 2 cm. thick (Fig. 86). Due to the high location of the growing fundus, their direction becomes vertical. The round ligaments contract synchronously with the uterus and serve to moor it to the pelvis during labor, although their effectiveness in this regard is relatively weak.

The *uterosacral ligaments* are attached to the posterolateral aspects of the cervix at one end and to the presacral fascia at the other, passing laterally to the rectosigmoid. They vary in size and they too are continuous with the uterine musculature and hypertrophy in pregnancy. During labor they contract with the uterus and aid to keep it in the proper axis of the pelvis.

The *broad ligaments* are the laterally anchoring structures lying within the two folds of peritoneum that encompass the uterus (anteriorly and posteriorly). Enhancement of their lowermost aspects results in the formation of the *cardinal* or Mackenrodt's ligament, which can be a fairly strong support for the growing uterus. They are also strengthened by the addition of muscular fibers around the arteries and veins. The two peritoneal layers are progressively separated by the growth of the gravid uterus, so that a much larger portion of its lateral surface becomes retroperitoneal in that it is unassociated with an intimate serosal peritoneal covering.

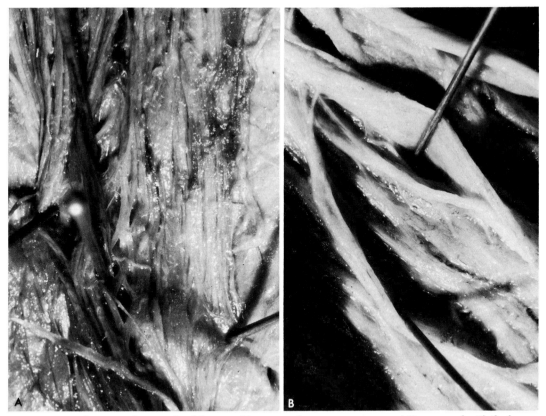

Figure 86 Fibromuscular strands of the round ligament, the nonpregnant state (*A*) compared with the hypertrophied condition that occurs during pregnancy (*B*). Both enlarged identically. (Courtesy of W. Langreder.)

THE PERITONEUM

The peritoneum grows with the uterus; a true hyperplasia occurs. Over the developing lower uterine segment the peritoneum becomes loose and movable. After delivery the peritoneum is wrinkled and lies loosely on the contracted uterus; its folds are fairly characteristic, corresponding to the course of the muscular fibers.

Retroperitoneally, the areolar tissue in the pelvis loses fat. The unstriped muscular fibers in it develop more abundantly. There is a serous imbibition in all the tissues, and the whole pelvis is congested and more succulent. The veins in and around the vagina and cervix enlarge, sometimes to a pathologic extent. The sides of the uterus bulge with large, soft venous swellings.

During pregnancy a phagocytic reaction takes place in the connective tissue around the cervix. It consists of monocytes and clasmatocytes and is increased by infection. Macrophages take part in local immune reactions.

THE UTERINE TUBES

In pregnancy the tubes are stretched and suspended almost perpendicularly at the sides of the uterus. There is no hypertrophy of the muscular fibers, but their vascularity and succulence are increased. A moderate decidual change of the mucous membrane has been observed even with intrauterine pregnancy.

THE OVARIES

The ovaries are enlarged, especially the one containing the corpus luteum of pregnancy. Nelson and Greene concluded that the corpus luteum actively flourishes and functions during the first six weeks of pregnancy. It deteriorates between the eighth and sixteenth weeks and is passively maintained from then on to the end of pregnancy (Table 2). After this it degenerates rapidly and becomes a corpus albicans (see Chapter 2).

Decidual cells similar to those within the endometrial stroma are present in most ovaries during pregnancy. Fibroblasts (or mesenchymal cells) of the connective tissue immediately beneath the germinal epithelium are undoubtedly precursors of these ectopic decidual cells. In 21 patients subjected to elective cesarean section at term, Israel et al. found velvety, reddish, gyriform ridges over the surface of the ovary; microscopically, these ridges were shown to be decidua-like reactions. The rough surface was present in all patients but the decidua-like change was found in only 90.5 per cent. That this formation represents a hormonal response produced by the chorionic elements of the placenta seems established. When endometriosis of the ovary exists, a decidual response of its stromal elements may be observed during pregnancy. In the ovary decidual reaction occasionally may also be present in the nongravid state. Decidual changes may also be encountered elsewhere, such as on the posterior surface of the uterus, the uterosacral ligaments, the round and broad ligaments and even on the appendix and the omentum.

THE VAGINA

The vagina increases in length and capacity by a truly eccentric hypertrophy. It becomes more distensible, the elastic fibers increase, the muscular fibers hypertrophy and the tissues become infiltrated with serum. The rugae deepen and the papillae swell, so that sometimes they are palpable as small granules. The epithelium thickens like a true rejuvenation (Fig. 87). The veins enlarge enormously, imparting to the surface a deep wine color (Chadwick sign of pregnancy, see p. 123). This engorgement may be attended by a pronounced leukorrhea, which is contributed to by increased secretions from the endocervical glands. Estrogens evoke these changes in the vaginal epithelium.

The upper portion of the vagina enlarges as pregnancy advances, so that in the later months it is usually easily possible to touch the sides of the pelvis with the examining fingers. When the uterus ascends, the vagina is drawn up; when the fetal head enters the pelvis in the last month of pregnancy, the vagina is pushed down and sometimes thrown into horizontal circular

---

TABLE 2   *SUMMARY OF THE CHANGES IN THE OVARY DURING PREGNANCY*°

	First Trimester	*Second Trimester*	*Third Trimester*
Corpus luteum			
Size	Large but decreasing		Small
Cavity	Large but decreasing		Small or absent
Connective tissue	Delicate and mesenchymal		Heavy and hyalinized
Granulosa cells	Large, plump, loosely arranged		Smaller, compact
Stellate	Present	Most numerous	Present
Prickle	Usually inner one third		None seen
Vacuoles		Prominent	Few
Colloid	Present	Most	Present
Calcium		Absent	Present
Theca cells	Prominent to readily noticeable		Few or absent
Theca lutein reaction	Moderate in about one half		Flourishing
Decidual reaction		Infrequent	Usually prominent

°From Nelson and Greene. (By permission of Surgery, Gynecology and Obstetrics.)

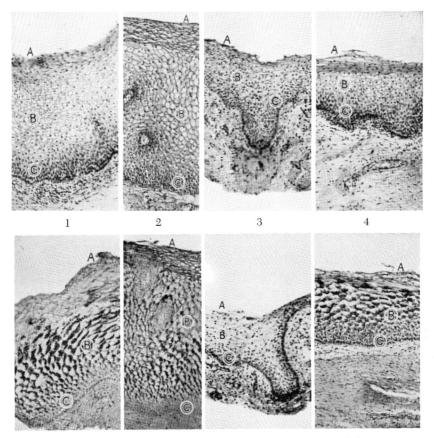

Figure 87 Histology of the vaginal mucosa during the course of pregnancy and the puerperium. *A*, desquamating, keratinized epithelium; *B*, maturing glycogen-containing epithelial cells; *C*, actively growing basal epithelial cells. Upper row stained with hematoxylin-eosin, lower row with Best's carmin for glycogen. *1*, The mucosa of midpregnancy showing moderate development of the glycogen-containing layer. *2*, Mucosa at 36 weeks illustrating profuse development of all layers and the production of much glycogen. *3*, Five days post partum with definite desquamation of the keratinized layer and essentially no glycogen present. *4*, Mucosa six weeks post partum with regeneration well under way as evidenced by the reappearance of glycogen.

folds. Changes on the vulva include softening, the appearance of varices, pigmentation, thickening, enlargement and increased glandular secretion.

The uterus throughout pregnancy is sterile. The portion of the mucus plug filling the upper part of the cervix contains neither leukocytes nor bacteria; the middle part of the plug has only leukocytes, but the part near the external os is full of both. The vagina shows increasing numbers of bacteria from the cervix downward with a maximum in the vestibule and vulva. These areas always contain organisms from the adjacent rectum, especially after defecation and coitus, and from bacteria introduced by the fingers. In the vagina Döderlein's bacillus predominates.

Along with other lactic acid–making bacilli, it transforms the glycogen present in the desquamated epithelium into lactic acid (Cruikshank and Sharman). During pregnancy there is a tendency for the vaginal secretion to reach its maximal acidity or lowest pH.

THE PELVIC FLOOR

The pelvic floor takes part in the general imbibition of the pelvis. The levator ani muscles hypertrophy, become less rigid and more distensible. The infiltration with interstitial fluid may cause a pronounced swelling and even sagging of the perineum.

THE BLADDER AND URETERS

In the early months of pregnancy the corpus uteri lies upon the bladder. Disturbing symptoms do not necessarily result. A certain amount of traction and pressure is exerted by the retropositioned cervix on the urethra and this, in association with the congestion, explains the frequency of urination experienced by women during this period of pregnancy. Cystoscopically, the broad indentation made by the corpus is easily identified. The color of the interior is darker, and one may suspect pregnancy from the appearance of the congested and newly vascularized bladder mucosa. After the uterus rises in the abdomen, the bladder soon becomes largely an abdominal organ in terms of its location. When distended it is flattened against the abdominal wall and it is saddle shaped, extending up to either side of the uterus—more toward the right. The urethra is lengthened. When the fetal head enters the pelvis in the last month, it may press directly on the bladder or distort its base, thus giving rise to urinary frequency and occasionally incontinence.

The ureters are enlarged early in pregnancy. Thickening is one of the diagnostic signs. They are displaced to the side of the pelvis. Their walls are hypertrophic and hypotonic. Comparable hypotonicity involves the uterus, the bowel, the ureters, the kidney pelves and the abdominal wall. This general condition may be due to a disturbance in the balance of sympathetic and parasympathetic systems, which in turn may be caused by progesterone. However, distention of the ureters may also result from compression at the pelvic brim by the growing uterus. Cystoscopically, the ureteral openings in the bladder appear elevated, thickened and deeply congested. Normal conditions are reestablished four to six days after delivery, unless urinary infection exists. Stasis of the urine is a predisposing cause of infection, and many otherwise normal pregnant women often have asymptomatic bacteriuria.

THE PELVIC GIRDLE

The tissues of the pelvic joints imbibe fluid, the capsules thicken, the vascularity is increased and there is an increase of synovia. The pubic, sacrococcygeal and sacroiliac joints are affected in the order named. Hartman and Straus observed relaxation of the pelvic joints in the monkey. These changes took place despite castration early in gestation or death of fetus. The basis of the relaxation in animals and human beings is probably hormonal. Whereas pelvic relaxation takes place in preparation for delivery, the degree of widening or mobility is so slight that it has an insignificant influence on the process of labor.

THE ABDOMINAL WALL

As pregnancy advances, the abdominal wall relaxes and becomes thinner, especially around the umbilicus. In primigravidas the abdominal wall is more tense and sags less than in women who have borne children.

Any tendency to umbilical, femoral, diaphragmatic or inguinal hernia may be aggravated by pregnancy, but usually the uterus causes the intestines to be pushed up so that they and the omentum are kept from the hernial openings, unless these are adherent to the sac.

Usually the skin is smooth, silvery, pearly white or has broad violet lines, called *striae or lineae gravidarum* (Fig. 88). The lines are curved, irregular, sometimes confluent and show a fine transverse fibrillation. They are arranged concentrically, sometimes radially, around the umbilicus and especially on the lower part of the abdomen. They occur on the buttocks and the thighs. The breasts also show them, arranged radially to the nipple. Blondes are more affected than brunettes, primigravidas more than multiparas, fat women more than thin ones and large

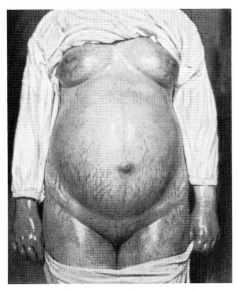

Figure 88 Illustration of striae gravidarum in a preeclamptic patient. Characteristic markings appear in a radiating pattern along the lower abdomen, outer thighs and lower breasts.

women more than small ones. Formerly, they were considered positive proof of preexisting pregnancy, but this is not true since they occur with rapid accumulation of fat at any period (as at puberty) and in Cushing's syndrome. The latter is evidence that striae are by no means solely, or even essentially, the result of overstretching of the skin. Hormonal rather than physical factors are suggested here as etiologic.

THE BREASTS

In the embryo of six weeks a line of cells extends along the *milk line* from the axilla to the groin. The breasts develop from the thoracic portion of this. An ingrowth of epithelial cells, which later become tubulated, marks the site of the mamma. In the fetus at five months the gland consists simply of a collection of ducts which open at one spot, the future *nipple*. At seven months the ducts are branched and at term they divide two or three times. These primitive ducts represent the future lobules. Hardly any acinous structure exists at birth, but the tubules are capable of secreting milk and colostrum. The growth of the gland is extremely slow until puberty.

Then acini develop in the primitive tubules; each becomes a tubuloracemose gland. Thus, the breast is made up of distinct lobules embedded in a fat cushion. Each lobe empties by a duct on the surface of the now prominent nipple. Before opening on the nipple, each duct dilates a little, producing the *sinus lactiferus*. There are 15 to 20 ducts.

The nipple is a muscular organ, is covered by delicate pigmented skin and is vascular. Its base is surrounded by unstriped muscular fibers which unite with those of the nipple itself to produce an erection of the nipple. For a varying distance around the nipple the skin is delicate, pigmented and raised from the fascia covering the mammary gland by soft connective tissue and fat. This is the *areola*. Embedded in the areola lie tiny milk glands, *Montgomery's tubercles*, each opening on the surface by a microscopic duct. Sebaceous sweat glands are also found.

With the advent of pregnancy the glands take on renewed growth, and as early as the second month a change may be noticed. The breasts increase in size and sensibility; the firm, tense character of virgin glands is usually lost. The lobules become more defined because of enlargement, development of acini in the periphery and softening of the connective tissue and fat around them. The acinous formation on the tubules in the center of the gland is especially pronounced during pregnancy, there being both hyperplasia and hypertrophy. The veins enlarge and are seen through the skin as bluish streaks, especially at the periphery. Striae often develop.

The nipples become more erectile. Both nipples and areolas become more deeply pigmented. The base of the areolas becomes puffy, raising the surface above that of the rest of the glands, and the glands of Montgomery enlarge prominently. Occasionally, a drop of secretion may be expressed from them. Around the primary areolas, especially in brunettes, a secondary areola, less pigmented, sometimes develops. Pigment-free spots are present in the secondary areola around the openings of sweat and sebaceous glands. From the early months a little clear, sticky fluid may be expressed from the nipple. Later this is

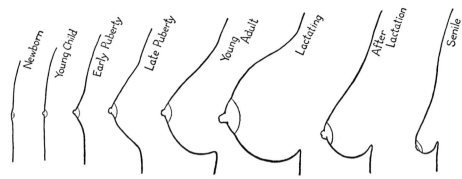

Figure 89   Breast development at different intervals of life according to coexistent hormonal activity shown diagrammatically in outline to demonstrate characteristic configurational changes. (From Patten, B. M.: Human Embryology. New York, Blakiston Division, McGraw-Hill Book Company, 1968.)

mixed with yellow material, *colostrum.* Often it oozes out and dries into branny scales on the nipple.

The shape of the breasts varies in women, and also at different periods of life. In young, nonpregnant women the breasts sometimes are hemispheric and prominent. In older women and in the later months of pregnancy they are pendulous (Fig. 89). Their size depends on the amount of gland tissue and fat. One breast is sometimes larger than the other.

The mammary glands may be considered modified skin glands, with embryonic origin similar to sebaceous glands (Fig. 90). Rarely, supernumerary glands and

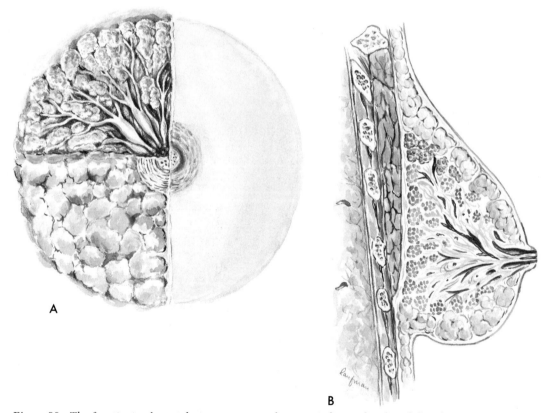

Figure 90   The functioning breast during pregnancy shown to indicate alveoli and duct formation in antero-posterior (*A*) and lateral cross sectional (*B*) views.

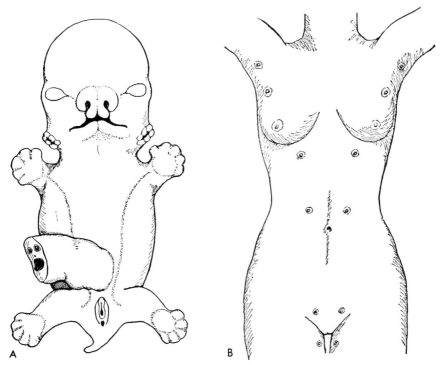

Figure 91 *A*, The location of the "milk line" as found in most mammalian embryos. *B*, The most common sites at which supernumerary nipples and mammary glands are found in adult women. (From Patten, B. M.: Human Embryology. New York, Blakiston Division, McGraw-Hill Book Company, 1968.)

nipples are found above and below the normal one. This is called *polymastia*. Accessory glands and nipples are usually found in the milk line, from the axilla to the abdomen (Fig. 91). The axilla is the most common site of aberrant mammary tissue, which may swell and become painful when lactation starts. The sweat glands in the axilla, too, are often enlarged and palpable, secreting freely. Rarely, the breasts enlarge immensely.

After the child has been delivered and lactation begins, the breasts reach their greatest development. The onset of lactation results from liberation of *prolactin*, an anterior pituitary hormone, which acts on the ducts and acini after they have been prepared during pregnancy by estrogen and progesterone, respectively. Milk ejection is mediated subsequently by the posterior pituitary principle, oxytocin, liberated by way of a reflex arc initiated by the stimulation of the infant suckling at the breast.

THE BONES

The skeletal system in pregnancy shows increased vascularity, especially the red marrow. The spinal column is straightened; the uterine contents, prominent in front, change the line of direction of the woman's figure. This line of direction tends to fall anteriorly to her base of support. Therefore the gravida throws her shoulders back and straightens her neck and head. The curve in the small of the back is exaggerated (Fig. 92); the pelvis is rotated slightly on the femurs. These changes in the skeletal dynamics give the patient a peculiar attitude and gait or strut. The softening of the pelvic joints gives the patient a waddling gait because of the resulting degree of pelvic instability. These changes in carriage require greater effort on the pregnant woman's part to maintain an erect position, and this unaccustomed change in body mechanics may cause backache by placing unusual strains

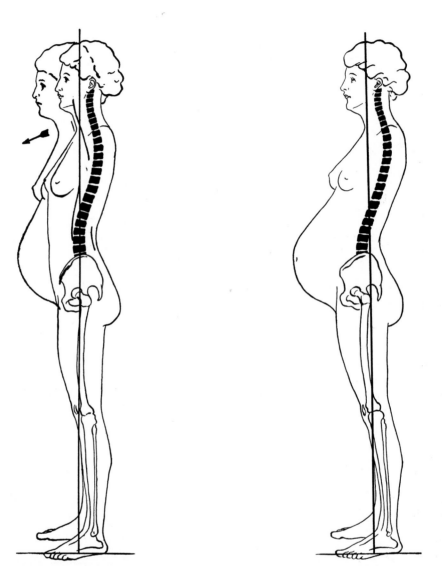

***Figure* 92**   Mechanical diagrammatic representation of the postural changes which take place during pregnancy. As the uterus grows, its weight disturbs the normal postural balance as shown by the arrow in the left diagram. The pregnant woman compensates by hyperextending her lower vertebral column, placing undue strain on the small muscles of the back (right).

on certain muscle bundles. With pendulous abdomens and with twins the changes in posture are exaggerated.

THE SKIN

Pigment is preferentially deposited in definite skin areas: the nipples, the vulva, the skin above the linea alba, the umbilicus and the face. Recent scars become heavily pigmented but old scars do not. The forehead, cheeks and nose are often covered with brown stains. When pronounced, they appear like a mask, the *mask of pregnancy* (Fig. 93). Brunettes are more affected than blondes. A peculiar darkening of the eyelids has also been observed. The actual cause of the deposit of melanin is unknown. The appearance of striae has already been mentioned (see above).

The sweat and sebaceous glands increase in activity. In some women hair growth increases, beginning about the third month of pregnancy. Sometimes a fine lanugo appears on the face and chest, disappearing two or three months post partum. The nails are thinner. The subcutaneous fat becomes thicker, the finer features of the face coarser. The complexion in the early months is sallow, in the later months florid.

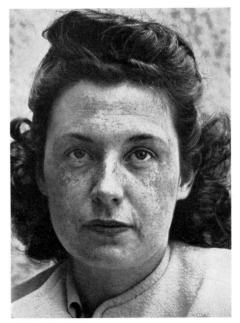

Figure 93 Illustration of characteristic chloasma, the mask of pregnancy, represented by a typical increased pigmentation in a butterfly pattern across the upper cheeks, bridge of the nose, and the forehead. (From Bookmiller, M. M., et al.: Textbook of Obstetrics and Obstetric Nursing. Philadelphia, W. B. Saunders Company, 1967.)

Anatomic and functional changes affecting other specific organ systems, including cardiovascular, pulmonary, renal and gastrointestinal, are reviewed in Chapters 41 and 43 to 45.

REFERENCES

Aschoff, L.: Zur Cervixfrage. Mschr. Geburtsh. Gynäk. 22:611, 1905.

Asplund, J.: Uterine cervix and isthmus under normal and pathological conditions. Clinical and roentgenological study. Acta Radiol. Scand. Suppl. 91:3, 1952.

Assali, N. S., Douglass, R. A., Jr., Baird, W. W., Nicholson, D. B., and Suyemoto, R.: Measurements of uterine blood flow and uterine metabolism. IV. Results in normal pregnancy. Amer. J. Obstet. Gynec. 66:248, 1953.

Borell, U., and Fernström, I.: The sphincter mechanism of the isthmus uteri: A radiological study. Acta Obstet. Gynec. Scand. 32:7, 1953.

Cruikshank, R., and Sharman, A.: Biology of vagina in human subject: Vaginal discharge of noninfective origin. J. Obstet. Gynaec. Brit. Emp. 41:369, 1934.

Danforth, D. N.: The fibrous nature of the human cervix and its relationship to the isthmic segment in gravid and nongravid uteri. Amer. J. Obstet. Gynec. 53:541, 1947.

Danforth, D. N.: The distribution and functional activity of the cervical musculature. Amer. J. Obstet. Gynec. 68:1261, 1954.

Danforth, D. N., and Chapman, J. C. F.: The incorporation of the isthmus uteri. Amer. J. Obstet. Gynec. 59:979, 1950.

Danforth, D. N., Buckingham, J. C., and Roddick, J. W., Jr.: Connective tissue changes incident to cervical effacement. Amer. J. Obstet. Gynec. 80:939, 1960.

Fluhmann, C. F.: The Cervix Uteri and Its Diseases. Philadelphia, W. B. Saunders Company, 1961.

Frankenhäuser, F.: Die Nerven der Gebärmutter und ihre Endigung in den glatten Muskelfasern; ein

Beitrage zur Anatomie und Gynäkologie. Jena, F. Mauke, 1867.

Friedman, E. A., and Sachtleben, M. R.: Placental oxygen consumption in vitro: I. Baseline studies. Amer. J. Obstet. Gynec. 79:1058, 1960.

Gillespie, E. C.: Principles of the uterine growth in pregnancy. Amer. J. Obstet. Gynec. 59:949, 1950.

Goerttler: Die Architektur der Muskelwand des menschlichen Uterus und ihre funktionelle Bedeutung. Morphol. Jahrbuch 65:45, 1930.

Harkness, M. L. R., and Harkness, R. D.: Changes in the physical properties of the uterine cervix of the rat during pregnancy. J. Physiol. 148:524, 1959.

Hartman, C. G., and Straus, W. L.: Relation of pelvic ligaments in pregnant monkeys. Amer. J. Obstet. Gynec. 37:498, 1939.

Hodgkinson, C. P.: Physiology of the ovarian veins during pregnancy. Obstet. Gynec. 1:26, 1953.

Israel, S. L., Rubenstone, A., and Meranze, D. R.: The ovary at term: Decidua-like reaction and surface cell proliferation. Obstet. Gynec. 3:399, 1954.

Ivy, A. C.: Functional anatomy of labor, with special reference to human beings. Amer. J. Obstet. Gynec. 44:952, 1942.

Joseph, J.: Cited in Nixon, W. C. W.: Uterine action, normal and abnormal. Amer. J. Obstet. Gynec. 62:964, 1951.

Knaus, H. H.: Zur Anatomie, Physiologie und Klinik der Uterus Muskulatur. Z. Geburtsh. Gynäk. 129:122, 1948.

Nelson, W. W., and Greene, R. R.: Collective review: The human ovary in pregnancy. Internat. Abstr. Surg. 97:1, 1953.

Nixon, W. C. W.: Uterine action, normal and abnormal. Amer. J. Obstet. Gynec. 62:964, 1951.

Plentl, A. A., and Friedman, E. A.: Lymphatic System of the Female Genitalia: The Morphologic Basis of Oncologic Diagnosis and Therapy. Philadelphia, W. B. Saunders Company, 1971.

Reynolds, S. R. M.: Physiology of the Uterus, ed. 2, revised. New York, Paul B. Hoeber, Inc., 1965.

Ullery, J. C., and Shabanah, E. H.: The cervical-mucus smear during pregnancy and the fate of conception. Obstet. Gynec. 10:233, 1957.

Youssef, A. F.: The uterine isthmus and its sphincter mechanism, a radiographic study: I. The uterine isthmus under normal conditions. Amer. J. Obstet. Gynec. 75:1305, 1958.

Zondek, B., Forman, I., and Cooper, K. L.: Placental insufficiency: Cervical mucus arborization as aid in diagnosis. Fertil. Steril. 6:523, 1956.

Chapter 8

Diagnosis of Pregnancy

The likelihood of pregnancy can be diagnosed with a fair degree of reliability. It is important, however, that the physician guard his statements because much may depend on a definitive diagnosis of pregnancy. Many legal, moral and ethical issues are involved. Errors can have serious consequences. It behooves the physician, therefore, not to take his responsibilities in this regard lightly.

Numerous examples of the kinds of sociologic dilemmas that may result from errors in diagnosis of pregnancy might be given, but such detail is probably superfluous. Although the stigma of illegitimacy is perhaps not so awesome today as it once was, it still carries a heavy burden of guilt and emotional stress. Of equal or at times overriding importance are medical or surgical implications of the diagnosis of pregnancy, particularly insofar as problems relating to altering management are concerned.

Sources of Error. In the early months there is no single sign or complex of signs that are specifically diagnostic of pregnancy in the absolute sense. The biological and immunologic tests (see p. 57) are about 95 to 98 per cent accurate. The typical physical characteristics of the gravid uterus can be mimicked by several other conditions. The pelvic examination may be unsatisfactory because the patient is too fat; she may have a coexistent pelvic tumor, a full urinary bladder or distended bowel, or she may hold the muscles of the abdominal walls and perineum so rigidly that the physician can discern very little in the pelvis. A not uncommon source of error results from the patient withholding information either because she may desire to conceal the possibility that she may be pregnant (perhaps to get the physician to perform an abortion inadvertently) or because of fear or shame. On the other hand, patients may feign the symptoms of pregnancy in order to obtain a positive statement from the physician for various reasons (some rather underhanded or overtly illegal, including blackmail, the institution of bastardy proceedings or acquisition of an estate).

It is unfortunate, but true nevertheless, that the physician cannot always accept the statements of a patient as true because she may even delude herself into believing she is pregnant. These are cases of *pseudocyesis*. Fried et al. reviewed 465 cases of pseudocyesis reported in the literature, including 22 of their own. The patients presented themselves with the common symptoms and signs of pregnancy. The first and most common symptom was a menstrual disturbance. Breast changes were frequent, especially enlargement, tenderness and secretion of milk or cloudy fluid (Fig. 94). Fetal movements were claimed to have been perceived by most of the patients. The cervix of many was reported to be soft. In no instance was the uterus actually enlarged to more than the size of a gestation of six weeks' duration. Moreover, the uterine or cervical changes were not entirely typical of any stage of pregnancy. Weight gain occurred and was usually greater than in normal pregnancies.

Etiology involved primarily psychic or endocrine disturbances. Psychogenic factors included either an intense desire for or a great fear of pregnancy. All but one of their group were childless and the wish factor was predominant. Many of the pseudopregnancies were apparently motivated subconsciously based on a number of definable mechanisms: (1) to bolster a failing marriage, (2) to satisfy reproductive cravings and thereby to become a complete

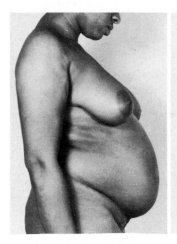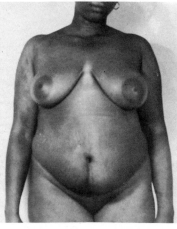

Figure 94 Lateral and anterior views of the abdominal contour and breasts of a patient with pseudocyesis showing changes indistinguishable from those of normal pregnancy. (From Fried, P. H., et al.: J. A. M. A. *145*:1329, 1951.)

woman, (3) to achieve parity with other women in terms of reproductive accomplishments, (4) to acquire a child as a love-object, plaything and companion, or (5) to effect masochistic self-punishment.

The approach to management of the patient with pseudocyesis is not simple. Telling the patient bluntly that she is not pregnant is ineffectual. After she has been gently advised of the true diagnosis, a psychiatric interview is appropriate. Extended psychotherapy will provide the patient with support and insight into the underlying basis of her condition and produces, in most instances, a complete reversal of the process without recurrence.

The findings in normal pregnancy may be divided into two groups: the subjective symptoms which the patient reports and the objective signs which the examiner himself discovers (see Table 3, p. 132). Reliance on objectivity is preferable because this will substantially reduce the chances of error. Moreover, the potentially ensnaring element of suggestion is avoided. We will deal with signs and symptoms of pregnancy as they appear during each of the three conventional divisions of pregnancy into trimester (three month) intervals.

FIRST TRIMESTER

Subjective Symptoms

Cessation of Menstruation. This is one of two important symptoms of pregnancy.

To be relevant and meaningful it must occur in a woman whose periods were previously regular. At least three pitfalls are inherent in this symptom insofar as its value for diagnosis of pregnancy is concerned.

First, pregnancy may occur following an indeterminate interval of amenorrhea (a) during lactation, (b) during debilitating diseases, such as tuberculosis or emotional crises, including the stress of war, or from no apparent cause at all, (c) after curettage, and (d) around the menopause; it may even occur prior to the time in puberty when menstruation has begun or has become established.

Second, vaginal bleeding essentially indistinguishable from menstruation may continue after conception. It is not rare for a woman to have one or two "periods" after she has conceived, but usually the bleeding is scant and otherwise abnormal. Bleeding after conception is the rule in monkeys (Hartman). Bleeding from the endometrial lining is possible because the two deciduas do not fuse until the fifth month. Instances in which apparent menstruation persisted during the nine months of pregnancy have been reported. Whether it is possible for the ovary to continue to function during gestation is highly unlikely in view of the feedback effect of placental hormones on the pituitary-ovarian axis (see Chapter 4). However, rare instances of superfetation and occasional occurrences of menstrual molimina (the characteristic premenstrual symptoms of the ovulating woman) during pregnancy challenge this concept. Rather than true menstruation, a bloody vaginal discharge during pregnancy is more likely due to a local pathologic condition, such as cervical erosion or polyp, or rupture of a varix in the cervix, vagina or vulva, or to some inherent defect of the pregnancy, such as threatening abortion or extrauterine pregnancy.

Third, other conditions may cause the amenorrhea: (a) Change of climate or environment, for example, in girls on holiday, away at school or relocated from abroad, is rather commonly coassociated with periods of amenorrhea. It seldom persists for more than three months. (b) Mental influence, a strong emotion or fear of conception, such as occurs after clandestine exposure, may have similar effects. (c) Debilitating conditions, such as tuberculosis, anemia, various endocrinopathies, as well as local conditions, such as vaginal atresia, may act likewise. (d) Some women are habitually irregular in their menstrual patterns, being amenorrheic for several months without apparent cause or ill health. Timing and intervals of menstrual flow are likely to be uncertain during lactation and near the menopause.

The woman who is menstruating normally and regularly can generally be regarded as not pregnant. By the same token, one who is apparently capable of conceiving and has been exposed by sexual intercourse and who suddenly ceases to flow can be presumed to be pregnant. Although one can never be certain on such evidence, there is reasonable safety in the deductions. Amenorrhea, therefore, is only presumptive evidence of pregnancy, but it is useful in fixing the date of conception and determining the probable time of labor.

Nausea and Vomiting. Many pregnant women have some nausea and vomiting in early pregnancy. These distressing symptoms usually make their appearance by the fifth week of pregnancy and may persist up to 12 weeks or more. Although morning nausea is rather typical, many women experience it at other times of the day. It is common after breakfast or while preparing meals. The patient generally will vomit and may experience no further recurrence during that day. There are many theories concerning its origin, but none is based on substantiated data. There is undoubtedly a large emotional factor, and it is likely that hormonal factors play a role as well (see Chapter 31).

Urinary Frequency. The anteversion of the corpus throws the cervix toward the hollow of the sacrum and stretches the base of the bladder. Pressure of the enlarging uterus on the dome of the bladder (Fig. 78) reduces the volume to which the bladder can fill. Distortion of the bladder base and diminished capacity makes the bladder irritable and causes considerable urinary frequency during the first trimester. Later, when the corpus grows so that it is supported by the abdominal wall, the symptom disappears.

Objective Signs

The Breasts. As early as the fourth week there may be some enlargement of the breasts, and often there is a tingling or burning sensation in them. The enlargement continues throughout pregnancy, though not evenly. The mammary signs have no value in an older multipara, as the breasts are enlarged and sometimes contain milk for years.

Mucosal Discoloration. The bluish, dusky hue of the vestibule and the anterior wall of the vagina in pregnancy was first discovered by Jacquemier in 1846, but Chadwick emphasized its importance. This sign, named after both men, is usually most definite around the urethral meatus and in the vestibule, extending up the anterior vaginal wall, and is of an opaque, bluish tint with a tendency to violet. It appears about the eighth to the twelfth week and becomes more pronounced as pregnancy advances. It is more definite in multiparas than in primigravidas. It often disappears if the conceptus dies or if abortion begins. The discoloration is essentially a manifestation of local venous congestion. It may, therefore, be stimulated by other conditions, for example, menstruation, rapidly growing pelvic tumors, obesity and heart disease. All these circumstances detract from the value of the sign, making it only presumptive of a diagnosis of pregnancy.

Softening of Cervix and Vagina. The

congestive hyperemia of the pelvis is manifested early in pregnancy by a softening of the vagina and the cervix, observed in primigravidas in the sixth week and even earlier in multiparas. The upper and lower portions of the cervix soften first and are associated at the same time with succulence of the vagina and an increase of the leukorrheal discharge. Goodell felt this sign had diagnostic value: if the cervix feels as hard as the cartilage of the nose, pregnancy is not likely to exist; if it feels like the mucous membrane of the lip, pregnancy is possible. The same shortcomings exist for this sign as for the blue discoloration and, therefore, it is also only presumptive. Sometimes one of the earliest pelvic signs is softening of the congenitally thin areas at the sides of the cervix, felt as shallow grooves on its lateral walls.

Hegar's Sign. Hegar's sign consists of softening and compressibility of the lower uterine segment (Fig. 95). It is elicited as follows: On bimanual abdomino-vaginal examination the isthmus uteri can be compressed between the two fingers in the anterior vaginal fornix and the hand on the abdomen behind the anteflexed uterus. In typical cases the fingers can be brought closely together so that the uterine tissue between them seems extremely thin. Another way of eliciting Hegar's sign is to place the fingers of one hand in the posterior vaginal fornix and the other on the anterior abdominal wall in front of the lower uterus, compressing the isthmus between them. The soft succulence of the affected tissues is most pronounced in the isthmus and permits the pressure exerted by the fingers to displace the conceptus toward the uterine fundus. Hegar's sign appears in multiparas at the sixth week and in primigravidas at the eighth week, but is seldom fully developed until the tenth week. It disappears when the uterus attains a size and height which make the part inaccessible.

When well defined and typical, the sign

6th week - multiparas

8th week - primigravida

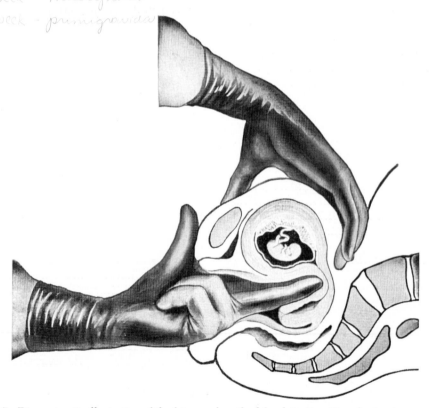

Figure 95 Diagrammatic illustration of the bimanual method for detecting Hegar's sign in pregnancy. The softened isthmus between the corpus and cervix uteri is readily compressed between the hand on the abdomen and the fingers inserted anteriorly to the cervix in the vagina.

is highly presumptive and the most reliable of the first trimester. The uterine isthmus may also be soft and compressible for weeks or even months after abortion or term delivery and just before menstruation. The findings may be imitated occasionally by a retroflexed uterus because the angle of flexion is soft or by a leiomyoma in the uterine wall. Indeed, the isthmus may be softened and elongated in such a way that the examiner may be deluded into thinking that the cervix is actually a nongravid uterus, while the gravid corpus is diagnosed as a tumor of the uterus or adnexa. On the other hand, even in pregnancy, Hegar's sign may be absent or slight or, because of fat or rigidity of the abdomen, may not be elicitable.

Changes in the Uterus (see Chapter 7). FORM. The change from the thin, pear shape of the never-pregnant uterus to the rounded, plump form of early pregnancy is decidedly noticeable. If the ovum is embedded in one or the other cornu near the entrance of one tube, that half of the uterus will develop first and cause asymmetry of the corpus. Symmetry is reestablished as the ovum develops. Early in pregnancy one lateral half tends to be thicker than the other (*Piskaček's sign*), or the anterior or the posterior wall of the uterus may bulge out more. Toward the end of the first trimester, the bulging of the corpus at the sides, above the relatively small cervix, may be determined with the examining fingers placed in the lateral fornices.

SIZE. Enlargement of the uterus should suggest pregnancy and its steady increase in size is one of the most valuable signs. However, at least two examinations, two to three weeks apart, are required. The same rapid rate of growth is not found with any other uterine mass. If a uterus that has been observed to have the usual rate of enlargement of pregnancy suddenly begins to grow too fast, hydramnios or hydatid mole should be suspected; if the growth is interrupted and the size decreases progressively, the conceptus almost certainly is dead.

If a gravid uterus is palpated or manipulated for long, it will usually contract and remain hard for a minute or so. This may give a false impression as to the true uterine size and as to the duration of pregnancy. When in doubt, one should examine the uterus again in a few minutes.

CONSISTENCY. An experienced physician can often make a diagnosis of early pregnancy from this one sign. A gravid uterus is spongy and soft, resembling dough. At the site of the ovum the corpus is a little softer than the rest of the uterus. Hicks called attention to the intermittent uterine contractions of early pregnancy. The uterus may contract as early as the eighth week and it may even contract unevenly in its different parts. A soft spot above the cervix in the early weeks (*Ladin's sign*) is a valuable sign.

POSITION. The strong anteflexion of the uterus, lying on the bladder, serves to draw attention to a possible pregnancy immediately on the introduction of the fingers into the vagina.

These four signs—changes in form, size, consistency and position—considered together by an experienced examiner, are sufficient to make a highly probable diagnosis of pregnancy.

Basal Body Temperature. A diagnostic procedure which can be of great help for diagnosing early gestation is the basal body or waking temperature. In fact, the diagnosis can be made by this means as early as, if not earlier than, it can be made from any other signs, symptoms or tests. Temperatures must be taken with the patient in a truly basal condition, before she arises from bed in the morning or has eaten anything. The expected thermogenic response to progesterone will be seen beginning around the time of ovulation. It will fall just prior to menstruation if fertilization does not occur (see Fig. 59). A level of 37.1° to 37.7° C. (98.8° to 99.9° F.) sustained for more than 16 days after ovulation is highly suggestive of pregnancy. Slight fluctuations not exceeding 0.2° C. (0.4° F.) in either direction may be observed and should not be misinterpreted as being significant. The diagnosis of pregnancy based on a persistently high basal body or waking temperature is correct in at least 97 per cent of cases (Palmer; Barton and Wiesner). This test can be applied only to those women who are recording daily temperatures before ovulation and continue to do so after conception occurs.

SECOND TRIMESTER

Subjective Symptoms

During the second three-month interval of pregnancy, the symptoms of nausea and vomiting and irritability of the bladder will usually subside, but the mechanical symptoms increase. A new subjective symptom develops as the patient feels the movements of the fetus.

Quickening. At about the sixteenth to the eighteenth week the woman begins to feel something in the abdomen, entirely unlike any previous sensation. It has been described as resembling the fluttering of a tiny bird in the hand. It usually takes the woman a week to determine that it is indeed the movement of the fetus. *Quickening* is the ancient term applied to the first perception of active fetal movements, a relic of a time when the fetus was considered inanimate until movements were first perceived.

Fetal movements are felt earlier by women who have experienced them before. Extreme instances are recorded of "feeling life" 10 weeks after conception, or the movements may not be felt until the sixth or seventh month, and rarely not at all throughout pregnancy. The movements, which are weak at first and stronger later, may be vigorous or sluggish throughout pregnancy. Emotional trauma may abolish the movements for a time. They may also cease, without apparent cause or consequences, for days or weeks. As a symptom of pregnancy, quickening is only of presumptive value.

Fetal movements are claimed in nearly every instance of pseudocyesis. Active intestinal peristalsis gives the patient the impression of fetal movements. Similarly, movements may be mimicked by contraction of the rectus muscles or a mobile tumor in the abdomen.

One may use the symptom with caution for diagnosis in intelligent women who have no cause for deception. It may serve as a check on the date of the last menses in determining the length of pregnancy. In primigravidas, one may count 22 weeks ahead to determine the probable date of delivery; in multiparas, 24 weeks.

Objective Signs

The diagnosis of pregnancy may be affirmed during the second trimester by the existence of clear-cut, positive, objective evidence.

Intermittent Uterine Contractions. As early as the tenth week the whole uterus can be felt to contract and relax intermittently without any perception of these events by the mother (Hicks). During contraction, the uterus assumes a pear shape. The contractions recur most irregularly. Brusque manipulation and active fetal movements cause contractions. Toward the end of pregnancy, the irritability of the uterus is such that even ordinary palpation causes it to become hard. Regular perceptible contractions may be present in the later weeks as *false labor* and may seriously disturb the mother's rest.

Fetal Movements. Active fetal movements felt, seen or heard by the obstetrician are a certain sign of pregnancy. In favorable cases, it may be determined as early as the twelfth week. One may see the slight movement of the abdominal wall or the passage of a limb under it. Sometimes the movements are so vigorous that they are visible through the clothes. Listening with the stethoscope, one hears a light tap or dull thump. With the hand laid on the abdomen, one perceives a weak knock or stroke, but sometimes quite tumultuous actions of the extremities. The sign is a positive one for ascertaining the presence of fetal life.

Fetal Ballottement. Owing to the flaccidity of the uterine wall and the presence of amniotic fluid, certain characteristic movements can be ascribed to the fetus; they have been called *ballottement* or *repercussion*. The sign is best elicited with the patient in the lithotomy position. With two of the examiner's fingers in the vagina, the head or breech of the fetus is felt just above the cervix; it is given a gentle push. One usually feels the fetus leave and quickly return to the fingers (Fig. 96). Ballottement is present from the sixteenth to the thirty-second week. Before this time the fetus is too small and afterward too large relative to the amount of amniotic fluid. Partial ballottement of the fetal head may be obtained on abdominal examination, especially in a breech presentation.

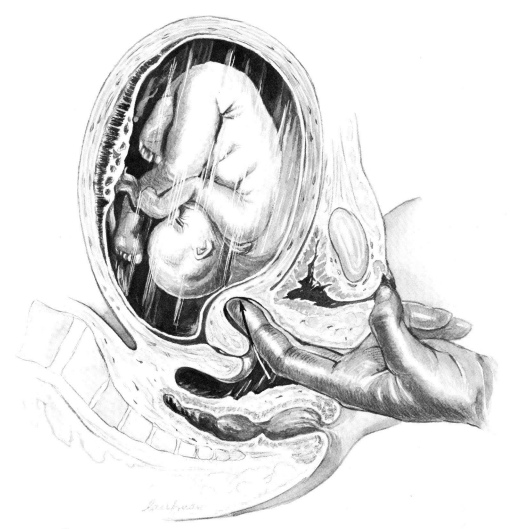

Figure 96   Illustration of the method by which ballottement is demonstrated *per vaginam*. The fetal head or breech is pushed gently so that it can be felt to move away and return quickly to the examining fingers.

Ballottement may be simulated by a leiomyoma or an ovarian tumor with a long pedicle, especially if ascites is also present.

Palpation and Identification of the Fetus.   On palpating an enlarged uterus the examiner may feel a hard mass within it with parts which resemble the head or extremities of a fetus. Hasty conclusions must be avoided. Leiomyomas of the uterus and neoplasms of the ovaries may assume shapes and positions which can mislead a casual observer.

Fetal parts may be felt as early as the fourth month. As the fetus grows they can be differentiated, so that later *large parts* (head and breech) and *small parts* (the extremities) may be distinguished. The absence of discernible fetal parts in a pregnancy in which they should be felt leads to the suspicion of a dead fetus, hydatid mole, hydramnios or a monster.

Auscultatory Signs.   Fetal Heart Tones.   Usually the heart tones are heard first between the sixteenth and the twentieth week of gestation. Faint at first, the beat becomes stronger as the fetus grows larger. The heart sounds may be missed because of an excessive amount of amniotic fluid or because the sounds are confused by a placenta lying on the anterior uterine wall, by the uterine bruit or by external noise.

The fetal heart tones resemble the tick-tock of a watch heard through a pillow. Characteristically, the pattern is a tick, short pause; then tock, long pause. The first sound is synchronous with the systole of the fetal heart and with the pulse in the umbilical arteries; the second sound is due to closure of the semilunar valves.

The rapidity of the beat normally varies from 120 to 160 per minute. Definite variations in the rapidity occur without cause. Rates above 160 are not uncommon; they do not necessarily indicate fetal distress. Fetal movements may sometimes accelerate the beat; palpation of the fetal body may do the same. Fever increases the rapidity of the heart. Pressure on the fetal skull may slow it momentarily.

The naked ear will suffice when no stethoscope is available and when rumbling exterior noises interfere, but this may be disagreeable to the patient and the examiner. A smooth towel should be laid between the ear and the patient's skin.

Best of all nonamplified stethoscopes is the head stethoscope shown in Figure 97. Noises imparted by the fingers holding the tubing of other kinds of stethoscopes are avoided. The head stethoscope also has the added advantage of bone conduction of the sounds.

Up to the fifth month the stethoscope should be placed in the median line at the edge of the pubic hair. When the fetus is palpable, one will be able to determine where the heart is located (best heard through the fetal back) and listen there. It may be necessary to push the fetus against the abdominal wall with the hand, so as to bring its heart nearer the stethoscope, but it is preferable if possible not to touch the abdomen and thereby add confusing noises. In the early months, if a diagnosis is imperative, one may lift the uterus up nearer the abdominal wall with fingers in the vagina.

Perhaps one of the most reliable signs for the diagnosis of pregnancy is auscultation of the fetal heart tones. Unless the mother's heart beat has the same rate, there is no question about the existence of pregnancy. The sign is easily verified by feeling the mother's pulse while listening over the uterus.

Recent technological advances have introduced ultrasonic methods for auscultation of the fetal heart. The approach has elevated detection of the fetal heartsounds to a very sophisticated state. It is possible to monitor the fetus as early as 10 weeks.

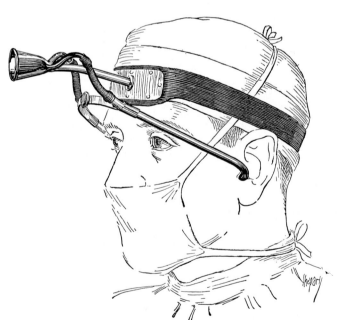

Figure 97 The DeLee-Hillis fetoscope showing method for obtaining optimal auditory acuity by way of air and bone conduction while simultaneously avoiding noises imparted by the examiner's fingers. Short rubber connectors are important so that the line of vision is not obstructed and the sound-damping effects of long connectors are reduced.

Fetal life can be regularly detected by 12 to 14 weeks rather definitively. The required equipment detects changes in the frequency of an emitted sound (Doppler effect) brought about by movement of particulate matter (like blood). It is most useful in ruling out fetal death *in utero*.

FETAL SOUFFLE. Sometimes called *funic souffle*, there is a characteristic sound heard that is caused by the rush of blood through the umbilical arteries, especially when they are subjected to pressure, torsion or tension. It is synchronous with the fetal heart sounds. The fetal souffle is a soft, blowing murmur heard with the first fetal heart sound, but it may be heard with both sounds or even with the diastolic alone. It occurs in about 15 per cent of pregnant women and is more common during labor. When present, this sign is diagnostic of pregnancy.

UTERINE SOUFFLE. Lejumeau de Kergaradec described a sound which he heard while listening at the sides of the uterus. He ascribed it to rushing of blood through the placenta and called it the *placental souffle*. It is a soft, blowing sound, synchronous with the maternal heart, and has a rushing character. It is similar to the bruit heard in an aneurysm or is like the French *vous* pronounced in a low, blowing tone, *voo*. During uterine contraction it is diminished and/or altered in quality. It is heard best at the left side of the uterus, low down, or occasionally on the right side. When the uterus is dextro- or sinistrorotated, the uterine souffle may be heard anteriorly and occasionally all over the uterus.

The origin of the sound is in the large anastomotic uterine arteries at the sides of the uterus. It is not located in the placenta because it has been heard even after the placenta has been removed, but it seems loudest near the placental site. In extra-uterine abdominal pregnancy, a pronounced uterine souffle may serve to indicate the location of the conceptus in the abdomen. It is present whether the fetus is alive or dead, but is usually diminished in intensity in the latter instance. As a diagnostic sign of pregnancy its value is limited. It may be heard in the presence of large vascular pelvic tumors.

Changes in the Uterus. The shape of the uterine mass, its size for the supposed length of gestation and its consistency and location all point to a diagnosis of pregnancy and are rarely imitated by other conditions. Usually, an experienced physician can obtain enough information with his fingers for a definitive decision (Fig. 98). Confirmation is available by determining the rate of the growth of the uterus when examined at intervals of three to four weeks. Together all these signs give a positive diagnosis of pregnancy.

Skin Changes. Characteristic increase in pigmentation, the mask of pregnancy, abdominal striae and a secondary areola on the breasts are all useful but not definite signs of pregnancy.

THIRD TRIMESTER

Amenorrhea continues into the third trimester of pregnancy. Any sign of vaginal bleeding must be considered either pathologic or a sign that labor is beginning. Nausea is absent. Its persistence or reappearance may be serious and indicates the necessity for a careful examination, particularly for evidence of toxemia. Active fetal movements are more pronounced.

The painless uterine contractions become more and more noticeable as the months go by until, toward the end of this trimester, the uterus often responds to the slightest stimuli. The cervix and other pelvic structures become prepared for the great dilatation they are about to undergo.

The examiner has no difficulty feeling the movements of the fetus. Ballottement is not elicitable unless there is a great deal of amniotic fluid (hydramnios). Partial ballottement may be accomplished, especially in breech presentations. Direct palpation of the fetal body is easy unless the placenta is implanted anteriorly. The fetal presentation and position may be diagnosed readily.

The fetal heart tones are louder and more constant. The funic souffle is more likely to be heard. The uterine bruit is more intense and more widely distributed. X-ray study will always disclose a fetus or parts of it.

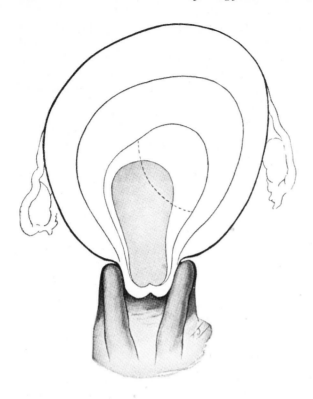

Figure 98 Examination of the vaginal fornices, illustrating how the examining fingers can determine the changes in the shape of the uterus, particularly as it encroaches laterally.

Lightening. Toward the end of pregnancy the patient may notice a disappearance of the pressure symptoms referable to the upper abdomen, an increase of pelvic discomfort and a change in the configuration of the abdomen when this occurs. It is fair to assume that *lightening* or dropping of the fetal head into the pelvis has occurred.

The diagnosis is definite if on internal examination the fetal head is low in the pelvic cavity. Lightening generally takes place about three weeks before the onset of labor at term in primigravidas; it may not occur in multiparas until labor is well under way. This phenomenon has real prognostic value. It means that the particular head can pass the particular pelvic inlet. Since many serious pelvic deformities are at the inlet, it usually predicts a successful delivery. Lightening may not occur under the following circumstances: contracted pelvis, a large fetus, twin pregnancy, hydramnios, malpositions, malpresentations, placenta previa and obstruction by tumors. In primigravidas, lack of lightening at term should be viewed as significant. Although the outcome is often favor-

[handwritten left margin: D. Dx. of absence of Lightning]

able, the possibility of a serious difficulty should be borne in mind when this situation is discovered.

Diagnosis of Fetal Life or Death. Without positive evidence to the contrary, a fetus is considered alive. The heart tones, the fetal souffle and active fetal movements are convincing evidence that the fetus is alive. The following are symptoms and signs of fetal death:

1. Cessation of fetal movements after they have been felt is presumptive evidence of fetal death.

2. The sudden cessation of nausea and vomiting, in the early months, is suggestive of fetal death.

3. If a woman gives a history of having lost several conceptuses at a certain month in pregnancy and now has identical symptoms, the information is suggestive. When a cause exists for anticipating fetal death, such as maternal diabetes, hypertension or renal disease, the diagnosis is rendered easier.

4. The absence of fetal heart tones is of value when auscultation by ultrasound (Doppler effect) is available. With only stethoscopic means at hand, the absence of

fetal heart sounds is acceptable evidence only after repeated prolonged examinations, under the most favorable conditions (quiet room and proper position). There is a characteristic ominous complete silence and stillness over the uterus.

5. The cessation of uterine growth is a valuable sign if confirmed by examinations every three weeks. The uterus, instead of growing larger, becomes smaller, harder and usually more evenly resistant. Unless carefully considered, this sign may be fallacious because sometimes the uterus seems to stop growing for a time or may become smaller, even with a living fetus.

6. A positive sign of fetal death is the palpation of the softened and macerated fetal head, with the bones freely movable on one another. This sign may be elicited through the vault of the vagina, through the cervical canal or, rarely, through the abdominal wall. Maceration of the fetus is usually so far advanced in a week to 10 days that softening of the skull may be discerned. Horner and, independently, Spalding called attention to overlapping of the bones of the skull seen by x-ray. This is not a definitive sign, however, because it has been observed in a living fetus. Combined with decided curvature or angulation of the spine and general crowding together of the skeleton, it is almost pathognomonic of fetal death (Schnitker et al.). This sign is best elicited with the patient erect.

7. Roberts called attention to the presence of gas in the fetal circulation seen in roentgenograms. Crick and Sims found this present in 12 of 30 fetal deaths, suggesting that gas is not a rare finding. The gas is almost entirely nitrogen. Its roentgen demonstration is not only pathognomonic of fetal death but probably occurs earlier than vertebral or skull deformities. To detect it, lateral views are necessary.

8. The discharge of dark, milky or bloody amniotic fluid is suggestive.

9. The fact that a fetus changes its presentation from head to breech or vice versa does not constitute proof of life.

10. The patient loses weight. This is significant only because it is an unusual event in late pregnancy.

11. The pregnancy tests offer some aid in the first half of pregnancy when chorionic gonadotropin levels are normally very high. Later, when levels are expected to be relatively low, falsely negative pregnancy tests may be encountered even though the conceptus is perfectly intact.

12. Fetal electrocardiography will reveal cardiac standstill. However, it may be difficult to detect the fetal electrocardiographic pattern under the best of circumstances, so that one cannot rely on its absence. Ultrasound detection is much more reliable in this regard.

Duration of Pregnancy and Delivery Date. Both the physician and the patient desire to know when labor will occur. Since the actual duration of pregnancy is variable even in different gestations in the same woman, the day when labor is to begin is never definite. Certain data can be supplied by the patient to help in predicting with some degree of accuracy. Clinical information will be discussed here; more objective laboratory techniques are taken up in Chapter 13.

DATE OF FRUITFUL COITUS. The date of conception based on a single occasion of coitus is reliable when it is known and documented. To determine the probable delivery date within a narrow range, one need merely count 266 days from the date of the single impregnating coitus. In about one-half of the cases this date will be accurate within seven days.

DATE OF ONSET OF THE LAST MENSTRUATION. Nägele's rule is based on an average interval of 280 days to delivery from the beginning of the last normal period prior to conception. One merely counts nine months and seven days from the first day of the last menstrual period. It may be easier to count back three months and add seven days. For example, if the patient's last menstruation began on March 1, December 8 will be the calculated day of labor. In about 60 per cent of cases this method is correct within eight days.

Knaus felt he could determine the onset of labor more precisely from the date of ovulation, thereby reducing the inherent variability in the length of gestation caused by the variation in menstrual cycle (or more precisely by variation from onset of menstruation to ovulation). Since precise timing of ovulation cannot be accomplished, his approach added little.

QUICKENING. It is customary to count ahead 24 weeks in multiparas and 22 weeks in primigravidas from the first recognition by the patient of fetal movement. Little reliance can be placed on this rule.

SIZE OF THE UTERUS. The height of the uterine fundus from the pubis or the umbilicus is a measurement of limited value. Many conditions may alter it, including the amount of abdominal wall fat, tumors, gas in the bowel, a full bladder or rectum, hydramnios, twins or a pendulous abdomen.

The McDonald rule uses the measurement of the contour of the abdomen from the upper margin of the symphysis to the fundus. The average height of the fundus at term is approximately 35 cm. McDonald's rule states that the length in centimeters divided by 3.5 gives the duration of the pregnancy in lunar months. This rule can only be applied after the sixth month. Bartholomew's *rule of fourths* is also helpful (p. 103) for approximating gestational age. Complications such as hydramnios, malpresentations and multiple pregnancy nullify the findings in both McDonald's and Bartholomew's rules.

SIZE OF THE FETUS. More certain information is obtainable by estimating fetal size, although large errors can be expected. Direct measurement of the fetal head, using an ordinary caliper, is possible through a thin abdominal and uterine wall. The position of the head with reference to the pelvis is first carefully determined and then the arms of the calipers are placed as nearly as possible in the biparietal diameter. One should deduct 1 to 2 cm. from this measurement for the thickness of the abdominal wall. Although the results obtained may be questioned, its value increases with experience.

A much more accurate and reliable technique is now available in the form of ultrasound (A mode or B scan) measurements. Serial determinations are particularly useful in assessing growth *in utero*. Precision of about 2 to 3 mm. can be expected. By inference, estimation of gestational age within two weeks is possible on this basis.

Palpation of the fetal body is of little value. Fetuses may vary in size at identical periods of pregnancy. It also seems that the fetus has periods of slower and quicker growth, similar to that which occurs after delivery. Therefore, estimations of the duration of pregnancy and of probable date of

TABLE 3   SUMMARY OF THE DIAGNOSTIC FEATURES OF PREGNANCY

First Trimester	
Cessation of menses	Presumptive
Nausea	Presumptive
Changes in the breasts	Presumptive
Chadwick's sign	Presumptive
Softening of cervix and vagina	Presumptive
Hegar's sign	Probable
Changes in form, size, consistency and position of uterus	Probable
Positive biologic, immunologic or serologic test	95 to 98 per cent certain

Second Trimester	
Absence of menses	Presumptive
Quickening	Presumptive
Intermittent uterine contractions	Probable
Active fetal movements observed by the physician	Certain
Ballottement	Certain (with limitations)
Direct palpation of fetal body	Certain (with limitations)
Fetal heart tones and fetal souffle	Certain
Uterine souffle	Probable
Changes in form, size, consistency and position of uterus	Probable
X-ray of fetal skeleton	Certain

delivery, based only on the size of the fetus, are often unreliable.

LIGHTENING. It is safe to expect delivery to occur within three weeks from the time the head settles into the pelvis in primigravidas.

PRELABOR PELVIC CHANGES. During the last few weeks of pregnancy, repeated vaginal examinations usually enable a physician to detect the approaching proximity of the onset of labor. In succeeding examinations he will find the cervix more and more effaced and dilated. If the patient is not near term, the cervix remains firm and undilated. On the other hand, labor is fairly imminent if the cervix becomes shorter and begins to soften and dilate.

REFERENCES

Barton, M., and Wiesner, B. P.: Waking temperature in relation to female fecundity. Lancet 2:663, 1945.

Chadwick, J. R.: Value of the bluish coloration of the vaginal entrance as a sign of pregnancy. Tr. Amer. Gynec. Soc. *11*:399, 1887.

Crick, A. F., and Sims, F. H.: Gas within the foetus indicating foetal death. J. Faculty Radiol. 5:126, 1953.

Fried, P. H., Rakoff, A. E., Schopbach, R. R., and Kaplan, A. J.: Pseudocyesis: A psychosomatic study in gynecology. J.A.M.A. *145*:1329, 1951.

Goodell, W.: Lessons in Gynecology, ed. 3. Philadelphia, D. G. Brinton, 1887.

Hartman, C. G.: Studies in reproduction of the monkey *Macacus (Pithecus) rhesus*, with special reference to menstruation and pregnancy. Contrib. Embryol. 23:1, 1932.

Hegar, A.: Diagnose der frühesten Schwangerschaftsperiode. Deutsch Med. Wschr. *21*:565, 1895.

Hicks, J. B.: On the contractions of the uterus throughout pregnancy: Their physiological effects and their value in the diagnosis of pregnancy. Tr. Obstet. Soc. *13*:216, 1871.

Horner, D. A.: Roentgenography in obstetrics. Surg. Gynec. Obstet. 35:67, 1922.

Jacquemier, J. M.: Manuel des accouchements et des maladies des femmes grosses et accouchées, contenant les soins à donner aux nouveaux-nés. Paris, Germer-Baillière, 1846.

Knaus, H. H.: Period of human gestation in light of modern research. Ciba Symposium 6:191, 1958.

Ladin, L. J.: Signs of early pregnancy, with special reference to Ladin's Sign. Med. Rec.*143*:294, 1936.

Lejumeau de Kergaradec, M. J. A., quoted by Fasbender, H.: Geschichte der Geburtshülfe. Jena, Gustav Fischer, 1906, p. 426.

McDonald, E.: Mensuration of the child in the uterus with new methods. J.A.M.A. *47*:1979, 1906.

McDonald, E.: The diagnosis of early pregnancy, with report of one hundred cases and special reference to the sign of flexibility of the isthmus of the uterus. Amer. J. Obstet. 57:323, 1908.

Nägele, F. C.: Erfahrungen und Abhandlungen aus dem Gebiethe der Krankheiten des weiblichen Geschlechtes. Nebst Grundzügen einer Methodenlehre der Geburtshülfe. Mannheim, T. Loeffler, 1812, p. 280.

Palmer, A.: Basal body temperature in disorders of ovarian function and pregnancy. Surg. Gynec. Obstet. 75:768, 1942.

Piskaček, L.: Über Divertikel des Uterus. Wien. Med. Wschr. 63:2689, 1913.

Roberts, J. B.: Gas in the fetal circulatory system as a sign of intrauterine fetal death. Amer. J. Roentgen. *51*:631, 1944.

Schnitker, M. A., Hodges, P. C., and Whitacre, F. E.: Roentgenologic evidence of fetal death. Amer. J. Roentgen. 28:349, 1932.

Spalding, A. B.: A pathognomonic sign of intrauterine death. Surg. Gynec. Obstet. *34*:754, 1922.

Chapter 9

Antepartum Care

In obstetrics, perhaps more so than in other branches of medicine, prevention is of greater importance and simpler than cure. Hence, physicians must familiarize themselves with the essentials of antepartum care. The objective of antepartum care is the proper investigation and supervision of a pregnant woman so that she will be able to go through pregnancy and labor without detriment to herself or to her baby. The great value of such care is well established in terms of significant reductions in maternal and fetal mortality and morbidity based on the detection and treatment of various medical disorders.

Ideally, every woman should be examined completely preconceptionally, that is, well before she plans to become pregnant. If this procedure were carried out routinely, many abnormal and potentially serious conditions would be detected and corrected before pregnancy is undertaken. Some of these conditions, if uncorrected, may lead to impairment or death of the mother or the fetus or both. Needless to say, if prepregnancy examination reveals a medical disorder serious enough to jeopardize the patient's life or health in the event pregnancy should occur, it is imperative that this information be imparted to the patient and to her husband. If the ailment can be cured or alleviated, measures should be instituted to accomplish this objective well before gestation occurs. Special attention is given the patient when pregnancy supervenes to prevent a recurrence or aggravation of the illness. Counseling of the patient in ill health is an important aspect of preventive care, particularly as regards advice on conception control (see Chapter 77).

TAKING A HISTORY

At the time of the patient's first visit certain information should be obtained for purposes of identification and proper record keeping, such as (1) the patient's full name, (2) date of the visit, (3) by whom she was referred, (4) her address and telephone number, (5) her age, and (6) if married, her husband's name and (7) the number of years she has been married. Additionally, details on important aspects of family and personal medical history are essential, including: (8) Family history of the childbirth experiences of the patient's mother and sisters, especially regarding contracted pelves, hemorrhages, toxemias, hypertensive disorders, obstetric accidents, twins and diabetes mellitus.

(9) Past history of medical, surgical and psychiatric problems, with special inquiry about abdominal operations, cardiac, hypertensive, renal, metabolic and pulmonary diseases. Drug allergies should be determined. A tactful query should be made concerning venereal disease.

(10) Menstrual history, including age of onset of menses, their frequency, regularity, duration and the amount of flow; if pain is experienced, the time of its occurrence, duration and character. The dates the last two periods began should be recorded and determination made as to whether or not they were normal.

(11) Obstetric history with a brief account of each pregnancy, abortion or labor, with dates; information about the type of deliveries, whether premature or full term; complications during pregnancy, labor or the puerperium, especially toxemia, hemorrhage and infection; weight

and condition of the babies; breast feeding.

(12) System review, concentrating on the patient's present condition and recording all her complaints. One should ask specifically about nausea, vomiting, bladder disturbances, constipation, edema, excessive weight gain, cough, dyspnea, dizziness, headache, visual disturbances, pain and vaginal bleeding in the present pregnancy.

(13) Probable date of confinement as calculated from the last menstrual period (Nägele's rule) and verified by uterine size, date of quickening and when the fetal heart tones are first heard (see Chapter 8).

PHYSICAL EXAMINATION

The patient is examined after the history is taken. A bimanual vagino-abdominal examination is performed to make certain that the patient is pregnant. When doubt exists, the patient should be asked to return two weeks later for another examination, or a pregnancy test may be made. The vaginal examination will aid in disclosing, if present, a retroflexed gravid uterus, ectopic pregnancy, leiomyoma, ovarian cyst or other neoplasm.

It is recommended that both male and female physicians undertake the physical examination in the presence of a female chaperone. At the general examination note should be made of the patient's body type—whether she is unusually tall or short, thin or obese. Her general health status should be surveyed, including whether she is younger or older than she appears and whether any gross medical, endocrine or other disturbance is manifest. Weight and height should be recorded. Blood pressure should be obtained with the patient supine and at rest and rechecked later if necessary. It may be preferable to delay obtaining the blood pressure until the end of the physical examination because it is well recognized that lower readings are seen if the patient is relaxed, less apprehensive and more comfortable with her environment and with the examiner.

A detailed, thorough general examination is made. Beginning at the head, the eyes are checked with attention paid to the eyegrounds. Ophthalmoscopic examination of the retina may reveal important manifestations of vascular and other disorders. The ear canals are checked and the condition of the tympanic membrane noted. One gives attention to the teeth and gums, noting the presence of caries and gingival hypertrophy. The thyroid is palpated for nodules, cysts or diffuse enlargement. The neck, axillas and groins are checked for enlarged lymph nodes. The heart and lungs are carefully examined by auscultation and percussion.

The breasts should be carefully and gently palpated and the nipples inspected. Then the abdomen is examined for masses, including an enlarged uterus, as well as for the presence of tenderness, hernias and scars. The size of the uterus should be accurately recorded for future comparisons. If the duration of the pregnancy is more than four months, an attempt should be made to hear the fetal heart tones. The lower extremities should be inspected for deformities, scars, varicose veins and edema. Deep tendon reflexes should be checked. The back should be inspected for deformities and tenderness, especially at the costovertebral angles.

For the vaginal examination the patient should be in the lithotomy position, properly draped with her legs comfortably supported in heel stirrups or other mechanism. Before being placed on the examining table, the patient should empty her urinary bladder. One of the first essentials of the vaginal examination is the Papanicolaou smear for cytologic study of vaginal and cervical cells. Since lubricants will distort the morphologic appearance of the cells to be examined, the smear should be done before the examiner's fingers are inserted and the speculum used should be unlubricated. The smear should be done regularly at the first antepartum visit of every patient without exception. After the cervix has been exposed, material is obtained for smears by scraping around the external os and using a cotton-tipped applicator that has been dipped in saline for the endocervical canal. Careful inspection of the cervix and vagina for erosions, polyps, lacerations or other lesions should be carried out at this time. Routine culture of cervical mucus for gonococci is probably of value in view of the relative silence of such infections in pregnancy and their dire effects to both the fetus and the mother after delivery. Silent gonorrheal infestations are being uncovered in large numbers in certain populations where routine cultures are being obtained.

Digital examination is done next. After the external genitalia are inspected for discoloration, varicosities, lacerations, edema, cysts or abscesses of the Bartholin ducts, vaginal discharge and congenital abnormalities, the labia are widely separated and the gloved fingers inserted gently and slowly into the vagina. Gentleness must be exercised throughout the examination. Bartholin glands and Skene's glands are palpated. The urethra is "milked" to see if it contains pus. The pelvic floor is depressed by pressure against the perineal body with the fingers in the vagina to determine its tonicity and the presence of any lacerations. The patient is asked to bear down to disclose any cystocele and/or rectocele.

The cervix is palpated to determine its size, shape, consistency, position and deformations. Following this, the adnexa and the body of the uterus are palpated bimanually for size, position, consistency and regularity. The hand on the abdomen must be used in unison with the fingers in the vagina for this procedure. The pelvic cavity is explored to determine its obstetric capacity. For details of this procedure see Chapter 12.

LABORATORY STUDIES

We have already alluded to the essentiality of Papanicolaou cytologic screening. This bears repeating and emphasis. Vaginal discharges should be investigated by use of smear, culture and hanging drop preparations to detect such offending organisms as *Neisseria gonococcus*, *Tricho-*

monas vaginalis and *Candida albicans*. The anus and rectum are examined for abnormalities, including hemorrhoids, fissures, polyps and any lack of normal tonus in the anal sphincter muscle.

For all patients a hemoglobin or hematocrit determination must be made and blood taken for a serologic test for syphilis. A serologic test is compulsory in some states. The test should be repeated, perhaps in another laboratory, if the reaction is positive or doubtful.

All pregnant women, primigravidas or multiparas, should have their blood typed and their Rh status determined. This information is absolutely necessary in the event that a blood transfusion is needed; moreover, knowledge of the Rh status is important as a warning that Rh isoimmunization may arise. If the patient is Rh negative, the Rh status of her husband should also be determined. If he is Rh positive, special tests must be made to determine whether he is homozygous or heterozygous (see Chapter 52). Routine screening for atypical antibodies is done in some areas to uncover less common sensitization phenomena.

Urinalysis is mandatory and should include specific gravity, protein, glucose, microscopic examination of the sediment for casts, pus and blood, and culture of a clean midstream specimen for bacteriuria. Where indicated, urobilinogen, acetone or porphyrins should be sought.

Recent evidence has suggested the wisdom of routine examinations for phenylketonuria, rubella titer and erythrocyte sickling. The last is especially pertinent in black women. Information obtained by these tests may be invaluable in the management of some pregnancies, particularly in regard to fetal well-being.

The patient should be tested for tuberculosis. It may be possible to avoid radiation in many patients by routine use of skin testing. If the Mantoux or Tine skin test is positive, the patient should have a roentgenogram of the chest of the conventional 14″×17″ size. This is preferable to a photofluorograph because the latter has limited accuracy and, if something suspicious is seen, the standard x-ray will be needed. Moreover, the amount of radiation received by the gonads from photofluorographs may be as high as 10 to 20 times that from conventional roentgenograms.

edema and glucosuria or symptoms such as headache, blurring of vision, dizziness or syncope.

SUBSEQUENT VISITS

At each visit, the blood pressure should be taken and the weight recorded. Hemoglobin or hematocrit should be repeated at least once late in pregnancy, at about 32 to 36 weeks. If the patient is anemic, blood counts and hemoglobin determinations should be made repeatedly after therapy is prescribed. In populations with high prevalence of gonorrhea, the cervical culture should be repeated at 36 weeks, regardless of what the earlier culture had revealed. Urine is examined at every visit for albumin and glucose. Repeat culture for bacteriuria is important, especially if significant numbers of bacteria were present earlier.

At each return visit an abdominal examination should be made and the fetal heart tones auscultated. Uterine size should be recorded. The presentation and position of the fetus, the size of its head in relation to the maternal pelvis and the possible presence of twins is noted.

Vaginal examination for the purpose of reevaluating the cephalopelvic relationships (see Chapter 12) should be done within the last two to three weeks before term. Some physicians do weekly vaginal examinations in the last month in order to detect the expected prelabor changes in the cervix. When effacement occurs in primigravidas, labor is not far off; similarly, beginning dilatation may often be encountered prior to labor in both primigravidas and multiparas.

Edema of the pretibial area should be checked for; other sites should also be examined for edema, including the face, sacral region and the fingers. The latter is reflected in a noticeable increase in the tightness of finger rings. Regular inquiry about it will uncover this important sign. Correlation of the observations made at each visit with earlier observations is essential. This holds especially for the appearance of acute weight gain, proteinuria,

ADVICE

Most of the advice given to pregnant women, both by lay and professional people, is based on our heritage of customary practice. Very few of the stringent restrictions sometimes imposed on pregnant women are based on substantive evidence. As a general rule, it is probably safe to say that most healthy pregnant women should be able to do just about everything they could do before they became pregnant without risk to them or to their fetus. Of course, this should not be carried to extremes. For example, faddistic diets are probably best avoided, and exhausting activities or potentially perilous sports are not advisable. The material that follows should serve as a guideline only. It should not be construed as rigid constraints, except where indicated.

Clothing. The manner in which an expectant mother dresses is important only in that comfort should not be sacrificed for appearance. Sufficient clothing should be worn for warmth during cold weather. Cleanliness should be stressed and the clothing kept laundered. No circular constrictions, such as garters, should be permitted so as to avoid obstructing venous and lymphatic return from the extremities. Underclothing is recommended. It should be changed and washed daily, or as often as possible, for purposes of personal hygiene.

The question of foundation supports is unanswered. Generally speaking, whether or not a patient should wear them will depend on her comfort. Backache is especially prevalent in pregnancy because of the changes in mechanical dynamics of weight bearing (see Chapter 7). It is sometimes alleviated by the support given by a properly fitted and well-constructed maternity corset. This applies especially to the obese woman with a pendulous abdomen. Despite the growing antipathy in our current culture to brassieres, many women find they need support of the breasts during pregnancy. As the breasts increase in size, undue strain is placed on Cooper's ligaments. The discomfort that ensues can be relieved by a good brassiere that provides elevation without constriction. Its use may help preserve the breast contours, an important consideration to women who are concerned about their appearance and figure.

Proper shoes are essential. It is fortunate that high heels are no longer in vogue because they seemed to increase backache, lower abdominal discomfort and fatigue. This was probably due to mechanical factors. Beyond this, women who wear high heels during pregnancy may be a bit unsteady on their feet and experience falls. Although the fetus is well protected against such trauma within the uterus, it is best to try to avoid such accidents. The best shoes for a pregnant woman are those which are comfortable and have low, broad heels. Rubber heels prevent slipping and tend to lessen the amount of jarring while walking. In the latter months of pregnancy the feet may enlarge somewhat; hence, slightly larger shoes may have to be worn for comfort.

Exercise. A pregnant woman should take a certain amount of exercise daily. Walking is especially recommended. The benefits ascribed to exercise are improvement in circulation, better appetite and digestion of food, better bowel function, restful sleep, and diversion from routine responsibilities.

The amount and kind of exercise for an expectant mother depend to a certain extent on the individual. However, she should never exercise to the point of fatigue. She should stop as soon as she begins to feel tired. Fatigue may come on very abruptly. Her tolerance will depend on the kind of life style she has led previously. Women who are accustomed to strenuous sports can generally tolerate more exercise than those who lead a sedentary life. Violent exercise should be avoided except perhaps for women who are accustomed to sports. However, moderation is probably a reasonable admonition.

Work. The American College of Obste-

tricians and Gynecologists has succinctly stated an acceptable policy based on a principle of individualization according to the patient's health, as follows: "It is desirable that the working woman see her physician during the first 2 or 3 months of pregnancy, both to verify the pregnancy and for a thorough initial examination. At this time recommendation can be made regarding work during the remainder of pregnancy. If the patient continues in good health, feels well, and the pregnancy proceeds normally, there is generally no reason why a normal working schedule cannot be continued until close to the expected date of delivery.

"The working woman, as all pregnant women, should maintain a good state of nutrition and get adequate rest and exercise. The patient and her employer should give consideration to these basic health needs in determining if a normal work schedule can be continued. Regular visits to the physician are an important part of good prenatal care and this should be taken into consideration. At these visits the patient and her physician can determine how long she should continue to work.

"Following delivery, adequate time should be allowed for complete recovery from the effects of childbirth before resuming a full work load. Six weeks is generally the time required for physiologic changes to return to normal but in individual instances a longer time may be required for this or for adjustment of feeding or other problems of baby care. A postpartum checkup is important and the physician can determine at this time if the patient is able to resume a normal work schedule."

Travel. Most women may safely undertake long journeys by train, automobile, boat or airplane without mishap. The chief drawback is that skilled obstetric care may not be available if it should become necessary during the journey or at its destination. The patient should not sit for long intervals in a car without stopping to stretch and walk about so as to avert venous stasis in the legs, thereby preventing thrombophlebitis. Similarly, aboard long air flights, the pregnant woman should walk the aisle at intervals. The hazards of hypoxia during air travel today are essentially nonexistent with pressurized cabins and the availability of oxygen in the rare event that the pressure fails.

Rest and Recreation. The prospective mother should learn to rest frequently, especially if she is continuing her business, professional or homemaking activities. Women who tire easily will find a short afternoon nap beneficial. Even if she does not actually sleep, complete relaxation in a reclining position proves refreshing. The mother with young children might take her siesta when the children take theirs. If exercise is taken during the day, there need be no fear that an afternoon nap will prevent sleeping at night. Patients who experience acute fatigue during the day will often find they will snap back quickly after a short nap or rest period.

There is no reason why patients may not continue to engage in or be spectators at various entertainments. Places of amusement may be visited, but those that are poorly ventilated, crowded or overheated are perhaps best avoided.

Bathing. Basic principles of personal hygiene should be observed. Skin care is important because its excretory function is increased in pregnancy. The gravida tends to perspire more heavily than when she is not pregnant, and at the same time she is more sensitive to odors. Daily bathing with soap and water is strongly recommended. This may take the form of a shower, sponge or tub bath in comfortably tepid water. Since the object of a bath is not only to cleanse the skin but also to stimulate the circulation of the skin, it is advisable to rub the whole body fairly vigorously. The skin may become dry and be itchy. Some women are relieved by the use of creams, such as cocoa butter, rubbed into the skin. The hair should be washed about once a week with a mild soap. There is no harm in having the hair processed, set or dyed. Care should be taken by the pregnant woman to prevent falling in the shower or tub.

Douching should be avoided during pregnancy unless required and prescribed by the physician for some local vaginal condition or infestation that calls for it.

Some women find an increase in vaginal discharge during pregnancy unassociated with any abnormality. No treatment is generally needed.

Sexual Intercourse. In general, coital activity during pregnancy should be unrestricted. Specific exceptions include those women who are threatening to abort or have a history of abortions or premature labors. Women who bleed vaginally during the current pregnancy may have to restrict or even abstain from intercourse, depending on the cause.

Routine recommendations against coitus during the final weeks of pregnancy are not well founded. Pugh and Fernandez were unable to show any untoward effects in 600 women studied. Goodlin et al., on the other hand, suggested that orgasm in late pregnancy may be associated with painful uterine contractions and with premature labor. This remains to be verified but conservative recommendations are perhaps advisable, particularly for women who have previously had premature babies. For others, full sexual activity is permissible up to term, unless the membranes are ruptured and provided the patient does not experience any discomfort during intercourse.

Mental Hygiene. The expectant mother should try, if possible, to avoid emotional turmoil. The kinds of stresses she may anticipate are detailed in Chapter 11. Many are unfortunately unavoidable, particularly those relating to marital, social and financial matters. Some, however, are possible to escape. The pregnant woman is well advised to avoid contact or conversation with friends and relatives who instill fear and anxiety by relating stories of obstetric problems and all sorts of misinformation and advice. Nowhere else is it more important for the physician to establish and maintain good communications with his patient. The patient should be made to feel she always has someone to whom she can turn for information and reassurance. She should be able to confide in her physician and discuss her every concern or fear with him.

It is recommended that the physician endeavor to discuss fully the important matters of medical costs with his patient.

Even where medical insurance covers some of the cost, the financial burden of pregnancy can be substantial, such as physician's fees, hospital charges, costs of layette and preparations at home for the new baby. The patient is well advised to be adequately prepared or to seek help from various social agencies, if necessary. Such supportive discussions with the physician can be of inestimable aid. Additional sociologic material that should eventually be covered includes marital and sexual relationships, as well as issues of responsibility, other children, in-laws and family planning.

If possible, arrangements should be made for the patient to tour the hospital facilities, especially the labor-delivery suite, nurseries and postpartum unit, so that she can become somewhat familiar with the surroundings and some of the personnel with whom she will come in contact when she delivers. Tours of this kind are conducted routinely in some hospitals and are well received. They go a long way toward allaying some of the fears encountered among pregnant women.

Symptoms. The symptoms that pregnant women complain about are many and varied. Fatigue is common as has already been discussed. Patients may suddenly become exhausted. They find that they snap back quickly after a short nap or brief rest period. This symptom starts early in pregnancy and may disappear as pregnancy advances. Frequently, it recurs in the last two or three months. Simultaneously, insomnia is not uncommon, particularly near term when physical discomfort of the enlarged uterus makes it difficult for patients to sleep. The fetus' kicking may also sometimes be quite disturbing.

The nausea and vomiting of early pregnancy are relatively common, occurring especially when the stomach is empty. This symptom generally abates by the end of the third month. Patients usually find that eating dry foods or taking smaller and more frequent meals may help. It is usually associated with excessive salivation, which can be annoying. Constipation is also quite common in pregnancy and may aggravate hemorrhoids. Heartburn is sometimes seen and may be difficult to relieve.

Various types of discomfort are frequently encountered, including backache, groin pain, and an assortment of acute, intermittent vaginal or abdominal stabbing pains. Pregnant women complain of leg cramps, particularly at night, recurrent in the calves. Urinary frequency and nocturia are common. Gravidas tend to be moody with wide swings in temperament ranging from elation to irritability to depression. Tears may appear with little provocation.

Generally, these symptoms are not manifestations of serious pathologic conditions and can be managed conservatively and symptomatically. The physician should be alert, however, to the possibility that persistent or progressive symptoms may herald the appearance of medical or surgical conditions that demand his attention. It is well to advise patients, if possible without causing undue alarm, that the following symptoms should be reported at once as possible indicators of serious problems that threaten the gravida and her fetus: any vaginal bleeding during the course of pregnancy; the appearance of puffiness of the face or tightness of the finger rings indicating digital and facial edema; headache, particularly if it is severe, continuous or unresponsive to usual analgesic agents; blurring of vision, double vision or spots before the eyes; dizziness or fainting spells; acute, persistent abdominal pain, intractable vomiting; chills or fever; pain on urination; loss of fluid from the vagina denoting the possibility of ruptured membranes.

The patient should be tactfully advised to avoid subjecting her fetus to potentially adverse effects of drugs she may take for a variety of symptoms. As a general rule, it is best to avoid any medications during pregnancy if it is at all possible. The full spectrum of effects of various pharmaceutical agents ingested by pregnant women is as yet unknown, but it is nevertheless appropriate to avoid any unnecessary risk. In prescribing medicines for the pregnant woman, the physician must continually bear in mind whether the benefits of the agent outweigh the theoretical hazards to the fetus. The fetus is also exposed to materials that are not as readily recognizable as pharmacologic agents, such as pollutants in the air, water and food, as well as material inhaled when the mother smokes. With regard to the latter, it is clearly demonstrated that smokers have smaller babies and it is advisable for women to curtail or stop smoking during pregnancy. However, it is generally accepted that the emotional strain to the gravida of such a program may exceed its benefits to the fetus. A nicety of judgment will be required on the part of the physician to permit him to make appropriate recommendations for individual patients.

REFERENCES

Goodlin, R. C., Keller, D. W., and Raffin, M.: Orgasm during late pregnancy: Possible deleterious effects. Obstet. Gynec. 38:916, 1971.

Pugh, W. E., and Fernandez, F. L.: Coitus in late pregnancy: A follow-up study of the effects of coitus on late pregnancy, delivery, and the puerperium. Obstet. Gynec. 2:636, 1953.

Chapter 10

Nutritional Considerations

Many social, cultural and familial factors influence the dietary habits of pregnant women. Aside from deficiencies that may result from special taboos and societal customs, various kinds of dietary fads are encountered from time to time. If dietary deficiencies are to be avoided, it is important that the physician try to uncover such eating habits. At the same time, it is imperative that he not contribute to the problem by unnecessarily constraining the patient with regard to arbitrary and perhaps unnecessary restrictions.

Although it is well established that increased nutritional requirements are imposed during pregnancy by the metabolic and physiologic demands of both maternal and fetal organisms, dietary restrictions in pregnancy have been introduced and accepted widely with essentially no supporting evidence to substantiate their benefits. Indeed, there is a growing body of information now available to support the opposite contention, namely, that fetal well-being, weight gain and long term outcome are all directly related to both prepregnancy weight and maternal weight gain during pregnancy.

Eastman and Jackson found that progressive increase in weight gain was paralleled by progressive increase in mean birth weight and concomitant decrease in the incidence of low weight babies. Independently, progressive increase in prepregnancy weight paralleled the progressive increase in mean birth weight and diminished incidence of low birth weight infants. The highest incidence of low weight newborn infants in their series occurred among patients with low prepregnancy weight under 120 lb. coupled with weight gains of less than 11 lb. Neonatal mortality was markedly increased in this group when compared with mortality rates for the series as a whole.

Recognizing that birth weight alone is not necessarily the single best indicator of reproductive success, Singer et al. confirmed that high maternal weight gain is related to higher birth weight and decreased prematurity rate, while also showing better growth and performance during the infant's first year of life. They proposed that doing away with the traditional obstetric practice of keeping weight gain during pregnancy to a minimum might significantly reduce the incidence of prematurity and its attendant mortality and morbidity.

This concept, of course, is completely contrary to widely held clinical obstetric practice which has emphasized the value of low weight gain during pregnancy. The basis for weight control admonitions in antepartum care apparently stems from the recognized significance of acute weight gain preceding or associated with onset of preeclampsia (see Chapter 36). It is apparent that there needs to be a clear-cut distinction between such acute weight gain on the basis of fluid retention and long-term pregnancy weight gain that is appropriate and reasonably expected according to the physiologic changes that occur during pregnancy. The controversy in this regard is unsettled at this time. However, there appears to be ample evidence to suggest that stringent weight restrictions during pregnancy are not necessarily a good practice, whereas moderate weight gain is by the same token not harmful.

It is probable that the normal average weight gain of a healthy patient in pregnancy, whose diet is wholesome, well balanced and unrestricted, is about 25 lb. This is consistent with the findings of the average weight gain in pregnancy of nor-

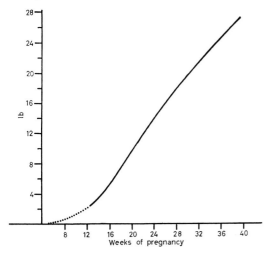

Figure 99 Progressive increase in mean weight during pregnancy of 2868 normotensive primigravidas showing essentially linear increase from the twelfth week to term and suggesting that the practice of stringent weight limitation is unphysiological. (From Thomson, A. M., and Billewicz, W. Z.: Cited in Hytten, F. E., and Leitch, I.: The Physiology of Human Pregnancy. Oxford, Blackwell, 1967.)

son). In relative terms, most of the increment attributable to the conceptus occurs in the second half of pregnancy, while maternal stores are laid down rather early. Much of this latter appears to be fatty tissue, especially in the area of the hips, as demonstrated by serial skinfold thickness measurements (Taggart et al.), and in central sites.

Recommendations against weight control probably apply to the issue of excessive weight gain during pregnancy insofar as it will result in the development of permanent obesity. Whereas many patients who gain excessively during pregnancy will lose it again spontaneously after delivery, most do not return to their normal weight unless they make strong efforts to do so. However, it is advisable not to attempt weight control or weight reduction during pregnancy because of the likelihood that nutritional deficiencies will result.

motensive primigravidas encountered by Thomson and Billewicz (Fig. 99). This can be accounted for approximately as follows: fetus 7 to 8 lb., placenta 1.5 lb., amniotic fluid 2 lb., increase in uterine mass 2 lb., blood volume 3 to 4 lb., and breasts 1 to 2 lb. Some of the remainder is undoubtedly accounted for on the basis of increased interstitial fluid.

Most of the normal weight gain occurs during the second half of pregnancy at a rate of about 1 lb. per week. The relative components of the weight gain change progressively with advancing pregnancy as shown in Figure 100 (Hytten and Thom-

CALORIES

Pregnancy is a period of metabolic and physiologic change for the mother, involving all organs and organ systems of the body. Requirements for dietary essentials are increased according to the additional demands made by changes within the mother and by the growing fetus. During intrauterine life fetal growth and development are at their most rapid of the entire life cycle. The only nutrient sources for them are the mother's diet and body stores. The ancient concept that the fetus

Figure 100 The relative increments in the components of weight gain during normal pregnancy, illustrating the relatively early deposition of maternal stores and late increase attributable to the fetus and placenta. (From Hytten, F. E., and Thomson, A. M.: In Assali, N. S. (ed.): Biology of Gestation. Vol. 1. New York, Academic Press, 1968.)

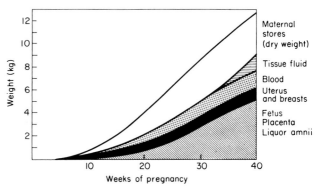

will take what it needs from the mother regardless of her nutritional status or deficiency has been shown to be invalid. Although it is true that the fetus is parasitic on the mother to the degree that it depends on her nutritional status and her diet during pregnancy for its resources, it has been amply demonstrated that the fetus may remain deficient when the mother is nutritionally depleted.

It is clearly inappropriate for the mother to "eat for two," but she does have increased demands on her during pregnancy. If such requirements are inadequately satisfied, her nutritional status and the condition of the fetus will be adversely affected.

Firm data on specific requirements are not available from experimental work, but certain general principles have been established and are accepted. It has been computed, for example, that the increased total calorie requirements for pregnancy should be around 80,000 kilocalories, of which half is accounted for by increased fat storage. This is based on the total extra nutritional requirement needed for the growth of the fetus, placenta and associated maternal tissues, on the increase in basal metabolic rate of the mother, and on the increased expenditure of energy by the mother involved in carrying an increased body weight during pregnancy.

Excluding the nonessential fat accumulation, the 40,000 kcal. essential requirement of pregnancy is represented by an additional daily increment of about 200 kcal. to the normal diet, or the equivalent of a total weight gain of 25 lb. This does not take into account the reduced physical activity that so commonly occurs with pregnancy, diminishing the energy requirements proportionally. It is probable that the healthy pregnant woman actually needs no additional intake of food because of the balance achieved by restricted physical activity. This, of course, does not apply to women whose socioeconomic state demands continued energy expenditures throughout pregnancy.

imately 950 gm. Balance studies show increased nitrogen retention of 200 to 400 gm. in excess of that needed by the fetus and reproductive organs. During the last half of pregnancy, a daily increase of 6 gm. appears necessary. The National Research Council (NRC) recommends a daily intake of 55 gm. for the nonpregnant adult and 65 gm. in pregnancy.

The biological value of a protein tends to be determined in terms of the relative components of amino acids it contains. It is generally agreed that animal proteins are better nutritional sources for the pregnant woman. Emphasis should be placed on adequate intake of eggs and milk, both of which may be considered valuable adjuncts to the diet. The relatively poor contribution of most plant proteins in this regard suggests the potential hazards of diets consisting almost entirely of such foodstuffs, whether this be the result of poverty, unavailability, custom, taboo or faddism.

Pregnancy requirements for nitrogen include: fetus 60 gm., placenta 19 gm., uterus 39 gm., breasts 17 gm., for a total of 135 gm. of nitrogen that is extracted from the diet from protein metabolism. This amount is equivalent to a daily utilization of 0.5 gm. in excess of that of nonpregnant adult females. Zuspan and Goodrich showed an average total storage in pregnancy of 515 gm., or 1.8 gm. daily, 80 per cent of which was stored after the fourth month of pregnancy. After the fifth month, the daily storage amounted to 3.5 gm.

On the basis of these data, the protein equivalents of 12.5 to 21.5 gm. should be added to the recommended levels of protein intake, bringing the total daily intake to 85 gm. In practice, however, such high-protein diets tend to result in high caloric intake owing to the increased amount of fat content. At the same time, because not all proteins contain all essential amino acids in appropriate relative proportion, it is sometimes recommended that an excess of proteins be taken to ensure adequacy.

PROTEINS

Protein requirements are clearly increased during pregnancy, totaling approx-

CALCIUM

The fetus acquires about 30 gm. of calcium, mostly during the third trimester.

During pregnancy, maternal metabolic adaptations result in mechanisms for absorbing and conserving calcium from the gastrointestinal tract in a more efficient manner. Exact quantitation of these adaptive mechanisms, however, has not yet been accomplished. It is estimated that the additional daily intake of 350 mg. of calcium that would be needed during the third trimester to supply the fetal requirements can be met with an additional maternal dietary intake of about 300 mg. NRC recommends a daily calcium intake of 1.2 gm., which is 400 mg. in excess of the nonpregnant adult requirements.

The total calcium needs of the pregnant woman constitute about 2.5 per cent of that which is in stores in her skeleton (Hytten and Leitch). There is little doubt that the fetal requirements can be met from the maternal stores, but with diminishing likelihood in successive pregnancies unless supplemented. Without replenishment, maternal osteomalacia and fetal rickets have been reported.

IRON

The total iron requirement of pregnancy is approximately 800 mg. This includes about 300 mg. of iron needed for the increase in total maternal circulating red cell volume, 300 mg. contained in the full-term fetus, 70 mg. in the placenta, and about 50 mg. or more in blood loss at delivery. There is about 150 mg. compensation in the reduced loss based on cessation of menstruation during pregnancy. Most of the iron demands occur during the second half of pregnancy.

Unfortunately, many women begin pregnancy with markedly reduced stores of iron. Indeed, more than 20 per cent have no storage iron at all (Monsen et al.). Since the average American diet provides between 5 and 15 mg. of iron daily, of which only about one-tenth is absorbed, it is quite clear that the iron requirements of pregnancy cannot be met without supplementation in women with depleted or absent iron stores.

The total increment of iron needs can theoretically be met with a daily intake of 6 mg. during the last half of pregnancy.

There is evidence that iron absorption is increased. The proportion of ingested iron absorbed is increased from the 10 per cent level of nonpregnancy to as high as 40 per cent (Hahn et al.). Therefore, the NRC recommendation that normal diets should be supplemented with 30 to 60 mg. of iron daily during pregnancy is defensible.

This can be supplied as ferrous sulfate, fumarate or gluconate in oral form. Usual doses may cause gastric distress, colicky pain and diarrhea, but these symptoms can be minimized if medication is administered just following meals. There is probably no truth to the claims made that gastrointestinal intolerance to some iron preparations is diminished, because such reactions are primarily a function of the total amount of soluble elemental iron per dose rather than related to the form in which the iron is administered (Goodman and Gilman). Use of various adjuvant substances to aid absorption and utilization, including ascorbic acid and emulsifying agents, tends to be rather ineffectual and costly.

FOLIC ACID

The folic acid requirements of pregnancy are not known with precision, although it has been suggested that the minimum intake of this substance necessary to maintain serum folate levels may be as high as 300 µg. daily. Overt folate deficiencies are rare in the United States, but there has been recent interest generated by the correlation determined to exist between subclinical maternal folate deficiency and obstetric disorders, including abruptio placentae, preeclampsia and anomalous infants (Strief and Little).

The relationship has not been verified by other investigators, nor have attempts to reduce pregnancy wastage by means of folic acid supplementation been successful. Nevertheless, serum folate levels do decline significantly, especially in the last trimester of pregnancy, with or without neutrophilic hypersegmentation and the appearance of megaloblasts in the peripheral circulation. Rarely will overt megaloblastic anemia develop.

Folates are ubiquitous in foodstuffs, appearing in relatively large amounts in yeast, liver and fresh green vegetables. Much of the folate content of foods is destroyed by protracted cooking or by canning. It is likely that pregnancy requirements are met by an adequate, well-balanced diet. Supplemental intake of as little as 0.1 mg. daily will maintain serum folate levels during pregnancy, while 1 mg. is adequate therapy even for severe megaloblastic anemia. Routine use of such supplements, although recommended by NRC, is not firmly founded. The NRC recommendation includes a daily supplement of 200 to 400 μg. of folic acid (0.2 to 0.4 mg. folacin), especially in instances where folate requirements are high, such as in chronic hemolytic anemia and multiple pregnancy.

IODINE

Iodine requirements are increased in pregnancy as evidenced by the high incidence of goiter in areas where this is endemic. The magnitude of the pregnancy demands for this element is unknown, but it is wise to ensure that iodinated salt, for example, is utilized by gravidas. This holds especially, of course, in areas where there is a deficiency in natural iodine sources and where goiter is prevalent. NRC recommends that 25 μg. iodine be given to supplement daily dietary intake, bringing the total to 125 μg. in such regions.

FLUORIDE

Fluoride supplements have not been demonstrated to be of any significance to the fetus. This is as might be expected in view of the very early state of development of fetal dentition *in utero*.

VITAMINS

Except for supplemental iron, there is essentially no substantive evidence to support the widespread prophylactic use of vi-

tamin and mineral preparations by pregnant women in the United States. NRC clearly states: "Vitamin and mineral supplements should not be routinely instituted as a means for correcting poor food habits. In considering the wisdom of recommending them, the relative cost, as compared to enhancing the nutrient intake with foods, should be taken into account, especially in caring for pregnant women with inadequate incomes."

Avitaminoses can result, however, from severe, prolonged dietary deficiencies. Vitamin A needs total 50 μg. daily during the last half of pregnancy to provide for the fetal stores of about 7000 μg. in its liver (Gopalan). This is an insignificant fractional increment over total normal daily requirement and intake of 750 μg., suggesting that no special dietary allowance is necessary under normal circumstances in pregnancy. The malnourished woman, however, does clearly need such supplementation.

Fetal storage of vitamin B_{12} is about 50 to 100 μg. which can be provided by an additional daily absorption of 0.1 to 0.2 μg. This can be assured by supplementation with 1 μg. of vitamin B_{12} daily. NRC recommends 3 μg. be added to the usual daily dietary allowance of 5 μg. Such supplementation is imperative in those regions where megaloblastic anemias are common to ensure that adequate levels are provided.

Quantitation of other dietary elements in terms of pregnancy needs is less certain in that there is little clear-cut evidence to support recommendations. Nevertheless, some items are sufficiently well documented that supplementation may be necessary where indicated. These latter include: vitamin D to ensure proper calcium absorption and utilization, especially in patients insufficiently exposed to sunlight; vitamin C, especially during lactation; as well as thiamine, riboflavin, niacin and pyridoxine. The NRC recommendations are summarized in Table 4.

SALT

Dietary restriction of salt intake will be discussed in Chapter 36. The evidence

TABLE 4 RECOMMENDED DAILY DIETARY ALLOWANCES*

	Nonpregnant	Pregnant
Calories (kcal.)	2000	2200
Protein (gm.)	55	65
Calcium (gm.)	0.8	1.2
Iron (mg.)	18	18†
Vitamin A (I.U.)	5000	6000
Thiamine (mg.)	1.0	1.1
Riboflavin (mg.)	1.5	1.8
Niacin (mg. equiv.)	13	15
Ascorbic acid (mg.)	55	65
Vitamin D (I.U.)	400	400

*For women aged 22 to 35 years, 58 kg. weight and 163 cm. height. Recommendations require modification according to body habitus, age, physical activity, environmental factors and preexisting deficiencies.
†It is recommended that diet be supplemented with 30 to 60 mg. iron daily.
From NRC Committee on Maternal Nutrition, 1970.

supporting this almost universal practice is meager and rather dubious. Moreover, when pursued in conjunction with diuretics, ostensibly to prevent preeclampsia, it is potentially hazardous. Continuation of this practice must be questioned because neither safety nor value appears to warrant it.

ADOLESCENT GRAVIDA

A special problem exists for the pregnant teen-ager. In addition to the nutritional demands of pregnancy, she presents needs of her own in terms of continuing growth. Thus, she cannot tolerate caloric deprivation well. It is imperative that there be no stringent caloric restriction in such patients, even if they are obese. Many pregnant adolescents are in poor nutritional state, whether because they have been pursuing a program of dietary restriction volitionally or because of socioeconomic constraints. Such patients are particularly vulnerable to the metabolic demands of pregnancy and may demonstrate deficiency states themselves or the results of such deficiencies in the fetus. Good dietary control with supplementation is usually necessary under these circumstances. Emphasis should be placed on caloric, protein and calcium requirements.

REFERENCES

Eastman, N. J., and Jackson, E.: Weight relationships in pregnancy: I. The bearing of maternal weight gain and pre-pregnancy weight on birth weight in full term pregnancies. Obstet. Gynec. Survey 23:1003, 1968.

Goodman, L. S., and Gilman, A.: The Pharmacological Basis of Therapeutics, ed. 4. New York, The Macmillan Company, 1970.

Gopalan, C.: Nutrition. In Phillip, E. E., Barnes, J., and Newton, M., eds.: Scientific Foundations of Obstetrics and Gynecology. Philadelphia, F. A. Davis, 1970.

Hahn, P. F., Carothers, E. L., Darby, W. J., Martin, M., Sheppard, C. W., Cannon, R. O., Beam, A. S., Denson, P. M., Peterson, J. C., and McClellan, A. S.: Iron metabolism in human pregnancy as studied with radioactive isotope Fe⁵⁹. Amer. J. Obstet. Gynec. 61:481, 1951.

Hytten, F. E., and Leitch, I.: The Physiology of Human Pregnancy. Oxford, Blackwell, 1967.

Hytten, F. E., and Thomson, A. M.: Maternal physiological adjustments. In Assali, N. S., ed.: Biology of Gestation, Vol. 1. New York, Academic Press, 1968.

Monsen, E. R., Kahn, I. N., and Finch, C. A.: Iron status of menstruating women. Amer. J. Clin. Nutr. 20:842, 1967.

National Research Council Committee on Maternal Nutrition: Maternal Nutrition and the Course of Pregnancy: Summary Report. Washington, National Academy of Sciences, 1970.

Singer, J. E., Westphal, M., and Niswander, K.: Relationship of weight gain during pregnancy to birth weight and infant growth and development in the first year of life. Obstet. Gynec. 31:417, 1968.

Streif, R. R., and Little, A. B.: Folic acid deficiency in pregnancy. New Eng. J. Med. 276:776, 1967.

Taggart, N. R., Holliday, R. M., Billewicz, W. Z., Hytten, F. E., and Thomson, A. M.: Changes in skinfolds during pregnancy. Brit. J. Nutr. 21:439, 1967.

Thomson, A. M., and Billewicz, W. Z.: Clinical significance of weight trends during pregnancy. Brit. Med. J. 1:243, 1957.

Zuspan, F. P., and Goodrich, S.: Metabolic studies in normal pregnancy: I. Nitrogen metabolism. Amer. J. Obstet. Gynec. 100:7, 1968.

Chapter 11

Psychologic Aspects

All pregnancies, probably without exception, are associated with emotional conflicts. This notwithstanding, doctors are all too often unaware of the importance of the psychologic problems attendant upon pregnancy, concentrating their attention almost entirely on prevention and treatment of somatic disorders. The physician who ignores the emotional stresses of his patients, or is unwilling or unable to discuss them, is not providing complete care. There is little doubt that one of the best services that a physician can provide to his patient is in this discipline. It is imperative that every physician who manages the care of pregnant women should be thoroughly versed and knowledgeable in such relevant psychiatric matters.

Many patients, regardless of whether or not the pregnancy was planned, develop intense feelings of resentment, fear or anger. Ambivalence is very common, taking the form of overt acceptance conflicting with an inward rejection. Feelings of guilt and shame are not unusual, especially among unmarried gravidas, but may even be present where social pressures do not exist. Some women look forward to their "ordeal" with great dread because they consider pregnancy, labor and delivery as terrifying prospects. Phobias relevant to pain, mutilation and death occur, as do anxieties concerning the fetus, particularly with regard to the possibility of its being defective. Moreover, even the most stable women express concern over what the pregnancy means to them in terms of increased economic burdens, especially if it signifies loss of the patient's own wage earning capabilities, and the new or increased personal responsibilities it will entail. The sensitive physician will be able to establish good rapport with his patient and provide her with sufficient security to permit her to speak to him on such subjects without fear of embarrassment or moralization.

Pregnancy constitutes one of life's major stresses. It tends to be a time of emotional crisis because of the kinds of complex motivations which are involved. Although it represents the fulfillment of the biological reproductive function, "The biological capacity for procreation does not imply that a woman's psychological makeup is in conformity with her condition" (Wengraf). Besides the potential for pregnancy to exacerbate or reactivate a preexisting mental illness, it is stressful even for women who have been functioning quite normally and who appear to have been in very good emotional health prior to conception. Some women may be motivated in a complex and bizarre fashion to conceive on the basis of the desire to cement their marriage or, in the case of the unmarried girl, to entrap. Others may be complying with social expectations or conceiving out of a sense of identification with their own mothers. In recent years, some pregnancies appear to have resulted from a desire on the part of the gravida to punish her parents. Deep hostility is manifested in such patients by outbursts of rage or other irrational conduct, or, where this is repressed, by nearly total incapacitation.

The sources of anxiety are manifold. Fears may be overtly expressed or hidden. It is important for the physician to try to uncover these and to discuss them openly. The woman who appears happy and carefree may be suppressing intense feelings of trepidation that should be allayed. Ambivalence may take the form of hostility against the fetus because it has caused the patient to become unsightly (in her eyes) and uncomfortable, and is threatening her sexuality or security. Anxieties may arise over the possibilities that activity or diet or medication may adversely affect the growing fetus. Conflicts may strain the patient's relationship with her husband or family or physician.

Moreover, most patients have pressing questions concerning pregnancy physiology and the development of the fetus, as well as an understandable interest in analgesia, anesthesia and the management of labor and delivery. Unless the physician is willing to give of himself in terms of interest, the patient's fears will not be alleviated. It is vital that he instill the kind of confidence that only a physician who does not appear to be too busy to talk can provide. Patients are very sensitive indeed to subtle signals from their physicians indicating that they are irritated or annoyed or bored and cannot be bothered with such trivia. It should be made quite apparent that these matters are worthy of full disclosure and discussion. They should not be brushed aside or ignored in a cavalier manner.

From the therapeutic point of view, there can be little doubt that the primary goal of our approach to obstetric patients is to establish strong rapport. This entails the development of an authoritative dependency to provide the patient with security for discussing any subject she has on her mind without fear of any kind. For the physician to be able to accept the responsibility that this dependency requires, it is essential that he comprehend the psychodynamics of the woman who is pregnant. One of the best available short discourses on the subject is that by Heiman to which the reader is referred for details of this mechanism from the psychoanalytic point of view. Fuller understanding of the psychologic processes affords the physician keen insight into the patterns of behavior of his pregnant patients. The greater his knowledge in this regard the better his patients will be cared for on the basis of his ability to deal with their behavioral problems.

Briefly stated, from the psychologic vantage point pregnancy is a state involving both maturation and regression. As a "maturational crisis," it is a critical phase leading to motherhood and all its attendant responsibilities and obligations. The woman is transformed from her own mother's child to her child's mother, a role she must assume at the conclusion of her pregnancy. This process involves an interval during which she may find that she must confront and try to resolve any earlier conflicts that she has had with her own mother.

At the same time, the situation is compounded by a regressive psychologic process. This takes the form of the patient identifying with her fetus so that she may begin to behave, feel and function in certain aspects like a child. The normal regression that takes place during pregnancy is emphasized by Heiman as a key to the understanding of a great many psychopathologic symptoms. The obstetrician should be thoroughly aware of the existence of regression in his patients, particularly so that he can comprehend and deal with the childlike fears that exist. Moreover, awareness that the pregnant woman is as suggestible as some children is of enormous benefit in terms of his ability to provide reassurance and security.

A clear understanding of these psychodynamic mechanisms will also permit the physician to understand and avoid contributing to problem manifestations. The commonly encountered admixture of ambivalent feelings toward pregnancy, for example, may be unwittingly promoted by the physician. On the one hand, he repeatedly and appropriately reassures his patient that childbirth is a normal, physiologic experience; on the other hand, he negates these reassurances by admonishing her concerning potential hazards and restrictions that may lead to significant danger to her and to her fetus.

It is obvious that the physician must individualize according to his patient's ego strengths. Most require and clearly deserve to be given full reassurance regarding specific and general matters that are of concern to them. In general, this seems to suffice, perhaps because of their increased suggestibility. On this basis it is the general experience that most phobias can be easily managed with simple, confident statements of assurance. Since most fears are entirely unrealistic, such authoritative assurances usually suffice. It is probably unwise to attempt to provide detailed scientific explanations or to discuss statistical probabilities under such circumstances, unless in response to specific questions.

With regard to unexpressed fears, most are perhaps based on deep-rooted fears of childhood, or, more prevalently, fear of the unknown. Concerning the latter, most women are readily relieved of such worries once they are thoroughly informed, making the situation considerably less stressful and more interesting to them. The effect of removing the fear response to stress as it relates to pain perception is the underlying basis for the psychoprophylactic approach to childbearing (see below).

The intensified suggestibility of women who have undergone pregnancy regression is probably the basis for the success of some authoritative physicians who deal with their patients' anxieties without ever having achieved insight into or knowledge of them. Such physicians, by their very authoritarian nature, engender confidence and a protective charisma. They dispel fears on a nonverbal level in patients who have developed deep trust in them. The regressed patients in their hands are treated much the same as they would treat children who derive assurance and self-confidence from their strength. Interestingly, it is the same childlike suggestibility that provides for the measure of success of psychoprophylactic techniques in allaying anxiety and pain (see below).

There are many varieties of manifestations that the emotional upheaval of pregnancy may take. They range from somaticized symptoms, such as ptyalism and hyperemesis, to palpitations, sleeplessness, confusion and/or malaise. The patient may be depressed or manic. She may express suicidal thoughts or the urge to destroy the fetus. Where reassurance and symptomatic treatment are ineffectual, psychiatric evaluation should be sought. The relationship of such serious manifestations to the issue of continuing the pregnancy or terminating it will be discussed at length in Chapter 35.

The common occurrence of depression during the immediate puerperium, the so-called blues, occurs at a time when the new mother must readjust to her separation from the fetus (analogous to the loss of a love object) and establish a new relationship with her newborn child. Puerperal depression constitutes an anticlimactic letdown. The patient tends to be irritable and unreasonable. She may burst into tears without provocation. She is moody and unresponsive. Generally, these episodes are mild and self-limiting, lasting no more than a few days. There is cause for concern only if they persist and are associated with unremitting lack of interest in the infant. They may be minimized or even averted by anticipatory discussions between physician and patient in which the patient can be forewarned appropriately and advised concerning their benignancy. Characteristically, the severely affected patient feels weakness, apathy, insomnia and loss of appetite and libido. Rare instances of psychotic decompensation that occur post partum are undoubtedly triggered to develop during this stressful time in a patient with underlying predisposition. It cannot be implied that the common postpartum depression is in any way generically related to organic psychopathology. The prognosis for the usually encountered minor case of blues is excellent.

The dependency relationship that frequently develops between doctor and patient is based largely on a transference phenomenon. The patient relates to her physician as she may have related to her mother or father or husband. This may provide salutary or harmful effects. She may come to rely upon him for security and relief of anxieties. This can be used very effectively by the informed physician as we have indicated above. On the other hand, deep affections may develop of a sexual nature that may threaten the physician's role in the community. It is imperative that the physician avoid such entanglements lest he destroy his effectiveness and endanger his career. Nevertheless, the dependency aspects of patients, when understood and accepted for what they are by the physician, can be used to advantage in caring for patients appropriately.

Above all, the doctor must act as a sounding board for his patient. He must be available to answer all her questions—voiced and unexpressed—to allay her fears, provide emotional support and inspire confidence. The physician can make it easier for the patient to be able to experience the difficult adjustment to pregnancy and its problems and responsibilities in this way. Her pregnancy can then be a fulfilling and highly rewarding experience to her. The patient who is thus able to take a positive attitude toward her pregnancy will most likely be able to relate well to the fetus both while it is within her womb and after it is born. A growing body of evidence suggests that poor mother-child relationships are detrimental to optimal development of the child. Such serious pathologic processes can have their origin in pregnancy based on the poor emotional preparation of the mother and her negativistic association with the fetus. The physician's role in correcting such attitudinal disorders is, therefore, of utmost importance.

PSYCHOPROPHYLACTIC PREPARATION

Psychologic preparation of women for childbearing has occupied much attention in recent decades. Its history has unfortunately been marked by exaggerated enthusiasm countered with vehement skepticism. There can now be little doubt that the approach has been demonstrated to be quite effective. It is its theoretical basis that remains unclear and controversial. The terminology is rather confused as well. Read, who introduced "natural childbirth" in 1933, later modified his designation to "childbirth without fear." The Neo-Pavlovian approach introduced by Velvovski in 1944 was called "psychoprophylaxis of the pains of childbirth." This latter has been modified to "psychoprophylactic preparation of pregnant women for childbirth," and has been superseded in practice by more than a dozen related names (Buxton). Its great popularity in Western Europe and belatedly in this hemisphere can undoubtedly be ascribed to Lamaze, who introduced it into France in 1952 after his visit to Russia. His name is still widely applied to the method he popularized. Although not entirely synonymous, we will use the various terms interchangeably.

All psychoprophylactic techniques appear to be based on essentially the same Pavlovian concept of conditioned reflex training. Painful sensations appear to be blocked by counterstimulus. There are various technical approaches in common use. Their differences tend to be minimal, all containing elements of didactic, physiotherapeutic and psychotherapeutic aspects. The psychotherapeutic factors are undoubtedly of most importance in effecting analgesia. Unfortunately, results are still rather difficult to evaluate in the absence of objective criteria for pain. Nonetheless, great enthusiasm has been generated by the many women and their physicians who have had good experiences in this area.

Read believed that childbirth pain was a pathologic response produced by fear, apprehension and tension. Although physiologically debatable (Chertok), this concept was the basis for his approach to the elimination of the pain of parturition through a mechanism of the correction of these psychologic attitudes. He felt it essential to teach the women anatomic and physiologic facts relating to the act of childbirth. Physical and mental relaxation were carefully taught, concentrating on respiratory exercises (Heardman). Both approaches are alleged to diminish pain by familiarizing the pregnant woman with the process of childbirth and by creating an atmosphere of confidence. Stressed above all is the essential requirement for the establishment of a good relationship between the doctor and the patient. Read openly stressed the dependency for success on "his patients' faith and his conscious or unconscious powers of suggestion."

It is easy to understand, on the basis of our earlier discussion concerning regression in pregnancy, that one could put the coassociated increased suggestibility of patients to good use in this way. It seems to be established that, although physical training is a useful adjunct, the Read method works best when it cultivates faith, dedication and trust both in the method and in the authoritative figurehead, whether it be monitrice (the instructor-guide-helper) or the physician.

There have been many modifications of Read's original approach. Introduction of the psychoprophylactic technique by Lamaze has further complicated the issue because of ostensible differences in approach. This has unfortunately created much confusion and controversy. In the overview, the conflict seems quite unnecessary because they share so many good features. There are differences insofar as theoretical basis and the technical details of exercise, respiration and relaxation are concerned, but the objectives are the same and they appear to have essentially equivalent effectiveness in terms of pain relief for individual patients.

Course material for childbirth preparation classes includes growth of the embryo, anatomy and physiology of the generative organs, adaptation to pregnancy, signs and symptoms of pregnancy, diet during pregnancy, signs and symptoms of onset of labor, the stages of labor, physiology and progress of labor and the process of delivery. Additionally, some courses deal with postpartum care, rooming-in, breast care and baby care.

The presence of the husband during labor and delivery is a matter of growing popularity, particularly in the setting of psychoprophylactic preparation. The enthusiasts hold that he may be of considerable psychologic assistance to the mother. Moreover, his presence may serve a useful function in producing closer marital ties, consolidating the family unit and providing for a warm and intensely meaningful experience at childbirth. The issue, however, is far from settled. Although it is likely that many husbands would indeed serve such contributory roles, others might not. Their presence can be emotionally upsetting to them, particularly if they are not properly prepared. Furthermore, if they faint, they may injure themselves or contaminate the area. Some women may insist that their husbands attend in order to ensure that they will share in their "suffering." These situations are quite clearly exceptional, however, and should not in any way be interpreted as deprecation of the practice. Most husbands can be very helpful in this psychologically trying situation. "The ideal joy, love and togetherness described as existing when the young father and mother achieve the actuality of those first moments with their newborn together is of course a beautiful and sublime aspect of parenthood" (Buxton).

Needless to say, psychoprophylactic preparation is not without its drawbacks. One of the most severe and probably justifiable criticisms is that all patients may be accepted into such programs with no preliminary screening. The results may be disastrous for psychiatrically disturbed individuals. The answer is, of course, that such patients might do just as disastrously, if not worse, without the education and preparation. In the absence of objectivity whereby one could appropriately evaluate the results of such programs, their enthusiastic acceptance is still without scientific substantiation. Reported results indicate a high proportion of effectiveness in terms of minimization of analgesia and anesthesia. These data serve as splendid testimonials to the method, but as yet cannot be considered to constitute proof. Many questions remain unanswered.

Second only to this is the misguided enthusiasm of some of its proponents. Concern is particularly applicable to those who willingly or inadvertently convince patients that labor is of necessity painless and analgesia or anesthesia, if it should become necessary to administer it, constitutes a failure on the part of the patient. This cultist attitude places some women, whose psyche may be somewhat unstable to begin with, in serious jeopardy with regard to the development of great feelings of anxiety and guilt. Such feelings will be magnified to pathologic levels if the infant is not completely normal. The essential mother-child relationship alluded to above may be adversely affected by such feelings. Severe depression under these circumstances can sometimes be expected.

Thus, it is imperative that the educational and training aspects of the psychoprophylactic programs be tempered with logic and reason. Extremism must be avoided. There can be no question that the woman who understands what is happening to her and is prepared emotionally for the process of parturition will do better than one who is not. Problems center on the woman who insists to the point of fanaticism on "natural childbirth" in the presence of a clear-cut need for analgesic or anesthetic intervention.

ROOMING-IN AND FAMILY-CENTERED CARE

A more recent outgrowth of "natural childbirth" programs are the concepts of rooming-in and family-centered care. A small but growing number of hospitals have an arrangement whereby the baby may room-in with the new mother. This requires special physical and nursing facilities, but its advantages are many. The mother can learn how to care for her infant and to acquaint herself with its habits before returning home. It allows for the development of natural mother and baby relationships.

Psychologically, separation of mother from baby may have disadvantages, particularly as it may interfere with certain essential psychologic needs of both mother and child. Imposition of a rigid visiting and feeding schedule does not properly consider the newborn's needs and developmental changes or the mother's particular stresses in her adjustments to her new role. In the rooming-in system the infant is on a demand feeding schedule so that mothers tend not to get as much rest in the hospital as they might otherwise. This small disadvantage is generally outweighed by its benefits in terms of the fostering of mother-child relationships.

Rooming-in units may consist of a two or four bassinet nursery adjacent to the patients' room. The mother can thus have her baby with her as much or as little as she desires. Such arrangements require that nursing and medical personnel understand and display the special attitudes of maternity care necessary for success of this important undertaking. The physical arrangement has as its objective the fostering of a more natural and healthy initiation of family life. The mother is promptly able to attend to the needs of her infant, especially if she desires to breast feed it. She quickly learns how to take care of her baby and what to expect of it. Similarly, the father is able to become intimately acquainted with the newborn infant. The atmosphere is conducive to learning in an informal, permissive and relaxed facility. The parents are encouraged to ask questions freely and to discuss them with nurses and physicians. The parents have leisure to observe and learn. There is ample opportunity for contact with the child so as to gain complete confidence in its care before returning home.

The fewer the rules and the fewer the unpleasant distractions the better. The constant presence of the baby in the mother's room or in the adjoining nursery will be reassuring. When she goes home she will not be caring for a delicate stranger. She will have developed some sense of togetherness and will have learned that the demands of her newborn infant are not very great. Although it has been stated that too early exposure to the child may create fear and tension for some women, this rarely actually takes place. Moreover, it is much better to uncover such problems in the hospital rather than to await their development at home where supervision, support and instruction are unavailable. Rooming-in may also serve to establish an earlier and easier father-child relationship. Parental relations are clearly better if both parents learn to know and to care for the infant during the first weeks of life. The child is most impressionable during this time and this is probably the optimal time to educate the parents concerning how to give the infant the love and security it will need during its formative years.

Family-centered care is a further modification recently introduced. It consists of inclusion of the husband as part of the puerperal unit. He is not considered a visitor, but is instead integrated into the postpartum care arrangement. In this way, the close husband-wife relationships established and fostered during labor and delivery may be maintained and further augmented. The husband participates in changing and feeding the baby (if it is bottle fed), thus developing some insight into his essential role in the family unit.

The goal of family-centered care programs is to ensure that the mother has the best possible experience during pregnancy, labor and puerperium, enabling her to share this experience with the baby's father, both returning home confident in their ability to care for the baby. The approach treats childbearing as a normal and healthy process and as a major family experience for all concerned. It provides the wherewithal for parents to get to know the new baby and to begin to function as a family unit under guidance and in the security of the hospital environment. Each mother may have her baby with her as much or as little as she desires (with constraints imposed during general hospital visiting hours). Fathers may be present at all times throughout the day to participate in baby care activities. They are afforded hospital courtesies, congeniality and good sound teaching. Thus, they leave the hospital having been provided an opportunity to gain confidence, security and a positive attitude toward parenthood.

Staff reeducation is generally essential before this type of approach can be introduced into a hospital unit in order to ensure success. Enthusiasm, cooperation and acceptance by nurses and physicians are prerequisites. The rewards in terms of improved patient care and attitudes are many and make the effort well worthwhile.

REFERENCES

Buxton, C. L.: A Study of Psychophysical Methods for Relief of Childbirth Pain. Philadelphia, W. B. Saunders Company, 1962.

Chertok, L.: Psychosomatic Methods in Painless Childbirth: History, Theory and Practice. London, Pergamon Press, 1959.

Heardman, H.: Relaxation and Exercise for Natural Childbirth. Edinburgh, E. & S. Livingstone, Ltd., 1955.

Heiman, M.: A psychoanalytic view of pregnancy. *In* Rovinsky, J. J., and Guttmacher, A. F., eds.: Medical, Surgical and Gynecologic Complications of Pregnancy, ed. 2. Baltimore, Williams & Wilkins Company, 1965.

Lamaze, F., and Vellay, P.: L'accouchement sans douleur par la méthode psychophysique: Premiers résultats portant sur 500 cas. Gaz. Méd. Franç. 59:1445, 1952.

Read, G. D.: Natural Childbirth. London, William Heinemann, Ltd., 1933.

Velvovski, I. Z.: Psychoprophylaxis of the pains of childbirth: A complex system. Pediat. Akush. Ginek. 3:18, 1951.

Wengraf, F.: Psychosomatic Approach to Gynecology and Obstetrics. Springfield, Ill., Charles C Thomas, Publishers, 1953.

Chapter 12

Evaluation of the Pelvis

Every patient who presents herself for obstetric care should have her pelvis evaluated to determine its adequacy for vaginal delivery. Digital pelvimetry is an integral part of the physical examination at the first visit. Pelvimetric evaluation is a requisite skill that must be developed by every physician who is engaged in obstetric care. The physical relationships of the pelvis, both in terms of shape and dimension, may be critical in determining the course of events that will transpire during labor. Moreover, the relationship between the pelvic anatomic features and those of the fetal presenting part may influence myometrial efficiency by means as yet undetermined.

External measurements bear essentially no relationship to the size and shape of the true pelvis. They are no longer done because they are generally considered invalid.

Some physicians prefer to delay the initial detailed internal examination of the pelvis until early in the third trimester at which time the patient may have developed more rapport with the physician. She tends to be less tense and more likely to cooperate. The perineal tissues are more elastic at this time and yielding. Therefore, more information may be obtained regarding the pelvic dimensions and contours, and the impressions thus gained may be more reliable.

A more popular practice is to evaluate the pelvis immediately at the first visit and to reevaluate it near term. In this manner, the fetal presenting part is also available so that vital data concerning presentation, status of cervix, engagement, and the cephalopelvic relationships may be ascertained.

CLINICAL PELVIMETRY

A great deal of information can be obtained by means of vaginal examination if it is carried out in such a manner that the essential features of the pelvis are studied carefully. A rather good assessment of the size and shape of the pelvis can be done in this manner. With the patient on a comfortably padded table in dorsal lithotomy position and well draped, the examiner inserts two well lubricated, gloved fingers between the widely separated labia gently into the vagina. In so doing, the topography of the levator ani muscles can be studied by pressing the fingers downward on either side of the vagina. These muscles may be broad and slinglike, especially in the nullipara, contracting tightly on a voluntary or involuntary basis. In the multipara, the introitus may gape and the levator ani muscles are represented by thick pillars at the side of the vagina, contracting poorly.

It is not important which aspects of the pelvis are examined first as long as the physician establishes some sort of routine so that he will not forget to check each landmark. One such suggested routine follows: The height of the pubis is measured and its inclination to the inlet determined. The forepelvic aspect of the inlet, behind the symphysis pubis and radiating posterolaterally, is next examined and its curvature envisioned. Moving down the sidewalls, the examining fingers determine the inclination of the sidewalls, that is, whether they are straight, convergent or divergent (see below). The fingers reach the ischial spines in the midsagittal plane and note their prominence. The sacrospinous ligaments are measured. The mo-

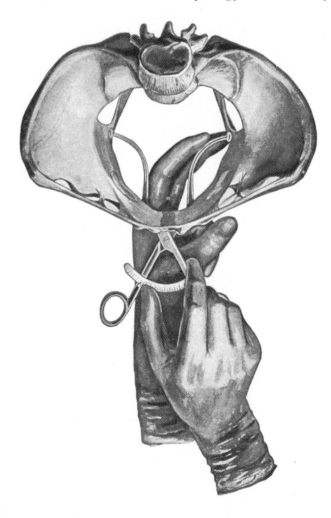

Figure 101 Method for instrumental mensuration of the interspinous diameter. The calipers are applied so that the distal knobs are pressed against the ischial spines and the measurement obtained by reading the scale externally.

bility of the coccyx is ascertained as is the inclination of the sacrum. The examining fingers move progressively up the sacrum in an attempt to reach the promontory. If reached, measurement is taken of the distance from the lower border of the symphysis pubis to the promontory. This is the so-called *diagonal conjugate.*

The interspinous diameter is measured digitally also. This may be estimated or measured by a special caliper designed for this purpose (Fig. 101). When utilized, the instrument is closed and passed with the scale upward along the examining finger until it has passed the levator ani. Then the blades are spread until one terminal knob rests on or just in front of the ischial spine. The blades are spread in the horizontal plane until they are arrested by both

ischial spines. The external caliper scale is read at this instant. If the vagina is soft and distensible, and if the examiner proceeds slowly and gently, this examination should cause little discomfort. No force should ever be used. Bear in mind that a measurement in excess of 10 cm. shows ample room. Therefore, it is unnecessary to get a full and accurate measurement if 10 cm. is already exceeded. Fortunately, in a contracted pelvis, it is generally quite easy to reach the spines.

To evaluate the slope of the sidewalls, the examining fingers may be placed at the base of the ischial spine as a landmark. The ischial sidewall can then be palpated above and below this point down to the ischial tuberosities to determine the inclination. The distance from the sacral tip to

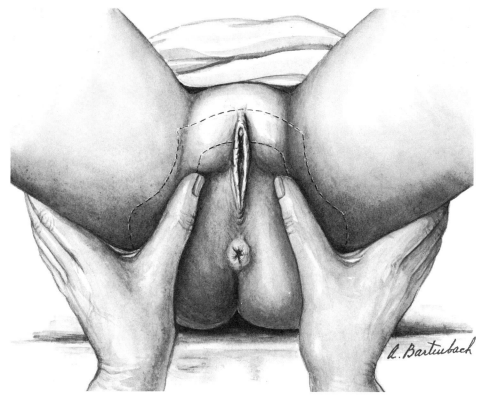

Figure 102 The shape of the subpubic arch is determined by applying the examining thumbs along the inferior rami of the pubic bone as indicated.

the underborder of the symphysis pubis, the anteroposterior diameter of the outlet, is directly measurable as a useful indicator of outlet adequacy. The measurement can be obtained by placing the tip of the extended middle finger of the examining hand on the sacrococcygeal joint and marking off the point on that hand corresponding to the lower border of the symphysis. The mobility of the coccyx can be readily determined by holding the coccyx between the examining fingers and attempting to move it backward and forward.

The shape of the pubic arch can be determined by external palpation of the inferior rami of the pubis (Fig. 102) by placing both thumbs along these structures pointed toward the symphysis. The intertuberous diameter can be measured instrumentally (Fig. 103) or with the examining hand. In the latter method, the clenched fist is apposed to the perineum to obtain an estimate of the distance between the ischial tuberosities (Fig. 104). Other information is also obtainable, including the

rather important observation that the pelvis is asymmetric.

The best determination of the diagonal conjugate diameter may be obtained by keeping the examining fingers and wrist straight and in line with the forearm. With the fingers deep in the vagina, the examiner's elbow is depressed toward the ground. The elbow may be rested against his own knee while he gently, but firmly, advances the fingers toward the sacral promontory. It may be necessary to keep steady pressure on the perineum for several minutes before the rigid muscles will relax sufficiently to allow this advancement. When the promontory is reached, the elbow is raised until the hand touches the lower border of the symphysis. This point is marked with a finger of the external hand (Fig. 105) and the internal hand withdrawn. An accurate measurement may then be obtained by using a caliper or other measuring device. Merely subtracting 1.5 to 2 cm. from this dimension, according to the estimated inclination of the

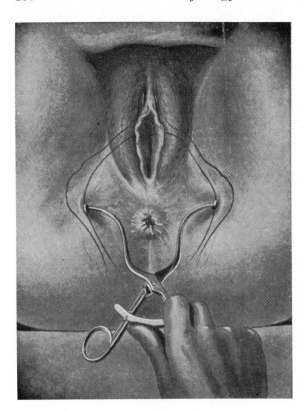

Figure 103   Caliper measurement of the intertuberous diameter. Compare with Figure 104.

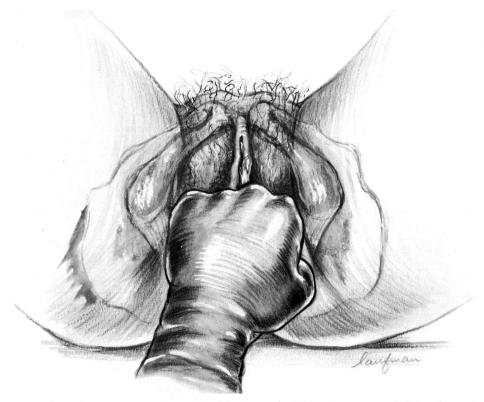

Figure 104   Manual measurement of intertuberous diameter utilizing the examiner's fist at the perineum.

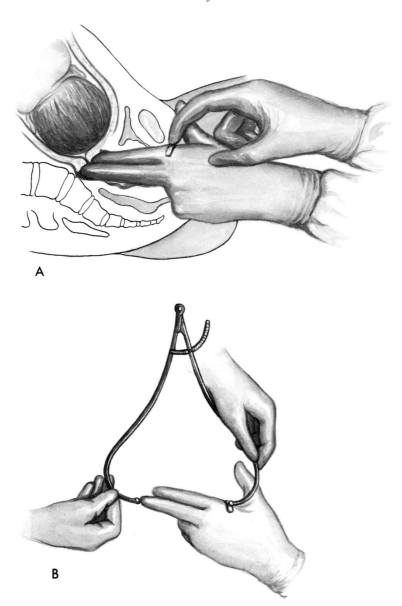

Figure 105 The diagonal conjugate is measured (A) from the sacral promontory to the lower border of the symphysis pubis. The point on the internal hand is marked at the symphysis. The calipers (B) then measure the distance between this point and the tip of the middle finger to determine the diagonal conjugate.

symphysis, will give an approximate length of the true conjugate.

On average, the diagonal conjugate diameter is at least 12.5 cm., the interspinous diameter 10.5 cm. and the intertuberous diameter 10.5 cm. Whereas usually 1.5 cm. may be deducted from the length of the diagonal conjugate to obtain the true conjugate, this may be an overestimate if the pubis is unusually high. Pubic height can be measured simply as shown in Figure

106. If it is 6 cm. or more, at least 2 or 2.5 cm. must be deducted from the diagonal conjugate dimension to obtain the true conjugate diameter. If the upper border of the pubis inclines more than usual toward the sacrum or is extremely thick, as much as 3 cm. may have to subtracted.

If it is found that the ischial spines are very prominent and associated with foreshortened sacrospinous ligaments, one can anticipate a midplane contraction. This is

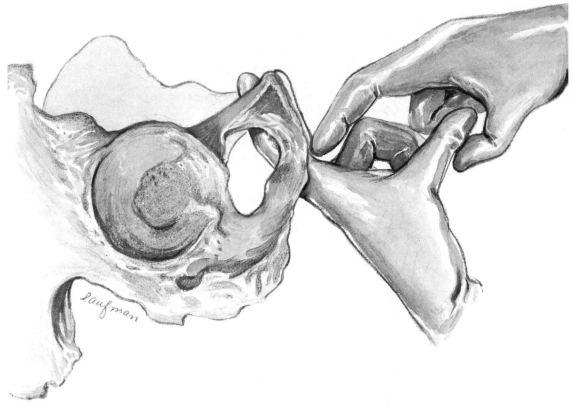

Figure 106   Height, angle of inclination and shape of the symphysis pubis can be determined digitally as shown.

not uncommonly seen in android and anthropoid pelves (see below). Similarly, convergent sidewalls suggest funneling and may be associated with midplane or outlet problems. Foreshortened sacrospinous ligaments may indicate forward inclination of the sacrum as well. Narrowing of the forepelvis of the inlet occurs in association with android and anthropoid pelves with constriction in the transverse diameters. A narrow subpubic arch is similarly suggestive. A foreshortened anteroposterior diameter or true conjugate implies the likelihood of a serious inlet problem. In order for the physician to interpret his findings in terms of the clinical prognosis, it is important to understand the typical characteristics of the various classic pelvic types.

CLASSIFICATION OF PELVES

A morphologic classification of the pelvis was introduced in 1933 by Caldwell and Moloy. They described four basic pelvic types: (1) gynecoid, (2) android, (3) anthropoid and (4) platypelloid. The shape of the inlet was the primary basis for these types. The gynecoid pelvis has a rounded or oval shape with a well-rounded anterior and posterior segment. It represents the normal female pelvis and is found in 45 per cent of women. The android pelvis is roughly wedge- or heart-shaped with the transverse diameter of the inlet approximately equal to the anteroposterior diameter, but with the widest transverse diameter located closer to the sacrum. The posterior segment of the android pelvis is short and flattened and the anterior segment or forepelvis is narrowed. Android pelves are found in about 15 per cent of women. The anthropoid pelvis has an elongated anteroposterior diameter characteristically. About 35 per cent of women have anthropoid pelves. The platypelloid pelvis has marked flattening of the anteroposterior dimension with relative widening of the transverse. It is seen in five per cent or less. Typical examples of these pelvic types are shown in Figures 107 to 110.

— GYNECOID —

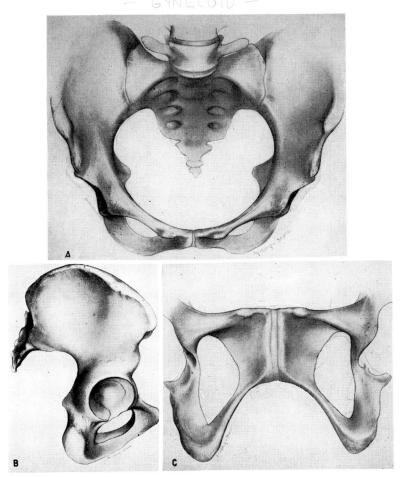

Figure 107 Inlet (A), lateral (B) and anterior (C) views of the typical gynecoid pelvis showing well-rounded inlet, average inclination of the sacrum, well-formed sacrosciatic notch, rounded subpubic arch and straight side walls. (From Steer, C. M.: Moloy's Evaluation of the Pelvis in Obstetrics. Philadelphia, W. B. Saunders Company, 1959.)

Pure types are rather unusual. Most often, admixtures of anterior and posterior inlet segment types occur (Fig. 111). Nevertheless, the typical characteristics of the pelvis tend to be retained. For example, generally gynecoid pelves have, in addition to the well-rounded inlet, straight sidewalls, well-formed sacrosciatic notches, good sacral curvature and inclination, moderately sized ischial spines, average sacrospinous ligaments and well-rounded subpubic arches. By contrast, the android pelvis has a narrow forepelvis with convergent sidewalls, prominent spines, forward sacrum, narrow sacrosciatic notch, foreshortened sacrospinous ligaments and narrowed subpubic arch. The anthropoid pelvis is elongated in the anteroposterior diameter and relatively narrow in the transverse with a backward, deeply curved sacrum, long sacrospinous ligaments and very prominent ischial spines, as well as a narrowed forepelvis and subpubic arch. The platypelloid pelvis has a characteristically foreshortened anteroposterior diameter with widened forepelvis, straight sacrum, wide subpubic arch, flat ischial spines and elongated sacrospinous ligaments. Thus, it is possible to reconstruct the inlet shape knowing some of the features of the lower pelvis even though the entire inlet cannot be palpated by the examining fingers.

Knowledge concerning the pelvic characteristics is important insofar as it provides information about the probable mechanisms of labor (see Chapter 18). In the gynecoid pelvis, the most common

— ANDROID —

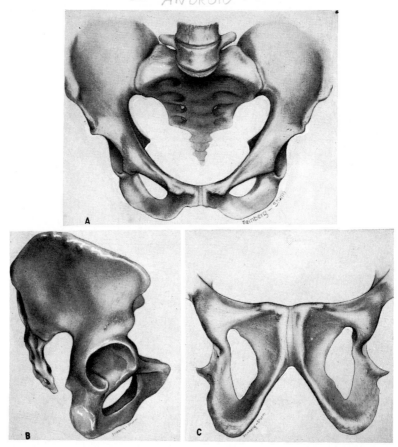

Figure 108   Comparable views of a typical android pelvis illustrating heart-shaped inlet with narrow fore-pelvis and widest transverse diameter located close to the sacrum. The sacrum is forward with a narrow sacro-sciatic notch. The subpubic arch is narrow and the sidewalls converge. (From Steer, C. M.: Moloy's Evaluation of the Pelvis in Obstetrics. Philadelphia, W. B. Saunders Company, 1959.)

mech.
of
labor
c̄
type
of
pelvis

position of the fetal head is obliquely anterior. In the android pelvis, posterior oblique positions are usually seen. It is generally accepted that anthropoid pelves are commonly associated with occiput posterior mechanisms, whereas occiput transverse is common in flat pelves. The inherent problems that result from these phenomena will be discussed in detail subsequently.

These classifications, of course, are based on configuration of the pelvis and do not take into account pelvic size as such. This latter aspect introduces another, equally important consideration. A third feature has to do with the dimensions of the fetal head. Obviously, these are critical considerations that are all too often ignored in evaluations of the pelvis. The pelvis that is deemed small may be quite ample for a small fetus. An average pelvis, by the same token, may be inadequate for a large fetus. Thus, it is important that the pelvis be evaluated late in pregnancy, perhaps most preferably in labor, when the fetal presenting part is available for critical comparison of its dimensions with the available space in the bony pelvis (see Chapter 16).

X-RAY PELVIMETRY

In terms of objectivity, there can be no question that x-ray pelvimetry has clear-cut advantages over digital pelvic measurements. However, because of the increasing awareness of the hazards of the radiation to both mother and fetus, its ap-

— ANTHROPOID —

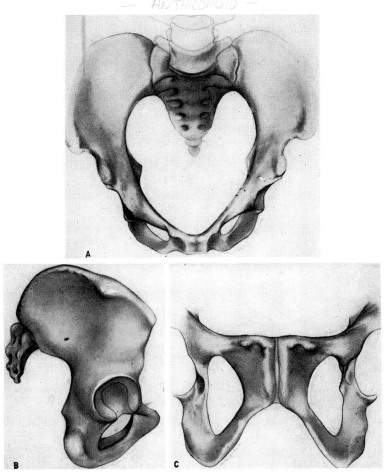

Figure 109 A pelvis showing typical anthropoid features including elongated anteroposterior diameter and narrowed forepelvis. The sacrum here has an average inclination, but the sacrosciatic notch is wide. The subpubic arch is rounded and the ischial spines are prominent. (From Steer, C. M.: Moloy's Evaluation of the Pelvis in Obstetrics. Philadelphia, W. B. Saunders Company, 1959.)

plication has become increasingly limited. The technique is reserved for those instances where it is clearly essential that it be done. Thus, it should be held in abeyance until the patient is well in labor and the course of labor has indicated the existence of a problem found coassociated with cephalopelvic disproportion (see Chapter 55). Exceptions to this interdiction include such situations as the nullipara with breech presentation in labor. Under these circumstances, the course of labor and its variations may not be sufficient to forewarn the physician of impending problems in fetopelvic relationships.

X-ray cephalopelvimetry is a valuable adjunct to the evaluation of labor progression. There are many recognized short-

comings which must be borne in mind. The technique is merely a laboratory aid and cannot be expected to provide irrefutable answers. Many techniques are currently in use and it is probable that none is particularly better than any other insofar as reliability, precision of measurement, degree of error and reproducibility are concerned (Weinberg and Scadron). Some do have technical disadvantages relating to specific requirements for very accurate positioning of the patient, precise location of special rules or grids, use of specially designed equipment or the capability to perceive stereoscopically. The Ball technique which we will describe here has the advantages of simplicity and almost complete absence of technical drawbacks.

— PLATYPELLOID —

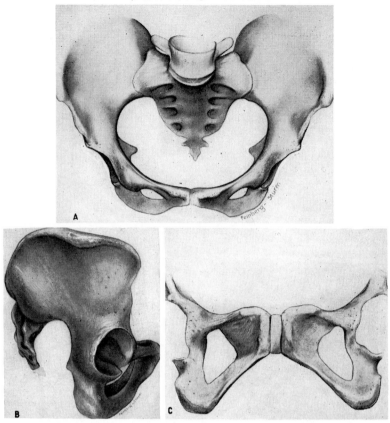

Figure 110 Typical platypelloid type of pelvis with wide transverse diameter, foreshortening in the antero-posterior diameter, narrowing of the sacrosciatic notch, forward inclination of the sacrum and broadening of the subpubic arch. (From Steer, C. M.: Moloy's Evaluation of the Pelvis in Obstetrics. Philadelphia, W. B. Saunders Company, 1959.)

Some reluctance has been encountered in its broad application and interpretation because of the mathematics needed for computing the corrections for measurements. Special nomograms and slide rules have been devised, but have not sufficiently simplified the calculations to provide universal appeal for practicing physicians who may not be mathematically oriented. The technique has recently been modified to reduce it to its maximum simplicity without affecting accuracy (Friedman and Taylor).

The Ball technique is based on the geometric theorem which states that the corresponding parallel sides of similar triangles are proportional to each other. Thus, simple mathematical corrections can be made for the distortion that results from the dispersion of x-rays from a point source at a set distance from the film. In order to correct the measurement of any apparent image obtained on an x-ray film so as to learn its true dimension, it is merely necessary to know the object-film distance and the distance from the x-ray tube source (anode) to the film. The film image (measured) and the object dimension (true) are the parallel sides of similar triangles corresponding proportionally to anode-film distance and anode-object distance, respectively. The anode-object distance is obtained by subtracting the object-film distance from the total distance of the x-ray source from the film. This is expressed (Fig. 112) by the simple proportion:

$$\frac{x}{a} = \frac{c}{d}$$

where x is the true dimension, a the measured dimension on the x-ray film, c the anode-object distance and d the anode-film distance. Since $c = d - b$ (where b is

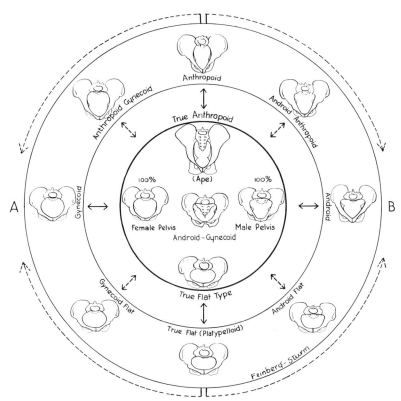

Figure 111 Composite morphologic classification according to Caldwell and Moloy illustrating gradations of change in pelvic configurations from the pure types to admixtures according to the inlet shape of the posterior and anterior segments, respectively. (From Steer, C. M.: Moloy's Evaluation of the Pelvis in Obstetrics. Philadelphia, W. B. Saunders Company, 1959.)

the object-film distance) and d can be readily standardized in any given institution, say at 100 cm., the above equation can be further reduced and simplified to:

$$\frac{x}{a} = \frac{100 - b}{100}$$

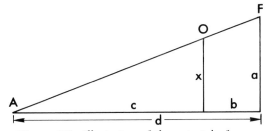

Figure 112 Illustration of the principle for correcting dimensions in the Ball cephalopelvimetric technique showing similar triangles with proportional sides. A represents the anode; O, the object to be measured; F, the film; x, true dimension; a, measured dimension; b, object-film distance; c, anode-object distance; and d, anode-film distance. (From Friedman, E. A., and Taylor, M. B.: Amer. J. Obstet. Gynec. *105*:1110, 1969.)

Thus, to correct for any given measured dimension, it is merely necessary to know the object-film distance for that particular plane in the patient. The Ball technique provides for ready accessibility to the latter information by means of correlative 90° angle films (anteroposterior and lateral, respectively), utilizing one film to obtain object-film distances for images measured on the corresponding film and vice versa.

Most other pelvimetric techniques are seriously limited in their intrinsic capability for measuring head size. With vertex presentation in which the sagittal suture is directed precisely anteroposteriorly or laterally, measurement and correction of the biparietal diameter of the fetal skull can be accomplished quite readily. However, this situation pertains in only a small minority of cases. In most instances accurate biparietal measurements are impossible to obtain. The Ball technique overcomes this major shortcoming by directing attention to the circumference of the fetal skull and, assuming the fetal head to be approximately spheroidal, converting this measurement to a corresponding volume. By the same token, each measured pelvic diameter can be converted to determine the circular area capable of accommodating a given spheroidal volume, that is to say its capacity. Circumference *(C)* and diameter *(D)* are both related to volume *(V)* by the expressions:

$$V = \frac{\pi D^3}{6} \text{ and } V = \frac{C^3}{6\pi^2}$$

The technical requirements are among the simplest and least complicated of all existing pelvimetric examination procedures. Two films are taken, both with the patient in standing position. The x-ray source is placed at a measured distance from the film, preferably 100 cm. An anteroposterior and a lateral x-ray centered at the pelvis on 14 × 17 in. (or 18 × 24 in.) film are obtained, using a 16:1 grid Potter-Bucky diaphragm.

The films obtained should be studied in depth to ascertain pelvic shape, abnormalities or pelvic architecture, fetal presentation and position, station of the fetal presenting part, degree of flexion, synclitism, molding, overriding of cranial bones, shape of inlet, prominence of the ischial spines, curvature of the sacrum, inclination of the sidewalls and the shape of the subpubic arch and sacrosciatic notch. Critical diameters (Fig. 113) include anteroposterior and transverse diameters of the inlet and interspinous diameters at the midplane. Additionally, the circumference of the fetal head should be measured on both anteroposterior and lateral views. Correcting diameters (object-film distances) include the distance from the midpoint (symphysis pubis) to the greater trochanter of the femur, the distance from the ischial spines to a vertical line passing through the posterior aspect of the sacrum and the distance from the point representing the widest transverse diameter of the inlet to the posterior sacrum. Corrections of pelvic and fetal head measurements are made using appropriate object-film distances as follows:

a. Widest transverse diameter of the inlet (measured on the anteroposterior

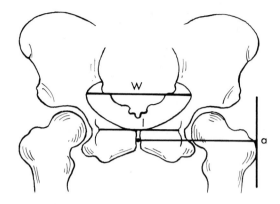

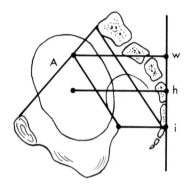

Figure 113 Diagram showing anteroposterior (above) and lateral (below) x-ray films of the pelvis. The dimensions shown are: W, widest transverse inlet diameter and *w*, its corresponding object-film distance; *I*, interspinous diameter and *i*, its object-film distance; A, anteroposterior diameter of inlet and *a*, object-film distance for it and for the circumference of the centrally located fetal head as measured on the lateral view; *h*, object-film distance for circumference of the head as measured in the anteroposterior film. (From Friedman, E. A., and Taylor, M. B.: Amer. J. Obstet. Gynec. *105*:1110, 1969.)

film): Corrected using the distance from the point representing the widest transverse diameter of the inlet (obtained by drawing a line parallel to the inclination of the sacrum through the ischial spines on the lateral x-ray view) to the posterior sacrum. To the latter measurement one should add an arbitrary figure of 4 cm. to take into account the distance from the posterior bony aspect of the sacrum through the gluteal soft tissues to the film-holding cassette.

b. Interspinous diameter (measured on the anteroposterior film): Corrected using distance from spine to posterior sacrum plus factor of 4 cm. (obtained from the lateral view).

c. Anteroposterior diameter of the inlet (measured on the lateral view): Corrected by using distance from midpoint to greater trochanter plus 4 cm. (obtained from anteroposterior view).

d. Circumference of fetal head as measured on anteroposterior film: Corrected using distance from midpoint of head to posterior sacrum plus 4 cm. (obtained from lateral view).

e. Circumference of fetal head as measured on lateral view: Corrected using distance from midpoint to greater trochanter plus 4 cm. (obtained from anteroposterior view). If the anteroposterior view of the fetal head is not in the midline, one uses the distance from the midpoint of the image of the fetal head to the appropriate greater trochanter. If the correct side is unknown, one measures to both trochanters independently and then uses only the measurement that approaches most closely that obtained after correcting the circumference of the anteroposterior view of the head.

The final step is conversion of the corrected diameters to capacities and conversion of circumferences to volumes. One is then in a position to compare capacities and volumes for the purpose of evaluating the cephalopelvic relationships. The following classification has proved to be useful: At the inlet, if inlet capacities are equal to or greater than fetal head volume, no disproportion exists. Cases in which the inlet capacities are smaller than the head volume by 50 ml. or less are deemed to have relative or borderline disproportion. Where the negative difference exceeds 50 ml. (head volume is more than 50 ml. larger than smallest inlet capacity), a high degree of disproportion may be considered to be present. For the midpelvis, if the interspinous capacity is up to 150 ml. smaller than the volume of the head, no disproportion exists; between 150 and 200 ml. negative difference, there is a relative midpelvic disproportion; if the negative difference exceeds 200 ml. at the midplane (head volume more than 200 ml. larger than interspinous capacity), an interpre-tation of a high degree of disproportion is warranted.

Clear-cut differences in outcome have been demonstrated by Schwarz et al. Cases deemed radiologically not to have disproportion required cesarean section in one per cent, borderline cases 33 per cent, and high degrees of disproportion 80 per cent. In the last group there were nearly 90 per cent with difficult deliveries, including cesareans, high forceps and midforceps. The value of this approach in terms of prognostication is thus demonstrated.

As indicated earlier, a nomogram is available for purposes of reducing the complexity of calculations (Fig. 114). The nomogram is a simple device that enables one to bypass complex or tedious mathematical computation to obtain the value of a dependent variable when the values of two or more independent variables are given. The independent variables here are the anode-film distance, the object-film distance and the measured dimensions. The dependent variable is the true or corrected dimension. The nomogram shown here is applicable when the anode-film distance is kept constant at 100 cm. The need to resort to use of tables or slide rules for converting diameters to capacities or circumferences to volumes can be eliminated merely by the expediency of providing appropriate scales directly on the nomographic axis representing the true dimension. No loss in accuracy has occurred by this approach. The error introduced is of the same order of magnitude as the error in the original measurement itself.

X-ray technique is also of value in determining fetal presentation and position and the presence of skeletal abnormalities, estimating fetal maturity and diagnosing fetal death, multiple pregnancy and abdominal pregnancy. However, its use in this regard is generally quite limited today because of the radiation hazards involved. Moreover, with the advent of ultrasonography, it is no longer appropriate to subject a patient and her fetus to radiation if other means are available that do not offer comparable risks. In locations where ultrasound techniques are not yet available for use, such risks may be undertaken provided the information to be obtained by x-ray study warrants it.

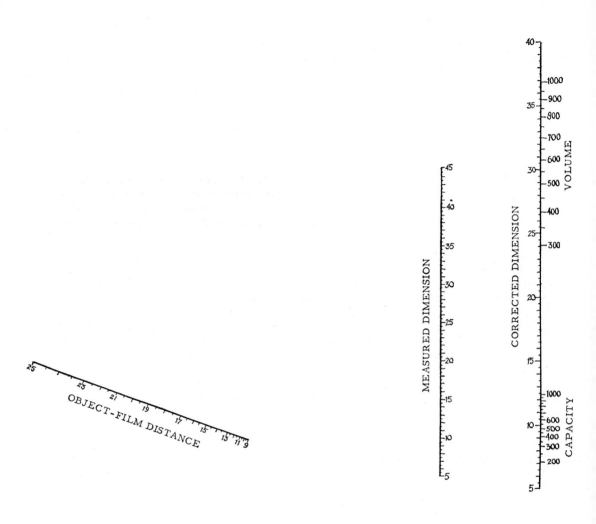

Figure 114   A nomogram for correcting the measured dimensions on films taken at 100 cm. from the anode of the x-ray tube. A straight-edged ruler aligned at the appropriate points on the independent axes of the object-film distance and measured dimension, respectively, will automatically cross the true dimension axis to provide both the corrected dimension and the corresponding head volume or pelvic capacity. (From Friedman, E. A., and Taylor, M. B.: Amer. J. Obstet. Gynec. *105*:1110, 1969 and *106*: 884, 1970.)

RADIATION HAZARDS

The value of x-ray pelvimetry in the management of labor must be counterbalanced by consideration of its potential hazards. It is generally agreed that totally eliminating this technique for the diagnosis of serious obstetric problems may result in more harm than good. One of the important objectives in this regard is to perfect techniques so that the least amount of radiation is used to obtain x-rays of quality suitable for establishing diagnosis in situations where indications are acceptable.

To reduce the radiation exposure to a minimum, certain technical principles should be observed: (1) Exposures should be taken as near to term as possible; (2) the smallest film possible should be used with proper coning and shielding so that only the field to be studied is irradiated; (3) filtration of the x-ray beam should be between 2 and 3 mm. of aluminum to eliminate the soft rays and reduce the amount of radiation reaching the skin; (4) positioning and exposure should be perfected to minimize reexposures; (5) high kilovoltage, high speed film and long tube-film distances should be used to reduce radiation needed for quality x-rays; (6) employing a technique that minimizes the number of exposures (e.g., the Ball technique which needs only two films) and reduces the chance of technical errors is recommended. It has been shown that good diagnostic x-rays can be obtained with a fraction of the radiation exposure that used to be commonly employed.

Reports dealing with exposure to fallout, medical x-ray, gamma rays and radiation from natural sources have indicated that the potential hazard is to the human germ plasm, by increasing the rate of mutations. Future generations may show the harmful effects of such mutations by a shortened life span, abnormalities and even death. In x-ray pelvimetry a certain amount of radiation reaches both maternal and fetal gonads. The fetus also receives some total-body radiation according to the technique used. Serious questions have recently been raised concerning the possibility of remote carcinogenic effects of such radiation.

The documented evidence to show that radiation in the dosage used for pelvimetry may be harmful to the fetus includes reports by MacMahon and by Stewart and Kneale indicating a 50 per cent increase in the risk of developing cancer in childhood after *in utero* exposure to diagnostic radiation by doses of 0.5 to 2 rads. Griem et al., on the other hand, could find no comparable increased risk in a large group exposed to 1.5 to 3 rads by routine diagnostic x-ray pelvimetry. The issue is still speculative, but it cannot be treated lightly.

The National Academy of Sciences has defined 10 roentgens as the maximum permissible accumulated dose of radiation any individual can receive up to age 30. Measurements of the radiation dose to the pelvis during x-ray pelvimetry (Berman and Sonnenblick) showed the total dosage administered averaged 0.7 roentgens per exposure. The technique used was one in which four films were obtained, including an inlet view which is now recognized to expose fetal gonads excessively. Moreover, no attempt was made to reduce the radiation dose to the absolute minimum by special procedures or precautions. It is probable that, with the improved equipment and precision techniques now available, the total radiation exposure could be reduced to one third or less of that administered without sacrificing the quality of the roentgenograms.

In considering the exposure to maternal ovaries and the fetal gonads, we should be concerned with how much radiation is absorbed by these organs. Estimations from experiments with phantoms and theoretical calculations are not entirely accurate and may be considered only as approximations. The maternal ovaries are not in line with the direct x-ray beam, as they are displaced laterally and well out of the pelvis, often into the upper abdomen, by the full-term uterus. Much of the radiation to the ovaries is probably derived from back scatter and oblique rays.

The fetal gonads are also not in the direct x-ray beam during exposure of anteroposterior and lateral films of the pelvis if the presentation is cephalic. The fetal gonads in breech presentations are radiated during pelvimetry. Under these circumstances, radiation to the gonads is chiefly indirect and the fetus is somewhat protected by the uterus, amniotic fluid and the abdominal wall of the mother. Therefore, the dosage to the fetal gonads is only a fraction of that reaching the mother's skin.

There are many advantages of properly indicated roentgenography in obstetrics. The roentgenogram is a permanent record of the conditions existing at the time of delivery. Its objectivity is useful in diagnostic problems relating to fetal lie, station and attitude and pelvic architecture, as well as fetopelvic relationships. The record is of inestimable aid for teaching purposes in correlating the outcome of labor with the x-ray and clinical findings. The benefits of accurate x-ray pelvimetric diagnosis in obstetrics probably outweigh its potential hazards where it is clearly indicated. No woman should be denied it if circumstances justify it.

REFERENCES

Ball, R. P.: Pelvicephalometry. Amer. J. Obstet. Gynec. *32*:249, 1936.

Berman, R., and Sonnenblick, B. P.: Intravaginal measurement of radiation dose incident to x-ray pelvimetry and hysterosalpingography. Amer. J. Obstet. Gynec. *74*:1, 1957.

Caldwell, W. E., and Moloy, H. C.: Anatomical variations in the female pelvis and their effect in labor with a suggested classification. Amer. J. Obstet. Gynec. *26*:479, 1933.

Friedman, E. A., and Taylor, M. B.: A modified nomographic aid for x-ray cephalopelvimetry. Amer. J. Obstet. Gynec. *105*:1110, 1969.

Griem, M. L., Meier, P., and Dobben, G. D.: Analysis of the morbidity and mortality of children irradiated in fetal life. Radiology *88*:347, 1967.

MacMahon, B.: Prenatal x-ray exposure and childhood cancer. J. Nat. Cancer Inst. *28*:1173, 1962.

Schwarz, G. S., Kirkpatrick, R. H., and Tovell, H. M. M.: Correlation of cephalopelvimetry to obstetrical outcome with special reference to radiologic disproportion. Radiology *67*:854, 1956.

Steer, C. M.: Moloy's Evaluation of the Pelvis in Obstetrics, ed. 2. Philadelphia, W. B. Saunders Company, 1959.

Stewart, A., and Kneale, G. W.: Radiation dose effects in relation to obstetric x-rays and childhood cancers. Lancet *1*:1185, 1970.

Weinberg, A., and Scadron, S. J.: Value and limitations of pelvioradiography in management of dystocia, with special reference to midpelvic capacity. Amer. J. Obstet. Gynec. *52*:255, 1946.

Chapter 13

Tests of Fetal Status

The clinical guidelines useful for determining the duration of pregnancy have been discussed in Chapter 8. All considered, they present serious limitations with regard to accuracy of dating gestational age and, still more pertinently, with reference to the functional maturity of the fetus. We will briefly review here means whereby the clinician can acquire relevant and meaningful information. Conditions which specifically call for the use of these procedures are discussed in greater depth elsewhere.

Additionally, we will list and characterize some of the newer objective investigative techniques that have been introduced for the purpose of determining the condition of the fetus, both with regard to its health and the functional status of the placenta. These important examinations constitute avenues of study of utmost significance in certain situations that have been appropriately designated *high risk* obstetric problems. Such problems will also be dealt with at length in those sections of this book that take up specific pathologic disorders. Furthermore, technical developments that permit one to disclose the presence of congenital anomalies and metabolic disorders of the fetus will be included.

The aim of this chapter is to catalogue testing procedures that will prove useful in the conduct of obstetric practices. Collectively, this battery comprises the laboratory backbone of the field of study that has been called *fetology* or *perinatal medicine*. It is understood that not all of these procedures will be available in every community by virtue of limitations in facilities, personnel and funding. However, where they are, it is recommended that those who are responsible for the care of gravid patients should become familiar with and utilize those tests that are indicated. They serve as valuable adjuncts to knowledgeable physicians in caring for pregnant women and their unborn fetuses. For tests dealing with placental localization, the reader is referred to Chapter 37. Similarly, the scoring systems for characterizing the condition of the newborn infant are detailed in Chapter 67.

TESTS OF FETAL MATURITY

Many difficult obstetric decisions depend on the availability of reliable means for assessing the maturity of the fetus. Practical problems of considerable importance demand that such information be available, particularly as regards clinical conditions that may require termination of pregnancy. Indirect objective measurements of gestational age have recently been introduced based on changing cytologic and biochemical characteristics of amniotic fluid. Also useful are x-ray and ultrasonography methods for detecting landmark changes in the growing fetus. Data obtained from several tests performed simultaneously tend to provide a more reliable prediction, thus giving rise to simple point-scoring systems which take into account biochemical, x-ray and cytologic features (O'Leary and Bezjian). The inherent advantage in any such system is that the techniques rely on signs of changing physiologic maturity of the fetus rather than actual gestational age. Thus, discrepancies may arise because not all physiologic functions of the fetus mature predictably and at the same time.

Cytologic Examination

Characteristic changes of the cells in the amniotic fluid when stained with Nile blue sulfate form the basis of an approach to determining fetal maturity. This was first recognized by Kittrich and later popularized by Brosens and Gordon. Cells containing lipid substances within amniotic fluid stained orange color with 0.1 per cent Nile blue sulfate. There is a sharp rise in the percentage of such cells after 38 weeks of pregnancy. This is believed to be related to the functional maturity of the sebaceous glands from which these cells may arise. Bishop and Corson found a prematurity rate of 85 per cent when there were less than two per cent of these cells in amniotic fluid as contrasted with no infants under 2500 gm. with fat cell counts exceeding 20 per cent.

The same orange-colored amniotic cells can be identified in vaginal smears for the diagnosis of ruptured membranes. Blystad et al. found that the numbers of squamous cells within the amniotic fluid increased progressively up to delivery. This observation was verified by Votta et al. who determined a correlation between cytologic patterns and fetal maturity in normal pregnancies. They discovered a good correlation among the total number of cells per cubic millimeter of amniotic fluid, the percentage of the various cell types and the duration of pregnancy. Amniotic cells, as contrasted with fetal cells, were found to disappear toward the end of pregnancy after 32 weeks. These were the small, round or oval cells with dense, vacuolated cytoplasm and vesicular nucleus. The fetal cells were large and polygonal either without a nucleus or with a small karyopyknotic or vesicular nucleus. This confirmed the work of Mandelbaum and Evans who found that parabasal and intermediate cells are virtually replaced by cornified and precornified squamous cells after 36 weeks.

Creatinine Concentration

Fetal age is reflected in the creatinine levels in amniotic fluid. Pitkin and Zwirek showed that the concentration of creatin-ine remained essentially constant up to about 34 weeks. A rather abrupt increase took place later in pregnancy with progressively rising concentrations. After the thirty-seventh week, 94 per cent of patients studied had creatinine levels in excess of 2 mg. per 100 ml. In a comparative study of amniotic fluid creatinine, bilirubin (see below) and percentage of fetal sebaceous cells, Droegemueller et al. found the creatinine concentration to be most reliable. Although most specimens with levels in excess of 1.8 mg. per 100 ml. correlated with gestational age over 36 weeks, exceptions were seen. Thus, it was possible to find high levels in association with small fetuses and low levels with large ones. These exceptions notwithstanding, the test was thought to be relatively reliable as an objective measure of gestational age.

Bilirubin Determination

By means of spectrophotometric analysis of amniotic fluid it has been possible to measure minute quantities of bilirubin and other breakdown products of hemoglobin according to the finding of an optical density peak at 450 mμ. This examination has been particularly beneficial in diagnosing the presence and the severity of Rh isoimmunization and erythroblastosis fetalis (see Chapter 52). Bilirubin pigment has also been found to be present in amniotic fluid in normal pregnancies, appearing as early as the twelfth week. Although the mechanism by which pigment appears in the amniotic fluid is unknown, it has been observed that relatively large amounts can be detected during midpregnancy under perfectly normal circumstances.

The progressive decreases which occur subsequently in late pregnancy have been used as a means for estimating fetal age by Mandelbaum et al., who showed that the 450 mμ peak disappeared by the thirty-sixth week in most instances. They felt this was probably the result of improved liver function in the fetus with consequent increase in its ability to conjugate bilirubin. None of their infants who delivered after a zero reading weighed less than 5 lb. or had other signs of prematurity. Moreover, neither diabetes nor toxemia affected the amniotic fluid analysis. However, both meconium and blood contamination negated its value and hydramnios reduced the readings by dilution. As indicated earlier, Droegemueller et al. were unable to verify this clear-cut correlation either by spectrophotometric analysis or chloroform extraction methods. Although their published data do show the expected trends, detectable bilirubin was present in their cases beyond 36 weeks and even at term.

Lecithin-Sphingomyelin Ratio

As the fetus matures, phospholipid protein material comes to line the alveolar surfaces for the purpose of ensuring adequate expansion of the alveoli for gaseous exchange after birth. This material, generically designated *surfactant,* is the essential prerequisite for expansion of the lungs and initiation of adequate respiratory function. It has been discussed briefly in Chapter 6. The appearance of this lipoprotein in the amniotic fluid reflects the maturation of the fetal lungs. Lecithin is its major component. Biosynthesis of lecithin takes place in the mature, stable alveoli.

By means of lipid extraction and examination by thin-layer chromatography, Gluck et al. discovered the existence of a sudden upsurge in lecithin concentration after the thirty-fifth week of pregnancy, heralding the maturity of the pulmonary alveolar lining (Fig. 115). Fetuses in which this was found were not subject to the respiratory distress syndrome (see Chapter 68) when they were born. The concomitant fall in sphingomyelin, another phospholipid fraction, serves as a further guideline, particularly if the ratio between lecithin and sphingomyelin is examined. Gluck et al. showed that the concentrations of the two phospholipids were essentially equal before the lung matured, while lecithin concentrations rose abruptly as the sphingomyelin fell beyond 35 weeks. Thus, the relative densities of these substances constitute a valuable measure of functional maturation.

X-ray Techniques

X-ray methods for determining maturity are based on (1) the appearance of specific epiphyseal centers of ossification, (2) the size of the fetal skull in terms of specific diameters or volume, and (3) measurements of total fetal length. Aside from the inherent risks of radiation to the fetus, all such methods possess intrinsic inaccuracies resulting from variations in growth rate and skeletal maturation. Indeed, there are wide variations in osseous develop-

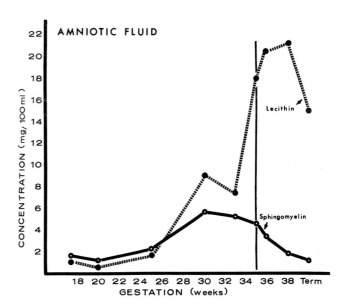

Figure 115 Relative concentrations of lecithin and sphingomyelin in the amniotic fluid at various gestational ages, showing the acute surge in lecithin concentration at 35 weeks in association with maturation of lung function. At the same time, sphingomyelin levels fall. This illustrates the usefulness of the lecithin-sphingomyelin ratio as a measure of the functional maturity of the fetal lung. (From Gluck, L., et al.: Amer. J. Obstet. Gynec. *109:*440, 1971.)

ment according to sex and race, and differences have been seen even in twins (Cope and Murdock). Bony development tends to be further advanced in female fetuses than in males and more advanced in blacks than in whites.

Christie et al. have defined the chronologic order of appearance of ossification centers as follows: calcaneum, talus, distal femoral epiphysis, proximal tibial epiphysis, cuboid, head of humerus, capitatum, hamatum, third cuneiform and head of femur. Hartley found the calcaneum ossified at 24 to 26 weeks and the talus at 26 to 28 weeks. These tend to be rather difficult to visualize, however.

The usual and more accurate x-ray identification of maturity concerns the appearance of the distal femoral epiphysis toward the end of the thirty-sixth week. It is visible as a small homogeneous shadow of less than 0.5 cm. diameter lying 0.5 cm. from the distal end of the femur. At 38 weeks the proximal tibial epiphysis usually becomes sufficiently ossified to be visible on x-ray.

An error of about 10 per cent was found to occur by Christie et al. when estimates of fetal maturity were based on the presence or absence of both the distal femoral and the proximal tibial epiphyses. When only the distal femoral epiphysis was observed, an error of 20 per cent was encountered. This latter suggests that the usual practice of observing only this landmark is less than satisfactory.

Measurement of the crown-breech length of the fetus has been reported by Zuppinger as a reliable index of fetal age, particularly when used in conjunction with measurement of the occipitofrontal diameter of the skull. He found the crown-breech length at 36 weeks, for example, to be 30 cm., corresponding to an occipitofrontal diameter of 11.5 cm.; at 40 weeks, 32 cm. and 12.0 cm., respectively. Although this technique is seldom used today and has been superseded by ultrasonographic cephalometry (see below), it appears to be useful where no other methods are available.

The patient is placed in the prone position so that the fetal body is relatively close to the film, with its vertebral column practically parallel with the table top. With the x-ray tube at least 100 cm. away from the film, distortion can be minimized and the measured crown-breech length corrected by multiplying it by 0.9. It should be pointed out that, because the fetal coccyx is not calcified until after birth, the lower point of measurement is taken at the proximal end of the femur.

The occipitofrontal and biparietal diameters of the fetal skull have long been used as means for estimating fetal age. The data gathered by Scammon and Calkins have served this purpose. They noted, for example, that fetuses of crown-heel length 450 to 500 mm., corresponding to about 37 weeks, had average biparietal diameters of 87.0 mm., ranging from 70 to 99 mm.; fetuses 500 to 544 mm. length or about 40 weeks had biparietal diameters averaging 94.0 mm., ranging from 85 to 102 mm. The suboccipitobregmatic diameters corresponding were found to be 83 to 109 and 94 to 110 mm.; the occipitofrontal diameters, 99 to 123 and 105 to 129 mm.

Reasonably clear linear relationships were established for these diameters and crown-heel lengths. These data in turn were then made available for use in estimating fetal age by means of x-ray measurements of the appropriate diameters. Techniques such as outlined in Chapter 12 were utilized to obtain moderately accurate data. The Ball technique which estimates head volume on the basis of measurement of its circumference carries about a 10 per cent error (Ball). The considerably more accurate and less hazardous ultrasound method is recommended instead.

Progressive growth of the fetal biparietal diameter has been documented by both x-ray (McDonald and Thomas; Crichton) and cephalometry (Willocks et al.), the latter showing a mean growth rate of 0.023 cm. per day. In general, however, estimation of fetal weight from these data has been shown to be rather inaccurate, although Willocks et al. suggest that estimates of fetal weight from ultrasonic measurements of biparietal diameter are accurate within a pound in two-thirds of infants. Kosar and Steer have clearly shown that the extremes of variation that exist between head size and body weight make it nearly impossible to predict accurately. This latter conclusion was based on study of newborn infants in an attempt to relate head size with body weight. A rough correlation was encountered but it was insufficient to be of clinical predictive value.

Ultrasonography

The introduction of ultrasound examination into obstetrics by Donald in 1958 opened new pathways for simple, apparently safe and reliably accurate diagnosis. The method is based on the reflection of pulsed ultrasound beams from interfaces between tissue media having different acoustic impedances. The reflected sound is detected by a piezo-electric crystal which generates electric potentials that can be displayed on an oscilloscope screen. One can calculate, based on the knowledge of how fast sound will travel in tissue, the distance to the reflecting surface by measuring the time it takes for the echo to return. Multiplying the speed of sound by half the time gives the distance.

Use of oscilloscopic display provides the same information by showing deflections of various echoes along a line that represents the time (and therefore the distance) from the ultrasonic transducer. The amplified pulses from the crystal are displayed as upward spikes along the line traced by the oscilloscope beam. The distance between two such spikes corresponds to the distance between two tissue interfaces which represent the sources of echoes. This is referred to as the A-mode. The walls of the fetal skull, for example, provide clear-cut interfaces for reflecting the ultrasound echo back to the transducer probe.

When the ultrasonic pulse beam is directed so as to traverse perpendicularly through the fetal head, the biparietal diameter may be measured directly from the oscilloscope screen (Donald and Brown). A cross-sectional or B-mode display can also be obtained by means of compound scanning whereby the oscilloscopic beam is coupled with the ultrasonic beam so that the echo dots yield a cross-sectional anatomic picture on the screen. The latter

requires much more sophisticated and expensive equipment but offers a means whereby more information of greater accuracy can be obtained. It has been shown to be capable of detecting intracranial lesions, recording changes in volume of the heart and movement of heart valves, defining intraocular tumors and distinguishing varieties of intraabdominal structures, including gallstones, foreign bodies, renal calculi, various cysts, abscesses and tumors, as well as normal pregnancy, twins, hydramnios, hydrocephalus and hydatidiform mole. Furthermore, and of most interest to us here, the echo technique has been found to be capable of measuring the biparietal diameter of the fetal skull with great accuracy.

A technical error may be introduced into ultrasonic echo measurements of the biparietal diameter when the beam is not directed in a precisely perpendicular manner to the fetal head. Willocks et al. have shown that, when the ultrasonic beam axis is at right angles to the reflecting surface, the opposing skull margins will produce simultaneous echoes of maximum amplitude. Thus, echo peaks of equal magnitude on the display screen are obtained only along the occipitofrontal or the biparietal diameters. Within this constraint, errors of 1 mm. or less were encountered in 73.5 per cent of biparietal measurements and 90 per cent were within 2 mm. Taylor et al. found that 80 per cent of biparietal measurements were correct within 2 mm.; 95 per cent within 3 mm.

Data are now available from ultrasonic measurements to help define the normal growth curve based on fetal biparietal diameters (Campbell and Newman). Such information may provide a means whereby intrauterine growth retardation may be detected from serial ultrasonographic determinations. Although not very useful for estimating fetal weight, Thompson et al. found that 91 per cent of fetuses with biparietal diameters of 8.5 cm. or greater weighed in excess of 2500 gm.; 97 per cent if more than 9 cm.

Some difficulty is obtained in measuring the biparietal diameter accurately when the fetal head is deeply engaged in the pelvis because there is interference in transmission of the sound beam from the maternal pelvic bones. In breech presentation, it may also be difficult to obtain a good measurement unless the fetal head is more or less fixed in one position sufficiently long to allow repetitive readings. Similar problems exist in the presence of hydramnios or marked obesity. Thus, in about 10 per cent of patients accurate measurements cannot be obtained (Thompson). Other sources of error have been emphasized by Hellman et al., including difficulty in locating the biparietal diameter, the presence of exaggerated biparietal bosses and technical failure to equalize the two pulsations in the A-mode. These potential limitations notwithstanding, ultrasonography appears to provide a reliability heretofore unobtainable by other means.

Hellman et al. also recently described use of serial ultrasonic measurements to evaluate placental growth. This may be a potentially important additional means for utilizing this technique in assessing fetal well-being.

TESTS OF FETAL WELL-BEING AND PLACENTAL FUNCTION

Amnioscopy

Saling introduced a simple endoscopic technique for observing the condition of the amniotic fluid during late pregnancy and in labor. By inspecting the forewaters through the intact membranes with an amnioscope introduced into the cervical canal, the physician can determine whether the amniotic fluid is clear or milky and flecked with *vernix caseosa* or whether it contains meconium. The latter finding is said to suggest that the fetus is at risk. The technique itself is quite simple. The amnioscope may be passed by aseptic technique either by touch or under direct vision. The color of the liquor amnii is best judged by observing it as reflected on a surface such as fetal skin or large flecks of vernix.

The significance of positive amnioscopy, that is, one which demonstrates the presence of meconium in the amniotic fluid, is unclear. Although meconium-stained amniotic fluid is sure evidence that the fetus has defecated, its cause is not necessarily demonstrated. Saling insists that "Almost all disturbances which compromise the foetus during the last weeks of pregnancy result in the passage of meconium." He theorizes this to be on the basis of oxygen-conserving adaptation by which the blood supply to organs such as the bowel diminishes preferentially in the presence of oxygen deprivation, thereby economizing oxygen use. This results in hyperperistalsis as a result of ischemia.

Whether meconium staining is a *sine qua non* of hypoxia, however, is rather doubtful. Kubli has shown that, although meconium staining of the amniotic fluid statistically increases the risk to the fetus, it is not necessarily associated with manifest fetal hypoxia. On this basis, he concludes that detection of meconium is not diagnostic of hypoxia and that amnioscopy serves merely as a screening procedure.

Passage of meconium may be minimal or absent particularly with premature fetuses, even in the presence of severe hypoxia, possibly because the autonomic nervous system is not yet sufficiently mature. Although it is unlikely that death of a mature fetus can occur without passage of meconium, cases have been documented. By the same token, meconium has been encountered rather frequently in association with perfectly normal fetuses who show no clinical signs of asphyxia at all. Moreover, clear amniotic fluid may be seen after known intrauterine death, suggesting that meconium may be absorbed over the course of time. Thus, amnioscopy may serve as a potentially useful screening device with somewhat limited diagnostic capability.

Endocrine Studies

Estriol. Serial determinations of urinary estriol excretion have provided useful information concerning the status of the fetoplacental unit in high risk pregnancies. It appears that biosynthesis of estriol within the placenta cannot occur without precursor substances produced in the fetal adrenal gland. Dehydroisoandrosterone sulfate is formed by the fetal adrenals from pregnenolone. This is converted in the fetal liver by 16-hydroxylation and finally aromatized to estriol in the placenta (Ryan). Where the fetal adrenal is atrophied, as in anencephaly, consistently low estriol excretion occurs (Frandsen and Stakemann).

Reasonably accurate and relatively reproducible colorimetric and gas chromatographic techniques are now available for routine assay of estriol levels in maternal urine. As pregnancy progresses, the low values of the first and second trimesters increase sharply during the last three to four weeks of pregnancy, falling dramatically after delivery. The range of normal values depends somewhat on the technique of the determination, but in general values below 12 μg. per 24 hours may be considered suspicious. Much more significant than absolute values, however, is progressive and dramatic fall in estriol levels. This latter strongly suggests impending fetal death.

Unfortunately, estriol excretion is influenced by other factors, including length of gestation and fetal and placental size, as well as multiple pregnancy. Moreover, there is poor correlation with fetal well-being in erythroblastosis fetalis. Low values are encountered in conjunction with some types of fetal malformation, such as anencephaly.

There are day-to-day variations in estriol excretion under normal circumstances in pregnancy. Estriol levels are also affected by maternal renal function. Adequacy of urine collection must be ascertained. Some laboratories routinely do creatinine determinations simultaneously both as a check on renal function and on adequacy of urine collection, reporting the estriol level as a ratio to creatinine content. This approach has much to recommend it.

Because of the difficulty sometimes encountered in interpreting urinary estriol levels, determinations of estriol content in amniotic fluid has been pursued (Berman et al.). Values less than 100 μg. per liter were consistently indicative of fetal jeopardy, but wide variations were encountered. Correlation with fetal well-being did not seem to be especially better than urinary determinations.

Plasma estriol assays, when more readily available, will undoubtedly prove to be more valuable in this regard. The technique is still rather complex and not widely used. Plasma estriol levels at term range from 9 to 22 μg. per 100 ml. (Ratanosopa et al.). The use of serial estriol assays to monitor patients with problems that threaten the fetus will be discussed at length in relevant chapters dealing with diabetes, preeclampsia, intrauterine growth retardation and placental insufficiency.

Placental Polypeptides. Determinations of chorionic gonadotropin (HCG) have been employed as tests of placental function for many years. Their value as a means for diagnosis of pregnancy has previously been discussed (Chapter 4). They are also critical in the management of hydatidiform mole and choriocarcinoma. Greene et al. reported finding increased excretion of HCG in association with diabetes mellitus, Rh isoimmunization and preeclampsia, suggesting that high levels encountered near term might be indicative of impending fetal death. In early pregnancy, the outcome of patients with threatened abortion appears to be well correlated with HCG immunoassay levels (Midgley). Here, falling levels are ominous. Use of HCG determinations as a means for assessing fetoplacental well-being is limited in terms of accuracy, dependability and significance.

The origin of human placental lactogen or *chorionic somato-mammotropin* (HPL) from the placenta has been discussed in Chapter 4. Its limited usefulness as a possible measure of placental function, particularly on the basis of information obtained by serial determinations, has been suggested (Spellacy et al.). Serum levels were found to be greater than 6.8 μg. per ml. in pregnancies over 32 weeks by Saxena et al., who reported good correlation with placental weight. They felt that the rate and direction of HPL change could serve as a sensitive indicator of placental function. Josimovich et al. found a linear increase in HPL levels with advancing pregnancy. Correlation with placental weight was verified, but they were unable to determine any meaningful correlation with outcome. Recent studies by Varma et al. show that serial monitoring of HPL is effective in allowing one to follow the progress of pregnancy and anticipate the hazards of placental failure. Applicable situations include diabetes mellitus, hypertensive disorders, isoimmunization, retarded intrauterine growth and threatened abortion. The controversy is as yet unresolved. It would appear that HPL measurement may be a useful adjunct to the study of placental function in coassociation with other examinations, such as urinary estriol excretion (see above).

Progesterone Metabolites. There is widespread use of measurements of urinary pregnanediol for evaluating pregnancy. The true clinical value of this approach is seriously limited (MacNaughton). The placenta produces large amounts of progesterone increasingly during pregnancy (see Chapter 4), and this is reflected in increasing levels of pregnanediol in the urine. Formation of this metabolite, however, takes place in the placenta even if the fetus is faring poorly or is dead. Continued use of pregnanediol excretion as a means for studying fetal well-being appears to be indefensible.

Hormone Cytology. The hormonal status of the pregnancy may be reflected in the morphologic appearance of desquamated vaginal cells. Normally in pregnancy one finds an abundance of large, basophilic intermediate cells with dense cytoplasm. Beyond the fourteenth week, small intermediate cells of the navicular type predominate, with basophilic cytoplasm and large yellow vacuolization. Near term, the numbers of navicular cells diminish and significant numbers of karyopyknotic superficial cells appear, totaling at least 15 per cent of the cell population.

An inverse relationship between the number of karyopyknotic cells and estriol levels has been demonstrated by Leeton. In threatened abortion associated with falling estrogen production, increase in karyopyknotic cells in the vaginal smear is seen. The risk of abortion appears to increase with rising karyopyknotic index, characterized by the disappearance of the navicular pattern and an increase in the number of superficial cells (Madsen et al.).

Late in pregnancy, after the karyopyknotic index has risen, death of the fetus is associated with diminished numbers of small cells and the appearance of parabasal cells in the smear. These large, rounded cells with vesicular nuclei tend to indicate fetal jeopardy. Persistence of the ferning pattern of the cervical mucus beyond the first two or three months of pregnancy is confirmatory of the poor prognosis one can anticipate under such circumstances. The inherent value of hormone cytology is improved considerably by serial observations.

Enzyme Studies

Diamine Oxidase. Interest has recently been revived in the study of plasma diamine oxidase (histaminase) by the development of specific radioimmunoassay techniques for its evaluation (Okuyama and Kobayashi). This enzyme is found in large amounts during pregnancy, levels increasing with advancing gestation up to about the twentieth week. It has been shown useful for accurate prognostication in the presence of threatened abortion (Southren et al.). Persistently low levels are seen with missed abortion. Weingold has shown that serial plasma enzyme titers within the normal range, that is, greater than 500 units per ml., consistently indicate that pregnancy will be maintained into the third trimester. This assay appears to be uniquely applicable to evaluation of pregnancy in the first and second trimesters, unlike estriol excretion which is useful only in the third trimester.

Alkaline Phosphatase. Consistent patterns of increasing levels of alkaline phosphatase are said to be encountered with advancing pregnancy on serial determinations beyond the thirty-second week. The source of this enzyme in pregnancy is not known precisely, although it is likely to be of fetal or placental origin. Placental alkaline phosphatase is heat stable at $56°$ C. for 30 minutes, as contrasted with the alkaline phosphatase derived from other tissues. Messer showed a partial correlation between levels of heat-stable alkaline phosphatase and fetal outcome. Good results were uniformly encountered with a normally progressive increase in enzyme levels; abnormal curves, on the other hand, were associated with both good and bad results. Thus, the test served merely as a useful screening device.

Cardiotachometry

Auscultation of the fetal heart is widely used as a method for assessing fetal condition. Bradycardia, particularly if persistent beyond the end of contractions, is generally felt to be indicative of "fetal distress." The lack of real correlation between such stethoscopic observations and neonatal condition, however, has been demonstrated by Benson et al. in a large series of patients studied quite critically. By the use of sophisticated instantaneous rate techniques, great strides have recently been made in the identification of fetuses truly at risk on the basis of fetal heart rate patterns.

The work of Hon and others has shown that it is possible to identify specific patterns of fetal heart rate response to uterine contractions. This requires continuous recording of instantaneous beat-to-beat rate and simultaneous measurement of intrauterine pressure changes. The former is obtained by the application of suitable silver-silver chloride electrodes to the fetal scalp. Uterine pressure recordings are obtained by use of an intrauterine amniotic fluid catheter attached to an external strain gauge or, less reliably, by means of an external tocodynamometer attached to the abdominal wall. Electronic instrumentation notes the interval between fetal heartbeats, ideally measuring from one fetal R wave on the electrocardiogram to the next. It converts this time interval to an instantaneous rate in beats per minute by the formula:

$$\text{rate} = \frac{60}{t}$$

where t is the beat-to-beat interval in seconds.

A less satisfactory method is that of averaging the number of beats per unit time, similar to that which is done by auscultation. This does not provide the same kind of valuable information one derives from the more sophisticated instantaneous

rate determinations. It is likely that phonocardiographic or ultrasonographic techniques will soon be perfected so that the "invasive" intravaginal use of scalp electrodes will no longer be required.

The precision afforded by such techniques far exceeds that of the human ear. It has been learned, for example, that clinically undetectable fluctuations in baseline rate are quite normal. This irregularity or variability reflects the balance between vagal and sympathetic tone, occurring at a frequency of about 3 to 5 cycles per minute with variations ranging up to 10 per cent of the baseline rate. The absence of this normal variability may result from immaturity of the autonomic system, as in the premature fetus, or from the pharmacologic vagal blocking action of drugs such as atropine. It may also be seen late in the course of developing hypoxia; the appearance of a fixed heart rate under such circumstances may be ominous.

Three patterns of periodic deceleration of the fetal heart rate according to their relationship to timing of the contraction have been recognized (Fig. 116). There is some confusion with regard to nomenclature: Hon's designation of early deceleration or head compression deceleration (HC) and variable deceleration or cord compression pattern (CC) encompasses Caldeyro-Barcia's type I dips. The type II dips include delayed examples of cord compression patterns. Caldeyro-Barcia et al. fail to designate the important specific disorder of late deceleration or uteroplacental insufficiency pattern (UPI) stressed by Hon. The Hon terminology will be used here.

Early deceleration patterns coincide with the onset of uterine contraction, returning to the base line as the contraction subsides. They are uniform in shape. They are believed to be innocuous and related to head compression during contraction. They may be elicited by digital or forceps pressure on the head. *Late deceleration* patterns are identical in form except that they begin some time after the uterine contraction has begun, usually reaching maximum bradycardia after the contraction has ended. This pattern is encountered in the presence of impaired uteroplacental exchange and is considered

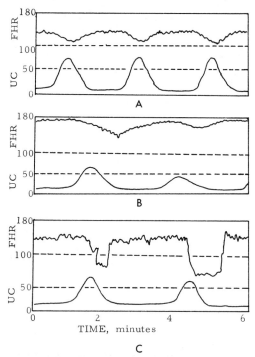

Figure 116 Typical fetal heart rate (FHR) deceleration patterns as related to uterine contractions (UC). FHR in beats per minute and UC in mm Hg. *A,* Early deceleration or head compression pattern with onset early in the course of contraction, symmetrical shape. *B,* Late deceleration or uteroplacental insufficiency patterns with late onset relative to contraction, symmetrical shape. *C,* Variable deceleration or cord compression pattern with variable onset, variable shape. (From Hon, E. H.: Biophysical studies of the human fetus. *In* Adamsons, K., ed.: Diagnosis and Treatment of Fetal Disorders. New York, Springer-Verlag New York, Inc., 1968.)

ominous in that it appears related to hypoxia. It is theorized that the uterine contraction impedes uterine blood flow, interfering with placental exchange and causing a transient drop in available oxygen to the fetus. Thus, the uterine contraction provides a periodic stress to the fetus. The fetal lack of reserve becomes manifest in the fetal heart rate pattern. *Variable deceleration* patterns are variable in onset with reference to uterine contractions and variable in shape. Typically, they are characterized by rapid fall in heart rate followed by a variable interval of acute bradycardia and terminated by rapid return to baseline levels. Unless persistent and prolonged, this pattern is not the ominous indicator of fetal distress it was once thought to be.

The value of the cardiotachometric approach to fetal monitoring may be considerable, particularly when used in conjunction with biochemical surveillance. The approach has recently been expanded to provide a form of "stress test" (oxytocin challenge test) to determine placental reserve (Ray et al.). By stimulating a series of uterine contractions using oxytocin infusion, adequacy of reserve is demonstrable in the resulting fetal heart rate patterns. The fetus that shows it cannot tolerate such contractions, by manifesting UPI patterns, for example, demonstrates a clear lack of placental reserve to maintain adequate oxygenation during labor and further shows clearly that it will probably not be able to tolerate intrauterine life much longer.

Correlation with outcome has recently been demonstrated by Schifrin and Dame, who studied cardiotachometric patterns within 30 minutes of delivery and related the appearance of abnormal patterns to Apgar scores. Aside from those with serious fetal anomalies, all infants delivered following a normal fetal heart rate pattern were in good condition, none showing neonatal depression. The correlation with abnormal patterns was less clear-cut, many infants being delivered in good condition despite the appearance of patterns suggesting intrauterine hypoxia. All depressed infants, however, had shown such patterns earlier. Thus, this approach is a most useful screening device. Among fetuses yielding abnormal heart rate patterns, the additional information potentially available by means of scalp blood sampling may be invaluable in distinguishing those truly in jeopardy from others.

Biochemical Assessment

Access to study of fetal acid-base status was achieved by Saling in 1961 with the introduction of a technique for sampling capillary blood in the fetal scalp transcervically during labor. Under endoscopic visualization, the fetal scalp is cleansed, made hyperemic by ethyl chloride spray, coated with a silicone gel to promote formation of a blood globule and incised with a small measured stab blade. The capillary blood is collected in a capillary tube. The sample is available for biochemical study.

Most clinical evaluations have been confined to blood pH measurements as indirect indices of oxygenation. The normal placenta functions efficiently to maintain acid-base balance by removing carbon dioxide and replacing free acid ions from the fetus with oxygen from the mother. Rapid equilibration is expected so that the pH determination is a reasonable measure of oxygen availability. If limited, fetal asphyxia will be revealed by rising pCO_2 and falling pO_2, pH and base excess, resulting in combined respiratory and metabolic acidosis. The fall in pH and base excess reflects breakdown of glycogen to pyruvate and lactic acid by anaerobic means. As lactic acid levels rise, pH falls.

Most workers in this field consider pH values below 7.20 to be critical. More importantly, confirmation of progressive fall in serial pH determinations is ominous. A single value may easily be misinterpreted, particularly since it may reflect maternal acidosis which is seen so commonly in prolonged labor. With the availability of microanalytic techniques, not only can pH be measured but other acid-base parameters as well. These latter provide additional information that may be of great importance in the management of the fetus at risk. There can be little doubt that fetal scalp blood sampling is a valuable addition to the diagnostic armamentarium relative to evaluation of fetal status. It is particularly applicable in those high risk pregnancy situations in which cardiotachometric monitoring indicates the presence of heart rate patterns seen in association with fetal hypoxia (see above).

INTRAUTERINE DIAGNOSIS

The past decade has seen rapid advances in our ability to diagnose various fetal problems during pregnancy. Several genetic disorders are readily detectable prenatally at this time because of the general acceptance of transabdominal amniocentesis as a procedure with real but acceptably minimal risks. Moreover, tissue culture techniques, microanalytic biochemical procedures and simplified chromosomal analyses have advanced to the point where this discipline is becoming widely available. Coupled with the pervading liberalization of attitudes toward abortion, facilities and expertise in the detection of the genetic and metabolic disorders offer much promise for the future.

Amniocentesis

In the first section of this chapter we alluded to utilization of information obtainable by study of amniotic fluid acquired by amniocentesis in determination of fetal maturity. Much additional insight is available from investigation of amniotic fluid. The detection, assessment and management of Rh isoimmunization, for example, is perhaps best known and most widely utilized (see Chapter 52). Other situations of interest center on the diagnosis of congenital and metabolic disorders. Antenatal determination of the sex of the fetus is useful in managing pregnancies where sex-linked recessive disorders may exist. Hemophilia, muscular dystrophy and Hunter's disease are examples of such conditions.

Examination of desquamated cells of fetal origin from its skin, buccal mucosa, vagina, umbilical cord or urinary bladder will reveal the presence or absence of sex chromatin. Although uncultured cells may be studied by cytologic techniques, tissue culture of amniotic fluid cells is recommended (Nadler and Gerbie). The condensed X chromosome is readily identifiable as a Barr body seen at the periphery of cells obtained from female fetuses. Such chromatin-positive cells are normally encountered in at least 20 per cent of such cells; they are absent in males.

Chromosomal abnormalities have been diagnosed *in utero* by karyotyping cultured fetal cells from amniotic fluid. Chromosomal translocations and trisomies have been diagnosed *in utero*, including Down's syndrome primarily. Although such major chromosomal defects can be recognized readily, minor variants are more difficult to detect. Biochemical analysis of both amniotic fluid and of cultured cells has aided considerably in this regard.

Various familial metabolic disorders have been diagnosed by examining amniotic fluid for excess or deficiency of characteristic substances. Among these are adrenogenital syndrome (increased 17-ketosteroids and pregnanetriol), Tay-Sachs disease (deficiency of hexosaminidase A), Pompe's disease (deficiency of α-1,4-glucosidase), and mucopolysaccharidosis.

Study of cultured amniotic fluid cells has been equally effective in uncovering similar disorders, as well as galactosemia, Niemann-Pick disease (deficiency of sphingomyelinase) and Fabry's disease (deficiency of ceramide trihexasidase). Mucopolysaccharide storage disorders and related conditions have been detected *in utero* by the demonstration of intracellular metachromatic granules in cultured amniotic fluid cells. Such conditions as Hurler, Hunter and Marfan syndromes, as well as cystic fibrosis and Gaucher's disease, have been discovered in this way. However, the reliability of such diagnoses based on metachromasia has been questioned, particularly from the point of view that heterozygosity cannot be determined. As time passes and greater sophistication is brought to bear in this area, other disorders of the fetus are being detected. A review of this subject and discussion of its sociologic implications in terms of selective abortion may be invaluable to the reader (Bergsma).

Transabdominal amniocentesis is not without risk to both mother and fetus. Fetal risks are those of trauma or induction of abortion or labor. Maternal hazards include primarily bleeding and infection. In experienced hands, however, reported risks are less than one per cent, justifying its utilization where clearly indicated.

If adequate laboratory support is available, it is now recommended that these studies be undertaken in certain high risk situations. These include the following: (1) one parent is a carrier of a known chromosomal aberration, particularly if the disorder is sex-linked recessive; (2) women who have previously delivered anomalous infants, particularly with trisomic Down's syndrome; (3) patients with known familial biochemical disorders.

The risk of conceiving a child with a chromosomal disorder, particularly Down's syndrome, in women beyond age 40 years is in excess of one per cent (Maegenis et al.). It would be impractical to recommend widespread initiation of screening programs for such patients in view of the limited facilities and expertise available as yet in most locations. It is likely, however, that in due course this important service will become available to a larger number of patients whose fetuses may be at risk.

Amniography

The popularity of amniography as a diagnostic technique for intrauterine diagnosis, although first introduced in 1930, became widespread in association with technical advancements relative to treatment of severe Rh isoimmunization. Menees et al. first utilized it to help localize the placenta. McLain has more recently popularized the approach utilizing nonirritating contrast media, such as Diodrast, Hypaque or Conray 400, in the amniotic sac. Amniography today is used in many different ways, some of which are being replaced by ultrasonography because of the radiation hazards recognized to be associated with amniography. The status of the fetus is readily demonstrated by showing its ability to swallow contrast medium. Moreover, motility of the gastrointestinal tract is readily displayed. Anomalies of the gastrointestinal tract, such as esophageal and duodenal atresia, can be shown. Other soft tissue and bony anomalies may be apparent. Monoamniotic or conjoined twins have been discovered by the use of this technique. Fetal ascites and scalp edema are well recognized in association with Rh isoimmunization. Hydatidiform mole is readily diagnosed and accurate placental localization is also possible. Similarly, hydramnios is readily visualized.

Ultrasonic Diagnosis

Earlier we discussed the use of ultrasonography for diagnosing fetal maturity and assessing fetal growth by repetitive measurement of the biparietal diameter of the fetal skull. Where B-scanning equipment is available, a great many diagnostic possibilities are opened to the clinician. Resultant two-dimensional pictorial representations of the scanned area give important insights into the anatomic variants in that cross section. Aside from its use in evaluating fetal development, it has been shown effective in detection of pregnancy as early

as the eighth week, in diagnosing multiple pregnancy, in documenting such fetal abnormalities as anencephaly and hydrocephaly, in demonstrating hydramnios, in placental localization, in diagnosing hydatidiform mole and in verifying fetal death. The reliability of this method in technically competent hands appears good and thus far there has been no demonstration of any fetal risk from the use of low intensity energy sources.

REFERENCES

Ball, R. P.: Roentgen pelvimetry and fetal cephalometry. Radiogr. Clin. Photogr. *11*:11, 1935.

Barr, M. L., and Bertram, E. G.: Morphological distinction between neurons of the male and female, and the behaviour of the nuclear satellite during accelerated nucleo-protein synthesis. Nature *163*:676, 1949.

Benson, R. C., Shubeck, F., Deutschberger, J., Weiss, W., and Berendes, H.: Fetal heart rate as a predictor of fetal distress. Obstet. Gynec. *32*:259, 1968.

Bergsma, D., ed.: Symposium on intrauterine diagnosis. Birth Defects 7:1, 1971.

Berman, A. M., Kalchman, G. G., Chattoraj, S. C., and Scommegna, A.: Relationship of amniotic fluid estriol to maternal urinary estriol. Amer. J. Obstet. Gynec. *100*:15, 1968.

Bishop, E. H., and Corson, S.: Estimation of fetal maturity by cytological estimation of amniotic fluid. Amer. J. Obstet. Gynec. *102*:654, 1968.

Blystad, W., Landing, B. H., and Smith, C. A.: Pulmonary hyaline membranes in newborn infants: Statistical, morphological and experimental study of their nature, occurrence and significance. Pediatrics 8:5, 1951.

Brosens, I., and Gordon, H.: Estimation of maturity by cytological examination of the liquor amnii. J. Obstet. Gynaec. Brit. Comm. 73:88, 1966.

Caldeyro-Barcia, R., Ibarra-Polo, A. A., Gulin, L., Poseiro, J. J., and Méndez-Bauer, C.: Diagnostic and prognostic significance of intrapartum fetal tachycardia and type II dips. In Mack, H. C., ed.: Prenatal Life: Biological and Clinical Perspectives. Detroit, Wayne State University Press, 1970.

Campbell, S., and Newman, G. B.: Growth of the fetal biparietal diameter during normal pregnancy. J. Obstet. Gynaec. Brit. Comm. 78:513, 1971.

Christie, A., Martin, M., Williams, E., Hudson, G., and Lassier, J.: Estimation of fetal maturity by roentgen studies of osseous development. Amer. J. Obstet. Gynec. *60*:133, 1950.

Cope, I., and Murdock, J. D.: The estimation of foetal maturity. J. Obstet. Gynaec. Brit. Emp. 65:56, 1958.

Crichton, D. J.: Intra-uterine growth of foetal head after thirty-sixth week of pregnancy. J. Obstet. Gynaec. Brit. Emp. *60*:233, 1953.

Donald, I., and Brown, T. G.: Demonstration of tissue interfaces within the body by ultrasonic echo sounding. Brit. J. Radiol. *34*:539, 1961.

Donald, I., MacVicar, J., and Brown, T. G.: Investigation of abdominal masses by pulsed ultrasound. Lancet *1*:1188, 1958.

Droegemueller, W., Jackson, C., Makowski, E. L., and Battaglia, F. C.: Amniotic fluid examination as an aid in the assessment of gestational age. Amer. J. Obstet. Gynec. *104*:424, 1969.

Frandsen, V. A., and Stakemann, G.: The site of production of oestrogenic hormones in human pregnancy. Acta Endocr. 38:383, 1962.

Gluck, L., Kulovich, M. V., Borer, R. C., Jr., Brenner, P. H., Anderson, G. G., and Spellacy, W. N.: Diagnosis of the respiratory distress syndrome by amniocentesis. Amer. J. Obstet. Gynec. *109*:440, 1971.

Greene, J. W., Jr., Duhring, J. L., and Smith, K.: Placental function tests: A review of methods available for assessment of the fetoplacental complex. Amer. J. Obstet. Gynec. 92:1030, 1965.

Hartley, J. B.: Radiologic estimation of fetal maturity. Brit. J. Radiol. 30:561, 1957.

Hellman, L. M., Kobayashi, M., Fillisti, L., and Lavenhar, M.: Sources of error in sonographic fetal mensuration and estimation of growth. Amer. J. Obstet. Gynec. 99:662, 1967.

Hellman, L. M., Kobayashi, M., Tolles, W. E., and Cromb, E.: Ultrasonic studies on the volumetric growth of the human placenta. Amer. J. Obstet. Gynec. *108*:740, 1970.

Hon, E. H.: Biophysical studies of the human fetus. In Adamsons, K., ed.: Diagnosis and Treatment of Fetal Disorders. New York, Springer-Verlag New York, Inc., 1968.

Josimovich, J. B., Kosor, B., Boccela, L., Mintz, D. H., and Hutchinson, D. L.: Placental lactogen in maternal serum as an index of fetal health. Obstet. Gynec. 36:244, 1970.

Kittrich, M.: Zytodiagnostik des Fruchtwasserabflusses mit Hilfe von Nilblau. Geburtsh. Frauenheilk. 23:156, 1963.

Kornacki, Z., Biczysko, R., and Jakubowski, A.: Amnioscopy as a routine obstetric examination in the later stages of pregnancy. Amer. J. Obstet. Gynec. *101*:539, 1968.

Kosar, W. P., and Steer, C. M.: The relation of body weight to the biparietal diameter in the newborn. Amer. J. Obstet. Gynec. 71:1232, 1956.

Kubli, F.: Amniotic fluid and the early detection of fetal hypoxia. In Huntingford, P. J., Hüter, K. A., and Saling, E., eds.: Perinatal Medicine. New York, Academic Press, 1969.

Leeton, J. F.: Relation between vaginal cytology and oestriol excretion in normal pregnancy. Aust. New Zeal. J. Obstet. Gynaec. 3:78, 1963.

MacNaughton, M. C.: Hormone excretion as a measurement of fetal growth and development. Amer. J. Obstet. Gynec. 97:998, 1967.

Madsen, M., Parks, W. S., Lang, G. H., Johnson, C. R., Guerriero, C. P., and Zimmerman, Y.: Vaginal cytology as an aid in predicting normal pregnancy. Acta Cytol. 10:156, 1966.

Maegenis, R. E., Hecht, F., and Milham, S.: Trisomy 13 (D₁) syndrome: Studies on parental age, sex ratio and survival. J. Pediat. 73:222, 1968.

Mandelbaum, B., and Evans, T. H.: Life in the amniotic fluid. Amer. J. Obstet. Gynec. 104:365, 1969.

Mandelbaum, B., LaCroix, G. C., and Robinson, A. R.: Determination of fetal maturity by spectrophotometric analysis of amniotic fluid. Obstet. Gynec. 29:471, 1967.

McDonald, C., and Thomas, S.: One thousand complete pelvimetries: Radiological and obstetrical analysis. Med. J. Australia 1:357, 1953.

McLain, C. R., Jr.: Amniography, a versatile diagnostic procedure in obstetrics. Obstet. Gynec. 23:45, 1964.

Menees, T. O., Miller, J. D., and Holly, L. E.: Amniography: Preliminary report. Amer. J. Roentgen. 24:363, 1930.

Messer, R. H.: Heat-stable alkaline phosphatase as an index of placental function. Amer. J. Obstet. Gynec. 98:459, 1967.

Midgley, A. R., Jr.: Immunoassay of human gonadotropins: Current status. Clin. Obstet. Gynec. 10:119, 1967.

Nadler, H. L., and Gerbie, A.: Present status of amniocentesis in intrauterine diagnosis of genetic defects. Obstet. Gynec. 38:789, 1971.

Okuyama, T., and Kobayashi, Y.: Determination of diamine oxidase activity by liquid scintillation counting. Arch. Biochem. 95:242, 1961.

O'Leary, J. A., and Bezjian, A. A.: Amniotic fluid fetal maturity score. Obstet. Gynec. 38:375, 1971.

Pitkin, R. M., and Zwirek, S. J.: Amniotic fluid creatinine. Amer. J. Obstet. Gynec. 98:1135, 1967.

Ratanosopa, V., Schindler, A. E., Lee, T. Y., and Herrman, W.: Measurement of estriol in plasma by gasliquid chromatography. Amer. J. Obstet. Gynec. 99:295, 1967.

Ray, M., Freeman, R., Pine, S., and Hesselgesser. R.: Clinical experience with the oxytocin challenge test. Amer. J. Obstet. Gynec. 114:1, 1972.

Ryan, K. J.: Metabolism of C-16-oxygenated steroids by human placenta: The formation of estriol. J. Biol. Chem. 234:2006, 1959.

Saling, E.: Foetal and Neonatal Hypoxia in Relation to Clinical Obstetric Practice. Baltimore, Williams & Wilkins Company, 1968.

Saxena, B. N., Emerson, K., and Selenkow, H. A.: Serum placental lactogen (HPL) levels as an index of placental function. New Eng. J. Med. 281:225, 1969.

Scammon, R. E., and Calkins, L. A.: The Development and Growth of the External Dimensions of the Human Body in the Fetal Period. Minneapolis, University of Minnesota Press, 1929.

Schifrin, B. S., and Dame, L.: Fetal heart rate patterns: Prediction of Apgar score. J.A.M.A. 219:1322, 1972.

Southren, A. L., Kobayashi, Y., Weingold, A. B., and Carmody, N. C.: Serial plasma diamine oxidase in first and second trimester complications of pregnancy. Amer. J. Obstet. Gynec. 96:4, 1966.

Spellacy, W. N., Cohen, W. D., and Carlson, K. L.: Human placental lactogen levels as a measure of placental function. Amer. J. Obstet. Gynec. 97:560, 1967.

Taylor, E. S., Holmes, J. H., Thompson, H. E., and Gottesfeld, K. R.: Ultrasound diagnostic techniques in obstetrics and gynecology. Amer. J. Obstet. Gynec. 90:655, 1964.

Thompson, H. E.: The clinical use of pulsed echo ultrasound in obstetrics and gynecology. Obstet. Gynec. Survey 23:903, 1968.

Thompson, H. E., Holmes, J. H., Gottesfeld, K. R., and Taylor, E. S.: Fetal development as determined by ultrasonic pulse echo techniques. Amer. J. Obstet. Gynec. 92:44, 1965.

Varma, K., Driscoll, S. G., Emerson, K., and Selenkow, H. A.: Clinical and pathologic evaluation of serum immunoreactive human placental lactogen (IR-HPL) in abnormal pregnancy. Obstet. Gynec. 38:487, 1971.

Votta, R. A., deGagneten, C. B., Parada, O., and Giulietti, M.: Cytologic study of amniotic fluid in pregnancy. Amer. J. Obstet. Gynec. 102:571, 1968.

Weingold, A. B.: Enzymatic indices of fetal environment. Clin. Obstet. Gynec. 11:1081, 1968.

Willocks, J., Donald, I., Duggan, T. C., and Day, N.: Foetal cephalometry by ultrasound. J. Obstet. Gynaec. Brit. Comm. 71:11, 1964.

Zuppinger, A.: Roentgen diagnosis in obstetrics. In Case, J. T., ed.: Roentgen Diagnostics. New York, Grune & Stratton, 1954.

SECTION TWO

PHYSIOLOGY AND CONDUCT OF LABOR

Chapter 14

Onset and Clinical Course of Labor

DEFINITIONS

Labor is the process by which the product of conception is expelled from the uterus through the vagina to the outside world. This definition excludes extraction by any other passage, as in cesarean section. Synonyms for labor are *delivery, parturition, travail, childbirth, accouchement* and *confinement*.

Abortion is the interruption of pregnancy before the fetus is viable. In most areas today *viability* is defined in terms of fetal weight as 500 gm. or in terms of gestational age as 20 weeks. It refers to the potential capability of the fetus to survive outside the uterus. The lay term *miscarriage* generally refers to any premature termination of pregnancy with death of the fetus.

Premature labor is the interruption of pregnancy after the fetus is viable, but before term. The expression premature labor is usually applied to the interruption of pregnancy between the twentieth and thirty-seventh weeks, or more commonly in association with the delivery of an infant weighing 500 to 2500 gm.

Postmature or *postterm* or *postdate labor* implies that labor occurs two weeks

or more after the expected date of confinement. This situation is difficult to evaluate since exact estimation of term is not easy to predict. The relationship of this condition to the more critical problems of placental insufficiency and fetal dysmaturity will be discussed in Chapter 54.

A *gravida* is a pregnant woman. A *primigravida* is one pregnant for the first time; a *nulligravida* has never been pregnant. A *multigravida* is one who has been pregnant several times. *Gravidity* refers to a pregnancy regardless of its duration.

A *primipara* is a woman who has had one pregnancy which resulted in a viable child, regardless of whether the child was living at birth and regardless of whether it was a single or multiple birth. Although the words "primigravida" and "primipara" are not synonymous, they are often erroneously used as if they were interchangeable. A *nullipara* is a primigravida or multigravida who has not yet been delivered of a viable infant.

A *multipara* is a woman who has had two or more children; *pluripara* is its synonym. The term *grand multipara* is usually reserved for the woman who has delivered many viable pregnancies; the qualifying number is variable, but is usually placed by convention arbitrarily at six or more.

The designation *para* refers to pregnancies that have continued to viability. A patient is a primigravida or *gravida I* and a nullipara or *para 0* during her first pregnancy. She becomes a primipara when she delivers a viable baby, whether the child is dead or alive at birth. During her second pregnancy she is a secundigravida or *gravida II* and at the same time she is a primipara or *para I*. If a patient had two abortions and then becomes pregnant she is gravida III, para 0. After she delivers a viable baby she is gravida III, para I, and so on. *Gravida* and *para* refer to pregnancies, not to babies. Hence, a woman who delivers twins in her first pregnancy is still a gravida I, para I.

In some clinics it is customary to summarize the past obstetric history of a patient by a series of four numbers, e.g., 4-1-2-4. The first digit refers to the number of full-term infants the patient has delivered; the second to the number of premature infants; the third to the number of abortions and the fourth to the number of living children. This example would indicate that the patient has had 4 full-term deliveries, 1 premature delivery, 2 abortions and 4 living children. This gives a more complete picture than the mere statement that she is a gravida VII.

A *parturient* is a woman in labor.

A *puerpera* is a woman who has just given birth.

Labor is divided into (1) normal labor or *eutocia* and (2) abnormal labor or *dystocia*.

The phenomenon of parturition must be considered in three parts: (1) the *powers*, by which the expulsion is accomplished; (2) the *passages*, which represent the course and the resistances encountered; and (3) the *passengers*, the fetus and the rest of the conceptus (placenta, membranes and amniotic fluid, collectively called *secundines*).

ONSET OF LABOR

The mechanism which triggers the onset of labor is unknown. Many theories abound, none of which is entirely satisfactory or proved. Reynolds held that parturition is initiated as a result of a gradually accelerating convergence of a number of factors — structural, humoral, nervous, nutritional and circulatory. At a specific time for each species and adapted to the morphologic conditions present in each, these factors lead to evacuation by the uterus of its contents. Among the various prevalent theories as to how this comes about are those that invoke modification of the regulatory mechanism of uterine contractility through (1) uterine volume, (2) autonomic nervous system, (3) endocrine balance and (4) fetal factors. No single, simple, integrated concept has as yet been evolved to satisfy all known facts relating to this phenomenon.

It is probably easiest to consider normal pregnancy a condition in which the intrinsic contractile potential of the uterus is kept in check until such time as the fetus is sufficiently mature to survive in the outside world. As we have seen (Chapter 7), the uterus enlarges greatly during pregnancy. Its muscle fibers hypertrophy markedly and increase their content of actin, myosin and adenosinetriphosphatase in response to stimulation by estrogens from the placenta. Estrogens also augment myometrial contractility ionically by altering the gradient across cell membranes, leading to high sodium and low potassium concentrations within the cells. As a result the uterus undergoes spontaneous activity. In the absence of some inhibiting factors, it is likely that pregnancy could not long continue.

Progesterone or an analogue of progesterone may constitute such an inhibiting factor. Csapo has elaborated a popular theory in this regard. Progesterone inhibits uterine activity by effecting hyperpolarization of the cell membrane and by blocking electrical conduction. The evolution of uterine activity to full-blown labor with efficient, coordinated contractions may be a consequence of progesterone withdrawal. The withdrawal is believed to be a local phenomenon, taking place near the placental site. As placental production of progesterone falls at term, its inhibiting effects are diminished progressively and synchronous contractions of the uterine muscular mass evolve as labor ensues.

Although progesterone effectively prevents the expected expulsion of fetuses in rabbits following oophorectomy, systemic administration of progesterone to human gravidas has not been shown to be effective as a means for inhibiting uterine contractions. Csapo postulated a local effect to explain this discrepancy, indicating that there must exist a very high concentration gradient such that the myometrial level of progesterone cannot be substantially augmented by systemic administration. Scommegna et al., however, were able to inhibit contractions using infusions of pregnenolone and adrenal steroid, which acts as the immediate precursor of placental progesterone. This observation has provided support for the "progesterone block" theory.

Specifically what causes the pregnancy-stabilizing factors to stop acting at a given time in pregnancy is not understood. If indeed it is a local inhibition due to absorption of progesterone from the placenta, it is possible that withdrawal is related to the degenerative or aging changes which take place in the placenta near term in association with disturbances of uterine and placental circulation. Unfortunately, there is no evidence yet available that local tissue levels of progesterone fall prior to the onset of labor.

Oxytocin may play a role in initiation of labor. Caldeyro-Barcia and Sereno have shown that the uterus is increasingly sensitive to exogenous oxytocin with advancing pregnancy. Circulating endogenous oxytocin levels do not appear to be increased in the course of pregnancy. However, concentrations in venous blood rise during labor (Coch et al.). The mechanism by which oxytocin causes myometrial contraction is unknown. It appears to act directly on the cell membrane to lower the membrane potential. A specific enzyme system, oxytocinase, has been found that hydrolyzes liberated oxytocin (Fekete). It is postulated that uterine activation may occur because this enzyme loses its potency or reduces its concentration at term, thereby allowing circulating oxytocin to become effective. However, there has been no experimental verification of a prelabor decrease. Moreover, the hypothesis cannot be considered valid for normal labors that begin and are maintained in the absence of an anatomic source of oxytocin, namely, where the pituitary is hypofunctioning or absent. That normal labor can normally occur under such circumstances speaks against the likelihood that oxytocin plays a primary role in this process. Nevertheless, recent investigation has shown that hormones previously believed formed in the pituitary may actually arise in the hypothalamus, which may in theory serve as an effective source for endogenous oxytocin in the absence of the pituitary gland.

Similar doubts exist with regard to the role of catecholamines and acetylcholine in initiating labor. Whereas the hyperpolarization of the cell membrane due to epinephrine inhibits contractility, norepinephrine appears to have an opposite effect as evidenced by the increase in basal tonus and frequency of contractility seen following its administration. The excitatory effect of acetylcholine, based on membrane depolarization, results in increased basal tonus of the uterine muscle. Epinephrine and its derivatives, isoxsuprine and isoproterenol, act to inhibit uterine activity but stimulate beta-receptors; norepinephrine stimulates uterine activity by its apparent effect on alpha-receptors. It has been conjectured that labor may ensue as a consequence of alterations in endogenous release of these substances (Sauter). Since blood levels before and during labor are unaffected, however, this concept is unsupported (Israel et al.).

Whether or not prostaglandins serve any function in the process of labor or its initiation is as yet unknown (see Chapter 4). Although apparently quite effective in inducing both abortion and labor, they have not been detected in the plasma of pregnant women prior to the onset of labor. They are present in amniotic fluid during labor. Further study in this potentially important area is clearly needed before the part played by prostaglandins in labor can be defined.

The fetus may also be involved in regulating onset of labor. It is a recognized characteristic of pregnancies associated with anencephalic fetuses, whose pituitary hypofunction results in retarded adrenal development, that onset of labor may be delayed and pregnancy prolonged. Post-term pregnancies result in about 40 per cent of these cases (Milic and Adamsons). The timing of onset of labor in sheep has been altered by Liggins by manipulating fetal adrenal function, either by hypophysectomy or adrenalectomy. He was also able to provoke premature labor by stimulating the fetal adrenals with ACTH. He postulated that the action of the fetal adrenal on labor is perhaps mediated by the glucocorticoid effect of cortisol, increased concentrations of which might inhibit progesterone production by the placenta. This in turn would result in withdrawal of the progesterone block referred to earlier.

A final consideration is the possibility that the duration of pregnancy is governed by intrauterine conditions. For example, in general, a greater degree of uterine distention predisposes to a shorter gestation. With greater uterine distention the intrauterine pressure and intramural tensions are necessarily higher and this in turn may be a contributing factor, perhaps through local ischemia, to aging of the placenta and regression of the placenta-stabilizing influences of gestation. Whether or not this is the case is unknown. It is clear, however, that increased stretching of the uterine wall has an enhancing effect on the irritability and contractility of the uterine muscle, as is true with all other muscle.

Parturition begins not merely because inhibitory influences on the uterus are withdrawn but also because a number of other factors stimulate the myometrium. These are not sudden in their onset as is attested to by the gradual development of spontaneous myometrial activity as pregnancy advances, by the gradual increase in sensitivity to exogenously administered oxytocin and by the gradual evolution within the uterus of conditions that predispose to constantly increasing irritability of the myometrium.

As pregnancy advances, the curvature of various parts of the uterus undergoes a progressive change in which the lower uterine segment and cervix are most involved. The tension in any part of the uterus is proportional to the principal radius of curvature at that part. As a result the tension at the fundus is more than three times that in the lower uterine segment and cervix. Therefore, the resistance to stretching of the lower uterine segment

must be less than that of the corpus uteri. Thus, at the onset of labor the uterine wall is in such a condition that the initiation of forceful, intermittent contractions retract the lower part of the uterus up toward the fundus. The lower uterine segment is essentially passive in this process and becomes progressively thinner.

The change in uterine shape with advancing pregnancy plus the factor of stretching may somehow influence when labor begins. That this is probably not singularly important, however, is suggested by the fact that uterine volume characteristically decreases just prior to onset of labor at term as the amount of amniotic fluid diminishes. Moreover, if the fetus should die, the volume shrinks, yet labor generally ensues in due course, usually well before it might have if the fetus had survived.

CLINICAL COURSE OF LABOR

In most nulliparas and many multiparas there is a *prodromal stage* preceding labor, but the symptoms may be so slight that they may be unnoticed and labor, therefore, seems to begin abruptly without forewarning. The prodromal signs include the following: (1) *Lightening*, with relief of pressure in the upper part of the abdomen and increase of pressure in the pelvis, together with a mucous discharge from the vagina. (2) *False pains* which manifest themselves as uncomfortable, intermittent uterine contractions in the latter weeks of pregnancy that often annoy the patient. They occur especially at night, subsiding toward morning. They indicate that labor may be imminent. Ordinarily, contractions are occurring at irregular intervals throughout pregnancy and are unnoticed. They are usually not painful until actual labor begins. Many women complain of drawing sensations in the pelvis similar to those experienced during menstruation, sometimes painful. The contractions which occur prodromally prior to the onset of true labor are the *Hicks contractions,* named after John Braxton Hicks who first described them; they often efface and dilate the cervix. (3) A discharge of mucus, often mixed with blood, may appear from the vagina. It is the plug which formerly filled the cervix, closing off the uterine cavity from the vagina. Separation from the cervical mucosa may result in slight bleeding, called the *show*. Show may not appear until labor has been in progress for some time. (4) Examination prior to labor often demonstrates the cervix to be soft and shortened, perhaps completely effaced. In nulliparas the external os may be sufficiently dilated to permit one finger to be inserted into the canal, indicating prelabor dilatation of 1 to 1.5 cm. In multiparas often two fingers may be inserted, indicating a 3 cm. dilatation. Exceptionally, the external and the internal os remain tightly closed until labor begins, but this is unusual. Occasionally, the cervix is dilated to a greater degree, perhaps 4 or even 5 cm. so that three fingers may be inserted, the result of insensible prelabor contractions.

The transition into labor is usually gradual, but we consider that labor has begun when the uterine contractions are perceived, usually as painful, and are recurring at regular intervals. However, if they subside, the condition denotes a *false labor*, a diagnosis generally made by hindsight alone. The time of the rupture of the membranes or "bag of waters" is variable. Labor is not assumed to have begun merely because there is a bloody show or the membranes have ruptured.

The process of parturition divides itself classically into three stages: The *first stage* extends from the beginning of regular uterine contractions until the external os is completely dilated and flush with the vagina, thus completing the continuous channel called the *parturient canal*. This is considered to be the *stage of dilatation*. The membranes usually rupture toward the end of this stage or during it.

The *second stage* extends from the end of the first stage until the expulsion of the baby is completed. This is called the *stage of expulsion*. In actuality, descent through the birth canal generally begins before the end of the first stage (see Chapter 15).

The *third stage* extends from the delivery of the child until after the placenta and membranes are expelled. This is the *afterbirth* or the placental stage.

By convention, a *fourth stage* is usually appended. This includes the first hour or two after delivery of the placenta during which recovery of uterine tone must occur so that acute bleeding may be averted or recognized promptly and treated effectively.

First Stage

When labor begins, the uterine contractions usually occur 5 to 15 minutes apart. They are often considered by the patient to be painful and, therefore, have been designated widely as "pains." The current emphasis on pain-fear relationships (see Chapter 11) is reflected in a growing taboo against use of this term, which is now preferably referred to merely as "contractions."

As labor progresses the contractions gradually become stronger and more frequent. Women regard labor pain differently. Strong, stoic women of quiet, even temperament bear up bravely, while nervous, hysterical or anxious parturients cry out even early in the first stage, demanding relief. It is conceivable that such women, through fear. inhibit the course of an otherwise normal labor. Patients may be cheerful between contractions or doze. As the contractions become stronger the intervals between are shorter.

The uterus begins to contract before the pain is felt and ends after the pain is over. During a contraction the uterus rises forward in the abdomen pushing against the anterior abdominal wall. It increases in diameter anteriorly and posteriorly and decreases laterally, assuming a pear shape (Fig. 117). It becomes sensitive and tense and the round ligaments stand out sharply. There is a stage of increment, of acme and of decrement with each contraction. On vaginal examination an increased resistance over the fetal head is felt with the fingers, as well as tenseness and a bulging of the membranes toward the external os. Striking changes occur in the cervix—its effacement and dilatation.

Changes in the Cervix. At the beginning of labor the cervix is considerably effaced and somewhat dilated in many women. The dilatation occurs during the

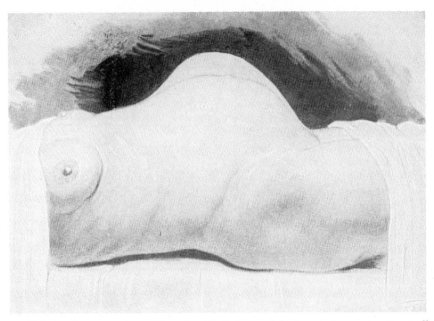

Figure 117   Abdominal contour viewed from the side before and during uterine contraction to illustrate how the uterus rises forward against the anterior wall.

last two or three weeks of pregnancy. The uterus is divided into two parts, an upper or contracting portion and a lower or dilating part. They are delineated by the *physiologic retraction ring* (Fig. 118). When contraction occurs, the amniotic fluid and the fetal head are pressed down toward the cervix. At the same time the membranes are impelled, pouchlike, into the cervical canal, pushing out the plug of mucus which had protected it during pregnancy. According to Stieve and others, the upper portions of the mucosa are expelled with the plug, leaving only the basal layers of the glands. The large veins, which impart erectile qualities to the cervix, are emptied and compressed; this provides considerable space in the passage. These factors help the lower uterine segment to develop fully and the cervix to unfold (Figs. 119 and 120). The completed passage from the external os to the retraction ring, when fully developed in labor, may be 7 to 12 cm. in length.

The cervix is completely *obliterated, effaced* or *unfolded* when it is so changed that only the external os remains. Dilatation now begins or continues as shown in Figures 120 and 121. When the external os is opened so wide that it is flush or nearly flush with the vagina, dilatation is complete and the fetus is able to pass through it. After the cervix is completely dilated it is pulled up in response to retraction by the upper active uterine segment until it is often out of reach of the examining fingers.

The comparison of the parturient passage to two funnels, one placed above the other, is quite apt. The fetus has to pass first through the upper funnel, the cervix, and then through the lower one, the pelvic floor. Effacement or obliteration of the cervix and dilatation occasionally occur simultaneously, especially in multiparas (Figs. 118 and 119). When the cervix is fully opened, the first stage of labor is ended and the second stage begins.

Forewaters.   Baudelocque defined the *bag of waters* as that portion of the membranes which pouched into the cervix during uterine contractions. Others apply this name to that portion which is uncovered by the dilating os, while still others call the whole amniotic sac the bag of waters. To avoid confusion we will use the term *forewaters* to designate that portion of the amniotic sac ahead of the fetal presenting part, and *amniotic sac* or *membranes* to refer to these specific entities.

At the beginning of labor the mem-

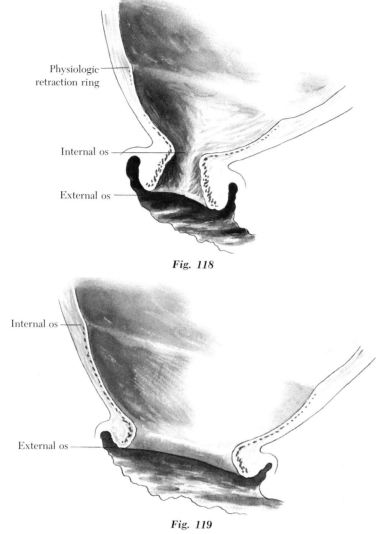

Physiologic retraction ring

Internal os

External os

Fig. 118

Internal os

External os

Fig. 119

Figures 118 and 119   Progressive effacement and dilatation of the cervix of a multipara showing that dilatation may occur even if effacement is incomplete.

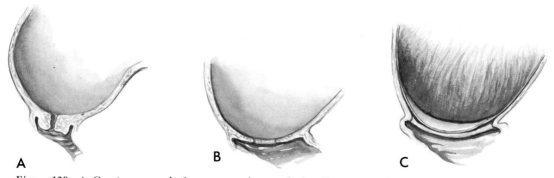

A

B

C

Figure 120   *A*, Cervix near end of pregnancy showing little effacement or dilatation. *B*, Cervix during first stage of labor with complete effacement but only partial dilatation. *C*, Cervix at end of the first stage illustrating complete effacement and dilatation, and intact membranes.

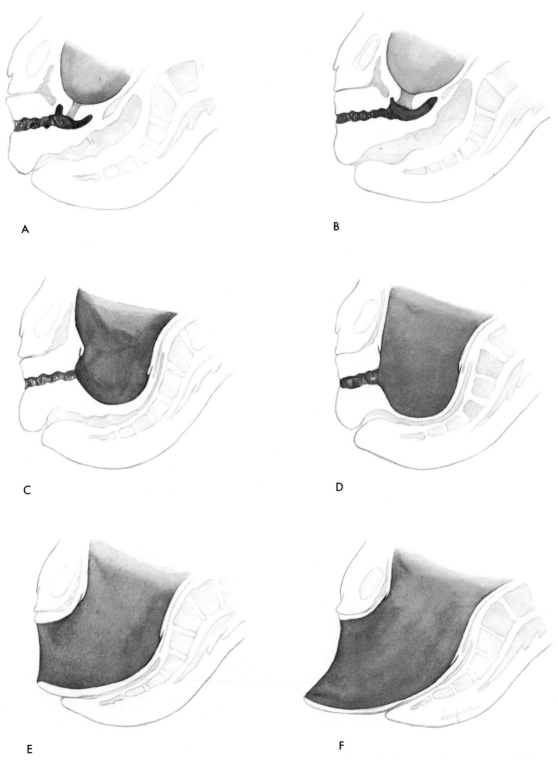

A

B

C

D

E

F

Figure 121   A, B and C, Effacement and dilatation of the cervix during the course of the first stage of labor. D, E and F, Stretching of the vagina and pelvic floor during second stage.

branes point into the cervix like a flat cone (Fig. 122). As dilatation progresses the forewaters assume the shape of a large watch crystal, projecting through the os (Fig. 123). If the membranes are soft and exposed to the entire pressure in the uterus, they bulge out into the vagina or they may rupture early. If the head fits the lower uterine segment closely and the membranes are firmly apposed to the head, the membranes do not protrude. With each contraction the membranes become tense, relaxing between contractions.

The membranes may rupture at any time, even before the contractions begin. If the chorion ruptures alone the amnion may be pushed out, covering the head of

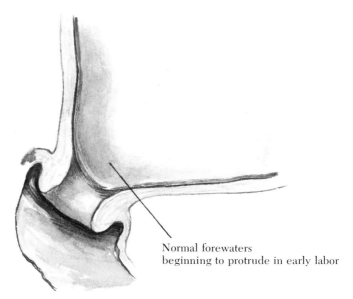

Normal forewaters
beginning to protrude in early labor

Fig. 122

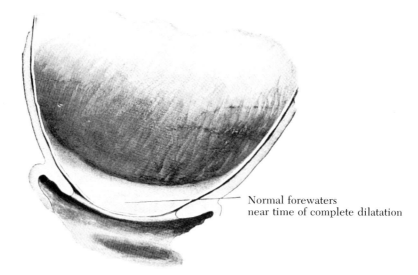

Normal forewaters
near time of complete dilatation

Fig. 123

Figures 122 and 123   Changes in shape of the forewaters as labor advances.

caul

the advancing fetus. The child may be delivered with the amnion intact covering its head. The child is then said to be born with a *caul.* The caul must be removed as soon as the head is delivered to allow the infant to breathe.

The membranes usually rupture centrally at the height of a strong contraction; the amniotic fluid escapes with a gush. The rupture may take place high up and then the water dribbles away during each contraction or even in the absence of contractions. Sometimes there is an accumulation of fluid between the amnion and the chorion; the chorion may rupture while the amnion remains intact giving the false impression that there are two amniotic sacs.

Coincidentally with these changes toward the end of the first stage, the fetal head descends lower into the pelvis, distends the vagina and may reach the pelvic floor. It presses on the nerves of the rectum and outlet muscles of the pelvis, and the parturient feels like bearing down. This bearing-down sensation usually heralds the onset of the second stage.

Second Stage

The contractions grow stronger, more frequent, recurring every two to three minutes, and become expulsive. The patient often utters a peculiar grunting cry. She feels there is something in the pelvis which she must expel; she closes the glottis, having fixed the chest in inspiration, braces her feet and by a powerful action of the abdominal and diaphragmatic muscles drives the fetal head against the perineum. During the contraction the uterus becomes boardlike. The process is indeed labor. The parturient's pulse is rapid, the veins of the neck stand out, the face is turgid and the body may be bathed in sweat.

Because the head presses on the sacral and obturator nerves, the patient may experience pains radiating into the legs and back. In general she is encouraged and hopeful, since now she can help and she feels that there is progress in the labor and the end is almost in sight.

The woman feels pressure on the rectum

and may insist on having a bedpan. Occasionally, there are feces in the lower bowel which are forced down by the advancing head, but more often the sensation is due to the head itself pressing on the rectum. After 10 to 20 minutes the anus begins to open and hemorrhoids swell if present. Soon the labia part during the height of a contraction, allowing the wrinkled scalp of the fetus to show. As the contraction subsides the elastic pelvic floor forces the head back. With the next contraction the perineum bulges more, the anus opens wider, the labia separate further and a larger segment of the scalp becomes visible. This is called *crowning* (Figs. 124 and 125). As the contraction disappears the head recedes. In the intervals between, the woman lies back exhausted, resting.

When the pelvic floor has relaxed sufficiently, the head rests in the vulva, the nape of the neck stemming behind the pubis. Now by a supreme effort, under great emotional exultation and powerful abdominal and diaphragmatic action, the head is forced out, the occiput coming from behind the pubis and then the forehead, face and chin rolling over the perineum (Figs. 126 and 127). After this there is usually a pause of a few minutes, then the contractions are renewed; the shoulders are delivered and finally the trunk and lower extremities in one long, hard, expulsive effort. The child gasps and soon cries vigorously.

A little blood and the rest of the amniotic fluid are discharged. Abdominally, the uterus has contracted to a ball-shaped mass. It still must expel the placenta and the membranes. The second stage is ended.

Third Stage

The strong compression exerted on the placenta by the first contractions of the third stage must drive some placental blood to the child. Moreover, even in the absence of such contractions, holding the infant so that its umbilicus is at a level below the mother's perineum allows some autotransfusion to take place passively from the placenta by gravity alone. It is,

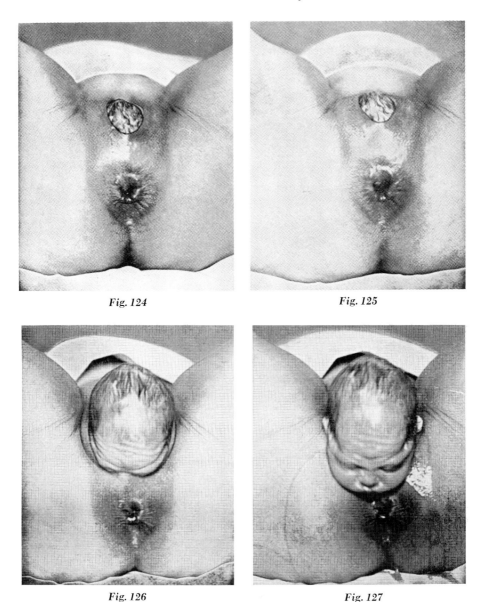

Fig. 124

Fig. 125

Fig. 126

Fig. 127

Figure 124 Head beginning to distend perineum, a process called "crowning." Note anus is flattened.

Figure 125 Perineum much distended and thinned. Note glistening surface of the stretched perineal skin. Anus is opened, showing anterior wall of rectum.

Figure 126 Perineum slipping back over face. Fetal head in process of being delivered by extension as the perineum slips back over the face of the fetus.

Figure 127 Fetal head is delivered and the perineum is retracted under the chin.

therefore, advantageous not to clamp the cord too soon after the birth.

The contractions of the third stage of labor separate the placenta and start its descent. The after-birth contractions are usually not too uncomfortable. Often the patient perceives only a slight drawing sensation, but the regular contractions can be felt every four to five minutes. After a while, usually a few minutes to an hour, the corpus rises high in the abdomen and changes shape from discoid to globular. At the same time the cord advances a few centimeters from the vulva. Some increase in vaginal bleeding may occur at this time. These signs indicate that the placenta has become separated from the uterine wall.

When this occurs, after a few minutes the placenta usually is expelled spontaneously by the combined efforts of the abdominal muscles and the uterus. Generally, the physician completes this process. The placenta is usually inverted like an umbrella and draws the membranes after it, peeling them off the uterine wall. Sometimes, it slides out without doubling up, the lower portion appearing first (Fig. 128). With the placenta, a quantity of blood is discharged. Now the uterus contracts into a hard mass, about the size of the baby's head.

It is common practice to expedite the

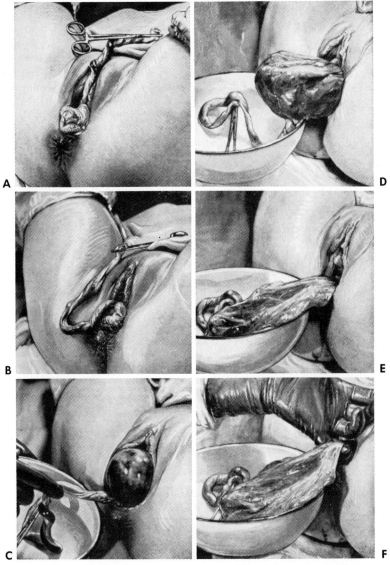

Figure 128 Delivery of the placenta. *A*, The cord has been clamped and cut; the clamped distal end is here laid on the mother's abdomen; a gauze sponge has been placed in the episiotomy wound. *B*, Cord advancing, forms loop showing that placenta has separated. *C*, Placenta with blood behind it appears; traction is not made on the cord. *D*, Part of placenta delivered. *E*, Only membranes still attached; note how basin is placed (not over anus) so that only the weight of placenta pulls on the membranes to effect their separation. *F*, Last part of membranes is aided with finger.

third stage with uterotonic agents. When oxytocin or ergonovine is administered after delivery the third stage is considerably altered. These drugs cause, in from two to five minutes, a powerful contraction which usually forces the placenta into the lower uterine segment and upper part of the vagina. Another contraction soon follows and the placenta appears. Thus, the third stage is usually shortened to perhaps five or eight minutes.

After the third stage is completed the *puerperium* begins and the patient becomes a *puerpera*.

The Discomfort of Labor

The uterine contractions are perceived variously from mere pressure at one extreme to intense pain at the other. Subjectively, they gain in intensity as labor progresses. Contractions are usually first felt in the back. Later they are felt more in the pelvis. In the first stage they result largely from the pressure of the presenting part on the nerves of the cervix and lower uterine segment, from the stretching of the cervix during the dilatation of the os by the presenting part, from the stretching of the peritoneum covering the uterus and the culdesac of Douglas or from the compression of the nerves in the wall of the uterus. Perhaps all four causes are combined. Women describe them as cramping, menstrual-like or similar to abdominal colic. The pain in the small of the back is due to radiation involving nerves of sacral and lumbar plexuses.

When the head passes into the vagina and begins to press on the perineum, discomfort results from stretching of these parts. Some women describe this as tearing. The patient bears down reflexly with the abdominal and diaphragmatic muscles. The greatest anguish is felt when the head goes through the vulva, although an occasional patient has characterized the delivery of the head through the vulva as orgasmic.

After the placenta and membranes are delivered, the after-pains disturb the first days of the puerperium and often medication is required. These occur most often in multiparas as recurrent cramps comparable to those of dysmenorrhea.

There is disagreement in regard to the degree of discomfort manifest in labors among women (Engelmann; Ploss; Freuchen). There is no factual basis for the myth that primitive women have babies with greater facility and less pain than modern women.

If the sensory nerves of the uterus are disrupted, as in transverse myelitis, paraplegia or after bilateral lumbar sympathectomy or presacral neurectomy, labor may be painless. Rysanek and Cavanagh reviewed 262 pregnancies after presacral neurectomy done mostly for unremitting dysmenorrhea. The onset of labor was insidious; the patient often did not recognize that she was in labor. First stage pains were attenuated in all patients and were entirely absent in two. Second stage pains also were reduced in intensity. The duration of labor was shorter than expected, but accurate timing was impossible in view of the difficulty in recognizing onset. Precipitate and unattended delivery at home is likely. The special needs of these patients must be understood by the obstetrician, who should clearly instruct them to call if in doubt about labor and to go immediately to the hospital in the event of ruptured membranes or bloody show. Such patients should be examined at frequent intervals during pregnancy so that the changes presaging imminent labor may be anticipated. Induction of labor (see Chapter 24) should be considered in patients with previous rapid labors if the fetal head is engaged and the cervix is ripe.

REFERENCES

Baudelocque, M.: L'Art des Accouchements. Paris, Chez Mequignon, 1789.

Caldeyro-Barcia, R., and Sereno, J. A.: The response of the human uterus to oxytocin throughout pregnancy. *In* Caldeyro-Barcia, R., and Heller, H., eds.: Oxytocin. New York, Pergamon Press, 1961.

Coch, J. A., Brovetto, J., Cabot, H. M., Fielitz, C. A., and Caldeyro-Barcia, R.: Oxytocin-equivalent activity in the plasma of women in labor and during the puerperium. Amer. J. Obstet. Gynec. *91*:10, 1965.

Csapo, A.: Function and regulation of the myometrium. N.Y. Acad. Med. *75*:790, 1959.

Engelmann, G. J.: La Pratique des Accouchements Chez les Peuples Primitifs. Paris, J. B. Baillière, 1886.

Fekete, K. v.: Beitrage zur Physiologie der Gravidität. Endokrinologie *7*:364, 1930.

Freuchen, P.: Arctic Adventure. New York, Farrar and Rinehart, 1935.

Hicks, J. B.: On the contractions of the uterus throughout pregnancy: Their physiological effects and their value in the diagnosis of pregnancy. Trans. Obstet. Soc. London *13*:216, 1872.

Israel, S. L., Stroup, P. E., Seligson, H. T., and Seligson, D.: Epinephrine and norepinephrine in pregnancy and labor. Obstet. Gynec. *14*:68, 1959.

Liggins, G. C.: The foetal role in the initiation of parturition in the ewe. *In* Wolstenholme, G. E. W., and O'Connor, M., eds.: Foetal Autonomy. London, J. & A. Churchill Ltd., 1969.

Milic, A. B., and Adamsons, K.: The relationship be-

tween anencephaly and prolonged pregnancy. J. Obstet. Gynaec. Brit. Comm. *76*:102, 1969.

Ploss, H. H.: Das Weib in der Natur und Völkerkunde, ed. 4. Leipzig, T. Grieben, 1895.

Reid, D. E., and Cohen, M. E.: Evaluation of present day trends in obstetrics. J.A.M.A. *142*:615, 1950.

Reynolds, S. R. M.: The Physiology of the Uterus, ed. 2. New York, Hafner Publishing Company, 1965.

Rysanek, W. J., Jr., and Cavanagh, D.: Presacral neurectomy and its effects on subsequent pregnancies. Amer. Surg. *24*:355, 1958.

Sauter, H.: Die motorische Innervation des menschlichen Uterus und die sich daraus ergebenden Schlussfolgerungen für die medikamentöse Geburtsleitung. Bibl. Gynaec. *12*:5, 1954.

Scommegna, A., Burd, L., Goodman, C., and Bieniarz, J.: The effect of pregnenolone sulfate on uterine contractility. Amer. J. Obstet. Gynec. *108*:1023, 1970.

Stieve, H.: Die menschliche Gebärmutter und der Geburtsweg während der Schwangerschaft, der Entbindung und des Wochenbettes. Med. Welt. *7*:1413, 1933.

Chapter 15

The Dynamic Forces of Labor

Uterine contractions are the main source of power in labor. They are the only source in the first stage, but during the second stage the abdominal and diaphragmatic muscles play an important ancillary role. The changes that take place in the uterus during pregnancy to prepare it for labor have been detailed earlier (Chapters 7 and 14).

A great deal of information has been acquired concerning uterine contractility by means of objective measurements derived from use of strain gauges attached to intraamniotic catheters (Caldeyro-Barcia) and other devices. Isometric pressure recordings produced during myometrial contractions have thus been studied extensively. It has been learned that there is a progressive increase in spontaneous uterine activity throughout pregnancy (Fig. 129). Prior to 30 weeks of gestation, one sees infrequent contractions of short duration and low amplitude, rarely attaining more than 20 mm. Hg intensity at their peaks. In addition, there are encountered minor fluctuations in the baseline pressure, or *tonus*, representing focalized and noncoordinated contractions of portions of the uterine wall. The larger and longer Hicks contractions are generally painless but readily perceived by the patient or the examiner. The uterine tonus is maintained throughout pregnancy at pressures of about 3 to 8 mm. Hg.

During the third trimester of pregnancy intensity and frequency of the Hicks contractions gradually increase and they become more rhythmic. At the same time, the small intervening contractions disappear. At term, only strong, coordinated and more or less rhythmic contractions are seen superimposed on a smooth basal tonus. Absolute rhythmicity and regularity are not characteristic of the spontaneous activity of the normal uterus, even in active labor.

There is no distinction whatsoever between contractile patterns recorded before and after the onset of labor. The transition is characterized by gradual and progressive increases in intensity, frequency and duration of the contractions from the patterns of late pregnancy through to delivery. The contractions of early labor average about 40 mm. Hg in amplitude, rising from a baseline tonus of 10 mm. Hg. As indicated earlier, there is a characteristic lack of strict rhythmicity so that contractions do not follow each other in a regimented fashion; moreover, they are not identical either in amplitude or duration with one another. This is not the case with labors stimulated with uterotonic agents, such as oxytocin, which usually demonstrate monotonous regularity in contraction patterns.

As labor progresses, the frequency and the intensity of contractions tend to progress also. In the second stage, for example, contractions tend to recur about every two minutes (measuring from the beginning of one to the beginning of the next) with amplitudes averaging 50 mm. Hg, but rising often to much higher levels, particularly with superimposed increase in intraabdominal pressure due to the voluntary and involuntary expulsive efforts of the abdominal and diaphragmatic muscles.

It is possible to evaluate contractions rather well with the examining hand, even in the absence of sophisticated intrauterine pressure recordings. Contractions are perceived by palpating the hardening of the uterine walls. The threshold of perception is affected by the degree of adipos-

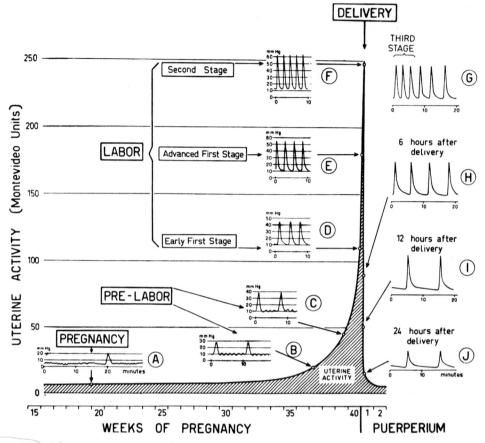

Figure 129 Schematic presentation showing evolution of uterine activity as it develops throughout pregnancy, in labor and the early puerperium. Typical tracings of intraamniotic pressure are shown (A to J), as well as a composite representation of activity expressed in Montevideo units (summation of peak amplitude of contractions per ten minutes in mm. Hg, shaded area). (From Caldeyro-Barcia, R., and Poseiro, J. J.: Ann. N.Y. Acad. Sci. 75:813, 1959.)

ity and muscular guarding of the abdominal wall, the intensity of the contraction itself and, of course, by the experience of the observer. Generally, contractions cannot be palpated as such unless the intraamniotic pressure rises at least 10 mm. Hg above the basal uterine tonus (Fig. 130). If the uterine tonus is abnormally elevated, above 12 mm. Hg, perception of the contraction by palpation becomes more difficult. It is generally impossible to detect contractions by palpation when uterine tonus exceeds 30 mm. Hg, as occurs with abruptio placentae (see Chapter 38).

The physician's perception of the contraction corresponds to an interval that is somewhat shorter than the true contraction as determined by intraamniotic pressure records (Fig. 130) because he cannot perceive the initial and terminal portion. Similarly, the patient's perception is still shorter, depending on her pain threshold, because she may not recognize the early increase in amniotic pressure until it is perhaps 15 mm. Hg or more of the above tonus.

The examiner can also estimate intensity. Contractions exceeding 40 mm. Hg in amplitude are very firm to the examining hand and generally the uterus cannot be readily indented. Those of 20 mm. Hg intensity or less are very easily indentable. In active labor strong contractions lasting 55 to 60 seconds and recurring every two to three minutes are common with associated inter-

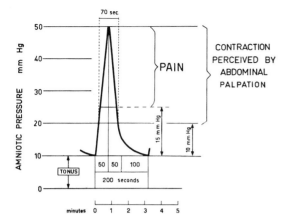

Figure 130 Graphic correlation between intrauterine pressure tracing and clinical objective findings by palpation as well as subjective perception by the patient. (From Caldeyro-Barcia, R.: Modern Trends in Gynaecology and Obstetrics. Montreal, Librairie Beauchemin Limitée, 1959.)

vals of uterine relaxation down to basal tonus between contractions. This interval of relaxation is most essential for fetal well-being because of the fact that myometrial contraction perforce results in partial or complete interference with uterine blood flow and placental exchange (see Chapter 4).

Objective study of uterine forces has provided much information concerning the physiology of labor. By obtaining simultaneous recordings of local activity using intramyometrial microballoons, for example, Alvarez and Caldeyro-Barcia were able to show that the contraction generated in the upper uterine segment began earlier and was of greater amplitude than contractions in the lower segment. On this basis they postulated that the contractile wave originates in a pacemaker site in one or the other cornu and spreads distally to the lower segment at a speed of 2 cm. per second, invading the entire uterus within 15 seconds. This has been termed a "triple descending gradient" because the uterine fundus in the vicinity of the pacemaker is demonstrated to have stronger contractions which occur earlier and are of longer duration than the lower parts of the uterus. Such descending gradients of propagation, duration and intensity are said to be essential for the production of cervical dilatation. In addition

coordination and incoordination of contractile waves have been described. A form of asynchrony has been demonstrated, apparently on the basis of separate and independent pacemaker sites acting asynchronously to produce ineffectual and disordered contractions.

The functional kinetic characteristics of myometrium have also been defined in detail by Csapo *in vitro* with regard to (1) the factors which determine the maximum tensile strength that the muscle is capable of developing, (2) the relationship between length and tension, (3) the correlation between the strength of the electrical stimulation and the duration of the resulting contraction, and (4) the relationship between the speed of muscle shortening and the weight of the load applied. He was able to document that the principles of myometrial contraction are quite comparable to those of skeletal muscle, but that there were significant differences in the kinetics of their reactions, particularly with regard to the rate of activity.

Many disparities appear to exist between the objective data obtained by such sophisticated techniques and the actual clinical course of labor. For example, it has been shown that only small increases in amplitude and frequency of uterine contractions occur as labor advances. Despite this, the pattern of cervical dilatation (see below) undergoes marked change, although unaccompanied by concomitant change in contractility pattern. Indeed, very small increments of activity are needed to produce the rapid cervical dilatation which takes place toward the end of the first stage of labor (Burnhill et al.).

CLINICAL CORRELATION

The clinical data that the obstetrician must interpret include the patterns of uterine contractility, cervical dilatation and descent of the fetal presenting part. Basic assessments of these phenomena have been well supported, as indicated above, by refinements of techniques and various physiologic tools. While these provide useful and accurate measures of ongoing activity, they have not yet offered means whereby normal labor can be distinguished from abnormal labor. They have not provided us with realistic methods for the study by practicing obstetricians and generalists of individual labors in progress. We, therefore, seek some other form of simple, practical and objective tool for the study by clinicians of individual labors in progress.

A method of clinical study is now available that concerns itself basically with the variations in cervical dilatation and descent with the time elapsed in labor (Friedman). Using this technique, we may simplify the relatively complex clinical art concerned with the dynamic nature of the changes that take place in labor. Cervical dilatation and station of the fetal presenting part can be periodically measured by means of simple digital examination. This information, when properly used, can be of inestimable aid to us in the management of the parturient. This is not meant to deprecate in any way or diminish the potential value of other modalities of study of the phenomenon of labor but only to point out that digital estimations of cervical dilatation and descent are available to all without accessory equipment or special knowledge.

It is through the utilization of the singular relationships between dilatation and time and between descent and time that new, clear-cut concepts of labor progression and its aberrations have been developed. The approach has been found useful for the study of individual labors in progress, for the study and teaching of the management of labor and for the study of the effects of various factors that may potentially influence the course of labor.

Conceptual Model

It is appropriate, albeit simplistic, to consider the laboring patient as a complex machine whose inner workings are largely unknown. We can carry this analogy quite far by illustrating the parallel between the uterus and other complex machines we are all familiar with, but whose internal operations we do not fully comprehend, such as the automobile. Our defective understand-

ing accepted, we can study both in great detail insofar as energy input, work output and factors that affect both are concerned. The inherent work demanded of a gravid patient consists of two components, cervical dilatation and descent. The energy sources for accomplishing these objectives also consist of two aspects, uterine contractions and expulsive efforts.

In Figure 131, we find a schematic representation of this situation, shown as a lever diagram. To the right, the box which represents work to be accomplished might be thought of as being full of some heavy objects. In order to lift the work output box (that is, to accomplish dilatation and descent), it is necessary to fill the empty energy input counterweight box on the left end of the lever arm. The "filling" material consists of effective uterine contractions and strong expulsive efforts. The efficacy of these latter may be enhanced as shown by the use of uterotonic agents, and more pertinently diminished by a variety of factors, including anxiety states, uterine anomalies, overdistention by multiple pregnancy and hydramnios, leiomyomata uteri, high parity and diverse debilitating conditions. Moreover, inhibitory agents may also adversely affect contractility, thereby reducing their influence on work output.

The burden of the work to be accomplished is lightened significantly if maternal soft tissues are adequately prepared prior to labor—i.e., by decreased inelasticity and resistance. Characteristically, prior vaginal delivery will have accomplished this. Pathologically, cervical incompetence may be looked upon as an unusual excess of prelabor soft tissue preparation in which there is negligible resistance to dilatation and descent. The work requirement is considerably augmented, on the other hand, by increased resistance and inelasticity, as in labors that begin with the cervix long, closed, rigid and unyielding. Factors that impose problems in fetopelvic relationships, including disproportion, tumor obstruction, malpresentation and malposition, considerably increase the job to be accomplished.

This very simple, mechanistic concept of the labor phenomenon allows us to consider as separate entities those factors relating to energy resources and those

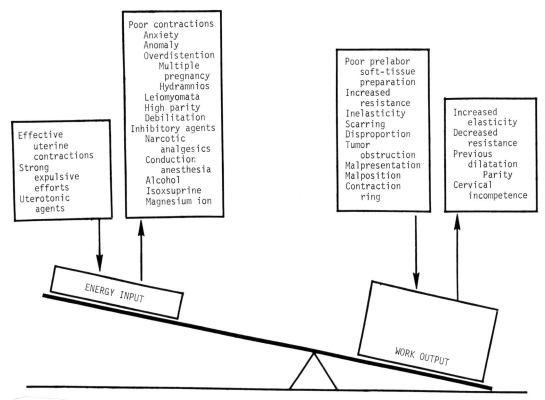

Figure 131 Mechanistic concept of the balance of forces and resistances in effect during the course of labor, shown as a lever diagram. The factors which increase or decrease the work to be performed are indicated together with factors which enhance or diminish effectiveness of the energy input.

contributing to or diminishing work requirements. Furthermore, the two ends of the lever diagram can also be interrelated. The physics of this relationship between energy input and work output is well defined, the ratio of one to the other being a measure of the *efficiency* of the mechanical device under study. The degree of efficiency, as we shall see, can be measured and utilized for the purpose of determining the presence or absence of labor abnormalities. The components of the efficiency equation for the laboring patient consist of the summation of contractile and expulsive forces counterbalanced by the composite resistance of maternal tissues to dilatation and descent.

Whereas the driving forces are readily measurable in great detail by available means today (see above), we have no way to measure resistance accurately. Thus, a direct measure of efficiency is unobtainable. A more indirect approach, however, is

readily at hand. The end results of all the forces of labor are apparent in the essential work that must be accomplished in order for labor to terminate normally, namely, progressive cervical dilatation and progressive descent of the fetal presenting part. Both must occur in the normal course of labor.

Estimates of cervical dilatation and of station have long been used as guides in evaluating the progress of labor. Single estimates, however, must be understood to represent only momentary observations within the framework of a constantly changing process. Alone, these give rise to a static concept of labor. The inadequacy of the picture portrayed by such isolated observations is apparent, since they cannot give an adequate overview of the entire process. Multiple observations, on the other hand, may be correlated with elapsed time in labor to provide a means whereby labors may be followed objectively and aberrations detected as they arise. The critical aspect here is the correlation of these observations with elapsed time in labor, affording us an appreciation of the dynamism inherent in the phenomenon we wish to study.

Whereas heretofore evaluation of progress in labor was synonymous with a fairly nebulous degree of change, we now have means whereby specific rates of change and the development of specific patterns of dilatation and descent can be made meaningful for diagnostic purposes. The inconsistencies in the measurable aspects of contractility, namely, the lack of correlation between progression and the frequency, intensity and duration of contractions, make them rather unreliable for evaluating labors in progress. The dilatation-time and descent-time functions, on the other hand, represent a meaningful summation and an ongoing measure of the complex labor process.

GRAPHIC DIAGNOSIS

When one plots the isolated observations of cervical dilatation in any particular labor against the time elapsed in labor, using a vertical axis of cervical dilatation in centimeters and a horizontal axis of hours in labor, one finds the characteristic sigmoid-shaped curve traced. This curve is seen in all normal labors (Fig. 132). A similarly characteristic hyperbolic curve is traced in all normal labors when station is plotted against elapsed time.

These rather simple visual patterns allow for quick interpretation and evaluation of the labor in progress. Each patient constructs her own unique clinical picture. This offers a reliable means for following the course of the normal labor and distinguishing it objectively from abnormal varieties. The characteristic normal dilatation and descent patterns are common to all patients and independent of other more variable and less reliable aspects of labor, including contractility patterns or soft-part resistance. They provide rather sure indications of changes in the quality of labor, the timing of delivery and the presence of abnormal factors.

The method entails recording of simple data that the physician would ordinarily gather in any event. Except for graph paper, it requires no special equipment and no specialized knowledge. Inasmuch as the shape of the pattern is the chief evaluative factor, it will be seen that minor inaccuracies of digital estimates are unimportant, provided they are consistent. Easily communicable, the method is readily grasped by novices and in their hands it rapidly becomes as reliable as the accumulated intuition and clinical impressions of physicians with many years of experience.

Any square-ruled graph will do for con-

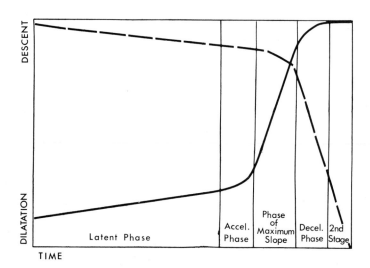

Figure 132 Graphic illustration of the composite dilatation-time and descent-time functions in normal labor. The first stage is divisible into a latent and an active phase; the active phase is composed of the acceleration phase, phase of maximum slope and deceleration phase combined. Descent is seen to begin concurrently with onset of phase of maximum slope of dilatation; descent reaches its maximum at the beginning of the deceleration phase of dilatation.

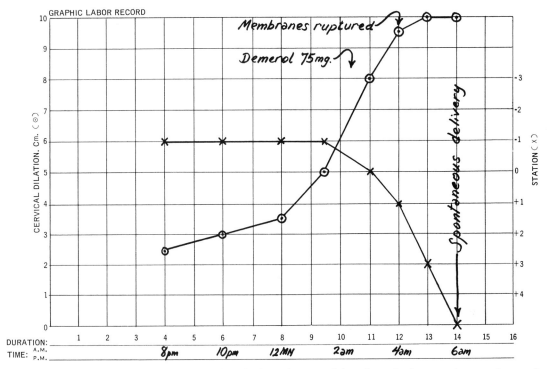

Figure 133 A typical graphic labor record with elapsed time in labor along the horizontal axis and cervical dilatation (left) and station of the fetal presenting part (right) on the vertical axis. Each observation of dilatation (circle) and station (cross) is entered sequentially to trace the course of labor.

struction of these graphs. Many institutions prefer to devise their own so as to incorporate this record into the hospital chart. A version used at our institutions is illustrated here (Fig. 133). The horizontal coordinates are numbered by hours of labor. The onset of labor is arbitrarily defined as the onset of regular uterine contractions as perceived by the patient. The left vertical coordinates are numbered in ascending order to represent centimeters of cervical dilatation. At the right, the same vertical coordinates are keyed in descending order with measurements denoting the station of descent, the level of the forward leading edge of the fetal bony prominence relative to the plane of the ischial spines. For convenience, an estimate of cervical dilatation is entered by a small circle and that of station by an *x*. Each subsequent observation is joined to the preceding notation by a straight line. The resulting graph furnishes a simple visual pattern for quick assessment of labor in progress.

The characteristic patterns allow us to measure the durations of the various distinctive portions of the first stage and to study the changes in cervical dilatation and in descent per unit time. The slope of the curve is seen to be a very accurate measure of the specific rate of change for a given labor. Careful study has revealed that this slope, within limits of error, is specific for each patient, but that it undergoes predictable changes during the course of normal labor. Moreover, it is now clear that the slopes of the curves of active dilatation and of descent are measures of the efficiency of the complex machine to which we referred earlier.

The physician is confronted by an enormous range of normality in terms of contractility patterns. At one extreme is the patient with negligible contractions, quietly dilating her cervix and perhaps precipitately delivering the baby while the physician is debating whether or not she is in labor. The rapid dilatation and descent that occur under these circumstances in the presence of minimal generation of labor forces bespeak a highly efficient unit. At the other extreme is the woman with contractions of great intensity and frequency that may continue for many hours before cervical dilatation becomes apparent. Here a great deal of energy is being expended to overcome considerable resistance and ultimately to accomplish the same objective. This represents an exceedingly inefficient laboring machine. These examples illustrate the paradoxical dissociation between contractile pattern and labor progression, emphasizing the importance of assessing the rates of dilatation and descent primarily as indices of normality.

Phases of Labor

Arbitrary subdivisions of the first stage of labor have permitted study in depth. The first stage is readily divisible into two parts: the *latent phase,* extending from the onset of labor to a point in time when the curve begins to change acutely; and the *active phase,* which begins with the upswing of the curve and terminates at full dilatation and full retraction of the cervix at the onset of the second stage. The active phase is further subdivided into an initial *acceleration phase,* a *phase of maximum slope* and a terminal *deceleration phase.*

The latent phase is an interval occupied with orientation of uterine contractions and softening and effacement of the cervix in preparation for subsequent active dilatation. The phase of maximum slope is that interval during which cervical dilatation proceeds at its most rapid rate in a constant, linear manner. Its slope is a measure of efficiency, the more steeply inclined, the more efficient the energy input in effecting work output. The deceleration phase merely represents the cephalad cervical retraction occurring at the end of the first stage.

The corresponding descent curve retains its latent aspects until the dilatation curve has entered the phase of maximum slope, at which time descent generally begins its active phase. Descent reaches its maximum slope concurrent with the onset of the deceleration phase of dilatation. From this point in time onward, de-

scent continues in a linear manner until the presenting part reaches the perineum. The slope of descent here is another measure of the efficiency of the energy source in accomplishing the work required of it.

Functional Divisions of Labor

One may arbitrarily subdivide labor into functional units based on dilatation and descent. This represents a departure from the classic concept of labor which considers the first stage to be the stage of dilatation and the second stage the stage of descent. Closer observation has shown that dilatation occupies only a small part of the first stage, while descent overlaps both stages, beginning and progressing well before the first stage terminates. Accordingly, we may consider labor to be divisible into three separate functional units.

These are important insofar as they represent distinctive intervals from physiologic, pathologic, therapeutic and prognostic points of view. Each of these separate, functional parts is easily recognizable, each affected by different factors, each responsive to various exogenous influences and each subject to its own disorders. The recognition and understanding of these differences, particularly as they relate to etiology, therapy and prognosis of disorders associated with the separate, functional divisions of labor, must be considered essential for the practitioner in this field. These divisions, termed *preparatory, dilatational* and *pelvic,* respectively, are based on the aforementioned cervical dilatation-time and descent-time patterns (Fig. 134).

Preparatory Division. The changes that take place during the preparatory division of labor are subtle. They include factors relating to orientation and coordination of myometrial contractility and softening and effacement of the cervix. Delayed evolution of effective contractility to overcome soft-part resistance will result in abnormal prolongation of the latent phase of the dilatation curve. This division is particularly sensitive to sedation and anesthesia. The poorly polarized uterine contractions are readily disturbed because myometrial function has not be-

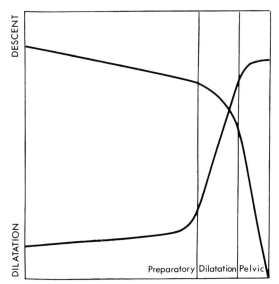

Figure 134 The functional divisions of labor as represented by the components of dilatation and descent as they interrelate. Total labor is divided into its functionally distinct parts: preparatory, dilatational and pelvic. (From Friedman, E. A.: Amer. J. Obstet. Gynec. *109*:274, 1971.)

come sufficiently coordinated to completely withstand inhibitory influences. Furthermore, the labor that begins with the cervix poorly prepared for later active dilatation will of necessity be characterized by a longer preparatory division. The latent phase in nulliparas averages 8.6 hr. and normally does not exceed 20 hr.; in multiparas it averages 5.3 hr. and usually does not go beyond 14 hr.

Dilatational Division. The cervix undergoes active dilatation only during a relatively short part of the first stage. All dilatation, except that which has occurred prior to the onset of labor and the small additional amount that takes place during the preparatory division, occurs in the interval span of time that terminates the first stage, the active phase. It is important to repeat that the inclination of the maximum slope of dilatation can be considered to represent a measure of the efficiency of a contractile pattern in overcoming resistance to dilatation. Disordered dilatation, particularly where protracted and dilatory, may result from unfavorable combinations of myometrial dysfunction and excessive soft-part resistance. The slope of active phase dilatation in nulliparas averages 3.0

cm. per hr. and is not less than 1.2 cm. per hr. under normal circumstances; in multiparas it is 5.7 cm. per hr. and is rarely less than 1.5 cm. per hr.

Pelvic Division. The beginning of the pelvic division is marked by the onset of the deceleration of dilatation and the simultaneous attainment of maximum rate of descent. Ordinarily, descent continues uninterruptedly from this time onward. The linear descent pattern constitutes another measure of the overall efficiency of the labor process, analogous to that of the linear active dilatation curve. The inclination provides a meaningful measure of the effectiveness of the motive force in producing the work required of it, namely, descent of the fetus through the birth canal. Disorders of this functional division will result from factors that interfere with descent, such as fetopelvic disproportion, malpresentations and disordered forces, including those secondary to exogenous factors or exhaustion. Slope of descent averages 1.6 cm. per hr. in nulliparas and is normally greater than 1.0 cm. per hr.; it averages 5.4 cm. per hr. in multiparas, exceeding 2.1 cm. per hr. in normal labors.

EFFECTS OF UTERINE FORCES

Effacement and dilatation of the cervix, distention of the lower uterine segment and descent and delivery of the fetus are the end results of all the forces of labor acting on the uterine contents and against the resistance of maternal structures. How these are brought about will be discussed here in terms of the dynamic forces involved.

Dilatation of the Cervix

These effects are brought about by intrauterine pressure and augmented in the second stage by intraabdominal pressure. Additionally, the upper uterine segment musculature shortens its myometrial cell components progressively, while thinning and retracting the more passive lower segment and cervix.

If one regards the uterine cavity as a hydrodynamically contained unit, the pressure generated within it is distributed uniformly throughout. This situation undoubtedly prevails until such time as the membranes are ruptured. During uterine contractions, the tension in the walls of the uterus increases also, but the distribution of tension is dependent on the topographical curvature of the inner surface (Reynolds). In a flexible spherical container, the tensile strain in the wall is represented by the equation $T = pr^2/2$, where p is the pressure acting perpendicularly to the surface and r the radius of curvature at the point under consideration. Thus, at any point the tension is proportional to the square of the radius of curvature. Since the ratio of the radii of curvatures of the fundus and lower segment is about 7:4, the tension in the fundus should be 49:16 or three times greater than in the lower segment. At the same time the fact that the fundic musculature is so much thicker than that in the lower segment comes into play. The uterus does not behave as a uniformly elastic system as a result of this difference in the structure of its walls. Reynolds has shown that in equilibrium the pull of one hemisphere of a sphere on the other is $2\pi rzt$, where t is the tension per square centimeter of surface area, r the radius and z the thickness of the tissue. If this relationship does indeed hold for the uterus in labor, one can derive a meaningful concept of the massive pull that the upper uterine segment exerts on the lower: each component of the expression rzt reflects this effect, radius 7:4, tension 3:1 as indicated above, thickness at least 3:1 and progressively increasing during labor. These data mirror the clinically demonstrable fact that resistance to pressure at the cervix is relatively small, resulting in dilatation. At the same time, the centrifugal forces from the upper segment myometrium pull directly on the passive lower segment and cervix to effect retraction (Fig. 135).

It is doubtful that it is really essential for there to be a "dilating wedge" present for dilatation to occur, at least in its early aspects. Examples of essentially normal beginning dilatation are documentable even with no forewaters or fetal presenting

part against the lower segment. It is a reasonable expectation that the terminal part of dilatation and retraction will not occur normally unless the fetal head or breech is presenting and descending well into the pelvis (see Chapter 55), but this is not a *sine qua non* for the evolution of the initial portion of the active phase of dilatation. The concept of the "dilating wedge" as essential for labor progression was once widely held and accepted as a simplistic way to explain the process of dilatation. Al-

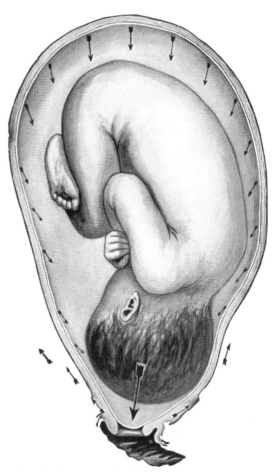

Figure 135 Composite representation of the forces by which dilatation and descent occur. The small intrauterine arrows indicate the increase in intra-amniotic pressure caused by myometrial contractions which act to dilate the cervix, the portion of the uterine wall offering least resistance to stretching. At the same time the outer arrows represent the cervix and lower segment being pulled up over the presenting part by the centrifugal or longitudinal traction exerted by the forceful contraction of the upper segment musculature.

though the presence of the fetal presenting part or the forewaters may be contributory to effective dilatation in some way as yet undetermined, it can no longer be considered to be the primary factor in this phenomenon.

The upper uterine segment progressively shortens and exerts traction on the cervix, causing its ripening, effacement and dilatation. The traction is transmitted by the lower segment, which also contracts but with less force than the upper segment. During the active phase of labor, after each contraction, myometrial bundles of the upper segment remain shorter and thicker, undergoing retraction, while the cervix becomes more effaced and dilated.

Each normal coordinated uterine contraction in the active phase causes the cervix to become tense and to dilate somewhat, perhaps as much as 1 to 3 cm. in diameter; this regresses slowly during uterine relaxation (Friedman and von Micsky). Progressive increments in dilata-

tion result when the transient dilatation exceeds the regression accompanying each contraction and relaxation cycle. The physiologic aspects of lower segment and cervical changes in labor are discussed in Chapter 7; the clinical progressions in labor as related to elapsed time have been outlined earlier in this chapter.

Descent

Because its cervical end is moored to the pelvis by the Mackinrodt's and uterosacral ligaments, shortening of the contracting myometrium reduces the uterine volume and pushes the fetus downward into the pelvis until it is born. The contractions of the round ligaments which occur synchronously with those of the upper segment tend to pull the uterine corpus in the same direction, thus contributing to fetal descent (Fig. 136). They also pull the corpus forward and bring its axis parallel with that

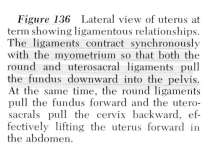

Figure 136 Lateral view of uterus at term showing ligamentous relationships. The ligaments contract synchronously with the myometrium so that both the round and uterosacral ligaments pull the fundus downward into the pelvis. At the same time, the round ligaments pull the fundus forward and the uterosacrals pull the cervix backward, effectively lifting the uterus forward in the abdomen.

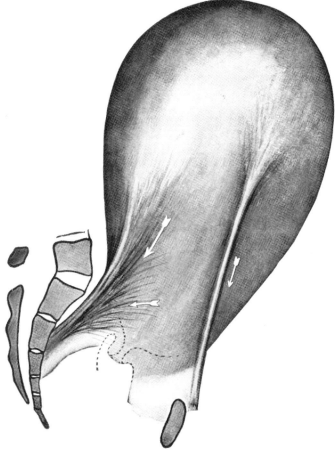

of the inlet, producing a condition in which the uterus rises up in the abdomen against the anterior abdominal wall (see Chapter 14). The contractions of the utero-sacral ligaments pull the cervix backward.

Although the most important part of fetal descent occurs during the second stage, this process starts much earlier during the active phase of the first stage (see above). As the fetus descends in the pelvis, the upper segment becomes still shorter and thicker after each contraction and the lower segment retracts further upward.

The descent of the fetal head is not uniform but is rather an oscillating phenomenon. The head progresses during each uterine contraction, distending the birth canal and later the perineum. When the uterus relaxes and expulsive efforts subside, the fetal head regresses somewhat because of the elastic retraction of the vagina and the perineum. Each of these progression-regression cycles leaves a positive balance so that the head remains a little lower in the pelvis and the birth canal is somewhat more distended than before.

The bearing-down efforts are superimposed on the uterine contractions as motive forces in this process. These are the result of strong contractions of the diaphragm (Agostoni and Rahn) and the rectus, oblique and transverse abdominal muscles. They are preceded by an inspiration or several deep ventilatory exchanges which tend to build up oxygen reserve and blow off carbon dioxide. Then the glottis is closed. Each bearing-down effort causes an acute, short rise of intraabdominal pressure of about 50 mm. Hg superimposed on the intrauterine pressure. The addition of the pressure developed by uterine contractions plus that of the bearing-down efforts raises the intrauterine pressure to 110 to 130 mm. Hg.

Normally, expulsive efforts are reflexly elicited by the distention of the vagina and the perineum, most especially of the levator ani muscles. They usually occur only during uterine contractions when the presenting part further distends and stimulates these structures. This reflex mechanism results in the efficient addition of the two pressures. If the patient should bear down when the uterus is relaxed, the efforts are ineffective and wasteful of her energy. Similarly, if she bears down before the cervix is fully dilated and completely retracted, it will have an adverse effect. Not only will such efforts be useless in producing descent but they may also impinge the lower segment between the two bony surfaces of the head and the pelvis. This may cause damage as a result of necrosis, or edematous swelling by occluding the venous and lymphatic drainage. One should try to ensure that no bearing-down expulsive efforts are made by patients before the second stage has been entered.

REFERENCES

Agostoni, E., and Rahn, H.: Abdominal and thoracic pressures at different lung volumes. J. Appl. Physiol. *15*:1087, 1960.

Alvarez, H., and Caldeyro-Barcia, R.: Contractility of the human uterus recorded by new methods. Surg. Gynec. Obstet. *91*:1, 1950.

Burnhill, M. S., Danezis, J., and Cohen, J.: Uterine contractility during labor studied by intra-amniotic fluid pressure recordings. Amer. J. Obstet. Gynec. *83*:572, 1962.

Caldeyro-Barcia, R.: Contractility of the pregnant human uterus and controlling factors. Proc. Internat. Congr. Physiol. Sci. *21*:7, 1959.

Csapo, A.: The mechanism of myometrial function and its disorders. *In* Bowes, K., ed.: Modern Trends in Obstetrics and Gynaecology. London, Butterworth and Company, 1955.

Friedman, E. A.: Labor: Clinical Evaluation and Management. New York, Appleton-Century-Crofts, 1967.

Friedman, E. A.: The functional divisions of labor. Amer. J. Obstet. Gynec. *109*:274, 1971.

Friedman, E. A., and von Micsky, L. I.: Electronic cervimeter: A research instrument for the study of cervical dilatation in labor. Amer. J. Obstet. Gynec. *87*:789, 1963.

Reynolds, S. R. M.: Physiology of the Uterus, ed. 2, revised. New York, Hafner Publishing Company, 1965.

Chapter 16

The Birth Canal

BONY PELVIS

The fetus has to traverse a curved passage which is partly bony and partly fibrous and muscular. The bony portion constitutes the composite structure made up of the confluence of ilium, ischium and pubis on both sides plus the sacrum. The pelvis is divided into two parts by a ridge called the *linea terminalis* (Figs. 137 and 138). The upper part is the *false pelvis* and is of little obstetric interest. It is made up of the flaring wings of the ilium at the sides and the spine behind; the strong abdominal muscles complete the circle anteriorly. The false pelvis is shaped like a flattened funnel. The shape and size of the false pelvis give the obstetrician essentially no real conception of the shape and size of the true pelvis.

The lower part is the *true pelvis* which is of immense obstetric importance since it supports the muscles of the pelvic floor and gives shape and direction to the parturient canal, itself being a part of it. The true pelvis can be considered to be a cylinder with a bluntly pointed exaxial lower end. It is slightly curved anteriorly much

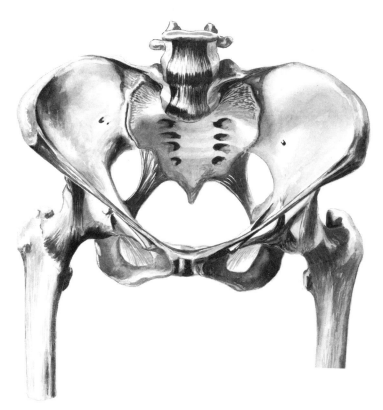

Figure 137 Normal female pelvis.

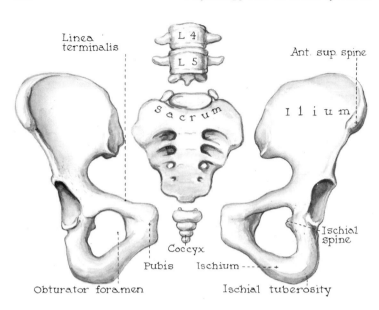

Figure 138 The component bony parts of the female pelvis. The paired innominate bone is made up of the conjoined ilium, ischium and pubis.

like a bent stovepipe. The entrance and outlet of the true pelvis are smaller than the middle portion and have, therefore, been called *straits* — the superior and inferior straits, respectively (Fig. 139). The region between, being large and roomy, is

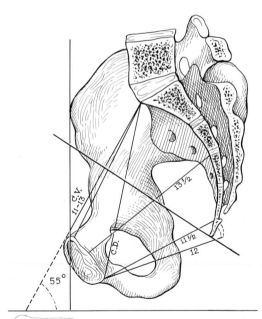

Figure 139 Sagittal section of the erect pelvis showing anteroposterior diameters. *C.V.*, true conjugate or conjugata vera; *C.D.*, diagonal conjugate. The pelvic inclination is shown as 55 degrees. (After Hodge, H. L.: The Principles and Practice of Obstetrics. Philadelphia, Blanchard and Lea, 1864.)

called the *excavation*. Anteriorly the canal is short, being only about 4.5 cm. in length, corresponding to the height of the symphysis pubis. Posteriorly, it is as long as the length of the sacrum and measures 12.5 cm. Laterally, the pelvic canal is longer, reaching from the linea terminalis at the superior strait down to the ischial tuberosities. The contour of the canal varies at different levels and it is customary to describe these variations by means of horizontal planes drawn at various levels in the pelvis. The planes were first described by Levret in 1753.

The *plane of the inlet*, or *superior strait* (Fig. 140), is bounded by the upper border of the pubis in front, the *linea innominata* or *linea terminalis* at the sides and the *sacral promontory* behind. This plane is usually a transverse ellipse on which the sacrum intrudes from behind. The classic varieties of pelvic architecture based on the Caldwell-Moloy classification of inlet planes has been detailed in Chapter 12. The shape of the superior strait defines the pelvic type as follows: rounded, gynecoid; heart-shaped, android; ellipse elongated anteroposteriorly, anthropoid; flattened ellipse, platypelloid.

The inlet is an extremely important area of the pelvis because contraction and distortion of the bones due to disease are likely to be pronounced. It plays a deter-

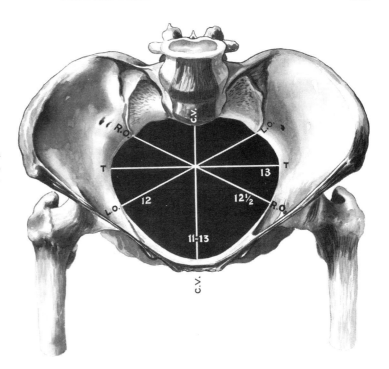

Figure 140 C.V., conjugata vera; *T.*, widest transverse; *L.O.*, left oblique; *R.O.*, right oblique.

minant role in normal labor. One critical diameter is the anteroposterior, pubosacral, *true conjugate* or *conjugata vera* (C.V.). It extends from the top of the symphysis pubis to the middle of the sacral promontory and measures 11 to 13 cm.

Except roentgenographically (see Chapter 12) it is impossible to measure the C.V. of the living human being satisfactorily. An approximate idea of its length can be had by measuring the distance from the undermargin of the pubis to the promontory as shown in Chapter 12 (Fig. 105). This diameter is called the *diagonal conjugate* or *conjugata diagonalis* (C.D.) (Fig. 139). In normal pelves, it measures about 12.5 cm. Transversely, the inlet measures about 13 cm. but may be as wide as 14 or 14.5 cm., while the two oblique diameters usually measure about 12.5 cm.

The *midpelvic plane* or *midplane* passes through the apex of the pubic arch, the ischial spines and the end of the sacrum. This is the smallest strait of the pelvis and is frequently the site of contraction. This plane is ovoid; its large end anteriorly and its smaller end posteriorly are formed by the sacrosciatic ligaments. Its most important diameter is that between the spines; the *interspinous diameter* generally meas-

ures 10.5 to 11 cm. The plane through an imaginary line drawn between the spines of the ischia is used to determine the *station* of the fetal head in the pelvis, an important means for assessing progressive descent in labor.

The *plane of the outlet* or *inferior strait* passes through the arch and the rami of the pubis, the ischial tuberosities and the top of the coccyx. The plane is the lower boundary of the bony outlet and is rarely the site of contraction. There are really two planes, roughly resembling triangles bent at their applied bases on the *intertuberous diameter*. During labor the coccyx is usually pushed back by the fetal head (Fig. 139), increasing the anteroposterior diameter to 12 cm. The transverse diameter of this plane is important; it measures 10.5 to 11 cm. (Fig. 141).

In the erect position the inlet makes an angle of about 55 degrees with the horizontal (Fig. 139). It may vary from 40 to 100 degrees depending on the degree of flexion of the pelvis which is primarily dependent on posture and carriage (see Chapter 7). This is called the *pelvic inclination*. A quick way to determine if this inclination is normal is to see if the anterior superior iliac spine and the pubis are on a

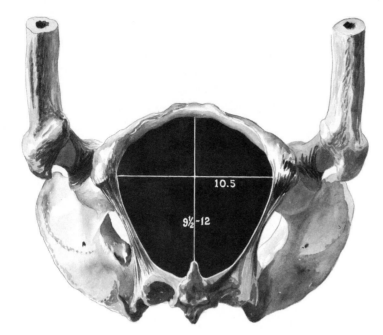

Figure 141 The pelvic outlet viewed from below. It passes through the arch of the pubic rami, the ischial tuberosities and the tip of the coccyx, forming two triangles bent at their mutually shared base, the inter-tuberous diameter.

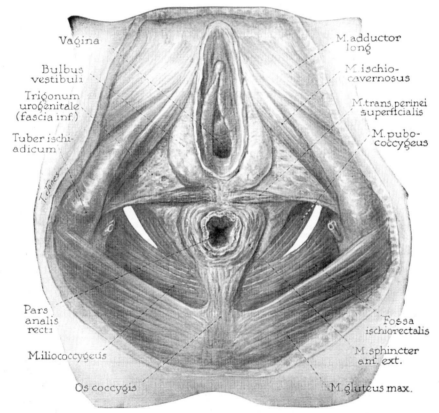

Figure 142 Female perineum. In the anal triangle the fatty tissue has been removed from the ischiorectal fossas to expose the pelvic diaphragm and the external anal sphincter. With removal of the fascial investment of the levator ani, the cleft between the pubococcygeal and iliococcygeal portion is evident. In the urogenital triangle the layers of superficial fascia have been removed to show the superficial perineal muscles. The integument of the labia minora and of the clitoris is intact. (From Curtis, A. H., et al.: Surg. Gynec. Obstet. 74:709, 1942.)

vertical plane. In the supine position the inlet inclines 25 degrees below the horizontal. The iliac crests practically parallel the plane of the inlet.

The pelvis is not a solid and fixed bony structure. The coccyx is easily pressed back by the advancing fetal head, enlarging the outlet. The pelvic joints are fixed by strong ligaments, but during pregnancy these soften and may impart a degree of mobility to the bones, although this is probably negligible from the functional standpoint.

SOFT PARTS

The cervix and the lower uterine segment have already been considered in Chapter 7. Of most obstetric interest is the pelvic floor. One can distinguish two diaphragms in the pelvic floor—an upper, stronger, muscular system and a lower, weaker system developed from the sphincter cloacae, which closes the orifices in the pelvic floor (Figs. 142 to 145).

The *pelvic floor* or *diaphragm* is made up of the levator ani muscles and the pelvic fascia. Anteriorly, the muscle is attached to the back of the pubic rami (Fig. 146). Thus, it extends on either side across the opening of the obturator foramen, being attached to the fascia covering the internal obturator muscle underneath a tendinous duplication of the superior levator fascia, called the *white line* or *arcus tendineus musculi levatoris ani*. On vaginal examination this arcus tendineus can often be felt.

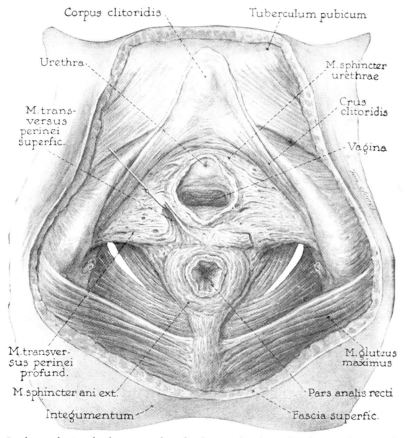

Figure 143 In the anal triangle the external anal sphincter has been freed somewhat in order to show the coccygeal extension of the urogenital diaphragm. In the urogenital triangle the superficial structures of the perineum have been removed. The medial portion of the superficial transverse perineal muscles is retained and the stump on the left elevated to demonstrate fusion at the central tendinous part of the perineum. (From Curtis, A. H., et al.: Surg. Gynec. Obstet. 74:709, 1942.)

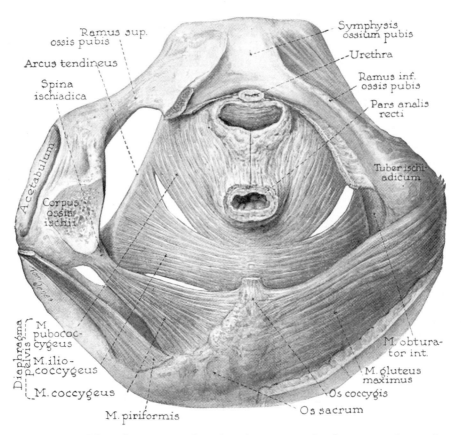

Ramus sup.
ossis pubis

Arcus tendineus

Spina
ischiadica

Acetabulum

Corpus
ossis
ischii

Symphysis
ossium pubis

Urethra

Ramus inf.
ossis pubis

Pars analis
recti

Tuber ischi-
adicum

M. obtura-
tor int.

M. gluteus
maximus

Os coccygis

Os sacrum

M.
pubococ-
cygeus

M. ilio-
coccygeus

M. coccygeus

Diaphragma pelvis

M. piriformis

Figure 144 Portions of the right innominate bone have been removed to demonstrate the attachments, form and relationships of the pelvic diaphragm. The following features are especially important: tendinous origin of the pubococcygeal and iliococcygeal divisions of the levator ani; the way the pubic division passes into the iliac division; the proximity of the urethra to the pubic symphysis; the distance between the vagina and anus; the complementary position of the coccygeus to the iliococcygeus (left); the manner in which it is covered by the gluteus maximus (right); the dorsal location of the piriformis. (From Curtis, A. H., et al.: Surg. Gynec. Obstet. 74:709, 1942.)

From their origin the fibers of the levator ani muscles pass downward and inward toward the median line. Posteriorly, they come together on the lower end of the sacrum and the coccyx. Anteriorly, they interlace in the median line behind the anus. They fuse into a slinglike hammock under the perineal curve of the rectum. Many of the medial fibers fuse with the upper border and sides of the sphincter ani and lower part of the rectum; a few fibers meet between the anus and the vagina in the perineal body (Luschka's fibers). Holl named the separate muscle bundles of the levator ani as follows: the muscular portion between the spine of the ischium and the coccyx, the *ischiococcygeus;* that from the arcus tendineus to the median raphé, the *iliococcygeus;* that from the posterior surface of the pubis, passing along the

urethra, vagina and rectum to its counterpart in the tendinous raphé extending from the tip of the coccyx toward the rectum, the *pubococcygeus;* and the strong slinglike band from the pubis around the lower part of the rectum, the *puborectalis.*

Through the pelvic diaphragm pass the urethra, vagina and rectum. The sides of the muscle slope together in the middle, form a V-shaped gutter and pass under the arch of the pubis. Figure 146 shows the distribution and action of the various portions of the levator ani muscles and the opposing action of the sphincter ani. When the levator ani contracts, the rectum and the vagina are pulled up against the pubis; when the sphincter ani contracts, the anus and the lowest portion of the rectum are drawn backward. The result of the two forces is to close the rectum.

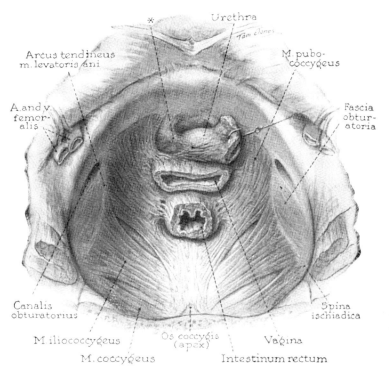

Figure 145 Pelvic floor viewed from above with the fascial layers removed and the viscera excised at a low level to demonstrate the muscular constituents and their relations to the viscera. The urethra has been pulled aside to show the levator fibers (asterisk) which are inserted into it. (From Curtis, A. H., et al.: Surg. Gynec. Obstet. 74:709, 1942.)

The puborectal portions of the levator ani can be felt easily as two roundish pillars at the sides of the vagina, displacing the examining finger to the pubis when they contract. Beneath the pelvic diaphragm lie the ischiorectal fossas, the perineal body, the urogenital diaphragm, the vulva and its glands. The *urogenital diaphragm* (Fig. 142) closes the genital hiatus. It is a three-cornered, musculofibrous septum, fitted into the pubic arch and extending backward to the anterior wall of the rectum. It is made up of the deep layer of the perineal fascia, enclosing

Figure 146 Lateral view to show levator ani from the side and its slinglike action. *a*, Vagina; *b*, rectum; *c*, posterior fibers of sphincter ani; *d*, anterior fibers of sphincter ani; *e*, levator ani, puborectal portion; *f*, musculus ischiococcygeus. (Modified from Luschka, H.: Das Becken, in Die Anatomie des Menschen in Rücksicht auf die Bedürfnisse der prakitschen Heilkunde. Tübingen, H. Laupp, 1864.)

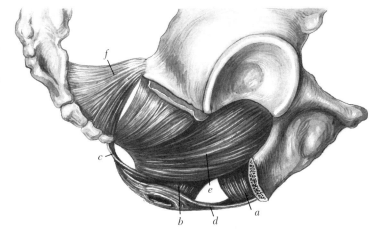

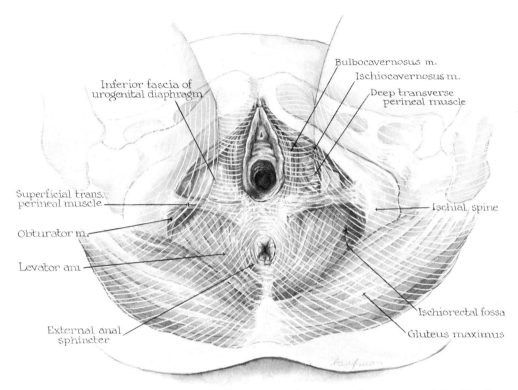

Figure 147   Topographic anatomy of the important perineal structures showing interrelationships between bony, muscular and visceral structures.

the fibers of the deep transverse perineal muscle and the compressor urethra. On this septum lie the bulbocavernosus (sphincter cunni), the ischiocavernosus and the superficial transverse perineal muscles. The *perineal body* consists of dense connective tissue located in the midline between the vulva and the anus.

The external sphincter ani lies between the skin and the pelvic diaphragm, surrounding the lower end of the rectum. It is attached posteriorly to the coccyx by the anococcygeal ligament and anteriorly to the perineal body. Most of its fibers encircle the anus, some continue into the bulbocavernosus and some mingle in the skin near the anal margin to become the cutaneous sphincter ani. The puborectal portion of the levator ani fuses with the sphincter at the sides and behind.

Figure 147 shows the important perineal structures in relationship to one another and also their relations to the bony structures, urethra, vagina and anus.

PELVIC FASCIAS

Pelvic fascias include the areolar tissue, fibroelastic connective tissue and muscular sheaths. The endoabdominal or endopelvic fascia extends downward over the brim of the pelvis where it splits into two layers. One covers the obturator internus muscle and one lies beneath it. About half way down the inner surface of the obturator internus the fascia thickens into a ridge or seam, the *white line*. Here the fascia splits again; one layer extends downward on top of the levator ani and the other continues underneath it. A short distance below the white line the superior levator fascia thickens into another ridge or mass of fibrous tissue in which the hypogastric vessels, the cervix and the fibers of the bases of the broad ligaments are found. This band of fibrous tissue, called *retinaculum uteri* (Martin), extends from the pubis around the pelvis to lose itself in the fascia over the piriformis muscle. From its

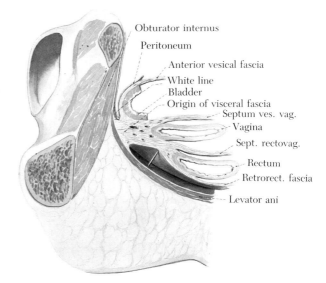

Figure 148 Coronal section of left half of the pelvis that shows the root or origin of the visceral fascia from the superior levator fascia and how it splits into four layers so as to ensheath the bladder, the vagina and the rectum.

Obturator internus
Peritoneum
Anterior vesical fascia
White line
Bladder
Origin of visceral fascia
Septum ves. vag.
Vagina
Sept. rectovag.
Rectum
Retrorect. fascia
Levator ani

inner border four layers of fascia arise. One extends anteriorly to the bladder, the second between the bladder and the vagina, the third between the vagina and the rectum and the fourth is retrorectal (Fig. 148).

The root stock of these four layers or leaves forms the bases of the *broad ligaments*. It rises from the inner surface of the superior levator fascia and supports the pelvic viscera; hence, it should be called the visceral layer of this fascia. Anteriorly, it is continued to the pubis to form the pubovesical ligaments, posteriorly to the sacrum to form the uterosacral ligaments and laterally to form the bases of the broad ligaments (Mackenrodt or cardinal ligaments originally described by Savage and by Kocks). This arrangement might be compared to a wheel with the cervix as the

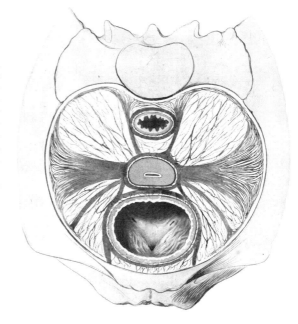

Figure 149 Semidiagrammatic representation of the pelvic fascia, illustrating how each pelvic organ has a sheath of fascia, the fibrous thickenings forming ligaments and fascial planes, supporting the organs and holding them in proper relation to each other and the pelvis, and the loose cellular tissue binding them all together. Note the resemblance of the cervix to the hub of a wheel, the ligaments being the spokes. (From Halban, J., and Tandler, J.: Anatomie und Ätiologie der Genitalprolapse beim Weibe. Vienna, Wilhelm Braunmüller, 1907.)

Fig. 150

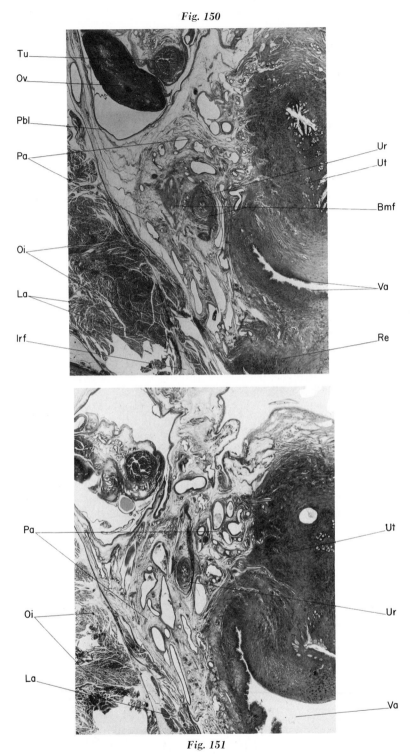

Fig. 151

Figures 150 and 151 Coronal tissue sections of pelvis through parametrium which show that the cardinal ligament is not actually ligamentous tissue but essentially a plexus of veins surrounded by loose connective tissue. *Bmf*, Bladder muscle fibers; *Irf*, ischiorectal fossa; *La*, levator ani muscle; *Oi*, obturator internus muscle; *Ov*, ovary; *Pa*, parametrium; *Pbl*, peritoneum of broad ligament; *Re*, rectum; *Tu*, tube; *Ur*, ureter; *Ut*, uterus; *Va*, vagina. (From Berglas, B., and Rubin, I. C.: Surg. Gynec. Obstet. 97:277, 1953.)

hub and the radiating ligaments the spokes. If one of the spokes is broken or stretched, the hub (cervix) will be displaced (Fig. 149). The fascias vary in strength and degree of support among women, and those of multiparas tend to be weaker and more stretched than those of nulliparas.

The superior levator fascia covers the free edge of the levator ani muscles, uniting with the deep layer of the fascia of the urogenital septum. Near the hiatus genitalis the fascia thickens into a ridge or strand of tough glistening fibers, called the *arcus tendineus fasciae pelvis*. On vaginal examination it can often be felt on each side as a sharp cord, coursing down the levator ani muscle. The fascia extends from one pillar of the levator ani to the one on the opposite side between the rectum and the vagina, forming part of the perineal body and fusing with the third layer of the visceral fascia. It is somewhat thicker here and holds the two pillars of the levator ani close together. It is important in the mechanism of labor and in the repair of lacerations of the pelvic floor. DeLee named it the *intercolumnar fascia* of the perineum.

These fascial planes and seams are of supreme importance in holding the cervix, bladder, vagina and rectum in their proper relation to each other and to the pelvis. When they are torn or stretched in labor they allow the pelvic organs to descend or to be displaced. These fascias, as shown by Goff, are more of the nature of areolar fascias and not the tough fibrous structures usually so called. Power found an unstriped muscle system in them. Contrary to this description, the histological studies by Berglas and Rubin of sections from female pelves with an intact relationship of vascular and connective tissue components failed to show a Mackenrodt ligament or a pubovesicouterine ligament. The bulk of tissue structures taken for these ligaments consists of plexuses of blood vessels embedded in loose areolar connective tissue (Figs. 150 and 151). There appear to be no true sheathlike condensations of the connective tissue surrounding the pelvic organs. Whether or not the fascial planes and condensations, to which obstetricians ascribe such great importance, actually exist is thus debatable.

FORMATION OF THE PARTURIENT CANAL

To be born the fetus must pass through three rings: the cervix, the opening in the levator ani and the hiatus genitalis (the vulva and perineum). Normally, the cervix is dilated and retracted around the fetal head before the head descends onto the pelvic floor, dilating the vagina progressively in its descent. Dilatation of the urogenital diaphragm occurs with that of the pelvic floor, and together they form a fibromuscular canal attached to the bony pelvic outlet. How the cervix is dilated until it is flush with the vagina has been described in Chapter 7. As the cervix and upper vagina dilate, adjacent fascias also participate. The retinaculum uteri in the parametrium, as well as the pubosacral and uterosacral ligamentous extensions of the endopelvic fascia, are all distended during parturition.

After the fetal head has passed through the cervix and rests on the pelvic floor, the levator ani begins to stretch. It is displaced downward and backward with all the soft parts of the pelvic outlet. Thus, these structures are displaced axially, in addition to being dilated radially. This lengthening of the soft parts is greater on the posterior than on the anterior wall, being only 2 or 3 cm. on the anterior and as much as 10 cm. on the posterior wall. The bundles of the levator ani are separated and drawn out so as to form a canal the circumference of which is equal to that of the head of the fetus—33 to 35 cm.

The urogenital septum lies flat on the outside of the canal and also undergoes some dilatation. However, it has little muscle or connective tissue and dilates poorly so that tears occur in the septum in full-term labors. These tears permit the anterior vaginal wall and urethra to sag in later years, causing prolapse in some instances.

The sphincter ani is stretched circumferentially in all directions. The anus, therefore, gapes widely as the head descends, exposing the anterior wall of the rectum. The rectum is flattened against the sacrum and levator ani. The vagina is dilated radially and axially to form a lining membrane for the canal. When the pelvic floor tears, the vagina usually does also.

The four layers of the visceral fascia (Fig. 148) are distended circularly and at the same time they are forced downward by the advancing head. As a result these semielastic fascial layers are thinned and may be torn. The vesicovaginal septum receives the first brunt of the attack, next the paracervical retinaculum, next the superior fascia of the levator ani with the arcus tendineus of the pelvic fascia, then the intercolumnar fascia gives way, which in turn allows the levator ani pillars to separate, and finally the urogenital septum.

In pathologic cases where delivery may be traumatic, the parametria and the root stock of the four layers of the visceral fascia are pushed off the superior layer of the levator ani fascia. Prolapse of the pelvic organs follows in due course.

The shape of the entire parturient canal may be depicted as shown in Figure 152, but the reader must understand that it does not exist as such, in its entirety, at any time during labor. The advancing head produces such a displacement of the surrounding structures only at the moment that it passes through them.

The parturient canal is straight until it reaches the midpelvic plane. Then it curves forward in a sharp angle centered at the symphysis pubis. If the arch of the pubis is narrow or if the fetal head is extremely large, the occiput stems on the pubic rami, forcing the pelvic floor farther back toward the sacrum, making a more obtuse angle. The axis of the parturient canal is, therefore, not a smooth curve such as that described by Carus and still bear-

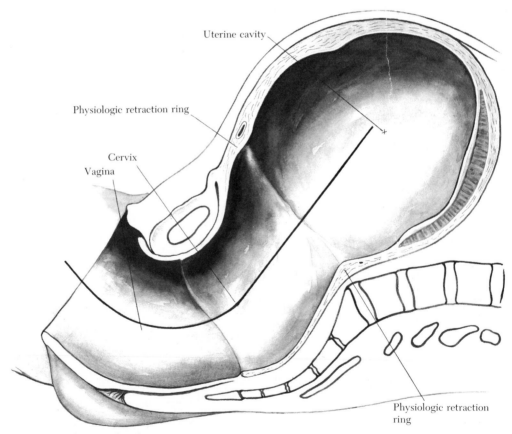

Figure 152 The completed parturient canal represented diagrammatically as if all its component portions remained maximally distended throughout labor. Central curved heavy line indicates the axis of the canal. Note sharp curve at the midpelvic plane. Above the retraction ring is the actively contracting portion of the uterus, below it the passively dilating portion.

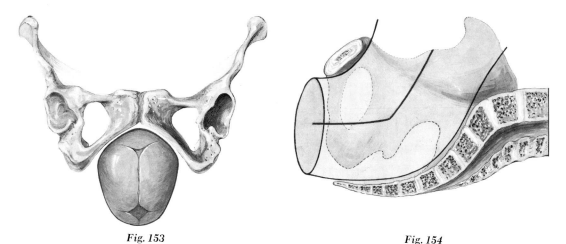

Fig. 153   Fig. 154

Figures 153 and 154   Normal sacrum and pelvic outlet giving proper curve to parturient canal. Note that all the available space under the pubis is utilized by the head.

ing his name. Rather it is a composite of a straight linear component bent at the mid-plane and curved below that.

In normal as well as pathologic labor, much depends on the curve of the sacrum and the angularity of the pubic arch. The angle of the parturient canal is slightly obtuse if the sacrum is sharply curved and the pubic arch broad (Figs. 153 and 154). The angle of the curve will be relatively straighter if the sacrum is not so deeply curved and the pubic arch is narrow (Figs. 155 and 156). This relationship may influence the mechanism of labor and affect the movement of the fetus along the birth canal.

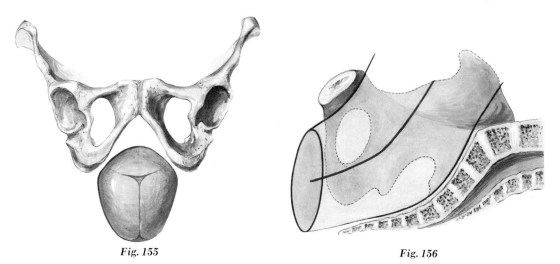

Fig. 155   Fig. 156

Figures 155 and 156   Obtuse angle given to parturient canal by abnormal pelvic configuration. Note that the head cannot utilize all available space under the pubis because of the narrow subpubic angle. As a consequence, more room is needed posteriorly and the head will therefore press the perineum backward.

REFERENCES

Berglas, B., and Rubin, I. C.: Histologic study of the pelvic connective tissue. Surg. Gynec. Obstet. 97:277, 1953.

Berglas, B., and Rubin, I. C.: Study of the supportive structures of the uterus by levator myography. Surg. Gynec. Obstet. 97:677, 1953.

Caldwell, W. E., and Moloy, H. C.: Anatomical variations in the female pelvis and their effect in labor with a suggested classification. Amer. J. Obstet. Gynec. 26:479, 1933.

Carus, C. G.: Lehrbuch der Gynäkologie. Leipzig, G. Fleischer, 1820.

Curtis, A. H., Anson, B. J., and Ashley, F. L.: Further studies in gynecological anatomy and related clinical problems. Surg. Gynec. Obstet. 74:709, 1942.

DeLee, J. B.: The Principles and Practice of Obstetrics, ed. 7. Philadelphia, W. B. Saunders Company, 1938.

Goff, B. H.: An histological study of the perivaginal fascia in a nullipara. Surg. Gynec. Obstet. 52:32, 1931.

Halban, J., and Tandler, J.: Anatomie und Ätiologie der Genitalprolapse beim Weibe. Vienna, Wilhelm Braunmüller, 1907.

Hodge, H. L.: The Principles and Practice of Obstetrics. Philadelphia, Blanchard & Lea, 1864.

Holl, M.: Handbuch der Anatomie des Menschen. Jena, v. Bardeleben, Abt. 2, 7:279, 1897.

Kocks, J.: Die normale und pathologische Lage und Gestalt des Uterus. Bonn, M. Cohen und Sohn, 1880.

Levret, A.: L'Art des Accouchements, ed. 1. Paris, Delaguette, 1753.

Luschka, H.: Das Becken, in Die Anatomie des Menschen in Rücksicht auf die Bedürfnisse der prakitschen Heilkunde. Tübingen, H. Laupp, 1864, vol. 2, pt. 2.

Mackenrodt, A.: Über die Ursachen der normalen und pathologischen Lagen des Uterus. Arch. Gynäk. 48:393, 1895.

Martin, E.: Der Haftapparat der weiblichen Genitalien. Berlin, S. Karger, 1911.

Power, R. M. H.: Unstriated muscle fiber of female pelvis. Amer. J. Obstet. Gynec. 29:834, 1939.

Savage, H.: The Surgery, Surgical Pathology, and Surgical Anatomy of the Female Pelvic Organs, ed. 3. London, J. & A. Churchill, 1876.

Chapter 17

Fetal Factors in Labor

The size, shape, compressibility and pliability of the fetus must be considered in order to understand the mechanisms of labor. The head is larger and more important than the trunk, and when it is pathologically enlarged it may give rise to dystocia. The face at term is small. The vault of the cranium forms the major portion of the head. Large squamous bony plates make up the cranial vault: the *parietal*, the *frontal* and the *occipital*. At the sides the *temporal* bones unite with the parietals. These bones are not solidly joined to each other. Their ossification halts at the lines of impingement. The bones are held in relation to one another by a membrane, the *chondrocranium*, in which ossification will take place later in life. The lines of impingement are called *sutures*. Rounding of the bony corners of the separate bones leaves junctional spaces filled by membrane. These spaces are the *fontanels*. These spaces are of vital importance because they serve as critical guideposts in providing information on the relation of the head to the maternal pelvis, the mechanism of labor and the application of the obstetric forceps.

Between the two parietal bones lies the *sagittal suture* (Fig. 157); between the parietal and the occipital bone is the *lambdoidal suture;* between the frontal bone and the parietal is the *coronal suture;* and between the two plates of the frontal bone lies the *frontal suture*. At the sides, where the parietal bones touch the temporals, lie the *lateral* or *temporal sutures* which are of little obstetric importance.

At the junction of the sagittal, frontal and two coronal sutures there is a lozenge-shaped space, the *anterior* or *large fontanel*. Its size and shape depend on the degree of ossification of the adjoining bones. With advanced ossification it becomes more nearly square. Four sutures fuse into the large fontanel, characterizing and distinguishing it from the others. Three of its angles are acute and one is obtuse. The obtuse angle points toward the occiput, or posterior pole of the head, and the longest acute angle points toward the face. This enables one to determine the position of the fetal head in the pelvis.

At the junction of the sagittal suture with the lambdoidal, there is a small triangular space, the *posterior* or *small fontanel*. Three sutures enter the small fontanel to characterize it. During labor it is obliterated as a space and these three lines join at a point like the letter Y. The stem of the Y is the sagittal suture and points toward the face.

Where the lateral sutures meet the ends of the coronal and lambdoidal sutures, spaces exist which are *lateral fontanels*. They are important because they may be

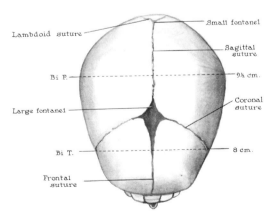

Figure 157 Top view of fetal skull, showing cranial bones, anterior (large lozenge shaped) and posterior (small triangular) fontanels and sutures. The two important diameters, *Bi P.*, biparietal and *Bi T.*, bitemporal, are also designated.

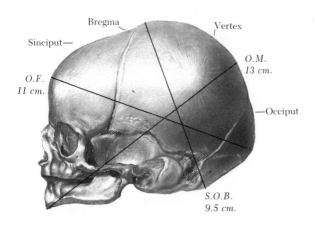

Bregma

Vertex

Sinciput—

O.M.
13 cm.

O.F.
11 cm.

—Occiput

S.O.B.
9.5 cm.

Figure 158 Lateral view of fetal skull showing cranial relationships, regional designations (reference points) and main diameters, including *O.F.*, occipitofrontal; *O.M.*, occipitomental; and *S.O.B.*, suboccipitobregmatic.

confused with the other fontanels and lead to serious diagnostic errors. The ear is close to the posterior lateral fontanel and the bony ocular orbit is next to the anterior lateral fontanel. *Wormian bones* are accessory centers of ossification which sometimes occupy the spaces of the fontanels; they have no obstetric importance. In the sagittal suture, occasionally a quadrangular space is found; it can be easily mistaken for the large fontanel and may cause errors in diagnosis. Confusion may be avoided by following the sagittal suture to its terminal fontanels.

The areas of the skull (Fig. 158) are distinguished by particular names. The *occiput* is that portion lying posterior to the small fontanel; the *sinciput* is that portion lying anterior to the large fontanel; the *bregma* is the area of the large fontanel; the *vertex* is the area between the two fontanels and extends to the parietal protuberances.

In shape the fetal head is irregularly ovoid—narrow in front, broad in back. The frontal bone is square, the result of the angularity of the frontal protuberances, and the parietal bones have a sharp prominence on each side—the *parietal bosses*. They mark the points at which the fetal head encounters the greatest resistance in passing through the pelvis. The size and shape of the head modifies the mechanism of labor and may cause dystocia.

The fetal head diameters vary considerably within normal limits. The molding of the head by labor shortens some diameters and lengthens others. Measurements taken at delivery will be modified four or

five days after birth, when the head has recovered its original shape. Circumferences measured around the occipitofrontal and the suboccipitobregmatic diameters average 34 and 31 cm., respectively. The suboccipitobregmatic circumference outlines the most important plane of a fetal head in labor (Fig. 158). Boys usually have larger heads at birth than girls.

The diameters of the fetal skull are critical. When discussing mechanisms of labor (Chapter 18), we will indicate the important adaptations the fetus makes to accommodate its most favorable head diameters to the limiting dimensions of the bony pelvis. Viewed coronally (Fig. 157), the biparietal diameter is of utmost importance; laterally (Fig. 158), the suboccipitobregmatic is clearly shorter than either the occipitofrontal or the large occipitomental diameter. Deflexion of the head thus results in a larger diameter presenting than strong flexion.

The trunk, while apparently larger, presents small diameters to the birth canal because it may be compressed to cylindric proportions. The mean bisacromial diameter across the shoulders of a newborn child is 11 cm.; the bisiliac diameter at the pelvis is 9 cm. The circumference of the upper trunk at the shoulders is 34 cm. and that of the chest is 32 cm.

By *attitude* or *habitus* is meant the relation of the various parts of the fetal body to one another. The normal attitude of the fetus, when there is adequate amniotic fluid, is one of moderate flexion of all the joints, making an ovoid figure of the fetus as shown in Figure 159. The back is

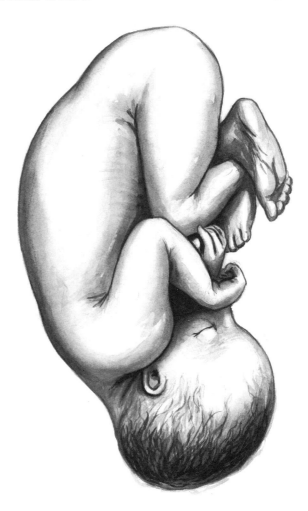

Figure 159 Attitude of fetus at beginning of labor. The so-called fetal position with extremities and head flexed on abdomen and chest. Prior to the onset of labor, if amniotic fluid is adequate in amount, the fetus has considerable freedom of movement.

curved outward, the head is slightly bent on the chest and the arms and legs are crossed anteriorly and flexed, although they remain free to move in all directions. Various attitudes are found at different times during pregnancy—flexion, deflexion and lateroflexion of the head, while the extremities may be placed in all conceivable positions. When the amount of amniotic fluid is scant, so that the fetus has insufficient space to stretch out, its attitude tends to be tightly flexed and cramped.

PRESENTATION AND POSITION

There is considerable confusion concerning the terms *presentation, presenting part* and *position*. By *presentation* or *lie* is meant the relationship that the long axis of the fetus bears to that of the mother. There are two basic lies or presentations—*longitudinal* and *oblique* or *transverse*. Longitudinal presentations occur in about 99 per cent of all labors. Either the head or the breech presents. When the head presents it is a *cephalic presentation;* when the breech or the lower limbs present it is a *breech presentation.*

Presenting part refers to that portion of the fetus which is bounded by the girdle of resistance during labor and touched by the fingers during an internal examination.

Position relates a given arbitrary reference point in the presenting part to the four quadrants of the pelvis. In occipital presentation the occiput is the reference point; in breech presentation, the sacrum;

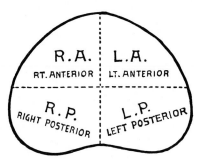

Figure 160 The four quadrants of the pelvis, viewed from below with patient in lithotomy position as encountered during vaginal or rectal examination.

in shoulder presentation, the scapula or acromial process; in face, the chin; in brow, the bregma.

All terms concerned with direction refer to the mother: anterior, the direction to the front of the mother; right, the right side of the mother, and so on. These terms have no relation to the fetus or the examiner and they are not changed by any position the mother may assume. By keeping this rule in mind confusion will be avoided.

For easy description the pelvis is divided into four quadrants: a left and a right anterior and a left and a right posterior (Fig. 160). The position of the presenting part is defined according to that quadrant in which its reference point lies.

Three general divisions of presentation are recognized:

1. Cephalic presentation and its varieties: vertex, brow and face. The vertex is the normal; the others are due to deflexion of the head. They are called *deflexion attitudes*.

2. Breech presentation and its varieties: frank or single, complete and incomplete breech, all referring to various placements of the lower extremities (see below).

3. Shoulder presentation, or transverse lie, includes shoulder, arm and any other part of the trunk.

The first two groups are longitudinal presentations because the axis of the fetus lies parallel to that of the uterus. In the last group the fetus lies more or less obliquely or perpendicularly to the axis of the uterus.

When the breech is incomplete, that is, when one or both feet have prolapsed or one or both knees are down, the sacrum is still the reference point. The designations

remain the same but qualifications, such as footling, knee and so forth, are added.

Each presenting part may so occupy the pelvis that its reference point may lie in any pelvic diameter; for example, the occiput may be to the right, to the left, behind, in front or at any intermediate point when labor begins. Eight main positions are recognized generally for each presentation, designated clockwise: direct anterior, left anterior, left transverse, left posterior, direct posterior, right posterior, right transverse and right anterior. Positions are designated for clarity in terms of (1) reference point, (2) right-left direction and (3) anterior-posterior direction. By common usage, the right-left designation has come to precede the reference point, and this convention will be continued here. Customary abbreviations as popularly employed are also included. The most common fetal position, for example, is left occiput anterior or L.O.A. (Fig. 161).

Two very important items are lacking in this discussion. How is the distance the fetus has advanced down the birth canal toward the vulvar outlet to be determined? How is the idea of the location or degree of progress of the presenting part in the birth canal to be conveyed? Müller suggested the word *station*. Degree of engagement is often used; the entry of the head into the pelvis is called *engagement*. DeLee devised designations of station by centimeters above or below the level of the ischial spines at the midplane. The designation "minus one" signifies that the forward leading edge of the presenting part is 1 cm. cephalad to this level; "plus two," 2 cm. caudad. Use of such station designations has proved very effective.

FREQUENCY OF PRESENTATIONS AND POSITIONS

In any large series of vaginal deliveries one would expect vertex presentations in 95 per cent and breech in four per cent. The remaining one per cent include about 0.5 per cent shoulder, 0.3 per cent face and 0.1 per cent brow. During the last few weeks of pregnancy both the presentation

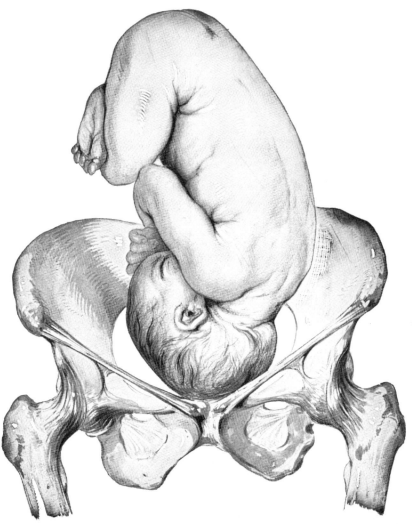

Figure 161 Fetus in left occiput anterior position, L.O.A. The head is well flexed on the chest and rotated 45° clockwise from the midline as viewed from the perineum.

and the position of the fetus may change, most frequently from breech to cephalic. Ordinarily, the presentation becomes fixed after the presenting part has engaged in the pelvis.

While changes of the long axis are frequent in pregnancy, changes in position are almost daily occurrences. Examination of women on successive days will at one time show the fetal back on one side and at another on the other side. In multiparas, because of their lax uterine and abdominal walls, mobility of the fetus is most pronounced. During labor the fetus often alters its position. This generally follows a set pattern, as will be discussed in Chapter 18 when we deal with the mechanisms of labor. For example, if a patient is examined early in labor, the position may be L.O.P.; a few hours later, L.O.T. and still later, L.O.A. or even R.O.A.

During pregnancy the fetus is mobile and accommodates itself to the position assumed by the mother. When she is erect, its back tends to fall forward; when she is lying on her side, it drops to the side on which she lies. This explains the frequency of transverse and posterior fetal positions in routine antepartum examinations prior to labor.

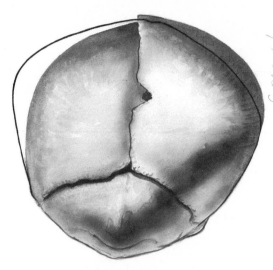

Figure 162 Rear view of skull molded in L.O.A. showing the right parietal bone overlapping the left. Line shows shape before molding.

CHANGES DURING LABOR

The head undergoes definite changes in labor. They vary with the presentation of the fetus and are caused by pressures exerted by the maternal structures. In ordinary cephalic presentations, with a moderately snug parturient passage, the face and the forehead are flattened, the occiput is drawn out and the bones overlap.

Usually the occipital bone is pressed under the two parietals; the frontal is also somewhat below the parietals. One parietal overlaps the other; the one that lies against the sacral promontory is the one that is depressed (Figs. 162 and 163).

The head thus offers a long narrow cylinder to the birth canal instead of a round ball. These changes in shape, or *molding*, are possible because of the softness of the bones and the loose connection they have with one another at the sutures. When this molding does not take place labor may be more difficult.

In long labors a soft, boggy circumscribed swelling appears on that part of the head which is most dependent and least subjected to pressure. In vertex presentations it is formed on one parietal bone. It is caused by the pressure of the uterus transmitted through the fetal body, acting below the girdle of resistance at the opening in the cervix, the vagina or even the vulva (Fig. 164). The effect is similar to that occurring distal to a tourniquet; the venous obstruction results in congestion with edema and extravasation. Small hemorrhages persist long after the edema is absorbed and define the site of the swelling, called *caput succedaneum*. It occurs in and under the scalp. Therefore it is movable on the skull. A distinction must be made between caput succedaneum and *cephalhematoma,* which is an accumula-

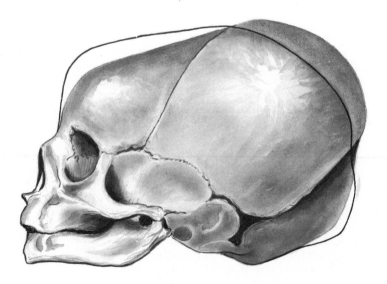

Figure 163 Side view of skull molded in R.O.A. with depression of the frontal bone where it was resting on the promontory of the sacrum. Line shows shape of skull before molding.

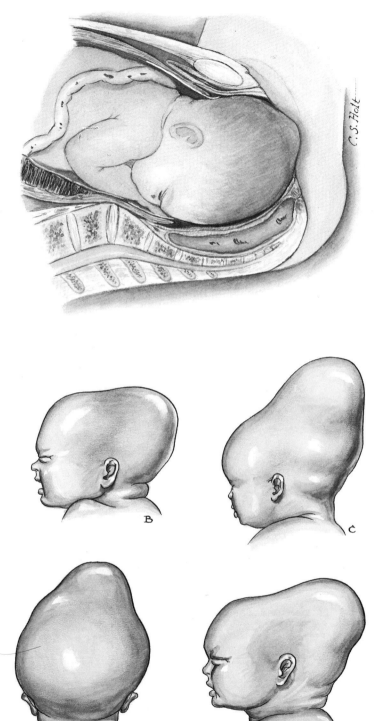

Figure 164 Lateral diagrammatic view showing how a caput succedaneum is formed over the most dependent and least supported part of the fetal head.

Figure 165 Various types of caput succedaneum and molding of infants' heads shown in outline. *A*, Head shape after delivery from the L.O.A.; *B*, breech presentation; *C*, persistent occiput posterior delivered by extension; *D*, persistent occiput posterior delivered by flexion; *E*, molding of head in flat pelvis; *F*, molding of head in generally contracted pelvis.

tion of blood under the periosteum (see Chapter 68) and is clearly delimited by the cranial sutures.

The caput exaggerates the obliquity of the head produced by the depression of the parietal bone by the promontory of the sacrum or the pelvic floor (Figs. 162 to 165). The caput is absorbed in 24 to 36 hours, and the asymmetry of the head disappears by the end of a week.

Sometimes the head occupies the pelvic cavity for the last three to five weeks of pregnancy and is permanently deformed and flattened by the levator muscles. The lateroflexion of the trunk shortens the sternocleidomastoid muscle, and during delivery the deformed muscle may rupture, causing hematoma, myositis and wryneck. However, most wrynecks are not the result of compression but are true congenital deformities, a developmental defect.

In breech presentations the head may be flattened by the long-continued pressure of the uterine fundus against it. In a nullipara with limited capacity of the abdomen, the flattening may begin in the later months of pregnancy and may be permanent.

REFERENCES

DeLee, J. B.: Principles and Practice of Obstetrics, ed. 7. Philadelphia, W. B. Saunders Company, 1938.

Müller, P.: Untersuchungen über die Verkürzung der Vaginalportion in den letzten Monaten der Gravidität. Beitr. Geburtsk. Gynäk. 5:191, 1868.

Chapter 18

Mechanisms of Labor

Understanding of the mechanisms of labor is essential for the practice of obstetrics. This subject deals with the sequence of movements that the fetus undergoes in accommodating itself passively to the birth canal during its descent and birth. It consists of a series of successive changes that reflect alterations in attitudes usually resulting in presentation of more favorable diameters to the particular portion of the pelvis in which the fetus is at that moment. Thus, the mechanisms are the results of the forces of labor as they affect the fetal presenting part which in turn is responding to the conditions prevailing in its vicinity, with particular regard for the bony pelvic configuration and the muscular and fascial resistances that it meets. In order for the clinician to comprehend the mechanisms of labor it is essential that he be familiar with the important anatomic features of the pelvis (Chapter 16) and of the fetal skull (Chapter 17).

The main features involved in labor mechanisms include (1) engagement, (2) flexion, (3) internal rotation, (4) extension, (5) restitution or external rotation and (6) delivery of the shoulders and expulsion of the remainder of the body of the infant. Confusion sometimes arises because descent is considered a separate and distinct mechanism when in fact it is a continuous concomitant phenomenon of the parturitional process occurring at the same time as the other mechanisms are evolving. Although we describe them as if they take place independently, some of these movements are actually going on simultaneously. Indeed, the main or cardinal movements could not take place unless descent were occurring. Moreover, there are additional fetal changes taking place,

namely, those of *attitude,* in which the vertebral column changes from its flexed condition to become straight or even lordotic in its cervical and thoracic portions. The course of descent as it relates to progression in labor has been previously detailed in terms of the advancement of the forward leading edge of the presenting part (that is, its *station* in the pelvis) in time sequence (see Chapter 15).

The pathway that the fetus follows is represented by the pelvic axis described in Chapter 16. Its direction is straight and perpendicular to the inlet plane until it reaches the midplane. At this point its axis becomes curvilinear, arching in an anterior direction toward the outlet. It is apparent from this description that the fetal presenting part must descend into the pelvis more or less in a straight line until it reaches the midplane, after which it must somehow adjust itself to turn toward the outlet. The cardinal movements constitute collectively the way in which this accommodation is accomplished.

ENGAGEMENT

In most instances (95 per cent) the fetus has adapted itself well before labor begins so that it occupies the longitudinal axis of the uterus with its head directed toward the pelvis, the breech in the fundus and the vertebral column strongly flexed. Under these circumstances, the fetal head will be found high above the superior strait, a condition termed *floating.* If the head has entered the superior strait but its widest diameters are still above the pelvic inlet, it is considered to be *dipping* into the inlet and can be shown to be still quite mobile so that its position may change considerably from one observation to another. The inlet is accommodated when the fetal head is fixed in the pelvis and its biparietal diameter or occipitofrontal plane is at or below the superior strait; this head may be said to be *engaged* and to have accommodated itself to the inlet by the process of engagement.

Engagement may occur gradually during the last few weeks of pregnancy, but as a rule, especially in nulliparas, it takes place rather acutely over a period of several hours or days about three weeks prior to onset of labor. In multiparas, on the other hand, the head may not be fixed into the inlet until after labor has been in progress for some time. Once the fetal presenting part has accommodated itself completely to the pelvis, its position is stabilized.

Inlet shapes have been detailed in Chapter 12 according to the Caldwell-Moloy classification. The position that the fetal head assumes during engagement depends largely upon this factor. In about 60 per cent of cases, the sagittal suture of the fetal head will be arranged transversely. Left occiput transverse and right occiput transverse positions predominate at the superior strait because of the fact that the more or less oval shape of the fetal head with its elongated occipitofrontal diameter accommodates itself to the oval inlet with its somewhat widened transverse diameter. In the platypelloid pelvis this is particularly true because the transverse diameter is so much longer than the true conjugate. By contrast, in the anthropoid pelvis with elongated anteroposterior diameters, the fetal head more often enters the pelvis with the sagittal suture aligned anteroposteriorly or obliquely. In the more common gynecoid pelvis, the position at engagement is most often transverse or oblique.

Engagement is clinically recognizable by two means: abdominal verification of fixation of the head in the pelvis and vaginal determination of the fact that the forward leading edge of the presenting part is at or below the level of the ischial spines or station zero (see Chapter 17).

Synclitism refers to the planar relationship between the occipitofrontal plane of the fetal head and the plane of the pelvis in which that fetal plane is located. When both fetal and pelvic planes are parallel or in concordance, the relationship is referred to as *synclitic* (Fig. 166). More often the head is flexed so that the two planes are *asynclitic* or not parallel. Synclitism can be recognized by finding the sagittal suture exactly midway between the symphysis pubis and the sacral promontory with both parietal bones equally prominent and exposed in the pelvis. Usually, the sagittal suture is encountered closer to the symphysis pubis and the posterior parietal bone more prominent and more deeply descended into the pelvis. This is called *posterior asynclitism* (Fig. 167). *Anterior asynclitism,* in which the sagittal suture lies closer to the sacrum and the anterior parietal bone is more prominent and more deeply engaged, is rather unusual under normal circumstances (Fig. 168). If encountered, one should search for some underlying bony factor causing dystocia.

In the normal course of events in labor, there is some posterior asynclitism at the time of engagement. The head gradually flexes itself laterally so that the sagittal suture comes to lie more and more toward the midline, becoming synclitic for a time, and then perhaps a slight further backward displacement of the sagittal suture occurs when engagement is complete. Usually, the fetal head is well flexed before labor begins, with the occiput much lower than the frontum and the posterior fontanel lower or at least at the same level as the anterior fontanel.

The head is sometimes not well flexed and the bregma may be lowermost in the inlet. Such positions are rather unstable and the head will generally become progressively more flexed as descent takes place. Rarely, the head will descend unflexed into the lower pelvis. Where both anterior and posterior fontanels are at the same level, the condition is a *sincipital presentation* or military attitude. If the anterior fontanel is lowermost, deflexion exists and brow presentation is likely. Normally, however, flexion takes place before or early in labor and the position of the fetal head can be characterized as decidedly stable during descent.

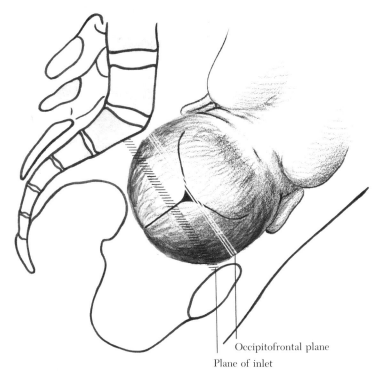

Occipitofrontal plane

Plane of inlet

Figure 166 Lateral representation of synclitism showing parallelism or concordance of the fetal occipito-frontal plane and the pelvic superior strait. The sagittal suture is in the midline of the pelvic axis.

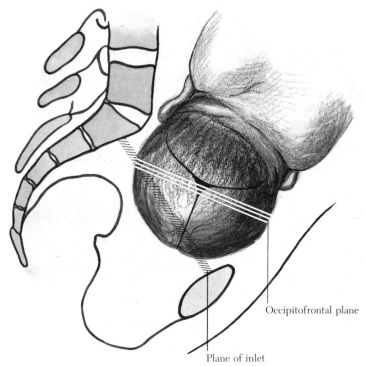

Occipitofrontal plane

Plane of inlet

Figure 167 Illustration of the common posterior parietal presentation or posterior asynclitism (Litzmann's obliquity), with the sagittal suture facing toward the symphysis pubis.

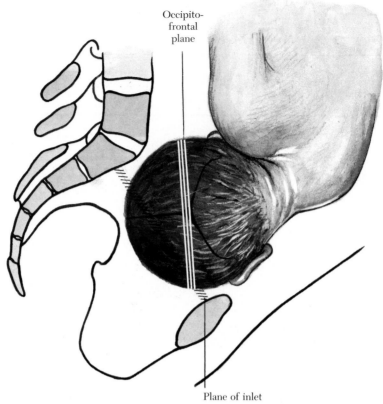

Occipito-
frontal
plane

Plane of inlet

Figure 168   The unusual anterior parietal presentation or anterior asynclitism (Nägele's obliquity), with the sagittal suture facing the sacrum.

FLEXION

Flexion is an important cardinal movement in the labor mechanism because it results in a significant reduction in the diameters that the fetus presents to the pelvis. If the head is deflexed, the occipitofrontal diameter of perhaps 12.0 cm. presents as contrasted with a 9.5 cm. suboccipitobregmatic presenting diameter of the well-flexed head (Fig. 169). When flexion takes place, the baby's chin comes to lie closely against its thorax.

Although the exact mechanism by which flexion occurs is unknown, it is likely the passive response of the head to the pelvic resistance it meets during descent. It is an attractive concept to consider the head as representing a type of lever such that the occipitofrontal plane is balanced at the foramen magnum, the junction with the vertebral column. Since the two arms of the lever are unequal, it follows that equivalent pressure on the longer anterior arm will exert more force to effect flexion than the forces on the shorter, counterbalancing posterior arm at the occiput. Thus, the fetal head will flex on its transverse axis normally whenever pelvic resistance is met during descent. Rydberg demonstrated by x-ray that fetal heads may be well flexed before engagement takes place. The essentiality of this mechanism must nevertheless be stressed because it so effectively reduces the presenting fetal skull diameters during the course of descent.

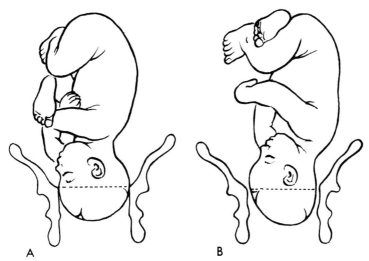

A   **B**

Figure 169   Reduction in the presenting fetal diameters as a result of flexion. The occipitofrontal diameter in a moderately deflexed sincipital presentation (A) is converted to the smaller suboccipitobregmatic in a well-flexed vertex presentation (B).

INTERNAL ROTATION

Internal rotation refers to the progressively changing fetal position in the pelvis as the head descends through the lower part of the birth canal. If the head has descended to the midplane in a transverse position, L.O.T. or R.O.T., internal rotation will result in the reorientation of the fetus to the corresponding occiput anterior position. Generally, internal rotation is not complete until the fetal head has advanced in its descent so as to begin to distend the perineum and to be visible at the vulva. There is no real demarcation between the cardinal movement of internal rotation and the concomitant ongoing descent and subsequent extension with delivery of the head over the perineum (Fig. 170).

Several contractions are necessary to effect complete internal rotation. It proceeds gradually during the alternating advance and recession of the head with each contraction. It may sometimes take place quite suddenly and be accomplished in one or two contractions. As the head turns in the pelvis, the shoulders and body usually follow suit but they may either turn incompletely or not at all.

It is likely that internal rotation is brought about by forces active in the birth canal to determine the position of the head at any given moment. As the head impinges on the wall of the lower pelvis, tensional forces are transmitted to the head by the elasticity in the wall. Rydberg has attempted to explain rotational movement on the basis of the interplay between the elastic forces at work and the shape of the head. He ascribed much significance to the anterior and upward convexity of the fetal skull in bringing about conformity between the wall of the birth canal and the surface of the head and neck along the region of contact.

Although this is probably correct, it does not explain the occasional instance when internal rotation will result in the occiput turning posteriorly toward the sacrum. This latter may occur especially in anthropoid pelves, where the sacral hollow is particularly roomy and will accommodate the relatively large posterior aspect of the fetal skull. This relationship suggests that internal rotation is more a matter of the fetal head accommodating itself passively to the space available for it, analogous to the accommodation which results in flexion during engagement and extension just prior to delivery over the perineum (see below).

It is probable that the trough formed by the levator ani muscles (Fig. 146) is a prime factor in effecting internal rotation.

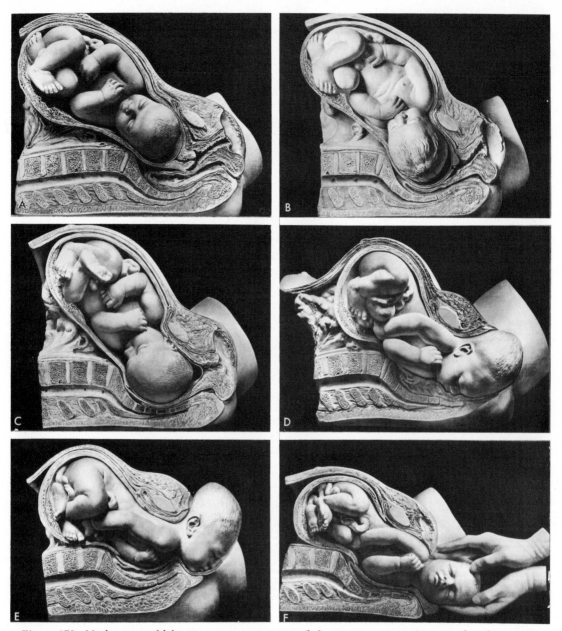

Figure 170 Mechanisms of labor in vertex presentation (left occiput transverse). *A*, Head at the superior strait. *B*, Engagement and flexion completed. *C*, Internal rotation in progress. *D* and *E*, Extension. *F*, External rotation and delivery of the shoulders. (From Birth Atlas, Maternity Center Association, New York.)

As the head descends below the midplane, this trough is reached and the leading edge of the head is carried forward, effectively turning the occiput toward the midline anteriorly. This results in a spiraling or corkscrew motion such that the part of the fetal vertex that first reaches the pelvic diaphragm will be directed along the pathway of least resistance to rotate anteriorly.

Internal rotation may be impeded by transverse constriction of the midplane due to prominent ischial spines or a foreshortened interspinous diameter. In a posterior mechanism, such as will occur in anthropoid pelves, the fetal head may descend with the occiput facing posteriorly and persist in this position until the head reaches the perineum because internal rotation may not be possible as a result of the constrictive transverse diameters in the midplane.

EXTENSION

As already indicated above, when the fetal head reaches the levator trough it begins to rotate internally and to extend along the anteriorly curved pelvic axis. This process takes place only when the head has reached the pelvic floor and the occiput is impinging upon the subpubic arch. Progressively, extension results in distension of the vulvar tissue by the advancing head as it is driven more and more anteriorly. The perineum becomes elongated, the vulva opens and the fetal scalp becomes visible between contractions. With further progression, the head is finally born over the anterior edge of the perineum (posterior fourchette). First the occiput appears under the symphysis pubis and advances through the vulvar opening until the bregma, forehead, nose, mouth and chin of the infant are successively born. Thus, the vertex, the brow and finally the face advance rapidly and appear in succession over the perineum.

Extension seems to be the resultant of progressive movement as influenced by the shape and resistive forces of the birth canal. The pelvic axis is directed in a curvilinear direction anteriorly (Fig. 152) and the pelvic musculature and perineum contribute the directional resistance to force the head in an anterior arc, effectively extending it under the subpubic arch and over the perineum itself.

RESTITUTION AND EXTERNAL ROTATION

After the head is delivered, it spontaneously rotates to its original oblique direc-

tion. This process, called *restitution,* signifies the realignment of the fetal head with its shoulders. In the course of internal rotation of the occiput to the anterior position, the shoulders may or may not follow. In the L.O.A. position, for example, the shoulders may persist in an oblique direction analogous to the left oblique diameter of the inlet (Fig. 140) and as a consequence the head will return to the L.O.A. position after it is delivered.

Subsequently, with further descent of the fetus in the birth canal, the shoulders undergo internal rotation as they accommodate to the pelvic dimensions and, simultaneously, the infant's head follows to complete *external rotation* to a transverse position. This occurs most often because the shoulders align themselves with the anteroposterior diameter of the lower pelvis by mechanisms which are undoubtedly the same as those that produce internal rotation of the fetal head.

DELIVERY OF SHOULDERS AND EXPULSION

At the completion of external rotation, the bisacromial diameter across the shoulder region has rotated to coincide with the anteroposterior diameter of the pelvis. The anterior shoulder moves forward to stem under the pubic arch. The perineum becomes distended once again as the posterior shoulder is carried forward by the advancing body, propelled by the combined expulsive forces of uterine contraction and voluntary bearing-down efforts. The posterior shoulder is generally delivered first over the perineum and the anterior shoulder follows easily under the symphysis. The rest of the infant is readily expelled thereafter.

Delivery of the shoulders can occur spontaneously, but it often requires manual aid to expedite it. Gentle depression of the fetal head without undue traction (for fear of injuring the brachial plexus) will help the anterior shoulder to stem under the symphysis. Then gently elevating the head will effect controlled delivery of the posterior shoulder (see Chapter 20).

OCCIPUT POSTERIOR MECHANISMS

We have already indicated that occiput posterior positions are common in association with anthropoid pelves. Because of the roomy posterior segment of such pelves and the deep scoop to the sacrum, the occiput tends to rotate internally toward the sacrum rather than anteriorly. Moreover, since the transverse diameters tend to be relatively short and the ischial spines prominent, anterior rotation is difficult to accomplish and posterior positions tend to be persistent throughout descent.

Engagement and early descent in labor in an oblique posterior position is probably more common than generally recognized. However, anterior internal rotation is quite prevalent with the occiput rotating through a long arc up to 180° in the course of descent.

The common cardinal movements describing the mechanisms associated with occiput posterior positions are analogous to those described earlier for transverse and anterior positions of the occiput. Engagement is associated with flexion. As the head descends to reach the pelvic floor, internal rotation takes place so that the oc-

ciput rotates all the way to the anterior position beneath the symphysis pubis.

In less than 10 per cent of patients with occiput posterior position, internal rotation will not take place or will result in rotation of the occiput directly to the sacrum. In others, anterior internal rotation will be attempted and will become arrested by impingement on the ischial spines. Persistent occiput posterior position and transverse arrest, when they are encountered, suggest the presence of pelvic abnormalities (see Chapter 63).

If anterior internal rotation is successful, subsequent extension and delivery of the fetal head over the perineum will occur as described earlier for anterior positions. Restitution may result in the fetal head rotating all the way back to its original position in alignment with the shoulders, so that the occiput may be directed posteriorly and the face upward.

In the persistent occiput posterior position in which anterior internal rotation has not occurred at all (Fig. 171), the delivery mechanisms are quite distinctive. The anterior curvature of the lower axis of the birth canal forces the head to flex strongly so that the chin is tightly against the chest. As the head advances against the pelvic floor, flexion is reinforced still more, if pos-

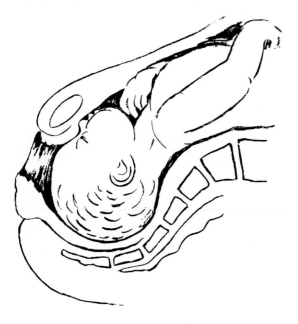

Figure 171 Direct occiput posterior position deeply engaged in the pelvis, illustrating the close conformity between the head and the birth canal.

sible. During actual expulsion, the brow and the face are stemmed anteriorly under the symphysis and the occiput markedly distends the perineum. Advancement proceeds until the occiput crosses the anterior margin of the perineum. This is followed in sequence by delivery from under the symphysis of the forehead, nose, mouth and chin.

This mechanism results in the presenta-tion to pelvis and perineum of much larger fetal dimensions than in occiput anterior mechanisms, namely, the occipitofrontal rather than the suboccipitobregmatic diameter, a difference of as much as 3 cm. The clinical implication of this phenomenon will be discussed in greater detail in Chapter 56 along with mechanisms and significance of other deflexion problems, such as brow and face presentations.

REFERENCES

D'Esopo, D. A.: The occipitoposterior position: Its mechanism and treatment. Amer. J. Obstet. Gynec. *42*:937, 1941.

Rydberg, E.: The Mechanism of Labour. Springfield, Ill., Charles C Thomas, 1954.

Rydberg, E.: Stereoscopic X-ray in Obstetrics: An Atlas and a Clinical Study. Aarhus, Universitets-forlaget, 1969.

Chapter 19

Preparations for Delivery

RESPONSE TO PATIENT'S CALL

The pregnant woman should be instructed to notify her physician immediately after she believes that labor has begun or if she thinks that something unusual is taking place. The physician should inquire if any symptoms other than contractions or leaking fluid are present before instructing the patient to go to the hospital. If there is any active bleeding, it is best to have the patient brought to the hospital expeditiously by ambulance.

It is a good policy for the physician to keep a small notebook in his pocket at all times; in it should be listed all the important data about every obstetric patient for whom he is responsible. Such information should include any known medical ailment, such as heart disease or diabetes, as well as the Rh factor, previous cesarean section, twins, anemia and other facts. Immediately after being notified that a patient is in labor, the physician must consult this notebook and any special fact should be telephoned to the nurse or resident physician at the hospital. On the way to the hospital the attending physician should review these facts and decide if it will be necessary to conduct labor in a special way. There should be a complete copy of every patient's antepartum record at the hospital four weeks before the expected date of delivery, and it must be carefully reviewed as soon as the physician reaches the labor room. However, conditions may have arisen after the antepartum record has been sent to the hospital and these must be listed in his book and transferred to the hospital record at the time of admission.

ASEPSIS AND ANTISEPSIS

The first consideration is the physician himself. Holmes in 1843 and Semmelweis in 1847 called attention to the *physician as a carrier of infection,* and the important role that he plays in this has been recognized ever since. In fact, it has been somewhat exaggerated, as the public has held him responsible even when he may not have been to blame. Infection will sometimes occur under ideal conditions and its cause must be sought perhaps in the woman herself, in her husband or in other hospital personnel.

The obstetrician should have clean personal habits and not soil his clothes by contact with patients who have a contagious disease. *In spite of the availability of antibiotics, he must scrupulously avoid getting infective material on his hands.* All contaminated items should be handled with forceps and rubber gloves.

Hospital shirt, trousers, shoe coverings, sterile gown, cap, mask and gloves should be worn during delivery procedures just as they are for surgical operations. DeLee believed, long before it was proved by Colebrook, White and others, that droplet contamination of puerperal wounds and sterile instruments, as unavoidably occurs during speaking, is a common source of infection. Scales of dried mucus may drop from the nose onto the sterile field. Moreover, spray contamination may still occur right through most cloth face masks.

Everything introduced into the vagina should be absolutely sterile. This requires repeated emphasis.

Next, we must consider asepsis as it relates to the patient herself. The cervix, vagina, vestibule and vulva are always contaminated with nonpathogens and sometimes with pathogenic bacteria. Why is autoinfection not more common? The reasons for its rare occurrence are not clearly known, but the following have been considered relevant: In the parturient, local and general immunities have developed against normal vaginal bacteria; the process of labor involves a continual washing out from above with amniotic fluid, a somewhat antibacterial liquid. Also, the bacteria may have an inherently low virulence during labor, acquiring invasive properties later in the puerperium when the wounds are covered by granulation tissue.

Bacteria will rapidly invade the body and cause puerperal infection if the natural immunities are broken down by hemorrhage, debilitation, anemia or shock. This will occur especially if a new virulent bacterium is introduced. If the physician in his manipulations transfers vaginal bacteria into the uterus or subjects the tissues to trauma or leaves necrotic tissue, serous or blood collections to serve as culture media, infection may arise.

Asepsis, therefore, consists mainly in the preservation of the patient's immunities by sustaining her strength, optimizing her general condition, procuring a normal course of labor, avoiding operative intervention, handling tissues with utmost gentleness and conducting necessary procedures with the least possible damage. The transfer of infective material from the vulva and vagina to tissues higher up in the birth passage should be stringently prevented.

Admission Toilet

The routine administration of a shower to all labor patients at the time of admission to the hospital has been largely abandoned in most areas. However, it may still be appropriate for selected patients to be washed thoroughly if necessary. Enemas are given in most obstetric units to empty the lower bowel thoroughly, but it is best to avoid this procedure if the fetal head is unengaged (risk of prolapsing the cord if the membranes should rupture while feces are being expelled) or if delivery is immi-

nent (hazard of precipitating delivery) and the head is deep in the pelvis (inability to administer the enema).

The practice of shaving the perineum is slowly vanishing. Its lack of benefit in preventing infection has been proved. The pubic region may be shaved or the hair is cut off closely with scissors. The pudendal area is scrubbed with soap and hot water using a washcloth and paying especial attention to the folds around the clitoris. Accumulated smegma is removed with olive oil, albolene or liquid soap.

Since bacteria with virulent possibilities are naturally present in the vagina of all parturients, it would seem logical to attempt to disinfect the vagina as is done before gynecologic operations, but experience shows that such attempts before labor are completely unsuccessful. Scrubbing the vagina robs the softened mucous membrane of its protective epithelium and any strong chemical antiseptic destroys the delicate cells as well as the bacteria. All that the treatment does is to remove some of the bacteria and the secretions, but a few hours later the bacteria are as numerous as they were before. The tissues, however, may have sustained some injury, and their natural immunities have been reduced.

EXAMINING THE PATIENT

On entering the labor room, the physician should notice the patient's general appearance and the frequency and strength of her contractions. He should inquire if she is suffering from pain other than that of labor. In addition to the special obstetric examination to be described, it is essential to ensure that there is no previously unrecognized or newly developed condition that warrants attention or will affect the management of the labor. The physician or a nurse should take the patient's pulse and temperature. The urine is examined for albumin, sugar and leukocytes. The hematocrit or hemoglobin is checked.

Is the woman in labor? The regular character of the contractions, the bloody show, the proved rupture of the membranes and the observation of the cervical changes on rectal or vaginal examination will help to determine this point. Only further progression with time will provide verification as the labor evolves.

Abdominal Examination

A definite plan which leads to accurate results and prevents omissions should be followed. After the size and shape of the uterine mass have been determined, the following five questions should be answered: (1) Is the uterine ovoid longitudinal or transverse? (2) What is over the inlet? (3) What is in the fundus? (4) Where is the fetal back? (5) Where is the cephalic prominence? These constitute Leopold's maneuvers.

1. *Ovoid—longitudinal or transverse?* The physician faces the patient, places his hands on either side of the abdomen and straightens the uterine mass between them, thus easily determining if the fetal ovoid lies parallel with the long axis of the mother (Fig. 172). If it is not parallel, the presentation is an oblique or a transverse lie.

2. *What is over the inlet?* The physician stands with his back to the patient's face. He gently presses his hands into the inlet of the pelvis from the iliac fossas (Fig. 173). If a hard, ball-shaped mass is felt, it is the head. If his hands almost meet above the inlet it means that (a) the head is very high, (b) the breech lies over the inlet and is likewise up high or (c) there is no part over the inlet but the shoulder is presenting and not engaged. If a soft, irregular mass is encountered by the fingers, it is the breech.

3. *What is in the fundus?* The physician again faces the patient and places his hands on the fundus (Fig. 174). Attempting to grasp the object in the fundus between his hands, he determines its hardness and shape. He differentiates between the hard, round head and the softer, irregular

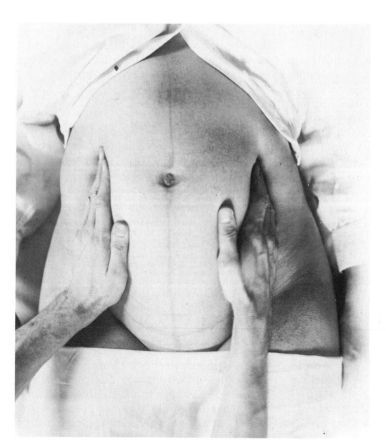

Figure 172 Is the ovoid longitudinal or transverse? Facing the patient's head, the physician applies his hands to the sides of the uterus to determine the fetal lie.

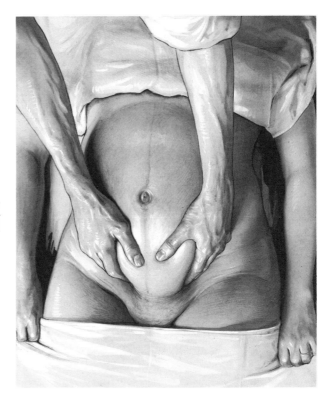

Figure 173 What is over the inlet? By pressing deeply into the pelvis on either side, one learns whether the hard fetal head or soft breech is presenting.

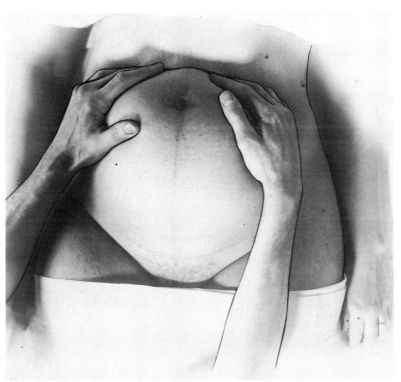

Figure 174 What is in the fundus? Palpation of the uterine fundus will disclose the presence of the breech or the head.

breech. It is usually easy to feel the small extremities of the fetus.

4. *Where is the fetal back?* The location of the back is determined by placing the hands on the abdomen, as for the first maneuver, and pressing alternately inward toward the umbilicus. The back offers more resistance and the hand cannot be pressed in as much.

5. *Where is the cephalic prominence?* Having thus mapped out the fetus, one should then determine its position and attitude. The head is studied first. Facing the patient's feet again, the physician presses both hands downward toward the linea innominata. Normally, with a flexed head, the occiput lies deeper in the pelvis; it is flatter than the forehead, nearer the midline and more difficult to outline. The forehead is reached sooner by the hand, is angular, farther from the midline and easier to outline (Fig. 175). Distinguishing these two points will clarify the position of the head. In flexion, the forehead forms the cephalic prominence. When the head is deflexed, the occiput is more prominent.

In partial deflexion (military position), the two portions of the head stand out equally. Another method, a single grasp to palpate the head, is illustrated in Figure 176.

The position of the fetal head is ascertained by the relation of the occiput and the forehead to the inlet. If the forehead is felt to the right side toward the posterior, and the hand, to reach the occiput, sinks deeply behind the left ramus of the pubis, the position is L.O.A. If the forehead or chin is over the left pubic ramus and the occiput is deep on the right side, the position is R.O.P.

A further method of determining position is by locating the shoulder. One hand is passed upward from the rounded head until a soft prominence, the shoulder, is contacted. If this is in the midline or to the right of it, when the back is on the left side, the position is L.O.A.; if the shoulder is to the left of the midline, the position is L.O.T. or L.O.P.

Passing the hand upward, one encounters a triangular space (Fig. 177) made by the side of the fetal trunk, the thigh

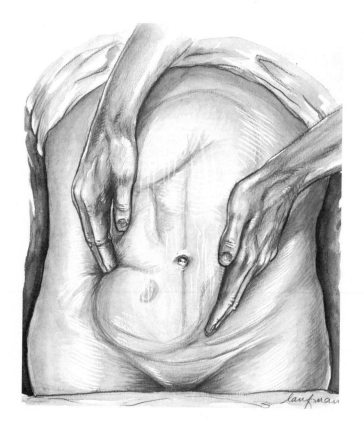

Figure 175 Method of determining the greater cephalic prominence, here shown on the mother's right side. As both hands are passed along the abdomen toward the pelvis, one is impeded by the fetal forehead and the other one descends until the occiput is reached. The forehead is the greater cephalic prominence in well-flexed vertex presentations, but in face and brow presentations the occiput is the greater cephalic prominence because the head is deflexed.

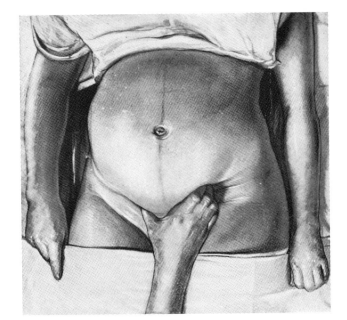

Figure 176 The fetal head is grasped with one hand. In R.O.P. positions, the thumb sinks deep to the occiput, whereas the fingers strike the forehead (greater cephalic prominence) over the left pubic ramus. Often the chin can be distinctly felt.

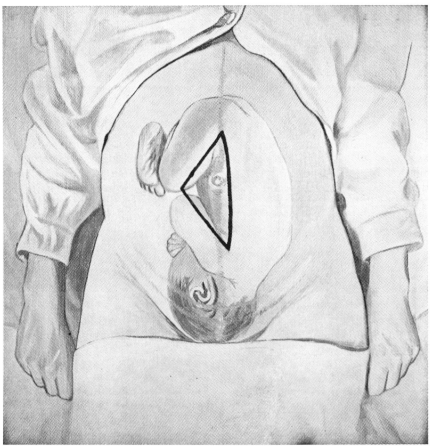

Figure 177 Fetal triangle. The arm is felt by pushing downward and the thigh by pushing upward. Four fingers on the right hand are placed in the broad base of the triangle and the side of the fetus is felt with the palm.

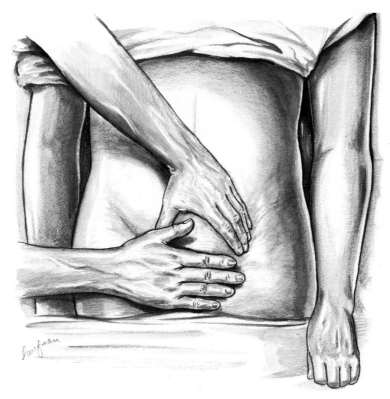

Figure 178 A method of determining overriding of the head. The head is grasped with one hand and pushed down toward the pelvic cavity, while with the other hand over the symphysis pubis it is determined whether the head sinks into the pelvic cavity or overrides the symphysis.

above and the arm below. The breech and trunk closely follow the movements of the head so that, for example, if the breech is in a position which it would occupy in L.O.P., the head will lie in this position and, by definitely outlining the breech, one may deduce the position of the head. The fundus is marked as a circle and divided into four quadrants. If the breech is found in the left anterior quadrant, the position is probably L.O.A.; if the breech is in the right posterior quadrant, the head is R.O.P. The back will offer similar information.

Determining Engagement. What is the station or degree of engagement? This important question must be answered frequently in every labor. First, place the two hands on the fetal head, as in Figure 173, and try to move the head from side to side. If movable, the part is not engaged. Second, how much of the head can be felt above the inlet, using the pubis as a landmark (Figs. 175 and 178)? If only the fore-

head is palpable, and that on deep pressure, the head is well engaged. Other information is obtained on internal examination (see below).

Tumors in the uterus or the abdomen and excessive or unusual tenderness should be noticed. Hydramnios and uterine and fetal anomalies, such as bicornuate uterus, anencephalus or hydrocephalus, may be detected.

Pelvic Examination

For a complete obstetric diagnosis, the internal pelvic measurements must be taken, the diagnosis of position and presentation confirmed along with the degree of effacement and dilatation of cervix; whether the membranes are ruptured, the station of the head, synclitism, flexion and other conditions must also be determined.

The relative advantages of vaginal versus rectal examinations are debatable.

There is no difference in mortality or morbidity when all the examinations are rectal as compared to when all examinations are vaginal. In any case of doubt about a rectal examination, there should be no hesitancy in making a vaginal examination. There is no set rule as to how many rectal or vaginal examinations should be made during labor. This depends on the progress of labor and the presence of any complications but, in general, the fewer the better. Peterson and Richey made bacteriologic studies during vaginal examinations and found no evidence to support the contention that rectal examinations are safer than vaginal ones. Vaginal examinations certainly are more comfortable for the patient. Nonetheless, many physicians limit their observations entirely to rectal examinations because of the firmly held belief that this approach will avert infection. In actual fact, digital examination of the cervix by way of the rectum introduces bacteria because the posterior vaginal wall is pressed into the cervical canal.

Rectal Examination. During the pregnancy and especially in labor the sphincter ani and the levator ani muscles soften and become more dilatable, permitting insertion of a finger without causing pain. The rectovaginal wall is so soft that it is easily compressed, and the amount of dilatation of the cervix and outlines of the presenting part are discernible. Furthermore, after the head has engaged, rectal examination gives accurate data because the parts of the cervix palpated may be steadied against the hard skull. After the cervix is thinned out and dilated, one can readily distinguish the cranial sutures or other landmarks on the presenting part, enabling one to diagnose its position.

The ischial spines are felt without difficulty and thus the station is more easily determined by rectal than by vaginal examination. Rectal examination may be repeated as frequently as necessary so that dilatation of the cervix and the descent of the presenting part may be accurately followed.

Any doubt about rupture of the membranes can be settled by pushing the presenting part up slightly and observing the escape of amniotic fluid. Vigorous displacement of the presenting part in the presence of ruptured membranes is not recommended because it may result in prolapse of the cord.

Breech, face and shoulder presentations, prolapse of the cord or extremities and tumors blocking the pelvis may be detected by rectal examination. An advantage over vaginal examination is that the cervix cannot be torn with the finger by inadvertent or ill-advised attempts to dilate it.

For a rectal examination a clean rubber or disposable plastic glove should be drawn on and the index finger coated with a suitable lubricant jelly. The patient is asked to bear down a little while the finger is introduced in order to relax the sphincter ani and the levator ani (Figs. 179 and 180). To avoid bruising the tender rectal mucosa, gentleness is imperative. The presenting part may be pressed down toward the finger in the rectum by the hand on the abdomen. The examination should be conducted in the same manner as the vaginal examination and the points elicited in the same sequence.

Vaginal Examination. The patient should be positioned so that her buttocks hang over the edge of the bed or table. The physician should wear a cap and mask and clean hospital clothing, not street clothes. Preparations vary widely, some using very little by way of precautionary measures other than sterile gloves and some antiseptic solution poured over or applied to the vulva. At the other extreme is the widely practiced full scrub preparation: The nurse disinfects the vulva while the physician scrubs. The parts are washed with soap, water and an antiseptic solution. The physician now draws on sterile gloves and washes off the starch or talcum powder on them by rinsing in the antiseptic solution. Then two fingers of one hand are placed on the vulva, separating the labia widely with the index finger and thumb. He then inserts two fingers of the other hand into the vagina (Fig. 181), passing them at once deeply and gently into the canal, after which the labia are allowed to close around the fingers (Fig. 182). In either technique care must be

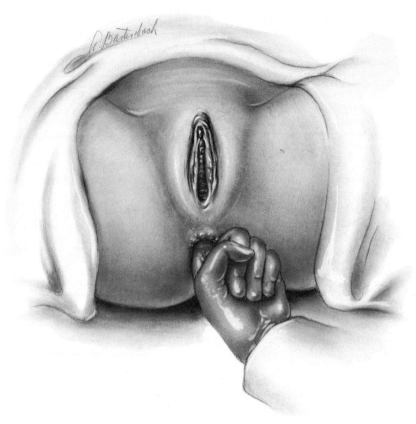

Figure 179　Ideal way of making a rectal examination. The introitus or the vulva must not be touched with the thumb.

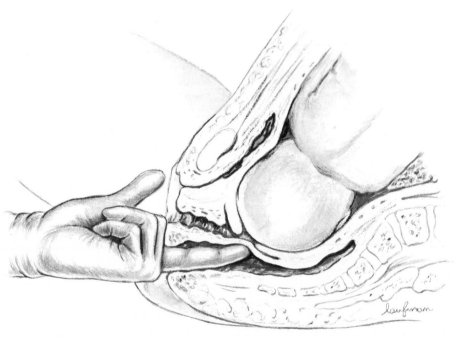

Figure 180　Lateral view of rectal examination showing the technique for palpating the cervical dilatation and station through the rectovaginal wall. The thumb here is precariously close to the introitus.

taken to avoid the anal area; the fingers should contact only the mucous membrane of the vaginal introitus. Although there are good theoretical reasons for taking all stringent precautions in doing vaginal examinations, it is difficult to find substantive data to defend the practice. Care is important at any rate. We continue to recommend the stated precautions for vaginal examinations, but there is no clear justification for so much preparation.

Six points should be determined during vaginal (or rectal) exploration done in labor: (1) condition of the cervix; (2) status of the membranes; (3) diagnosis of presentation and position; (4) station of the pre-

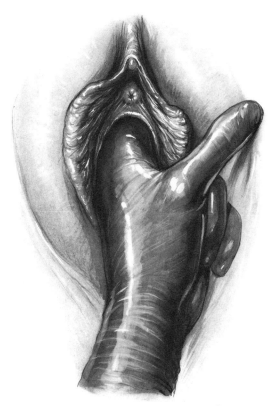

Figure 182 Vaginal examination with fingers inserted, wrist straight and elbow sunk, to allow fingertips to point toward umbilicus.

senting part; (5) evaluation of spatial relations; and (6) presence of any abnormalities.

DEGREE OF EFFACEMENT AND DILATATION OF THE CERVIX. The fingers are passed to the cervix, noting its consistency, whether the external os is open and whether the cervical canal is obliterated. The varying degrees of effacement and dilatation have been described and illustrated in Chapter 7. Physicians speak of the cervix as being *effaced* or *obliterated* totally or a percentage, according to what one estimated the uneffaced cervix to have been (e.g., 50 per cent effaced). It is preferable instead to record the actual thickness of the canal (e.g., 1.5 cm.) so that one can use this objective measure to follow progressive effacement as labor advances. The os is measured in centimeters of dilatation, although many still use the less meaningful and more variable fingerbreadth measurements.

HAVE THE MEMBRANES RUPTURED? If the membranes are of watch-crystal form,

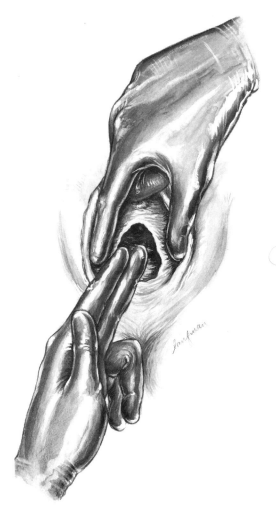

Figure 181 Method of making vaginal examination using sterile gloves. The labia are spread widely so that the examining fingers may be inserted without touching surrounding vulvar structures. Care must be exercised to avoid touching the anus.

the tense membranes a short distance below the head are felt during a contraction. In the interval between contractions the membranes are relaxed. If the membranes are pressed tightly against the head like a cap and are intact, it may be possible, by pushing the head up only a little, to notice amniotic fluid flowing between the membranes and the head; no fluid will escape alongside the fingers. If, however, the membranes have ruptured, pushing the head up will release a flow of fluid which can be felt by the fingers in the vagina and also can be seen at the vulva. An experienced physician can distinguish the smooth chorion from the rough, hairy scalp. The discharge of amniotic fluid, vernix caseosa or flakes of meconium will confirm the diagnosis of ruptured membranes.

Determining whether the admixture of amniotic fluid renders the vaginal secretion neutral or slightly alkaline may be helpful (Berlind). Nitrazine paper is a very effective means for determining pH quickly (Baptisti). A sterile cotton-tipped applicator is inserted deeply into the vagina, withdrawn and the cotton tip touched to a strip of nitrazine paper. Then the color of the paper is compared with a standard nitrazine color chart. A neutral or alkaline pH, with blue discoloration of the nitrazine paper, indicates that the membranes have probably ruptured. False positive readings may be obtained when there is an unusual amount of bloody show or the vaginal secretions are contaminated with alkaline urine. However, the test is accurate in the early stages of labor.

Vaginal smears may be stained and examined for vernix, fetal squamous cells and lanugo. Other examinations are also helpful, including study of the vaginal discharge for ferning which is normally absent in late pregnancy but which returns soon after rupture of the membranes. The test is of limited value, however, because the ferning is disturbed by blood and inflammatory discharge (Smith and Callagan). In doubtful cases, the vagina may be opened with a broad speculum or with the fingers, and the presence of the membranes over the head determined visually. Errors here involve rupture of the membranes higher up alongside the head; these cannot be seen. All methods considered collectively, the reliability of diagnosis of ruptured membranes is poor.

DIAGNOSIS OF PRESENTATION AND POSITION. It is usually impossible to outline the sutures and fontanels through the lower uterine segment. If there is some dilatation of the cervix, the intact membranes do not hinder palpation of the sutures and fontanels. After it is determined that the hard, presenting part is the vertex, the sagittal suture is sought and followed until the fontanels are felt and definitely identified. The position of the head can almost always be determined with ease, but in doubtful cases, especially when a caput succedaneum interferes with clear recognition of the landmarks, it is well to search for an ear. The position of the ear will disclose the position of the head. However, there must be considerable cervical dilatation to permit palpation of an ear. The tragus points to the face.

STATION AND DESCENT. By external and pelvic examinations the degree of engagement or station of the head can be determined with fair accuracy. The head is *floating* when it is freely movable above the inlet. It is *dipping* when it has entered the inlet but is still somewhat mobile. It is *fixed in the inlet* when moderate pressure from below will not dislodge it, but its parietal bosses have not yet passed the inlet.

The head is *engaged* when its greatest horizontal plane has passed the pelvic inlet. In vertex presentation this is the biparietal plane. *Engagement* is usually shown clinically by the lowest part of the skull having reached or passed the interspinous line. The head is in the midplane when the lowest part of the cranium lies below the plane of the ischial spines; it is at the pelvic outlet when the two parietal bosses have passed the ischial spines and the lowermost part of the head comes well down on the perineum, lying in the distended vagina and vulva. To express the station of the head exactly, DeLee devised the following plan: A coronal plane is imagined passing through the ischial spines. This is the reference plane. Parallel planes at 1 cm. intervals above and below the reference plane are numbered as shown in Figures 183 and 184. The interspinous plane is zero-station. The centi-

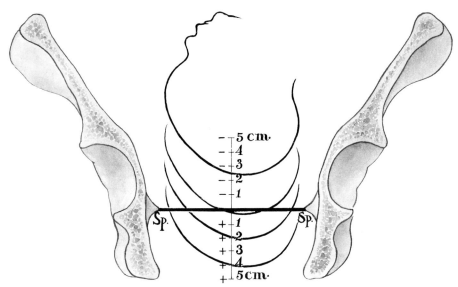

Figure 183 Diagrammatic presentation of the station or degree of engagement of the fetal head. The location of the forward leading edge or lowest part of the head is designated by centimeters above or below the plane of the interspinous line.

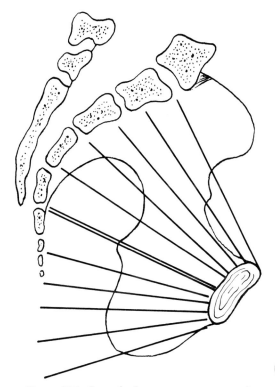

Figure 184 Lateral planar representation of station designations comparable to those in Figure 183 along the pelvic axis. Each line shows the location of the leading edge of the fetal head above or below the interspinous plane (double line). Station lines are spaced 1 cm. apart at their midpoints.

meters above are designated minus; those below are plus. If the lowest part of the head has reached the spines (that is, just engaged) the head is at station zero. If it is higher, it is not engaged; it is at station −2 if its forward leading edge has descended to a plane just 2 cm. above the spines. If it has passed the spines, it is engaged; it is at station +1 if located 1 cm. below the interspinous plane.

By first touching the top of the head then passing the fingers to the ischial spines on the sidewalls of the pelvis, one may easily determine the relation of one to the other.

Too great emphasis cannot be laid on the importance of accurately defining the station of the head in the birth canal repeatedly during the course of labor. Following the descent pattern can be most useful in uncovering serious labor disorders (see Chapter 55). Before one performs a forceps operation, this information is absolutely essential.

INTERNAL PELVIMETRY AND SPATIAL RELATIONS. Passing the fingers slowly over the bony walls, one can determine the general size of the cavity and the size and sharpness of the ischial spines and palpate the sacrum and coccyx. Then the relations of the head to the pelvis, as described in Chapter 12, are elicited. The diagonal conjugate is measured with the fingers if the head is not too low.

ABNORMALITIES. The presence of the umbilical cord or fetal parts in the vagina, tumors, excessive rigidity of the perineum and other conditions are determined. Conditions that may adversely affect the course of labor or alter one's management may be detected at this time.

The physician now completes the patient's hospital record, entering all relevant features of the examination as outlined above. After all the foregoing information has been obtained, the various points are weighed and considered. The size of the fetal head is balanced against the size of the pelvis and both are evaluated in light of the contractility pattern.

The anxious patient will undoubtedly ask, "Is everything all right?" It is a good general policy to answer this in the affirmative, with a word of encouragement. If some abnormality is found or anticipated, the husband must be informed for the physician's own protection. The patient should be spared any alarm until it becomes necessary to intervene. At that time it is essential that the problem be explained to her gently, kindly and tactfully. A second query, "How long will it last?" should be answered with care. The clock will very often contradict the statement if a certain hour for the delivery of the child is set, and the parturient will lose faith and courage. One should usually reply that the length of the labor will depend on the strength and frequency of the contractions, but that everything is in good order. The patient may have to be reminded that, for her own safety and her baby's, the process should not be hastened.

ATTENDANCE OF THE PHYSICIAN

Ideally, every woman in labor should be continuously attended by a physician from beginning to end. If the physician must leave the patient, he should do so only after assuring himself that the presentation and position of the fetus are normal, that the pelvis is adequate, that the cervix is dilating normally, that the mother is not threatened with a potentially serious medical or obstetric disorder and that the fetus is in perfect condition. The nurse or assistant must observe contractions and listen to the fetal heart tones at least every half hour, and report at once any unusual happening. Only accurate observation of many labors will give the physician that knowledge that will enable him to determine if it is safe for him to leave the parturient, when and for how long; even with such knowledge he will occasionally return to find the child delivered, the contractions having suddenly become very strong. In a nullipara it is best to remain with the patient after the cervix is dilated 7 cm. One must not leave a multipara after the cervix is dilated 4 cm., if the contractions are strong and progress is rapid or if her previous labors were rapid.

REFERENCES

Baptisti, A.: A chemical test for the determination of ruptured membranes. Amer. J. Obstet. Gynec. *35*:688, 1938.

Berlind, M. W.: Test for ruptured bag of waters. Amer. J. Obstet. Gynec. *24*:918, 1932.

Colebrook, L.: Prevention of puerperal sepsis. J. Obstet. Gynaec. Brit. Emp. *43*:691, 1936.

DeLee, J. B.: The Principles and Practice of Obstetrics, ed. 7. Philadelphia, W. B. Saunders Company, 1938.

Holmes, O. W.: The contagiousness of puerperal fever. New Eng. Quart. J. Med. Surg. *1*:503, 1842–1843.

Peterson, W. F., and Richey, T. W.: Routine vaginal examinations during labor: Comparative study with bacteriologic analysis. Illinois Med. J. *122*:35, 1962.

Semmelweis, I. P.: Die Aetiologie, der Begriff und die Prophylaxis des Kindbettfiebers. Wien, C. A. Hartleben, 1861.

Smith, R. W., and Callagan, D. A.: Amniotic fluid crystallization test for ruptured membranes. Obstet. Gynec. *20*:655, 1962.

White, E.: On possible transmission of haemolytic streptococci by dust. Lancet *1*:941, 1936.

Chapter 20

Management of Labor

THE FIRST STAGE

Having determined that everything is in order, that the parturient can be delivered vaginally and that there is no immediate or projected danger threatening the mother or fetus, the obstetrician should remind himself that the treatment of the first stage is one of intelligent expectancy. His duty is to observe the efforts of nature, and not to intervene until the patient has indicated or proved herself unequal to the task. Meddlesome midwifery has cost thousands of lives. Attempts to hasten dilatation of the cervix, either manually or by having the woman bear down before dilatation is complete, must not be made. Premature bearing-down efforts tire the mother and may cause the cervix to become edematous. Furthermore, they may be distinctly harmful to supporting structures, causing the broad ligaments to be overstretched and the foundation perhaps laid for future prolapse of the uterus.

Let the parturient walk about the labor room, not getting too far from her bed in the event the membranes should break and the cord prolapse, although the likelihood is very small unless the head is floating above the inlet. She may rest at intervals in a chair or on the bed, lying preferably on her side.

Frequent external and occasional rectal or vaginal examinations may be made to determine the progress of labor, and the fetal heart tones should be listened to at least every half hour. The probable value of electronic fetal heart rate monitoring has been outlined in Chapter 13 and is here recommended where the expertise is available to evaluate patterns. The patient's temperature and pulse should be taken and recorded every four hours. If labor is protracted, the physician should try to ensure that the patient gets some rest and relief from her anxiety and discomfort. Exhaustion and anxiety are more common than most physicians think. They do not appreciate with what misgivings and dread most young mothers approach labor (see Chapter 11). Add to these the reported sufferings of the first stage, the sleepless vigil, the dehydration and insufficient nourishment, the termination of the process by racking pain, the loss of blood in the third stage and the possibility of an obstetric operation—and anyone will understand why some women suffer after delivery and are slow to regain their strength.

Diet

During labor, women should not eat or drink because gastric motility is retarded and emptying time significantly prolonged once labor begins. If food and liquids are taken during labor and an inhalation anesthetic becomes necessary for delivery, resultant vomiting may lead to aspiration pneumonitis. In fact, if the patient has eaten up to eight hours prior to the beginning of labor, the stomach should be regarded as probably not emptied. Fluid, electrolytes and nourishment must be given intravenously in prolonged labor.

The Bowels

After the admission enema, the lower bowel may require additional evacuation after 12 to 24 hr., but no enema should be

255

given if delivery is imminent because of the danger of liquid feces accompanying the birth of the infant. If feces accumulate in the rectum, obstructing delivery, an enema may be needed. During labor, both the physician and the nurse should take precautions against contaminating the vulva with fecal discharges.

The Bladder

The bladder should be emptied regularly, preferably by encouraging spontaneous voiding, but if necessary aided by catheterization. A full bladder may be an obstacle to delivery and inhibit uterine action (Fig. 185).

Rupture of the Membranes

If the membranes rupture, the patient is put to bed, lying on her back or side. A rectal or vaginal examination is made to determine the size of the cervical opening and to verify that prolapse of the cord has not occurred, especially if the head was high before the membranes ruptured. Auscultation of the fetal heart is impor-

tant. One can also ascertain if the labor is sufficiently advanced so that the head is ready to be delivered, in which event everything is prepared for delivery.

THE SECOND STAGE

Bearing-down efforts do not always indicate that the second stage has begun, nor does rupture of the membranes. The latter may occur before the contractions start and sometimes not until after the head is visible. From the actions of the parturient, an experienced attendant may usually deduce that the cervix is fully dilated. A few particularly sharp pains attended by a show of bright blood usually indicate that the head is slipping through the cervix.

The patient often feels as if her bowels are about to move, but she must not be permitted to use the toilet. Usually this sensation is due to pressure of the head against the rectum. The patient should be given a bedpan if she must defecate. Five main points are considered during the second stage: (1) asepsis, (2) analgesia and anesthesia (discussed in Chapters 21 and 22), (3) preservation of well-being of the fetus,

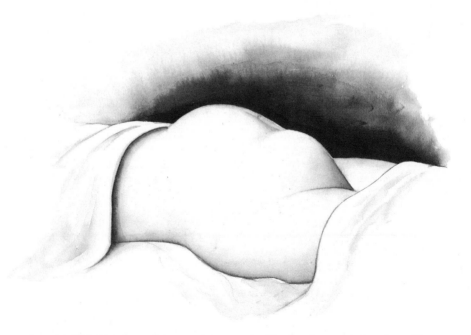

Figure 185 A full bladder during labor can be recognized by the characteristic soft swelling suprapubically.

(4) preservation of the perineum and (5) various complications which are discussed elsewhere.

Asepsis

If the area of the vulva is kept clean with antiseptic solutions, if the gloves are kept sterile and if the few objects that must necessarily be introduced into the vagina are aseptic, one can conduct even difficult and prolonged obstetric manipulations with minimum morbidity.

Preservation of Fetal Well-being

Even normal labor carries dangers for the fetus and, when complications occur, they may compromise its life. Asphyxia from interference with placental exchange or cord compression is a serious consideration. Trauma from excessive molding, as well as cerebral edema and hemorrhage from prolonged compression of the head, are also dangers.

The means currently available for discovering peril to the fetus have been outlined in Chapter 13, including fetal heart rate monitoring and scalp blood sampling. Auscultation of the fetal heart sounds is a substitute with limited value, but serves as the only source of information where the newer and more sophisticated monitoring techniques and requisite consultative expertise are not available. The head stethoscope is indispensable and with it one should listen to the fetal heart tones every two or three minutes, or, in the second stage, at least after every contraction or more often, especially if the heart tones are not of proper frequency and regularity.

In general, labor is to be conducted so as to prevent the natural powers from injuring the fetus, and one must not goad the normal natural powers with oxytocics. Too strong contractions may have to be moderated by narcotics if needed. Prolonged compression of the fetal head should be avoided, but this is not meant to imply that one should substitute a potentially more traumatic operative delivery in order to accomplish this objective.

Preservation of the Perineum

Examination of the pelvic floor after delivery often shows evidence of injury. The connective tissue may be torn in many places, the layers of fascia loosened, the levator ani muscles lacerated more or less, the urogenital septum ruptured, the perineal body torn and all the tissues bruised, showing hemorrhages and suggillations. The long-term results of these macroscopic and microscopic injuries may be relaxation and prolapse of the urethra, vagina, bladder and uterus.

Efforts should be exerted to preserve the levator ani muscles and the vesicovaginal septum; also, some attention should be given to the perineum itself. A perineal tear may extend through the anus into the rectum causing fecal incontinence; fresh tears may form the atria of bacterial invasion. The hymen tears; 70 per cent of nulliparas have tears of the fourchette. Most of these are *first degree lacerations,* which by definition are mucosal tears only. Perhaps 25 per cent of nulliparas and 10 per cent of multiparas have lacerations extending well into the perineal body and, in many, injury may expose the sphincter ani; these are *second degree lacerations.* In difficult operative cases a *complete* or *third degree laceration,* a laceration through the sphincter ani or one extending through the rectal mucosa (in some areas termed *fourth degree* laceration), may occur.

Factors Responsible for Perineal Trauma

Laceration of the perineum cannot always be prevented. The pelvic outlet may be weakened by edema, varicosities, lack of elasticity from scars or from previous operation, age or constitution. In some women the perineum tears like wet blotting paper. A narrow subpubic arch favors laceration by forcing the head back onto the perineum and not allowing the occiput to crowd up close to the arcuate ligament. The necessity for fairly rapid delivery, as in breech presentations and when the fetus is threatened with asphyxia, often forces one to disregard the perineum. In such deliveries the perineum is unprepared for the rapid dilatation and it is difficult or even unwise to take the usual due caution in effecting slow stretching. Exit of the head in unfavorable attitudes, such as face, brow and posterior rotation of the occiput, frequently causes lacerations because the most favorable fetal diameters are not presented to the canal. A large fetus also overstretches the outlet. In all of these instances a timely, adequate and well-placed episiotomy will minimize the damage.

Prevention of Perineal Injury. The levator ani muscles and the investing fascia above and below them can be spared serious injury only by slow dilatation. If the contractions and the bearing-down efforts are tumultuous, an anesthetic may be given to inhibit them. The most common injury is a separation or tearing of the two levator ani pillars at or near the raphé attached to the coccyx. Finally, the whole pelvic floor, muscles and fascias may be more or less disintegrated by overstretching. This occurs when the head is forced rapidly through the passage.

The two operating principles to be kept in mind for protecting the perineum are: (1) slow delivery, developing to the ultimate the elasticity of the pelvic floor, and (2) delivery of the head in forced flexion, thereby presenting to the parturient passage its smallest circumferences. The head should be well flexed until its larger part has escaped from the vulva. If the head were to come out in partial extension, the occipitobregmatic, occipitofrontal and occipitomental diameters and corresponding circumferences would be presented to the girdle of resistance. If the chin is forced down on the sternum and flexion maintained until the nape of the neck fits closely into the pubic arch, the diameters and circumferences which have to pass the ring of the outlet are the suboccipitobregmatic, suboccipitofrontal and suboccipitomental, which are 1.5 to 3 cm. smaller on average.

Delivery of the Infant

The physician, masked, scrubbed, gowned and gloved, stands at the side of the patient, who is lying on her back with her knees raised and abducted. Every two or three minutes he lifts the sterile towel from the patient's abdomen and listens to the fetal heart tones with the head stethoscope. Unless the patient is bearing down too much and the head is advancing too rapidly, he does not intervene until about 4 cm. of the scalp is visible. The rapidity of the descent of the head may be determined by pressing the fingers upward and inward along the ramus of the pubis (Fig. 186). The hard resistance of the presenting part can be felt if the part is low in the pelvis. The location of the anus also indicates the degree of dilatation and downward displacement of the levator ani. If the physician considers that the head is coming through too fast, he asks the woman to cease bearing down, to breathe through her mouth in short, rapid respirations until the force of the effort is expended. *The head should never be held back forcibly under any circumstances no matter what the reason.* An unruly patient may need anesthesia.

With each contraction the head is allowed to come down to distend the perineum a little more. A warning against overzealousness must be given. It is possible for a fetus to be damaged irrevocably because the attendant is overanxious to deliver the woman "without stitches." The fetus may be injured by pressing on the head too forcibly. If the uterine and abdominal efforts are violent and the fetus is not allowed to be delivered, the uterus may rupture as it does under other circumstances of obstruction.

In gentle fashion the head is permitted to descend until its greatest periphery distends the vulva. If at all possible, the head is now delivered in the interval between contractions. It is gently restrained at the height of the bearing-down effort and the woman is asked to breathe through her mouth, while the physician tucks the clitoris and labia minora behind the occiput under the pubis. An anesthetic alleviates the pain of this stage and lessens too violent bearing-down efforts. After the contraction has ceased, the woman is asked to bear down and during this effort the distended perineum is slipped back over the baby's forehead, face and chin.

During this maneuver, the head is main-

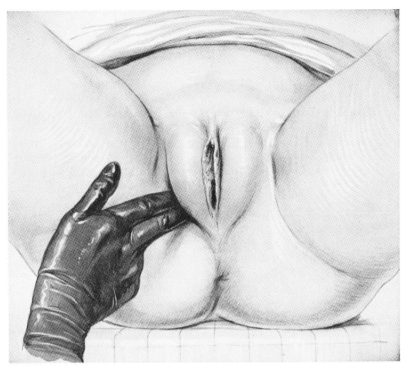

Figure 186 Determining rate of descent of the head at the outlet by palpating the fetal skull through the perineal tissues.

tained in a state of flexion, not by pressure on the forehead through the perineum, but rather by manipulation of the part that is accessible to the fingers. During two or three contractions, a gentle attempt is made to lead the suboccipital part under the pubis by pressing the head back onto the perineum with the finger on the occipital protuberance. When the head has descended far enough to be held, the fingers are applied right at the edge of the frenulum and are used to press the head up under the arch of the pubis. As the head finally rolls up onto the pubis, the flexion is maintained by very gently pressing the part of the head that has been delivered against the pubis.

If the head does not deliver easily by this approach, a *modified Ritgen maneuver* may be used; this is the only manipulation advised at this stage, except cleansing the parts. The extended fingers of one hand are placed on the vertex to control forward motion and the fingers of the other hand, covered with a sterile towel, grasp the fetal chin through tissues posterior to the rectum to prevent recession between contractions. This maneuver provides a delicate kind of control to allow the physician to effect delivery of the fetal head optimally.

When the head is on the perineum, some physicians resort to the Kristeller expression, meaning that the hands of the obstetrician or an assistant are spread over the fundus and pressure is exerted in the axis of the inlet. Kristeller expression can be effective, but does carry recognized risks: bruising of the abdominal and uterine muscles, abruptio placentae, rupture of the uterus and injury to the abdominal viscera. Carried out with gentleness, such complications can be minimized. Distribution of the pressure points can be accomplished by using a broader surface, such as the forearm rather than the hands or fists; this modification is of theoretical advantage in averting traumatic damage.

As soon as the face is delivered, the mucus and amniotic fluid are squeezed out of the nostrils and wiped out of the mouth with a finger or aspirated with a rubber bulb to prevent aspiration of the foreign matter and the development of atelectasis or bronchopneumonia, while permitting the establishment of an airway.

The physician now feels for the presence of the cord around the neck. He notes its location and determines if it is tight and as such might constitute an obstacle to delivery. If the cord is around the neck and cannot be slipped over the head or the shoulder, it should be doubly clamped and cut. A cord that is too short, or relatively so, may tear or pull on the placenta, unless cut, and cause disorders of the third stage.

Delivery of the Shoulders. The temptation to hurry delivery of the shoulders should be resisted. If the child's face is not cyanotic and the circulation is adequate to return flow to an area on the scalp that has been momentarily blanched by finger pressure, one may wait for the renewed action of the uterus. After a minute or two, with another contraction, the patient gently bears down until the anterior shoulder becomes visible just behind the pubis. Now the physician lifts the head up gently and brings the posterior shoulder over the perineum in a slow, controlled manner. If the child's hand is accessible, the arm is drawn out gently, being very careful not to injure the long bones. Then the head is depressed as the anterior shoulder emerges from behind the pubis. It is sometimes easier to effect delivery of the anterior shoulder first, aiding in the process by which the anterior shoulder stems under the symphysis by first pulling the head down (Fig. 187) followed by delivery of the posterior shoulder as described by pulling up (Fig. 188). Now the rest of the body follows in one long contraction. The child must not be dragged out. It is best if the natural powers force it out, the physician only aiding the process. Unless proper care is exercised, the perineum may be torn by the shoulders, a clavicle broken or the nerve plexuses and muscles of the neck overstretched and damaged.

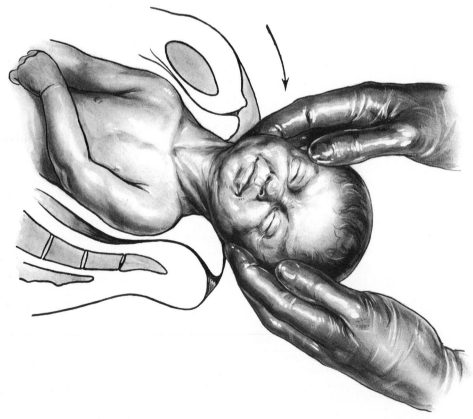

Figure 187 Depressing head gently toward the sacrum for delivery of the anterior shoulder. Care should be taken not to overstretch the neck and thereby cause Erb's paralysis.

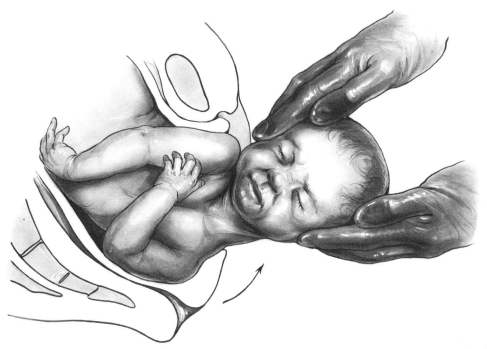

Figure 188 Lifting the head for delivery of the posterior shoulder after the anterior shoulder has been stemmed under the symphysis pubis. Greatest gentleness should be exercised to avoid injury to the baby.

If the delivery of the shoulders is delayed because the natural forces are inadequate or the shoulders are too broad, the woman is asked to bear down. If this fails, their passage can be aided by pressure just above the pubis or by slipping a finger under the pubis into the anterior axilla and pulling it down gently, care being taken not to injure bladder or urethra. Sometimes the shoulder can be forced into the oblique diameter and delivered by a spiral or corkscrew movement. The neck should never be stretched because Erb's paralysis may result (see Chapter 68).

Episiotomy

When a tear of the perineum appears inevitable, one must decide whether or not to substitute a clean, well-placed surgical incision for it. By use of an *episiotomy* one can direct damage away from the sphincter ani. Many obstetricians perform the operation, preferring a clean cut to a jagged tear. The incision may be made in two acceptable ways: *median* in the midline raphé and *mediolateral* at a 45° angle from the midline toward one or the other ischiorectal fossa. Episiotomy consists of an incision of skin and vaginal mucosa, urogenital septum, constrictor cunni, transversus perinei muscle, intercolumnar fascia and a few of the anterior fibers of the puborectal portion of the levator ani muscle.

The indications for the usual episiotomy are: resistant perineum causing delay in the exit of the head through the vulva; some pathologic condition of the vulva, such as scars; a large fetus or abnormal mechanism causing mechanical disproportion; the delivery of a premature fetus to save its head from pressure; the necessity for rapid extraction when the perineum cannot be accorded time to dilate; and diversion of a laceration away from the anus when it seems certain that the perineum will tear. Episiotomy should be performed before the intercolumnar fascia is destroyed and the levator ani pillars are torn, after which there is little of the pelvic floor to save.

For a mediolateral episiotomy, one blade of a pair of straight scissors is laid on the vaginal mucous membrane and the other rests on the skin of the perineal body, midway between the anus and the tuberosity of the ischium. The cutting angle of the scissors is at the posterior fourchette in the midline above the median raphé (Fig. 189). With a finger in the vagina and a thumb on the perineum, the sphincter may be pressed out of the bite of the scissors. With appropriate anesthesia, either in the form of general inhalation or regional or local block, the tissues are usually cut with one motion. It may require several more "bites" to complete it properly, especially to ensure that the vaginal mucosa (Fig. 190) is adequately severed. Bleeding is checked by pressure with gauze sponges.

The same technique applies for a median episiotomy, except that the scissors are directed straight down the median raphé toward the anus, avoiding if possible the sphincter ani and rectal mucosa that

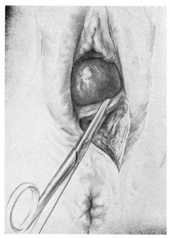

Figure 190 Second step of the mediolateral episiotomy, cutting vagina and subvaginal fascia.

may tent up close to the vaginal mucosa a few centimeters within the vagina.

Usually, the head is delivered quickly after the incision is made and the bleeding subsides. However, it is important to remember that, if it does not, a firm tamponade may be necessary or, more properly, one may have to resort to direct clamping and ligation of any large bleeding arteries and veins. The physician should not permit bleeding from an episiotomy wound because considerable blood can be lost. According to Odell and Seski, the average amount of blood lost from an episiotomy wound is 253 ml. Therefore, constant pressure must be applied or vascular ligation undertaken in the interim before the wound is sutured.

The techniques of repairing both median and mediolateral episiotomies are detailed in Chapter 65. The end results of these episiotomies are about the same. There is a growing school of adherents for the median episiotomy. Accepting its inherent added risk of sphincter and rectal injury, proponents feel it is generally more comfortable for the patient during her puerperium; it is easier to repair well, and it heals better with fewer complications. Even when the sphincter and rectal mucosa are cut, and this is sometimes done quite deliberately to provide adequate room for delivery, repair is not difficult and healing almost invariably good. Most do

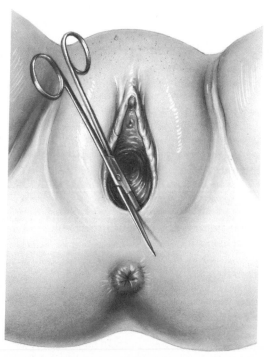

Figure 189 Left mediolateral episiotomy showing scissors prepared to incise skin, vaginal mucosa, fourchette and urogenital septum. This cut exposes the fascia over the left pillar of the levator ani muscle, which may or may not have to be incised according to the size of the fetus, the length of the perineum and the distensibility of the tissues. The incision may be made on the right side, if preferred.

not repair the episiotomy wound until after the placenta has been delivered because occasionally it is necessary to remove the placenta manually and the repaired wound may be damaged in the process and require resuturing.

Care of the Child

Immediately after the baby is delivered, it should be held below the level of the vulva for a few minutes or placed in a warm container the level of which is considerably below the mother's buttocks. The purpose of keeping the baby at this level is to permit the blood in the placenta to get to the baby. If the placenta separates while waiting, the same purpose is accomplished by expressing it from the uterus and holding it elevated for two or three minutes. The widespread practice of placing the newborn infant on its mother's abdomen immediately after birth before the cord is clamped, therefore, cannot be condoned.

If the baby is held below the level of the placenta, it may gain in one minute 80 ml. of blood by autotransfusion from the placenta (Yao and Lind). If the baby is held above the level of the placenta, blood from the baby flows into the placenta between uterine contractions. Therefore, care should be taken to assure that no blood is drained from the baby, since profound hemodynamic changes take place in the baby after birth.

DeMarsh et al. showed that infants whose cords were not clamped until the placenta had separated from the uterus had an average of 0.56 million more erythrocytes per cubic millimeter and 2.6 gm. more hemoglobin per 100 ml. during the first week than those whose cords were clamped immediately. Wilson et al. found that infants whose umbilical cords were clamped immediately after birth had a lower mean corpuscular hemoglobin at 8 and 10 months of age than those whose cords were clamped after the placenta had separated from the uterine attachment. Thus, early clamping of the cord may lead to an iron deficiency during the first year of life.

McCausland et al. advise stripping the cord and placental blood into the infant because it is harmless if done gently and because term babies receive about 100 ml. of extra blood. Such babies have higher erythrocyte counts, higher hemoglobin values, higher initial weights and less initial weight losses. It is theoretically possible that, in premature infants or in those with subsequent neonatal hemolytic disease, the additional erythrocytes will account for an increase in bilirubin from hemoglobin destruction. Moreover, in such small infants it may be possible to overload the circulation by this technique and cause congestive failure.

The cord is doubly clamped about 6 to 12 inches away from the baby's abdomen; the clamps are placed about 1 inch apart and the cord is severed between the clamps with scissors. This is done after about three minutes or after the cord vessels stop pulsating and collapse. If it is obvious that the baby will require resuscitation, one should clamp and cut the cord at once so that the necessary resuscitative procedures can be initiated. As soon as possible after delivery any mucus in the air passages must be removed with a soft rubber bulb, a tracheal catheter or a laryngoscope. Resuscitative principles and measures are discussed in Chapter 67.

Tying the Cord. After pulsation in the exposed cord has ceased, the cord is severed. Later, with a piece of linen tape, a special plastic or metal clip or any sterile strong string, the cord is ligated close to the cutaneous margin of the umbilicus, making sure that there is no umbilical hernia which might allow a loop of intestine to be caught in the grasp of the ligature. Double ligation is an additional precaution, leaving a space of 1 cm. between the ligatures. As little as possible of the cord is left to be cast off except with an erythroblastotic baby when it should be left long for obtaining blood for study and for possible catheterization of the umbilical vessels for exchange transfusion. The knot is made secure by tightening the thread or string slowly and interruptedly, permitting Wharton's jelly to escape from under the thread.

A piece of dry gauze is laid over the cord, and the infant, wrapped in a sterile receiving blanket, is laid in a safe, warm bassinet. Someone should watch it and see that it breathes naturally.

Care of the Baby's Eyes. Legislation in many states requires antiseptic treatment of the eyes of the newborn using either the Credé silver nitrate method (see below) or penicillin. There are, unfortunately, many people who become blind through the lack of proper precautions at birth. Such blindness, due to *ophthalmia neonatorum,* is caused by a purulent inflammation of the conjunctiva and cornea. It is preventable and even among populations of patients with high prevalence of gonorrheal vaginitis, it has been almost entirely eradicated. The bacteria reach the eyes during the passage of the head through the vagina; they may also be washed into them by the attendant or wiped into them by the mother. While the gonococcus is usually the causative agent, pneumococcus, diphtheria bacillus and other organisms may also cause serious conjunctivitis. Rarely, a child may be born with the disease already well advanced.

Any patient known to have gonorrhea during pregnancy should be treated adequately with penicillin or other effective antibiotic. Introduction of routine culture at the first antepartum visit (see Chapter 9) frequently uncovers silent cases requiring such treatment. Repeat culture late in pregnancy may disclose new infection, recurrence or reinfection. During labor, penicillin retreatment may be found necessary. During all vaginal examinations the eyes of the fetus (for example, in face presentation) must not be touched so as to avoid introducing infection inadvertently. When there is purulent vaginal discharge or if there are condylomas on the vulva, the precautions are redoubled; the aim is to prevent any possibility of maternal inflammatory secretions entering the eyes of the fetus. The same principle is carried out after the head is born; the vaginal mucus is removed at once from and around the eyes and great care taken to prevent infection.

When gonorrhea is suspected, the old Credé method is used: a drop of two per cent silver nitrate solution is instilled in each eye and neutralized immediately with saline solution. In addition, penicillin should be instilled in the baby's eyes every three hours during the first 24 hours. When gonococcal ophthalmia is present, a full course of parenteral penicillin or other appropriate antibiotic should be given.

Greenberg and Vandow determined the relative rates of gonococcal ophthalmia after various prophylactic regimens in large series of cases: no prophylaxis, 25.5 per 100,000; silver nitrate, 6.6; saline, 7.4; antibiotic ointments, 11.2; parenteral penicillin, none. They questioned whether the single application of any drug to the eyes of an infant actually exposed to infection could invariably prevent gonococcal ophthalmia, but it is clear that the disease may arise more frequently when prophylaxis is omitted. Complete prevention by local measures is doubtful. Reliance must be placed on early recognition and definitive antibiotic therapy of this potentially serious problem when it arises in the newborn infant. If caught early, blindness will not occur.

REFERENCES

Credé, C. S. F.: Klinische Vorträge über Geburtshülfe. Berlin, August Hirschwald, 1853.

De Marsh, Q. B., Alt, H. L., Windle, W. F., and Hillis, D. S.: The effect of depriving the infant of its placental blood on the blood picture during the first week of life. J.A.M.A. *116*:2568, 1941.

Greenberg, M., and Vandow, J. E.: Ophthalmia neonatorum: Evaluation of different methods of prophylaxis in New York City. Amer. J. Publ. Health *51*:836, 1961.

McCausland, A. M., Holmes, F., and Schumann, W. R.: Management of cord and placental blood and its effect upon the newborn. California Med. *71*:190, 1949.

Odell, L. D., and Seski, A.: Episiotomy blood loss. Amer. J. Obstet. Gynec. *54*:51, 1947.

von Ritgen, F.: Über ein Dammschutzverfahren. Mschr. Geburtsh. Gynäk. 6:321, 1855.

Wilson, E. E., Windle, W. F., and Alt, H. L.: Deprivation of placental blood as cause of iron deficiency in infants. Amer. J. Dis. Child 62:320, 1941.

Yao, A. C., and Lind, J.: Effect of gravity on placental transfusion. Lancet *1*:505, 1969.

Chapter 21

Analgesia for Labor

The current trend in obstetric analgesia for labor is one of moderation. One should individualize according to the patient's needs and consider the inherent risks involved. In addition, it is important to avoid impeding the course of labor. Moreover, the prevailing emotional and physiologic status has to be taken into account. The ideal analgesia program is elusive and perhaps does not yet exist. A means is sought to relieve the discomforts of labor, which are sometimes not inconsiderable, and at the same time to avoid influencing the fetal welfare deleteriously.

Ideally, the patient should be comfortable, alert and cooperative; the course of labor and delivery should be uneventful, and the fetus left entirely free of central nervous system depression. There are sufficient numbers and varieties of sedative, analgesic, hypnotic, amnesic and ataractic drugs so that the pain of labor can be readily diminished. It is clear, however, that all pass across the placental barrier and may depress vital centers of the fetus. The reciprocally incompatible relationship between complete pain relief and safety to mother and fetus has been well expressed by Waters and Harris with the couplet: more safety, less pain relief; more pain relief, less safety.

The objectives of pain relief in labor may be achieved in one of several ways: (1) psychologic preparation, (2) combinations of exogenous analgesic agents and (3) intermittent or continuous anesthetic techniques (Chapter 22).

PSYCHOPROPHYLACTIC PREPARATION

The basis for this approach has been discussed in Chapter 11. The need for analgesia during labor is highly variable and appears to depend largely on the patient's subjective pain threshold. Emotionally stable, stoic gravidas require little analgesic support. High-strung, emotionally keyed patients in general require a great deal. "Natural childbirth" can be made a stimulating emotional and educational experience. Although labor is generally accompanied by discomfort, it is usually a normal physiologic phenomenon ending with the gratification of accomplishment in the birth of a healthy child.

Unfortunately, some of its strongest proponents have occasionally misinterpreted the basic principles to insist that patients must strive for labor devoid of analgesia at all costs. The controversy over the psychoprophylactic methods stems largely from unfounded lay exaggeration which insists that any medication during labor may influence the baby's neurological and developmental outcome.

Consequently, the patient who desires and receives sedation and anesthesia considers herself inadequate in her role as a functioning female. She suffers pangs of conscience because of the potential harm she imagines she may be inflicting on her unborn fetus. The effect of the overemphasis of these techniques in interdicting analgesia and anesthesia is to frighten the patient unnecessarily. Major problems may arise relating to guilt feelings in patients who fail to achieve this objective. Short of this sadistic-masochistic complex, which should be decried, the attitude toward psychologic preparation for childbirth should be a flexible one.

The theoretical consideration that fear exaggerates pain, although not clearly defined on a physiologic basis, appears to be valid from the clinical purview. Whether one can attribute all of the pain of labor to fear, however, is highly debatable. Assuredly, the patient who is emotionally well prepared for labor is relaxed and may require only minimal analgesia and anesthesia. She may present a state of exhilaration and animation that is maintained throughout a portion of early labor, particularly the latent phase. If emotionally supported by the nursing staff and her physician, she will retain confidence well into the active phase, and occasionally the second stage. The great sense of accomplishment these patients feel is a tribute to their ability to retain their self-composure, minimize their fears, reduce their needs for medication and be awake to participate in and observe the culmination of their efforts at delivery.

In practice the patient attends a series of classroom exercises designed to acquaint her with the physiology of pregnancy and labor, thereby to eliminate the fear of the unknown and to train her in exercises designed ostensibly to aid her in relaxing, in muscle control and in breathing so that she may be cooperative and efficient in performing her function as a parturient.

Unsubstantiated claims for these methods include shortened labor, absence of discomfort, diminished number of operative procedures, decreased pelvic or perineal damage, reduced blood loss and improved condition of the baby. Apparently justified claims include diminished use of drugs for analgesia and anesthesia, accomplishment of a sense of achievement and happiness and establishment of a strong mother-child relationship. Objective studies have not indicated any alteration in the course of labor by these techniques (Davis and Morrone). Nevertheless, the psychologic aspects of pregnancy are well recognized and the obste-

trician is well advised to provide emotional as well as physical support to the patient in labor. This involves insight and empathy on his part as well as understanding and patience.

HYPNOSIS

The autosuggestion implicit in the psychoprophylactic techniques is undoubtedly related in some way to the effects obtained with hypnosis. The interest in this field stems from several reports suggesting that the hypnotic trance produces comfortable, painless labors without any apparent detriment to mother or fetus (Winkelstein). Similarly, posthypnotic suggestion appears to reduce fear, tension and anxiety, and, as a consequence, raises the pain threshold (Kroger). Despite these reported successes and its increasing use, psychiatrists believe the technique to be unsuitable as a routine procedure because of occasional severe psychotic and psychoneurotic reactions after its use.

It is rare for the obstetrician to have the necessary psychiatric training to use hypnotherapy with safety. It is recommended that hypnosis be avoided in patients who may represent poor psychiatric risks, including those who are obviously unstable or immature, who have doubtful past histories or family histories, who are carrying an unwanted fetus, whose husband or mother is demanding and domineering or those who are otherwise insecure. In addition, psychiatrists warn against the likelihood of activating underlying, previously unrecognized psychoneuroses, personality disorders or psychoses. The casual therapist should not undertake this procedure without acquiring an adequate background in the knowledge of psychodynamics of the unconscious (Giffin).

Nevertheless, the infant demonstrates a condition comparable in biochemical terms to that of the infant delivered with regional block anesthesia (Moya and James). The technique, therefore, when properly used and in competent hands, can effectively reduce or even alleviate pain in labor without affecting the infant's biochemical status adversely.

There are two major disadvantages to its use: (1) A disproportionate amount of time is necessary to train the patient and ultimately to produce an adequate hypnotic state of sufficient depth to be effective. (2) Only a small number of patients are willing to accept or are suitable for the technique. It has been suggested that the susceptible patients are those who would do well in an aggressive natural childbirth program of preparation. This technique is acknowledged to be useful, but it presents apparent obstacles and limitations that prevent it from gaining widespread popularity.

AMNESIC AGENT

Scopolamine is a naturally occurring alkaloid of belladonna that inhibits effector organs innervated by postganglionic cholinergic nerves. It has been used widely with analgesic medications for preanesthetic and obstetric medication. As a preanesthetic agent it has a potent inhibitory effect on secretions, much like atropine. In addition it depresses the central nervous system, thereby reducing excitement and fear preoperatively. This tranquilizing effect, however, is not seen in association with pain. On the contrary, the manifest idiosyncrasy of many patients to the drug is expressed by marked excitement or even delirium, particularly when sufficient pain relief does not accompany its administration. Scopolamine appears to be relatively harmless for the fetus.

The major therapeutic usefulness of this drug in obstetrics is its ability to produce profound amnesia, although this cannot always be relied upon in clinical usage. In therapeutic doses it produces drowsiness, euphoria, fatigue and dreamless sleep. Not infrequently, however, excitement, hallucinations and restlessness result instead. These may be counteracted or averted by the concomitant administration of narcotics in sufficient doses. The initial therapeutic dose is 0.4 mg.; this may be repeated in doses of 0.2 mg. every two to four hours as needed to produce amnesia. Overdosage may produce toxic effects and even lead to death. Symptoms of overdo-

sage include tachycardia, rapid, weak pulse, dilated pupils with almost completely obliterated iris, blurred vision, disturbed speech, hot, dry skin characterized by its scarlet color, ataxia, restlessness, delirium and finally coma. The drug should be treated with respect. The trend away from its use is encouraging.

ANALGESIC AGENTS

The popular analgesic agents in current common use include the phenanthrene alkaloids of opium, especially morphine, and the synthetic narcotic, meperidine (pethidine, Demerol). In addition to their major use—for the relief of severe pain in labor—they variably produce central nervous system depression of a selective nature. Most notably, they depress the respiratory center.

Morphine. Morphine also produces euphoria. In excessive doses, respirations become very slow and shallow; pupils are constricted; there is constipation, nausea and vomiting, coma and finally respiratory failure.

The drug passes across the placenta readily and effectively depresses the respiratory center of the fetus. If the baby is born during this time, depression will be manifested by apnea requiring artificial ventilation and oxygenation. Premature fetuses are particularly susceptible. It is imperative, therefore, that morphine be avoided within the terminal four hours prior to delivery, if at all possible.

In general, except for its occasional use in abnormal labor states, morphine has been supplanted largely by other agents because of its undesirable properties, including fetal depression, maternal nausea and vomiting, interference with gastrointestinal function, urinary retention, respiratory depression, stupefaction, occasional allergic reaction, tolerance, physical dependence and addiction liability.

Meperidine. Meperidine is today perhaps the most widely used analgesic agent for labor. It is a synthetic piperidine derivative. It is about one-tenth as potent on a dosage basis as morphine for relieving pain. Sedation occurs only after large doses, and the ratio of analgesic to hypnotic potency is greater than that of morphine. Its action is depressant on the central nervous system in usual pharmacologic doses. It augments the action of anesthetic agents necessary to produce surgical anesthesia. Respiratory depression occurs. Overdosage is characterized by incoordination, tremors and convulsive movements, mydriasis, disorientation and hallucinations; these are followed by terminal respiratory depression and coma.

Meperidine reaches the fetus very rapidly after administration to the mother and produces significant depression of the baby at birth if circulating levels are high at the time of delivery. However, its action on the fetus is somewhat less than that produced by morphine. This is especially true in the susceptible premature fetus, although quantitation is difficult. The real problem perhaps is not the direct effect of the depressant drug but rather its potentiating effect on an already existing abnormal state. The delivery process appears to reduce the exchange of oxygen and carbon dioxide between mother and fetus, resulting in relative biochemical asphyxia in the fetus (James). The additive factor of the mildly depressant action of a drug such as meperidine may aggravate the asphyxic state already existing to produce permanent irreversible damage. The obstetrician must be continually mindful of this possibility when administering analgesic agents late in labor. It is important, therefore, to avoid or to minimize their use when delivery is imminent. The action of meperidine lasts about four hours. This should serve as a guide in managing the analgesic needs of the patient in labor.

Alphaprodine (Nisentil). This agent is a close congener of meperidine. Its pharmacologic properties are similar to those of other narcotics. Its analgesic potency is between that of morphine and meperidine. The duration of action is somewhat shorter. Its advantage over meperidine in obstetrics has not been established.

The effect of narcotic-analgesic agents on the course of labor has not been clarified. It is believed that uterine contractions can be reduced significantly with adequate amounts of narcotics, especially morphine. Objective studies have shown inhibition of the course of labor by meperidine (Friedman; Gordon and Pinker), Nisentil (Ekelman and Reynolds) and morphine (Snyder and Geiling). Significant depression of neonatal cord blood oxygen levels has been shown to occur from meperidine given to the mother (Shields and Taylor). This corroborates the objective demonstration of transmission of meperidine across the human placenta (Apgar et al.).

In practice, meperidine is administered in doses of 50 to 100 mg. after labor is well under way, preferably in the active phase. If tranquilizers (see below) are used synergistically, dosages may be cut to 25 to 50 mg. It has been shown that the latent phase is particularly sensitive to narcotics (Friedman). These drugs should be avoided, if possible, until the active phase. The drug is administered intramuscularly and reaches a therapeutic effect in about one-half hour. It may be administered intravenously if a more rapid action is necessary, but it must be given very slowly because a sudden drop in blood pressure may follow rapid intravenous administration. The drug may be repeated at four-hour intervals as needed.

NARCOTIC ANTAGONISTS

The morphine antagonistic properties of *nalorphine* (N-allylnormorphine), a semisynthetic congener of morphine, and *levallorphan* (the levorotatory isomer of 3-hydroxy-N-allylmorphine) have been demonstrated experimentally and inconsistently on clinical grounds. They appear to antagonize the respiratory depressant and analgesic effects of morphine and its congeners, as well as the effects of the synthetic narcotics. In the nonmedicated individual, these drugs act much like morphine, but their actions are less intense. In the nonaddicted individual, however, the most striking property of nalorphine and levallorphan is their marked ability to prevent or to abolish many of the actions of morphine and other narcotics.

The adult dosages are 5 to 10 mg. of nalorphine or 1 to 2 mg. of levallorphan. The same effect may be produced in the newborn infant depressed by narcotics with the intravenous (umbilical vein) administration of 0.1 to 0.2 mg. of either drug. The action, however, is quite inconsistent and unreliable. It is obvious that these drugs cannot be relied on to counteract the effect of indiscriminate administration of massive doses of narcotics to the mother in labor (Gordon and Pinker). They cannot be used as a substitute for tempered conservatism.

The latest addition to this group of agents is the promising drug, *naloxone,* which is similar in chemical structure to nalorphine except for a methyl group in place of the allyl radical. Naloxone appears to be unique in having no depressant or additive narcotic effects of its own while having 10 to 30 times the antagonistic potency of nalorphine (Goodman and Gilman). If this proves to be correct, naloxone may become an invaluable aid in clinical practice.

Recent evolution of the concept suggesting the combined administration of a narcotic and its antagonist simultaneously has not proved satisfactory in clinical practice to date (Eckenhoff et al.). In general, it is felt that they should not be used routinely. Indeed, the simultaneous presence of a nonnarcotic depressant such as ether facilitates the appearance of synergistic additive depressant effects. Similarly, the problem may be compounded by aggravation of the depression when it is due to factors such as prematurity or cerebral trauma (Greene). It appears that these agents should be used rather sparingly and with studied judgment because (1) a substantial number of narcotized mothers give birth to depressed babies, (2) the incidence and management of neonatal asphyxia is not improved significantly by routine use, and (3) with general anesthesia there is a tendency to prolong neonatal depression. These agents are not effective in counteracting depression due to ether, cyclopropane or barbiturates.

HYPNOTIC-SEDATIVE AGENTS

The barbiturates are widely used in obstetrics for their hypnotic, sedative, anesthetic and anticonvulsant action. All available barbiturates exert a depressant action on the central nervous system. They differ mainly in speed of onset of action, in duration and in intensity of effect. They are not analgesic in the ordinary sense. They lack significant ability to obtund pain sense without definite impairment of consciousness. Administered early in labor, the short-acting barbiturates, such as *secobarbital* (Seconal) and *pentobarbital* (Nembutal), are useful to allay apprehensions and fears, and in sufficient dosage they produce somnolence and sleep for three or more hours. They may be administered in doses of 100 to 200 mg. orally.

The placenta allows prompt passage of these drugs to the fetus with significant depression of its respiratory center. It is imperative, therefore, to avoid using these drugs late in labor in order to prevent dangerous depression in the newborn. The course of labor is apparently uninfluenced by barbiturates in moderate therapeutic doses. However, sizable doses, especially if anesthetic levels are reached, appear capable of prolonging labor. It is most important to remember that there are no antagonists available to counteract the action of these drugs in the newborn.

ATARACTICS

The most recent development in the field of analgesia for labor consists of the phenothiazine derivatives. These tranquilizing drugs appear to exert their primary action subcortically, inducing therapeutic pseudohypnotic states. Those in current use include chlorpromazine (Thorazine), promethazine (Phenergan), promazine (Sparine), prochlorperazine (Compazine), diazepam (Valium), hydroxyrine (Vistaril), triflupromazine (Vesprin) and perphenazine (Trilafon). These vary as to potency as antiemetic, tranquilizing and antipsychotic agents. Their essential uses in labor are: (1) potentiating effect on narcotic agents, (2) relief of anxiety and apprehension, and (3) reduction of postanesthetic nausea and vomiting. There appear to be differences in their degree of synergistic action in combination with narcotic agents, but they do have a uniform calming effect that reduces the need for analgesia or anesthesia significantly. These drugs have successfully prevented or relieved the anxiety, apprehension and restlessness that exist so frequently in the parturient. They appear in general to be well tolerated by the mother and to have relatively little, if any, effect on the newborn infant. They help to produce a state of relaxation in obstetric patients, thereby increasing cooperation during labor. Similarly, the restlessness that may follow scopolamine and barbiturates is often reduced when an ataractic is used concomitantly.

Objective studies have indicated that effect occurs within 15 minutes and lasts three to four hours. Tranquilizers appear to cross the placenta readily, but are seemingly not harmful to the fetus (Potts and Ullery). There is no reduction in the quality of clinical labor (Benson and Benson; Stewart). Diminution in uterine contractions has been reported with large doses (Hershenson et al.), but this has not been verified (Vasicka and Kretchmer).

A variety of untoward effects has been reported, including intensification of psychologic disturbances, fatigue, weakness and aggravation of depressive reactions. Somnolence may occur, and high doses have induced tachycardia, palpitation, constipation, headaches and pyrexia. A sympatholytic effect occurs, not uncommonly manifested as postural hypotension with faintness or actual syncope. Jaundice of the cholestatic type with obstruction of the interlobular canaliculi has been reported in conjunction with chlorpromazine, but this appears to be reversible. Agranulocytosis also occurs rarely.

Use of these agents has effectively reduced the need for narcotizing levels of analgesic agents in labor in the majority of patients. As to their relative efficacy, in the absence of clear-cut significant differences between these drugs, it is difficult to make specific recommendations. Additional study and experience appear to be necessary, but they are obviously valuable adjuncts in our armamentarium.

PLACENTAL TRANSFER OF DRUGS

The fundamental mechanisms of placental transfer have been dealt with at length in Chapter 4. Developments of recent years have indicated that nearly all systemic agents cross the placental barrier and may in turn affect fetal welfare. It is quite apparent, therefore, that drugs that depress the maternal central nervous centers simultaneously depress those of the fetus. The classic concept of the placenta as a simple, passive, semipermeable filter, however, is no longer tenable in light of present knowledge (Moya and Thorndike). It appears that the important issue is the rate and mechanism of transfer (Page) and not whether a given substance passes the placental barrier. In other words, penetration of the placenta occurs in nearly every instance unless the drug is destroyed or altered in transit or its rate of transfer is so slow as to render it physiologically inactive or pharmacologically undetectable.

In general, it may be said that substances are transferred across the placental barrier in an undissociated or nonionized form most readily. Ionized molecules appear to penetrate only with difficulty. At the same time lipid solubility also influences transfer. The higher the fat solubility, the more rapid is the rate of transfer. Thus, nonionized drugs with high fat solubilities are transferred most rapidly, while ionized materials and those with low lipid solubility penetrate very poorly if at all. This does not appear to hold for very small molecules; substances with a molecular weight of less than 100 penetrate readily almost without regard for fat solubility or ionization factors.

These observations explain the clinical and experimental findings of low penetration by drugs with high degrees of dissociation or low lipid solubilities, including succinylcholine, *d*-tubocurarine and tris buffer. At the other end of the spectrum, fat-soluble nonionized drugs penetrate extremely rapidly, achieving prompt equilibrium between maternal and fetal blood levels. These drugs include most of the analgesic, sedative, hypnotic and ataractic drugs in common use. It would appear reasonable, on the basis of similarities between the blood-brain and blood-placental barriers, to expect materials that act on the maternal brain centers to cross the placenta to the fetus and exert similar influences in the fetal brain. The search for substances that will relieve maternal pain by central action but not affect the fetus simultaneously is, therefore, probably doomed to failure (Moya and Thorndike).

ABDOMINAL DECOMPRESSION

An interesting development is the device used by Heyns for relieving pain in the first stage of labor. Its use has since been expanded as an aid in the second and third stages (Heyns et al.). A rigid, enclosed, airtight chamber is fitted over the lower part of the thorax, abdomen and legs. On evacuation of the air from the suit by suction, a negative pressure is developed of between 20 and 50 mm. Hg. The patient may be either supine or sitting. Examination is possible through an access opening or by removing the apparatus. The relative vacuum created causes the abdominal wall to bulge forward, permitting the uterus to elevate itself anteriorly at the fundus without encountering the usual resistance of the abdominal wall. In practice, the patient applies the negative pressure voluntarily during painful contractions. Both the timing and the amount of negative pressure are controlled by the patient.

Ostensibly, there is said to be a decided reduction in the subjective appreciation of pain. The reasons proposed by Heyns include a reduction of the forces resisting the change of the shape of the uterus from oblate to spheroid. When the abdominal wall is drawn forward, the uterus is permitted to become spherical during a contraction instead of being contained in its ovoid form. When spherical, the uterus is in its optimal contracting position, mechanically speaking. Thus, theoretically, pain is relieved.

Claims are unsubstantiated that decompression speeds labor (Quinn et al.; Scott and Loudon; Loudon) and improves fetal oxygenation (Heyns et al.). Since it appears to be harmless to the fetus and may be beneficial to some women in terms of pain relief, however, it deserves further study.

REFERENCES

Apgar, V., Burns, J. J., Brodie, B. B., and Papper, E. M.: The transmission of meperidine across the human placenta. Amer. J. Obstet. Gynec. *64*:1386, 1952.

Benson, C., and Benson, R. C.: Hydroxyzine-meperidine analgesia and neonatal response. Amer. J. Obstet. Gynec. *84*:37, 1962.

Davis, C. D., and Morrone, F. A.: An objective evaluation of a prepared childbirth program. Amer. J. Obstet. Gynec. *84*:1196, 1962.

Eckenhoff, J. E., Helrich, M., Hege, M. J. D., and Jones, R. E.: The combination of opiate antagonist and opiates for the prevention of respiratory depression. J. Pharmacol. Exp. Ther. *113*:332, 1955.

Ekelman, S. B., and Reynolds, S. R. M.: Effect of the analgesic Nisentil on uterine contractions: Considered by parity, stage of labor, and status of membranes. Obstet. Gynec. *6*:644, 1955.

Friedman, E. A.: Primigravid labor: A graphicostatistical analysis. Obstet. Gynec. *6*:567, 1955.

Friedman, E. A.: Labor: Clinical Evaluation and Management. New York, Appleton-Century-Crofts, 1967.

Giffin, M. E.: Hypnosis in obstetrics. Minn. Med. *40*:238, 1957.

Goodman, L. S., and Gilman, A., eds: The Pharmacological Basis of Therapeutics, ed. 4. New York, The Macmillan Company, 1970.

Gordon, D. W. S., and Pinker, G. D.: Increased pethidine dosage in obstetrics associated with the use of nalorphine. J. Obstet. Gynaec. Brit. Emp. *65*:606, 1958.

Greene, B. A.: Role of N-allylnormorphine in the prevention and treatment of narcotic depression of the newborn. Amer. J. Obstet. Gynec. *70*:618, 1955.

Hershenson, B. B., Koons, C. H., and Reid, D. E.: Chlorpromazine as a sedative in labor. Amer. J. Obstet. Gynec. *72*:1007, 1956.

Heyns, O. S.: Abdominal decompression in first stage of labour. J. Obstet. Gynaec. Brit. Emp. *66*:220, 1959.

Heyns, O. S., Roberts, W. A. B., and Smulian, H. G.: Decompression: New aid in second and third stage of labor. J. Internat. Coll. Surg. *34*:333, 1960.

Heyns, O. S., Samson, J. M., and Graham, J. A. C.: Influence of abdominal decompression on intra-amniotic pressure and foetal oxygenation. Lancet *1*:289, 1962.

James, L. S.: The effect of pain relief for labor and delivery on the fetus and newborn. Anesthesiology *21*:405, 1960.

Kroger, W. S.: Psychosomatic Obstetrics, Gynecology

and Endocrinology, Including Diseases of Metabolism. Springfield, Ill., Charles C Thomas, 1962.

Loudon, J. D. O.: Extra-abdominal decompression in labour. J. Obstet. Gynaec. Brit. Comm. 69:1049, 1962.

Moya, F., and James, L. S.: Medical hypnosis for obstetrics. J.A.M.A. *174*:2026, 1960.

Moya, F., and Thorndike, V.: Passage of drugs across the placenta. Amer. J. Obstet. Gynec. *84*:1778, 1962.

Page, E. W.: Transfer of materials across the human placenta. Amer. J. Obstet. Gynec. *74*:705, 1957.

Potts, C. R., and Ullery, J. C.: Maternal and fetal effects of obstetrical analgesia: Intravenous use of promethazine and meperidine. Amer. J. Obstet. Gynec. *81*:1253, 1961.

Quinn, L. J., McKeown, R. A., Moore, T., and Dorr, H. P.: Abdominal decompression during the first stage of labour: A preliminary report. Canad. Med. Ass. J. 83:1192, 1960.

Scott, D. B., and Loudon, J. D. O.: A method of abdominal decompression in labour. Lancet *1*:1181, 1960.

Shields, L. V., and Taylor, E. S.: Serial oxygen saturation studies of newborn infants following obstetric complications, difficult deliveries, and cesarean section. Amer. J. Obstet. Gynec. *73*:1011, 1957.

Snyder, F. F., and Geiling, E. M. K.: Action of morphine in obstetric analgesia. Amer. J. Obstet. Gynec. *45*:604, 1943.

Stewart, R. H.: Phenothiazine derivatives in labor and delivery: A study of four drugs. Obstet. Gynec. *17*:701, 1961.

Vasicka, A., and Kretchmer, H. E.: The effect of prochlorperazine on uterine contractions: A clinical and experimental study. Obstet. Gynec. *14*:500, 1959.

Waters, R. M., and Harris, J. W.: Factors influencing the safety of pain relief in labor. Amer. J. Surg. *48*:129, 1940.

Winkelstein, L. B.: Routine hypnosis for obstetrical delivery: An evaluation of hypnosuggestion in 200 consecutive cases. Amer. J. Obstet. Gynec. 76:152, 1958.

Chapter 22

Anesthesia for Delivery

The optimal anesthetic agent or technique does not exist. If it were available, it would relieve all the discomforts of labor without affecting its course (that is, without altering uterine contractility, cervical dilatation, voluntary expulsive forces and fetal descent) and also without deleteriously influencing the fetus in any way. It is essential to realize that every effective anesthesia has some significant drawbacks, reflected in increased maternal and fetal hazards.

Anesthesia persists as one of the leading causes of maternal mortality. It ranks fourth after hemorrhage, infection and toxemia, and is notable as the single cause of death in this list showing the least improvement in recent years. Undoubtedly responsible for this phenomenon is the fact that between 40 and 60 per cent of all obstetric anesthesias in the United States are administered by people without adequate training in anesthesiology (Phillips and Frazier; Shnider). The situation is no doubt worse abroad, although it is recognized that relatively fewer mothers receive anesthesia for delivery.

Aside from the shortage of trained physician anesthetists around the world, the problem is compounded by a general negativism on the part of many anesthetists for this activity. This lack of interest is based largely on a pervading feeling that there is little challenge to obstetric anesthesia. It is further increased by inadequate exposure during training and minimum experience in practice. It is vital that the importance of and critical problems inherent in this discipline be stressed in anesthesia training programs and that physician anesthetists be encouraged to participate actively in obstetric care.

At the same time, because so many anesthesias are being administered by untrained personnel, it is necessary for all physicians who are engaged in delivery care to become thoroughly familiar with anesthesia principles. Particularly important in this regard is a complete understanding of the indications and, more importantly, contraindications of various anesthetic techniques, as well as the recognition and management of their complications.

To this end we recognize that an intensive grounding in the principles and practice of obstetric anesthesia cannot be acquired through the medium of a vehicle such as this chapter, which can only provide the most superficial overview. The physician who is desirous of acquiring a meaningful foundation for his practice would do well to spend time in a preceptorial program, supplementing practical experience with extensive reading in such excellent resources on the subject as those by Moore and by Bonica. He should acquire wide knowledge concerning the placental transfer of drugs (Chapter 4), fetal pharmacology (Chapter 51), analgesia in labor and preanesthetic medication (Chapter 21), as well as extensive competence in resuscitation of the newborn (Chapter 67).

PREANESTHETIC PREPARATION

A complete history and comprehensive physical examination are essential before any anesthetic agent is administered. It is essential that drug allergies and idiosyncrasies be uncovered, as well as any inherent preexisting medical or psychologic problem that might affect the choice of anesthetic agent or technique. These include upper respiratory infection, anemia, hypertensive disease, acute anxiety, apprehension and similar conditions.

No food or liquids should be taken orally from the onset of labor until after delivery. Gastric emptying time is markedly diminished in labor and it can be assumed that any food taken during labor or shortly before its onset will remain in the stomach throughout labor. Aspiration of vomitus during or after anesthesia is a very serious condition and may be fatal. Every precaution should be taken to ensure that it will not occur. Parenteral feeding and hydration during labor should be managed to provide fluid, electrolyte and nutritional needs by means of intravenous infusions.

Laboratory studies, if not already done, may be necessary for ascertaining the patient's suitability for anesthesia in terms of the possible existence of unrecognized problems, such as anemia or renal dysfunction.

The requirements of preanesthetic medication are often fulfilled in the course of the management of the pain of labor. Narcotic-analgesic and tranquilizing agents are frequently administered in adequate dosages to allay fear and apprehension. If not, additional amounts of drugs, such as meperidine 50 mg. and promethazine 25 mg. intramuscularly, may be given as needed about 20 minutes prior to anticipated delivery. If general anesthesia is to be employed, a belladonna alkaloid should be used to diminish upper respiratory secretions. Atropine 0.4 mg. intravenously usually suffices.

The essential prerequisites for anesthesia include availability of suction apparatus, oxygen supply, appropriate airways, endotracheal tubes and a functioning laryngoscope. The patient should be adequately monitored with observations of vital signs, including blood pressure determinations. An intravenous infusion should be started, if not already in progress, so as to have available an open access to the vascular system for administration of drugs or blood or volume expanders in the event these should become necessary on an emergency basis. The availability of cardiac monitoring equipment, including an easily applied oscilloscopic display of the electrocardiogram and a defibrillator, is strongly recommended.

Medicolegal precautionary preparations include (1) obtaining signed consent for the anesthesia and the obstetric procedure from the patient or someone responsible for her, (2) a detailed, complete anesthetic chart and (3) appropriate predelivery and postanesthetic evaluations and follow-up examinations, fully recorded in the patient's hospital chart. Good medical practice as well as medicolegal constraints make these essential.

SELECTING THE ANESTHESIA

There is no routine anesthetic technique or practice which is universally applicable to all obstetric patients. It is mandatory that close intercommunication be maintained between anesthesiologist and obstetrician so that the optimal anesthetic will be selected on an individual basis for each patient. Factors which determine such selection are many and varied. They include (1) the physical condition of the patient, (2) coexistent medical disorders, (3) pregnancy and labor complications, (4) the condition of the fetus and (5) limitations imposed by availability of personnel, technical proficiency and equipment.

Patients with cardiac disease, especially those with little reserve or already decompensated, may fare poorly under general inhalation anesthesia. A well-conducted regional block anesthesia, particularly one that can be maintained continuously over long periods of time for both the pain relief required during labor and for the delivery itself, such as continuous caudal or lumbar epidural anesthesia, may prove most satisfactory for these patients. On the other hand, patients with neurologic disorders, such as multiple sclerosis and poliomyelitis, are at risk if given spinal or peridural anesthesia and, therefore, should preferably have general anesthesia instead. Patients with active disease of the spinal nerves should not have conduction anesthesia because it is possible that the disease will become aggravated or a neurologic sequela could result from or be attributed to the anesthetic technique (Bonica). Patients with aortic stenosis or cyanotic heart disease cannot tolerate the transient hypotension of spinal or peridural anesthesia and may be more effectively and safely managed by use of local, pudendal or paracervical block or carefully managed general anesthesia.

As to complications of pregnancy, hypovolemia secondary to dehydration or blood loss, or the anticipation of blood loss, are relative contraindications to regional block anesthesia. Obstetric conditions in which the risk of acute hemorrhage is great include placenta previa and abruptio placentae. Labor associated with hypertonic contractions, on the other hand, can be effectively treated with general anesthesia. Where progression in labor is abnormally slow or disordered, spinal or peridural anesthesia may serve as a deleterious factor, inhibiting progress still further. When one anticipates that intrauterine manipulation will be necessary, as for example in internal podalic version, uterine relaxation can be obtained only through the use of appropriately deep general anesthesia; by contrast, conduction anesthesia may enhance uterine tonus and make the procedure more difficult and potentially more traumatic to both fetus and mother.

The presence of food or liquid in the patient's stomach has already been mentioned as a relative contraindication to general anesthesia because of the risks of aspiration of vomitus. Should it become necessary to give general anesthesia under these circumstances, preventive measures, such as endotracheal intubation during the induction of the anesthesia (the so-called crash intubation), should be used to avoid this serious complication.

The fetal condition may also dictate proper choice of anesthesia. General inhalation anesthesia adversely affects the premature infant, for example, in much the same way as narcotic-analgesic agents by depressing its respiratory centers. However, conduction anesthesia can augment hypoxic states in the infant by diminishing the available oxygen supply to the fetus as a result of reduced uterine blood flow secondary to hypotension. When it is necessary to effect delivery of the fetus because it is in jeopardy, demonstrating evidences of distress (see Chapter 13), urgency dictates the use of general anesthesia. The depressive effect of such anesthesia on an already compromised infant is recognized and usually cannot be averted under such circumstances.

Insofar as the training and capability of personnel administering the anesthesia are concerned, limitations must be taken into account. It is mandatory that no form of analgesia or anesthesia be given unless the person giving it is thoroughly knowledgeable on matters relating to prevention and treatment of complications and, moreover, all equipment, drugs and facilities are also available and at hand for carrying out appropriate prevention and treatment programs. Selection of a given anesthetic on the basis of maternal or fetal condition, therefore, may have to be considered in this light and a less preferable technique chosen as dictated by the prevailing constraints imposed by limited facilities or inadequately trained personnel. The latter may clearly be an overriding factor.

GENERAL INHALATION ANESTHESIA

Inhalation techniques have several special advantages over other forms of anesthesia. The patient can be put to sleep very quickly so that acute obstetric emergencies can be handled expediently. The depth of anesthesia can be controlled delicately and its duration adjusted accordingly. The effects of the agents used are rapidly dissipated from both mother and infant. It is possible to effect uterine relaxation when it is necessary to do so for purposes of performing procedures requiring intrauterine manipulation. As stated above, it is the anesthesia of choice for the patient who is hypovolemic or in whom acute blood loss is anticipated.

The techniques involved can be taught easily. However, the subtle nuances of the pharmacokinetics of the agents used, particularly with regard to uptake, distribution and elimination, as well as recognition of the different stages of anesthesia and appreciation of principles relating to oxygenation and the maintenance of cardiovascular status, are all acquired with considerably greater difficulty.

There are disadvantages as well. Emesis with aspiration is a serious problem related to persistence of undigested food within the stomach during labor. The newborn infant is depressed by the agent used because rapid equilibration of blood concentrations takes place between maternal and fetal circulations. Thus, infant resuscitation is often required and must be instituted promptly and expertly. It is inappropriate for the anesthetist who is giving general anesthesia to the mother to be called upon to resuscitate a depressed infant, although he is sometimes the only individual available to do so. The special technical skill required in the use of delicate, complicated (and expensive) machines for administration of many inhalation agents constitutes a relative disadvantage which increases in importance when anesthesia must be administered by personnel who are not fully trained. The inflammatory nature of some inhalation agents must also be stressed.

It is important to recognize the stages of anesthesia. *First stage* is the stage of analgesia, extending from the onset of induction to loss of consciousness. Pain is obtunded and there may be some amnesia, but the patient is usually oriented and cooperative. *Second stage* refers to the stage of delirium. The patient may struggle, vomit and hold her breath; respirations are irregular. *Third stage* is the stage of surgical anesthesia, generally subdivided into four planes. *Plane 1* is light surgical anesthesia adequate for most obstetric procedures and is recognized by regular respirations and presence of ocular movement; pupils are constricted, and swallowing and lid reflexes are gone. *Plane 2* is associated with loss of eye movements, but intercostal muscle function is retained. Corneal and gag reflexes vanish. Moderate uterine relaxation occurs. *Plane 3* is deep general anesthesia with intercostal paralysis, partially dilated pupils, obtunded light reflex, and muscular relaxation, including the uterus. Respiratory assistance is essential. *Plane 4* is never needed in obstetrics. It is accompanied by intercostal and diaphragmatic paralysis, dilated pupils, respiratory lag and flaccid uterus. *Fourth stage* is the stage of medullary paralysis. It is associated with progressive cardiovascular collapse terminating in cardiac arrest and must be avoided.

Nitrous Oxide

Nitrous oxide may be used in 40 to 50 per cent concentrations with air or oxygen as an effective intermittent analgesic agent late in labor, allowing the patient to remain awake and cooperative and apparently without affecting the fetus (Shnider et al.). The gas mixture is administered as soon as the uterine contraction begins rather than waiting for it to develop to its acme. To do so will generally result in failure of the technique to effect any analgesia. It is imperative that hypoxia or cyanosis be avoided. The gas is withdrawn as the contraction subsides. In the second stage, when the patient is bearing down reflexly, she can be instructed to take three or four deep breaths of the gas mixture, to hold the last breath and then to bear down. If analgesia is not obtained by this technique, the number of breaths may be increased.

Adequate surgical anesthesia cannot be obtained with nitrous oxide without exceeding a concentration of 85 per cent. Since this will invariably result in a hypoxic state for both mother and fetus, it is contraindicated in obstetrics. Lesser concentrations of 75 per cent with 25 per cent oxygen can be made adequate as an anesthesia for episiotomy, delivery and repair when used in conjunction with other agents. It may be used in conjunction with moderately heavy narcotic-analgesic sedation or, more preferably, with a combination of muscle relaxant and thiopental (see below). The thiopental provides a means for rapid induction of anesthesia; the muscle relaxant assures that the patient will not move, and the nitrous oxide provides the anesthesia.

The advantages of nitrous oxide over other agents include its ability to produce a rapid and nonirritating induction and recovery; it is nonexplosive and inexpensive, and it does not disturb the general physiology a great deal, although it may be synergistic in producing respiratory depression when used in conjunction with narcotic agents and thiopental. Pertinently, it is important to avoid diffusion anoxia (Fink) at the conclusion of the anesthesia by administering 100 per cent oxygen at high flow rates for 5 to 10 minutes. The problem appears to result from a dilution of alveolar oxygen caused by rapid elimination of the nitrous oxide and relatively slow uptake of nitrogen from the inspired air.

When properly administered, nitrous oxide has no demonstrable effect on uterine contractility or the course of labor. It passes rapidly to the fetus, but analgesic mixtures have no clinical or biochemical effect (Shnider et al.; Romney et al.). In hypoxic concentrations, as needed for anesthesia, the newborn may develop significant degrees of metabolic acidosis (Rooth). On this basis, the practice, although widely used, cannot be condoned. Hypoxia must be avoided and a concentration of oxygen in excess of 25 per cent maintained. Proportionately more oxygen is required at elevated altitudes (for example, 30 per cent is the minimum necessary at 1 mile altitude to maintain alveolar oxygen tension of 100 mm. Hg).

Ethylene

Ethylene is very similar to nitrous oxide in potency and pharmacodynamics. Its use in obstetrics has been limited by its unpleasant odor and inflammable nature, even though it is perhaps somewhat more potent. Concentrations of 25 to 35 per cent ethylene produce effective analgesia and 75 to 80 per cent are needed for first plane anesthesia. As with nitrous oxide, however, hypoxic concentrations are necessary for adequate surgical anesthesia.

Ethylene is somewhat more emetic than nitrous oxide. It does not affect uterine contractions, but may interfere with coordination of bearing-down efforts in the second stage by its disorienting effect on the mother. It crosses the placenta readily but ordinarily does not depress the fetus unless used in conjunction with other agents such as narcotics or barbiturates.

Cyclopropane

Cyclopropane is a potent inhalation anesthetic agent, capable of providing a rapid, pleasant induction in the presence of high concentrations of oxygen. It does have some serious drawbacks, including its flammability and explosiveness, its ability to evoke cardiac arrhythmias when used concurrently with uterotonic agents or epinephrine and its depressant effects on maternal and fetal respiratory function. Moreover, a prerequisite for its use is expertly qualified personnel.

This powerful gas produces effective analgesia in concentrations of three to five per cent (Shnider et al.). In these concentrations, it does not interfere with uterine function or labor progress and produces no apparent ill effect on the fetus. In some women, analgesic levels result in amnesia as well.

When concentrations of cyclopropane exceed 10 per cent, surgical anesthesia occurs. Uterine contractility is inhibited and fetal depression can occur. Its effect on the newborn is directly related to the depth and the duration of the maternal anesthesia prior to delivery (Apgar et al.). However, there is poor correlation between levels of cyclopropane anesthesia and neonatal condition, ostensibly attributable to its ability to potentiate the depressant effects of agents or conditions acting concurrently, such as other anesthetic or narcotic agents and obstetric conditions that may in themselves produce hypoxia (Moya). It is important to bear this in mind because cyclopropane anesthesia, when used in conjunction with such factors, can adversely affect the newborn infant.

Cyclopropane should not be used to supplement regional blocks if epinephrine has been used, because of the risk of cardiac arrhythmias. Similarly, one should avoid combinations of cyclopropane and oxytocin or ergot preparations. Ventricular arrhythmias have also been reported during cyclopropane anesthesia from the administration of atropine or succinylcholine (after the first dose). This tendency is aggravated by hypercarbia. The blood pressure may increase during cyclopropane anesthesia and be augmented further by hypoventilation and hypercarbia, enhancing the sympathetic hyperactivity. This effect can be minimized by adequate alveolar ventilation.

Nausea and vomiting are seen frequently following cyclopropane anesthesia, but the incidence is less than that seen with ether anesthesia.

Cyclopropane is highly flammable and explosive in all concentrations. It is absolutely essential that it never be administered unless all appropriate precautionary measures have been taken. These include appropriate ventilation, high humidity, spark-proof apparatus and electrical switches, proper grounding of all personnel and equipment, regular testing of conductivity, elimination of materials that generate static electricity, interdiction of any open flame or cautery unit and the proper storage of all flammable gases.

Cyclopropane is particularly advantageous for use when rapid induction is necessary on an emergency basis for purposes of vaginal or abdominal delivery. This holds even in the presence of hypovolemic states, such as may result from acute hemorrhage associated with abruptio placentae or uterine rupture. Under these circumstances, adequate anesthesia can be obtained with high oxygen concentrations and the anesthesia will not enhance the hypotensive condition (contrary to the effect sometimes seen from regional block anesthesia).

Ether

Diethyl ether is widely used in obstetrics because it is fairly easy to administer by the relatively safe open drop technique. It has a wide margin of safety and low cost. Its potency is such as to be useful when it is necessary to relax the uterus for specific kinds of intrauterine manipulation and operative obstetric procedures. Induction tends to be slow and rather unpleasant to the patient. Ether is quite irritating to the lungs and mucous membranes of the tracheobronchial tree, causing marked increase in secretions; thus, it is contraindicated in patients with respiratory problems. Nausea and vomiting are common in conjunction with ether anesthesia.

A major disadvantage is its explosive potential.

Induction of anesthesia requires an inspiratory mixture of 5 to 10 volumes per cent; anesthesia can be maintained with 3 to 4 volumes per cent ether-air mixture. Induction of anesthesia is carried out with minimal concentrations at the outset and increased slowly in order to avoid irritating the respiratory tract to the point where the patient begins to cough, thereby delaying and complicating the induction. It is because of this latter feature that the use of ether alone has fallen into disfavor in institutions and areas where personnel and facilities permit the use of other, more preferable agents and techniques.

Ether anesthesia inhibits uterine contractility. During deep surgical anesthesia (Stage III, plane 3) contractions may be almost entirely abolished and the ability of the myometrium to respond to uterotonic agents and other exogenous stimuli obtunded. This effect is particularly useful when it becomes necessary to relax the uterus which is undergoing tetanic contractions or, as indicated above, when uterine relaxation is necessary for intrauterine manipulation, such as internal podalic version (see Chapter 74). Chloroform and halothane are equally effective in this regard. The inhibition of myometrial contractility may persist post partum, resulting in atony and coassociated uterine hemorrhage.

Ether crosses to the placenta rapidly and fetal blood levels equilibrate quickly with those of the mother. Neonatal respiratory depression correlates closely with circulating ether levels. The longer the duration and the deeper the ether anesthesia of the mother, the more severe and prolonged the neonatal depression.

Divinyl ether (divinyl oxide, Vinethene) is a potent inhalation anesthesia used primarily for induction by open drop technique. Its action is more rapid and it is less irritating than diethyl ether, but unless carefully given it will result in excessively deep planes of anesthesia. It is seldom used in obstetrics today because of its rapid action and potency as well as the fact that hepatic necrosis may result from prolonged administration.

Chloroform

Although highly potent, chloroform can be used for analgesia. It requires a precision vaporizer to deliver concentrations of 0.5 per cent air mixture (Moya). The degree of pain relief and the amnesia produced compare favorably with nitrous oxide. Moreover, in analgesic concentrations, the effects on mother and fetus are negligible.

Anesthesia is readily induced with chloroform in concentrations of 1 to 1.5 per cent. This is generally adequate to produce a depth of anesthesia sufficient for most obstetric procedures (Stage III, plane 1). Deeper anesthesia, as is required for intrauterine manipulation, can be induced with higher concentrations around 1.5 to 2 per cent or more for short periods. Maintenance of anesthesia requires inspired mixtures of 0.5 to 1 per cent. If concentrations of 1.5 to 2 per cent chloroform are continued for too long, respiratory paralysis will result. Overdosage, therefore, must be stringently avoided. This can be accomplished by use of a precision vaporizer which requires expert administration.

There are several significant hazards associated with the use of chloroform. Both cardiac and hepatic damage may result. Cardiac arrhythmias are not uncommon and cardiac arrest may also occur due to vagal inhibition and ventricular fibrillation. Chloroform, particularly in combination with hypoxia and hypercarbia, sensitizes the myocardium to the effects of epinephrine. Myocardial depression may also result from overdosage. Chloroform is recognized as hepatotoxic, causing toxic hepatitis from central necrosis.

Its effect on labor is profound, readily inhibiting or even eliminating uterine contractility. This effect may be seen with light surgical anesthesia, but tends to be enhanced at deeper levels as a result of myometrial depression (Van Liere et al.). This action makes chloroform especially useful when it is necessary to relax the uterus.

Fetal blood concentrations of chloroform rapidly equilibrate with levels in maternal blood. This occurs because chloroform is lipoid soluble and of low molecular weight, therefore readily crossing the placenta (see Chapter 4). Although the effects of analgesic concentrations on the fetus are negligible, anesthetic levels may produce severe neonatal depression, aggravating preexisting fetal hypoxia or contributing to the effect of other deleterious factors.

Chloroform is not flammable and quite inexpensive. It can be administered by open drop technique, but it has a narrow margin of safety. Therefore, calibrated vaporizers are advisable. Because of the special expertise necessary and its potential toxicity, chloroform is seldom used today in obstetrics.

Trichloroethylene

Trichloroethylene is used primarily for obstetric analgesia during labor. It is commonly self-administered by the patient in hand-held Duke or Cyprane inhalers. These devices allow the patient to deliver a 0.5 per cent vapor concentration to herself beginning at the onset of contractions. As she loses consciousness, the inhaler falls from her face. A wrist strap is useful in this regard. The gas mixture concentration can be adjusted, if needed, so that pain relief becomes more effective. The fact that the patient holds the mask herself is an automatic safeguard against overdosage.

Trichloroethylene (Trilene, Trimar, TCE) inhalation produces a smooth induction and is generally considered to have a pleasant odor. Light planes of surgical anesthesia may be produced by using higher concentrations, but only poor muscular relaxation can be achieved. Limits of safety are exceeded when attempts are made to effect deep surgical anesthesia.

Although analgesic concentrations appear to be innocuous, deep anesthetic levels may produce cardiac arrhythmias, especially in association with epinephrine or hypercarbia. Moreover, hepatotoxicity and nerve damage have been reported. The latter is associated with use of equipment containing soda lime for carbon dioxide absorption. Convulsions, encephalopathy and cranial nerve palsies may result.

Prolonged use may diminish the rate and intensity of uterine contractions somewhat. Similarly, severe depression of the newborn may result from use of this agent in anesthetic concentrations or for prolonged periods of time. The gas may be synergistic with other depressant agents and augment a preexisting hypoxic state in the fetus.

Use for anesthesia is generally avoided. Complications of trichloroethylene can be avoided by restricting its use to analgesic concentrations and a total time duration of no more than four hours.

Halothane

Halothane (Fluothane) is a potent, rapidly active agent capable of inducing anesthesia smoothly and pleasantly. It is nonirritating and nonflammable. It is very effective in relaxing the tetanically contracted uterus and allowing the obstetrician to perform intrauterine manipulations. It is so effective in relaxing the uterus that uterine atony and hemorrhage, often unresponsive to uterotonic agents, may result.

Halothane is not useful for analgesia. However, it is a very effective agent for inducing any desired depth of anesthesia in concentrations of 0.5 to 3 per cent; anesthesia levels can be maintained at 0.5 to 1.5 per cent. It is often combined with nitrous oxide and oxygen to increase uptake and decrease the required concentration of halothane. Because of its potency, halothane must be administered with special vaporizers by fully trained, expert personnel.

Maternal respiration may be severely depressed with halothane anesthesia. Respiratory acidosis will occur if ventilation is not assisted. The blood pressure will fall in proportion to the depth of anesthesia. Similarly, cardiac output is diminished owing to myocardial depression and decreased venous return. Cardiac arrhythmias have been reported, especially in association with respiratory acidosis or the administration of epinephrine. The hepatotoxic effect of halothane is widely recognized, but this complication is rare as shown by the National Halothane Study.

The effect of halothane on uterine contractility is very marked. Contractions are diminished in first plane anesthesia and essentially abolished completely in the second plane. Myometrial depression is so effective that the uterus will not respond to oxytocin. Subsequent occurrence of postpartum atony and bleeding, as mentioned above, may be a serious problem. The action of halothane on the uterus is much more rapid than ether; similarly, recovery is also faster (Vasicka and Kretchmer). Halothane crosses the placenta readily and may depress the newborn infant, particularly when higher concentrations are used or deeper anesthesia achieved. Because of its potency and the risk of possible complications associated with its use, halothane is generally reserved for selected obstetric patients in whom very rapid uterine relaxation is required.

Methoxyflurane

Methoxyflurane (Penthrane) is becoming a popular agent in obstetrics for both analgesia and light anesthesia. It has a wide margin of safety, producing a slow, smooth and pleasant induction with little irritation of the upper respiratory tract. It is also nonflammable. When necessary, it can be used to relax the uterus. Both induction and recovery from anesthesia are quite slow so that patients may persist in a drowsy state for a long time.

Concentrations of methoxyflurane necessary to produce effective analgesia range from 0.3 to 0.6 per cent. Light anesthesia requires 1 to 1.5 per cent for induction and 0.4 to 0.6 per cent for maintenance. It can be self-administered by a Duke or Cyprane inhaler in the same manner as Trilene (see above).

In analgesic concentrations, methoxyflurane has little effect on either mother or fetus. Anesthetic concentrations, however, decrease respiratory minute volume and produce respiratory acidosis. Bradycardia and decreased cardiac output occur as blood pressure falls in a manner similar to that of halothane. It has a depressant effect on the myometrium, and deep methoxyflurane anesthesia can relax the uterus. Prolonged and deep anesthesia will also depress the neonate.

This agent may be administered in one of several ways, including open drop technique which has the advantages of simplicity, portability and adaptability. It has the additional advantages over ether of being nonexplosive and relatively nonirritating. Compared with chloroform, it has a much greater margin of safety. Most often, however, methoxyflurane is administered in a semiclosed system utilizing a calibrated vaporizer, a method which requires considerably greater expertise but achieves more rapid induction of anesthesia under better conditions of control and safety.

INTRAVENOUS ANESTHESIA

Ultra-short-acting barbiturates can be administered to obstetric patients as basal hypnotic agents and as useful adjuvants for induction of anesthesia. Thiopental (Pentothal) is the most widely used of these agents; also available are thiamylal (Surital) and methohexital (Brevital). Induction is smooth and pleasant, requiring minimal equipment and producing no respiratory tract irritation or stimulation of secretions. They are nonflammable and entirely compatible with epinephrine and uterotonic agents.

On the debit side, ultra-short-acting barbiturates are not true analgesic agents, they cause respiratory depression and are unable to produce muscular relaxation. Extravascular extravasation may result in the administration of excessively high doses to maintain anesthesia and will cause local sloughing and neuropathy. They are contraindicated in the presence of respiratory or bronchial disease, porphyria, diabetes, renal acidosis, adrenal insufficiency, cardiac decompensation and hypovolemia. Moreover, there is a lack of control inherent in the use of intravenous anesthetic agents because, once injected, they cannot be retrieved.

Barbiturate anesthetics are very powerful respiratory depressants. However, they do not obtund laryngeal reflexes until the patient is deeply anesthetized. Therefore, stimulation of the tracheobronchial tree may produce coughing, bucking, laryngospasm or bronchospasm, especially in patients with bronchial asthma or chronic bronchitis. Marked arterial hypotension may occur during induction of anesthesia with thiopental as a result of central vaso-

motor depression, peripheral vasodilatation and myocardial depression. This response is seen especially in patients with hypovolemia and in those with vasomotor paralysis from concomitant regional block anesthesia.

In the usual therapeutic doses, intravenous barbiturate anesthetics do not appear to affect uterine contractions, although excess doses may depress the myometrium somewhat. Because barbiturates pass through the placenta very quickly, one can anticipate significant levels in the fetal circulation promptly. There is no verification of the popular misconception that the fetus delivered within a given interval after injection, usually stated to be eight minutes, will not be affected. Similarly, injection during a contraction does not protect the fetus by reducing transfer to it. In fact, it is likely that the longer the interval between injection and delivery, the lower the fetal level and the less the resultant respiratory depression. Most infants do well after thiopental induction of anesthesia unless there is some preexisting hypoxic condition that is aggravated by the thiopental (Moya and Thorndike).

Thiopental is best used as an adjunct in the induction of anesthesia. The basal hypnotic dose of no more than 150 to 250 mg. is given intravenously. As the patient becomes drowsy, this dose is supplemented with nitrous oxide-oxygen mixture (4:2 ratio) together with a muscle relaxant, such as succinylcholine or *d*-tubocurarine, as needed. These latter and other muscle relaxants should not be used unless the anesthetist is entirely familiar with them. They provide means to relax the patient without deepening the anesthesia, allowing use of lighter planes of anesthesia regardless of the agent employed. They are ineffective for relaxing the uterus and produce no analgesia or anesthesia of their own. Cumulative effects result from repeated doses, and antidotes are not always reliable.

It is essential that the anesthetist maintain artificial ventilation when paralytic doses are used; therefore, he cannot leave the patient to help in resuscitating the infant. Use of muscle relaxants is contraindicated in such situations as myasthenia gravis and patients with potassium deficiency, atypical cholinesterase levels and respiratory obstruction (Adriani). They do not cross the placenta. It is essential that muscle relaxants not be given unless one can be assured the patient is amnesic or unconscious; otherwise, she will experience all the discomforts of the procedure and be entirely unable to indicate her distress because of the muscle paralysis. The effect of this situation on the patient's emotional state may be quite serious.

REGIONAL BLOCK ANESTHESIA

Regional anesthesia is most often selected for delivery of the healthy gravida who is not hypovolemic, provided she does not have some neurologic disorder that contraindicates it or have some emotional objection to it. It is preferred because the infant is seldom affected by the anesthesia. The patient usually does not have any secondary nausea or vomiting from it; recovery is usually quite smooth; there is no problem with regard to use of flammable or explosive agents, and the equipment and drugs are not expensive. Some continuous forms of regional anesthesia can also be used to provide pain relief during much of labor. The anesthetist who has administered a regional block is available for resuscitation of the infant, if this should prove necessary.

Certain disadvantages are also recognized. Neurologic sequelae and systemic toxic reactions to the agent used have been reported. The block may not always be successful. Toxic reactions result from rapid absorption of the anesthetic drug itself or of the vasoconstrictor agent used with it. Hypersensitivity, in the form of urticaria or anaphylactic shock, is a rare cause of systemic reactions (Moore). More often central nervous stimulation will result from high blood levels, including cortical symptoms of excitement, disorientation, incoherency and convulsions, or medullary symptoms with increased pulse and respiratory rate, hypertension, nausea and vomiting. Central nervous depression may be manifest by syncope, hypotension, tachycardia and apnea. Peripheral effects

include myocardial depression with bradycardia or local vasodilatation.

Treatment of such systemic reactions includes maintaining an airway, avoiding aspiration, administering oxygen and supporting ventilation, keeping an intravenous line open so as to be able to combat cardiovascular collapse, if it should occur, and stopping convulsions (with muscle relaxants or short-acting barbiturates). Closed chest cardiac massage must be instituted immediately in the event that cardiac arrest or ventricular fibrillation occurs.

Vasoconstrictor agents are commonly used in conjunction with local and regional anesthetic drugs to slow their absorption and thereby prolong their action. Vasoconstrictors may also prevent secondary hypotension resulting from an effective regional block anesthesia. Systemic reactions to the vasoconstrictor may include palpitation, hypertension and headache.

Sensory Pathways

The nerve supply of the uterus is reviewed in Chapter 7. The sensory fibers are traced from the spinal cord through the sacral nerves by way of Frankenhäuser's ganglion into the uterus and upper vagina. Sensory fibers from the uterus that transmit the pain of uterine contractions travel primarily in the eleventh and twelfth thoracic nerve roots; those from the upper vagina and cervix traverse the second, third and fourth sacral nerve roots; those of the lower vagina and vulva are transmitted by way of the pudendal and ilioinguinal nerves. Thus, the discomforts of the first stage may be relieved by bilateral paravertebral block of the eleventh and twelfth thoracic nerves or of the second lumbar sympathetic ganglia, by bilateral paracervical block, by peridural block involving dermatomes T-10 through S-4, or by a subarachnoid block from T-10 down. The discomfort of the second stage results from distention of the vagina, vulva and perineum and may be relieved by local infiltration, pudendal nerve block, low subarachnoid or peridural block. The nerve pathways and sites for pain relief are illustrated in Figure 191.

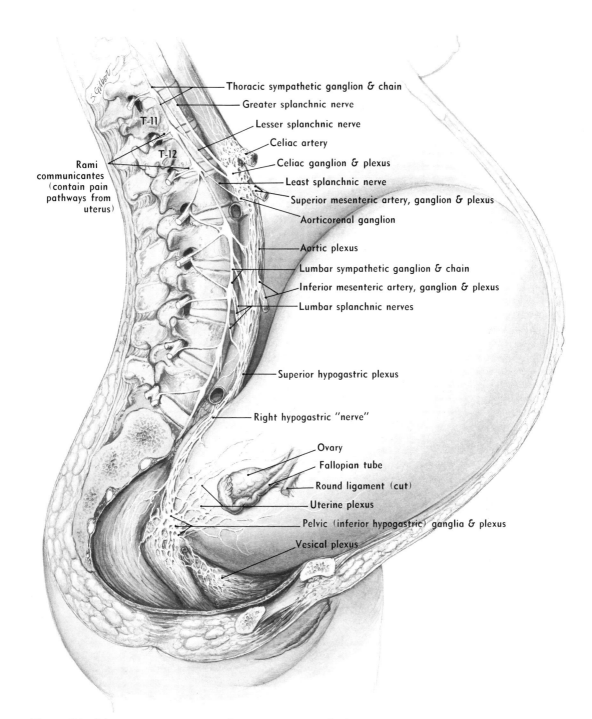

Thoracic sympathetic ganglion & chain

Greater splanchnic nerve

Lesser splanchnic nerve

Celiac artery

Celiac ganglion & plexus

Least splanchnic nerve

Superior mesenteric artery, ganglion & plexus

Aorticorenal ganglion

Aortic plexus

Lumbar sympathetic ganglion & chain

Inferior mesenteric artery, ganglion & plexus

Lumbar splanchnic nerves

Superior hypogastric plexus

Right hypogastric "nerve"

Ovary

Fallopian tube

Round ligament (cut)

Uterine plexus

Pelvic (inferior hypogastric) ganglia & plexus

Vesical plexus

T-11

T-12

Rami communicantes (contain pain pathways from uterus)

Figure 191 Schematic representation of uterine nerve supply showing nerve routes arising from thoracic and lumbar spinal nerves and traversing through the lumbar sympathetic chain to the aortic plexus, superior hypogastric plexus and pelvic plexus. (From Bonica, J. J.: Principles and Practice of Obstetrical Analgesia and Anesthesia. Philadelphia, F. A. Davis Company, 1967.)

Local Block

Local infiltration of the episiotomy site is readily accomplished to provide pain relief for making and repairing the incision. It is especially useful in patients who are delivering by psychoprophylactic methods entirely without benefit of other forms of anesthesia. The technique consists of infiltration of an anesthetic agent subcutaneously. The drugs listed in Table 5 may be used. The area is prepared as a sterile field and a skin wheal is raised using a 25-gauge hypodermic needle; infiltration is carried out through this site with a 3-inch, 22-gauge needle.

The same technique can be used for purposes of infiltrating the abdominal wall and uterus for cesarean section. In addition to intracutaneous and subcutaneous infiltration, it is necessary to inject local anesthetic agent into the rectus fascia, parietal and visceral peritoneum and into either the uterine wall or paracervical regions bilaterally. In order to slow the absorption of the agent and prolong the anesthesia, epinephrine is usually added to the infiltrating solution in concentrations of 1:200,000 or less.

This is a very useful technique but often goes wrong because obstetricians are sometimes deluded by the apparent simplicity of this approach. Failure generally results from impatience in allowing the anesthetic agent to take effect or misdirected injection of the agent itself.

Hazards involve use of excess volume and concentrations of agent to yield systemic toxic reactions. Mild reactions include palpitation, vertigo, cephalagia, apprehension, excitement, confusion, nausea and vomiting with tachycardia, hypertension and muscular twitching. This may progress to loss of consciousness, convulsions, coma, hypotension, respiratory depression and bradycardia. It is essential in this regard to avoid accidentally injecting material intravascularly or aiding its rapid absorption by use of spreading agents such as hyaluronidase. One must use the weakest concentration and the smallest total amount necessary to produce the results. Local toxic effects may also occur because of tissue toxicity from high concentrations of the local anesthetic agent. This may affect healing or produce residual neurologic problems persisting for a variable time.

Pudendal Block

Pudendal nerve block is an effective means for providing regional analgesia for purposes of relieving pain during the second stage, delivery and the third stage. It is very popular because of its simplicity and almost complete lack of side effects when properly performed. Because it does not relieve the discomforts caused by uterine contractions, it is often combined with paracervical block (see below). Properly done, pudendal block is usually sufficient to effect adequate perineal anesthesia for spontaneous or low forceps delivery as well as for performing and repairing an episiotomy.

Satisfactory anesthesia by this technique depends almost entirely on the skill used in administering it and a thorough knowledge of the relevant pelvic anatomy. Proper placement of small amounts of an-

TABLE 5   CHARACTERISTICS OF LOCAL ANESTHETIC AGENTS

Drug	Concentrations (Per Cent)	Dose Limits (mg.)	(mg./kg.)	Duration of Anesthesia (hr.)
Procaine (Novocain)	0.75–2.0	1000	14	0.7–2.0
Tetracaine (Pontocaine)	0.05–0.25	200	1.5	1.5–6.0
Lidocaine (Xylocaine, Lignocaine)	0.5 –2.0	500	7	1.5–2.5
Mepivacaine (Carbocaine)	0.5 –2.0	500	7	1.5–2.5
Piperocaine (Metycaine)	0.5 –2.5	1000	10	1.0–1.5
Chloroprocaine (Nesacaine)	0.75–2.0	1000	20	0.7–1.0
Propitocaine (Citanest)	0.5 –2.0	1000	10	1.5–3.0

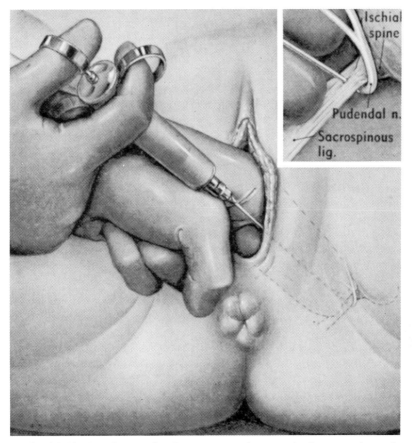

Figure 192 Pudendal block technique by the transvaginal approach showing relationship of pudendal nerve to the ischial spine and sacrospinous ligament (inset) and the method by which the needle is guided by the fingers in the vagina and advanced through the sacrospinous ligament to block the nerve. (From Bonica, J. J.: Principles and Practice of Obstetrical Analgesia and Anesthesia. Philadelphia, F. A. Davis Company, 1967.)

esthetic agent is essential both for successful results and minimization of systemic toxic reactions from overdosage. When the pudendal nerves are blocked bilaterally in this manner, neither mother nor fetus is adversely affected in any way.

The anatomic relationships of the pudendal nerve are illustrated in Figure 192. The nerve is a branch of the pudendal plexus, carrying somatic fibers from the anterior primary divisions of the second, third and fourth sacral nerves. Its constant location posterior to the ischial spine, between the sacrotuberous and sacrospinous ligaments where it enters Alcock's canal, makes it particularly amenable to infiltration at this point. Subsequently in its course, the pudendal nerve divides into the perineal nerve, the dorsal nerve to the clitoris and the inferior hemorrhoidal

nerve, each contributing to the sensory supply of the perineum. The superficial branches of the perineal nerve (posterior labial nerves) supply the skin of the perineum and the labia majora and minora. The deep branch of the perineal nerve supplies various deep and superficial muscle bundles of the perineum, including the superficial and deep transverse perineal, bulbocavernosus, ischiocavernosus and urethral sphincter and the anterior aspect of the levator ani and sphincter ani muscles. The inferior hemorrhoidal nerve supplies both muscular and cutaneous branches for the perianal region and the external sphincter.

It is important to recognize the proximity of the pudendal nerve to the ischial spine for purposes of skillful nerve block. Moreover, it is necessary to recognize the anatomic relationship of the nerve to both the pudendal and the inferior gluteal vessels, which may be injured or serve as the channels by which inadvertent intravenous injection may occur. Great care must be taken to avoid these problems.

The anesthetic solutions used for pudendal block are listed in Table 5. Most commonly, lidocaine (Xylocaine) or mepivacaine (Carbocaine) is used in concentrations of 0.8 to 1.0 per cent, maximum volume 10 ml. on each side, to deliver 160 to 200 mg. of the drug in all. If it is anticipated that more than a total of 25 to 30 ml. of solution will be required (for example, where lack of skill exists), lower concentrations of anesthetic agent should be used. Epinephrine in concentrations of 1:200,000 is useful for prolonging the duration of anesthesia.

Pudendal blocks may be administered transvaginally or by way of the perineum. The transvaginal approach is now used almost exclusively because it is simpler, quicker and more direct. A 5-inch needle is used, attached to a 10 ml. syringe filled with the anesthetic solution. The needle is guided into the vagina and directed 45° laterally and 45° posteriorly until the tip of the ischial spine is reached. The needle is then advanced through the vagina mucosa, traversing the sacrospinous ligament near its attachment to the ischial spine. As the needle pierces the ligament and enters the space in which the pudendal nerve passes, one feels a sudden release of resistance. This occurs at a depth of 1 to 1.5 cm.

Another reliable method for ensuring that the needle is properly placed is to apply constant pressure on the plunger of the syringe; as the space is entered, the resistance encountered in the ligament will suddenly vanish. Careful aspiration should be performed next to ensure that the needle has not entered a blood vessel. If blood is obtained, the needle is withdrawn or advanced a few millimeters until blood is no longer obtainable by aspiration. Then 3 to 5 ml. of solution is injected into the space. The needle is advanced 1 cm. and, if no blood is obtained on reaspiration, an additional 3 to 5 ml. is given. The opposite side is then injected in the same manner.

An assortment of needle guides are available for use with this technique, including the Iowa trumpet, the Kobak guide, the Kohl instrument and even a simple plastic straw. These guides serve as protective sheaths to prevent the needle point from catching the vaginal mucosa as the needle is advanced into the vagina; they also aid in controlling the depth of penetration accurately. The plastic drinking straw makes an effective and disposable needle guide; it can be cut to accommodate either a 5-inch or 6-inch needle so as to allow the needle to extend no more than 1.5 cm. beyond the end of the guide, thereby ensuring that the needle cannot penetrate more deeply. Sterilization can be accomplished by gas or other cold sterilization procedure.

Perineal anesthesia is usually obtained within 5 to 10 minutes after the block is given. The anesthetized area involves the vulva, perineum and perianal region. Using lidocaine or mepivacaine, one can expect the anesthesia to last at least one hour and, with epinephrine, as much as 2.5 hours. Unilateral anesthesia can be corrected by reinjection on the unanesthetized side, provided toxic levels are not thereby exceeded.

Paracervical Block

Paracervical blocks anesthetize the inferior hypogastric plexus and ganglia to provide relief of the pain of cervical dilatation during the first stage of labor. The procedure is usually initiated as the labor enters the active phase of dilatation (see Chapter 15). It can be combined with bilateral pudendal block to provide anesthesia for second stage and delivery.

There are usually no maternal side effects from paracervical block, but it is possible for the large uterine veins in the vicinity to be injured with development of a hematoma; it is also possible for there to be systemic toxic reactions from rapid absorption of the anesthetic agent used. Uterine contractility may be inhibited for a short time, but generally the rate of cervical dilatation is not substantially affected. In this regard it is probably best to avoid the use of epinephrine in paracervical blocks because of its known inhibitory effects on the myometrium.

Transient fetal bradycardia occurs in association with paracervical block. The mechanism by which it arises and its significance are incompletely understood. It is possibly due to the toxic effect on the fetus of the rapidly absorbed anesthetic agent. Fetal and neonatal depression may be a consequence of such rapid absorption into the fetal circulation. Until this issue is clarified, one must consider paracervical block not to be an entirely innocuous procedure insofar as the fetus is concerned. It is strongly recommended that, where continuous fetal monitoring is available, it be instituted and carefully observed before and during the course of the paracervical block.

The technique involves injection of 10 to 15 ml. of local anesthetic solution in each lateral fornix of the vagina. Using the same kind of sheath or guide described under pudendal block, the operator inserts the needle transvaginally to a point just lateral to the cervix. The needle is then advanced through the mucosa 1 to 1.5 cm. If aspiration fails to yield blood, 10 ml. of solution is injected. The procedure is then repeated on the opposite side.

By means of the use of indwelling plastic catheters, it is possible to provide for repeated reinjection of this area for continuous paracervical block over long periods of time (Tafeen et al.). This technique permits the use of smaller amounts of anesthetic solution repeated in increments of 5 ml. for each paracervical space, reinjected as needed according to when the pain returns. With use of mepivacaine (Carbocaine), for example, reinjections may be required as often as every 45 minutes.

As the cervix nears full dilatation and the vagina and perineum begin to be distended by the descending fetus, it will become necessary to consider other forms of anesthesia. At this time, the addition of bilateral pudendal nerve block may be very effective.

Spinal Anesthesia

Spinal or subarachnoid block is still the most frequently used regional anesthetic technique for both vaginal delivery and cesarean section. Generally, for vaginal delivery anesthesia is limited to the low spinal (to a level of T-10 dermatome) or saddle block (below T-12) distribution. For cesarean sections, anesthesia up to T-6 or T-8 is essential. This form of anesthesia is very popular because it is a simple technique to learn and master. It is associated with a relatively low failure rate and, when properly used, has minimal side effects. It does have some disadvantages, however, including hypotension, postspinal headaches and the rare occurrence of complications due to excessively high levels, particularly when administered without regard for the possible effect on intrathecal pressure of the uterine contractility and changes in intraabdominal pressure.

The subarachnoid space appears to be diminished somewhat during pregnancy because of the engorgement of epidural veins. Thus, a given dose of anesthetic agent will produce a higher spinal block in gravidas than in the nonpregnant woman. Factors which alter the cerebrospinal fluid pressure, such as the Valsalva maneuver during the expulsive efforts of the second stage, will increase the level to which the anesthesia will spread intrathecally.

Spinal anesthesia is contraindicated in the presence of severe hypovolemia, whether caused by hemorrhage, dehydration or malnutrition, and severe hypo- or hypertension. Thus, the patient with placenta previa or abruptio placentae in whom one anticipates the possibility of an acute blood loss should not be given spinal anesthesia under ordinary circumstances. Central nervous system disease also contraindicates spinal anesthesia, as does the presence of infection over the puncture site. It should also not be given to the patient who is fearful or otherwise emotionally unprepared or unsuited. As for all other varieties of anesthesia, spinal anesthesia should not be administered unless the physician is skilled in the technique and in the management of its complications.

Although saddle block has no apparent adverse effects on mother or fetus, higher levels of subarachnoid anesthesia may alter maternal function, impede labor and have some deleterious effects on the fetus. Some degree of increase in respiratory dead space, accompanied by decrease in vital capacity and total lung volume, is seen in association with spinal anesthesia that is sufficiently high to influence function of the lower intercostal and abdominal muscles. Although there is usually adequate compensation for this effect by the diaphragm and upper intercostal muscles, pulmonary ventilation may be affected by uterine interference with diaphragmatic motion or by central respiratory center depression due to narcotic-analgesic agents.

Hypotension may also occur as a result of decreased cardiac output secondary to decreased peripheral resistance and venous return. Its onset is usually abrupt, occurring within 5 to 10 minutes after the anesthesia is given. The decreased peripheral resistance is the result of vasodilatation due to interruption of preganglionic vasomotor segments by the anesthesia. The degree of hypotension is augmented when the patient is supine and the large pregnant uterus rests on the inferior vena cava to further reduce cardiac return. This problem is immediately correctable by turning the patient on her side or merely displacing the uterus laterally to the left off the inferior vena cava. The supine hypotension syndrome, which this represents, is encountered rather commonly in late pregnancy unrelated to subarachnoid block (see Chapter 41).

The effect of spinal block on labor is fairly well documented. The contractility of the uterus is entirely unaffected as to frequency, intensity and duration of contractions regardless of the anesthetic level attained, provided maternal blood pressure remains normal (Vasicka and Kretchmer). Hypotension is associated with markedly diminished contractility. Spinal anesthesia does obtund the perineal reflex so that patients do not exhibit the spontaneous urge to bear down during the second stage. This results in diminished effectiveness of expulsive efforts. Normal descent mechanisms may be interfered with as a consequence and require operative intervention in the form of forceps delivery.

Babies born under spinal anesthesia tend to be less depressed than those delivered of mothers who receive general anesthesia (Apgar et al.; Moya and Smith). In general it may be said that spinal block has no apparent direct effect on the fetus. This constitutes a major advantage of this technique over inhalation anesthesia. However, it must be reemphasized that the hypotension so commonly associated with spinal anesthesia may indirectly result in fetal hypoxia. This complication, particularly if it is handled inexpertly, may have lasting adverse effects on the fetus. It has recently been suggested that use of vasopressor agents to correct the hypotension may indeed decrease uterine blood flow and augment the fetal hypoxic problem rather than correct it (Crawford). The longer the delay in delivering the fetus under these circumstances, the greater the asphyxia in the newborn.

The spinal block may be administered with the patient in either the sitting position or the lateral decubitus with the knees flexed tightly against the abdomen. The sitting position is essential for saddle block in order for the hyperbaric solution to gravitate downward. After properly positioning the patient and preparing the skin area as a sterile field with appropriate drapes, a skin wheal is raised over the third or fourth lumbar interspace with local anesthetic solution. Great care must be taken to maintain sterile technique.

The double needle technique is especially useful in that it allows a very fine gauge (25- or 26-gauge needle) to be used for the dural puncture after the intraspinous ligament has been traversed by the prior introduction of a 20- or 21-gauge spinal needle. Using this approach, the incidence of postspinal headache is reduced. The introducer needle is first passed through the skin wheal into the interspinous ligament and carefully advanced until it is felt to pierce the ligamentum flavum. Once this needle has entered the epidural space, the smaller needle is introduced through the larger one and advanced further until it can be felt to "pop" through the dura and enter the subarachnoid space.

When the stylet is withdrawn, spinal fluid will appear at the hub of the needle. After free flow of spinal fluid has been obtained, the appropriate amount of anesthetic solution is injected, care being taken not to displace the needle from its position. During the course of the injection and at the time of its conclusion, one should withdraw a small amount of spinal fluid to ensure that the needle point is still located within the subarachnoid space. After the injection, both the spinal needle and the introducer are withdrawn.

A great variety of local anesthetic agents are available for use in subarachnoid block. For vaginal delivery, 1 to 1.5 ml. total volume usually suffices. If dibucaine (Nupercaine) is used, the amount should be limited to 2.5 mg. (1 ml. of 0.25 per cent solution). This hyperbaric material will gravitate downward if injected intrathecally in the patient who is kept sitting for 30 seconds to produce an effective saddle block. For higher levels of anesthesia for vaginal delivery, 50 mg. of lidocaine (1 ml. of five per cent Xylocaine) is effective if the patient is immediately placed in the supine position. Spinal anesthesia for cesarean section requires 2 to 2.5 ml. total volume. Usually, tetracaine (Pontocaine) 7 to 8 mg., lidocaine 50 mg. or mepivacaine 50 mg. is given.

The anesthetic solution is administered slowly and, once completed, the patient is turned gently onto her back with a pillow beneath her head. Caution should be taken to avoid increasing intraabdominal pressure which may cause spreading of the anesthetic agent above the desired level. Changing the position, if done within two to five minutes after administration, can be used to adjust the dermatome level of anesthesia. After about 10 minutes, further position changes will not affect the level of anesthesia.

Should hypotension develop, either the patient is turned on her left side or the uterus is displaced to the left off the inferior vena cava, while at the same time the legs are elevated. Vasopressors are required only if the hypotension does not respond and the mother or fetus demonstrates evidences of distress. They are given with the understanding that they may augment fetal hypoxia by further reducing uterine blood flow.

Generally, oxygen is administered to the mother throughout the procedure both to maintain adequate ventilatory exchange and to aid in preventing nausea and vomiting. Since hypotension is such a common

complication of subarachnoid block and treatment must be given promptly, it is essential that an intravenous infusion be started and running well before the block is administered so that there will be immediate and easy access to a vein. We feel it is essential to stress that, despite the fact that spinal block may be deceptively simple to administer, physicians should not be deluded into using it under circumstances that are less than optimal in terms of adequate, knowledgeable personnel and all facilities for the management of its complications.

Peridural Anesthesia

Peridural or extradural anesthesia, administered by either caudal or lumbar epidural techniques, is effective in providing pain relief throughout the course of labor and delivery. It is frequently administered as a continuous block to control pain over long periods of time during the active phase of dilatation and the second stage of labor. This approach has become increasingly popular since it was first introduced for use in obstetrics by Edwards and Hingson in 1942.

Peridural anesthesia is especially useful in premature labors in which it is advisable to avoid the depressant effects of narcotic-analgesics and inhalation anesthesias. Maternal conditions, such as heart and pulmonary diseases, hypertensive states of pregnancy and diabetes, also warrant the use of peridural anesthesia to relieve the pain and anxiety associated with labor without putting undue burden on the cardiovascular system. It is contraindicated in the presence of severe hypovolemia or where hemorrhage is anticipated, in the presence of local infection over the site of puncture or with central nervous system disease, and in patients who are emotionally unsuitable for the technique.

Considerable skill is required in its administration. The incidence of unsuccessful blocks is directly dependent upon the technical skill of the physician who gives it. Aside from the greater technical difficulty involved in mastering peridural anesthesia, pain relief is slower and less predictable than with inhalation or spinal anesthesia. Much more anesthetic agent is used than in spinal anesthesia, greatly increasing the hazards of systemic toxic reactions. Accidental intrathecal injection of such large amounts may be extremely hazardous.

The risk of broken needles or sheared polyethylene catheters must be kept in mind at all times. If the catheter should break or shear off, surgical treatment to remove it is not warranted. The catheter material is essentially inert and can be expected to do no harm. However, it is best to try to avoid this embarrassing complication. Although the risks to the patient's well-being are negligible, this problem does carry medicolegal overtones and, therefore, should be guarded against.

Lumbar epidural block has certain advantages over caudal in that it usually carries a greater chance of success, requires smaller amounts of anesthetic solution and is associated with somewhat more rapid onset of pain relief. On the other hand, it does present considerably greater risk of accidental subarachnoid injection.

Properly used, the effects of peridural anesthesia on the mother, her labor and the fetus are negligible. Interference with pulmonary ventilation can occur with high peridural blocks only if there is concomitant hypotension or narcotic-induced depression of the respiratory center. By interrupting sympathetic vasomotor fibers, peridural anesthesia will decrease peripheral resistance and venous return to effect hypotension, particularly in a patient who is susceptible to the supine hypotensive syndrome. This latter is quickly correctable by turning the patient on her side or moving the uterus to the left off the inferior vena cava while elevating the legs.

Peridural anesthesia, properly administered, appears to have little effect on uterine contractility in the active phase and the progress of dilatation is essentially normal. In multiparas, there is a slight, but clinically unimportant, prolongation of the deceleration phase (Friedman and Sachtleben). The effects of such deleterious factors as excessive sedation, cephalopelvic disproportion and fetal malposition are augmented by peridural anesthesia in terms of their effects on cervical dilatation and descent of the fetal presenting part.

Thus, proper administration includes withholding it until the active phase of labor has been entered, not preceding it with an excess of sedative-analgesic agents and avoiding its use in the presence of documented or suspected bony or positional dystocia. The inhibitory effects on the course of labor caused by peridural anesthesia under such circumstances can be readily corrected by allowing the anesthesia to wear off or by administering oxytocin infusion.

By obtunding the perineal reflex, peridural anesthesia may interfere with efficient expulsive efforts so that the terminal aspects of descent do not progress well. Internal rotation is felt to be impaired so that the incidence of persistent occiput posterior and transverse fetal positions may be increased. Although this impression is not verified, if it is true, it is counterbalanced by the marked perineal relaxation which renders operative obstetric rotation and delivery very easy (see Chapter 73).

There seems to be no direct effect of peridural anesthesia on the fetus. In general, babies born after this type of anesthesia fare better than those subjected to the depressant effects of inhalation anesthesia. This is particularly so for those with associated prematurity or placental insufficiency. It should be emphasized, however, that severe maternal hypotension may adversely affect the fetus. It has been shown (Schifrin) that characteristic fetal heart rate patterns of uteroplacental insufficiency may occur in nearly one-fourth of patients who are given peridural anesthesia during labor. With documentable hypotension, the incidence of late deceleration patterns rises to 72 per cent. The diminished uterine blood flow that appears to result as a consequence of peridural anesthesia is apparently correctable by means of rapid hydration, turning the patient on her side and administering oxygen. It is clear that, unless the problem is promptly recognized and such corrective measures instituted, the fetus may be adversely affected. It follows that continuous fetal heart monitoring, where available, should be carried out in advance of and throughout the course of the anesthesia.

Caudal Anesthesia. Caudal anesthesia requires insertion of a needle into the sacral canal by way of the sacral hiatus. It

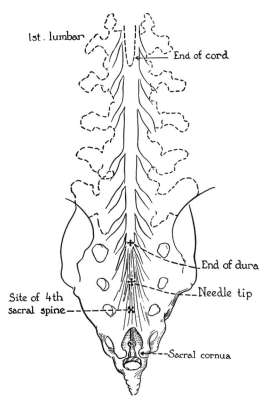

1st. lumbar

End of cord

End of dura

Needle tip

Site of 4th sacral spine

Sacral cornua

Figure 193 Schematic of the anatomic landmarks of the lumbar and sacral vertebrae, illustrating the characteristic shape of the sacral hiatus and the sacral cornua and showing the relationship between the end of the spinal cord, the end of the dura and the location of the tip of the needle inserted as for caudal anesthesia.

is mandatory that detailed anatomy of this area be learned before undertaking this procedure. The topographic landmarks and anatomic configurations are shown in Figure 193. The typical sacral hiatus is U-shaped, overlying the middle of the fourth sacral vertebra and bounded on either side by the raised prominent sacral cornua. It is readily identified by means of palpation.

With the patient in the knee-chest position or in the lateral decubitus position, the area is prepared and draped as a sterile field. An intradermal skin wheal is raised overlying the sacral hiatus and the subcutaneous tissue, and the periosteum is infiltrated with a local anesthetic agent. For single-dose injection a 3-inch, 20-gauge spinal needle is required; for continuous block, either a malleable needle or, preferably, an 18-gauge, thin-walled needle

with stylet which will accommodate a long plastic catheter is used.

Whichever method is chosen, the needle is advanced at an angle of 70 to 80° through the skin into the sacral hiatus until the sacrum is contacted with the point. The needle hub is then depressed toward the skin to an angle of 35 to 45° and the needle further advanced into the sacral canal for a distance of 2 to 3 cm. Aspiration should be done after the stylet is removed to ensure that no blood or spinal fluid is obtained. If spinal fluid appears, the procedure should be discontinued at once; if blood, the needle can be advanced a short distance. If one rapidly injects 3 ml. of air through the needle while palpating over the sacrum, one can detect crepitation indicating improper placement of the needle. Major resistance to injection indicates subperiosteal placement.

Injection of 3 ml. of anesthetic solution is given as a test dose for single-dose caudal anesthesia. Vital signs are observed carefully and after a full five minutes have elapsed, testing is done to determine the extent of hypesthesia. If there are no systemic manifestations of toxic reaction and no evidence of spinal block, the full therapeutic dose is administered very slowly. The needle is then withdrawn and the patient is turned to the supine position. A variety of agents can be given (Table 5) in amounts dependent upon the level of anesthesia one wishes to obtain. Usually, 8 to 10 ml. will provide a low block affecting dermatomes S-1 to S-5; 20 to 30 ml. will anesthetize sensory fibers of spinal nerves T-10 through S-5 in the patient of average height. Typically, 30 ml. of one per cent lidocaine or mepivacaine will provide adequate pain relief for delivery. The addition of epinephrine in concentrations of 1:200,000 will cause vasoconstriction, delay absorption and prolong the duration of the block.

Continuous Caudal Anesthesia. The technique for continuous caudal block is essentially the same as for single-dose block except that, once the needle has been placed and its position verified, a plastic catheter is threaded through the needle and advanced about 15 cm. into the sacral canal (Fig. 194). At no time should the plastic tubing be withdrawn through

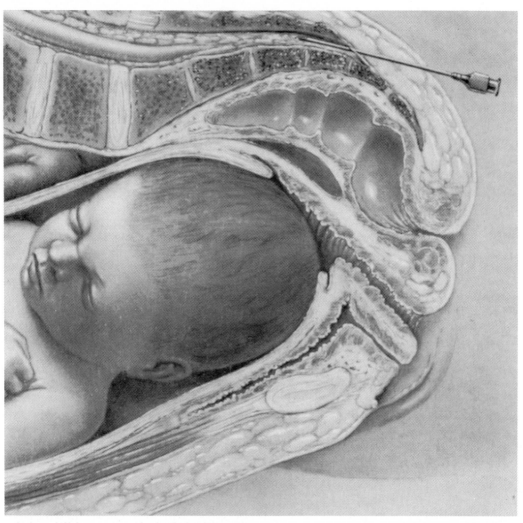

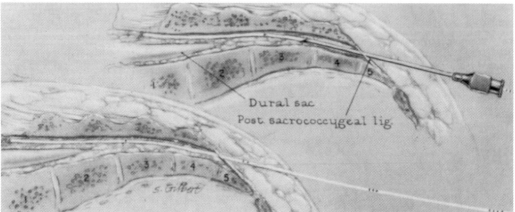

Dural sac

Post. sacrococcygeal lig.

Figure 194 Continuous caudal block anesthesia technique showing needle in sacral canal (top), with plastic catheter threaded through it (middle) and with the needle withdrawn (bottom) leaving the catheter in place for purposes of administering anesthetic solution. (From Bonica, J. J.: Principles and Practice of Obstetrical Analgesia and Anesthesia. Philadelphia, F. A. Davis Company, 1967.)

the needle; to do so might cause the plastic tubing to be sheared off by the sharp beveled point of the needle. If advancement of the catheter is impeded, it is best to withdraw the needle and catheter together as a unit and begin again.

When the catheter has been properly placed, the needle is slipped out over the catheter and a Tuohy adapter or 23-gauge needle is attached. Aspiration is repeated to detect blood or spinal fluid and the catheter securely taped in place. The patient is then returned to the supine position. The test dose of anesthetic solution is given and the patient is monitored for five minutes as described above. At the end of this time, if there are no reactions and no evidence of spinal anesthesia, an additional 15 to 20 ml. of anesthetic solution is given slowly through the catheter.

Reinforcing doses of about the same amount will be required every 45 to 90 minutes according to the type of agent used and the presence of epinephrine. The patient should be watched carefully for at least 20 minutes after each injection. Tachyphylaxis may occur if reinforcing doses are delayed to the point where the anesthetic level has fallen considerably; the results are the development of tolerance to the agent and reduction in the effectiveness of the block as time elapses. With the catheter tip placed high in the sacral canal at L-5 or S-1, smaller amounts of anesthetic agents are required to produce the same effect; for example, 20 ml. of one per cent lidocaine will usually suffice.

Lumbar Epidural Anesthesia. Lumbar epidural block requires insertion of a short-bevel or Huber-tip needle through the ligamentum flavum of the second, third or fourth lumbar interspace into the epidural space. Proper skin preparation and draping is necessary. A skin wheal is raised with a short, fine needle and the area infiltrated with local anesthesia to anesthetize the subcutaneous tissue, supraspinous and interspinous ligaments. The epidural needle is then advanced 2.5 to 3.5 cm. into the interspinous ligament. A 5 or 10 ml. syringe containing normal saline is attached to the needle at this time. It will be used to identify the peridural space accurately by applying constant pressure on the syringe barrel and noting

the moment that resistance is lost when the point of the needle enters the peridural space.

This is a most important consideration because of its reliability, its delicate control so that the dura is not perforated, and the extra safety inherent in the jet of saline pushing the meninges away from the needle point. The right-handed operator grasps the hub of the needle with the index finger and thumb of his right hand while the other fingers and dorsum of that hand rest firmly against the patient's back to guard carefully against sudden advancement of the needle. Pressure is exerted against the plunger of the syringe with the left hand and the needle advanced slowly. Great resistance is met during the time the needle lies within the substance of the interspinous ligament or ligamentum flavum. With constant unremitting pressure on the syringe plunger, the needle is advanced until there is a sudden lack of resistance, at which time the saline within the syringe can be injected easily. Advancement of the needle is halted immediately at this point.

Careful aspiration is done while rotating the needle to detect blood or spinal fluid. If none is encountered 2 to 3 ml. of anesthetic solution is injected into the epidural space as a test dose. After a full five minutes, examination is done to determine whether there is evidence of subarachnoid block by testing the level of anesthesia and checking the vital signs. For the single-dose block technique, an additional therapeutic dose is slowly injected at this time, the needle is withdrawn and the patient placed in the supine position. Usually, 10 to 12 ml. injected at the fourth lumbar interspace will be satisfactory for most vaginal deliveries.

Continuous Lumbar Epidural Anesthesia. The continuous lumbar epidural block requires threading a plastic catheter through the needle in much the same fashion as for a continuous caudal block (see above). The catheter is advanced only 3 to 5 cm. beyond the point of the needle. It is important to reemphasize that one must never withdraw the catheter through the needle once it has passed the needle tip to avoid shearing off a portion of the catheter within the peridural space. Once the catheter is in place, the needle is withdrawn.

The catheter is securely taped to the patient's back, the test dose is given and a full five minutes is allowed to elapse to safeguard against inadvertent subarachnoid block. Subsequently, 10 to 12 ml. of anesthetic solution is given to provide a full therapeutic level. Smaller doses, of the order of 5 to 6 ml., should be used when it is necessary to effect segmental block only to relieve uterine pain during the first stage of labor. After delivery, the catheter is withdrawn.

COMPLICATIONS

Vomiting and Aspiration

Vomiting during anesthesia can be a very serious problem and may be unnoticed. It can occur with both general and regional block anesthesia. It is most dangerous if it occurs at the time when the patient cannot expel the vomitus by reason of depressant drugs or anesthetic agents. The patient may present with signs of acute respiratory obstruction or, after she awakens, chest pain, respiratory embarrassment, cyanosis, fever and tachycardia. Aspiration pneumonia (Mendelson's syndrome) is thus manifested.

Treatment consists of placing the patient in head-down Trendelenburg position so as to use gravity to advantage in effecting drainage. One must make every effort to clear the vomitus from the mouth and pharynx by adequate suctioning. Visualization of the larynx and insertion of an endotracheal tube or bronchoscope may be helpful in removing large particulate material, if any, from the trachea and bronchi. Oxygen should be given. Any form of bronchial lavage has been found to be quite ineffectual. Wide spectrum antibiotics should be given to combat secondary pneumonitis. Large doses of corticosteroids may aid somewhat and should be given together with intermittent positive pressure ventilation as required. The supportive care of a pulmonary intensive care facility, if available, may sometimes be lifesaving under these circumstances.

Hypotension

The causes of hypotension during anesthesia are many and varied. Most commonly, it will reflect hypovolemia due to blood loss. Rising pulse and falling central venous pressure will usually precede the fall in arterial blood pressure. Definitive treatment for hemorrhagic shock is whole blood replacement. Oxygen is useful. Regional anesthesia should be avoided, if feasible. Temporizing measures must be used if blood is not immediately available, including blood volume expanders, such as albumin or dextran, and vasoconstrictor agents.

One must bear in mind the common supine hypotensive syndrome which results from pressure of the gravid uterus on the vena cava when the patient assumes the supine position. Partial occlusion of the vena cava will reduce venous return to the right side of the heart; this in turn reduces cardiac output and causes a dramatic fall in arterial blood pressure. Typically, the patient who is awake complains of syncope and turns herself onto her side unless constrained. Under anesthesia, one need merely pull the uterus to the left side off the vena cava to raise the blood pressure back to normal.

Hypotension may also result from widespread vasodilatation due to narcotic-analgesic drugs, deep inhalation anesthesia and major regional blocks. It is quite commonly seen in association with spinal, lumbar epidural and caudal anesthesias. Careful monitoring of both maternal and fetal vital signs is essential. Treatment should be instituted when the maternal systolic pressure falls more than 30 per cent below its preoperative level or when signs of fetal hypoxia occur. Elevating the patient's legs to effect autotransfusion is sometimes effective. Use of vasoconstrictor drugs, such as ephedrine sulfate, may be indicated. Ephedrine is given in doses of 15 to 25 mg. and, if needed, repeated in two to three minutes.

Other causes of hypotension include those resulting from surgical manipulation under light general anesthesia. This is usually due to traction reflex when the viscera or peritoneum are manipulated. Deeper anesthesia will usually correct this problem. Sudden postural changes under anesthesia may also produce hypotension, particularly in conjunction with regional block. It can be corrected with vasoconstrictors and oxygen. Use of large doses of tranquilizers may effect sufficient ganglionic block to supplement the sympathetic block from regional anesthesia to produce shock. Vasoconstrictors tend to reverse this effect.

One must also bear in mind the possibility that the pregnant patient may have experienced some vascular catastrophe, including pulmonary embolus, myocardial infarction or cerebrovascular accident. Correct diagnosis is essential, but admittedly very difficult during the course of the anesthesia. Supportive therapy, therefore, should be given to correct the hypotension and to relieve the underlying cause, if possible.

The complications that may occur during the course of obstetric anesthesia are of such serious nature that no one should undertake to provide anesthesia unless he is completely knowledgeable in preventing, detecting and managing all possible complications.

REFERENCES

Adriani, J.: The Pharmacology of Anesthetic Drugs, ed. 4. Springfield, Ill., Charles C Thomas, 1960.

Apgar, V., Holaday, D. A., James, L. S., Prince, C. E., Weisbrot, I. M., and Weiss, I.: Comparison of regional and general anesthesia in obstetrics, with special reference to transmission of cyclopropane across the placenta. J.A.M.A. 165:2155, 1957.

Bonica, J. J.: Principles and Practice of Obstetrical Analgesia and Anesthesia. Philadelphia, F. A. Davis Company, 1967.

Crawford, J. S.: A comparison of spinal analgesia and general anesthesia for elective cesarean section. Amer. J. Obstet. Gynec. 94:858, 1966.

Edwards, W. B., and Hingson, R. A.: Continuous caudal anesthesia in obstetrics. Amer. J. Surg. 57:459, 1942.

Fink, B. R.: Diffusion anoxia. Anesthesiology 25:364, 1964.

Friedman, E. A., and Sachtleben, M. R.: Caudal anesthesia: The factors that influence its effect on labor. Obstet. Gynec. 13:442, 1959.

Kobak, A. J., and Sadove, M. S.: Transvaginal regional anesthesia simplified by a new instrument. Obstet. Gynec. 15:387, 1960.

Kohl, G. C.: Transvaginal pudendal nerve block with an improved instrument. Obstet. Gynec. 11:314, 1958.

Mendelson, C. L.: Aspiration of stomach contents into the lungs during obstetric anesthesia. Amer. J. Obstet. Gynec. 52:191, 1946.

Moore, D. C.: Anesthetic Techniques for Obstetrical Analgesia and Anesthesia. Springfield, Ill., Charles C Thomas, 1964.

Moya, F.: Use of a chloroform inhaler in obstetrics. New York J. Med. 61:421, 1961.

Moya, F., and Smith, B. E.: Spinal anesthesia for cesarean section. Int. Anesth. Clin. 1:849, 1963.

Moya, F., and Thorndike, D.: Passage of drugs across the placenta. Amer. J. Obstet. Gynec. 84:1778, 1962.

National Halothane Study, Summary of: J.A.M.A. 197:775, 1966.

Phillips, O. C., and Frazier, T. M.: Obstetric anesthetic care in the United States. Obstet. Gynec. 19:796, 1962.

Romney, S. L., Kaneoka, T., and Gabel, P. V.: Perinatal oxygen environment. Amer. J. Obstet. Gynec. 84:32, 1962.

Rooth, G.: Influence of nitrous oxide on the acid-base balance of the cord blood. Amer. J. Obstet. Gynec. 85:48, 1963.

Schifrin, B. S.: Fetal heart rate patterns following epidural anesthesia and oxytocin infusion during labour. J. Obstet. Gynaec. Brit. Comm. 79:332, 1972.

Shnider, S. M.: Training in obstetric anesthesia in the United States. Amer. J. Obstet. Gynec. 93:243, 1965.

Shnider, S. M., Moya, F., Thorndike, V., Bossers, A., Morishima, H., and James, L. S.: Clinical and biochemical studies of cyclopropane analgesia in obstetrics. Anesthesiology 24:11, 1963.

Tafeen, C. H., Freedman, H. L., and Harris, H.: A system of continuous paracervical block anesthesia. Amer. J. Obstet. Gynec. 94:854, 1966.

Van Liere, E. J., Bell, W. E., Mazzocco, T. R., and Northup, D. W.: Mechanism of action of nitrous oxide, ether, and chloroform on the uterus. Amer. J. Obstet. Gynec. 90:811, 1964.

Vasicka, A., and Kretchmer, H.: Effect of conduction and inhalation anesthesia on uterine contractions. Amer. J. Obstet. Gynec. 82:600, 1961.

Chapter 23

The Third Stage

Two mechanisms are involved in delivering the placenta: its separation and its expulsion. The term *secundines* refers to all the products of conception other than the fetus. Third stage involves evacuation of secundines.

Separation of the placenta in most normal deliveries generally occurs as the fetus leaves the uterus (Leff). However, at cesarean section the placenta remains adherent to the uterus during the first moments of contraction of the muscle. The uterine wall is thick everywhere except at the placental site, where it is somewhat thinner, though nearly as thick as it was before delivery (Fig. 195).

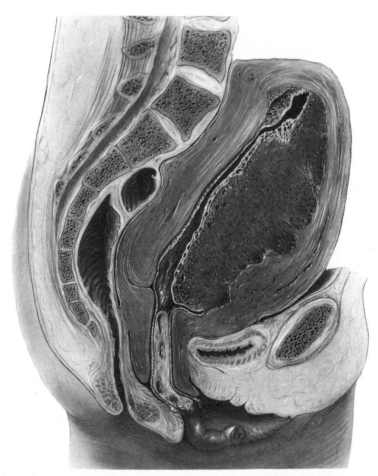

Figure 195 Sagittal section showing the uterus with fetus recently delivered and the placenta still attached. Note thin uterine wall at placental site. Frozen section. (From Couvelaire.)

During the second stage the placenta shrinks to accommodate itself to the diminishing size of its area of attachment. After delivery, if it has not separated, the first uterine contraction causes such a diminution of the surface area that separation is inevitable by shearing forces alone. It was formerly believed that separation of the placenta was brought about by the development of a retroplacental hematoma, but the retroplacental hematoma is instead the result of placental separation and not the cause of it.

Expulsion of the placenta begins when its separation is complete. The uterine contractions force it into the lower uterine segment and finally through the cervix into the vagina. The patient, if awake, bears down; if this fails to deliver the placenta, it is expelled by the physician with gentle pressure on the uterus. The placenta usually turns inside out like an umbrella; the fetal surface comes out first, the cord leading the way and the membranes containing blood following (Figs. 196 to 199). Less commonly, it may slide out with the maternal surface foremost.

The membranes are mechanically drawn off the wall of the uterus by the descending placenta, but the firm contraction of the muscle also helps in their separation. After the placenta is outside of the vulva, the membranes, if completely separated, follow by the weight of the placenta or, if necessary, by gentle traction. Normally, the membranes are expelled still adherent to each other. Microscopically, separation of the placenta and membranes usually occurs in the glandular layer of the decidua. The soft, pink, incomplete layer of tissue on the maternal surface of the chorion is decidua vera and capsularis. The gray translucent covering is decidua basalis. Some of the broken, adherent veins and arteries of the placental site are evident.

Hemorrhage from the large sinuses of the placental site is controlled by (1) contraction and retraction of the uterine muscular fibers and lamellae and (2) by clotting in the blood vessels. The retraction phase causes the muscle bundles to act as "living ligatures" around the thin-walled vessels coursing through the uterus. The shifting of the layers of muscle and shortening of the fibers compress, twist and bend the thin-walled vessels so that they are no longer pervious.

The uterus becomes a small, round organ lying low in the abdomen during the placental phase (Macpherson and Wilson). The corpus descends in an uninterrupted manner. There is no evidence that it actually elevates itself after the placenta enters the lower segment and the vagina. The placenta can be delivered safely and quickly often without aid of oxytocic agents. Indeed, it is commonly ready for delivery within five minutes of the end of the second stage. Clinical signs of descent of the placenta (change in uterine shape from discoid to globular, elongation of the exposed cord and appearance of increased bleeding) frequently lag behind actual separation. This discrepancy has been verified radiologically. On the other hand, the signs may appear even though a small part of the placenta is still attached in the upper segment. The generally accepted clinical signs are, therefore, not entirely reliable.

MANAGEMENT

More women die from accidents of the third stage than at any other time in labor. The proper conduct of this stage will avert postpartum hemorrhage, ensure the expulsion of the complete secundines, vouchsafe smooth convalescence during the puerperium and avoid potentially serious threats to the patient's subsequent health. Postpartum hemorrhage may well be fatal or may leave the woman invalided. Therefore, knowledge of the physiology of the third stage and its proper conduct are imperative.

After delivery of the baby, the physician palpates the abdomen to assess the condition of the uterus. In order to avoid contaminating the gloved hands, this is done through a sterile towel. Massage is not used. With the hand simply resting on the uterus, one notes its firmness and varying consistency, due to contraction and relaxation. After the cord has been divided, a fresh, sterile sheet is laid under the patient

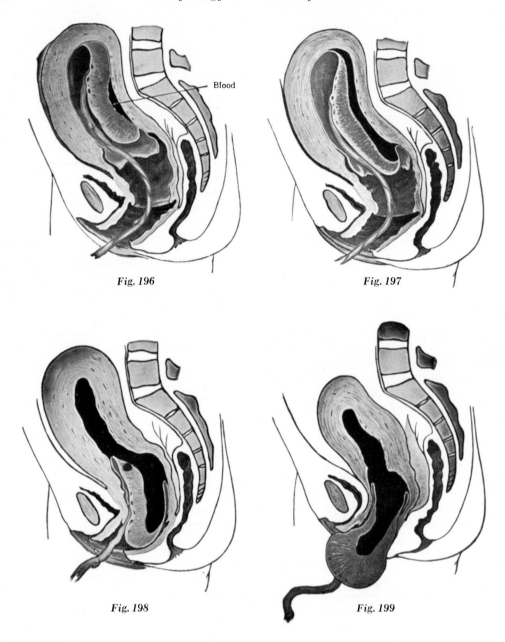

Fig. 196

Blood

Fig. 197

Fig. 198

Fig. 199

Figures 196 to 199 Sequence of usual mechanism of expulsion of placenta. Early central separation with formation of retroplacental hematoma shown progressing to inversion of the placenta and expulsion with fetal surface leading, followed by membranes and blood that has accumulated.

and a sterile basin or bedpan is held against the perineum. One must take precautions not to soil the vulva with feces. The free end of the cord is drawn up over the thigh (Fig. 128). The episiotomy wound is kept compressed with a gauze sponge or, if bleeding is heavy, large bleeding vessels are clamped and ligated.

The physician now sits or stands at the side of the patient or facing the perineum and waits. With the hand on the uterus, the frequency and strength of the contractions and the degree of advancement of the placenta are determined. The amount of blood accumulating in the basin is observed. Nothing is done if the uterus remains firm and does not balloon with blood and if there is no external bleeding. Gentle massage is practiced if the uterus softens and there is associated external bleeding. With four fingers, gentle circles are made on the posterior wall of the corpus while the thumb rests in front. As soon as the uterus becomes firm, the oozing will cease and the massage is discontinued. Meanwhile, inspection of the vulva, vagina and cervix will show whether the hemorrhage comes from a tear of the vulva or clitoris or from a higher point in the parturient canal. In pathologic cases abnormalities in the separation of the placenta cause hemorrhage and then the treatment of the third stage has to be altered (see Chapter 66).

The physician waits for the signs which indicate that the placenta has been expelled from the upper to the lower uterine segment. Strong uterine contractions, together with advancement of the cord, indicate this as the uterus assumes a globular shape, although, as indicated earlier, these may be unreliable. These signs are apparent in a few minutes. When the placenta is out of the cavity of the uterus and has moved into the vagina, there is no need for waiting longer for its delivery; in fact, it is perhaps best to express it at this time so as to minimize blood loss.

After the placenta has separated and before one proceeds, it is important to ascertain that the bladder is not overdistended and that the uterus is firmly contracted and in the midline. The woman is asked to bear down so as to determine whether she can expel the placenta herself. If she cannot, the uterus is grasped in the whole hand with the thumb in front (Fig. 200) and gently, *without squeezing,* is pushed down on the placenta in the axis of the inlet. The uterus is used simply as a piston to exert pressure on the placenta lying in the vagina.

As the placenta distends the vulva, the woman usually bears down reflexively and expels it into the basin. It should be allowed to fall the short distance into the basin by gravity and drag the membranes after it. It is best to allow the membranes to come out by their own weight. If they do not, one may exert gentle, steady traction

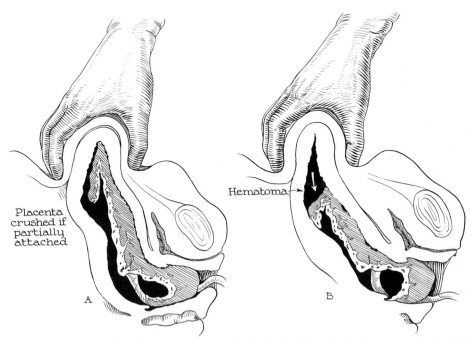

Figure 200 Expression of the placenta (A) incorrectly, by the Credé method of squeezing the fundus before separation, a dangerous and therefore inadvisable procedure, and (B) correctly, by using the corpus as a piston after the placenta has separated and entered the vagina.

on them without twisting. One grasps the membranes near the vulva from above to avoid contact with the possibly infected perineal and anal areas. If the membranes begin to tear, their proximal end should be grasped with two hemostats or other suitable clamps. These are progressively placed higher and higher as traction is made.

Some obstetricians still perform the Credé expression. It differs from simple expression in that the uterus, when it is forced down into the pelvis, is also squeezed from all sides so that its contents are expelled "like the stone from a cherry." The Credé maneuver is unphysiological and potentially dangerous and, therefore, should not be used (Fig. 200). Even the common method using the corpus as a piston is not completely without danger.

The physician should never hurry the separation of the placenta. It is safer to remove the placenta manually than it is to squeeze and maul the uterus in an effort to effect its separation. Manual removal of the placenta (see Chapter 66) may have to be done if excessive bleeding occurs and separation cannot be effected by simple external means. There is much to commend its use even on a routine, "prophylactic" basis, a practice of growing popularity. Its advocates feel it ensures complete removal of secundines, prompt termination of the third stage, reduced blood loss and thorough uterine exploration (see below); it does require adequate anesthesia and there is at least a theoretical risk of increased infection, but its apparent advantages may outweigh these.

A popular method to aid expulsion is the Brandt technique. After waiting a few minutes for the placenta to separate, the physician gently grasps the cord near the vulva with the left hand (but he does not pull it) and places his right hand on the abdomen suprapubically so that the palmar surfaces of the fingers are over the anterior surface of the uterus, approximately at the junction of the corpus and the lower uterine segment (Fig. 201). By gently pressing toward the patient's back and slightly upward with the right hand, the corpus is pushed up into the abdomen. If the placenta has separated from the corpus, the cord in the left hand will not follow the upward movement of the uterus. Having ascertained this, the physician stops the upward pressure on the uterus and begins instead to press downward on the lower uterine segment toward the vulva. As this is being done, gentle traction is made on the cord to bring forth the placenta and membranes.

It is true that the placenta may also be delivered by continued gentle traction on the cord while the corpus is being pushed up and back, but excess traction is risky because the placenta may be pulled away incompletely, the cord may tear away or the uterus may become inverted. This last is a very serious problem (see Chapter 66). If the placenta is still attached to the corpus or it is being held back by a constriction of the lower segment, this can be detected by an upward pull on the cord occurring while the corpus is being pushed up and back. In such cases one must wait and repeat the maneuver a few minutes later, after the placenta has separated or the lower segment has relaxed.

An important function of the obstetrician is to conserve the woman's blood. Women who have lost very little blood recuperate much faster, have less infection, nurse their babies better and are more healthy and vigorous than those with significant hemorrhage, including many with so-called physiologic blood losses.

Pritchard et al. studied blood loss objectively and found the average loss after vaginal delivery was 505 ml.; elective cesarean section, 930 ml.; cesarean-hysterectomy, 1435 ml. An average of 80 ml. of blood was collected from the vagina between the first hour and 72 hours after vaginal delivery. In normal pregnant women the loss of 20 per cent of blood volume as a result of typical bleeding at delivery produces little change in the hematocrit during the puerperium. The blood volume drops to approach the nonpregnancy level and the hematocrit remains relatively stable. Similar loss in nonpregnant women results in hemodilution and an appreciable fall in the hematocrit. Women during and after parturition appear to be able to tolerate the loss of much of the blood added to the circulation during pregnancy (see Chapter 41).

Routine use of uterotonic agents after delivery of the placenta is widely prac-

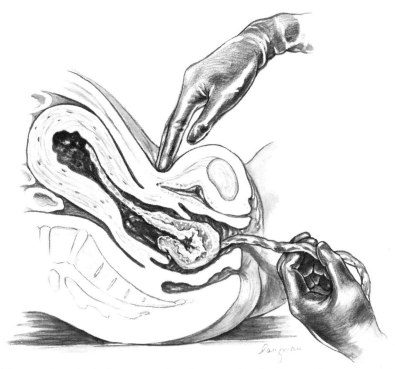

Figure 201 The Brandt method of expressing the placenta. After the placenta has separated from the uterus, the cord is held in one hand. The other hand is placed suprapubically as shown. By gently pressing backward and slightly upward on the corpus, one can easily determine if separation has occurred. Once this is verified, the placenta and membranes are easily extracted. (From R. B. Nicholls.)

ticed. It has been shown that blood loss can be reduced in this way. When not used, about 22 per cent of patients will develop uterine atony with hemorrhage (Friedman). Both oxytocin (10 I.U. of Syntocinon) and ergot preparations (0.2 mg. ergonovine maleate or tartrate) are equally effective when given intramuscularly. Ergonovine has some disadvantageous side effects, such as hypertension in sensitive individuals, and therefore is less preferable. Neither should be given directly intravenously in a bolus: oxytocin causes hypotension and electrocardiographic changes; ergot produces severe hypertension and emesis. Administration of a uterotonic agent routinely with the delivery of the anterior shoulder, another widely practiced custom, cannot be recommended because it may endanger an unrecognized second twin or entrap a placenta that does not separate promptly.

Exploration of the uterine cavity should be done whenever necessary. It can be helpful in detecting and removing pieces of membrane and placenta left behind.

Routine inspection of the placenta after it is delivered (see below) may well fail to reveal missing pieces. Occasionally, a uterine anomaly is found. One must also search for possible lacerations, particularly after difficult deliveries. Whatever hazards there are to a properly executed exploration of the uterine cavity (anesthesia, infection, trauma), they are counterbalanced favorably by the benefits.

EXAMINATION OF THE PLACENTA

A minute and systematic inspection of the placenta should be made as soon as it is delivered, while the gloves are still sterile and the patient is still on the table. Under a good light and after gently rubbing the blood clots off the maternal surface with a piece of gauze, the physician carefully inspects each cotyledon separately and successively. A gray, smooth surface (decidua basalis) is positive indication that the surface is intact at that spot and that a portion of the placenta is not missing; a roughened place without covering decidua basalis requires careful attention. If the torn and roughened surfaces fit smoothly without forcing the cotyledons together and if the broken and jagged edges of the thin decidua basalis mortise into each other perfectly, it is likely that nothing is missing from that area. One can wash every roughened portion of the placenta with water to ascertain that villi from deep within the placenta are freely floating; finding this confirms that a portion of cotyledon is missing and probably still attached to the uterine wall.

The fetal surface is next scrutinized for the distribution of the blood vessels. The possibility that an extra placental lobe or cotyledon has been retained must always be borne in mind because even the most minute examination of the placenta may fail to uncover such an occurrence. The following circumstances are highly suggestive: if the membranes are torn from the edge of the placenta, leaving the edge jagged, thick and rough; if a blood vessel runs to the edge of the placenta and breaks off sharply; if not all the vessels of a velamentous insertion are accounted for, and if the placenta is smaller than one would expect on the basis of the baby's size (fetoplacental ratio too large). Whenever doubt exists, the uterine cavity should be explored.

The membranes also must be examined. If the opening through which the infant came is round and complete, this usually indicates that all the membranes have been delivered. If the membranes are in shreds, one cannot be certain and the uterus should be explored.

All pieces of membrane and retained placental tissue should be removed manually by an experienced physician. Inept handling of this problem may lead to serious complications (see Chapter 66).

EXAMINATION FOR INJURIES

The tissues of the birth canal must be inspected carefully after the third stage. Blood is sponged away and the labia are gently separated. This is done under good light for proper visualization of the vagina and perineum. In all operative deliveries, as well as in breech births and precipitate deliveries, there should be a careful exploration of the whole parturient canal, including the uterine cavity, the vagina and the perineum, to determine the integrity of all the structures involved in labor. Generally, bladder catheterization should precede such examinations.

The cervix should be inspected and repaired if necessary. Inspection of the cervix is recommended as a routine. After inserting two right angle retractors into the vagina, one grasps the cervix with a sponge forceps or other appropriate blunt instrument at 12 o'clock and gently pulls the anterior lip of the cervix into clear view. Another sponge forceps then grasps the cervix at 2 o'clock and the first instrument is removed and replaced at 4 o'clock. In this way the physician advances the forceps stepwise around the cervix, inspecting every portion most carefully. The common areas of injury and accompanying bleeding at 3 and 9 o'clock are examined especially well.

For at least an hour after delivery the uterus should be palpated from time to time to ensure that it remains contracted, but it should not be squeezed or massaged unless there is bleeding. The physician or a competent agent or assistant must stay with the patient during this critical interval after the placenta is delivered. This time may be profitably spent watching for internal bleeding and other complications.

The records and birth certificate are completed and after-care instructions given. Before leaving the patient, the physician must assure himself on these points: (1) the uterus is firm and remains so; (2) there is no hemorrhage from the uterus and vagina and no internal bleeding; (3) the placenta and membranes are intact; (4) the bladder is not distended; (5) all tears are repaired and there is no hematoma; (6) the child is in good condition, and (7) the mother is well with normal pulse and blood pressure, without headache or vomiting, and has fully recovered from any anesthesia.

If all hospitals had a recovery ward in which recently delivered patients could be kept under observation as long as necessary postpartum, some lives would be saved. Immediately after delivery, the obstetric patient must be carefully watched for a minimum of one hour, and usually more time is needed before her condition is stable enough so that she can be returned to her hospital room. If the observation time is shorter, occasions will regretfully arise when, only a short time later, the patient will be found to have had a profuse hemorrhage or a convulsion, or to be in shock.

In a recovery ward, there should be a nurse in attendance at all times and a physician immediately available. This nurse's sole duty should be to watch the women carefully. Skin color, respirations, pulse, blood pressure, condition of the uterus and vaginal bleeding are observed frequently. The perineum is inspected for a possible hematoma. Medications are administered as needed, and intravenous fluids and blood transfusions given. Every obstetric unit should have a recovery ward or room functioning in this manner and suitably staffed at all times with knowledgeable, competent personnel.

REFERENCES

Brandt, M. L.: Mechanism and management of third stage of labor. Amer. J. Obstet. Gynec. 25:662, 1933.

Credé, C. S. F.: Klinische Vorträge über Geburtshülfe. Berlin, August Hirschwald, 1853.

Friedman, E. A.: Clinical evaluation of postpartum oxytocics. Amer. J. Obstet. Gynec. 73:1306, 1957.

Leff, M.: Management of third and fourth stages of labor based on 11,000 deliveries. Surg. Gynec. Obstet. 68:224, 1939.

Macpherson, J., and Wilson, J. K.: A radiological study of the placental stage of labour. J. Obstet. Gynaec. Brit. Emp. 63:321, 1956.

Pritchard, J. A., Baldwin, R. M., Dickey, J. C., and Wiggins, K. M.: Blood volume changes in pregnancy and the puerperium: II. Red blood cell loss and changes in apparent blood volume during and following vaginal delivery, cesarean section, and cesarean section plus total hysterectomy. Amer. J. Obstet. Gynec. 84:1271, 1962.

Chapter 24

Induction of Labor

It is a common current practice to initiate labor artificially at or near term for various medical and obstetric reasons and even more commonly without clear-cut indication. The popularity of *elective induction,* as this last is called, has resulted from its advantages to both patient and physician in terms of convenience. The pros and cons of elective induction are still debated and the issue is not yet settled.

ADVANTAGES

Elective induction is said to have many advantages, although some may constitute rationalization: (1) the patient is well rested; (2) she is psychologically prepared for labor; (3) her stomach is empty because oral intake has been restricted, thus limiting anesthesia risk; (4) her bowel is emptied; (5) she has avoided last minute transportation difficulties and those attendant on disposition of other children; (6) she avoids the risk of excessively rapid labor and (7) possible delivery at home or en route; (8) she has the advantage of the generally better equipped and staffed daytime hospital services (Tafeen et al.). Elective inductions of labor prevent uncontrolled delivery outside the hospital, ensure peace of mind, prevent anesthetic accidents, assure constant physician attendance, maintain orderly hospital occupancy and allow the patient sufficient time to organize family responsibilities (Fields et al.).

Some advocates of elective induction state that the only valid contraindication to elective induction is the inadvisability of labor itself (Crosby and Page). Others vehemently condemn this procedure (Wrig-

ley). Neither extreme seems appropriate. Frequencies of elective induction as high as 30 per cent have been reported in some institutions (Hellman et al.). Experience has shown that inductions may be undertaken electively without apparent risk provided certain ideal conditions exist and relative contraindications are absent.

PREREQUISITES AND CONTRAINDICATIONS

The dangers of elective induction of labor may be minimized if certain strict rules are observed (Bishop): (1) there are adequate numbers of trained personnel; (2) suitable facilities are at hand; (3) the patient is emotionally and physically prepared; (4) the attending physician is present at all times. There are relative prerequisites to ensure a successful attempt at induction: (1) the patient is near term by date and estimated fetal size (see Chapters 7 and 8); (2) the cervix is soft and yielding (particularly at the internal os) with a moderate amount of effacement and dilatation; (3) the vertex is presenting (rarely the breech) and (4) engaged or at least fixed in the pelvic inlet; and (5) cephalopelvic disproportion is not present.

The contraindications are those incompatible with safe and conservative obstetrics. Most contraindications are based on the fear of overstimulation of the uterus. The associated reduction in uteroplacental circulation leads to fetal hypoxia or may cause uterine rupture (Crosby and Page). Contraindications include (1) fetopelvic disproportion, (2) previous cesarean section or extensive myomectomy, (3) fetal distress, (4) malpresentation, (5) grand multiparity, (6) placenta previa and (7) uterine overdistention. These restrictions are based on isolated case reports of catastrophic results usually associated with uterine overstimulation. Conservatism dictates that these be observed except under unusual circumstances.

INDICATIONS

Aside from elective inductions, which are by far the most frequent, indications include conditions in which it is necessary to terminate the pregnancy before the life or health of mother or fetus is jeopardized. A partial list follows: (1) preeclampsia, (2) other hypertensive and renal disorders, (3) diabetes mellitus, (4) erythroblastosis, and (5) abruptio placentae. Prolonged pregnancy is a frequent indication for induction of labor (and even cesarean section) in some European centers (Nixon and Smyth) on the assumption that postmaturity is associated with placental insufficiency and fetal hypoxia. The validity of this indication is doubted unless one can demonstrate failing placental function (see Chapter 13).

Rarely, habitual death of the fetus before term in otherwise healthy women may also be a reasonable indication for induction of labor. These cases must be individualized; each situation should be considered on its own merit, the indication essentially being rather nebulous unless placental insufficiency is documentable.

COMPLICATIONS

Among complications reported with induction of labor are those associated with uterine overstimulation, including (1) tetanic contractions, (2) rupture of the uterus, (3) abruptio placentae, (4) amniotic embolism, (5) postpartum hemorrhage, (6) cervical laceration, (7) fetal distress, (8) anoxemia, (9) birth injuries, as well as (10) fetal and maternal deaths. In addition, less apparent ill effects attending induction of labor include (11) maternal anxiety (often associated with underlying fears and accompanying failure of induction), (12) prolonged labor, (13) prolapsed cord, (14) pelvic infection, (15) prematurity, (16) hypofibrinogenemia and (17) antidiuretic water intoxication. Aside from obvious reduction in maternal-fetal exchange associated with uterine tetany as a result of overstimulation, fetal heart rate patterns of hypoxia are sometimes encountered in oxytocin-stimulated labors (Hon and Wohlgemuth). In most reported series the incidence of fetal loss is not excessive (Hellman) except in association with prematurity (Keettel et al.). The hazard of prematurity in induction is a real risk based on our fallibility in correctly assessing fetal weight and size by clinical means. Objective measures for assessing fetal maturity are detailed in Chapter 13.

Additional risks include those secondary to the pharmacologic action of the oxytocic drugs used. Protein hypersensitivity to oxytocin, resulting in circulatory failure and death, is not likely to be encountered now that all commercial oxytocin is synthetic (Pitocin, Syntocinon). When oxytocin is given in large doses intravenously, marked transient hypotension and tachycardia occur with associated T-wave and S-T segment changes in the electrocardiogram (Lipton et al.). Cardiovascular collapse results from cardiac dysfunction due to coronary spasm or anaphylaxis. In addition to a decided fall in blood pressure, lasting one-half to three minutes, the patient may feel fullness in the head, severe abdominal and retrosternal throbbing, frontal headache and anxiety (Mayes and Shearman). Arrhythmia and death from oxytocin have occurred in connection with cyclopropane anesthesia. Concomitant use of oxytocin and vasoconstrictor drugs may produce severe hypertension (Casady et al.).

It has been suggested that the risks of induction may be minimized by better selection of patients, more careful screening to avoid prematurity, detailed knowledge of the procedures utilized and their potential hazards, and the constant presence of experienced personnel (Fields). Selection of patients by objective criteria of readiness for induction is a valid approach.

A scoring system such as that devised by Bishop is recommended. It consists of

TABLE 6   PRELABOR STATUS EVALUATION SCORING SYSTEM°

Factor	Score 0	Score 1	Score 2	Score 3	Factor Score
Dilatation (cm.)	Closed	1–2	3–4	5 or more	
Effacement (per cent)	0–30	40–50	60–70	80 or more	
Station	−3	−2	−1, 0	+1, +2	
Consistency	Firm	Medium	Soft		
Cervical position	Posterior	Midposition	Anterior		
Total score is equal to sum of factor scores					

°Modified from Bishop, E. H.: Obstet. Gynec. 24:266, 1964.

evaluation of relevant factors: (1) cervical dilatation, (2) effacement, (3) consistency of the cervix, (4) station of the fetal head and (5) position of the cervix in relation to the vaginal axis. Scoring of each factor is done as shown in Table 6. The higher the score, the more inducible the labor. Friedman et al. encountered no failures with scores of 9 or greater; 4.8 per cent failure if the score was 5 to 8; 19.5 per cent failure with 0 to 4 scores.

Ensuring that the uterus relaxes well between contractions and preventing overstimulation during oxytocin infusion are recognized as essential to the welfare of the fetus (Vasicka and Hutchinson). It is recommended that minute doses of oxytocin be given in drip fashion or, more preferably, by a delicately controlled infusion pump. Continuous "titration" of the dose-effect relationship is essential so that overstimulation is avoided.

METHODS

Amniotomy

Induction by artificial rupture of the membranes or amniotomy is probably the most popular method in use today. Its success in initiating labor depends largely on the preparedness of the cervix, especially when the cervix is effaced and partially dilated and the head is fixed deeply in the pelvis (see above). The drawbacks of this technique include the possibilities of infection with ascending amnionitis and of prolapsed cord. Care should be taken to maintain asepsis. One must avoid the procedure if the head is not fixed in the pelvis.

The most commonly encountered problem is failure to initiate active labor. Failure rates of 10 per cent have been reported (Manly) in some series. If the membranes are ruptured and labor does not ensue within a reasonable period of time, one runs the risk that infection will develop. The risk of failure and its associated complications can be accepted when it is performed for medical reasons, but it is a large price to pay when the amniotomy is done for elective induction of labor.

Technique.   The perineum and vulva are prepared as a sterile field with soap or antiseptic solution. Sterile gloves are used. Spreading the labia widely, the physician inserts two fingers into the vagina and then into the cervix. The membranes are separated from the lower uterine segment by a gentle sweeping motion. Then the membranes are ruptured by one of several instruments—an Allis clamp, toothed forceps, stylet, or another suitable amniotome. The instrument is guided through the cervix by the fingers until the membranes are reached. The membranes are punctured and the opening enlarged with the fingers. When done during labor, amniotomy is best performed between contractions to avoid the potential risk of cord prolapse as the amniotic fluid gushes out. Amniotomy under direct vision using an amnioscope (see Chapter 13) or speculum is also effective and has the added advantage of providing information on the presence of meconium or forelying umbilical cord. In the rare event that a loop of cord is visualized or palpated (see Chapter 59), the membranes should be left intact and appropriate measures taken to handle this serious problem.

The fetal heart tones should be checked

immediately before and after the membranes are ruptured so as to determine what effect, if any, the procedure may have on fetal oxygenation. Thus, if a previously undetected low-lying cord is compressed as the head descends, this can be detected promptly by the sudden persistent bradycardia that results. It can be relieved by gently elevating the head with the fingers in the vagina. It is imperative, therefore, for the physician to keep his fingers in the vagina until the head has descended against the cervix and he has been assured that the fetal heart rate is stable. If heart rate and uterine contractility monitoring is available, its use is highly advantageous in the course of stimulation of labor because it will detect subtle and early manifestations of hypoxia and overstimulation.

High rupture of the membranes is a common practice abroad involving the introduction of a long Drew-Smythe catheter between the membranes and the uterine wall. The membranes then are punctured above the level of the head. The success rate by this method is the same as by low amniotomy (Manly) and the infection rate is also similar (Eton). The possibility of injuring the placenta or the uterine wall with high rupture seems to be greater.

Stripping Membranes

A compromise method that has been advocated involves merely stripping the membranes by separating the chorioamniotic membranes from their loose areolar attachment to the lower uterine segment (Swann) without actually rupturing them. The technique has just been described above as a step preceding amniotomy. It has several advantages: The cervix does not have to be "ripe" and the fetal station is not critical. Other methods can be used if stripping the membranes fails. The patient does not actually need to be hospitalized.

Its disadvantages are its unpredictability, an apparent increase in morbidity, the danger of encountering previously unrecognized placenta previa or low implantation of the placenta and the possibility of accidentally rupturing the membranes with all its attendant risks, especially prolapse of the cord. Nevertheless, it has been shown to be moderately successful in selected patients and does not "burn one's bridge" by requiring that the membranes be ruptured.

The theoretical considerations as to why this technique works were first evolved by Ferguson, who demonstrated that dilatation of the cervix in rabbits increased myometrial activity in the opposite uterine horn. It has been shown that dilatation of the cervix in certain lower animals acts as a stimulus mediated by way of the hypothalamus to cause release of oxytocin. The increased secretion of oxytocin then evokes contraction of the uterine muscle that in turn causes further dilatation of the cervix. Thus, cyclic stimulation is initiated. Whether a similar reflex exists in man is not yet proved.

Uterotonic Agents

Pharmacologic agents are available and in wide use for induction of labor, including primarily synthetically prepared oxytocin and the alkaloid sparteine sulfate. Prostaglandins may soon prove worthy of clinical use also (see Chapter 4). There appears to be no way to predict the sensitivity of the individual gravid uterus to the agent administered. Certain patients may have a sustained tetanic contraction without forewarning when given minimal dosages. It is imperative, therefore, that stringent precautions be taken during the administration of these drugs. Minimal standards of care have been set forth by the American College of Obstetricians and Gynecologists as a guide for administering oxytocic agents:

Oxytocin: Pitocin and Syntocinon are valuable drugs under certain definite fixed precautions. Otherwise, they are dangerous by any mode of administration. They should be given only on the written order of the physician, in specified dosage and dilution.

1. When oxytocin is administered by hypodermic injection, the patient should be observed for at least thirty minutes thereafter by her physician.

2. When oxytocin is administered by intravenous drip, the patient should be under constant observation. This means that a physician

must be in the room with the patient at all times. If it becomes necessary to leave the patient alone, the drip should be stopped before the observer leaves the room and be resumed when he returns. The following should be checked regularly by routine technique: fetal heart sounds, frequency and character of contractions, blood pressure, rate of flow, stability of intravenous insertion, and other vital signs.

Oxytocin Sensitivity Test. A test for determining the readiness of the uterus for induction by minimal oxytocin stimulation has been devised by Smyth. It permits a forecast of the probable outcome of labor induction. It determines the response of the uterus to the intravenous injection of a standardized minute amount of oxytocin. After a preliminary period of about 15 minutes, during which the patient is at rest and the basic uterine activity is recorded by external tocography, 0.01 international unit of synthetic oxytocin is given intravenously. This is repeated every minute for 10 doses or until the uterus responds with a strong contraction. Readiness for induction is shown if response occurs with 0.02 unit or less. It has been determined (Husslein et al.; McCarthy and Fugo) that all patients responding to 0.01 unit will be in labor within 48 hours.

Extensions of this test have been suggested (Van den Driessche and Reygaerts) for determination of the approach of labor, assessment of prolonged pregnancy, diagnosis of false labor, detection of threatening premature labor, evaluation of the effect of sedation on the uterine muscle, prediction of whether delivery is imminent in the presence of a ripe cervix, forecast of the possibility of precipitate labor and ascertainment of the minimal doses of oxytocin sufficient for effective labor without hypertonicity. It seems likely that this technique will find wide application.

Oxytocin Administration. The recommended physiologic dosage of oxytocin for the initiation of labor varies from 0.2 to 0.5 mU. per minute (Theobald) to 1 to 8 mU. per minute (Caldeyro-Barcia et al.). The accepted technique for administering oxytocin is by intravenous infusion. A solution is prepared of 500 ml. of five per cent dextrose in water to which has been added 5 international units of oxytocin. The needle is inserted into a forearm vein. The infusion is begun at a very slow rate of 6 to 8 drops per minute. The patient is observed carefully for an interval of 15 minutes, checking pulse, blood pressure, respiration and fetal heart. The uterine response is watched to determine frequency, duration and intensity of contractions. Subsequently, the rate of drip is increased by about 4 drops per minute at 15 minute intervals and the observer is constantly alert for changes in vital signs and uterine reaction until strong, active labor is simulated. The optimal clinical features to look for include moderate to severe contractions recurring every two to three minutes and lasting 45 to 60 seconds. The uterus should relax completely between contractions. At no time should the patient be unattended during the oxytocin infusion.

A two-bottle technique may be used in which the first infusion is a solution of dextrose in water without oxytocin; the second bottle contains the aforementioned oxytocin concentration and is connected in a secondary fashion (perhaps by a Y connection) to the tubing of the first bottle. In this manner the oxytocin can be discontinued without disturbing the intravenous infusion. It enables the obstetrician to leave the patient if it should become necessary.

The rate of infusion may be more critically controlled by the use of infusion pump devices which are strongly recommended. The drip rate of standard gravity infusion is usually difficult to maintain. It requires intense vigil and constant readjustment. The amount of solution actually infused into the patient may also be affected by the positional factors or by obstructing venous flow. These variables are eliminated by use of an infusion pump which is capable of administering a set amount of solution at a predetermined rate continually over long periods of time without need for readjustments. Thus, one can avoid the occasional dangerous overdosage that may result from variations of infusion flow.

Overstimulation can usually be avoided by careful titration of the infusion according to the patient's needs by the technique outlined. The question of what constitutes the limit of rate of infusion is often asked. Many place arbitrary limits of 30 to 60 drops per minute. These limitations are not critical. They are based on the experience that inductions requiring greater speeds of infusion often fail. In actuality, the amount of oxytocin needed to produce good uterine contractions may occasionally be large, particularly when induction is carried out before the cervix is ripe as, for example, when there is a strong medical indication prior to term. The uterus in these patients is relatively insensitive to oxytocin. Since this situation may exist even at term, the limit of dosage should be considered merely the rate of infusion that produces good contractions. It will be understood that the more required, the less likely success. The risk of overstimulation is not increased in these insensitive patients despite the relatively large doses of oxytocin used.

As to duration of infusion, most patients become rather exhausted after eight hours. Generally, the patient's trial should not be extended beyond this unless urgency dictates. If necessary, the procedure may be repeated at daily intervals until labor supervenes.

It is imperative to discontinue the infusion at once if contractions exceed 90 seconds in duration or if evidence of fetal hypoxia occurs. The latter is especially apparent if heart rate monitoring has been used (Chapter 13). Stopping the infusion usually allows the tetanic contraction to subside promptly. Perhaps the only other measure consistently effective in alleviating uterine tetany is surgical anesthesia with open drop ether, chloroform or halothane (see Chapter 22). Unfortunately, these measures are not always immediately available or effective. By the time they are instituted, the contraction has usually spontaneously subsided. The concentration of oxytocin in the blood falls very rapidly as soon as the drip is stopped; its half life is about three minutes.

Tetanic contractions secondary to oxytocin given intramuscularly, however, may persist for a long duration as the circulating oxytocin is replenished from the intramuscular pool. The bad name that pituitary extract received when it was first introduced was due largely to the uncontrolled administration of excessive amounts of oxytocin by intranasal and intramuscular routes. Overstimulation and its consequences resulted. On the basis of such effects, intramuscular oxytocin should not be used.

In recent years there has been a resurgence of interest in administering oxytocin by sublingual, transbuccal and intranasal means. Oxytocin taken orally is deactivated in the stomach (Knaus). It is absorbed through the oral and nasal mucosa, on the other hand, but, because the amount is limited and not consistent, it produces weak and variable uterine contractions. Nevertheless, overdosage is possible, and tetanic contractions have occurred. Further evaluation of these modalities is in order before they can be accepted in clinical practice.

Sparteine Sulfate. Sparteine is a naturally occurring organic compound related to the lupanine alkaloids. It has uterotonic properties and is effective for inducing labor (Plentl et al.; Plentl and Friedman). Its pharmacologic action is similar to that of coniine and nicotine, with primary effect on the central nervous system. In large doses it may produce slight dizziness, palpitations and tingling of the hands and fingers. Its overall effect on the cardiovascular system is a depression of the myocardium qualitatively like that of quinidine. It causes slowing of the heart rate with an associated reduction in contractility, preventing or arresting auricular fibrillation and abolishing ventricular extrasystoles. The gravid uterus responds selectively to much smaller doses than those used in cardiac diseases. Sparteine, in clinically effective uterotonic doses, has no apparent cardiovascular or central nervous system effect (Gray and Plentl).

Sparteine is given intramuscularly as a sulfate in doses of 75 mg. every hour until labor is established, for an average of three doses. Hypertonicity cannot be as readily controlled as with oxytocin given intravenously. Quantitative comparisons with oxytocin show that 35 mg. of sparteine sulfate has an oxytocic action approximately equivalent to 1 international unit of oxytocin. There are isolated reports of tetanic contractions (Bedrosian and Gamble) and uterine rupture (Boysen) coincident with or after its administration. Since response can be variable and unpredictable, sparteine sulfate must be used with caution, even though the incidence of complications appears to be small.

REFERENCES

Bedrosian, L., and Gamble, J. J.: Uterine tetany and fetal distress coincidental with administration of sparteine sulfate: Report of a case. Obstet. Gynec. *21*:400, 1963.

Bishop, E. H.: Dangers attending elective induction of labor. J.A.M.A. *166*:1953, 1958.

Bishop, E. H.: Pelvic scoring for elective induction. Obstet. Gynec. *24*:266, 1964.

Boysen, H.: Sparteine sulfate and rupture of the uterus: Report of a case. Obstet. Gynec. *21*:403, 1963.

Caldeyro-Barcia, R., Sica-Blanco, Y., Poseiro, J. J., Gonzales-Panizza, V. H., Mendez-Bauer, C., Fielitz, C., Alvarez, H., Pose, S. V., and Hendricks, C. H.: A quantitative study of the action of synthetic oxytocin on the pregnant human uterus. J. Pharmacol. Exp. Ther. *121*:18, 1957.

Casady, G. N., Moore, D. C., and Bridenbaugh, L. D.: Postpartum hypertension after use of vasoconstrictor and oxytocic drugs. J.A.M.A. *172*:1011, 1960.

Crosby, W. M., and Page, E. W.: The clinical observation of an oxytocin infusion. Obstet. Gynec. *18*:60, 1961.

Eton, B.: Evaluation of low rupture of the membranes as a method of induction of labour with special reference to its advantages over high rupture. J. Obstet. Gynaec. Brit. Emp. *66*:462, 1959.

Ferguson, J. K. W.: A study of the motility of the intact uterus at term. Surg. Gynec. Obstet. *73*:359, 1941.

Fields, H.: Complications of elective induction: Prevention and management. Obstet. Gynec. *15*:476, 1960.

Fields, H., Grieve, J. W., Jr., and Franklin, R. R.: Intravenous Pitocin induction and stimulation of labor: A study of 3754 cases. Obstet. Gynec. *13*:353, 1959.

Friedman, E. A., Niswander, K. R., Bayonet-Rivera, N. P., and Sachtleben, M. R.: Relation of prelabor evaluation to inducibility and the course of labor. Obstet. Gynec. *28*:495, 1966.

Gray, M. J., and Plentl, A. A.: Sparteine: A review of its use in obstetrics. Obstet. Gynec. *11*:204, 1958.

Hellman, L. M.: Is perinatal loss increased as a result of the induction of labor? New York J. Med. *62*:2506, 1962.

Hellman, L. M., Kohl, S. G., and Schechter, H. R.: Pitocin—1955. Amer. J. Obstet. Gynec. *73*:507, 1957.

Hon, E. H., and Wohlgemuth, R.: The electronic evaluation of fetal heart rate. Amer. J. Obstet. Gynec. *81*:361, 1961.

Husslein, H., Baumgarten, K., and Hoshansl, W.: Der praktische Wert des Oxytocin-Sensitivity Testes. Zbl. Gynäk. *82*:49, 1960.

Keettel, W. C., Randall, J. H., and Donnelly, M. M.: The hazards of elective induction of labor. Amer. J. Obstet. Gynec. *75*:496, 1958.

Knaus, H. H.: The action of pituitary extract administered by the alimentary canal. Brit. Med. J. *1*:234, 1926.

Lipton, B., Hershey, S. G., and Baez, S.: Compatibility of oxytocics with anesthetic agents. J.A.M.A. *179*:410, 1962.

Manly, G. A.: Induction-delivery interval following artificial rupture of the membranes. Lancet *2*:227, 1956.

Mayes, B. T., and Shearman, R. P.: Experience with synthetic oxytocin: The effects on the cardiovascular system and its use for the induction of labour and control of the third stage. J. Obstet. Gynaec. Brit. Emp. *63*:812, 1956.

McCarthy, C. J., and Fugo, N. W.: The oxytocin sensitivity test. Obstet. Gynec. *17*:531, 1961.

Nixon, W. C. W., and Smyth, C. N.: Old and new methods for induction of labor and premature labor. Amer. J. Obstet. Gynec. *77*:393, 1959.

Plentl, A. A., and Friedman, E. A.: Sparteine sulfate: Clinical evaluation of its use for induction of labor. Amer. J. Obstet. Gynec. *85*:200, 1963.

Plentl, A. A., Friedman, E. A., and Gray, M. J.: Sparteine sulfate: A clinical evaluation of its use in the management of labor. Amer. J. Obstet. Gynec. *82*:1332, 1961.

Smyth, C. N.: The oxytocin sensitivity test for surgical induction of labor. Sandoz Triangle *3*:150, 1958.

Swann, R. O.: Induction of labor by stripping membranes. Obstet. Gynec. *11*:74, 1958.

Tafeen, C. H., Freedman, H. L., and Harris, H.: Elective induction of labor. Obstet. Gynec. *8*:720, 1956.

Theobald, G. W.: The separate release of oxytocin and antidiuretic hormone. J. Physiol. *149*:443, 1959.

Van den Driessche, R., and Reygaerts, J.: Test de sensibilité à l'ocytocine. Bull. Soc. Roy. Belg. Gynéc. Obstét. *28*:227, 1958.

Vasicka, A., and Hutchinson, H. T.: Fetal response to induction, augmentation and correction of labor by oxytocin. Amer. J. Obstet. Gynec. *85*:1054, 1963.

Wrigley, A. J.: Oxytocin drip: Some further experiences and observations. Lancet *1*:5, 1962.

PHYSIOLOGY AND CONDUCT OF THE PUERPERIUM

Chapter 25

Changes in the Puerperium

Labor ends with the completion of the third stage. After the placenta is delivered, the puerperal state or the puerperium has begun and the patient is considered to be a *puerpera*.

The *puerperium* starts after delivery of the infant, placenta and membranes and ends when the mother's internal and external genital organs return to their nonpregnant state. It lasts from six to eight weeks.

In the puerperium there are retrogressive changes which cause the mother's reproductive organs to return to their original condition. Also, progressive mammary changes occur and the breasts begin to function in the nourishment of the child. The retrogressive genital changes are grouped under the general heading of *involution*.

THE UTERUS

Immediately after delivery of the placenta the uterus shrinks to below the level of the umbilicus, and comes to rest on the sacral promontory (Fig. 202). Owing to its previous displacement, its ligaments and vaginal attachments are so loose that it may be easily displaced to any part of the abdomen or it may be pushed down so that the cervix hangs out of the vulva. The uterus now resembles a flattened pear. It is about 15 cm. long, 12 cm. wide and 8 to 10 cm. thick, being about as large as a baby's head. It weighs about 1000 gm. The full bladder displaces the uterus so that it usually rises toward the right side. Vaginal examination immediately after labor shows that the cervix is soft and succulent, hanging down from the hard contracted muscular uterus in folds like the cuff of a garment's sleeve. The cervix is bruised, sometimes almost black with suffused blood, edematous and frequently torn. It is about 1 cm. thick and 3 to 6 cm. long.

The physiologic retraction ring marks the point at which the thick upper uterine segment joins the thin lower uterine segment and cervix. A blood clot sometimes fills the cavity of the uterus or the walls lie apposed to each other. At first, the uterine wall at the placental site is thinner than elsewhere; after a few contractions have occurred, it becomes thicker. The location of the placenta is recognized by the roughened, raised surface. The thickness of the uterine wall varies from 3.5 to 5 cm.

The uterus may appear to rise in the ab-

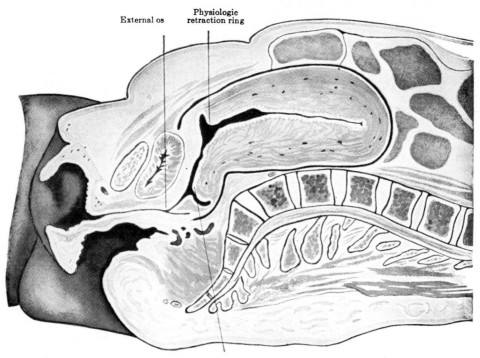

External os

Physiologic
retraction ring

Physiologic retraction ring

Figure 202   Frozen section of a primipara who died from hemorrhage one hour after delivery showing the size, position and relationships of the uterus following labor. (From Stratz.)

domen during the first day of the puerperium as the bladder fills. From then on a steady daily decrease occurs in all its diameters (Fig. 203).

On the first day the uterus is 12 to 15 cm. above the pubis; on the fifth day, 7 to 10 cm., and correspondingly narrower across the fundus; by the twelfth day it is acutely anteflexed and has sunk below the inlet so that it is no longer easily palpable through the abdomen.

By the end of the first week the uterus weighs about 500 gm. At the end of the second week it weighs 350 gm. In the eighth week it has returned to the size of a nongravid uterus, about 60 to 80 gm.

The placental site contracts rapidly, presenting a raised, rough surface about 7.5 cm. in diameter at first. It is sometimes mistaken for a piece of adherent placenta. By the fourteenth day it is about 35 mm. in diameter and in six weeks it may still be recognized by its elevated, though no longer roughened, surface which is about 24 mm. across.

The uterine serosa, in spite of its elastic-ity, cannot shrink to follow the receding uterus. It lies in fine wrinkles on the uterine surface. These wrinkles disappear within a week.

The serous infiltration of the cervix disappears rapidly. Within 18 hours the cervix regains its form, quickly shortens and becomes harder. By the third day, two fingers can still be passed easily into the uterus; on the twelfth day the endocervical canal will admit only one finger to the internal os, but the finger cannot be advanced through the os. In the fourth week the external os is a small transverse slit.

The Endometrium.   During pregnancy the glandular layer of the decidua vera and basalis undergoes the changes described in Chapter 3. Separation of the placenta and membranes from their attachment to the uterine wall takes place in this layer. Therefore, when the uterus is emptied, its mucosal surface is denuded and exposed. This denuding extends almost to the muscle at the placental site. The interior of the uterus is one large wound surface with large venous sinuses containing superfi-

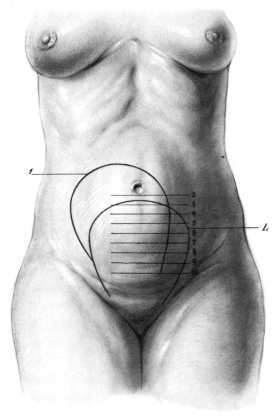

Figure 203 Frontal view of the abdomen indicating progressive changes in the height of the uterus post partum with the bladder empty. *L*, Immediately after labor; *1* to *10*, fundal height on each successively numbered day.

cial thrombi at the placental site. Leukocytes invade the decidua, forming a layer of granulation which separates the necrosing, autolyzing, sloughing surface decidua from the healthy, deeper layer of decidua. At first, the endometrium varies from 2 to 5 mm. in thickness. The surface is rough, with shreds of degenerating decidua, blood clots and bits of fetal membrane. By the third day, as the result of degeneration, this debris has softened so that it may be wiped off with the finger. The remaining decidual cells return to their original condition.

The epithelium from the stumps of the basilar glands proliferates rapidly, growing out on the surface of the endometrium and covering the new mucous membrane. Thus, a large part of the endometrium is cast off, and regeneration takes place from the epithelium of the deepest portions of the uterine glands.

At the placental site similar processes occur. Williams showed that six to seven weeks are required for the complete disappearance of the placental site. The site is not affected by absorption *in situ* but by a process of exfoliation, brought about through undermining of the placental site by the growth of endometrial tissue. This is effected in part by extension and overgrowth of endometrium from the margins of the placental site. Additionally, there is the development of endometrial tissue from the glands and stroma left in the depths of the decidua basalis after separation of the placenta.

Such a process of exfoliation can be regarded teleologically as a mechanism for ridding the uterus of the organized thrombi and obliterated vessels at the placental site. If these were to remain *in situ*, they would convert part of the mucosa into scar tissue, progressively increasing with each succeeding pregnancy. Instead, this area is effectively sloughed in due course. Throughout the process fragments of tissue are cast off. The discharge of tissue lasts many days.

The obliterated arteries of the placental site reflect changes that are present in the arteries deep in the myometrium (Williams). They show the characteristic picture of sclerosis. Certain of the distal vessels are recanalized or replaced by smaller ones; others become obliterated and are soon absorbed. In many women some of these vessels persist and afford an objective demonstration of a preexistent pregnancy.

THE VAGINA AND EXTERNAL GENITALS

After labor the vagina may be swollen, blue, bruised and pouting into the vulva. The tonicity of the perineum is reestablished with surprising rapidity. Perineal tears that looked large and deep at delivery are relatively small the next day. A peculiar consistency of the vagina and perineum persists for weeks after delivery.

The tissues are distensible to only a certain degree, the blood vessels are friable and surgery during the puerperium is likely to be complicated by troublesome capillary oozing. The vagina and the mucous surface of the vulva have a deep red, velvety appearance.

The pelvic floor, containing muscle, fat and fascia, is infiltrated with blood and serum and is full of small suggillations. The muscular fibers are often torn and overstretched. Absorption of the blood and serum takes place quickly, but many minute and larger scars are left. Coalescence of such tissue defects may result in atrophy and a weakened pelvic floor.

Gradually, the parts regain their tone and after four to eight weeks they are firmer. The closure is better so that the vulva gapes very little, unless a laceration has not healed well.

PUERPERAL WOUNDS

The hymen always tears in labor. The residua of this injury are a row of mucous membrane tags, called *carunculae myrti-formes*. There may be lacerations, ecchymoses and scraped surfaces around the clitoris, in the labia minora, the vaginal introitus, the vagina and the cervix. These occur especially in primiparas. They usually heal by primary union. Although the healing process in the skin is good, sometimes the damaged perineal body does not unite well. This is important physiologically. Lacerations of the vagina usually heal readily, but scar formation may distort the base of the bladder and contribute to the development of stress urinary incontinence.

Infected cervical tears do not heal well, but may give rise to potentially serious cellulitis in the adjacent broad ligaments. In the absence of infection these cervical wounds heal with little inflammatory reaction. The surface is covered with a light gray exudate. Underneath this, pink granulations appear, the surface sloughs off, epithelization occurs rapidly and by the eighth day healing is usually nearly completed.

LOCHIA

Another striking phenomenon of the puerperium is the appearance of *lochia,* a discharge from the vagina. At first it is bloody, then serous. It ceases in 10 days to 6 weeks. On the first day the lochia contain blood and tissue debris only, called *lochia rubra.* It is normally not mixed with clots. Clots are abnormal and their cause must be determined (see Chapter 66). This is followed by a flow of bloodstained serum; then the discharge becomes thicker, of a maroon color and creamy consistency, with a characteristic odor, *lochia serosa.* Gradually, the bloody component disappears, the leukocytes increase, and the lochia resemble cream, *lochia alba.*

Lochia rubra contain blood, shreds of decidua, and occasionally vernix caseosa, lanugo and meconium.

Lochia serosa contain mostly serous exudation, leukocytes, erythrocytes, shreds of decidua in a state of degeneration, cervical mucus and microorganisms.

Lochia alba are full of decidual cells, which are large, mononucleated, irregular, round or spindle-shaped cells in the process of degeneration, as well as leukocytes, flat and cylindric epithelium, fat and debris from the uterus and the puerperal wounds, mucus, cholesterin crystals and many bacteria.

The duration of lochia is variable and the amount and quality vary from day to day. Smith reported that lochia rubra continued on average for two to two and one-half weeks post partum and lochia serosa for an additional two to two and one-half weeks. Postpartum bleeding persists for about four and one-half weeks whether or not a woman is nursing. Bernstine and Bernstine found that the discharge of lochia rises rapidly to peak between 80 and 120 hours, subsiding subsequently. Afterwards the discharge subsides to from 2 to 5 gm. During the night the discharge is much less than during the day. The average total amount of lochia discharged is about 225 gm. Sometimes lochia rubra persist for several weeks or reappear on the occasion of unusual exercise, or the lochia may cease as the result of obstruction. This almost always is associated with fever which subsides when drainage is re-established.

The odor of lochia varies from day to day. It varies with the patient and with the kind of bacteria present in the vagina. Normally, the odor is not offensive. Decomposing clots, membranes, infection or a retained surgical sponge or gauze packing impart a foul odor to the lochia.

Bacteriology of the Lochia. By the end of the second postpartum day all uteri are contaminated by vaginal bacteria. Why infection does not develop in every woman during the puerperium is explained on the basis of the time sequences and on the relatively nonvirulent nature of the organisms. Unless labor has been prolonged, bacteria do not reach the raw surface of the uterus until perhaps the second or third day. By this time the protecting granulation barrier has formed in the endometrium. Infection is inevitable, however, if any manipulation or instrumentation causes a break through this protecting wall of granulation.

Of equal importance is the fact that the bacteria are of weak virulence or the puerpera possesses natural immunities against infection. When her general health is poor, as a result of hemorrhage, debilitation, exhaustion or shock, or if local resistance is lowered through injury, bacteria may invade. A phagocytic defensive mechanism against bacterial invasion is formed in pregnancy at the bases of the broad ligaments (Hofbauer). It consists of collections of round cell infiltrates. These may be effective in mobilizing local defenses against infection and serve the function of clearing away tissue debris.

INVOLUTION

The process by which the uterus returns to its prepregnancy state during the puerperium is called *involution.* The foregoing changes are part of involution. The most prominent manifestation of involution, however, is the reduction in the size of the uterus. Infection stops or inhibits the process of involution.

One of the essential features of involution is the shedding of the decidua. This resembles the cleansing of a granulating surface. In addition, the uterine wall shrinks in all dimensions. This comes about as a result of the reduction in size of the myometrial cells which had hypertrophied so extensively during pregnancy under estrogen stimulation (see Chapter 7). Tissue edema and vascularity subside as well.

Sometimes, involution is prolonged and is continued beyond the point at which the uterus has resumed its prior size. One may find the uterus to be extremely small at the tenth week. This is *superinvolution,* sometimes called *lactation atrophy* because it only occurs in nursing mothers. Often menstruation does not reappear during the course of lactation in these patients. The atrophy reaches its maximum by about the fourth month. If nursing is stopped, the uterus normally regenerates in six to eight weeks. If continued, actual atrophy of the uterus may occur although this is exceedingly rare and usually suggests the probability of other coexisting disorders, particularly those of endocrine, nutritional or psychiatric origin.

RETURN OF MENSTRUATION AND OVULATION

The reinstitution of menstruation is quite variable following delivery. Lactation tends to delay the onset. It is generally stated that menstruation begins about six weeks post partum. However, Sharman showed this to occur in only 24.7 per cent; within 12 weeks, 61.1 per cent; within 24 weeks, 77.7 per cent. At 12 weeks, about one-third of lactating primiparas were menstruating as compared with 91 per cent of nonlactating primiparas. Once reestablished, menstruation was regular in 72.5 per cent of lactating women and in 92.2 per cent of those not lactating.

Based on evidence obtained by endometrial biopsies, Sharman was unable to show ovulation during the first six weeks; during the next six weeks, 56 per cent of the biopsies showed ovulation, and during the following 12 weeks, 86 per cent ovulated. About 42 per cent of first menstruation had been preceded by ovulation. Once a woman ovulated, subsequent cycles tended to be ovulatory also.

It is a popular superstition that breast feeding prevents conception. Robinson studied mothers who conceived during lactation. They had no return of menstruation. They did not recognize a superimposed pregnancy until they felt fetal movements. By this time the fetus was 18 to 20 weeks old and the last born baby at least 7 months. This observation indicates that ovulation and conception can occur during lactation. Moreover, lactation can be quite adequate even in the presence of a new pregnancy.

THE ABDOMINAL WALL

In many women the musculature of the abdominal wall regains its previous tonicity slowly and imperfectly. A great deal depends on the amount of its distention during gestation, but mostly on the individual's constitution. Sometimes the abdominal wall is so weakened that the rectus muscles are attenuated and separated in the midline. This is called a *diastasis recti*. The abdominal wall is thinned where the muscle bundles are separated and the contents of the peritoneal cavity, including the uterus, are easily palpated.

THE BREASTS

The major change in the breasts post partum is the establishment of lactation. A good supply of milk after delivery depends on the proper functioning of four hormones. During pregnancy the duct system proliferates extensively in response to stimulation by estrogen. Likewise, the alveolar system undergoes pronounced growth from the effects of progesterone. Therefore, estrogen and progesterone prepare the mammary glands for the function they are to assume during the puerperium.

If the breasts are not properly acted on during pregnancy by these two hormones, the supply of milk will be limited or absent.

Soon after the baby is born there is a secretion from the breasts, but for the first few days this is *colostrum* (see below) and not milk. Milk is not actually produced (galactopoiesis) until prolactin, a hormone from the anterior pituitary, has had its effect on the mammary glands previously prepared by estrogen and progesterone. Finally, milk is not ejected from the alveoli where it is produced unless the myoepithelial cells contract to propel the milk through the ducts to the nipple (galactokinesis). The milk ejection factor is oxytocin, which is produced by the posterior pituitary gland in response to the suckling stimulus. Hence, all four hormones are essential for the normal function of the mammary glands.

On the third day after delivery, the breasts become harder, the veins prominent and the whole organ fuller and heavier. The patient describes a prickling or burning sensation. Soon the swelling reaches a considerable degree. The individual milk ducts can be felt as hard strings and the lobes as hard lumps. The breasts feel hot to touch. Rarely, they become reddened and sometimes there is a bluish turgescence of the surface.

The symptoms associated with the milk coming into the breasts are much more distressing in primiparas than in multiparas. In multiparas, the breasts do not become active so suddenly, but lactation begins more gradually and seldom do the breasts swell so that the skin is as tightly stretched over them as in primiparas.

Even though the breasts show the classic signs of an inflammatory process, including tumor, dolor, calor and rubor, the phenomenon is not a true inflammation. The patient usually has no fever. Although transient single temperature spikes of 101° F. have been attributed to "milk fever" in the past, focal or systemic sources of infection are more likely the real cause.

The first milk, colostrum, resembles the serous secretion that may be expressed from the nipple in the latter part of pregnancy. It is clear or only slightly cloudy, sticky, and contains yellow streaks.

Colostrum is made up of fat globules, a watery fluid and the so-called colostrum corpuscles. Colostrum corpuscles are round, ovoid or stellate cells with one to three nuclei. They sometimes show ameboid movement. They contain numerous fine fat globules and are believed to be altered gland epithelium, leukocytes or mast cells which have phagocytized fat globules. They persist for four to six days. Colostrum contains nearly 15 per cent of lactalbumin and lactoglobulin, with much fat; it possesses little, if any, casein.

Robinson described the normal lactating cycle in three phases: (1) The *period of filling* lasts 10 to 30 minutes. During this time the mother becomes increasingly aware of a sense of heaviness. (2) The *period of emptying* usually lasts five to seven minutes, rarely 10 minutes. Emptying of the breasts is brought about by the rhythmic pumping out of the milk by myoepithelial cell contractions at the rate of 40 to 60 jets per minute. (3) A *refractory period* sets in after emptying and lasts two and one-half to three hours. During this time manual expression produces only small beads of milk on the nipple.

Human milk has a characteristic odor and sweetish taste. Its specific gravity varies from 1.026 to 1.036. It is neutral or alkaline. On microscopic study innumerable fine, fat droplets and occasionally a glandular epithelial cell or a leukocyte are observed.

The composition of human milk varies from day to day and from hour to hour. It contains 87.5 per cent water and 12.5 per cent solids. Of the solids 6.2 per cent is milk sugar, 3.8 per cent fat, 2.3 per cent proteins (lactoglobulin 1.3 per cent, and casein 1 per cent) and 0.7 per cent salts. Breast milk is a vital secretion that contains all nutrient requirements for the infant, ready for immediate absorption, as well as antibodies against infection. Its quantity and quality vary considerably. Many drugs ingested by the mother will appear in the milk. Some have been reported to have adverse effects on the nursing infant. The spectrum of agents found in the milk has been reviewed by Sapeika.

He noted that, among central nervous system depressants, alcohol, barbiturates and bromides were excreted in the milk. Generally, the amounts are too small to affect the infant, although bromides may cause skin eruptions. Morphine is not found in the milk, even among addicts. Autonomic drugs, such as atropine and nicotine, appear in the milk and may affect both lactation and the child. Milk flow is diminished. Phenolphthalein, among the purgatives, crosses into the milk in small amounts but has no overt effect on the infant's bowel function. Many antibiotic agents are found in the milk. Sulfonamides appear in both free and conjugated form for days after administration has stopped, but toxic effects are negligible. Iodine and fluorine are excreted in the milk. Ergot alkaloids may cause toxic effects. Radioactive substances pass to the milk according to the molecular size of the molecule. Both radioactive sodium and iodine, for example, are found in the milk soon after administration and may still be recoverable four to five days later. In general, it is wise to review the mother's drug intake at the time lactation is undertaken.

AFTER-PAINS

In the absence of infection or traumatic injury most women feel well during the puerperal period. A multipara is likely to be annoyed by *after-pains*. These are uterine contractions which occur more or less regularly for one to three days after the delivery. They tend to occur especially when the child is being nursed. They are most pronounced when foreign matter, such as pieces of membrane, placenta or blood clots, have been left in the uterus. Women who have had overdistention of the uterus by twins or hydramnios are likely to suffer with after-pains.

TEMPERATURE

In normal parturients the temperature should not be above 37.2° C. (99° F.). The temperature may rise 0.5° F. after labor, but falls to normal within 12 hours and then shows the physiologic diurnal variations, but these do not exceed 1° F. If the temperature rises above 37.2° C. (99° F.) there usually is some cause for it, perhaps infection. *Milk fever*, or the transient febrile spike sometimes seen on the third day post partum, is probably due to genital infection and not to breast engorgement.

PULSE

In general, the pulse during the puerperium ranges from 68 to 80 per minute. Higher rates sometimes occur, even in healthy women.

A peculiar phenomenon is sometimes observed in healthy puerperas. The pulse rate immediately after delivery may be as low as 40 per minute. The cause is not known. It is probably the result of a combination of factors, including the patient's horizontal position in bed, her emotional sense of relief and satisfaction, the enforced rest after her long period of strenuous activity in labor and during delivery, the diminished food intake and the great excretion of liquid in milk, lochia and perspiration. It is of great prognostic significance because a slow pulse indicates that all is well.

A rapid pulse, in the absence of fever, points to hemorrhage, recovery from severe hemorrhage or cardiac disease. One must be careful about diagnosing cardiac disease during pregnancy and the puerperium, however, because murmurs are common. During the puerperium, the pulse rate is very labile. It fluctuates with the after-pains and with any excitement.

BLOOD

There is an impressive increase in blood volume post partum as a persistent reflection of the increase which took place during pregnancy (see Chapter 41). McLennan and Thouin found the plasma volume at term increased about 40 per cent and the total blood volume was 32 per cent greater than in normal control patients. The erythrocyte volume, on the other hand, rose only about 20 per cent. If major hemorrhage occurred at the time of delivery, corresponding reductions in red cell mass are encountered. Within a week after delivery, the blood volume returns virtually to the prepregnancy level.

KIDNEYS AND URINARY TRACT

In the first twelve hours after delivery retention of urine may occur, based on the patient's inability to void. This is due to some loss of detrusor tone or a general lack of elasticity of the bladder, inability of many patients to urinate in the horizontal position, edematous swelling of the vulva and urethra, reflex spasm of the urethral muscle from pain due to stitches in the perineum and injury to the bladder trigone and urethral orifice. However, most puerperas urinate spontaneously, especially if allowed out of bed.

Cystoscopic examination of the bladder after labor shows the effect of the sustained pressure and trauma of the natural forces of delivery or those of manual or instrumental manipulation. Edema may be present together with ecchymosis of the surface mucosa or underlying muscularis. The bladder trigone and the urethral orifices especially are edematous and show minute blood extravasations. Laceration of the urogenital septum and of the connective tissue around the base of the bladder causes the anterior wall of the vagina to prolapse, carrying the urethra and neck of the bladder with it.

Proteinuria occurs in about 40 per cent of women after labor, but it usually disappears before the third day. Organic causes, such as cystitis, pyelitis, nephritis and preeclampsia, must be considered, particularly if accompanied by suggestive symptoms or objective signs. To avoid confusion from admixture with lochia, only "clean" midstream or catheterized urine specimens should be examined.

INTESTINAL TRACT

The puerpera is thirsty and drinks a great deal, but usually her appetite is poor for the first three days. Loss of fluids during labor and in the lochia, urine and sweat explains the thirst.

Immediately after labor, the abdomen is flat, and may even be slightly concave. Moderate tympany is normal in the puerperium and is due to reduced intestinal peristalsis.

Spontaneous defecation is rare during the first few days. The causes of the obstipation are several: (1) The woman eats little and the excretion of fluids is so rapid that the intestinal contents are relatively dry. (2) The abdominal and perineal muscles, because of overstretching, are ineffectual in performing their work. (3) Perineal pain may serve as an inhibiting factor.

WEIGHT

The patient's weight undergoes decided changes during and after labor. The average loss in labor and delivery is about 5.8 kg. or nearly 12 lb. (Dieckman and Stout; Stander and Pastore). Most of this loss consists of the fetus and secundines together with urinary and insensible water loss. Continued loss may occur irregularly throughout the puerperium, ranging on average from less than 1 kg. to as much as 2.3 kg. (Chesley). However, many patients do not continue to lose weight. By the fourth day as many as 63 per cent show a gain over their immediate postpartum weight. The difference is probably due to early ambulation and early return to a normal diet.

REFERENCES

Bernstine, J. B., and Bernstine, R. L.: Lochia: A quantitative study. West J. Surg. 59:312, 1951.

Chesley, L. C.: Weight changes and water balance in normal and toxemic pregnancy. Amer. J. Obstet. Gynec. 48:565, 1944.

Dieckmann, W. J., and Stout, F.: Insensible and total weight changes during labor and delivery and gynecologic operations. Amer. J. Obstet. Gynec. 59:1021, 1950.

Hofbauer, J.: Defensive mechanism of parametrium during pregnancy and labor. Bull. Johns Hopkins Hosp. 38:255, 1926.

McLennan, C. E., and Thouin, L. G.: Blood volume in pregnancy: A critical review and preliminary report of results with a new technique. Amer. J. Obstet. Gynec. 55:189, 1948.

Robinson, M.: Failing lactation: Study in 1100 cases. Lancet 1:66, 1943.

Sapeika, N.: Excretion of drugs in human milk: A review. J. Obstet. Gynaec. Brit. Emp. 54:426, 1947.

Sharman, A.: Menstruation after childbirth. J. Obstet. Gynaec. Brit. Emp. 58:440, 1951.

Sharman, A.: Ovulation after pregnancy. Fertil. Steril. 2:371, 1951.

Smith, A. A.: The lochia has changed. J. Med. Ass. Georgia 51:532, 1962.

Stander, H. J., and Pastore, J. B.: Weight changes during pregnancy and puerperium. Amer. J. Obstet. Gynec. 39:928, 1940.

Williams, J. W.: Regeneration of uterine mucosa after delivery with special reference to placental site. Amer. J. Obstet. Gynec. 22:664, 1931.

Chapter 26

Postpartum Care

After delivery of the placenta the puerperal period begins. It does not end until all the organs of reproduction have returned to normal. This period of six to eight weeks or longer is generally divided into a strictly *lying-in interval* of two to five days and a further interval of five to seven weeks during which the patient gradually resumes her usual activities.

LYING-IN INTERVAL

Immediately after delivery the mother requires rest. This should be assured even if it is necessary to prescribe a sedative. Most patients are exhausted and fall asleep promptly, especially if they have been sedated during labor or have been given general inhalation anesthesia for the delivery. Others are exhilarated and require some form of tranquilization, sedation or analgesia. This ensures relative freedom from pain for a few hours and permits the patient to sleep or rest. If the patient is awake and not nauseated, oral medication may be given, perhaps in the form of codeine. Recent evidence showing the deleterious effect of aspirin on platelet function suggests we should stop its routine use during this time.

It may be necessary to bar visitors, draw the window shades and disconnect the telephone. It is wise to sequester the baby in the nursery for at least the first six to eight hours to ensure that the mother will get sufficient rest. For psychologic reasons, the mother and baby may be in the same room throughout hospitalization (see Chapter 11).

Vulvar pads are not necessary. If used, they should be applied loosely and changed after each urination and bowel movement and whenever soiled from any other cause. Douches should never be given.

The patient should be encouraged to urinate as soon as she is refreshed, and every effort should be made to avoid catheterization of the urinary bladder because of the real risk of infection. Usually sitting straight up in bed or, if necessary, at the bedside or on the toilet will permit spontaneous micturition. There is no harm in getting the patient out of bed to sit on a bedpan placed on a chair. Better still, she may walk to the bathroom with assistance.

Catheterization should be carried out as often as necessary, but only when necessary. Only a lubricated soft rubber catheter should be used; a glass or metal catheter may injure an already edematous or ecchymotic area. After the patient begins to void spontaneously, it may become necessary to ensure that emptying is complete by means of catheterization. This can be done immediately after a spontaneous urination to determine residual volume. Under normal circumstances, less than 60 ml. of urine is obtained. The use of prophylactic antibiotics to prevent urinary tract infection from intermittent catheterization is not defensible. Needless to say, however, infection should be treated vigorously when it arises.

Episiotomy pain is effectively treated with mild analgesics. Exposing the perineum to a heat lamp or sitting in a tub of tepid water for 30 minutes several times a day is most helpful for painful episiotomy wounds.

Normal bowel function should be resumed by the fourth day. Proper diet and a mild laxative may help. There is usually no necessity for giving a laxative until the third or fourth day after delivery. Rectal suppositories will eliminate the need for enemas in most instances. If obstipation occurs, it may be necessary to prescribe an enema. Rarely, one may be required to break up a fecal impaction digitally.

Diet during this interval will depend on the patient's tolerance. Usually, patients are thirsty because of relative dehydration and, therefore, they should be given primarily liquids on the first day. Others are hungry, particularly patients who have not been given narcotic-analgesics or inhalation anesthesia. No restrictions should be imposed on these patients with regard to diet.

The breasts do not usually require special care during the lying-in period. Before each nursing, the breasts and nipples should be cleansed with soap and water. No antiseptics need be placed on the nipples unless they are cracked. Some women find the nipples very sensitive at first. Tolerance to suckling may be increased by daily rubbing with cocoa butter during the last month or so before delivery. The baby should be put to breast only for a few minutes at a time at the beginning, gradually lengthening the time at each breast.

During the first 24 hours, the baby is nursed two to three times if the patient has had sufficient rest. Otherwise, the baby should be withheld from the breast until the patient has rested. After the first 24 hours, the child may be nursed every three to four hours or irregularly "on demand." It does not matter which schedule is followed. The child should not be permitted to pull on the nipple after the breast is empty because cracks and infection may result. The mother should be advised not to watch the baby constantly while it is at the breast; this not only strains her eyes and produces headache but also strains the muscles of the neck and back. She may sit up leaning against a back rest or lie down to nurse her baby. Generally, the baby should not be permitted to nurse for more than 10 minutes at each feeding.

Heavy pendulous breasts should be supported with a breast binder or good maternity brassiere. Engorgement may be relieved by a snug-fitting breast binder, ice bags and analgesics.

For the mother who does not wish to nurse her baby, suppressive measures are available. Fluid restriction is of no value at all (King) and may only result in dehydration. Tight supportive breast binders, snugly applied before engorgement begins, and continually readjusted as the breast size and configuration change, are very effective. The additional use of local ice packs and analgesic agents is generally sufficient. The binder should be worn day and night, except during showers, and maintained for several days after engorgement has subsided.

Hormonal suppressants of lactation, although widely used, are not entirely satisfactory. Estrogens do not actually interfere with lactation, but rather seem to prevent breast engorgement in about 25 per cent of nonnursing mothers. To counterbalance this potential benefit is the undesirable effect of withdrawal uterine bleeding sometimes seen. Long-acting preparations, such as estradiol valerate, appear to be superior to the short-acting preparations for the control of postpartum breast manifestations (Gold et al.). Whether the expense and the risk of bleeding, albeit a small risk, are warranted when other means are apparently just as effective is a matter for the individual physician to decide.

Fissured nipples should be treated immediately with tincture of benzoin and an antibiotic ointment. For the nursing mother, the breast pump should be used to obtain milk for the baby for 24 to 48 hours. In this way, lactation will be maintained and the fissure given an opportunity to heal.

Patients should be encouraged to nurse their babies. The practice is slowly gaining in popularity again as more and more women begin to understand and appreciate its real benefits, especially in terms of personal gratification, the establishment of meaningful and lasting mother-child relationships and its beneficial influence on the psychologic development of the infant.

Sedatives such as codeine and butazolidine should be given for after-pains. Retention of clots or placental tissue or infection should be suspected if very severe after-pains occur. Barbiturates should be given if needed so the mother may get sufficient sleep. Persistent insomnia is an important symptom because it may be a forerunner of puerperal psychosis (see Chapter 11).

Visitors should be limited in number during the first week and certainly all visitors with colds or infections should be barred. When making rounds at a hospital, the physician should first visit all his "clean" obstetric patients, keeping those with infections for last. He should wash his hands well before and after seeing each patient.

All patients with infection should be isolated immediately. The perineum should always be inspected when fever develops. If infected stitches are present, they should be removed. A vaginal examination should be made if necessary, but with great gentleness. Antibiotics may have to be prescribed as indicated.

If the perineal wound becomes red and swollen, one or more sutures should be removed even if there is no elevation of temperature. An infected perineum should be opened for drainage as soon as the infection is detected.

Bleeding during the lying-in period is usually due to subinvolution, retention of secundines and/or infection. Treatment consists of rest in bed and ergonovine by mouth. If hemorrhage is severe, the uterus should be curetted.

An abdominal binder is generally not necessary, but may be used especially in multiparas with relaxed abdominal walls. It should be applied loosely because all it does is relieve the feeling of emptiness and help steady the uterus when the patient moves in bed during the first few days.

The normal patient is encouraged to ambulate from the first day on. This favors drainage from the uterus, permits spontaneous urination and prevents thrombosis and embolism. She is assisted at first, and as soon as feasible is permitted to walk around and go to the bathroom. This applies even to those women who have had cesarean section. No adverse effects are seen from this procedure. However, a patient who bleeds should not get out of bed until the bleeding has been controlled. Shower or tub baths should be taken daily once the patient is fully ambulatory.

Patients without complications may go home, on average, two to five days after delivery. Local practices vary widely in this regard, depending on costs, demands for bed utilization and availability of home care facilities.

RECUPERATIVE PERIOD

On her return home the patient should go to bed to rest there for a half hour. During the next two weeks or so, activities should be gradually increased. It is important that the patient not be allowed to overtire herself. If she is feeling well, arbitrary restrictions are not applicable. Most women find it difficult to resume full household activities for at least two weeks, sometimes longer. It is probably wise for them not to tax themselves in this regard. Riding and walking outdoors should be minimized during this interval also. Baths should be taken daily.

During the recuperative period, a tactful attempt should be made to keep away oversolicitous friends and relatives. After the second week, the patient should spend at least one or two hours each day sitting, walking or riding in the open air, especially when the sun is shining. Normal activities are resumed gradually. Social functions should be reduced to a minimum.

During the first few weeks the patient's mental condition should be watched because of the common mild depression that occurs (see Chapter 11). Intercourse should be avoided until the perineal and uterine wounds are healed, an interval of at least four weeks. Contraception is advisable. Hyperthyroidism, pulmonary tuberculosis and cholecystitis may flare up after childbirth. If the history or symptoms suggest such preexisting conditions, close observation should be made during this interval.

POSTPARTUM EXAMINATION

The patient should return for an examination when the baby is six to eight weeks old. At this time the physician should determine the condition of the breasts and nipples, abdominal wall, perineum, bladder and rectal supports, adnexa and broad ligaments, size and position of the uterus, presence of any exudates and tone of the sphincter ani. The cervix should be palpated and inspected. Laceration, eversion, so-called erosion, cyst, leukorrheal discharge and any other abnormality should be observed. Appropriate diagnostic and therapeutic measures should be undertaken as indicated. A troublesome vaginal discharge may be treated. Contraceptive advice should also be given at this time.

If bleeding occurs during the recuperative period, it is usually due to uterine subinvolution. Rest in bed and ergonovine by mouth usually suffice to check this bleeding. If bleeding persists, the cause is likely to be retained secundines and curettage will be necessary.

The patient should be warned that the first menses may be profuse. Rest in bed and application of a cold pack to the lower abdomen are sometimes helpful.

If the cervix is red and granular, or excessive or irritating discharge is present, Papanicolaou smears should be obtained before initiating treatment. If negative, either electrocautery or cryosurgery is effective in clearing up the problem. If cytologic examination is positive or suspicious, however, it is mandatory that appropriate diagnostic measures be taken, including biopsies, to rule out malignancy.

POSTPUERPERAL PERIOD

The examination made six to eight weeks after delivery is too often considered "final." This is unfortunate because both the physician and the patient regard this as the last contact until a new pregnancy begins. While most women are in such good condition that they need not return until a new pregnancy occurs, some women, unfortunately, are not in this category. They have cervical lesions, pyelitis, hypertension, nephritis, heart disease and other complications which require continued observation and treatment.

It is gross negligence not to ensure that follow-up care is being given. The physician himself may provide such ongoing care or he may wish to refer the patient to a generalist or to a specialist with a wider experience in the management of the problem. Observations and treatment usually must extend over months or even years. Women should be educated to come for routine examination, especially of the breasts and pelvic organs, at least once, preferably twice, a year. Were this a universal custom, much invalidism would be prevented and many deaths from cancer of the breasts and uterus avoided. All women, pregnant or nonpregnant, young or old, should have Papanicolaou smears made at least once a year.

It should be emphasized that, just as prepartum care saves the lives of thousands of women and babies each year, postpartum care, if conscientiously carried out, results in the cure of many abnormal conditions and in the prevention of many others. Most older gynecologic patients come to physicians with ailments which are directly attributable to childbirth, and a large proportion of these women would have been spared their annoying illness had they received proper postpartum attention.

REFERENCES

Gold, J. J., Soihet, S., Hankin, H., and Cohen, M. R.: Hormone therapy to control postpartum breast manifestations. Amer. J. Obstet. Gynec. 78:86, 1959.

King, A. G.: Prevention of puerperal breast engorgement with large doses of long-acting estrogen. Amer. J. Obstet. Gynec. 78:80, 1959.

SECTION FOUR

PATHOLOGY OF PREGNANCY

Chapter 27

Minor Disturbances in Pregnancy

There is a wide spectrum of variegated symptoms experienced by women during pregnancy. Most are negligible in their manifestation and transient; others are severe, even to the point of incapacitation. They may reflect insignificant or minimally important pathologic conditions, but are of sufficient intensity to warrant our discussing them in some detail.

LEG CRAMPS

Acute, intensely painful cramps in the lower extremities, involving strong, unremitting contraction of the gastrocnemius muscles, occur especially during the night in many pregnant women between the twenty-fourth and thirty-fourth week of pregnancy. The cause is unknown, although many theories abound, particularly relating to calcium intake. If excessive quantities of milk or dicalcium phosphate are ingested, patients are said to be predisposed to muscular tetany (Page and Page). Whether or not reducing milk intake will help is doubtful, however.

Most patients soon learn that they can abort an attack by sharply stretching the involved muscle. They find that they have a moment or two warning, even if they are asleep, during which they can get out of bed and stand up, placing the heel on the floor and pulling the foot up, thereby averting the acute contracture of the calf muscle. Once the cramp has occurred, gentle kneading is effective.

SYNCOPE AND DIZZINESS

Often pregnant women have attacks of fainting or dizziness. It is especially prevalent among anemic patients. The condition is not serious; hence, there is no cause for alarm. As soon as a woman feels faint, she should lie down on a couch or bed or gently slip down to the floor and lie flat; sitting down and lowering the head between the knees is equally valuable. The faintness will pass in a few minutes. If the attacks are frequent, it is wise to keep spirits of ammonia or smelling salts within easy reach. The cause is undoubtedly related to the cardiovascular changes of pregnancy coupled with increased vagal responsivity. Because anemia aggravates the intrinsic tendency toward syncope, it is important that these patients be studied hematologically.

BACKACHE

Most multiparas and some nulliparas complain of backache, usually due to relaxation of the sacroiliac joints, change in posture because of shifting of the center of equilibrium (see Chapter 7) and other factors. Adhesive strapping over the low back region and sacroiliac joints will give immediate relief, but a few days after its removal the backache usually returns. In most instances a tightly fitting corset or abdominal support will relieve the backache. Warmth from a hot water bag or electric pad will provide symptomatic relief. A bed board placed beneath the mattress to ensure a firm sleeping surface will also help considerably.

VARICOSE VEINS

Varicose veins develop in most pregnant women to a greater or lesser degree (Fig. 204). Dilatation of the venous system appears to take place in a widespread distribution, affecting not only the legs but also the vulva, the pelvis, the abdominal wall and the breasts (Fig. 205). The cause is unknown. The commonly accepted view is that lower extremity varicosities result from venous engorgement due to the pressure on the iliac veins by the enlarged uterus. However, in many women varices develop in the first few weeks of pregnancy, well before pressure on the iliac veins can have occurred. Indeed, occasionally a woman knows she is pregnant before she has missed a menstrual period by the appearance or aggravation of varicose veins. This observation suggests an endocrine cause for increasing the intravascular volume while producing generalized venous stasis and passive dilatation of the venous wall. Heredity is undoubtedly a primary factor in many instances.

As a rule, varicose veins develop toward the end of the first trimester and progressively become aggravated until delivery. Both the greater and lesser saphenous systems are involved and can be palpated as tense cordlike tortuosities. Occasionally, numerous spider varices develop on the

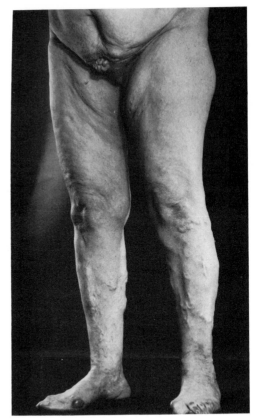

Figure 204 Typical appearance of lower extremity varicose veins in an elderly multipara. This patient also had varicosities in the vagina and on the vulva.

skin; they are disfiguring and may resemble diffuse hemangiomas. The vulvar veins may also enlarge and become varicosed, since the superficial external pudendal vein may empty into the greater saphenous vein in the groin. A feeling of heaviness in the legs and edematous ankles are the usual symptoms. When the vulvar veins are also affected, there may be considerable discomfort. Added to this is the mental anguish associated with the cosmetic disfigurement of the legs.

Fortunately, most of the enlarged veins disappear after delivery, sometimes completely. Many remain and enlarge progressively with each succeeding pregnancy and often without a subsequent pregnancy. Usually, supportive elastic stockings relieve the discomfort and prevent excessive enlargement. Lying down for short periods several times during the day with

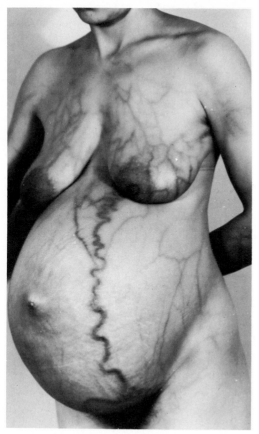

Figure 205 Distribution of anterior abdominal wall and breast venous distention in late pregnancy in a patient who also has large varicose veins on the vulva, in the vagina and in both lower extremities.

the legs elevated on pillows usually prevents or corrects edema. Sclerosing injections or surgery is unnecessary and should be avoided in most pregnant patients. Aside from the fact that many of the varices disappear after delivery, the results of treatment after delivery are better and more permanent. Active therapy during pregnancy may be necessary under the following complicating circumstances: the discomfort is severe; vulvar veins are so greatly enlarged that delivery may be expected to be complicated; the varices are so thin-walled that there is danger of rupture and hemorrhage; spreading superficial thrombophlebitis occurs, or a varicose ulcer develops. These complications occur infrequently and usually can be prevented by supportive stockings and by periodically elevating the legs.

Surgical stripping of varicose veins is probably inadvisable on an elective basis during pregnancy. Those with severe varices of legs and vulva, especially with intense symptoms, can be considered for the operation (Weismann and Jenkins). Even after stripping, however, recurrences are seen in subsequent pregnancies. It is advisable to delay venous stripping until 8 to 12 weeks post partum (McCausland et al.).

THROMBOPHLEBITIS

Antepartum venous thrombosis is rare but occasionally may involve either the superficial or the deep veins. Most thrombi in the superficial veins are inflammatory thrombophlebitic in character. In this type there is usually pain, local heat, tenderness and redness, as well as fever. Embolic phenomena are uncommon because the inflammation which precedes their formation causes the thrombi to adhere to the vein wall from the start.

Deep vein thrombosis is also infrequent during pregnancy, but of much more serious potential consequences. Many thromboses are mild and involve only the lower leg. They are usually unilateral. The patient complains of slight discomfort and pain in the leg on walking. She may notice enlargement of the ankle and leg. On examination there is measurable edema of the involved extremity and pain on pressure over the deep veins in the calf. Dorsiflexion of the ankle will cause pain in the calf in about 40 per cent of the cases (Homans' sign). Pulmonary emboli may occur when the deep veins are involved, especially when the thrombus has propagated itself as high as the thigh. Usually, this can be recognized when there is edema above the knee and tenderness on pressure over the deep veins in the thigh, but all too often there are no clear-cut signs to indicate the actual extent of the disease.

Superficial thrombosis is treated by conservative methods: bed rest, elevation of the leg and application of heat. Because of the local tenderness, bedclothes may not be tolerated. A cradle may be fashioned to support the sheets and blankets so that they do not come in contact with the legs. Under no circumstances must the leg be massaged.

Use of anticoagulant agents is generally reserved for deep vein thrombosis. They are very effective in preventing propagation and the very serious complication of pulmonary embolization. Anticoagulation in pregnancy is warranted under these circumstances, but the practice is not without risk. The coumarins readily cross the placenta and may cause fetal hemorrhage with ensuing damage or death. Heparin, being a larger molecule, will not traverse the placenta and is, therefore, not likely to affect the fetus. Heparin is the preferred anticoagulant agent in pregnancy, although it is more difficult to use because it requires periodic administration by injection. Bleeding and clotting time prolongation should be maintained at a minimum to avoid hemorrhage. At term or in labor, the anticoagulation should be discontinued until after delivery. It is advisable to start anticoagulant therapy after delivery in all patients who have had a thrombotic venous complication during pregnancy.

Pulmonary embolus may occur rarely in the presence of thrombophlebitis, even while the patient is on anticoagulant therapy. Such uncontrolled conditions demand a more aggressive approach. Vena cava ligation may be required. Newer methods are available with use of partially occlusive "filters" across the vena cava; these devices avert the severe edema and stasis that can occur after ligation. Superimposition of infection to produce septic thrombophlebitis complicates the problem greatly and requires special measures (see Chapter 70).

HEMORRHOIDS

Analogous to other venous disturbances, many pregnant women are troubled by hemorrhoids. They are more common in multiparas than in nulliparas. The usual symptom is bleeding during defecation. Pain may be present. Hemorrhoids are always aggravated by constipation and by straining during defecation. Hence, proper care of the bowels is most important in their prevention and treatment. When hemorrhoids bleed, the patient should take a stool softening agent, such as Metamucil, once or twice a day. If the hemorrhoids are swollen and painful, ice or cold witch hazel compresses held firmly against the anus for a few minutes may help considerably. Opium ointment or suppository relieves pain very effectively. With a lubricated finger, using great care and gentleness, edematous hemorrhoids can be pushed back into the rectum. If force is necessary, the hemorrhoids should not be replaced. A thrombosed hemorrhoid causes considerable pain; the clot can be easily removed under local anesthesia.

NOSEBLEED

Slight bleeding from the nose is frequent during pregnancy. Nothing need be done in most instances because the epistaxis is scant. Occasionally, pressure on the nostril from which the bleeding issues is necessary. If the bleeding is persistent or profuse, the patient should be examined for local ulcerations, polyps or other sources of bleeding, most particularly the arterial plexus on the medial wall that is so commonly subject to traumatic bleeding. This site, called Kiesselbach's plexus, is located on the anterior aspect of the cartilaginous nasal septum, where small superficial vessels may spontaneously rupture. Packing or cauterization may be necessary, but direct pressure alone usually suffices.

URINARY FREQUENCY

This is common during the second and third months and again in the last few weeks of gestation. There is no treatment needed. It is caused by pressure of the enlarging uterus on the urinary bladder in conjunction with concomitant pelvic congestion. If the patient has nocturia, disturbing her sleep, it is perhaps advisable for her not to drink any fluids after her evening meal. A soporific agent may have to be prescribed. Coassociated dysuria suggests the likelihood that cystitis requiring diagnosis and treatment is present.

HEADACHE

Headache occurs frequently in pregnancy. It seems to be considerably more common among women who wear glasses. There is no need to have the eyes examined because a change of glasses seldom helps. Mild symptomatic treatment is generally effective. Severe, persistent headache demands urgent attention because it may represent a premonitory sign of preeclampsia (see Chapter 36).

INSOMNIA

Some pregnant women have difficulty in falling asleep and others who fall asleep wake early in the morning or even after only one or two hours without any apparent reason. These patients should be reassured. If at all possible, they might be advised against thinking about serious problems after they retire, acknowledging that anxious women will find this difficult to accomplish. Such mental processes interfere with sleep. A hot tub bath will induce sleep in some women. The occasional use of tranquilizing agents is very effective and is probably not harmful.

DROWSINESS

Many pregnant women feel sleepy a great deal of the time and they tire easily. Sometimes this symptom discloses an unsuspected pregnancy. As a general rule, the patient should be assured and instructed merely to respond appropriately by resting whenever she feels tired. As to cause, it has been conjectured that perhaps the somnolence and drowsiness are due to the progesterone produced in such large amounts during pregnancy (see Chapter

4). Pharmacologically, progesterone produces anesthesia when given intraperitoneally in animals (Selye).

EDEMA

Moderate swelling of the feet and ankles is probably universal in pregnancy, appearing especially during hot weather. Pronounced swelling of the feet and ankles or other part of the body should make one suspect preeclampsia (see Chapter 36), particularly if it arises acutely. However, mild edema unassociated with other characteristic signs or symptoms of this disorder is of no special significance. It is the result of venous and lymphatic stasis; it is probably contributed to by changes in osmotic pressure in blood and tissue fluids and by altered capillary permeability. It is generally relieved by periodic elevation of the legs during the course of the day. Although transiently improved by diuretic agents, it promptly returns. The risks inherent in the use of powerful diuretics do not warrant their administration for correcting such a mild and inconsequential symptom as dependent edema.

VAGINAL DISCHARGE

Some pregnant women complain of a vaginal discharge. A search should be made for *Trichomonas vaginalis, Candida albicans* and gonococci (see Chapter 40). Often no specific organism can be found to explain the discharge. Here the discharge may reflect only an increase in accumulated vaginal secretions, a condition called *hydrorrhea gravidarum*. Treatment is ineffectual for this annoying symptom.

PALPITATION

A fluttering in the sternal area occasionally occurs and often frightens a pregnant woman. Thyroid function should be determined if it occurs often or if the tachycardia is persistent. Reassurance that there is nothing wrong with the heart helps immensely. A mild sedative or tranquilizer taken for a few days at a time may be helpful.

PICA

Cravings and pica for substances that are not ordinarily considered part of the diet during pregnancy are fairly common, approaching pathologic proportions in some women. There is a wide range of items called for, some apparently based on cultural or ethnic considerations. Generally, such cravings are of no real significance, but at times patients may satisfy their yearnings almost to the exclusion of adequate dietary intake. Iron deficiency anemias have been reported to be a common coassociated phenomenon in starch pica (Keith et al.). Posner et al. found carbohydrates to be the most common craving in 86 per cent of their patients, including Argo starch, sweets, fruits and juices. In the series studied by Harries and Hughes, the preponderant craving was for fruit, vegetables, candy, pickles and raw cereals. Mud, clay, chalk, ice and coal constitute other substances for which patients express pica.

REFERENCES

Harries, J. M., and Hughes, T. F.: Enumeration of the "cravings" of some pregnant women. Brit. Med. J. 2:39, 1958.

Keith, L., Evenhouse, H., and Webster, A.: Amylophagia during pregnancy. Obstet. Gynec. 32:415, 1968.

McCausland, A. M., Hyman, C., Winsor, T., and Trotter, A. D., Jr.: Venous distensibility during pregnancy. Amer. J. Obstet. Gynec. 81:472, 1961.

Page, E. W., and Page, E. P.: Leg cramps in pregnancy: Etiology and treatment. Obstet. Gynec. 1:94, 1953.

Posner, L. B., McCottry, C. M., and Posner, A. C.: Pregnancy cravings and pica. Obstet. Gynec. 9:270, 1957.

Selye, H.: Personal communication.

Weismann, R. E., and Jenkins, E. W.: Saphenous vein stripping for varicose veins during pregnancy. J.A.M.A. 161:1459, 1956.

Chapter 28

Pelvic Displacements

PENDULOUS ABDOMEN

Normally, the gravid uterus is anteverted. During the first few months it lies on the bladder but it is soon directed upward into the abdomen by the pubis. Later in pregnancy it is always anteverted. When the anteversion becomes pathologic so that the uterine corpus protrudes acutely against the anterior abdominal wall, or more often through a diastasis recti, it is called *pendulous abdomen* (Fig. 81). It is a rare occurrence in nulliparas. Causative or contributory factors include defective abdominal wall, such as with diastasis recti, and contracted pelvis or kyphosis.

During pregnancy a pendulous abdomen causes a sense of weight and distention, dragging pains in the loins and the abdomen and at the costal insertions of the rectus muscles. Intertrigo of the lower abdomen and thighs occurs and, occasionally, there are varices and edema of the vulva.

During labor, a pendulous abdomen may cause serious dystocia. The uterus is thrown so far forward that its axis forms an acute angle with the pelvic axis. The cervix is pulled up into the hollow of the sacrum, sometimes even above the sacral promontory, dilatation is delayed and the posterior uterine wall is overstretched. These conditions may combine with obstructed labor to lead to rupture of the uterus. Malpresentations, such as shoulder and breech presentations, and malpositions, especially anterior parietal bone presentation, are particularly prone to occur.

The pendulous abdomen can be corrected effectively with an abdominal corset as soon as the uterus rises out of the

pelvis. During labor a binder may be worn. In some patients it may be necessary to push the pendent uterus upward during each contraction until the fetal head enters the pelvis. After the head engages, cervical dilatation usually proceeds rapidly. Delay in descent is common in the second stage, and the terminal mechanisms of labor (see Chapter 18), especially internal rotation, are often arrested. The exaggerated lithotomy position is especially useful at this stage of labor. Midforceps operation may be necessary under these circumstances, if such conservative measures are ineffective, and must sometimes be undertaken to prevent uterine rupture.

UTERINE RETRODISPLACEMENTS

Retroversion of the uterus (Fig. 206) is common in pregnancy, usually spontaneously correcting itself as the uterus enlarges. Unless the displacement of the uterus is complicated by adhesions, there are no symptoms because the uterus unfolds as it grows out of the pelvis. Sometimes there is a sensation of fullness in the pelvis or there may be pain radiating from the sacral and lumbar plexuses. When the uterus is adherent, which is rare, bladder symptoms will arise before the end of the third month. Urinary frequency, dysuria and urinary retention occur, and patients have the feeling that the bladder has not been emptied completely. The bladder becomes enormously distended. Constant dribbling may occur as a result of retention with overflow, the so-called *paradoxic incontinence*.

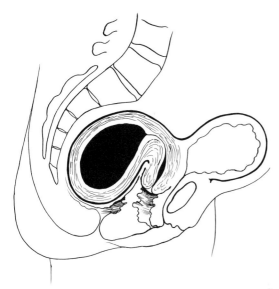

Figure 206 Diagrammatic representation of sagittal section showing retroflexed gravid uterus. As the uterus grows, the cervix rises behind the symphysis to obstruct the urethra and cause urinary retention.

There are four courses possible for symptomatic retroversion: (1) spontaneous rectification, (2) abortion, (3) partial correction or (4) incarceration.

1. Spontaneous correction is the rule during the third month as the corpus rises past the sacral promontory and falls forward.

2. Abortion is an infrequent termination of a retroflexed uterus. It is not certain why this occurs, but activity may be initiated as the uterus grows because of disturbances in the uterine circulation.

3. Incomplete correction may result in part of the corpus being retained in the pelvis while the anterior wall expands to accommodate the growing conceptus. The condition is due to persistent adhesions or tumors. Such patients may deliver normally at term, but abortion or premature labor or incarceration may occur.

4. Incarceration of the growing uterus in the pelvis is rare but serious. Bladder symptoms may demand intervention because the bladder cannot be emptied properly. The cause of urinary retention is compression and distortion of the urethra by the anteriorly displaced cervix. Sometimes there is edema of the neck of the bladder. Paradoxic incontinence may excoriate the vagina and thighs. Cystitis develops commonly. Hemorrhages or necrosis of the bladder wall may occur. Prolonged, unrelieved incarceration may lead to abortion or infection of the uterine contents, rupture of the uterus and peritonitis.

Diagnosis is seldom difficult. Every pregnant woman with sudden onset of dysuria or dribbling of urine should be examined for retroflexion of the uterus. Abdominally, the distended bladder is felt as an elastic mass. After the bladder has been emptied by catheterization, the change in the abdomen is striking. Vaginally, the cervix is pressed anteriorly and upward against the pubis or even above the pubis, and the culdesac is filled with the softly enlarged uterus bulging into the vagina.

The condition must be distinguished from pregnancy coexistent with uterine and extrauterine pelvic masses, such as leiomyomata uteri and an ovarian tumor. The availability of ultrasonographic B-scan techniques has simplified this difficult differential diagnostic problem (see Chapter 13). Clinical means for differentiation are suggested in Table 7.

As to treatment, if retroversion is discovered early, one should wait to see what nature will accomplish, because spontaneous correction is usual. However, an effort must be made to elevate the uterus gently if the retroversion persists after 12 weeks of gestation or if the patient begins to have bladder or other distressing symptoms. The attempt should be made by bimanual vaginoabdominal manipulation. If the uterus is successfully elevated, a pessary should be inserted into the vagina and left *in situ* for about four weeks. Afterward, it may be removed because the uterus will be too large to drop back. If the uterus cannot be raised by gentle bimanual efforts, more strenuous measures must be employed.

To accomplish this maneuver, first the bladder must be emptied. This is not easily done when the uterus is incarcerated because the urethra is long, flattened, distorted and edematous. A soft catheter should be used and one must avoid producing a false passage. Aids to catheterization include placing the patient in Sims or

TABLE 7　*DIFFERENTIAL DIAGNOSTIC CLINICAL FEATURES*

Pregnancy in a Retroflexed Uterus	*Pregnancy with Ovarian Tumor*
Bladder symptoms are pronounced.	Bladder symptoms are absent or inconsiderable.
The mass in question is symmetric and soft.	The tumor is often asymmetric, hard and tense.
There is no other mass above the pelvis.	Often the uterus can be felt above a tumor and to one side.
Moving the cervix imparts an impulse to the mass.	The upper mass (the uterus) can be moved independently of the ovarian tumor.
The mass in the culdesac usually contracts.	There are no contractions in the tumor.
Fetal parts may be distinguished.	Fetal parts are not present in the tumor.
Ultrasound distinguishes only one cavity with a fetus.	Ultrasound shows two separate cavities.

knee-chest position and, while pushing the corpus up or the cervix back with two fingers in the vagina, inserting a No. 12 to 15 French catheter with thorough lubrication, gentleness and patience. If the retention has been extreme and prolonged, the bladder may be greatly overdistended and it should be drained at a relatively slow rate of flow over the course of a few hours so as to avoid the sudden release of the abdominal distention and peritoneal stretching that may cause acute hypotension. Replacement of the uterus is usually easily accomplished once the bladder is emptied. It is aided by the knee-chest position, by pulling the cervix down with a vulsellum while simultaneously pushing the corpus upward and to the side. Anesthesia may sometimes be necessary. Gentleness is essential because too great force may rupture the uterus, tear vascular adhesions, cause hemorrhage into the bladder or rupture it and may even initiate abortion. Bladder necrosis may become manifest after replacement, the damage having occurred before the attempt at manual correction.

PROLAPSE OF THE UTERUS

Prolapse of the gravid uterus is rare (Fig. 207). A total of 256 cases have been reported in the world literature. Suzuki and Shane recently reported prolapse in a nullipara, a unique event. Patients with this condition can be carried through pregnancy safely with proper use of vaginal pessaries, bed rest and the prevention of infection by the employment of antiseptic measures for the protruding cervix. The management of labor is conservative and

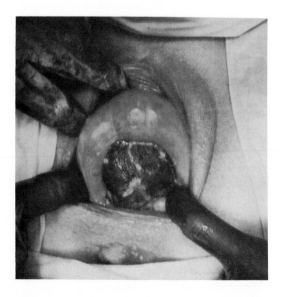

Figure 207　The presenting part and the edematous cervix are shown during labor between contractions in a patient with uterine prolapse.

needs no special intervention because spontaneous delivery is usual. Labor may actually be shorter than usual, requiring that care be taken in anticipation of precipitate delivery with resultant cervical lacerations. The latter are common. After the puerperium, if prolapse persists, it may be corrected surgically.

During pregnancy, extrusion of a cystocele or rectocele is an especially annoying condition. Rest in the supine position and maintaining cleanliness of the area are advised. Eversion of the vaginal walls may occur in multiparas in the second stage during the strong bearing-down efforts, especially if the patient begins to bear down before the cervix is fully dilated and retracted above the fetal head. The cervix may appear outside the vulva, as in association with uterine prolapse, and may not go back under pressure. It may become necessary for an assistant to hold the edges of the cervix and the everted vagina back with retractors to aid delivery.

Acute enlargement of the cervix due to edema is a rare occurrence during pregnancy (Fig. 208), but may occur in obstructed labor. During labor, when the head is arrested high in the pelvis, it may

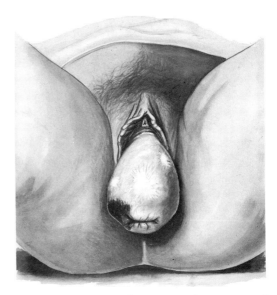

Figure 208 Acute elongation and protrusion of the cervix at eight months of gestation.

impinge the cervix between the fetal skull and the pelvic bony inlet. When this occurs, the cervix becomes swollen and may prolapse as a dark blue, hemorrhagic, edematous mass (Fig. 209). The protuber-

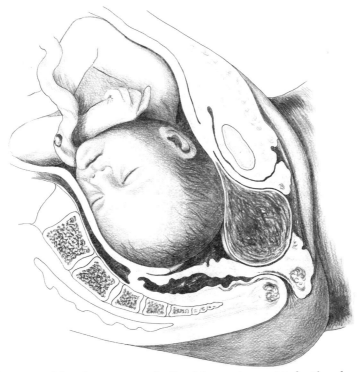

Figure 209 Illustration of the edematous anterior lip of the cervix associated with and possibly contributing to dystocia.

ant cervix may be gently pushed up and held in place during contractions. In the absence of cephalopelvic disproportion, the head will usually slip quickly past the elevated cervix in the course of its descent as labor progresses further. If it does not do so, obstructed labor should be suspected. Under these circumstances cesarean section is probably much more preferable than traumatic forceps operations and use of Dührssen's incisions of the cervix (see Chapter 73).

REFERENCES

Suzuki, K., and Shane, J. M.: Uterine prolapse in the pregnant primigravida. Amer. J. Obstet. Gynec. *112*:303, 1972.

Yellen, H. S., and McNeill, D. B.: Uterine prolapse and pregnancy: Report of two cases. Obstet. Gynec. *4*:235, 1954.

Chapter 29

Malformations

Embryologically, the uterus and vagina are formed by the fusion of the two paramesonephric ducts. The union takes place from below upward. Partial or complete lack of fusion or rudimentary development explains most anomalies. The uterine fundus may be indented in the middle to form the characteristic *uterus arcuatus* (Fig. 219), the most common uterine anomaly involving the line of fusion of the two ducts.

The two sides of the uterus and vagina are not always equally developed. Gradations from complete development of the two halves to almost entire absence of one paramesonephric duct are observed. The gamut of anomalies is illustrated in Figures 210 to 220. The rudimentary uterine horn may appear to be an appendage to the

well-developed uterine horn, but since its canal commonly does not communicate with the vagina, hematosalpinx and hematometra may occur as a result of repeated menstrual flow without egress.

Malformations of the urinary tract often accompany genital deformities and should be searched for whenever a uterine or vaginal anomaly is discovered.

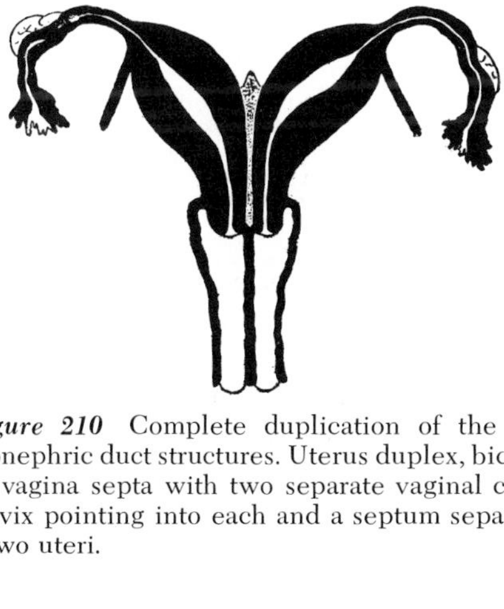

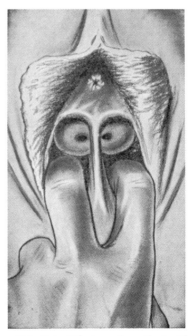

Figure 210 Complete duplication of the paramesonephric duct structures. Uterus duplex, bicornis, cum vagina septa with two separate vaginal canals, a cervix pointing into each and a septum separating the two uteri.

Figure 211 Introital view of a patient with uterus and vagina duplex who has a pregnancy in each horn.

335

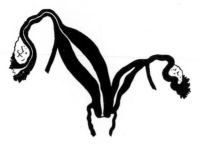

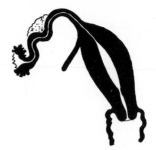

Fig. 212   *Fig. 213*

Figure 212   Uterus with a closed rudimentary horn. Menstrual blood will accumulate in it, causing hematometra.

Figure 213   Uterus unicornis, in which one paramesonephric canal failed to develop. Women with such a uterus may bear children without difficulty.

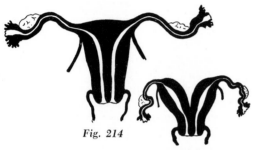

Fig. 214

Fig. 215

Figure 214   Uterus septus duplex or uterus bilocularis with one vagina and two cervices with a falciform ridge between them.

Figure 215   Uterus duplex bicornis, a variant of uterus septus duplex in which the septum intervening between the corpus cavities is divided.

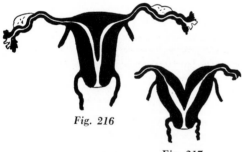

Fig. 216

Fig. 217

Figure 216   Uterus subseptus unicollis containing a simple septum in an otherwise single uterus.

Figure 217   Uterus bicornis unicollis, a variant of the subseptate uterus in which the corpus is split into two separate units, communicating with one cervical canal at or above the internal os.

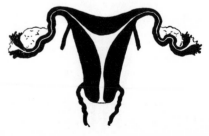

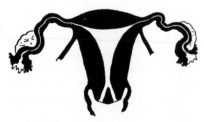

Figure 218   Uterus subseptus unicorporeus consisting of a septate cervix. The rest of the uterus is essentially normal. This condition may be imitated by a cervicovaginal fistula.

Figure 219   Uterus arcuatus, the simplest and most common uterine anomaly. Coassociated pregnancy often causes difficulty in differential diagnosis from ectopic gestation and cornual pregnancy. It is frequently associated with shoulder and breech presentations.

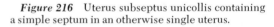

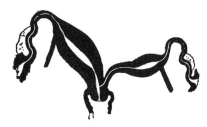

Figure 220 Uterus bicornis unilaterale rudimentarius. It is of great clinical importance because pregnancy may occur in the rudimentary horn. It is usually confused with ectopic pregnancy.

DUPLEX UTERUS AND VAGINA

Complete duplication of the paramesonephric ducts results in the situation depicted in Figures 210 and 211. Coitus is rarely interfered with because the vaginas are ample. Menstrual blood issues from both uteri simultaneously, but sometimes only from one at a time. Pregnancy may occur in one or both horns. If each horn contains a conceptus, the two pregnancies may theoretically have been conceived at different impregnations and be delivered at different times, thus suggesting (but not proving) superfetation.

When pregnancy occurs in one horn, it usually develops undisturbed. The uninvolved side grows and forms a decidua similar to that in ectopic gestation (see Chapter 32). The decidua of the empty side may be cast out while the pregnancy continues on the other side. The clinical picture of this event resembles an abortion. Unless the existence of a double uterus is known, the physician may proceed to evacuate the uterus and unwittingly destroy a living conceptus. Usually, the decidua in the empty horn sloughs away with the lochia during the puerperium.

Greiss and Mauzy manually explored 161 uterine cavities immediately after delivery and found 3.3 per cent with uterine anomalies. They analyzed published reports of 701 patients with genital anomalies; these women had 1290 pregnancies. From this collected material they concluded that, with specific exceptions, the physiologic capabilities of the anomalous

uterus are closer to normal than previously recognized. Uterine anomalies are associated with an increased abortion rate. Pregnancy and labor in these patients can be managed in the same manner as in normal women. Operative intervention need be invoked only when complications demand it.

Two minor anomaly types, namely, those involving simple longitudinal and transverse vaginal septa, present problems because of the obstruction offered to delivery through the vagina. Excision of the septum at the first delivery will provide a permanent cure.

Jones et al. studied 34 women with double uteri. They had had 100 pregnancies, most of which were successful. However, almost one-third of them experienced pregnancy wastage, including abortion or perinatal deaths in premature and term births. Salvage of term infants depends on careful management of labor and delivery, just as with term pregnancies in normal uteri. Similarly, reduction of losses due to prematurity and abortion depends on finding and correcting, as far as possible, those factors responsible for premature termination of each pregnancy. The incidence of disordered labor is not appreciably increased.

Jones and Jones emphasize that about one in four women with a double uterus has some serious reproductive problem, namely, premature labor or repeated abortion, or no living children. In such women surgical unification of the double uterus may be followed by term delivery of a living child provided prior investigation of both husband and wife reveals no other cause for the difficulty.

The Strassmann procedure involves a fundal uterine incision transversely from cornu to cornu, incision of the septum and closure in the anteroposterior midplane of the uterus. Jones recommended a procedure in which the muscular septum is excised by triangular incision. This results in a final vertical midline incision and has the additional advantage of avoiding injury to the cornua. Strassmann reviewed 128 plastic unifications of a double uterus. The indications were habitual abortion, sterility, severe dysmenorrhea and menometrorrhagia. There were no maternal deaths or uterine ruptures in 83 pregnancies after such operations; 61 full-term babies were delivered vaginally and only 10 by cesarean section. The percentage of full-term pregnancies in untreated cases of double uterus was about 25 per cent; this rose to 85.6 per cent after operation.

RUDIMENTARY UTERINE HORN

The clinical picture of pregnancy in a rudimentary horn resembles ectopic gestation (see Chapter 32). Perhaps 100 cases have been described. Mulsow found only nine reported since 1911. There were no deaths but there were many complications. The cavities of the two uterine horns usually do not communicate with each other. The rudimentary horn is hypoplastic and incapable of expanding beyond a critical limit. Rupture of the gestational sac usually occurs during the middle of pregnancy and profuse abdominal hemorrhage ensues. Since there is no communication from the rudimentary horn to the vagina, pregnancy results if the spermatozoa cross transperitoneally from the opposite side or if the ovum from the open side wanders over to the closed horn before or after fertilization.

The diagnosis of pregnancy in a rudimentary horn is rarely made before operation. Usually, the surgery is undertaken for rupture of a supposed extrauterine pregnancy. After the specimen is excised, it is easy to find the connecting band between the rudimentary horn and the spindle-shaped larger horn. One can easily determine that the round ligament and the tube arise from the outside of the gestational sac rather than proximally as in ectopic pregnancy. Analogous to changes that may occur with tubal pregnancy, the fetus may die *in situ* and ultimately become absorbed. When this takes place, the preoperative diagnosis is usually a leiomyoma or an ovarian cyst. Contractions in the sac of the tumor may suggest the clue to a correct diagnosis.

Treatment is the same as for extrauterine pregnancy. At laparotomy, the whole sac should be removed, if possible.

UTERINE SACCULATION AND DIVERTICULUM

There is a vast difference between a sacculation and a diverticulum of the uterus. A *sacculation* of the uterus is a functional malformation present only during pregnancy. It is a transitory pouch or saclike structure developing from a portion of a gravid uterus. The wall of the sacculation is composed of all three layers of the uterine corpus with an excessively thinned out layer of myometrium that is continuous with the normal myometrium of the remainder of the corpus. The aperture connecting the cavity of the sacculation with the main endometrial cavity may have a wide or a narrow mouth. In many cases the sacculation contains the placenta or fetal parts. A sacculation disappears after involution of the uterus.

A *diverticulum* is a permanent anatomic defect present even in the nonpregnant state. It may be congenital or acquired. It may become more apparent during pregnancy because of the excessive thinning of its wall. After involution of the uterus, its presence can be detected by physical examination or by means of a hysterosalpingogram.

The diagnosis of sacculation is usually made when the abdomen is opened for a suspected ectopic pregnancy and a normal gravid uterus is found. The pregnancy should not be disturbed if a sacculation is found because the pregnancy will usually continue normally. No ruptures of the uterus have been reported as a consequence of sacculation. Oxytocin, if indicated, may be used with impunity, observing the same care and precautions as with an intact uterus (see Chapter 24).

Sacculation has been diagnosed at the time of cesarean section. The uterus is seen to be very thinned out at the site of the sacculation. The uterine sac collapses after the baby is delivered. No special care of the defect is needed. It must be differentiated from a partial dehiscence of a uterine scar from previous surgery, such as cesarean section, myomectomy or hysterotomy. The latter is potentially much more serious and requires appropriate handling (see Chapter 65) in terms of either repair or sterilization measures to prevent future pregnancy.

TORSION OF THE UTERUS

The gravid uterus normally rotates on its own longitudinal axis. Commonly, dextrorotation is encountered with the left tube and ovary occupying a position anterior to the uterus, sometimes even reaching the midline. Extreme rotation beyond this, or *torsion*, may occur in association with partial or complete interference with uterine blood flow. The resulting acute clinical picture of uterine pain and shock is similar to that seen with abruptio placentae (see Chapter 38).

This may take place in a variety of conditions. Torsion of the human gravid uterus has been reported in 107 patients by Nesbitt and Corner. In 20 per cent the pelvic structures were normal; in 30 per cent there were associated leiomyomas and in 15 per cent uterine anomalies. Other coassociated factors were ovarian cysts, adhesions, prior uterine suspensions, fetal malpresentations and anomalies, as well as abnormalities of the spine and pelvis.

The diagnosis of torsion of the uterus is seldom established prior to laparotomy. The treatment of symptomatic torsion is immediate laparotomy. Contrary to prevalent opinion, hysterectomy may not always be necessary except in the most advanced degrees of torsion. Simple detorsion with corrective measures to eliminate the principal etiologic factor appears to be sufficient, especially during the earlier months of pregnancy. However, hysterectomy should be undertaken whenever it is clear that the long-standing, extreme torsion has left the uterus irreparably damaged.

There is considerable maternal risk with torsion of the gravid uterus after the fifth month of gestation, but improvements in anesthesia and acute care of shock states have been accompanied by improvements in this regard. There has not been any associated appreciable decrease in perinatal mortality, however. The fetal outcome is particularly poor with advanced degrees of torsion because of extreme fetal anoxia associated with obstruction of uterine blood flow. About one-third of fetuses succumb.

REFERENCES

Greiss, F. C., Jr., and Mauzy, C. H.: Genital anomalies in women: An evaluation of diagnosis, incidence and obstetric performance. Amer. J. Obstet. Gynec. 82:330, 1961.

Jones, H. W., Jr., and Jones, G. E. S.: Double uterus as an etiological factor in repeated abortion: Indications for surgical repair. Amer. J. Obstet. Gynec. 65:325, 1953.

Jones, H. W., Jr., Delfs, E., and Jones, G. E. S.: Reproductive difficulties in double uterus: The place of plastic reconstruction. Amer. J. Obstet. Gynec. 72:865, 1956.

Jones, W. S.: Obstetric significance of female genital anomalies. Obstet. Gynec. 10:113, 1957.

Mulsow, F. W.: Pregnancy in a rudimentary horn of the uterus. Amer. J. Obstet. Gynec. 49:773, 1945.

Nesbitt, R. E. L., and Corner, G. W., Jr.: Torsion of the human pregnant uterus. Obstet. Gynec. Survey 11:311, 1956.

Strassmann, E. D.: Plastic unification of double uterus: A study of 123 collected and five personal cases. Amer. J. Obstet. Gynec. 64:25, 1952.

Chapter 30

Tumors of Pelvis and Breast

LEIOMYOMA UTERI

Leiomyomas (fibromas, leiofibromas or fibroids) may coexist with pregnancy. The incidence is at least 0.5 per cent (Gainey and Keeler). They participate in uterine enlargement, especially during the first half of pregnancy. There is little proliferation of the smooth muscle fibers or hyperplasia of the connective tissue stroma within leiomyomas during pregnancy (Randall and Odell; Parks and Barter). Edema is the primary change and can explain the enlargement of leiomyomas during gestation.

There is an increase of necrosis, hyalinization and fibrous tissue stroma in leiomyomas during the third trimester of pregnancy (Lamb and Greene). Both the leiomyomatous and the myometrial cells enlarge. The cellular size in the leiomyoma increases during early pregnancy. The increase in myometrial cellular diameter lags during the first trimester, but in the third trimester it significantly surpasses that of the leiomyoma cells. Both respond to estrogen stimulation, and the difference in response may be explained by changes in blood flow reaching the tumor. Leiomyomas participate relatively little in the increased blood flow available to the myometrium.

Usually, leiomyomas do not interfere with growth of the conceptus during gestation (Fig. 221). *Red or carneous degeneration* is one of the most serious changes in leiomyomas. It is associated with pain, fever, leukocytosis and rapid sedimentation time. Dislocation and change in the shape of the tumors is another common event in pregnancy. Leiomyomas located in or attached to the cervix respond to the upward traction of the corpus late in pregnancy or in labor. Fortunately, they usually rise out of the pelvis; if not, they might obstruct delivery.

Subserous leiomyomas may become twisted and necrotic. They may also prolapse into the culdesac and later obstruct labor. Submucous leiomyomas, which are rare, are likely to become polypoid and may then be extruded through the cervix during the puerperium. During labor, leiomyomas may be traumatized by the advancing head or by attempts at delivery. On the other hand, in rare instances, the

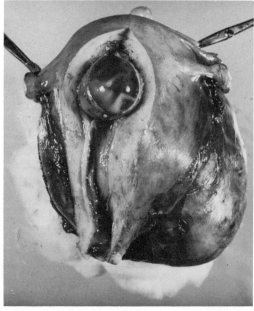

Figure 221 Gross specimen of an intact pregnancy in a leiomyomatous uterus. The leiomyoma occupies the entire posterior wall and protrudes subserosally. The anterior wall has been opened by a vertical incision to demonstrate the fetal sac *in situ*. (Courtesy of J. E. Fitzgerald.)

340

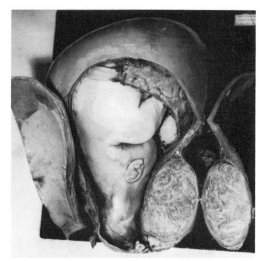

Figure 222 The anterior wall of the uterus has been opened by a frontal incision to show the fetal relationship to the cervical leiomyoma, demonstrating excessive compression of the fetal head by the leiomyoma. (Courtesy of M. Dekaris.)

head of the fetus may be compressed by a leiomyoma (Fig. 222). In the puerperium, leiomyomas usually involute with the rest of the uterus. Necrosis and infection of the tumors are unusual.

The effects of leiomyomas on pregnancy are variable. Abortion occurs in women with leiomyomas, particularly when the tumors are submucous, but how much more often than in a normal uterus is not clear. Intramural leiomyomas have less effect, and subserous ones, unless large or near the cervix, essentially none. Leiomyomas usually do not cause complications in labor unless they are impacted, adherent in the pelvis or attached to the placenta. A subserous impacted leiomyoma causes difficulty because it is not likely to be elevated above the pelvic brim by the contracting and retracting uterus (Fig. 223).

Leiomyomas may influence the mechanism of labor. Contractions are usually normal, but they may sometimes be weak or atonic. Abnormalities of position and presentation are prone to occur.

In the third stage, hemorrhage is common because the distorted uterus cannot effectively compress the vessels supplying the placental site.

During the puerperium, leiomyomas may obstruct the lochial flow. They may delay involution and predispose to phlebothrombosis. Infection may result when they are gangrenous.

Diagnosis

The diagnosis of pregnancy in a woman known to have leiomyomas is not difficult. Menstruation stops and there is rapid enlargement of the uterus. The uterus is irregular in consistency with softened areas, undergoing periodic contractions. Fetal heart tones can be perceived in due course. Fetal heart tones may be inaudible if leiomyomas are interposed between the fetus and the anterior abdominal wall. Ultrasound can be very useful under these circumstances both for detecting the fetal heart (Doppler effect) and for clarifying the differential diagnosis (see Chapter 13). It is usually easy to determine when leiomyomas and pregnancy coexist, but twins, ovarian tumor, double uterus, hematoma and abdominal wall adiposity have been mistaken for uterine tumors. During labor, leiomyomas become prominent when the uterus contracts. Unless obscured by an obese abdominal wall or located primarily on the posterior wall of the uterus, they are almost always discernible.

The differential diagnosis between a large symmetric intramural leiomyoma and pregnancy is sometimes difficult. Aside from the absence of the signs and symptoms of pregnancy, lack of fetal heart sounds and negative pregnancy tests, the cervix tends to be hard and displaced high in the pelvis in association with leiomyomas. If observed at laparotomy, the round ligaments and adnexa are seen to be located anomalously. The pregnant uterus is characteristically a dark color with congested, thickened tubes and ligaments. Congestion especially involves the round ligaments. One finds a large corpus luteum in one ovary. Ballottement of the fetus is possible and uterine contractions are palpable.

Prognosis

The dangers of leiomyomas complicating pregnancy are misrepresented, proba-

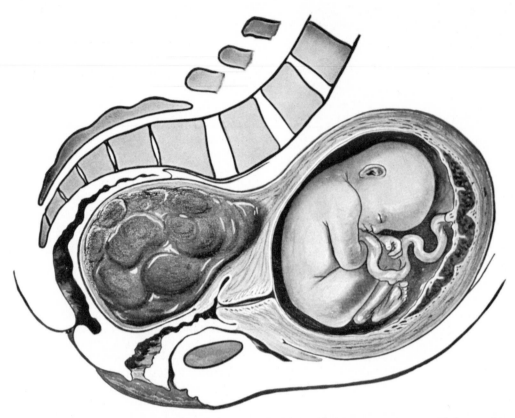

Figure 223 Diagrammatic view of sagittal section showing midtrimester pregnancy with large subserous leiomyoma uteri occupying the culdesac of Douglas, where it will undoubtedly cause obstruction in labor.

bly because only the severe cases are published. Except when the tumor obstructs delivery, there are few serious complications.

Treatment

The mere presence of leiomyomas in pregnancy does not warrant therapeutic abortion, myomectomy or hysterectomy because most women with leiomyomas go to term and through labor without difficulty.

A laparotomy may have to be performed in early pregnancy for red degeneration if there is a great deal of pain, especially if it is unresponsive to mild analgesics or is becoming aggravated. Moreover, impaction of the leiomyomas, extremely rapid growth of the tumors or excessive bleeding may warrant surgery. Under such conditions, it is best to remove the specific tumor causing the problem. This should

be done, if possible, leaving the pregnancy undisturbed, unless a special reason exists for removing the uterus. The reasons for hysterectomy include extensive degeneration of one or more tumors or excessive bleeding during operation.

Abortion or premature labor may follow in some patients after myomectomy. At times it may be best just to close the abdomen and leave the pregnant uterus and the tumors intact. The leiomyomas can be dealt with at some future date, after delivery and puerperal recovery. The morbidity of myomectomy or hysterectomy done on a nongravid uterus is considerably less than it is during pregnancy.

Leiomyomas in term pregnancies rarely interfere with labor. Most women so affected may be expected to deliver vaginally. Obstruction of the parturient passage due to leiomyoma is serious. In addition to the obvious problem inherent in the obstruction to descent, sloughing of the tumor may result from crushing, avulsion or trauma during spontaneous or operative delivery. Should a cervical leiomyoma be so large or so firmly fixed that it clearly will not be able to be retracted above the pelvic brim during dilatation, thereby completely blocking delivery, cesarean section should be performed.

When labor has been in progress for a long time and there is overt, objective evidence of infection, the condition is even more serious. With antibiotics a uterus that contains infected leiomyomas may sometimes be saved. Most patients will deliver uneventfully and will defervesce in due course if suitably treated with appropriate antibiotics. In this regard, it is essential to obtain cultures of the cervical discharge before antibiotic therapy is instituted. Cesarean section may be necessary if vaginal delivery cannot be accomplished. Undue delay in effecting delivery in the presence of infection may unnecessarily complicate the problem (see Chapter 70).

If cesarean section is undertaken for obstructed labor under these circumstances, one should consider whether or not hysterectomy is in order. Since many of the women with large leiomyomas are elderly, it may be justifiable to proceed with removing the uterus at this time. If the patient is young and desirous of retaining her childbearing function, conservative treatment may be tried, recognizing that it may become necessary to remove the uterus at a later date if the infection cannot be controlled medically. Myomectomy is less preferable because it leaves a raw, contaminated myometrial surface as a potential site for abscess formation. Myomectomy can be done with little risk if the offending tumor is a pedunculated subserous leiomyoma.

OVARIAN TUMORS

During pregnancy ovarian tumors are rare (Creasman et al.). Although pregnant women have no special propensity to develop ovarian cysts, they are by no means devoid of them. Grimes et al. found 6 cm. or more cystic ovarian enlargement in 1:274 pregnancies. Most women appear to experience no problem during their pregnancies, going to term without any knowledge of the tumor. The growth of benign cysts is not accelerated. Torsion of the pedicle and hemorrhage into the cyst occur occasionally (Beischer et al.).

Labor exerts no influence unless the mass lies in the pelvis, exposed to the trauma of delivery, when it may rupture, be crushed or have its pedicle torn. The puerperium has no special influence, but complications are likely if the tumor has been traumatized. Torsion is a more frequent event than in nonpregnant women.

Cysts are harmful in labor only when they are incarcerated in the pelvis and block the descent of the fetus. The puerperium is sometimes stormy because of trauma to the tumor, necrosis, hemorrhage, infection or suppuration. Tumors which adhere to the rectum are likely to be infected with coliform bacilli.

Diagnosis

Ultrasonic B-scan techniques (Chapter 13) are helpful in diagnosis. Benign cystic teratomas (dermoids) can be detected in roentgenograms if they contain calcified teeth or bone.

In the early months it is usually easy to differentiate the gravid uterus from the rounded, movable, pedunculated tumor lying at its side. When the tumor is intraligamentous, that is, between the peritoneal leaves of the broad ligament, or prolapsed in the pelvis behind the uterus, it must be differentiated from ectopic gestation or a retroflexed gravid uterus. Leiomyomas and a displaced kidney must be ruled out as well. Torsion of an ovarian cyst simulates ruptured ectopic pregnancy and appendicitis.

In the later months and during labor, difficulties may be encountered in locating the tumor. If adherent to the uterus, one may suspect twins, leiomyomas or double uterus. Tumors incarcerated in the pelvis are discovered easily during labor but their nature and origin are rarely clear. A cyst compressed during labor changes its characteristics and may become quite firm.

Treatment

Most obstetricians strongly favor removing ovarian tumors as soon as they are discovered. Patients require surgery if they have adnexal tumors larger than 6 cm. (because they may represent a malignancy), if they show the signs of infection or the symptoms of acute torsion. The danger of abortion is negligible, even if the tumor contains the corpus luteum of pregnancy (see Chapter 33). However, it is advisable, if possible, to delay the operation until the end of the third or beginning of the fourth month of pregnancy, because of the risks to the fetus of hypoxia that may occur during anesthesia. Such hypoxia during the first two months may affect embryogenesis adversely.

Whenever surgery is done, the gravid uterus must be handled as little and as gently as possible. If benign, the cyst can be removed, preserving as much as one can of the normal ovarian tissue.

During labor normal progression and vaginal delivery should be expected provided the ovarian cyst is not blocking the birth canal. A laparotomy should be performed if the cyst is ahead of the presenting part. The fetus should be delivered by cesarean section and then the cyst extirpated. The other ovary should always be inspected to determine whether or not another cyst requiring removal is present.

CARCINOMA OF THE CERVIX

Cancer of the cervix is rare in pregnancy, but potentially very serious when it occurs. There were 174 cervical cancers among 422,951 pregnancies collected from the literature by Waldrop and Palmer, an incidence of 4.1 per 10,000 or 1:2439 obstetric cases. At the Roswell Park Memorial Institute, among 6000 patients with cervical carcinoma there were 3.1 per cent who were either pregnant at the time of this diagnosis or had been pregnant within one year before the diagnosis. There is no evidence that pregnancy enhances growth of cervical carcinoma (Fogh; Peller).

Intraepithelial lesions and small inva-

sive cancers are generally asymptomatic. More advanced, ulcerated tumors may present with hemorrhage and necrosis with putrid leukorrhea. Labor may disrupt the tumor, and lacerations cause hemorrhage, infection and rapid extension of the neoplasm. In the puerperium these changes become evident quickly.

Invasive cancer of the cervix has an adverse effect on pregnancy, labor and the puerperium. Abortion is frequent because of infection, hemorrhage and restriction of uterine growth by tumor bulk. Labor is obstructed primarily by the rigidity of the cervix. If the tumor is small and soft, the cervix will easily dilate and allow the fetus to descend. If the whole cervix is involved in a hard mass, obstruction will result. If the cervix gives way, it may tear. The tear may extend into the parametrium. Profuse hemorrhage will occur. It cannot be stopped by suturing because the tissues are friable. Only bilateral internal iliac artery ligations will be effective. The risks of disseminating an invasive carcinoma by allowing vaginal delivery through the cancerous cervix are unknown, but on an intuitive basis most oncologists are agreed that the practice is best avoided. Cesarean section should be undertaken instead. Infection is common in the puerperium.

Diagnosis

Every pregnant woman should unfailingly have a Papanicolaou smear for cytologic study at her first antepartum visit (see Chapter 9). If positive or suspicious, appropriate biopsies are essential for definitive diagnosis. Every gravida who bleeds or has purulent or putrid leukorrhea should be examined for cancer of the cervix. Although most are silent, advanced cancers become manifest in almost 90 per cent of cases by vaginal bleeding as the first symptom. Any lesion on the cervix should be biopsied and the tissue examined histologically.

Women who exfoliate abnormal or suspicious cells, as determined by Papanicolaou smears, should be followed repeatedly until the source is discovered by means of biopsy or completely negative smears are obtained. When a lesion is visible on the cervix, it should be excised for biopsy whether the patient is pregnant or not. There have been some complications from punch or cone biopsies in pregnancy (Lieberman). Few abortions have occurred, but substantial hemorrhage can result and care must be taken to secure hemostasis by adequate suturing.

Hellman et al. observed proliferation and hyperplasia of the reserve cells of the cervix as well as adenomatous and atypical hyperplasia during pregnancy. Varying degrees of atypism can be marked and are sometimes difficult to distinguish histologically from *carcinoma in situ*. However, there is no evidence that they bear any direct relationship to cervical carcinoma. Greene et al. verified that metaplasia and hyperplasia of glandular elements are more common and more prominent during pregnancy and that the stratified squamous epithelium of the cervix grows rapidly during pregnancy, sometimes with an increase in the thickness of the basal cell layer. However, these changes should not be confused with the specific criteria for the diagnosis of preinvasive carcinoma.

Treatment

If intraepithelial carcinoma is discovered in pregnancy and one can ensure by conization that there is no focus of invasion, the pregnancy can be allowed to continue to term. Vaginal delivery is acceptable and does not increase the risk of disseminating the disease. After the puerperium, repeat conization is in order to ensure that the cancer has not become invasive. This is followed by simple hysterectomy in most instances, unless the woman's childbearing needs are unfulfilled. In the latter case, no further immediate therapy need be undertaken, but the patient must be advised of the risks and the need for close, frequent follow-up examinations. The end results of cervical carcinoma associated with pregnancy are as good as those in the nongravid state.

Invasive cancer demands immediate, definitive and aggressive treatment (Creasman et al.). The optimal program will depend on the stage of the disease. If

strictly limited to the cervix (Stage I), equally good results accrue to either radical surgery or effective radiation therapy. For more advanced cancers, radiotherapy is more effective, except for the special group of Stage IV lesions that invade the bladder and/or rectum, for which exenterative procedures may be indicated. The Catholic Church permits extirpation of a cancerous gravid uterus or radium therapy because the primary objective is to remove the neoplasm and not to produce an abortion (Burke). In most patients treated by radiation during early pregnancy, abortion follows. However, if the fetus should survive, it will probably be severely damaged (Goldstein and Murphy). Therefore, if possible, pregnancy should first be terminated if radiotherapy is to be the mode of treatment for the cancer.

In general, the fetus can be ignored when undertaking treatment. Abortion may be induced in advance, if desired and acceptable, in early pregnancy; if the fetus is viable, cesarean section is warranted in an attempt to salvage it.

Choriocarcinoma will be dealt with in detail in Chapter 53. Other types of pelvic tumor are exceedingly unusual in pregnancy. Cancer of the endometrium almost precludes pregnancy, eight proved cases having been reported (Nestarez and Assali). Similarly, there are only seven reported cases of uterine sarcoma in pregnancy (Hesseltine).

CARCINOMA OF THE BREAST

The discovery and diagnosis of early breast cancer may be difficult during pregnancy and lactation because of the physiologic enlargement and engorgement of the breasts. White says carcinoma of the breast complicates pregnancy in about 3 per 10,000 pregnancies, while pregnancy occurs in three per cent of women with breast carcinoma. Gross five-year survival rate is about 59 per cent and ten-year survival rate 47 per cent. These data are comparable to the gross survival rates of nonpregnant patients, although there is a widely held clinical impression that pregnancy accelerates the course of this disease. It is possible that this impression is based on the more advanced nature of breast cancer when discovered in pregnancy or the puerperium. This is due perhaps to the inevitable delay that results from our inability to detect small breast nodules in pregnancy.

For the treatment of mammary carcinoma, radical mastectomy or a combination of simple mastectomy and radiation therapy should be performed immediately after a definite diagnosis is made, even if the condition is found during pregnancy or lactation. It is a frequent practice to terminate pregnancy during the first or second trimesters. However, abortion cannot clearly be shown to have a favorable effect on the course of the disease. As to prophy-

lactic surgical castration, there is insufficient evidence to prove that it delays or prevents metastases or improves the chances of survival.

Patients who desire to become pregnant after radical mastectomy should wait at least three years if axillary metastases were not present at the time of operation, and five years if axillary metastases were present.

Any hope for improved prognosis of carcinoma of the breast during pregnancy lies in early diagnosis when the growth is still clinically operable. For this reason physicians should examine the breasts of their patients carefully and at frequent intervals, beginning with the first antepartum visit and including the postpartum examination.

REFERENCES

Beischer, N. A., Buttery, B. W., Fortune, D. W., and Macafee, C. A.: Growth and malignancy of ovarian tumours in pregnancy. Aust. New Zeal. J. Obstet. Gynaec. *11*:208, 1971.

Burke, E. F.: Acute Cases in Moral Medicine. New York, The Macmillan Company, 1922.

Creasman, W. T., Rutledge, F. N., and Fletcher, G. H.: Carcinoma of the cervix associated with pregnancy. Obstet. Gynec. *36*:495, 1970.

Creasman, W. T., Rutledge, F. N., and Smith, J. P.: Carcinoma of the ovary associated with pregnancy. Obstet. Gynec. *38*:111, 1971.

Fogh, I.: Cancer colli uteri and pregnancy. Cancer *29*:114, 1972.

Gainey, H. L., and Keeler, J. E.: Submucous myoma in term pregnancy. Amer. J. Obstet. Gynec. *58*:727, 1949.

Goldstein, L., and Murphy, D. P.: Microcephalic idiocy following radium therapy for uterine cancer during pregnancy. Amer. J. Obstet. Gynec. *18*:189, 1929.

Greene, R. R., Peckham, B. M., Chung, J. T., Bayly, M. A., Benaron, H. B. W., Carrow, L. A., and Gardner, G. H.: Preinvasive carcinoma of the cervix during pregnancy. Surg. Gynec. Obstet. *96*:71, 1953.

Grimes, W. H., Jr., Bartholomew, R. A., Colvin, E. D., Fish, J. S., and Lester, W. M.: Ovarian cyst complicating pregnancy. Amer. J. Obstet. Gynec. *68*:594, 1954.

Hellman, L. M., Rosenthal, A. H., Kistner, R. W., and

Gordon, R.: Some factors influencing the proliferation of the reserve cells in the human cervix. Amer. J. Obstet. Gynec. *67*:899, 1954.

Hesseltine, H. C.: Sarcoma of uterus diagnosed 19 days after normal full-term delivery: Case report. J. Iowa Med. Soc. *20*:560, 1930.

Lamb, E. J., and Greene, R. R.: A microscopic study of the growth of leiomyomas of the uterus during pregnancy. Surg. Gynec. Obstet. *108*:575, 1959.

Lieberman, B. A.: Cone biopsy in pregnancy. S. Afr. J. Obstet. Gynaec. 9:13, 1971.

Nestarez, O. B., and Assali, N. S.: Algunos aspectos do cancer do endometrio sua associacão com prehez. Obst. Ginec. Latino-Amer. *4*:161, 1946.

Parks, J., and Barter, R. H.: The myomatous uterus complicated by pregnancy. Amer. J. Obstet. Gynec. *63*:260, 1952.

Peller, S.: Der Geburtstod. Vienna, Franz Deuticke, 1936.

Randall, J. H., and Odell, L. D.: Fibroids in pregnancy. Amer. J. Obstet. Gynec. *46*:349, 1943.

Waldrop, G. M., and Palmer, J. P.: Carcinoma of the cervix associated with pregnancy. Amer. J. Obstet. Gynec. *86*:202, 1963.

White, T. T.: Carcinoma of the breast in the pregnant and nursing patient: Review of 1,375 cases. Amer. J. Obstet. Gynec. *69*:1277, 1955.

White, T. T.: Prognosis of breast cancer for pregnant and nursing women: Analysis of 1,413 cases. Surg. Gynec. Obstet. *100*:661, 1955.

Chapter 31

Hyperemesis Gravidarum

Nausea and vomiting occur in many pregnant women and are considered normal (see Chapter 43). These symptoms may be so severe, however, as to become serious and deserve the appellation *pernicious vomiting*. The disease has been designated by various terms, but *hyperemesis gravidarum* is the one generally used. The condition is now rare because ambulatory care of the "normal" nausea and vomiting of pregnancy with use of antiemetic tranquilizing agents is so effective.

ETIOLOGY

Uncontrollable vomiting is more common in neurotic women. A functional disturbance of the nervous system is intimately coassociated in most cases of hyperemesis. If the pregnancy is abhorrent or fearful to a woman, she may express her negativism by vomiting. Proper suggestion will often result in a cure. The pregnant woman's great vulnerability to suggestion has been stressed in Chapter 11.

Patients studied by clinical interview method and the Rorschach technique exhibited well-defined emotional psychopathology which was most prominent during the period of vomiting and not relieved prior to delivery (Harvey). Although the genesis of hyperemesis gravidarum is not entirely in the psychologic sphere, there is a large psychiatric component almost invariably present. Whether hormonal or neuronal factors are also at play is not known. The increased chorionic gonadotropin levels found associated are probably based on dehydration, although circumstantial evidence suggests a correlation. In hydatidiform mole, for example, both high chorionic gonadotropin levels and hyperemesis occur together.

There are a number of organic conditions which are usually associated with vomiting, even in the nonpregnant state. Unfortunately, when pregnancy is added, the vomiting is erroneously diagnosed as hyperemesis gravidarum and both diagnosis and treatment of the underlying pathologic state are delayed unnecessarily. Such diseases include gastric and duodenal ulcer, cholecystitis and cholelithiasis. Pyelonephritis is frequently a cause of vomiting in pregnancy. Our discussion here deals with the nonorganic variety or true hyperemesis gravidarum.

SYMPTOMS

Typically, the disease begins in the second month, usually within a week or two after the first missed period. If it first appears after the third month, some other cause, such as pyelonephritis, should be suspected. It usually lasts several weeks and disappears as abruptly as it began, generally at about the end of the twelfth week.

At first little attention is paid to the gravida's complaints because nausea and vomiting are such frequent occurrences in the early months. When intolerance for all liquid and solid food develops and the patient begins to lose weight and become dehydrated and ketoacidotic, the condition is serious. Anorexia may be manifest by an actual loathing of food. Nausea, associated with retching, may occur at the mere mention, sight or smell of food. Hiccup may be a troublesome symptom, as may heartburn. Thirst is harassing. The patient complains of a constant boring or burning pain in the upper midabdomen or lower chest and of soreness of the ribs and adjoining muscles. Marked ptyalism with profuse salivation is occasionally coassociated. Constipation is the rule, but sometimes diarrhea may be present.

The vomitus at first is composed of undigested food, mucus and a little bile. Later, it is mostly mucus and bile, and finally it becomes bloody. The blood may come from the mouth, pharynx or stomach. It is ominous only if it is of gastric origin. The urine, at first normal, becomes scanty and highly concentrated as a result of dehydration. As the disease progresses, the urine will reflect the acidosis by yielding acetone. Later, the urine may contain albumin, casts and sometimes blood, bile and glucose. Increased blood concentration (rising hematocrit) and electrolyte imbalance are seen from the substantial unreplaced fluid and electrolyte losses in the vomitus. There is often also a decreased concentration of serum protein. Anemia may develop on a nutritional basis.

Examination shows the skin to be pale, waxy and sometimes icteric. The patient becomes emaciated; the severely affected patient may die, if untreated, even before emaciation is pronounced. Usually, there are hemic murmurs. The pulse is weak and rapid at 100 to 140 beats per minute, but the blood pressure is variable. The abdomen is scaphoid. Great tenderness is elicited over the cardia and sometimes over the liver.

The irritating vomitus erodes the lips and lower part of the face; the gums are reddened and covered with sordes; the tongue is red, dry, brown in the middle and cracked and it sometimes bleeds; the pharynx is dry, red and sometimes infiltrated with minute hemorrhages; the breath is fetid and may have a penetrating or mild, fruity odor characteristic of ketoacidosis.

In the final stages, mental aberration, delirium, headache, somnolence, stupor and coma occur. The vomiting usually ceases about this time, raising false hopes, but the pulse increases in frequency, the myocardium fails, the general prostration rapidly augments, icterus and cyanosis appear and the patient dies.

DIAGNOSIS

The patient who does not respond promptly to conservative measures aimed at correcting the mild, common nausea and vomiting of early pregnancy should be suspected of having hyperemesis. This must be considered to be present when the stomach rejects everything and the anorexia is complete. The diagnosis is not simple. It consists of diagnosing pregnancy, which is not always easy in the first trimester, and of ruling out any organic cause for the vomiting.

PROGNOSIS

Occasionally, either spontaneously or as a result of treatment, the patient suddenly ceases to vomit, retains food and recovers rapidly. More often the disease subsides slowly or may not subside fully until after delivery. If the fetus dies or abortion occurs, recovery usually begins, but not always. Hyperemesis may recur in subsequent pregnancies.

TREATMENT

The prophylaxis consists of prompt conservative management of mild pregnancy vomiting. Reassurance is appropriate. Frequent, small, essentially carbohydrate meals should be prescribed. Patients tolerate bland, dry foods best during this time. One should restrict fluids to the periods between meals. Regular bowel movements help considerably. The most effective drugs for this symptom are the tranquilizers. A wide variety are available and effective, including meclizine and dimenhydrinate, both of which are used extensively with good results. Patients who do not show prompt response run risks of becoming severely dehydrated and, therefore, require more aggressive in-hospital management. Fortunately, nearly all patients respond well and the severe disease progression described above is almost never seen any longer.

When a patient has hyperemesis, she should be hospitalized and cared for by competent and tactful nurses. All visitors, including her husband, should be barred. Oral intake is stopped. Parenteral rehydration is carried out according to demonstrated needs, including supplementary electrolytes and glucose to correct acidbase imbalance and acetonemia. Fluid intake, urine output and the amount of the vomitus should be measured. Sedatives and tranquilizers should be given in large amounts to control emesis quickly. Bland, easily tolerated and digestible solid food may be started after 48 hours if all symptoms have subsided. Intravenous supplementation may still be needed at first. Small amounts of fluid should be given between meals. If all food given by mouth is retained, a normal diet, omitting fats but including an abundant supply of liquids, may be resumed gradually and all other treatment stopped. Ambulation can be initiated as soon as the condition is entirely under control. However, tranquilizers should be continued for a few days longer or until it is clear that they can be discontinued without the symptoms returning. Psychiatric evaluation and care may be most helpful.

If the patient's condition does not improve, one must try to determine with certainty that an organic cause has not been overlooked. The rare instance of hyperemesis that does not remit on this aggressive regimen warrants consideration of terminating the pregnancy. Abortion is indicated if, despite all therapy, the patient's condition becomes worse and persistent tachycardia, jaundice, fever, fall in blood pressure or psychosis develops or she continues to lose weight persistently. Since general anesthesia may be dangerous for these patients because of their tenuous condition, local or regional block anesthesia is recommended. The abortion can be performed by a simple suction curage or dilatation and curettage; if the pregnancy is advanced beyond the third month, it may be done by intrauterine injection of hypertonic saline (see Chapter 35). Hyperemesis is now an extremely rare indication for terminating a gestation because it can nearly always be prevented or cured by the program outlined above.

REFERENCE

Harvey, W. A.: Psychological findings in patients with vomiting during pregnancy. J. Nerv. Ment. Dis. *115*:457, 1952.

Chapter 32

Ectopic Pregnancy

Ectopic and extrauterine pregnancy are terms used interchangeably to designate a gestation outside of the uterine cavity. An ovum may be fertilized and implant at any point along its passage from the ovary through the tube to the uterus (Fig. 224), as well as at various sites in the peritoneal cavity. The most common sites are within the tubal lumen. The rarest variety is the *primary ovarian* and *primary abdominal pregnancy*. Implantation has occurred in the stump of a tube after partial salpingectomy, in a closed accessory horn of the uterus and on the fimbria ovarica of the uterine tube.

As the implanted ovum continues to grow, other structures are encroached on, adhesions form and the topography of the gestation is modified. In *tubal pregnancy*, when the tubal wall ruptures and the conceptus escapes into the abdominal cavity or into a mass of preformed adhesions, it may occasionally reimplant or continue to grow *in situ* as a *tuboabdominal pregnancy* or *secondary abdominal pregnancy*.

If the rupture occurs in the lower portion of the tube, between the folds of the broad ligament, an *intraligamentous sac* is formed. An *interstitial pregnancy* is one which is implanted in the interstitial portion of the uterine tube located within the myometrium. If the sac which is formed in an interstitial pregnancy burrows into the uterus (a rare occurrence), it results in a *tubouterine pregnancy*. If a tuboovarian pregnancy goes to term, it almost always becomes *ovarioabdominal*. These forms are difficult to distinguish one from the other clinically as well as anatomically.

The sites of 1225 ectopic pregnancies reviewed by Jarcho were as follows: ampulla 47 per cent, isthmus 21.6 per cent, fimbria 5.8 per cent, interstitial 3.7 per cent, infundibular 2.5 per cent and smaller frequencies in the various other parts of the tube, the abdomen, the broad ligament, the ovary, the uterine cornu and a rudimentary horn. The right tube seems to be preferentially affected nearly twice as often as the left (Beacham et al.). Double

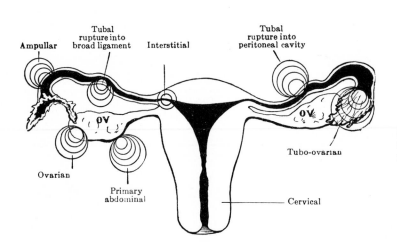

Figure 224 Composite diagram of uterus and adnexa showing possible implantation sites of ectopic pregnancies.

tubal gestation and two gestational sacs in one tube have been observed (Loh and Loh). Twins and even triplets have been found in one sac. Hoerner reported 110 bilateral simultaneous tubal pregnancies.

Some ruptures of the sac or tubal abortion with spontaneous recovery undoubtedly occur, often diagnosed as appendicitis, especially in women who have had antecedent pelvic disease. Repeated extrauterine pregnancies are believed to occur in three to four per cent of patients with ectopic pregnancies, but since many women who have had a tubal pregnancy cannot conceive again, either in the uterus or in a tube, the absolute incidence of repeated ectopic pregnancies in fertile women is much higher. Järvinen and Kinnunen found that ectopic pregnancy recurred in one of every four of their patients who became pregnant after an ectopic pregnancy. Grant reported that less than one-third of such patients succeed in bearing a live baby during the rest of their reproductive lives. The cause of this subsequent sterility is mainly tubal in origin.

HETEROTOPIC AND COMPOUND PREGNANCIES

The coexistence of intrauterine and extrauterine pregnancy is unusual. It is important to differentiate *combined* (heterotopic) from *compound* intrauterine and extrauterine pregnancy. *Combined* intrauterine and extrauterine pregnancy means the coexistence of simultaneous pregnancies, whereas *compound* pregnancy refers to the superimposition of an extrauterine pregnancy on a preexisting intrauterine pregnancy, generally a lithopedion, or vice versa.

The treatment is operative. The majority of patients come to the attention of the surgeon early in pregnancy because of tubal abortion or rupture. Even at operation, the diagnosis of intrauterine and extrauterine pregnancy is not always easy. Unless the uterine enlargement is pronounced, the abdomen is usually closed without detecting the coexisting intrauterine gestation. A sign that is helpful for diagnosing double pregnancy is the presence of two corpora lutea in the ovaries,

suggesting the possibility of two conceptions.

Extrauterine and intrauterine pregnancy offers a serious prognosis. The catastrophic events accompanying rupture of the ectopic sac may result in the subsequent abortion of the uterine ovum. The mother's life is in jeopardy from internal hemorrhage or from infection.

If the ectopic pregnancy is successfully removed, the intrauterine one may progress to term normally. Very rarely, if development is uninterrupted, both infants may be born alive at term. Intrauterine fetal survival rate in association with heterotopic pregnancy is about 54 per cent (Fleisher and Seaman). Burkhart et al. found 502 cases of combined intrauterine and extrauterine pregnancies reported up to 1961; 64 patients progressed into the third trimester and 24 were delivered of live twin infants.

The preferred method of delivery of the late ectopic pregnancy is by the abdominal route, removing the extrauterine fetus from its sac without disturbing its implantation site. If near term, the intrauterine fetus is readily delivered at the same time by cesarean section in the usual manner (see Chapter 76). The placenta of the extrauterine gestation should not be disturbed at laparotomy, unless it is attached only to nonvital and easily removable organs, for fear of initiating extensive uncontrollable hemorrhage and of traumatizing important structures, especially bowel and bladder. Roentgenograms that show the fetal spine overlapping the maternal spine are helpful in diagnosing abdominal pregnancy. Ultrasonography using B-scan technique (see Chapter 13) will reveal the gestational sac separate from the uterine mass.

TUBAL PREGNANCY

Etiology

The known causes of ectopic pregnancy include a variety of disorders that partially obstruct the uterine tube or alter its physiology so that ovum transport is adversely affected. These include (1) salpingitis, (2) pelvic adhesions, (3) infantile tubes with imperfect development of cilia, (4) excessively long tubes, (5) diverticula and accessory tubes, (6) spasm of the tube, muscular insufficiency and antiperistalsis and (7) endometriosis of the tube.

The incidence of ectopic pregnancy is 1:87 births (Breen) and appears to be increasing nationwide (Webster et al.), perhaps as a result of more widespread venereal disease with pelvic inflammatory complications (Fontanilla and Anderson). In some parts of the United States, the frequency of ectopic pregnancy has doubled since the advent of antibiotics. If this relationship is correct, it may be conjectured that treated salpingitis leaves the tube patent to allow conception, but sufficiently damaged to foster ectopic implantation. Many such patients would have had blocked tubes prior to the availability of effective treatment.

Recent support for the concept that ectopic pregnancy may be the result of post-abortal tubal inflammation comes from a study by Panayotou et al. They determined that patients with tubal pregnancy had more than twice the incidence (58 versus 24 per cent) of prior induced abortion than carefully matched control patients. This very significant difference in prior experience points to a tenfold relative risk that induced abortion predisposes to subsequent ectopic pregnancy.

Pathology

Early Changes.   Tubal pregnancy is the most common form of ectopic pregnancy.

The trophoblast produces cytolysis of the cells of the tubal mucosa, and the ovum then burrows into the muscular wall of the tube. Usually, islands of decidual reaction are present in and near the implantation of the ovum and even in the other tube. There is also a decidual change in the uterine endometrium. As the ovum grows, it bulges the wall of the tube inward, occluding its lumen; the cells of the opposing surfaces necrose and the capsularis, if there is one, fuses with the opposite side of the tube.

Conditions in the wall of the tube are different from those in the uterus. In the uterus, the ovum develops in the thick decidua which acts as a protective wall against the advancing erosion of the trophoblast. On the other hand, there is little decidua in the tube and the advancing trophoblast rapidly pierces its way into the muscular fibers and blood vessels (Figs. 225 and 226).

Usually, the hypertrophy of the muscle of the tube is insufficient to accommodate the growing ovum, and the wall at the placental site becomes weakened. Any trauma, such as straining at stool, coitus or a bimanual examination, causes a slight hemorrhage at this site. Later, the tube bursts from overdistention of the thinned, necrosed wall and the villi penetrate the peritoneum. This is called *extracapsular rupture*. Bleeding naturally follows. Blood usually flows into the peritoneal cavity, forming a *hematocele*. When the tube bursts into the broad ligament, a *hematoma* develops. Rupture of the tube is the usual termination of isthmic and interstitial pregnancy, and it almost always occurs

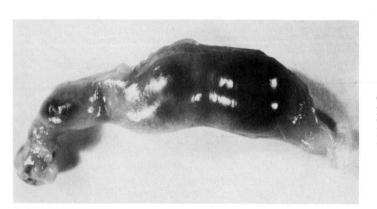

Figure 225 Gross specimen of excised unruptured ampullary tubal pregnancy illustrating its characteristic location, distention of the lumen and suffusion of tubal wall with blood.

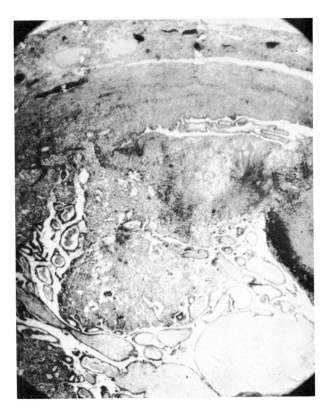

Figure 226 Photomicrograph of a histological section of an early unruptured tubal pregnancy demonstrating intact chorionic villi, decidual reaction in the stroma and hemorrhagic collections in the tubal muscularis. (Low power.)

in the second or third months after conception.

When the ovum is in the ampulla, the developing gestational sac may grow somewhat larger because of the distensibility of the ampullary part of the tube. Rupture may ultimately occur, but generally it takes place somewhat later than isthmic or interstitial pregnancy. More often, it may point in the direction of the fimbriated end of the tube and terminate as a *tubal abortion*.

The course of tubal abortion closely resembles that of uterine abortion. First, a hemorrhage occurs in the placental site, loosening the ovum from its bed. The blood fills the overdistended tube. The ovular sac may rupture and the embryo escapes among the clots. This is called *intracapsular rupture*. The ovum and clots are extruded through the open end of the tube into the peritoneal cavity and are absorbed, unless the hemorrhage has been so profuse as to cause shock and, thereby, demand surgical intervention.

Interstitial pregnancy is the growth of the fertilized ovum in the interstitial portion of the tube (Fig. 227). Frequently, this term is used interchangeably with *cornual pregnancy* and *angular pregnancy*. Reported cases (Grusetz and Polayes) terminate by rupture and abortion similar to tubal gestations. Rarely, abortion may occur into the uterus. Since only a corner of the uterus is being developed, it distorts the organ. Rupture occurs late because the uterine wall is capable of more distention and hypertrophy than the tubal wall. The embryo may die as a consequence of the rupture or it may develop to maturity within the broad ligament.

The clinical picture of rupture of an interstitial pregnancy may be similar to that of rupture of the uterus with profuse hemorrhage and shock. Interstitial pregnancies have occurred after homolateral salpingectomy (Simpson et al.) and even after salpingectomy or salpingectomy with cornual resection. Simple salpingectomy with careful peritonization appears to offer just as good results as cornual resection in this regard. Therefore, salpingectomy is pref-

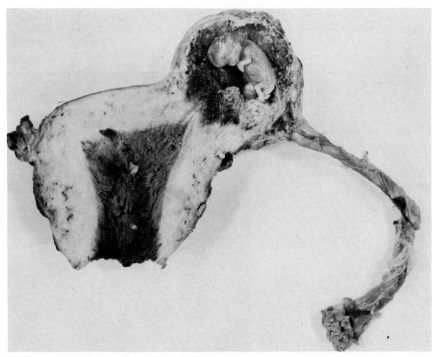

Figure 227   Gross view of excised uterus and left tube of a patient with an unusually large interstitial pregnancy. The site of rupture is seen. Both the endometrial cavity and the rest of the uterine tube are intact and undisturbed. (Courtesy of A. J. Kobak.)

erable to cornual resection, especially when dealing with a ruptured tubal pregnancy.

Late Changes. If a tubal pregnancy terminates by abortion without enough intraperitoneal bleeding to require an immediate operation, the extruded clots and the embryo are rapidly absorbed. During rupture, the placenta usually becomes detached, torn or disorganized, and the embryo dies and is absorbed. Chorionic gonadotropin production by the villi ceases soon after their oxygen supply from the mother is severed, but it may take three to seven days before circulating maternal levels fall sufficiently for the pregnancy test to become negative.

Sometimes the conceptus reimplants in a new site on the peritoneal surface. If this happens, the fetus may continue to develop among the intestines or on the broad ligament to form a *secondary abdominal pregnancy*. When the sac has ruptured, a new sac may take its place. Its wall may be made up of fibrin, adherent intestines, omentum, uterus, broad ligament and other tissue, depending on its location.

The placenta is spread out and implanted over the tissues adjacent to its first point of development and is usually thin. The blood vessels around the placenta are enormously dilated and many new ones are formed.

A secondary abdominal pregnancy may go to term. Spurious labor sets in. The fetus may die as the result of hemorrhage into or separation of the placenta, but it may not die until later. The contractions of the uterus will ultimately expel the decidua, usually with slight bleeding. The sac may rupture at any time.

After the fetus dies, if not removed, it first becomes *macerated,* then the amniotic fluid is absorbed, the sac attaches itself to the body, granulations fill the interspaces and the soft parts of the fetus are absorbed or *skeletonized.*

Another kind of event after death of the fetus is *mummification*. The fetus dries up and becomes leathery *(fetus papyraceus)*. In this state it may be found years later. After a few years, calcium salts are deposited in and around the fetus to form a *lithokelyphos* or *lithopedion* ("stone child").

Uterine Changes. In response to the estrogen stimulus of pregnancy, the uterus hypertrophies, but not as much as if it were carrying the embryo itself, and contracts intermittently. A decidua develops in it, presenting all the characteristics of a decidua of an intrauterine pregnancy, except that it contains no chorionic villi. At the time of spurious labor or spurious abortion the decidua may be sloughed in one piece, as a cast of the uterine cavity, or in large shreds or plaques. The uterus shrinks. Whereas decidua without chorionic villi is suggestive evidence of ectopic pregnancy, this does not exclude normal intrauterine gestation or abortion.

The integrity of the decidua is correlated with the histological appearance of the trophoblast (Speert). The decidua reflects the hormonal influence of pregnancy, dissociated from any local action of the trophoblast or pressure effect of the fetal sac. The thickness of the decidua varies widely, but is unrelated to the stage of pregnancy or the viability of the trophoblast. By the twelfth week, most of the gestational glands have undergone secretory exhaustion. The decidua consists chiefly of a broad sheet of transformed stroma. The integrity of the decidual stroma is maintained until full term or until death of the trophoblast.

Vaginal bleeding in ectopic pregnancy may be regarded as the counterpart of the physiologic bleeding of intrauterine pregnancy; both probably result from the same vascular phenomena that produce the bleeding of menstruation. Thus, vaginal bleeding in ectopic pregnancy does not necessarily signify fetal death.

Romney et al. examined 115 endometrial linings in patients with proved ectopic pregnancies and found 39.1 per cent to be secretory, 30.4 per cent to be proliferative and 6.1 per cent to be menstrual in type, all indistinguishable from comparable phases of normal menstrual cycles. Decidua without chorionic villi was present in only 19.1 per cent. Therefore, failure to find decidua in endometrial curettings does not rule out an existing ectopic pregnancy.

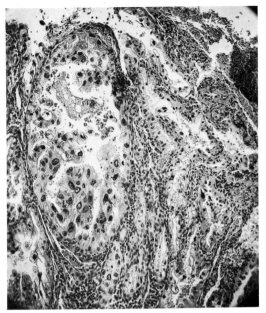

Figure 228 Histological appearance of a curettage specimen exhibiting atypical epithelial changes in the gland (Arias-Stella). These bizarre shaped, hyperchromatic, enlarged nuclei are associated with a loss of cellular polarity. The abnormal nuclei tend to occupy the luminal portion of the cell. Cytoplasmic vacuolization is occasionally present. The focal nature of these changes is shown. (Magnification × 168.) (Courtesy of R. B. Pildes.)

Changes in the endometrial epithelium are seen which consist primarily of nuclear and cellular hypertrophy (Fig. 228). These findings were first described by Sturgis and Meigs in 1936 (Sturgis) and later rediscovered independently by Arias-Stella. They appear to be due to excessive secretory activity in pregnancy. They are also found after incomplete abortion as well (Pildes and Wheeler).

There are as yet no reliable diagnostic laboratory procedures which definitively establish or exclude ectopic pregnancy. Ectopic pregnancy must be considered in any female in the childbearing period who presents a bizarre pelvic diagnostic problem.

Clinical Course

Rarely are the first weeks of an ectopic gestation without pelvic symptoms. Usually, the patient misses a menstruation, has the ordinary concomitant symptoms of early pregnancy and soon complains of pains in the lower part of the abdomen, especially on the affected side. After a few weeks, an irregular bloody vaginal discharge appears, simulating threatening abortion. On the occasion of a strain, coitus or an examination, the patient feels a sudden severe pain on one side; she feels faint or dizzy and may vomit or be nauseated. Symptoms of shock may appear. The pain continues and a piece or all of the uterine decidua may be discharged.

The physician may conclude that an abortion has taken place. The first internal hemorrhage is rarely severe. Usually, the hemorrhage recurs in a few hours or days. If the patient is not operated on, nature may effect a cure; the sac is sealed off by firm adhesions and the clots are slowly absorbed.

The symptoms of rupture of the sac are pain on the affected side, sometimes excruciating, sudden and spreading over the lower part of the abdomen, with or without associated nausea, vomiting and diarrhea, but with evidences of internal hemorrhage and shock. Extreme pallor with slight cyanosis about the lips, yawning and sighing, together with a fast, weak pulse and extreme weakness, are indicative of shock from blood loss.

Vaginal examination will usually reveal a large uterus and later, when the blood has clotted and a hematocele is forming, a mass in the culdesac can be outlined. Movement of the cervix or touching the culdesac usually elicits severe pain. A soft bulging of the culdesac may be felt. The pain is intense when the rupture has taken place into the broad ligament. This may be suspected in the presence of a firm mass to one side of the uterus. Shock is out of proportion to the anemia because the peritoneum is being stretched.

The symptoms are less stormy and much less characteristic if the rupture or the tubal abortion occurs gradually. After the ovum escapes into the peritoneal cavity or the broad ligament, if it continues to develop, symptoms of peritoneal irritation arise, including direct, rebound and referred pain, soreness, nausea, vomiting, diarrhea, constipation, bladder disturbances and invalidism. The signs and symptoms of pregnancy continue. Fetal movements become pronounced and are sometimes painful. The mass continues to grow. If the fetus dies, the symptoms of pregnancy disappear, but subfebrile temperature elevation, rapid pulse, anorexia and loss of weight may appear.

If the sac forms into a lithopedion, involution of the uterus occurs, and the irritation of the peritoneum subsides. Such patients recover completely and may even have children subsequently. The symptoms and the course of a pregnancy in a rudimentary horn of the uterus are similar to those of ectopic gestation.

Diagnosis

Ectopic gestation is rarely diagnosed before the tube ruptures or hemorrhage takes place because the tube is soft and difficult to palpate. It may, however, be extremely tender. No pelvic condition gives rise to more diagnostic errors. A high index of suspicion is essential.

First Trimester. Whenever a woman in the reproductive period complains of unilateral cramping pains in the lower part of the abdomen in association with any menstrual irregularity, ectopic pregnancy should be suspected. If sudden, excruciating pelvic pain occurs, with dizziness, faintness or collapse, the diagnosis is almost certain and is confirmed by finding an extrauterine adnexal mass. Pain in the shoulders may occur when blood reaches the diaphragm. After 24 to 48 hours, the hematocele becomes readily palpable and displaces the uterus. The hematocele is usually retrouterine.

A broad ligament hematoma can be more easily diagnosed from the stormy beginning of the clinical picture with severe pain running down the leg and a firm, tender tumor at one side. Other occasional symptoms are rectal pressure, frequent desire to defecate, tenesmus, pain, irritability of the bladder and a tender pelvis. Usually, the examination is painful and the utmost gentleness must be used to avoid rupturing the sac. Cullen's sign, or the ecchymotic blue skin discoloration tint at the umbilicus, may appear later (Merrill).

DIFFERENTIAL DIAGNOSIS. Ectopic pregnancy may readily be confused with spontaneous abortion, angular pregnancy, pregnancy in a retroflexed, incarcerated uterus, acute appendicitis and with an ovarian cyst that is undergoing twisting or rupture.

Before every curettage for abortion, it is wise to rule out extrauterine pregnancy by a careful bimanual examination. Should collapse occur during such an examination, rupture of an ectopic sac must be suspected.

If a hematocele or a hematoma becomes infected, the condition cannot be differentiated from a pyosalpinx, pelvic cellulitis or perimetritis, unless operation, laparoscopy or culdocentesis shows the hemorrhagic nature of the pelvic tumor. Jaundice is an important sign, but may not appear for several days, since it usually accompanies resorption of degenerating blood.

In the early months of a normal intrauterine pregnancy, confusion is often caused by a long cervix softened at its upper part. The cervix, which is hard, is mistaken for the uterus, and the corpus is thought to be the ectopic sac. By straightening out the uterus, one can make the correct diagnosis.

Except by means of laparoscopy or culdoscopy, it is usually not possible to differentiate a bleeding corpus luteum cyst or corpus hemorrhagicum from a ruptured tubal pregnancy. Similarly, angular pregnancy (Fig. 229) cannot be differentiated from interstitial pregnancy except by its clinical course. Therefore, it is best to hospitalize the patient for observation. Angular pregnancies remain quiescent, while an interstitial pregnancy may develop a catastrophic clinical picture.

A pregnancy in the uterus that is complicated by ovarian or other cystic pelvic tumors may be diagnosed as an ectopic gestation. The biological tests for pregnancy in the presence of intact ectopic pregnancies yield practically the same degree of accuracy as in intrauterine pregnancies. This is not true after rupture, however.

In rare instances rupture of a gestational sac with collapse must be differentiated from rupture of a pyosalpinx, the twisting of an ovarian tumor, ovarian hemorrhage, painful ovulation, bursting of an appendiceal abscess or of the gallbladder, gastric or duodenal perforation and ureteral stone.

Acute appendicitis has often been mistaken for extrauterine pregnancy; with coexisting pregnancy, the differential diagnosis cannot always be made. Whenever

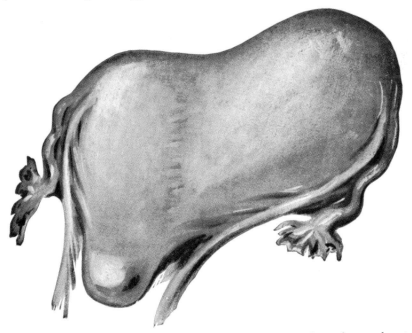

Figure 229 Angular pregnancy, implanted in the left cornual angle of the endometrial cavity simulating ectopic gestation. Note marked uterine asymmetry.

the diagnosis is uncertain, the patient should be hospitalized for observation and have a pregnancy test. Occasionally, curettage will yield valuable information. If chorionic villi are found, an intrauterine pregnancy is certain but, of course, an ectopic pregnancy may also be present. However, a large, thick, rough decidual membrane without chorionic villi expelled from the uterus, giving a more or less complete cast of the cavity, or clean decidua without villi obtained at curettage, is almost pathognomonic of ectopic gestation. It may be expelled after the operation. Heaney pointed out that the near absence of endometrium, or a dry

scrape, is highly suggestive that an ectopic pregnancy is present.

Hemoglobinemia and hematin are present with long-standing rupture, particularly in patients with jaundice (Whitacre) as a result of reabsorption of lysed blood products from the peritoneal cavity.

Culdocentesis is a relatively harmless and often helpful procedure (Fig. 230). Errors may arise by drawing blood from a vein, by getting a dry tap and by passing the needle into the amniotic sac, the lumen of bowel or an ovarian cyst. If one obtains blood containing minute clots (partially lysed old clotted blood), or bloody fluid that does not clot (totally lysed), one

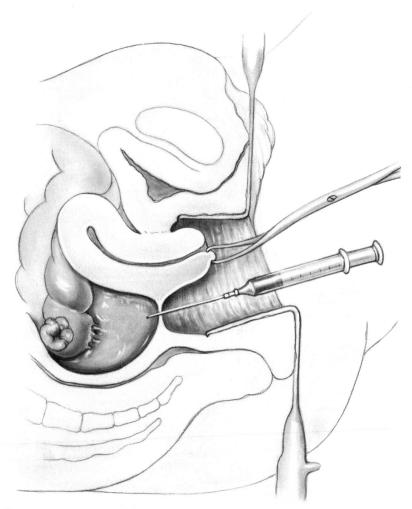

Figure 230 Diagnostic puncture of culdesac or culdocentesis. The cervix is exposed and steadied with a vulsellum attached to its posterior lip. A sharp, long 16-gauge needle is passed gently through the posterior fornix into the culdesac of Douglas. If the first tap is dry, the needle is withdrawn a little and passed into another position in the midline.

has added assurance of earlier intraperitoneal bleeding.

Posterior colpotomy is very useful in the diagnosis of both intact and ruptured ectopic pregnancy. In the former, the unruptured tube may be brought into view and often it can be removed through this opening. If this is not feasible, the gravid tube can be removed by laparotomy after the colpotomy wound is closed. In patients with rupture, this diagnostic approach may be superfluous and the additional time needed for the procedure may contribute to blood loss. The surgeon should perform a laparotomy.

A helpful procedure in suspected ectopic pregnancy prior to laparotomy is *culdoscopy* or *laparoscopy*. Culdoscopy permits visualization of the organs by way of the posterior vaginal fornix. Laparoscopy accomplishes even better visualization transabdominally. Not only may a definite diagnosis of tubal pregnancy be made but the diagnosis may also be clearly excluded and a laparotomy obviated.

Prognosis

The prognosis is relatively good for patients in whom ectopic pregnancies rupture early. Even when the correct diagnosis is not made, an operation is nearly always done in due course because the intensity and progression of symptoms will demand intervention. If delayed, shock is common and may even be fatal. In a national survey of maternal deaths occurring in a five-year interval in the United States, Breen found 6.5 per cent were due to ectopic pregnancy, ranking it seventh among causes.

Some patients recover completely without an operation because the disturbed ovum is absorbed. On the other hand, when an ectopic pregnancy ruptures, reimplants and becomes a secondary abdominal pregnancy, the condition becomes quite serious. Some women die despite surgery. A large proportion of the fetuses are deformed; few babies survive. The surgical removal of an unruptured ectopic pregnancy carries no more risk than the hazards of anesthesia and laparotomy.

Treatment

There is no expectant treatment for a growing ectopic gestation. The conceptus must be removed as soon as possible. If the diagnosis is made before tubal rupture or during tubal abortion, the procedure of choice is removal of the tube with the ovum, by laparotomy or, occasionally, by posterior colpotomy (see above). Some have recently recommended preserving reproductive function by doing a salpingotomy instead, shelling out the contained pregnancy and securing hemostasis. While this conservative approach is worth considering in a patient whose other tube has already been removed or is hopelessly diseased, it should be borne in mind that, following salpingotomy, recurrent ectopic pregnancy is likely in the same tube at some future time.

Tubal Rupture and Tubal Abortion. When the diagnosis is clear, the situation requires emergency care. The hospital is notified to have the operating room ready and the patient is transported in an ambulance just as any patient who is bleeding extensively. Entrance formalities are waived except for a very cursory check of the heart and lungs and vital signs. The patient is taken to the operating room and anesthetized, while simultaneously blood is drawn for typing and cross-matching; whole blood transfusion is given as quickly as possible (that is, as soon as blood is available), when needed to replace the loss due to intraperitoneal hemorrhage. The abdomen is opened with the utmost dispatch. The intestines, floating in blood, are pushed away. With one grasp the uterus is located, is pulled up and a clamp is placed on the mesosalpinx of the affected side. The sac is brought into view and a clamp is placed on its uterine side. A salpingectomy is performed; the stump is sutured and covered with peritoneum; the ovum, usually found near the site of the rupture, and the clots are removed (Fig. 231). The opposite tube and ovary should be inspected for possible disease and the rest of the abdominal cavity should be thoroughly explored.

One should not hesitate to operate while the patient is in shock, but blood should be given during and after the operation.

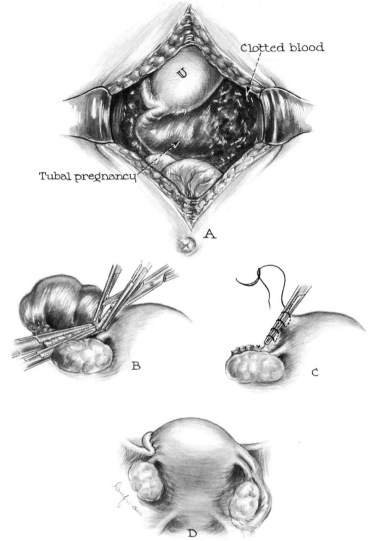

Figure 231 *A*, Pelvic findings at laparotomy for ruptured tubal pregnancy showing displaced uterus (*U*), mass of fresh and old blood and distended tube containing gestational sac and blood. *B*, Clamping and dividing tube at junction with uterus and mesosalpinx. *C*, Peritonization. *D*, Round ligament used to cover site.

Usually, the blood pressure will rise immediately after the arterial bleeder is clamped.

In interstitial pregnancy, if the sac is not too large, the cornua may be excised and the wound closed. This is the operation of choice if the patient is seen early and is in good condition. Total hysterectomy is indicated when cornual resection is not technically feasible.

Pelvic Hematocele or Hematoma. If asymptomatic and not progressive, expectancy is indicated for pelvic hematocele or broad ligament hematoma. Serial hematocrit determinations will be helpful in ascertaining whether or not the condition is stable. The blood is eventually absorbed along with the ovum. If fever, chills, rapid pulse, pain and symptoms of peritonitis develop, they suggest infection. This will require drainage as soon as possible. Suppurating hematoceles are opened through the posterior culdesac and a rubber drain inserted, without any attempt to remove clots and without irrigation. Cultures are obtained and then antibiotics should be given.

Abdominal Pregnancy. As the pregnancy advances beyond the fourth month, the fetus acquires considerable bulk. The adhesions of the sac to the adjacent organs become extensive, firm and vascular, especially in the placental region. Any operation may be formidable. It is best to intervene as soon as the diagnosis is made and not wait for the fetus to become viable. Exceptionally, or because of religious beliefs, the patient may demand delay to save the fetus; in this event, she might have to be hospitalized to await the time of operation at or after the thirty-sixth week. The operation may prove very difficult and should be undertaken only by a skilled surgeon because serious complications, especially hemorrhage, are common.

The abdomen must be opened carefully because fetal sac, omentum, intestines and placenta are netted with large and fragile blood vessels, some of which may lie just underneath the abdominal wall. It is most important to locate the placenta; this may not be possible until the sac has been opened and the fetus delivered. After the delivery of the child, the placenta may be found near the site of the rupture or original implantation of the placenta, spreading over the sides of the pelvis, the rectum, the sigmoid, the cecum and their mesenteries. Usually, in abdominal pregnancy, the safest thing to do is to ligate the umbilical cord as close to the placenta as possible after removing the fetus and to leave the placenta *in situ* undisturbed. This avoids hemorrhage which can be fatal. Some recommend drainage of the fetal sac to allow the degenerating tissues to exit. Others feel this is unnecessary and possibly dangerous because secondary infection may result.

If the fetal sac is already infected, part of the membranes should be marsupialized by suturing them to the abdominal wall to permit sloughing of the placenta. Antibiotics should be administered. Extrauterine pregnancy after 28 weeks' duration is not rare (Ware). Suter and Wichser found that only about one-fourth of extrauterine pregnancies diagnosed after the fifth month of gestation result in living viable babies. About one-third of these babies have deformities incompatible with life.

Intraligamentary pregnancy, also known as *intraligamentous, broad ligament* and *extraperitoneal pregnancy,* is one in which the embryo grows between the peritoneal folds of the broad ligament. It must be distinguished from the usual intraperitoneal type of abdominal gestation. Champion and Tessitore reviewed 70 cases in which the pregnancies lasted seven or more months. They called attention to the relationship of the ovisac to the pelvic organs. The medial boundary is the uterus; the lateral boundary is the wall of the pelvis; inferiorly is the pelvic floor and superiorly, the uterine tube. The round ligament is frequently prominent on the anterior surface of the sac.

Intraligamentary pregnancy is very rare indeed. Kobak et al. reported three cases of intraligamentary and 27 abdominal pregnancies among 932 ectopic gestations associated with more than 87,000 pregnancies.

The placenta develops retroperitoneally within the ovisac. If it is within the redundant areolar tissue of the broad ligament, it can be removed without too much risk. Care must be taken to ensure that there is no attachment to or distortion of the major pelvic vessels or the ureter. If it is attached to the uterus, hysterectomy will facilitate hemostasis.

RUDIMENTARY HORN PREGNANCY

It is difficult to distinguish between a tubal pregnancy and a rudimentary horn pregnancy, a very rare condition. Because the uterine cornu is thick and vascular, rupture is likely to occur later than with tubal gestation and hemorrhage is usually greater. Most ruptures of the uterine horn occur in the second trimester instead of in the first. About 10 per cent of rudimentary horn pregnancies go to term.

The clinical picture of rupture of a rudi-

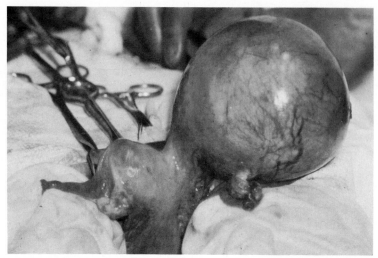

Figure 232 Photograph taken at surgery showing a pregnancy in an unopened rudimentary horn. Note intact tube and ovary attached inferolaterally. (Courtesy of S. L. Naor.)

mentary horn is exactly the same as that of a ruptured ectopic pregnancy. Differentiation between a tubal pregnancy and a rudimentary horn pregnancy can be made if the round ligaments can be felt (see above). Treatment consists of total removal of the gravid horn or, if necessary, hysterectomy (Fig. 232).

OVARIAN PREGNANCY

Ovarian pregnancy (Fig. 233) is another rare form of ectopic gestation. To establish the anatomic certainty of an ovarian pregnancy, certain criteria must be fulfilled (Spiegelberg): (1) the tube on the affected side must be intact; (2) the fetal sac must

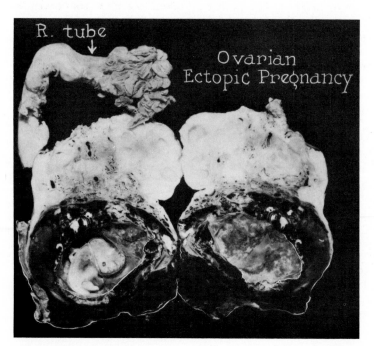

Figure 233 Right tube and ovary, fixed and transected, with an ovarian pregnancy *in situ*. Note presence of ovarian tissue and intact uterine tube. (Courtesy of A. J. Kobak.)

occupy the position of the ovary; (3) the fetal sac must be connected with the uterus by the utero-ovarian ligament, and (4) definite ovarian tissue must be found in the sac wall.

Ovarian pregnancy pursues the same course as a tubal one. The impregnation of the ovum by the spermatozoon takes place before the ovum leaves the ovary, where implantation occurs. The pregnancy is pedunculated because the fetal sac grows out into the peritoneal cavity from its implantation site in the ovary. It is generally easy to remove, but it does form adhesions with the surrounding structures. If the ovum was implanted near the hilum, the gestational sac may become intraligamentous, growing between the peritoneal leaves of the mesovarium. Rupture of the sac, with hematocele, is the usual termination, with or without fetal death. A laparotomy must be performed as in other forms of ectopic pregnancy.

CERVICAL PREGNANCY

This extremely rare type of gestation results when a fertilized ovum becomes implanted and develops in the cervix. Some of these pregnancies are unrecognized because the products of conception are expelled as abortions early in their development. It is usually necessary to intervene surgically because of hemorrhage with or without rupture of the amniotic sac or perforation of the cervical wall. Suggestive of cervical pregnancy are enlargement and expansion of the cervix accompanied by bleeding in the early months of pregnancy and the detection of the corpus uteri characteristically surmounting the cervical mass. Supravaginal rupture of the cervix must be treated by hysterectomy. Intravaginal bleeding from the cervical canal can sometimes be treated conservatively by curettage and local suturing. If ineffectual, hysterectomy will be required.

Duckman and Amico differentiate *cervical pregnancy* from *cervical abortion* (Chapter 33) as follows: (1) the corpus that surmounts the distended cervix is usually larger in cervical abortion than in early cervical pregnancy; (2) in cervical abortion both internal and external os are dilated, whereas in cervical pregnancy the internal os is practically closed; (3) in cervical abortion placental tissue can be palpated attached to the uterine wall above the internal os; (4) until the abortion is well advanced, the external os is usually closed in cervical abortion; it is this resistance to dilatation of the external os that is believed to be responsible for the cervical abortion. In cervical pregnancy the external os is usually partly or well dilated.

REFERENCES

Arias-Stella, J.: Atypical endometrial changes associated with presence of chorionic tissue. Arch. Path. 58:112, 1954.

Beacham, W. D., Collins, C. G., Thomas, E. P., and Beacham, D. W.: Ectopic pregnancy. J.A.M.A. 136:365, 1948.

Breen, J. L.: A 21 year survey of 654 ectopic pregnancies. Amer. J. Obstet. Gynec. 106:1004, 1970.

Burkhart, K. P., Mulé, J. G., Begneaud, W., and Kohen, J.: Combined intrauterine and extrauterine gestations progressing to viability. Obstet. Gynec. 22:680, 1963.

Champion, P. K., and Tessitore, N. J.: Intraligamentary pregnancy: A survey of all published cases over seven calendar months, with discussion of an additional case. Amer. J. Obstet. Gynec. 30:281, 1938.

Duckman, S., and Amico, J.: Cervical abortion: Report of a case. Obstet. Gynec. 10:240, 1957.

Fleisher, A. A., and Seaman, I.: Heterotopic pregnancy: The effect of shock on the first-trimester fetus. Obstet. Gynec. 18:763, 1961.

Fontanilla, J., and Anderson, G. W.: Further studies on the racial incidence and mortality of ectopic pregnancy. Amer. J. Obstet. Gynec. 70:312, 1955.

Grant, A.: Problems in fertility and sterility due to ectopic pregnancy: A study of 259 cases. Med. J. Australia 2:817, 1953.

Grusetz, M. W., and Polayes, S. H.: Interstitial pregnancy, with report of case of full-term gestation. Amer. J. Obstet. Gynec. 48:379, 1944.

Heaney, N. S.: Diagnostic errors in intra-uterine pregnancy. Med. Clin. N. Amer. 22:213, 1938.

Hoerner, M. T.: Bilateral simultaneous tubal pregnancy: Review of literature and report of case. Amer. J. Surg. 91:385, 1956.

Jarcho, J.: Ectopic pregnancy: I. With special reference to abdominal pregnancy. Amer. J. Surg. 77:273, 1945.

Järvinen, P. A., and Kinnunen, O.: The treatment of

extrauterine pregnancy and subsequent fertility. Int. J. Fertil. *2*:131, 1957.

Kobak, A. J., Fields, C., and Pollack, S.: Intraligamentary pregnancy: Extraperitoneal type of abdominal pregnancy. Amer. J. Obstet. Gynec. *70*:175, 1955.

Loh, W. P., and Loh, H.-Y. C.: Unilateral tubal twin pregnancy with intraperitoneal rupture: Report of a case. Obstet. Gynec. *19*:267, 1962.

Merrill, J. A.: Cullen's sign: A historical review and report of histologic observations. Obstet. Gynec. *12*:317, 1958.

Panayotou, P. P., Kaskarelis, D. B., Miettinen, O. S., Trichopoulos, D. B., and Kalandidi, A. K.: Induced abortion and ectopic pregnancy. Amer. J. Obstet. Gynec. *114*:507, 1972.

Pildes, R. B., and Wheeler, J. D.: Atypical cellular changes in endometrial glands associated with ectopic pregnancy. Amer. J. Obstet. Gynec. *73*:79, 1957.

Romney, S. L., Hertig, A. T., and Reid, D. E.: The endometria associated with ectopic pregnancy: A study of 115 cases. Surg. Gynec. Obstet. *91*:605, 1950.

Simpson, J. W., Alford, C. D., and Miller, A. C.: Interstitial pregnancy following homolateral salpingectomy: A report of six new cases and a review of the literature. Amer. J. Obstet. Gynec. *82*:1173, 1961.

Speert, H.: The uterine decidua in ectopic pregnancy: Its natural history and some biologic interpretations. Amer. J. Obstet. Gynec. *76*:491, 1958.

Spiegelberg, O.: Zur Casuistik der Ovarialschwangerschaft. Arch. Gynäk. *13*:73, 1878.

Sturgis, S. H.: Arias-Stella phenomenon (letter). Amer. J. Obstet. Gynec. *116*:589, 1973.

Suter, M., and Wichser, C.: The fate of living viable babies in extrauterine pregnancies. Amer. J. Obstet. Gynec. *55*:489, 1948.

Ware, H. H.: Observations on thirteen cases of late extrauterine pregnancy. Amer. J. Obstet. Gynec. *55*:561, 1948.

Webster, H. D., Jr., Barclay, D. L., and Fischer, C. K.: Ectopic pregnancy: A seventeen-year review. Amer. J. Obstet. Gynec. *92*:23, 1965.

Whitacre, F. E.: Discussion of Williams, P. E., and Corbit, J. D.: An analysis of 101 fatalities from ectopic pregnancy. Amer. J. Obstet. Gynec. *48*:841, 1944.

Chapter 33

Spontaneous Abortion

Spontaneous abortion is a common phenomenon, probably accounting for the termination of one in every five to seven pregnancies conceived. Hospital figures are not representative because only recognized instances and complicated cases of abortion are sent to hospitals. Furthermore, many abortions occur in the first weeks after conception and are considered to be delayed or profuse menstruation. Finally, it is likely that many abortions are deliberately concealed.

NOMENCLATURE

Terminology in this area is confused. *Miscarriage* is a totally unsatisfactory term used by the laity for every interruption of pregnancy before term, and the word *abortion* carries a distinct stigma implying an instrumental or criminal process. Abortion should be used to apply only to the process of expulsion of a nonviable fetus and not to the fetus itself, which should be called an *abortus*. By convention, abortion refers to pregnancies terminating up to 20 weeks' gestational age or delivering a fetus weighing less than 500 gm.

The various designations of abortion, most of which are dealt with in greater detail later in this chapter, include the following terms, all referring to pregnancies under 20 weeks:

1. Spontaneous abortion, occurring without evidence of willful or inadvertent interference.
2. Threatened abortion, associated with transcervical bleeding with or without recognizable uterine contractions and pain, but without cervical dilatation or expulsion of the conceptus.

3. Inevitable abortion, with bleeding, uterine contractions and progressive cervical dilatation.
4. Incomplete abortion, in which there is expulsion of only part of the products of conception.
5. Complete abortion, involving total expulsion of the uterine contents.
6. Missed abortion, the retention of the fetus in the uterus for eight weeks or more after it has died.
7. Habitual abortion, the occurrence of three or more consecutive spontaneous abortions.
8. Infected or septic abortion (see Chapter 34).
9. Induced abortion, the deliberate interruption of an intact pregnancy (see Chapter 35).
10. Tubal abortion, the termination of an ampullary ectopic pregnancy (see Chapter 32) by extrusion through the fimbrial ostium.

ETIOLOGY

Fetal Causes

The causes of most spontaneous abortions are unknown. Abnormal uterine environment (Mall) and intrinsic germ plasm defect have been conjectured to be causative. Abnormalities in the very earliest stages of human development are common (Hertig and Rock).

Hertig analyzed 1000 consecutive patients with abortions, most of which were spontaneous. Although 13 patients gave a history of trauma prior to the time they aborted, it could be demonstrated that the embryo was absent, dead or malformed in every one of these at the time of trauma. Hence, abortion clearly resulting from trauma is an extremely uncommon phenomenon, although it is possible, of course.

Rock et al. studied 36 fertilized ova discovered in 185 fertile, potentially pregnant women whose uteri were removed prior to the first missed menses. Among the 36 conceptuses, aged 36 hours to 17 days, 13 were abnormal. Hence, about 20 per cent of these fertile women, all of whom had been exposed to pregnancy at the time of ovulation, became pregnant. This gives some index of fertility for any given menstrual cycle in patients with known fertility. The incidence of abnormality in these early human pregnancies was 36 per cent, which is about the same as the incidence of abnormalities in experimental animals (Corner).

Huber et al. found an abnormal fetus in 76 per cent of 90 intact specimens among 314 abortions. In 40 per cent there were hydropic changes in the chorionic tissue. These changes were always associated with an abnormal fetus.

The clinical incidence of spontaneous human abortion is usually quoted as 12 per cent, which is comparable to some lower animals (Ingalls). As indicated above, the true rate for humans is probably higher, many not being recognized or diagnosed as such. The fertilized zygote in the presence of a demonstrably normal uterine environment can be intrinsically defective in a substantial percentage of pregnancies.

Among 1000 consecutive spontaneous abortion specimens studied by Javert and Barton, 297 had umbilical cords sufficiently complete for analysis. Of this number, 35 per cent were abnormal, in contrast to 4.8 per cent in a control group of therapeutic abortions. Approximately 64 per cent of the fetal disorders were congenital and 36 per cent were acquired. Most of the cord complications were such as to compromise the fetal circulation and produce death *in utero*. The incidence of cord lesions was 56 per cent of all the pathologic fetuses, indicating abnormality of the cord as an important associated cause of the pathologic fetus. Cord compli-

cations were observed in 24 per cent of macerated, degenerated and mummified fetuses in contrast to only six per cent with normal fetuses.

Carr has shown that chromosome abnormalities are about 40 times more frequent in spontaneous abortuses than in full-term babies. Hence, genetic factors at the chromosome level are a significant cause of spontaneous abortions.

Blighted ova, that is ova without an embryo, constituted about half of the abortuses examined by Hertig and Rock. None of the patients in whom abnormal ova were found showed any clinical or pathologic evidence that maternal environment alone played any pathogenetic role. The defective fertilized ovum in this type of case results from an intrinsic germ plasm defect rather than from its environment. Faulty germ plasm is a major cause of spontaneous abortion.

Levine showed a large proportion of hydatidiform moles in women of advanced age. A correspondingly higher incidence of spontaneous abortions and congenital malformations occurs in this same age group. The increase in incidence of these conditions commences at the beginning of ovarian failure. In women who have had a hydatidiform mole, the incidence of abortion is 36 per cent as compared with an expected 15 to 20 per cent. There is a striking histological similarity between typical hydatidiform moles and the hydropic changes seen in many abortions.

Maternal Causes

Some spontaneous abortions may be due to a decrease in the amount of progesterone produced by the corpus luteum of the ovary associated with a simultaneous lag in the production of this hormone by the placenta. The resultant inadequate progesterone support will not favor early implantation and development. Later, if the amount of progesterone secreted is insufficient, the sensitivity of the uterus is perhaps increased and this may result in coordinated contractions of the uterus and expulsion of the ovum.

Acute infections frequently cause the

death of a fetus and its expulsion from the uterus. These are due to (1) transmission of bacterial toxins from the mother to the fetus, (2) passage of microorganisms from the mother to the fetus, (3) high temperature which frequently stimulates the uterus to contract while at the same time increasing both placental and fetal oxygen demands, or (4) hypoxia secondary to increased metabolic needs or decreased resources, as occurs in the cyanosis associated with pneumonia.

Diseases and abnormalities of the decidua are the second most frequent causes of abortion in the early months of pregnancy. Williams found histological evidence of acute or chronic decidual endometritis in 70 per cent of his specimens of abortion. However, in many instances it is likely that the endometritis was a secondary phenomenon, resulting from the abortion and not causing it. After both normal and abnormal labor, the uterus contains numerous harmless and pathogenic bacteria by the second day of the puerperium. Similar invasion by bacteria occurs after abortions.

Rarely, incarcerated retroflexion causes abortion. The interruption of pregnancy is due to the changes in the decidua, which result from disturbances in uterine circulation, and not merely to the malposition of the uterus. Cervical defects constitute a rare cause of abortion and premature labor.

The severest mental and physical injuries are sometimes inflicted on the gravida without disturbing the uterus. Operations, too, usually do not affect the pregnancy even when performed on the uterus. This is not meant to condone nonessential surgery during pregnancy. Ovarian tumors have repeatedly been extirpated safely, even in the early months. Appendicitis may cause abortion, probably because of the infection. Anesthesia does not cause fetal death. However, it is imperative to avoid hypoxia (see Chapter 22). There is no proof that any lack of a vitamin or a group of vitamins or other food substances in women results in sterility or abortion.

In some patients there is documented thyroid dysfunction that may affect both fertility and the ability of the patient to carry the pregnancy to viability. Medical or surgical correction is effective in preventing some abortions and fetal deaths.

There may also be paternal causes which are difficult to document. Without doubt the spermatozoa of some men are inadequate to give the ovum the necessary generative impulse.

Habitual Abortion

The patient with habitual abortion is one who has had at least three successive pregnancies interrupted spontaneously at about the same period of development prior to viability. In most of these women no cause can ever be found. Germ plasm defects may be the underlying reason. In some, uterine leiomyomas, anomalies or incompetent cervix may be discovered to be etiologic (see below).

MECHANISM OF ABORTION

Uterine action accomplishes nearly all the work of abortion except the expulsion of the loosened ovum from the vagina which is done by the abdominal muscles. The bony passages never come into consideration.

In the first six to eight weeks, the whole ovum is usually delivered, covered by the decidua (Figs. 234 and 235) or expelled naked (Fig. 236). Should the external os offer resistance and not dilate, the ovum is arrested in the distended cervix. This is *cervical abortion* (Fig. 237).

Several courses may be taken by the abortive process during the third and fourth months. First, the whole conceptus may be expelled with the fetus in an intact sac attached to the placenta. This offers the best prognosis for the mother since hemorrhage is usually minimal, the process is self-limiting and intervention is not always necessary.

Second, the membranes may rupture and the fetus be extruded. The cervix may close and the placenta be retained. The uterus later makes a second effort to expel

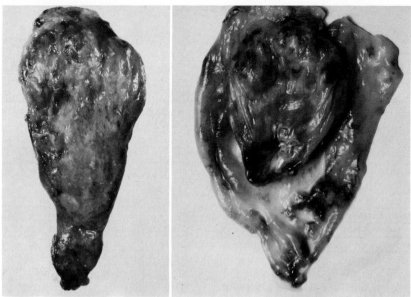

Fig. 234   **Fig. 235**

Figure 234 Complete decidual cast of the uterus. (From Potter, E. L.: Pathology of the Fetus and the Infant, ed. 2. Chicago, Year Book Medical Publishers, Inc., 1961.)

Figure 235 Decidual cast opened to show attached ruptured chorionic vesicle. The embryo was expelled several days before the decidua and chorionic sac. (From Potter, E. L.: Pathology of the Fetus and the Infant, ed. 2. Chicago, Year Book Medical Publishers, Inc., 1961.)

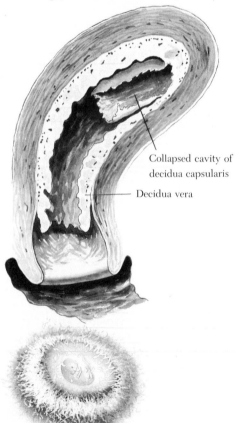

Collapsed cavity of
decidua capsularis

Decidua vera

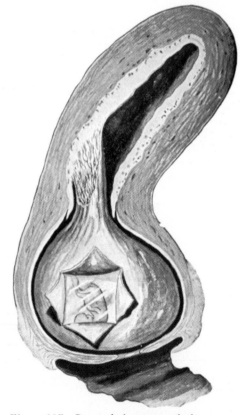

Figure 236 The naked ovum is shown in the lower illustration having been expelled from the ovular sac in early incomplete abortion.

Figure 237 Cervical abortion with the conceptus still adherent at its base protruding into the dilated cervical canal. External os not yet opened.

368

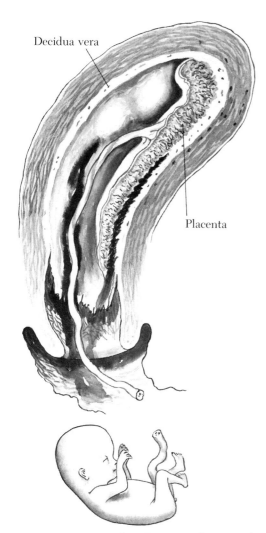

Figure 238 Incomplete abortion at three months. When only the fetus is expelled, all the secundines remain in the uterus. Compare with Figure 236.

After-pains occur sometimes, and even lactation occasionally.

SYMPTOMS

There are five terms applied to clinical patterns of abortion: *threatened, inevitable, incomplete, complete* and *habitual.* Characteristic symptoms include: uterine contractions, uterine hemorrhage, softening and dilatation of the cervix, and expulsion of all or part of the ovum. Another form, *missed abortion,* is discussed at the end of this chapter.

Threatened abortion usually presents with bloody vaginal discharge. Pelvic pains similar to menstrual cramps are often associated. The blood may gush or ooze out or appear as brownish staining of mucus. The uterus may be inconstantly harder than normal because it is contracting. Softening and dilatation of the cervix

the secundines (Figs. 238 and 239). During the interval, due to partial separation of the placenta, hemorrhage may become profuse, making intervention essential.

Third, the decidua capsularis and the chorion may break, allowing the fetus in the amniotic sac to escape. The uterus still contains the placenta and the chorion. Bleeding may or may not occur until such time as placental separation begins.

In abortion, the uterine contractions act the same as they do in labor. Dilatation of the cervix also is produced in the same way. After delivery of its contents the uterus contracts and involution begins.

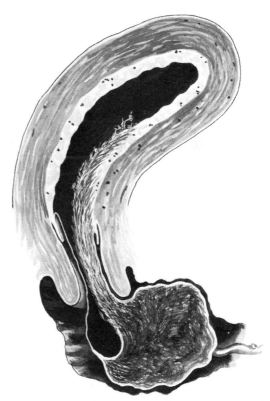

Figure 239 Placenta protruding into vagina and partly attached, inviting infection. The thick decidua is still in the uterus.

seldom occur. The clinical picture may persist and an abortion may appear threatening for days and weeks. In some patients the pregnancy may go to term. In others profuse hemorrhage may occur suddenly, acute and progressive uterine pains develop and the process becomes inevitable.

Abortion in progress or *inevitable abortion* presents the same symptoms in aggravated form. The bleeding is more profuse and the pains are stronger and more regular, resembling those of labor. Softening and dilatation of the cervix occur.

If the whole conceptus is expelled, the bleeding is usually moderate and the pains cease as soon as the ovum escapes from the cervix. In multiparas, because the cervix is more elastic and less resistant, the abortion tends to be easier and quicker than in nulliparas. The decidua is sloughed and expelled in the profuse lochial discharge.

If the membranes rupture and the fetus is discharged, the remaining membranes and placenta are usually expelled after minutes or hours. If they do not follow spontaneously, profuse hemorrhage may necessitate emptying the uterus.

Incomplete abortion means that the process has started but that the uterus has not entirely emptied itself of the whole conceptus. Incomplete abortion is dangerous because of its immediate and remote sequelae: (1) After the escape of the fetus, the retained parts of the placenta, membranes and decidua gradually break down and are discharged in the lochia. The lochia of such patients are profuse, bloody and sometimes odorous. Chronic endometritis and even sepsis may result from such a process. (2) An interval may follow during which there may be complete cessation of symptoms until, after hours or days, the uterus suddenly expels its contents. (3) A placental polyp may be formed.

Complete abortion signifies that all the products of conception have been expelled spontaneously.

DIAGNOSIS

Threatened Abortion

If a pregnancy is known to be present, uterine bleeding and pains signify that interruption of gestation threatens. Bimanual examination shows the enlarged, contracting and relaxing uterus, the beginning softening and unfolding of the cervix and the bloody discharge. One should consider every uterine hemorrhage after a period of amenorrhea in a woman capable of reproduction as a threatened abortion. Microscopic bleeding is common in pregnancy. Speert and Guttmacher found erythrocytes in vaginal smears in 18 per cent of pregnant women during the second month. Macroscopic bleeding may be of large proportions, even simulating a menstrual flow, perhaps explaining the disparity that sometimes appears between the duration of pregnancy calculated on the basis of the last menstrual period and a disproportionately large baby. In another series of patients who did not abort, the incidence of macroscopic vaginal bleeding up to the twenty-eighth week was reported to be 21.8 per cent.

Nesbitt et al. have demonstrated that vaginal cytology (see Chapter 13) permits one to make prognostic deductions concerning the outcome of a pregnancy. Only 8.9 per cent of 504 women who ultimately aborted did so in the presence of a normal smear, and only 1.3 per cent of those with a good smear ultimately aborted. Only three per cent of the patients who carried to term did so in the presence of a poor smear.

Inevitable Abortion

This condition is more easily characterized. The cervix is shortened and its angle with the corpus is straightened. The external os is dilated so that the conceptus can be felt with the finger or seen through a speculum. Pieces of the conceptus are expelled. Bleeding is more profuse. The membranes rupture and the patient experiences painful uterine contractions. It is important to study all expelled tissue microscopically to differentiate abortion of intrauterine pregnancy from ectopic or molar gestation. If villi are present in the tissue expelled, the abortion is incomplete. In women who expel decidua alone, an ectopic pregnancy must be suspected. There are instances of double uterus in which the decidua from one side is discharged while the other side contains a normal intact pregnancy. Rupture of the membranes may be simulated by a benign, but annoying condition known as *hydrorrhea gravidarum,* a periodic discharge of accumulated secretions.

Incomplete Abortion

It is important to know if the uterine cavity is empty. Even when the expelled parts have been examined by a competent observer, it may still be in doubt. If a woman who has had an abortion continues to have irregular bleeding or prolonged bloody lochia with occasional clots or bits of tissue, it is likely that something is left in the uterus. Examination reveals an enlarged, soft, subinvoluted uterus, which sometimes contracts, with a succulent, patulous cervix through which shreds of placenta or clots may occasionally be felt or observed through a speculum. Microscopic examination of discharged or curetted pieces of tissue may show chorionic villi. Verification of whether or not the uterus is empty may be impossible without curettage. A positive pregnancy test may persist in incomplete abortion as long as part of the placenta is adherent and functioning.

PROGNOSIS

Rarely, women die from hemorrhage during abortion. Death may more often result from an infection introduced by instrumentation performed under suboptimal conditions by the patient or an abortionist. Aggressive treatment of this serious complication is essential (see Chapter 34).

TREATMENT

Threatened Abortion

Hormone treatment of threatened abortion is controversial and unproved for all practical purposes. Diethylstilbestrol, the use of which was based on the claims of Smith et al., is now interdicted for use in pregnancy because it may somehow be related to later development of vaginal clear cell carcinoma among female offspring (Herbst et al.). This serious shortcoming may end the controversy by default, but for completeness it should be noted that Dieckmann et al. insisted that stilbestrol does not reduce the incidence of abortion.

Treatment for threatened abortion is at best empirical and based largely on dogmatism rather than substantiation. Since many abortions are associated with blighted ova, no treatment can be expected to be effective. Most physicians prescribe bed rest and abstinence from coitus. Neither can be supported by evidence (Diddle et al.), but both are acceptable recommendations because they are harmless (although they impose needless disability and economic hardship).

One may perform a pregnanediol test. If it is normal, there is no reason for giving progesterone. If the test shows a lack of or low pregnanediol excretion, progesterone is given by some obstetricians. Reifenstein reviewed the use of 17-α-hydroxyprogesterone caproate (Delalutin) in habitual abortion, showing 68.3 per cent total salvage with treatment as compared with 11.3 per cent in previous pregnancies. Goldzieher and Benigno considered that the results of progestin therapy could be achieved by chance alone.

Moreover, Wilkins observed fetal masculinization in 70 female infants whose mothers were given progestins orally because of habitual or threatened abortion. Labioscrotal fusion occurred only when administration of either 17-α-ethinyltestosterone (ethisterone) or Norlutin (norethindrone) was begun before the twelfth week of gestation. Phallic enlargement results when androgenic activity is exerted over a sufficient period at any time during fetal or postnatal life. These compounds are sufficiently potent when they cross the placenta to masculinize the relatively sensitive end-organs of the developing fetus, even though bioassays show that they have relatively weak androgenic effects in adults.

Goldzieher observed several instances of clitoral hypertrophy in newborn infants whose mothers did not receive any hormone therapy. Masculinization of female infants has been reported when mothers received only stilbestrol. Such observations argue more for spontaneous occurrence than for any causal relationship. Therefore, anomalies of infants whose mothers were treated with synthetic progestins perhaps reflect the current therapeutic vogue rather than any causal relationship between the steroid and the anomaly.

There should be no hesitancy about performing a bimanual vaginal and speculum examination when abortion is suspected. An erosion, polyp or even cancer is occasionally found to explain the bleeding. If fetal parts protrude through the cervix and the uterine size is 12 weeks' gestational age or less, the uterus should be emptied immediately by suction aspiration or curettage.

If restricted activity has been prescribed but does not relieve bleeding and cramps, the patient should be allowed up all the time. Nearly all such pregnancies are abnormal and the sooner the gestation is terminated the better. The uterus should be emptied if bleeding has continued and the pregnancy has failed to enlarge to the size expected for the duration of pregnancy. Pregnancy tests provide little help because they may be negative in the presence of a normal healthy gestation and a positive result does not prove that the embryo is living, but only that the chorionic ectoderm is still active.

McCord asserts that there is no proof that abortion or bleeding is more likely at the time of a missed menses. Until such proof is obtained, the time of the missed menstrual period should be considered no more important than any other time.

Inevitable Abortion

For inevitable abortions up to twelve weeks when the cervical canal is dilated only slightly, suction aspiration or dilatation and curettage is the simplest and most satisfactory procedure. If the pregnancy is more advanced and the cervical canal is not open, one should await further spontaneous developments or attempt to stimulate evacuation by nonoperative means. These latter include use of uterotonic agents or hypertonic saline (see Chapter 35).

When the cervix is open enough to admit one finger, the uterus can be emptied easily. The uterine cavity is evacuated by gentle curettage or vacuum curage.

Habitual Abortion

In all women with a history of habitual abortion, a hysterogram should be made before a new pregnancy is contemplated to rule out a submucous leiomyoma or a uterine abnormality as a possible cause of the repeated abortions. In hysterograms done on 56 habitual aborters, Halbrecht found 22 congenital malformations and submucous leiomyomas in six. Studies should be made to decide whether a clinical thyroid disorder exists.

Incompetent cervix may also cause habitual abortion, especially in the midtrimester of pregnancy. Incompetent cervix requires a careful evaluation of a history of repeated pregnancy losses. Characteristically, silent cervical dilatation precedes the abortion and the fetus is normal, albeit not capable of surviving. Hysterography is also useful in the diagnosis (Figs. 240 and 241). Treatment is surgical between pregnancies or when the cervix begins to efface and dilate. The simple Shirodkar encirclage procedure is shown in Figures 242 to 249.

Ovular factors were found causative in 43 per cent and maternal factors in 15 per cent of 100 habitual aborters studied by Wall and Hertig. Pathologic ova were the most common etiologic factors, accounting for 62 per cent of the 58 abortions. The more often these patients aborted, the more likely the same causative factor was involved. Among 82 patients with two consecutive abortuses, the same cause was found in 52.4 per cent. In 16 patients with three consecutive abortuses, the same cause was present in 81.2 per cent. It is important that every abortus be thoroughly examined for pathologic changes to provide information for future reference in the event the patient should abort again.

The gloomy prognosis usually given women with a history of three or more consecutive abortions (Malpas) has been

(*Text continued on page 376.*)

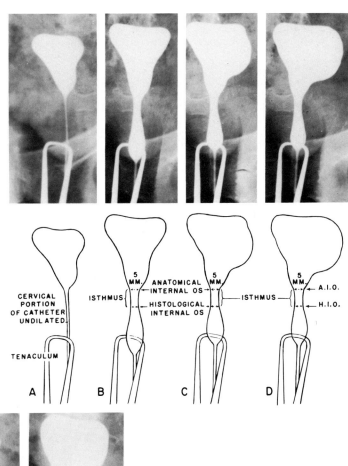

Figure 240 Film and film tracings illustrate cervical competency by the simple intrauterine balloon technique. Film and tracing (*A*) reveal the balloon filling the uterus. With an increased amount of dye injected, myometrial resistance raises the pressure within the balloon to a critical level (approximately 250 mm. Hg) at which point the neck of the balloon, lying in the upper reaches of the isthmus and cervix, expands (*B*). With the introduction of additional dye, there is increased pressure evidenced manometrically and, in this particular illustration, by adaptive regional hypotonia of the corpus (*C*). Despite increased pressure, the isthmus, particularly the anatomic internal os, does not dilate, as do the corpus and lower part of the cervix. Instead, the width of the isthmus remains narrow and constant, reconfirming cervical competency (*D*). (Courtesy of E. C. Mann.)

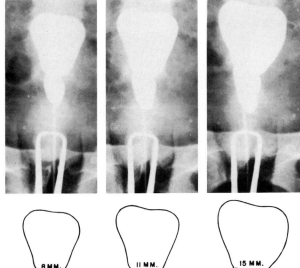

Figure 241 Film and film tracings illustrate cervical incompetency. *A*, Expansion of the balloon within the uterus results in expansion of the neck of the balloon within the isthmus and upper part of the cervix. The lower boundary of the isthmus in cervical incompetency loses its functional identity and only the anatomic internal os remains. With increasing amounts of dye and concomitant increases in pressure, the anatomic internal os progressively and abnormally widens (*B* and *C*), revealing cervical incompetency. (Courtesy of E. C. Mann.)

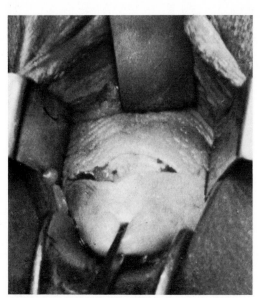

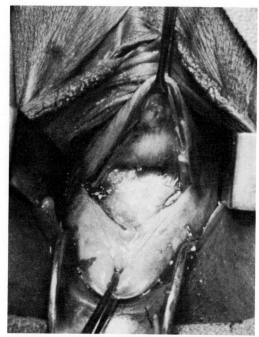

Fig. 242   *Fig. 243*

Figure 242   Shirodkar operation for incompetent cervix (Figs. 242 to 249). Adrenalin in saline is injected at the sides of the cervix, under the bladder and posteriorly where the incision is to be made. Then an incision is made on the anterior wall of the cervix. (Courtesy of V. N. Shirodkar.)

Figure 243   The bladder and anterior vaginal wall are dissected away from the cervix exposing the region above the external os.

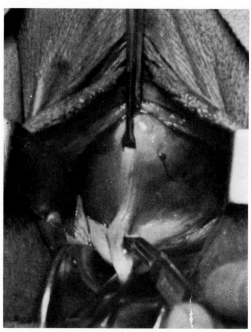

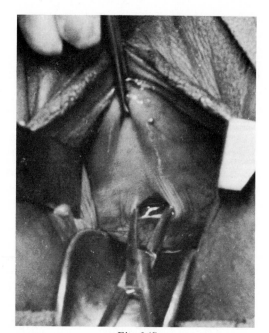

Fig. 244   *Fig. 245*

Figure 244   The cervix is pulled anteriorly and a fold of posterior vaginal wall is made prominent by pulling with Allis forceps. A vertical incision 1.5 cm. in length is made by a stab incision.

Figure 245   A curved artery forceps is introduced into this incision and the tissue stretched.

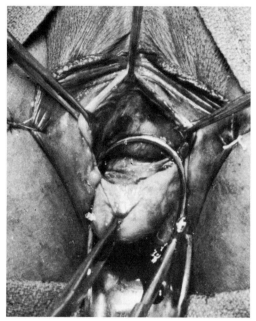

Fig. 246

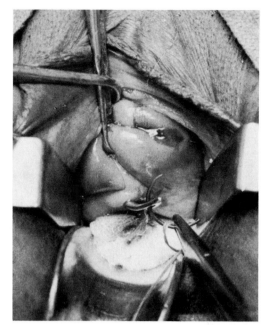

Fig. 247

Figure 246 A blunt ligature carrier (right) is introduced in and under the right pillar of the bladder. It is pushed in and backward beneath the mucosa toward the posterior incision.

Figure 247 Linen thread holding one end of a fascial strip (or Mersilene tape) is mounted on a Mayo needle and is passed through the eye of the ligature carrier. This is done in order to facilitate threading the eye. It is difficult to do this with the hands alone when the cervix is deep.

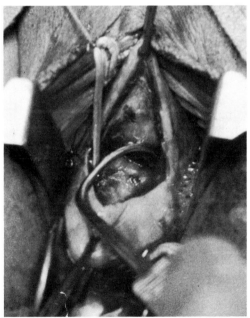

Fig. 248

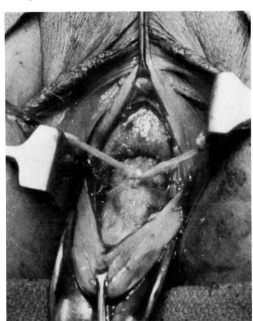

Fig. 249

Figure 248 The right end of the fascial strip has been pulled forward and the ligature carrier is introduced under the left bladder pillar to be pushed back and out of the posterior incision as was done on the right side.

Figure 249 Both ends of the fascial strip are tied into a reef knot. The knot is transfixed with a fine linen or silk suture. The surplus ends on each side are sutured to the circular part of the fascial strip to prevent slipping.

seriously doubted by Speert, who found that 81 per cent of 121 habitual aborters carried subsequent pregnancies to viability. A woman with three consecutive abortions had a better prognosis in a subsequent pregnancy than a woman with more than three consecutive abortions. Hormone therapy was of no apparent value in the treatment of these sequential aborters.

It is only after four consecutive abortions, according to Goldzieher and Benigno, that the subsequent abortion rate changes appreciably. The prognosis is significantly influenced by the past obstetric history and by urinary pregnanediol excretion. In threatened abortion, the prognostic significance of a low pregnanediol excretion is grave. They claimed a benefit from the use of progesterone therapy in these patients.

Bevis reported that 81 per cent of 32 women who had had three or more abortions gave birth to live children. He maintains that a great part of his success was due to the psychologic support he gave his patients.

In this regard, obstetricians can detect many serious emotional factors which might somehow be responsible for habitual abortion. Thorough history and analysis of patients' problems are useful. However, many will require referral to a psychiatrist for proper diagnosis and treatment (Greenhill).

CURETTAGE

The size and shape of the uterus must be determined by bimanual examination and an ectopic pregnancy ruled out before any instrument is passed into the uterus. Before inserting a curet, the uterus is to be pulled down with a vulsellum on the anterior lip of the cervix. This straightens the cervix and the uterus. Then a blunt sound is passed to determine the length of the cavity. The curet is gently introduced up to the uterine fundus. Exerting only slight pressure on the scraping edge of the curet, the instrument is drawn down and out of the cervix with a single slow, even, gentle sweep. The curet is cleaned in sterile sa-

line solution or on gauze, then reinserted and the process repeated, first over the posterior wall, then the anterior, then the corners of the uterus and finally the fundus from one tubal opening to the other. No to-and-fro movements are made; each stroke of the curet must be from above downward and out. The broadest curet that will pass into the cervix is to be used; a smaller one may be needed for cleaning out the cornua. The utmost gentleness is essential at all times. Vacuum curage is equally effective and less traumatic (see Chapter 35).

If the patient bleeds freely during curettage, ergonovine 0.2 mg. may be injected intravenously or 5 international units of oxytocin injected intramuscularly or into the cervical muscle. This will contract the uterus, reduce the bleeding and give a firm base for the curet.

Perforation of the uterus occurs occasionally (Fig. 250). It is usually due to ignorance of the dangers of curettage and rough handling, but it may also occur in the hands of the most skillful physician because the uterine wall is sometimes pathologically soft and friable. This is especially true in septic cases and during the puerperium. The placental site feels rough and the fissures in it allow the curet to pierce the muscle, giving the impression that there is a piece of adherent placenta. The cervix and lower uterine segment may be ruptured with dilators and a piece of uterine wall grasped and torn off with polyp or ovum forceps. A perforation can be diagnosed by the excessive freedom of movement of the end of the curet and the depth to which it disappears in the uterus.

A single small perforation of the uterus requires no treatment if there is no undue bleeding. Careful postoperative observation is essential to detect signs of continuing intraperitoneal bleeding. Evidence of progressive peritoneal irritation or falling hematocrit is critical. At any suggestion of injury to the bowel or omentum, the abdomen must be opened immediately and all damage repaired. Injured intestines must be repaired or resected as necessary. Perforation of the uterus is particularly serious when it occurs in the presence of a septic abortion. Evaluation and treatment are outlined in Chapter 34.

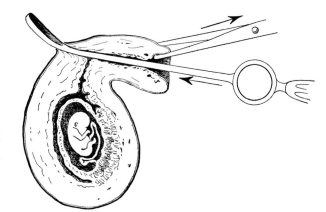

Figure 250 Diagrammatic representation to show how the retroflexed uterus is readily perforated by the inappropriately placed curet, sound or dilator.

Decker and Zaneski report that among 10,105 curettements there were 51 accidental perforations, an incidence of 0.5 per cent. The responsible instruments were curets in 29, uterine sounds in 18, cervical dilators in two, ovum forceps in one and the instrument was unknown in one.

RETURN OF OVULATION

Sullivan found that ovulation will occur in four to six weeks after abortion in 90 per cent of women prior to the first menses, whether or not a curettage was performed. In 50 per cent, the first ovulation after spontaneous abortion will have a shortened secretory phase.

MISSED ABORTION

Missed abortion is a condition signifying that the abortus has been dead for at least eight weeks and is retained in the uterus. This is indicated by cessation of uterine growth or by actual diminution in size; the absence of fetal heart tones after they have been heard is also definitive, especially if observed by ultrasound (Doppler effect) as described in Chapter 13. Ultrasound B-scanning is also useful in demonstrating this condition.

Changes in the Conceptus

If the fetus dies in the early weeks, the chorion and the decidua, nourished by maternal blood, may continue to grow. Hemorrhages in the decidua are common and the whole periphery of the conceptus may be involved. The cavity of the amnion is crowded together or the blood may, in rare cases, break into the conceptus itself. This is called a *blood mole*. It is called *fleshy mole* when it is older, organized and decolorized. These moles (not to be confused with hydatidiform mole) usually cause repeated bleeding until expelled or the physician intervenes. Later in pregnancy, after the fetus has developed, changes similar to those of a dead ectopic fetus are observed. This is *missed abortion* and it is not rare. In missed abortion, the fetus degenerates before the placenta (Greenhill).

The changes generally observed after the death of the fetus are (1) *maceration,* (2) *mummification,* (3) *lithopedion* formation and (4) *septic infection. Maceration* is most common, the fetus imbibing the dissolved blood pigments to become a *fetus sanguinolentis.* Its tissues are soft; the bones are loose; the brain is liquefied; the skin is flabby; large patches of epidermis are missing and thus the deep-red corium is exposed. The cord is thick and blood-stained; the placenta, which may continue to grow even after fetal death, is pale and soft. *Mummification* occurs more rarely. The fetus dries up, becomes leathery and may give considerable trouble in removal by morcellation. The amniotic fluid is absorbed or represented by a thick yellow or greenish paste; the placenta is a tough, white, infarcted mass. This condition occurs most often in twins when one of the fetuses dies in the early months and is

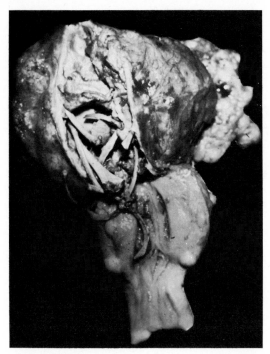

Figure 251 Abdominal pregnancy with lithopedion formation.

pressed against the uterine wall by the growing twin, producing a *fetus compressus* or *papyraceus* (Kindred). *Lithopedion formation* (Fig. 251) is exceptional in the uterus itself, being seen more often as a late consequence of ectopic gestation, the result of calcium deposition. *Septic infection* of the uterine contents is common in ordinary abortion but rare in missed abortion, unless instrumental interference has been practiced (see Chapter 34). Septic infection may occur even after months.

Symptoms

Missed abortion seldom produces symptoms. The breasts and pelvic organs retrogress toward the nonpregnant state. The uterus ceases to grow and assumes a nonresilient consistency. A brownish, sometimes fetid, vaginal discharge appears. The diagnosis of missed abortion is made by bimanual examinations at two- to four-week intervals. The uterus becomes smaller and harder. It is best to wait at least four to six weeks before deciding that

the fetus is dead because the uterus may not enlarge at a regular rate in normal pregnancies. From the history one learns that the signs and symptoms of pregnancy have retrogressed. Pregnancy tests may become negative after the fetus dies, but positive reactions usually persist until all chorionic activity within the uterus has ceased. This may require weeks or months.

Treatment

The best results are obtained when the uterus is emptied spontaneously. Interference by dilatation and curettage or other operative procedures frequently results in considerable morbidity. Serious hemorrhage from alterations in the blood clotting mechanisms may occur with prolonged retention of a dead fetus (Weiner et al.), usually seen if it is retained for more than five weeks. Immediately after delivery there may be excessive bleeding from the uterus or other sites. The principal defect seems to be a critical reduction in blood fibrinogen secondary to intravascular coagulation.

Beginning with the third week after apparent fetal death, the concentration of fibrinogen should be determined weekly. Heretofore, it was recommended that the uterus be emptied promptly if the concentration of fibrinogen falls below 150 mg. per 100 ml. When termination is undertaken in these circumstances, it is necessary to have whole compatible blood and fibrinogen available for administration. Recently, it has been shown possible to prevent intravascular consumption of fibrinogen by the administration of heparin intermittently by subcutaneous injection. Even after the fibrinogen has begun to fall, the process can be reversed through the use of anticoagulation. Once the intravascular clotting has been arrested, the patient's liver is capable of restoring fibrinogen levels quickly to normal in a matter of a day or so by synthesis.

Labor and vaginal delivery, with or without oxytocin stimulation, will not result in any significant change in the concentration of circulating fibrinogen, even if hypofibrinogenemia is present. The optimal termination mechanism in missed abortion is spontaneous evacuation. Second only to this is the use of intraamniotic injections of hypertonic saline (see Chapter 35).

REFERENCES

Bevis, D. C. A.: Treatment of habitual abortion. Lancet 2:207, 1951.

Carr, D. H.: Chromosome studies in abortuses and stillborn infants. Lancet 2:603, 1963.

Corner, G. W.: Ourselves Unborn: An Embryologist's Essay on Man. New Haven, Yale University Press, 1944.

Decker, W. H., and Zaneski, B. W.: Accidental perforation of the uterus. Amer. J. Obstet. Gynec. 66:349, 1953.

Diddle, A. W., O'Connor, K. A., Jack, R., and Pearce, R. L.: Evaluation of bed rest in threatened abortion. Obstet. Gynec. 2:63, 1953.

Dieckmann, W. J., Davis, M. E., Rynkiewicz, S. M., and Pottenger, R. E.: Does the administration of diethylstilbestrol during pregnancy have therapeutic value? Amer. J. Obstet. Gynec. 66:1062, 1953.

Goldzieher, J. W.: Synthetic progestational steroids: Their significance and use. Texas J. Med. 57:962, 1961.

Goldzieher, J. W., and Benigno, R. B.: The treatment of threatened and recurrent abortion: A critical review. Amer. J. Obstet. Gynec. 75:1202, 1958.

Greenhill, J. P.: Histological study of a fetus and implantation site in a case of missed abortion. Amer. J. Obstet. Gynec. 2:188, 1921.

Greenhill, J. P.: Emotional factors in female sterility. Obstet. Gynec. 7:602, 1956.

Halbrecht, I.: Role of anatomic changes of uterine cavity in pathogenesis of habitual abortion. Gynaecologia 131:1, 1951.

Herbst, A., Ulfelder, H., and Poskanzer, D. C.: Adenocarcinoma of the vagina: Association of maternal stilbestrol therapy with tumor appearance in young women. New Eng. J. Med. 284:878, 1971.

Hertig, A. T.: Prematurity, Congenital Malformation and Birth Injury: Traumatic Abortion and Prenatal Death of the Embryo. New York, Association for the Aid of Crippled Children, 1953.

Hertig, A. T., and Rock, J.: A series of potentially abortive ova recovered from fertile women prior to the first missed menstrual period. Amer. J. Obstet. Gynec. 58:968, 1949.

Huber, C. P., Melin, J. R., and Vellios, F.: Changes in chorionic tissue of aborted pregnancy. Amer. J. Obstet. Gynec. 73:569, 1957.

Ingalls, T. H.: Prematurity, Congenital Malformation and Birth Injury: Principles Underlying Experimentally Induced Anomalies. New York, Association for the Aid of Crippled Children, 1953.

Javert, C. T., and Barton, B.: Congenital and acquired lesions of the umbilical cord and spontaneous abortion. Amer. J. Obstet. Gynec. 63:1065, 1952.

Kindred, J. E.: Twin pregnancies with one twin blighted: Report of two cases with comparative study of cases in literature. Amer. J. Obstet. Gynec. 48:642, 1944.

Levine, B.: The early trophoblast: A review including theoretical considerations. Obstet. Gynec. 17:769, 1961.

Mall, F. P.: A study of the causes underlying the origin of human monsters. J. Morph. 19:1, 1908.

Malpas, P.: A study of abortion sequences. J. Obstet. Gynaec. Brit. Emp. 45:932, 1938.

McCord, J. M.: The myth of the missed menstrual period. Obstet. Gynec. 11:704, 1958.

Nesbitt, R. E. L., Jr., Garcia, R., and Rome, D. S.: The prognostic value of vaginal cytology in pregnancy. Obstet. Gynec. 17:2, 1961.

Potter, E. L.: Pathology of the Fetus and the Infant, ed. 2. Chicago, Year Book Medical Publishers, Inc., 1961.

Reifenstein, E. C., Jr.: Clinical use of 17-α-hydroxy-progesterone 17-n-caproate in habitual abortion. Ann. N.Y. Acad. Med. 71:762, 1958.

Rock, J., Mulligan, W. J., and Hertig, A. T., cited by Hertig.

Shirodkar, V. N.: Contributions to Obstetrics and Gynaecology. Edinburgh, E. & S. Livingstone Ltd., 1960.

Smith, O. W., Smith, G. V., and Schiller, S.: Estrogen and progesterone metabolism in pregnancy: Spontaneous and induced labor. J. Clin. Endocrin. 1:461, 1941.

Speert, H.: Pregnancy prognosis following repeated abortion. Amer. J. Obstet. Gynec. 68:665, 1954.

Speert, H., and Guttmacher, A. F.: Frequency and significance of bleeding in early pregnancy. J.A.M.A. 155:712, 1954.

Sullivan, C. L.: The return of reproductive capacity following spontaneous abortion. Amer. J. Obstet. Gynec. 63:671, 1952.

Wall, R. L., and Hertig, A. T.: Habitual abortion: A pathologic analysis of 100 cases. Amer. J. Obstet. Gynec. 56:1127, 1948.

Weiner, A. E., Reid, R. E., Roby, C. C., and Diamond, L. K.: Coagulation defects with intrauterine death from Rh isosensitization. Amer. J. Obstet. Gynec. 60:1015, 1950.

Wilkins, L.: Masculinization of female fetus due to use of orally given progestins. J.A.M.A. 172:1028, 1960.

Williams, J. W.: Obstetrics, a Textbook for the Use of Students and Practitioners. New York, D. Appleton-Century Company, 1930.

Chapter 34

Septic Abortion

Until recently, septic abortion was one of the leading causes of maternal death. In localities where hospital abortions have been readily available because of the existence of liberalized legislative attitudes, such as New York and California, there has been a remarkable decline in both the absolute numbers of documented cases of septic abortion and the numbers with coassociated endotoxin shock (Evrard). It is expected that this trend will become more widely applicable as optimal abortion services are made accessible to all on a national scale as a consequence of the recent United States Supreme Court ruling which effectively nullifies almost all preexisting legislative constraints in this matter.

The seriousness of septic abortion was first brought to our attention in 1956 by Studdiford and Douglas, who reported on seven patients with second trimester infected abortions, all of whom became hypotensive after admission. Four of these patients died, their hypotension having been treated as hypovolemic shock.

Subsequently, it was appreciated that the problem was secondary to a toxic depression of peripheral resistance rather than to blood volume loss primarily. It was also learned that evacuation of the uterus or hysterectomy, in conjunction with support of the cardiovascular system and aggressive antibacterial therapy against the infection, was sometimes lifesaving.

Many deaths have been associated with endotoxin shock, and in view of the alarming risks attending this condition, the management of septic abortion has undergone a notable tendency toward more aggressive medical and surgical therapy.

DIAGNOSIS

Diagnosis can be made on clinical grounds. The minimal criteria include fever (although this is variable, particularly in the shock state) and objective evidence of pregnancy and of a pelvic origin of the infection. Most patients present uterine and adnexal tenderness, purulent cervical discharge and infected products of conception.

Characteristically, the patient is frequently a multipara (only one in six is nulliparous), with an average age of 27 years, very commonly with previous abortions, and frequently from a rather poor socioeconomic background. Most patients are in their first trimester. About one-third admit or strongly imply active interference with the pregnancy, usually in the form of instrumentation, either self-inflicted or performed by a criminal abortionist. It is probable that many others were similarly involved.

These patients commonly seek medical aid rather late in the course of their condition, usually after widespread infection, and after the condition has become complicated by dehydration, impressive blood loss and frequently by cardiovascular instability. The clinical picture often includes precedent chills and high fever (many patients experience them for a long time prior to admission), unstable blood pressure or frank shock, evidence of local endomyometritis, adnexal spread or generalized peritonitis. Septicemia, as evidenced by spiking fever and frank chills, may be present in many of these patients.

Laboratory findings include anemia, leukocytosis with marked shift to the left in the polymorphonuclear leukocytic differential count, and positive cervical and blood cultures. Mixed enterococci and *Escherichia coli* are the most frequent organisms grown in cultures; other organisms, including *Clostridium welchii,* may also be present.

MANAGEMENT

In a survey of the trends in management (Neuwirth and Friedman), more aggressive handling was noted. Also demonstrated was the paradoxic fact that the outcome was not influenced. This appeared to be based on a general lack of distinction between patients requiring aggressive management (a relatively infrequent occurrence) and those who might more profitably be handled conservatively. It was found, for example, that early curettage while the patient was still febrile frequently resulted in the production of operative sepsis and hypotension, the very situation one was trying to avert.

A low-risk group can be identified. Patients with infected abortion, a relatively small uterus, infection localized to the uterus, low level of fever and normal, stable blood pressure do not warrant aggressive intervention. An effective, conservative, expectant program in these patients includes the use of bactericidal agents according to the organism detected, uterotonic agents to effect evacuation of the uterine contents spontaneously and fluids and electrolytes as required. Only after a suitable time to permit defervescence, perhaps 24 to 48 hours, should surgical evacuation of the uterus be performed by curettage.

This program of management presupposes that the patient's condition will remain stable. More urgent definitive therapy is obviously necessary if any extenuating or emergency situations arise or if the infection rapidly progresses despite the measures used and becomes complicated by hemorrhage, hypotension, ileus, oliguria, abscess formation or other dire consequence. It is strongly emphasized that any complicating situation takes urgent precedence and alters the conservative approach accordingly. Prompt, aggressive measures must be pursued if the patient fails to respond or if her condition becomes worse during this trial period, with evidence of spread of infection or signs of advancing cardiovascular instability with rising pulse rate and falling blood pressure or oliguria.

The high-risk patient is one with overt evidences of endotoxin shock, characterized by hypotension, rapid, thready pulse, pallor, spiking fever, chills, a large uterus (beyond 12 weeks' gestational age) and evidence of extensive infection, including generalized peritonitis. This is an ominous situation, but it is a relatively rare complication of infected abortion, occurring in about six per cent. The growing interest in this condition has tended to magnify it and to place it apart from the general picture of the more common uncomplicated case (Knapp et al.).

The pathogenesis of *endotoxin shock* is not completely known, but sudden circulatory failure associated with overwhelming infection, most commonly Gram-negative bacteria, is well documented. The sudden dispersion of large numbers of bacteria, or more specifically toxic lipopolysaccharide liberated at the time of the lysis of bacteria, will produce shock. The injection of this material into laboratory animals produces fever, profound hypotension, hyperglycemia and leukopenia. Subsequently, there is leukocytosis as a secondary phenomenon based on plasma loss (Thomas). There is simultaneously liberation of heparin, histamine and serotonin. The condition is marked by severe arteriolar and venular constriction in the visceral circulation. This results in severe tissue hypoxia and acidosis. Eventually, cell death occurs. Intravascular coagulation is a serious coassociated phenomenon.

It is interesting to note that antibiotic therapy has occasionally precipitated shock in patients with bacteremia, apparently by killing the bacteria and liberating endotoxin (Weil). Nevertheless, it is imperative to arrest bacterial growth with antibiotics in these patients, and this theoretical constraint should not be considered a sufficient reason for withholding this essential treatment.

Evaluation of the patient on an ongoing basis is vital. The peripheral resistance is reflected in the condition of the skin. Cold extremities suggest restricted peripheral circulation. Central venous pressure is invaluable as an indirect measure of blood volume and is useful as an index of cardiopulmonary function and as a guide to fluid replacement. Cardiac output is reflected in pulse pressure. Tissue perfusion can be followed by observing urinary output hourly. Blood pressure is a notoriously poor index of the shock state.

The high-risk therapeutic regimen consists of antibiotics, vasopressors, corticosteroids, whole blood, oxygen, early curettage and, if necessary, laparotomy. Attention to acid-base balance and fluid requirements is most important because acidosis enhances the shock state and diminishes response to therapy. In order to combat the hypovolemic aspects of endotoxin shock, maximum fluid replacement is essential, using the central venous pressure as a guide. Plasma expanders, such as dextran, or mannitol are especially recommended. If these measures are ineffective, digitalis may help, ostensibly because it combats the direct toxicity of endotoxin on the myometrium.

The choice of antibiotic depends largely on the organism, but it is usually imperative to begin therapy empirically before accurate identification can be made. Accordingly, cervical smears and Gram stains help in a rough manner so that a preliminary choice may be made. It is essential to treat aggressively. Deane and Russell have expressed preference for streptomycin and chloramphenicol. When giving streptomycin, the potential dangers of toxicity due to renal failure, which permits the accumulation of this drug to toxic levels, must be recognized. Chloramphenicol may be administered intravenously in total daily dosage of 2 gm. Others prefer penicillin in daily doses varying from 20 million (Stevenson and Yang) to 30 million units (Weil) in continuous intravenous drip. Changes or adjustments can be made in the type and dosage of antibiotics administered after bacteriologic identification and sensitivity studies have been made.

In *Clostridium welchii* septicemia, further complicated by jaundice, oliguria and hemoglobinuria, antitoxin may be used additionally. Dialysis by extracorporeal exchange, using an artificial kidney, may be required when oliguria or anuria becomes a significant problem. Hemodialysis is clearly indicated when the serum potassium levels rise to 6 mEq. per liter or higher. Polyvalent gas gangrene antitoxin, 40,000 to 100,000 units intravenously at four-hour intervals, may aid (de Alvarez and Wolter).

It is appreciated that the value of vasopressor agents in this condition is debatable; nevertheless, it is imperative that the irreparable damage that may result from prolonged hypotension be avoided if possible by maintaining relatively normal levels of blood pressure. The sympathomimetic amines, metaraminol (Aramine) and norepinephrine (levarterenol, Levophed), may be very effective. These appear to act by preventing pooling in the splanchnic bed, by peripheral vasoconstriction and by increasing cardiac output and venous return. Metaraminol in doses of 200 mg. per liter or norepinephrine (2 mg. per liter of five per cent glucose in water) may be used to advantage. The rate of drip and the dosage level in the infusion bottle is adjusted according to the patient's response so that the minimal amount necessary to maintain the arterial pressure at or below normal levels is given. Blood pressure should be maintained at levels sufficient to maintain a urinary output of 30 to 50 ml. per hour. The dosage is reduced as the patient's general condition improves. The risks implicit in the use of vasopressors, including vasoconstriction leading to permanent organ or tissue damage, must be accepted in seriously ill patients.

Blood replacement is obviously essential in the presence of blood loss and superimposed hypovolemic shock. It should be emphasized that pressor amines may produce a false sense of security in the presence of shock due to blood loss. The use of whole blood transfusion or blood volume expanders (such as albumin or dextran) in acute emergencies is necessary in these situations, but the dangers of overtransfusion must be kept continually in mind. This may readily produce cardiac decompensation and further complicate an already tenuous situation. Using venous pressure as a guide during blood administration forestalls impending circulatory overloading.

The use of corticosteroids in endotoxin shock has been encouraging. They must be given early and in large doses, but should be reserved for the treatment of the shock state and not used prophylactically. Their mode of action is not yet completely defined.

In the absence of demonstrable degrees of adrenocortical insufficiency, pharmacologic actions are presumed, including the blocking of the intense sympatholytic effect of endotoxins, restoring peripheral vascular tone, decreasing clinical toxicity (Madsen and Tieche), increasing the response to vasopressors and protecting tissues against endotoxin effect perhaps through alterations in cell membrane physiology. Very large doses of hydrocortisone (Solu-Cortef) or its equivalent in a bolus of 50 to 70 mg. per kilogram of body weight intravenously, for example, may be used with good effect in endotoxin shock. The response when corticosteroids are given late in the course of the disease, after other measures have been shown to be inadequate, is relatively poor. Because the prognosis is extremely grave, it is recommended that all measures be used early.

Timely surgical intervention is an unresolved problem. The superimposition of an anesthesia and a surgical procedure on an already jeopardized cardiovascular condition may be fatal. However, it is sometimes equally imperative to empty the uterus of its infected contents so that there is no longer a source for bacterial showers and the further production of endotoxin. Furthermore, surgical intervention may indeed be lifesaving in the presence of hemorrhage, bowel injury or other intraabdominal complication. Above all, astuteness and individualization must prevail.

REFERENCES

de Alvarez, R. R., and Wolter, D. F.: Management of postabortal sepsis and acute renal failure due to Clostridium welchii. Obstet. Gynec. *11*:280, 1958.

Deane, R. M., and Russell, K. P.: Enterobacillary septicemia and bacterial shock in septic abortion. Amer. J. Obstet. Gynec. *79*:528, 1960.

Evrard, J. R.: The impact of abortion on maternal and perinatal mortality rates. Amer. J. Obstet. Gynec. *113*:415, 1972.

Knapp, R. C., Platt, M. A., and Douglas, R. G.: Septic abortion: Five-year analysis at New York Hospital. Obstet. Gynec. *15*:344, 1960.

Madsen, P. R., and Tieche, H. L.: Hydrocortisone therapy for bacterial shock in septic abortion. Obstet. Gynec. *20*:56, 1962.

Neuwirth, R. S., and Friedman, E. A.: Septic abortion: Changing concepts of management. Amer. J. Obstet. Gynec. 85:24, 1963.

Stevenson, C. S., and Yang, C.-C.: Septic abortion with shock. Amer. J. Obstet. Gynec. 83:1229, 1962.

Studdiford, W., and Douglas, G. W.: Placental bacteremia: A significant finding in septic abortion accompanied by vascular collapse. Amer. J. Obstet. Gynec. *71*:842, 1956.

Thomas, L.: The physiological disturbances produced by endotoxin. Ann. Rev. Physiol. *16*:467, 1954.

Weil, M. H.: Endotoxin shock. Clin. Obstet. Gynec. 4:971, 1961.

Chapter 35

Induced Abortion

Terminologic confusion is avoided by using the all-inclusive term *induced abortion* to refer to all willful terminations of pregnancy before the fetus has reached viability. This includes *therapeutic abortions* done on clear-cut medical or psychiatric indications as well as legalized *abortions on demand. Criminal abortion,* on the other hand, refers to unsanctioned procedures done illegally and usually under suboptimal and clandestine circumstances.

MEDICOLEGAL CONSIDERATIONS

The approach to the subject of the interruption of a pregnancy prior to viability is clouded by legal, emotional, moral, ethical and theological overtones. There can be little doubt that the fetus is in fact an entity, but the Supreme Court declared on January 23, 1973 (Roe vs. Wade) that, since a consensus on the issue of when life may be considered to begin cannot be reached by physicians, philosophers and theologians, it was inappropriate for the judiciary to speculate about it. In legalistic terms the unborn child is not a "person" for purposes of constitutional protection (Curran). Moreover, the Court struck down almost all constraining abortion control laws as unconstitutional because they invaded the privacy of the pregnant woman. It asserted that the decision regarding abortion and its performance in the first trimester was strictly a matter of medical judgment between the woman and her physician. In the second trimester and up to viability, defined as seven months' gestational age, the state is permitted to enact laws dealing with standards of medical care to protect the health of the mother. Only after viability is the state justified in limiting abortion decisions to those instances in which it is necessary to preserve the life or health of the mother.

In another equally important decision (Doe vs. Bolton), the Court declared invalid such unconstitutional invasions of privacy as legislative requirements that abortions be done only in accredited hospitals, only after approval by a specially constituted hospital abortion committee, only if appropriate concurrence by consultants is obtained and only on bona fide state residents. It also upheld a Georgia law which states that the physician's decision be based on his best clinical judgment that pregnancy termination is necessary. This rested on the broadest interpretation of health needs, encompassing relevant physical, emotional, psychological, familial and socioeconomic factors (United States vs. Vuitch). By the same token, hospitals may refuse to do abortions and physicians or hospital employees may likewise refuse to participate in these procedures on moral or religious grounds. Curran's discussion of these issues is especially recommended to the interested reader.

Despite this attitude of liberality, induced abortion even under the most ideal circumstances is not without danger and should not be approached lightly. The incidence of serious complications has been reported in the range of 1 to 19 per cent, depending on the technique used (Berthelsen and Østergaard; Kolstad; Tietze and Lewit). The lowest complication rates occur with suction or curettage; there is about a threefold increase with use of hypertonic saline injection, and a further threefold increase with hysterotomy. Death rates range from 6 per 1000 to 6 per 100,000 (Mehlan).

Interruption of pregnancy dates back to antiquity. Methods are described in early Chinese and Egyptian writings and severe punishments are cited in ancient Assyrian, Inca, Visigoth and Hebrew laws (Gebhard et al.). The Greco-Roman liberal attitude toward abortion, amounting to social condonement, was superseded and interdicted by the Pythagoreans and subsequently by the early Christian Church.

The Catholic view still holds firmly to the thesis that abortion is murder, and therefore the Church does not sanction therapeutic abortion even though the mother's life might be saved. An exception exists, however, in that "indirect" abortion is licit. This has reference to the inadvertent or incidental termination of pregnancy in the course of therapy, such as radiation or hysterectomy, for a disorder like uterine cancer. This condition demands therapy to effect cure, and the treatment is permitted provided it cannot be deferred safely until the fetus is viable (Rosen). In the strictest sense of moral and ethical correctness, there can be very little argument against this approach.

INDICATIONS AND PREREQUISITES

Besides the need to abide by local health care regulations and hospital policies that are applicable in these matters, other worthwhile precautions include properly executed statements of permission and release signed by the patient and the physicians immediately concerned. The need for these statements cannot be overemphasized. If the patient is married, it is recommended that one get the husband's signature as well, but it is generally conceded that it is really not legally essential.

The numbers of induced abortions performed annually in this country have been rising astronomically. Aside from those done "on demand," psychiatric indications are diminishing in number, while medical reasons appear to be almost vanishing. The continued decrease in the number performed for medical reasons is perhaps related to improved methods of managing the medical conditions indicated. Indeed, medical therapy has improved so significantly that it is rare for organic disorders to be aggravated in properly managed pregnancies.

Nevertheless, there are several widely acceptable specific indications for therapeutic abortion. These include: (1) severe chronic hypertensive and renal disorders, especially those complicated by diminishing or failing cardiac, hepatic or renal function; (2) cardiac disease with recent atrial fibrillation or decompensation, or those in which failure occurs early in pregnancy; (3) malignancy involving the breast or the cervix; and (4) psychiatric disorders from which serious impairment of function or life may be expected to occur.

Psychiatrists do not agree as to the standards to be used for determining the indication for this procedure. Some interpret their role liberally and require merely the absence of contraindications (Bolter). Others limit it to acute depressions or anxieties, especially when they occur in immature, borderline or disordered personalities. The fixed psychoses with associated suicidal tendencies and related major mental disorders should be included.

The fetal indications often evolve into psychiatric polemics supporting and justifying interruption on the basis of the potential effect on the mother's emotional stability while carrying a fetus whose chances of surviving or of being normal are extremely slim. These controversies include mothers with rubella in the first trimester of pregnancy, in which the probability of a congenital defect of the fetus is high. Recently developed approaches to accurate intrauterine diagnosis (see Chapter 13) have simplified such decisions by sometimes providing clear-cut answers on whether or not the fetus is affected by a suspected disorder.

TECHNIQUES

Transcervical Evacuation

Various medical and surgical techniques exist for the termination of pregnancy prior to viability. The generally accepted approach in gestations of less than 12 weeks is dilatation of the cervix and evacuation of the uterus either by vacuum (preferably) or curettage. Under suitable anesthesia, either general inhalation or paracervical block with supplemental analgesics, careful bimanual examination is made to verify the presence of an intrauterine pregnancy and to determine the position of the uterine corpus with reference to the cervix.

The cervix is grasped with a tenaculum and is dilated slowly with Hegar dilators of increasing size. A specially constructed hollow plastic or glass tube of appropriate dimension is chosen. Usually, it is the same number of millimeters internal diameter as the weeks of gestation, e.g., 10 mm. for a 10-week pregnancy. It is attached by way of a glass trap to a vacuum source capable of generating at least one atmosphere negative pressure. With the vacuum off (controlled merely by a finger occluding or opening the tube lumen to the air), the tube is inserted into the uterus, the vacuum is applied and the tube gently withdrawn. Fetal and placental parts are seen being evacuated into the vacuum trap. The procedure is repeated until the uterus is empty and contracted. Recently, it has been suggested that dilatation of the cervix is not always necessary, especially in abortions under 10 weeks, because smaller bore evacuation tubes may be adequate and can often be inserted without dilatation.

Alternatively, the uterine contents are removed with ovum forceps. The uterus is then progressively denuded of adherent placental tissue with a dull or (less preferably) a sharp curette.

Blood loss by either method may be a problem, so that suitable preparation for replacement should be available. Uterotonic agents, especially ergot, in this procedure are often helpful in reducing blood loss.

The simple technique of inducing abortion merely by artificial rupture of the membranes has been utilized extensively (Bengtsson and Kullander), but subsequent complete spontaneous expulsion of the fetus and placenta has not been consistent.

Recent reintroduction of an old technique for dilating the cervix is gaining popularity (Newton). It involves inserting a cylinder made of the stem of a seaweed *(Laminaria digitata)* or other suitable material, called a *laminaria tent,* into the cervix beyond the internal os. As the hygroscopic tent expands to three to five times its original diameter, the cervix is dilated. Use of unsterile, Clostridia-bearing preparations in the hands of the uninitiated has in the past given this approach a bad reputation. Modern gas sterilization techniques have reduced this hazard. However, tents are not wholly innocuous as shown by Hanson et al., who routinely inserted them 12 hours before therapeutic abortion to aid cervical dilatation. They encountered intrauterine migration of the device rendering removal difficult; it was necessary to split the cervix by anterior trachelotomy to evacuate the tent from the uterus.

Intrauterine Hypertonic Solutions

With pregnancies of 12 weeks' duration or more the situation is much more treacherous. Use of hypertonic solution injected intraamniotically is the preferred approach. Injection of a 40 per cent formalin solution for interrupting pregnancy was first advocated in 1935 (Boero). This method has been used widely in South America. Its inherent danger involves the possibility of injection of formalin into the uterine wall or peritoneal cavity. The less dangerous use of hypertonic saline was first reported in 1938 (Aburel) and has since been investigated by others (Stamm and de Watteville; Bengtsson and Csapo; Jaffin et al.). The current modification of the method consists of withdrawing 100 to 250 ml. of amniotic fluid and replacing it with an equal quantity of 20 per cent sodium chloride solution. Good results have also been claimed by the instillation of saline extraovularly into the uterus by way of the cervical canal (Svane).

It has been shown (Bengtsson and Stormby) that severe damage results to the placenta with edema and necrotizing placentitis. Fetal death appears to be based on osmotic damage to the trophoblast. The systemic absorption of the hypertonic saline has occasionally resulted in headache, thirst, paresthesia, changes in blood pressure and hemolysis (Amris and Jepsen). On the other hand, serious complications have not been reported with 50 per cent glucose (Brosset; Wood et al.); one report indicates that 20 per cent saline and 50 per cent glucose are equally effective, although the risk of infection is probably greater with glucose.

Intraamniotic aspiration of amniotic fluid and replacement with hypertonic solution is an acceptable procedure for midtrimester abortion after about 14 weeks with minimal serious harmful effects. This is not meant to imply that the procedure is without risk. On the contrary, serious problems have been reported, especially if inadvertent injection into the vascular system is accomplished. Deaths, as well as neurologic and cardiopulmonary damage, have been reported (Wagatsuma). If undertaken, precautionary measures are advisable. The injections are far simpler than hysterotomy, which has hitherto been the usual treatment for interruption of pregnancy in midtrimester.

The patient should be fasted overnight to ensure that she will have an empty stomach. Sedation is not ordinarily given, but may be needed if the patient is apprehensive. Preinjection evaluation is important to safeguard the patient. The essentials of this technique include the preparation of the abdominal wall with antiseptic solution after the patient has voided. With the patient in a moderate Trendelenburg position, a 4-inch, 20-gauge needle with a trocar is introduced with a single swift thrust through the abdominal wall into the uterus.

The site selected should be about midway between the symphysis pubis and the umbilicus and one inch lateral to the midline on the side toward the fetal limbs. When the size of the gravid uterus is less than 20 weeks, a midline puncture is made about one inch below the top of the uterine fundus. Anesthesia is usually unnecessary, but some prefer to infiltrate the puncture site locally with an anesthetic agent (one per cent lidocaine). Sterile disposable exchange transfusion sets are useful adjuncts to this procedure. No more than 200 ml. of amniotic fluid is withdrawn and replaced with an equal amount of 20 per cent pyrogen-free sodium chloride solution.

In order to ensure that no saline is injected into the myometrium, peritoneal cavity or the venous system (all serious errors capable of giving rise to major complications), it has been suggested that methylene blue be injected first (Alpern et al.) and, at intervals during the course of the saline instillation, the amniotic fluid be withdrawn to recheck the position of the needle. If the blue-colored fluid is not seen, the injection is immediately discontinued. Similarly, one stops immediately if the patient complains of headache or thirst, symptoms suggestive of direct intravenous injection. Coagulopathy has also been reported with diminished circulating fibrinogen, platelets and factor V activity (Beller et al.), although few with these laboratory changes manifest the coagulation defect with overt hemorrhage.

Other Methods

One may approach the problem of midtrimester abortion by the less preferable method of dilating the cervix and rupturing the membranes with a curette or Allis forceps. Intracervical packing preliminary to dilatation and evacuation has also been advocated. Subsequent use of uterotonic agents may aid in the spontaneous expulsion of the uterine contents. If expulsion does not occur or is not complete within 24 hours, the uterus may then be emptied with ovum forceps and curette, but this is very risky in a uterus larger than 12 weeks' gestational size. The potential dangers in this approach are infection and hemorrhage. The large gravid uterus has a very soft, easily perforated wall, and traumatic injury during instrumentation is not uncommon.

The uterus containing a fetus more than 12 weeks of age may also be emptied by either vaginal or abdominal hysterotomy. The procedure is shown in Figure 252. Ab-

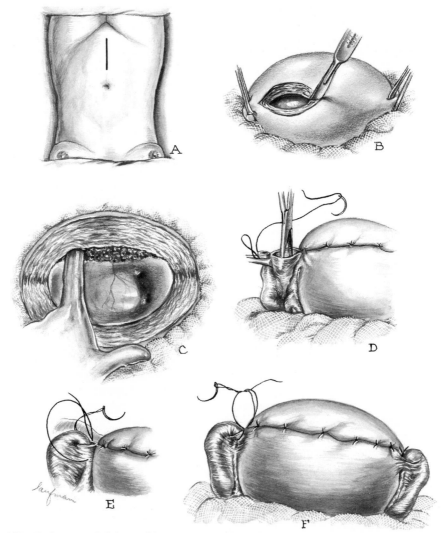

Figure 252   Technique of abdominal hysterotomy and sterilization. *A*, Abdominal incision may be a vertical midline as shown here or a Pfannenstiel incision. *B*, Incision across fundus. *C*, Separation of placenta and membranes followed by removal of the fetal sac. *D*, The fundus has been closed with interrupted surgical gut sutures in two layers. The tube has been cut from the uterine cornu and the folds of the broad ligament are separated. *E*, The distal end of the tube is buried between the folds of the broad ligament and sutured there. *F*, The tube is sutured to the fundus. The opposite tube is treated in the same manner. (Modified from Titus, P.: The Management of Obstetric Difficulties, ed. 5. St. Louis, C. V. Mosby Company, 1955.)

dominal hysterotomy is preferred if sterilization by tubal ligation is to be done simultaneously. However, two lesser procedures may be substituted, namely, intraamniotic hypertonic saline injection and subsequent tubal coagulation by laparoscopy, because they are associated with fewer complications.

Among abortifacient agents, very little consistent effect has been reported with quinine, pituitary extract or ergot prepara-

tions. The partial effectiveness of controlled synthetic oxytocin infusion in large doses has been demonstrated (Kumar and Russell; Burnhill et al.) as a method of inducing abortion in the midtrimester. The technique involves injection of copious unphysiologic amounts of oxytocin while the abdominal contractility is monitored by intraamniotic pressure determinations.

The folic acid analogues (pteroylglutamic acid) have not been found to be completely reliable abortifacients (Goetsch). They block the important actions of folic acid in nucleic acid metabolism and cytopoiesis, and seriously interfere with embryogenesis; their site of action is the embryonic mesenchyme. Early embryos are very susceptible. These drugs cannot be relied on to produce the desired effect. Although fetal death may occur, it cannot be guaranteed. Serious toxic effects may ensue in the mother.

Similarly, irradiation of the gravid uterus has resulted in varying degrees of success. It appears to be most suitable in early pregnancies and may be used when radiation for other therapeutic reasons (such as for cancer of the cervix) is being done. Generally speaking, however, termination of the pregnancy by vacuum curage or by curettage followed by radiation would probably be preferable in most instances. The risk of damaging the fetus, which may then be carried to term, must be kept in mind if irradiation should be ineffectual in actually terminating the pregnancy.

The injection of soaps, pastes and various other irritating solutions (unfortunately, often with criminal intent) into the uterine cavity has long been used to produce abortion; in general they are dangerous measures. Deaths due to air, soap, fat or paste embolization and widespread intravascular thrombosis have been reported. The serious consequences, including death, associated with the use of abortifacient intrauterine pastes were stressed by Greenhill. These techniques are mentioned only to be condemned.

REFERENCES

Aburel, E., cited in Cioc, M.: Le déclenchement du travail par la méthode d'Aburel. Gynéc. Obstét. 47:224, 1948.

Alpern, W. M., Charles, A. G., and Friedman, E. A.: Hypertonic solutions for termination of pregnancy. Amer. J. Obstet. Gynec. 100:250, 1968.

Amris, C. J., and Jepsen, O. B.: Intravenous infusion as a complication in therapeutic abortion by the intrauterine extraovular hypertonic saline method. Danish Med. Bull. 9:143, 1962.

Beller, F. K., Rosenberg, M., Kolker, M., and Douglas, G. W.: Consumptive coagulopathy associated with intra-amniotic infusion of hypertonic salt. Amer. J. Obstet. Gynec. 112:534, 1972.

Bengtsson, L. P., and Csapo, A. I.: Oxytocin response, withdrawal, and reinforcement of defense mechanism of the human uterus at midpregnancy. Amer. J. Obstet. Gynec. 83:1083, 1962.

Bengtsson, L. P., and Kullander, S.: Legal abortion induced by artificial rupture of the membranes. Acta Obstet. Gynec. Scand. 38:227, 1959.

Bengtsson, L. P., and Stormby, N.: The effect of intra-amniotic injection of hypertonic sodium chloride in human midpregnancy. Acta Obstet. Gynec. Scand. 41:115, 1962.

Berthelsen, H. G., and Østergaard, E.: Techniques and complications in therapeutic abortion. Danish Med. Bull. 6:105, 1959.

Berthelsen, H. G., and Østergaard, E.: Lethality and incidence of complications in therapeutic abortion in Denmark, 1953–1957. Danish Med. Bull. 6:110, 1959.

Boero, E. A.: Interruption de la grossesse incompatible avant la viabilité foetale: Nouveau concept et nouvelle méthode opératoire. Gynéc. Obstét. 32:305, 1935.

Bolter, S.: The psychiatrist's role in therapeutic abortion: The unwitting accomplice. Amer. J. Psychiat. 119:312, 1962.

Brosset, A.: The induction of therapeutic abortion by means of hypertonic glucose solution injected into the amniotic sac. Acta Obstet. Gynec. Scand. 37:519, 1958.

Burnhill, M. S., Gaines, J. A., and Guttmacher, A. F.: Concentrated oxytocin solution for therapeutic interruption of midtrimester pregnancy. Obstet. Gynec. 20:94, 1962.

Curran, W. J.: Abortion law in the Supreme Court. New Eng. J. Med. 285:30, 1971.

Curran, W. J.: The abortion decisions: The Supreme Court as moralist, scientist, historian and legislator. New Eng. J. Med. 288:950, 1973.

Doe vs. Bolton: Supreme Court 93:739, 1973.

Gebhard, P. H., Pomeroy, W. B., Martin, C. E., and Christenson, C. V.: Pregnancy, Birth and Abortion. New York, Harper & Brothers, 1958.

Goetsch, C.: An evaluation of aminopterin as an abortifacient. Amer. J. Obstet. Gynec. 83:1474, 1962.

Greenhill, J. P.: Abortifacient pastes: The exploitation and dangers of pastes sold for producing therapeutic abortion. J.A.M.A. 98:2155, 1932.

Greenhill, J. P.: World trends of therapeutic abortion and sterilization. Clin. Obstet. Gynec. 7:37, 1964.

Hanson, F. W., Niswander, K. R., and Trelford, J. D.: Cervical migration of laminaria tents. Amer. J. Obstet. Gynec. 114:835, 1972.

Jaffin, H., Kerenyi, T., and Wood, E. C.: Termination of missed abortion and the induction of labor in midtrimester pregnancy. Amer. J. Obstet. Gynec. 84:602, 1962.

Kolstad, P.: Therapeutic abortion: A clinical study based upon 968 cases from a Norwegian hospital,

1940–53. Acta Obstet. Gynec. Scand. *36*:1 (Suppl. 6), 1958.

Kumar, D., and Russell, J. J.: Controlled oxytocin infusion as a method of therapeutic abortion in early pregnancy. Bull. Johns Hopkins Hosp. *109*:141, 1961.

Mehlan, K. H.: Internationale Abortsituation, Abortbekaempfung, Antikonzeption. Leipzig, Georg Thieme, 1961.

Newton, B. W.: Laminaria tent: Relic of the past or modern medical device? Amer. J. Obstet. Gynec. *113*:442, 1972.

Roe vs. Wade: Supreme Court 93:705, 1973.

Rosen, H.: Therapeutic Abortion: Medical, Psychiatric, Anthropological and Religious Considerations. New York, Julian Press, Inc., 1954.

Stamm, O., and de Watteville, H.: Étude expérimentale sur le méchanisme d'avertment par hydramnios artificiel. Gynéc. Obstét. *53*:171, 1954.

Svane, H.: Interruption of pregnancy by intrauterine instillation of saline. Danish Med. Bull. 7:51, 1960.

Tietze, C., and Lewit, S.: Legal abortions: Early medical complications. Family Planning Perspectives 3:6, 1971.

Titus, P.: The Management of Obstetric Difficulties, ed. 5. St. Louis, C. V. Mosby Company, 1955.

United States vs. Vuitch: Supreme Court *91*:1294, 1971.

Wagatsuma, T.: Intra-amniotic injection of saline for therapeutic abortion. Amer. J. Obstet. Gynec. *93*:743, 1965.

Wood, C., Booth, R. T., and Pinkerton, J. H. M.: Induction of labour by intra-amniotic injections of hypertonic glucose solution. Brit. Med. J. 2:706, 1962.

Chapter 36

Hypertensive States of Pregnancy

There is much confusion in obstetric circles concerning the group of diverse pregnancy disorders usually considered together under the misnomer *toxemia of pregnancy*. The trend away from the use of this all-encompassing, ill-defined and altogether inappropriate term should be encouraged. Henceforth herein we will designate the collective group of diseases whose manifestations are so similar as *hypertensive states of pregnancy* (accepting the recommendation of the American College of Obstetricians and Gynecologists in this regard) and use the term *preeclampsia* to refer only to the specific syndrome uniquely encountered in late pregnancy.

Hypertensive states of pregnancy constitute one of the leading causes of maternal death and contribute significantly to perinatal mortality as well. Differentiation of these disorders is difficult, even by hindsight. Classification tends to be arbitrary. Diagnostic criteria are uncritical. Etiology and pathogenesis are entirely conjectural. Treatment is empirical. Experimental study of these conditions has been almost impossible because of the lack of a suitable animal model or comparable disease states in any species other than man. Investigation in the human has been hampered because there are no acceptable, uniform and verifiable standards of definition and diagnosis.

Despite these humbling and disheartening observations, however, the incidence of these conditions, considered collectively, has steadily declined during this century and the associated maternal mortality has fallen markedly from 52.2 per 100,000 live births in 1940 to 6.2 per 100,000 in 1970. This dramatic change is attributable in part to improved antepartum care, early detection and aggressive management. Other less apparent but probably more significant determinants undoubtedly play a major role, including factors of general health, nutrition and socioeconomic status for the gravid population at large.

CLINICAL CRITERIA

Edema

During some or all of pregnancy, most normal gravidas can be shown to have postural edema of the lower extremities which disappears characteristically after bed rest or merely elevating the legs for a brief interval. A gain of weight exceeding 500 gm. in one week signifies acute water retention and may be a manifestation of occult edema. Pitting edema of the abdominal wall, face, hands and sacral area may also indicate abnormally excessive retention of water. However, these changes may occur even in otherwise unaffected pregnant women (Hytten and Leitch) and, therefore, they cannot be considered pathognomonic. There are no available standards for detecting, evaluating and reporting edema.

Dependent edema of the lower extremities appears to be universal in pregnancy based on mechanical factors relating to gravity, increased venous pressure and lymphatic obstruction. These latter factors should not apply for edema appearing in the face and the hands, where such mechanical factors are not operative. This distinction has assigned edema of the hands and face a more important role as criteria of

391

the existence of a pathologic condition manifested by generalized edema. However, Hytten and Leitch showed that edema of the hands and face may occur in pregnancies which are normal in every other way. In a large series of normotensive primigravidas, they encountered it in 4.7 per cent; a small series undergoing special investigation and being followed very closely showed these manifestations in 29.4 per cent. Thus, it appears possible for widespread edema to occur in pregnancy unassociated with hypertensive states; similarly, edema need not be present invariably in these conditions.

Proteinuria

In many normal pregnant women, there is occasionally a trace or more of protein in voided specimens of urine associated with orthostatic albuminuria or contamination of the specimen by vaginal discharge. Determinations of total protein in 24-hour collections are required for accurate evaluation. Although limits of normal are arbitrarily designated, it is generally agreed that the maximum daily excretion of protein should not exceed 300 mg. in normal gravidas. In single specimens, concentrations greater than 1 gm. per liter (or more than 1+ by standard turbidometric methods) are considered significant when encountered in two or more random urine specimens collected at least six hours apart.

Because the appearance of protein in the urine is perhaps the most common manifestation of renal disease, there is widespread clinical agreement that proteinuria in pregnancy is ominous. However, as noted above, protein may be found in the urine of normal gravidas. The quantity of protein in the urine fluctuates widely and rapidly with time. Certain circumstances tend to enhance the amount of protein that appears in the urine, including violent exercise, hard work, exposure to cold, cold showering and various autoimmune and hypersensitive states. Orthostatic or postural proteinuria occurs in 5 to 20 per cent of young adults. Vaginal discharge or bleeding readily contaminates urine specimens that are obtained casually and will yield falsely high levels of protein. The need for clean, midstream voided or catheterized specimens is, therefore, apparent.

Hypertension

An elevation of 30 mm. Hg or more in the systolic and 15 mm. Hg or more in the diastolic pressure is considered abnormal in pregnancy regardless of the absolute levels observed. Levels in excess of 140 mm. Hg systolic and/or 90 mm. Hg diastolic by convention are hypertensive levels in pregnant women. It is recognized that such blood pressure levels in females of reproductive age are much too high to constitute meaningful criteria for detecting significant disease. Recent data from the Collaborative Project (Friedman) showed that pressures in excess of 125/75 prior to 32 weeks were associated with significantly increased fetal risk, as were levels over 125/85 at term. The blood pressure must be abnormal on at least two occasions with at least a six-hour interval between the two determinations.

CLASSIFICATION

Because clinical diagnoses are suspect (see below) and difficult to verify even in retrospect, any classification must of necessity be arbitrary. It has been shown (Vollman) that diagnoses based on such classifications are not necessarily valid, as evidenced by wide variations in incidence figures between institutions and with the passage of time, even though the criteria for making diagnoses were defined in a standardized fashion throughout. These limitations notwithstanding, the American College of Obstetricians and Gynecologists Committee on Terminology (Hughes) has recently updated its classification as follows:

Gestational Edema: Gestational edema is the occurrence of a general and excessive accumulation of fluid in the tissues of greater than 1+ pitting edema after 12 hours' rest in bed, or a weight gain of 5 pounds (sic) or more in one week due to the influence of pregnancy.

Gestational Proteinuria: Gestational proteinuria is the presence of proteinuria, during or under the influence of pregnancy, in the absence of hypertension, edema, renal infection or known intrinsic renovascular disease.

Gestational Hypertension: Gestational hypertension is the development of hypertension during pregnancy, or within the first 24 hours post partum, in a previously normotensive woman. No other evidence of preeclampsia or hypertensive vascular disease is present. The blood pressure returns to normotensive levels within 10 days following parturition. Some patients with gestational hypertension may in fact have preeclampsia or hypertensive vascular disease, but they do not satisfy the criteria for either of these diagnoses.

Preeclampsia: Preeclampsia is the development of hypertension with proteinuria, edema or both, due to pregnancy or the influence of a recent pregnancy. It occurs after the twentieth week of gestation, but it may develop before this time in the presence of trophoblastic disease. Preeclampsia is predominantly a disorder of primigravidas.

Eclampsia: Eclampsia is the occurrence of one or more convulsions, not attributable to other cerebral conditions, such as epilepsy or cerebral hemorrhage, in a patient with preeclampsia.

Superimposed Preeclampsia or Eclampsia: Superimposed preeclampsia or eclampsia is the development of preeclampsia or eclampsia in a patient with chronic hypertensive vascular or renal disease. When the hypertension antedates the pregnancy, as established by previous blood pressure recordings, a rise in the systolic pressure of 30 mm. Hg, or a rise in the diastolic pressure of 15 mm. Hg, and the development of proteinuria, edema or both are required during pregnancy to establish the diagnosis.

Chronic Hypertensive Disease: Chronic hypertensive disease is the presence of persistent hypertension, of whatever cause, before pregnancy or before the twentieth week of gestation, or persistent hypertension beyond the forty-second postpartum day.

Unclassified Hypertensive Disorders: Unclassified hypertensive disorders are those in which information is insufficient for classification. They should compose a minority of the hypertensive disorders in pregnancy.

It is important to be able to distinguish between mild and severe forms of preeclampsia on a clinical basis. The reasons for such distinction are the differences in prognosis and response to therapy. The severe variety manifests itself with blood pressures exceeding 160 mm. Hg systolic or 100 mm. Hg diastolic observed on two or more occasions at least six hours apart with the patient at rest in bed; proteinuria of 5 gm. or more in 24 hours or 3 to 4+ turbidometric analysis of single specimens; oliguria with urine production of less than 400 ml. in 24 hours or 30 ml. per hour; cerebral or visual disturbances, including blurring, diplopia, scotomata or blindness; cyanosis or pulmonary edema; epigastric pain. If none of these is present, the case is classified as mild preeclampsia; if one or more is encountered, it is severe preeclampsia.

ACCURACY OF CRITERIA

The designation of hypertensive states of pregnancy is limited to preeclampsia, eclampsia, chronic hypertensive vascular disease and superimposed preeclampsia or eclampsia, but the available clinical criteria for making distinctions between these conditions are not specific, as already indicated. Histological evidence of chronic renal disease was found on renal biopsies obtained at the height of the disease and was the only histological finding in 30 per cent of previously normal primigravidas fulfilling all the clinical criteria for preeclampsia. At the same time, there was chronic renal disease in 25 per cent of gravidas diagnosed clinically as chronic hypertensive vascular disease with superimposed preeclampsia (McCartney).

These findings clearly illustrate the shortcomings of clinical diagnostic criteria for differentiating the various types of disorders in this group. Moreover, they suggest that chronic renal disease plays a more important role in the hypertensive states of pregnancy than current statistics indicate. Therefore, all data pertaining to the hypertensive states of pregnancy must be interpreted with caution when clinical criteria alone are the bases for their differentiation. It is reasonable to assume that some of the contradictory data pertaining to preeclampsia are attributable to the heterogeneity of the groups of patients being studied.

INCIDENCE

The incidence of preeclampsia is about six to seven per cent among obstetric patients admitted to hospitals in the United States, while eclampsia is encountered once in every 2000 pregnancies. During the past decade the incidence of preeclampsia has decreased 25 to 50 per cent and eclampsia 60 to 95 per cent. Up to 90 per cent of all hypertensive states of pregnancy are attributed to preeclampsia. Wide variations in incidence result from differences in both clinical criteria and classification standards.

The proportions of types of hypertensive states of pregnancy are influenced by the ethnic composition of an obstetric population. For example, there is a higher incidence of chronic hypertensive cardiovascular and renal disease among black gravidas than among white. Based on renal biopsy studies it is estimated that the clinical diagnosis of preeclampsia is incorrect in 30 per cent and that chronic renal disease occurs 25 times more often than diagnosed (McCartney).

PREECLAMPSIA AND ECLAMPSIA

Preeclampsia is unique to human gestation, being encountered almost exclusively in the third trimester. It is characterized by rapidly progressive, profound biological changes which regress rapidly after delivery. It is associated with a low incidence of residual damage and rarely recurs in subsequent pregnancies.

Its special features include generalized vasospasm and excessive retention of sodium and water. A characteristic renal lesion has been described by electron microscopy. Clinical manifestations include excessive weight gain, edema, hypertension and proteinuria. These develop most frequently in young primigravidas who were previously normal. Visual, cerebral and gastrointestinal symptoms, together with oliguria or anuria, characterize the severe, progressive disorder. The latter may advance to convulsions and coma, designated eclampsia.

This entity is limited to the last 20 weeks of gestation, appearing most often during the last 10 weeks. There is an increased incidence among patients with hydatidiform mole and with twins. In association with these conditions, typical preeclampsia may even appear prior to the twentieth week of pregnancy. Hydramnios is encountered four to five times more often in patients with preeclampsia than in other gravidas, but it is generally considered to be a concomitant of the disorder and not a predisposing factor.

Etiology

The etiology is entirely unknown. Functioning trophoblastic tissue is required for its initiation and maintenance, but the presence of a fetus is not apparently essential. Age and parity (classically, it is a disease of the young nullipara), length of gestation (characteristically, the third trimester), twins and hydatidiform mole are predisposing factors. Incidence varies according to geographical location, the highest frequency of occurrence and mortality being seen in the southern states.

Socioeconomic factors are believed to play a role, but verification is not at hand. Baird was unable to show any particular differences in the incidence of preeclampsia among the social classes in Scotland. However, there is little doubt that the mortality is higher in impoverished areas. Racial differences are also in doubt. Although it is generally felt that black women are more prone to develop preeclampsia, supportive data are not available. Also, although it is true that chronic hypertension occurs nearly three times more often in black women than in comparable whites, this relationship does not appear to hold for preeclampsia.

The increased mortality associated with hypertensive states of pregnancy based on geography and socioeconomic status is undoubtedly a reflection of the quality of antepartum care. Whether nutrition and climate are also predisposing factors cannot be determined. Indeed, they may be interrelated. The increased frequency of eclampsia in areas where dietary deficiencies are common, such as in China, the Philippines and our own southern states, is suggestive. Davies studied this problem carefully and showed a somewhat poorer intake among preeclamptic patients than normal controls, largely on the basis of reduction in food intake secondary to the disease process. The proof of dietary deficiency as causative is wanting.

The multiple and reversible biological changes which occur in preeclampsia indicate that there are widespread aberrations in cellular function, suggesting that it is a metabolic disease. Abnormalities in steroid metabolism have been postulated, but not proved. High chorionic gonadotropin levels are occasionally seen in these patients, but the levels are not related to the severity of the disease process.

Innumerable hypotheses have been expressed concerning the etiology of preeclampsia. None affords a logical explanation for the predisposition in nulliparas and in patients with multiple pregnancy or hydatidiform mole, for its appearance in certain geographic areas and in impoverished populations, its appearance late in pregnancy, its tendency not to recur in subsequent pregnancies and its improvement after fetal death.

The hypothesis currently favored is that of uterine ischemia. It is postulated that mechanical factors in or about the uterus fail to allow the blood flow to adapt to the requirements of the uterus and the products of conception. Reduced uterine blood flow yields a situation that favors production of pressor polypeptides, thromboplastin or thromboplastin-like substances by an ischemic placenta or by ischemia-induced decidual degeneration. These substances in turn produce the clinical manifestations characteristic of preeclampsia.

Increased myometrial tension (as in multiple pregnancy or in the course of labor) and excessive amounts of trophoblast (as in the presence of hydatidiform mole) are suggested as mechanical factors augmenting uterine ischemia. In primigravidas, deficient vascular hypertrophy and hyperplasia are advanced as causes of the failure of circulatory adaptation. It is also believed that arteriolar sclerosis precludes adequate circulatory adjustment in patients with acute preeclampsia superimposed on chronic hypertensive disease. These hypothetical changes are suggested as the basis for exacerbation of chronic renal and vascular diseases during gestation, the high incidence of preeclampsia in primigravidas and in patients with twins and with hydatidiform moles, and for the failure of the disorder to recur in subsequent pregnancies after the first.

Assali et al. reported a 40 per cent decrease in measured uterine blood flow in hypertensive patients. Browne and Veall determined the rate of uptake of radioactive sodium from the placental lake and myometrium and found it decreased 60 per cent. Hunter and Howard reported finding pressor polypeptides in blood, amniotic fluid and decidua of patients with acute preeclampsia.

There is reason to believe that there are comparable degrees of uterine ischemia in many gravidas with chronic hypertensive cardiovascular and renal disease who do not develop either the clinical or the renal histological changes of preeclampsia. Therefore, there is no conclusive evidence that uterine ischemia is the specific cause of preeclampsia. It is possible that the decreased uterine blood flow, as well as the pressor substances observed in body fluids of patients fulfilling the clinical criteria for preeclampsia, is a result rather than the cause of the disorder.

McKay recently reviewed the evidence supporting the contention that disseminated intravascular coagulation is a major mechanism in eclampsia. Pathologic evidence is available in the form of demonstration of platelet-fibrin thrombi in the microcirculation of various organs, including the brain, kidney, heart, lung and placenta. The constellation of clinical signs and symptoms of consumption coagulopathy is shown to be quite similar to the manifestations of eclampsia, including secondary hypotension, bleeding tendency, oliguria, anuria, hematuria, convulsions and coma, abdominal pain, dyspnea and cyanosis.

Water and Electrolyte Metabolism

Total body water and exchangeable sodium are greater in patients with preeclampsia than in normal gravidas or patients with chronic hypertensive disease (Gray and Plentl; Hutchinson et al.; McCartney et al.). Dieckmann found that patients with preeclampsia failed to excrete sodium loads at the normal rate for the duration of their pregnancy. Page attributed this to a lowered glomerular filtration rate with unchanged tubular reabsorption of sodium. However, Chesley showed enhanced tubular reabsorption of sodium. The mechanism by which this comes about is unknown, but various factors may be at play, including estrogens and aldosterone, both of which are diminished in preeclampsia.

Plasma and extravascular fluid volumes are increased in preeclampsia (Freis and Kenny). There is also an increase in the capacity of the colloid of connective tissue to bind sodium and water (Friedberg).

In severe preeclampsia, there is a shift of fluid from the vascular compartment. This is manifested by a rising hematocrit, an elevation of serum proteins and often by increased edema. The cause of this phenomenon is unknown, but a transient reversal of the shift and temporary clinical improvement are usually obtained by administering albumen or hypertonic crystalloid solutions. Failure of these measures to produce hemodilution is a grave prognostic sign.

There is conflicting evidence concerning whether or not the volume of intracellular fluid is increased in preeclampsia. Muscle biopsies have shown a decrease in the concentration of sodium but unchanged potassium and water content.

Blood Chemistry

No pathognomonic changes occur in the concentrations of electrolytes, crystalloids or proteins in preeclampsia. Serum potassium, sodium, calcium and chloride are usually within the normal range. Some patients have hyponatremia because of an increase in serum lipids. Although serum sodium may fall below 130 mEq. per liter of serum, osmolality is normal and the relative sodium level per liter of diminished serum water is essentially normal. Thus, these patients do not have physiologic hyponatremia and they do not require the administration of sodium.

Blood sugar, plasma bicarbonate and pH are within the limits for normal pregnancy in preeclampsia. In eclampsia increased muscular activity and abnormal pulmonary exchange during seizures cause the blood sugar to rise transiently; blood lactic acid and total organic acid are increased as well and the plasma bicarbonate is decreased. The pH is often reduced immediately after a convulsion, but tends to return to normal when adequate ventilatory exchange is reestablished. Uncompensated acidosis may ensue when there are repeated convulsions.

Increase in the tubular reabsorption of urate, the result of decreased clearance, causes hyperuricemia in patients with preeclampsia (Chesley and Williams). Uric acid levels are inconstantly elevated, however. Moreover, use of thiazide diuretics may be associated with high levels of serum uric acid, thereby obtunding the value of this examination.

In preeclampsia the concentrations of creatine and creatinine are normal. Nonprotein nitrogen is also usually normal unless there is oliguria or anuria. Total serum protein, the albumin-globulin ratio and the oncotic pressure of the plasma are reduced in normal pregnancy and tend to be further reduced in preeclampsia except in the most severe cases when hemoconcentration occurs (see above). Since the concentration of serum proteins and the oncotic pressure of plasma are lowest in the immediate puerperium when the edema is subsiding and the diuresis is at its height, it must follow that hypoproteinemia is not the cause of the edema in preeclampsia. However, it is possible that this factor is contributory to some degree.

In normal pregnant patients at term there is a substantial increase in the concentration of plasma fibrinogen. In patients with preeclampsia, levels are further increased. The prothrombin time is generally within the limits for normal pregnancy. The coagulation time, which is usually shortened in normal pregnancy, is decreased further in preeclampsia. Clotting times of less than one minute have been observed in some patients with eclampsia. Increased coagulability sometimes makes it difficult to obtain blood from these patients. McKay reported eclamptic patients with acquired thrombocytopenia associated with multiple coagulation factor deficiencies, including fibrinogen and prothrombin.

Renal Function

Renal function in pregnancy is detailed in Chapter 44. In patients with preeclampsia there is retention of nitrogen when oliguria or anuria ensues. Unless there is tubular or cortical necrosis, the azotemia is mild and regresses rapidly after delivery. When deprived of water for 18 to 24 hours, patients with preeclampsia will not concentrate urine more than specific gravity of 1.022. This inability to concentrate maximally is believed to be mediated either by an intrinsic renal defect or by extrarenal factors, such as increased endogenous osmotic clearance and volume regulation necessitated by rest-induced mobilization of extracellular fluid.

The maximal urinary sodium concentration is about 1.9 per cent; in pregnancy it falls to 0.5 per cent (ranging from 0.1 to 0.9 per cent); in preeclampsia, the average is 0.16 per cent (Dieckmann). In normal pregnant patients the urea clearance is 102 to 104 per cent of normal, in contrast to an average range of 50 to 70 per cent for patients with preeclampsia.

Preeclamptic patients have decreased renal blood flow, decreased glomerular filtration rate, lowered glomerular filtration fraction and apparently increased resistance of the afferent glomerular arteries. The glomerular capillary lumina are narrowed because of an increase in the cytoplasm of the endothelial cells. It has been postulated that the decreased renal blood flow and the lowered glomerular filtration rate are due in part to this morphologic change.

Renal tubular function is not impaired in preeclampsia. The tubular capacity for reabsorption of sodium appears to be increased. Renal abnormalities are reversible. Persistent alterations in renal structure and function should not be expected to occur as a consequence.

Circulatory Changes

Hypertension in preeclampsia may precede the proteinuria, but usually both are encountered concurrently. Little is known about the mechanism of the hypertension. Assali et al. asserted that humoral substances primarily mediate the increased vascular resistance encountered. It is not known whether there are quantitative or qualitative changes in the circulating pressor substances or an increase in the reactivity of effector cells produced by electrolyte and other physicochemical changes, or whether there are multiple aberrations in the complex mechanism regulating peripheral vascular resistance.

Dieckmann reported that the vascular tree of patients with preeclampsia had a greater reactivity to parenterally administered hypertonic saline solutions and vasopressin than does the vascular tree of normal gravidas or patients with chronic hypertensive disease. Page showed the response to angiotensin to be enhanced. These observations suggest that the reactivity of the effector cells is increased.

Serotonin is a component of human plasma with vasoconstrictor properties. Carter et al. found that patients with preeclampsia have variable increased concentrations of this amine. Their studies suggested that in patients with either true preeclampsia or chronic hypertensive cardiovascular disease there is an increase in the urinary secretion product of serotonin, 5-hydroxytryptamine. The concentration of serotonin plasma and whole blood of patients with preeclampsia has not been correlated with the severity of the disease. Therefore, there is no conclusive evidence that an elevated concentration contributes significantly to the vasospasm of this disorder.

The cardiac output is increased in preeclampsia. Transient electrocardiographic changes attributable to myocardial damage have been reported. In the severe disorder the cardiac load is increased significantly because of increased peripheral vascular resistance, elevated viscosity of the blood in association with hemoconcentration and metabolic disturbances.

Uterine blood flow is decreased in the gravidas with hypertension (Assali et al.). This observation indicates that impairment of uteroplacental blood flow is the principal cause of fetal death and the tendency for infants to be small for their gestational ages.

McCall reported that cerebrovascular resistance, which is elevated in hypertensive states of pregnancy, is further increased in eclampsia. Nevertheless, cerebral blood flow and oxygen consumption in patients with preeclampsia or with chronic hypertensive disease are within the usual pregnancy range. Cerebral consumption of oxygen is reduced only in patients with eclampsia.

Capillary Permeability

There are no demonstrable differences in the capillary permeability of normal gravidas or those with preeclampsia. In preeclampsia the rate of flow of fluid into the interstitial space and the concentration of protein in the interstitial fluid are unchanged. There is, therefore, no evidence that the primary cause of edema in this disease is increased capillary permeability.

Plasma Enzymes

Determinations of the activity of plasma enzymes in normal and abnormal patients have shown increased alkaline phosphatase, amylase, glutamic-oxaloacetic transaminase and lactic dehydrogenase; cholinesterase activity tends to be decreased; the rates of enzymatic inactivation of histamine, angiotonin, oxytocin and antidiuretic hormone are increased. There are no consistent differences in the activities of these enzymes.

Hormonal Changes

Hormone levels have been studied extensively in preeclampsia, but no correlations can be made. Increases in the concentration of chorionic gonadotropin in the blood and in the amount excreted in the urine are seen inconsistently. There may be diminished quantities of estrogens and both free and conjugated pregnanediol excreted in the urine. It has been postulated that these changes are secondary manifestations of placental insufficiency. Patients with these findings may exhibit a high incidence of intrauterine fetal death (see Chapter 13).

Total corticoid excretion in preeclampsia tends to be increased. The excretion of 17-ketosteroids is often enhanced. Excretion of unconjugated aldosterone has been reported to be increased, although total aldosterone is within the range for normal pregnancy; however, decreased levels are also encountered.

There is no conclusive evidence to support the view that an increased rate of production or a decreased rate of inactivation of antidiuretic hormone is the primary cause of water retention in preeclampsia. The ability of the plasma to inactivate antidiuretic hormone is increased in normal pregnant patients. This enhanced inactivation, mediated by a specific enzyme, is not impaired in patients with preeclampsia.

Hepatic Function

Dieckmann et al. found abnormal thymol turbidity in three times as many preeclamptic patients and twice as many chronic hypertensives as in normal pregnant patients in the last trimester. The cephalin flocculation was abnormal in more than half of those with preeclampsia or with chronic hypertensive disease. The direct serum bilirubin was normal in gravidas with chronic hypertensive disease, but was elevated in one-third of those with preeclampsia. The indirect serum bilirubin was elevated in one-sixth of those with preeclampsia or with chronic hypertensive disease. Urinary bilirubin was not elevated in pregnant patients with chronic hypertensive disease, but was sometimes increased both in normal gravidas and in preeclamptics.

Retinal Changes

In preeclampsia one finds retinal edema, localized spasm or generalized constriction of one or more of the retinal arteries, and rarely, flame-shaped hemorrhages and cotton-wool exudates. Finnerty has observed a generalized retinal sheen in patients with preeclampsia. This sheen resembles the glistening of a normal tympanic membrane and is attributed to retinal edema. However, it is not specific for preeclampsia since it is present in acute glomerulonephritis and in the nephrotic stage of chronic glomerulonephritis. Moreover, a sheen limited to the temporal region of the fundus is commonly observed in normal children and young adults.

Arteriosclerotic retinopathy denotes antecedent vascular disease. It is not present in preeclampsia unless it is superimposed on preexisting long-standing hypertensive cardiovascular or renal disease.

Severe degrees of retinal angiospasm are indicative of severe preeclampsia irrespective of the level of the blood pressure, the amount of proteinuria or the degree of edema. Nevertheless, normal fundi or minimal vasospasm do not necessarily denote mild preeclampsia or preclude this condition.

Unilateral and bilateral retinal detachments may occur infrequently in preeclampsia. It is associated with sudden blindness. Detachment is caused by intraocular edema and is an indication for prompt termination of the pregnancy. Usually, there is spontaneous reattachment of the retina within two days to two months after delivery. Significant permanent visual impairment is rare.

Visual Disturbances

Scotomata, diplopia and amblyopia in patients with preeclampsia are serious symptoms indicative of imminent eclampsia. They are attributed to circulatory changes in the visual cortex or in the retina.

Amaurosis, rare in preeclampsia, is reported in one to three per cent of patients with eclampsia. It is caused most often by functional changes involving the optic nerve or the visual cortex, but may be caused by retinal detachment (see above). Blindness of central origin may persist for a few hours or may last for several weeks. Normal vision is usually regained within a week. Homonymous hemianopsia, initiated by reversible changes in the visual cortex, has been reported in eclampsia.

Pulmonary Edema

Pulmonary edema (see Chapter 45) is a major cause of death in preeclampsia and eclampsia. This complication has been attributed to left heart failure most commonly, but may be associated with right heart failure caused by pulmonary hypertension as well as to an increased permeability of the alveolar epithelium or to a combination of these abnormalities. In many patients, the injudicious administration of parenteral fluids which overloads an already constricted cardiovascular system may initiate this problem. Monitoring the central venous pressure may be of considerable aid in avoiding this potentially fatal complication.

Histological Changes

The anatomic changes in the acute hypertensive states of pregnancy are nonspecific. There are visceral hemorrhages, necrosis and infarction of tissue and thrombosis of small vessels encountered in fatal cases. These changes may be focal or diffuse and numerous or few. Their distribution varies widely. Hepatic, cerebral, mucosal and adrenal hemorrhages are seen, together with necrosis of the anterior pituitary, bilateral renal cortical necrosis, red and white splenic infarcts, focal hemorrhages and myocardial necrosis. Anemic infarcts of the liver (Fig. 253) and gross morphologic changes in the brain, heart,

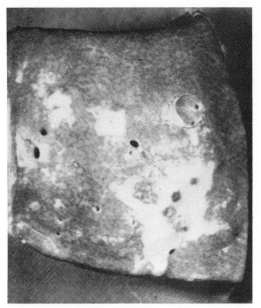

Figure 253 Characteristic appearance of anemic infarcts of the liver in a patient who died of eclampsia.

and small arteries, most pronounced in the kidney, range from concentric overlapping of normal smooth muscle cells to overt necrosis. Many of the vessels within foci of necrosis contain thrombi. Fibrin is believed to be deposited within the arterioles and capillaries of the systemic and pulmonary circulation and within the hepatic sinusoids (Schmorl; Fahr; McKay et al.). Arterial and arteriolar hypertrophy and fibrosis are indicative of antecedent vascular disease. They are seen in most pronounced form in the kidneys.

Hemorrhage, tissue necrosis, fibrin deposition and vascular thrombosis characterize the visceral lesions. In the liver these focal and diffuse changes arise in the periportal area and extend into the central zone (Fig. 254). They tend to be more pronounced in the right lobe of the liver. Petechial hemorrhages in the basal ganglia, pons and cerebral hemispheres are also composed of these elements. Massive cerebral hemorrhages are sometimes seen; they have been attributed to vascular degeneration, but their origin is not fully understood. In patients who die of this disease, there are hepatic lesions and, less frequently, lesions in many other organs.

The acute visceral changes are probably the direct result of intensive endarteriolar vasospasm. Recent studies suggest that intravascular deposition of fibrin is a critical factor in the pathogenesis of these lesions.

kidneys, adrenals and spleen are inconsistently encountered. Subcapsular hemorrhages of the liver of varying magnitudes are common in patients who die of this condition. In rare instances, the cause of death is massive hepatic hemorrhage. Aspiration during convulsions or in the postictal state may result in pneumonitis.

Histological changes in the arterioles

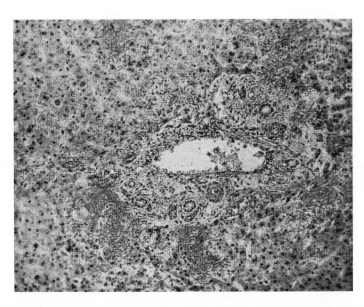

Figure 254 Photomicrograph of the liver in an eclamptic patient showing periportal hemorrhage and necrosis. (Magnification × 140.)

It has been postulated that placental metabolic aberrations initiate the intravascular deposition of fibrin and the fibrin thrombi in turn cause the periportal hemorrhage and necrosis.

A disseminated fibrin deposition, necrosis of the anterior pituitary and bilateral renal cortical necrosis have been described by McKay et al. in gravidas dying from endotoxin shock and from complications of acute hypertensive disorders. They have postulated that these phenomena are the human counterpart of the generalized Schwartzman reaction mediated by bacterial endotoxins in the first instance and by products of decidual degeneration in the second.

Renal Morphology. The renal changes in preeclampsia are inconsistent and include membranous glomerulonephritis, deposition of lipid in the glomeruli and tubules, hyaline thrombi within the glomeruli, swelling of the internal elastic lamina, necrosis and thrombosis of afferent glomerular arterioles and nonspecific changes in the tubular epithelium. Additionally, precipitates of hemoglobin and red cell casts are seen within the tubules, and there are interstitial hemorrhages, arteriolar sclerosis, lesions of chronic renal disease and cortical infarction.

Under light microscopy (Figs. 255 and 256), renal biopsy shows acute membranous glomerulonephritis. Electron microscopy (Fig. 257), on the other hand, demonstrates no proliferation of components in contact with the glomerular capillaries. The foot processes of the epithelial cells are distinct and there are no diffuse changes in the basement membrane. The cytoplasm of the endothelial cells is increased and exhibits a variety of changes, including vacuolization, hyaline droplet formation, membrane condensation, as well as increased particulate matter and cytoplasmic strands that approach the basement membrane but are separate from it. The glomerular capillary lumina are narrowed as a consequence of an increase in the cytoplasm of the surrounding epithelial cells (Altchek; Spargo et al.). Changes in the small renal arteries and arterioles are inconsistent and the tubular changes are nonspecific. It is doubtful that any permanent glomerular damage results, although Pollack and Nettles have reported it to have occurred.

Placenta. Bartholomew et al. found an increased number and severity of true placental infarcts, but others have been unable to substantiate their findings. Nevertheless, it is agreed that degenerative

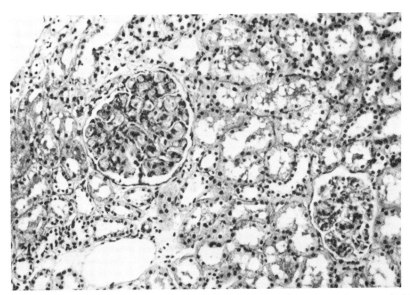

Figure 255 Histological appearance of the glomerular lesion in preeclampsia as shown on light microscopy. Hematoxylin and eosin. (Magnification × 170.)

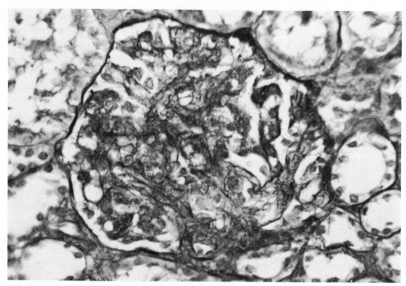

Figure 256 High-power light microscopic appearance of the glomerular lesion in preeclampsia. PAS stain. (Magnification × 425.)

changes in the trophoblast are consistently accelerated. There is little doubt that rapid diminution in placental function occurs in severe hypertensive disorders.

Clinical Course

Except when associated with hydatidiform mole or multiple pregnancy, the triad of hypertension, proteinuria and edema is limited to the last 20 weeks of gestation. Most often it makes its appearance in the last month. Preeclampsia is a progressive disease and may be rapidly fulminating, but initially all patients with this disorder have mild signs and symptoms. There is occult edema manifested by a weekly weight gain in excess of 500 gm. Subsequently pitting edema of the lower ex-

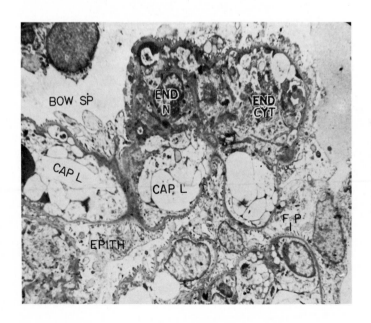

Figure 257 Capillary endotheliosis typical of the preeclamptic glomerular lesion seen on electronmicrography. *BOW SP*, Bowman's space; *END N*, endothelial cell nucleus; *END CYT*, endothelial cell cytoplasm; *CAP L*, capillary lumen; *EPITH*, epithelial cell; *FP*, foot process. (Courtesy of B. Spargo, C. P. McCartney and R. Winemiller.)

tremities, persisting after bed rest, appears in association with mild hypertension and slight proteinuria.

Progression from mild to severe manifestations may take place quickly over a matter of a few hours or slowly over an interval of weeks. In the rapidly progressing clinical syndrome, eclampsia is likely to ensue with convulsions, coma and death in rapid succession. Severe preeclampsia is associated with rapid progression in the above manifestations together with other ominous signs, including persistent blood pressure in excess of 160/110 mm. Hg, excretion of 4 gm. or more of protein in 24 hours, oliguria, anuria, hemoconcentration, azotemia, jaundice, evidence of cardiac impairment, headache, visual disturbances, clouding of consciousness, hyperactive reflexes, nausea and vomiting.

Progression of the disease may be manifested by progressive rise in blood pressure, increasing proteinuria, decreasing urinary output or the appearance of cerebral, visual or gastrointestinal signs and symptoms. In most patients there are signs of severe preeclampsia for several days and indications of progression before seizures occur, but eclampsia may develop in some patients who appear to have a relatively mild form of the disease.

Preeclampsia or eclampsia may arise during labor or post partum. Postpartum eclampsia usually appears during the first 12 hours of the puerperium. Rarely, it may appear subsequently, but other convulsive disorders are more likely to be the cause. Fairly well-documented eclampsia has been reported up to about five days post partum.

Patients with progressive disease invariably retain excessive quantities of sodium and water. Most have edema of the extremities (Fig. 258), abdomen, back and face. They may also have some ascites, although this is not usually detectable clinically. The sudden appearance of edema with rapid accumulation of interstitial fluid is ominous, although the disease may progress to convulsions in about 10 per cent of patients without demonstrable pitting edema. Characteristically, patients with fulminating preeclampsia have puffiness about the face, especially the eyelids, and edematous fingers. In terms of weight gain, a sudden rapid increment in weight

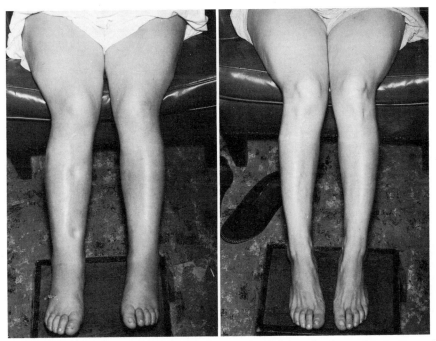

Figure 258 Acute peripheral pitting edema of the lower extremity in a patient with severe preeclampsia at term (left) and seven days post partum (right).

over a period of several days or a week is particularly significant; distribution of the same weight gain over the course of the pregnancy is of no particular importance in this regard (see Chapter 10).

Convulsions and Coma. Eclamptic seizures are generalized tonic and clonic contractions resembling grand mal usually followed by coma during the postictal state. Prodromes include progressive and unremitting headache, apprehension, disorientation, somnolence, nausea and vomiting, epigastric distress, visual disturbances and hyperactive reflexes. Focal prodromal spasms often involve the muscles of the face, neck or upper extremities, and generalized tonic and clonic contractions and coma follow in sequence. Anuria or oliguria occurs and there is an associated increase in proteinuria and usually a rise in the blood pressure. In some patients, however, there may be a precipitate fall in blood pressure and other signs of impending circulatory collapse. Hypotension under these circumstances is very ominous indeed.

During the tonic phase, the body is thrown into opisthotonos, the limbs are rigid and extended, respirations cease, the veins of the neck become engorged and cyanosis develops. The clonic state ensues. There are violent intermittent contractions of the muscles of the head, limbs and trunk, and the tongue may be bitten (Fig. 259). The patient is usually incontinent of urine during this time.

A period of coma follows; respirations are stertorous; frequently, there are rhonchi heard. In some patients vomitus is aspirated. The duration of coma is variable and tends to be related to the severity of the disease.

There may be only one seizure or the patient may have multiple convulsions, lapse into persistent coma and ultimately die. The eclamptic patient who regains consciousness is usually disoriented and restless for a time. Labor, if it should ensue, often enhances this agitation.

Causes of Death. The most frequent causes of death in preeclampsia and eclampsia are congestive heart failure, cerebral hemorrhage and the complications of operative obstetrics. Dieckmann reported that, among 50 fatalities from eclampsia, 29 resulted from congestive cardiac failure, 8 from cerebrovascular accidents, 5 from obstetric procedures, 4 from hemorrhagic shock and afibrinogenemia, 2 from acute hepatic failure, 1 from respiratory paralysis and 1 from bilateral pyelonephritis. Over the years, fewer and fewer eclamptic deaths are seen. This is perhaps the result of changes in management of the disorder and of its complications.

Regression of Signs

After delivery, the pathophysiologic changes tend to regress rapidly. Diuresis appears most often during the first 12 hours, but is sometimes delayed for as long as 72 hours. It is often the first manifestation of recovery and a valuable prognostic sign. Usually, edema and proteinuria diminish progressively and are gone by the fifth postpartum day. The blood pressure returns to normal quite promptly, sometimes within hours, but may take a week or two. In some patients there is moderate hypertension for as long as six months after delivery; when this occurs, it is rather likely that there is some other underlying and preexisting cause.

On recovery, the majority of women with eclampsia have some retrograde amnesia and are unaware of the events that transpired during the acute stage of their illness.

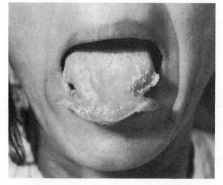

Figure 259 Posteclamptic patient showing evidence of damage to the tongue bitten during convulsive seizure. (Courtesy of O. Agüero.)

Differential Diagnosis

When there are no findings pathognomonic of chronic hypertensive cardiovascular or renal disease, the past history, the course of the disease and the vascular-renal status six or more months after delivery are used to help differentiate the hypertensive states of pregnancy retrospectively. History of hypertensive disease, evidence of arteriosclerotic retinopathy and persistence of hypertension after delivery raise serious doubts about the process being true preeclampsia, although exacerbations of hypertensive diseases are clinically indistinguishable late in pregnancy.

It is helpful if the disease occurs in a multipara, arises before the twenty-fourth week of pregnancy, is associated with very high systolic pressures and is recurrent in sequential pregnancies, because these features are characteristic of chronic hypertensive cardiovascular or renal disease and are not generally seen in association with preeclampsia alone. However, there are appreciable errors in diagnosis based on these criteria. As noted earlier, renal biopsy validation of the clinical diagnosis showed that 30 per cent of patients fulfilling the clinical criteria for preeclampsia actually had chronic renal disease and not the toxemic glomerular lesion of capillary endotheliosis believed to be pathognomonic of the disorder.

When seizures occur during pregnancy, other criteria must be fulfilled to warrant a diagnosis of eclampsia. Eclampsia must be distinguished from epilepsy, hypertensive encephalopathy, cerebral neoplasm, cerebral abscess, meningitis, encephalitis, cerebral vein thrombosis, sagittal sinus thrombosis, cerebral embolism, ruptured cerebral aneurysm, cerebral trauma, uremia, diabetic coma, insulin-induced hypoglycemia, tetany, poisoning, scleroderma, porphyria, hepatic disease, sickle cell crisis and drug encephalopathy.

Prognosis

Maternal Mortality. The maternal mortality for preeclampsia is nearly three times that for obstetric patients in general, and for eclampsia there is an overall mortality of seven per cent with an institutional range of up to 17 per cent. During the past 20 years the maternal mortality for preeclampsia has decreased 85 per cent; for eclampsia, 35 per cent, and for all hypertensive states of pregnancy, 75 per cent. Currently, 48 per cent of all deaths in this group are attributed to eclampsia. A further decrease in deaths is anticipated in the near future because, with few exceptions, this complication is probably preventable.

Infant Mortality. In preeclampsia the average perinatal mortality is 10 per cent; in the severe form it is 35 per cent and in the mild form, five per cent. Prematurity is the major cause of infant mortality. Incidence of prematurity with hypertensive disorders is at least twice that for normal gravidas. The mortality rate for these premature infants is about 22 per cent.

Prognostic Criteria. The appearance of the convulsive state is a major prognostic criterion. Maternal mortality is greatly increased when it occurs. About seven per cent of patients with eclampsia die. There are several features suggesting that the clinical picture is degenerating. They serve as forewarnings of a poor outcome and include such ominous occurrences as a sequence of more than 10 convulsions; coma for six hours or more; temperature of 39° C. (102.2° F.) or greater; pulse rate of 120 per minute or more; respiratory rate of 40 or more; cardiovascular decompensation manifested by pulmonary edema, rising central venous pressure, cyanosis, falling arterial oxygen tension, low or falling blood pressure and low pulse pressure; electrolyte imbalance; and failure of aggressive management to stop convulsions, to maintain urinary output of 30 ml. per hour and to effect some hemodilution as evidenced by a 10 per cent decrease in the hematocrit or the serum protein level (Eden).

Renal Damage. The kidneys of some patients who had preeclampsia many years earlier show the changes of chronic renal disease. These findings coupled with the appearance of hypertension following pregnancy in patients with unknown prepregnancy blood pressures have been cited to support the widely held belief that permanent renal damage may be a sequel of preeclampsia. Chesley et al. and Tillman both showed that permanent residual hypertension does not develop in preeclamptic patients who were normotensive before they conceived. Moreover, serial renal biopsies demonstrated the reversibility of the glomerular lesion believed to be pathognomonic and emphasized the error in retrospective autopsy studies (McCartney). Therefore, permanent renal damage can no longer be considered to be a sequel of preeclampsia or eclampsia.

Prevention

Whether or not one can prevent preeclampsia is a moot question. The incidence is declining, but no single factor or combination of factors can be shown to have been instrumental in this phenomenon. Antepartum care has been given most of the credit for alerting physicians to the earliest premonitory signs so that the disorder can be detected at its beginnings in the mild and more readily treatable forms. Thus, it can be credited with reducing the incidence of the severest forms of preeclampsia and eclampsia and thereby reducing the morbidity associated with them. However, there is no evidence that any feature of routine antepartum management in any way alters the overall incidence of the disease.

This applies both to dietary salt restriction and to the use of thiazide diuretics, neither of which is of any documentable value in preventing hypertensive states of pregnancy. Similarly, weight control during pregnancy is of no value in this regard either. In fact, it is possible that all three may, under certain circumstances, actually be detrimental. Electrolyte imbalances of such severity as to be fatal have been reported with combinations of restricted sodium intake and prolonged use of diuretics. Not only is the efficacy of salt restriction in doubt despite the prevailing practice but increased salt intake may even be beneficial. Robinson relieved early manifestations of preeclampsia in patients by increasing salt intake. Others have verified the benefit of this heterodox approach (Kumar et al.; Palomaki and Lindheimer).

There is a positive sodium balance in normal pregnancy. Increased renin levels in plasma are probably the result of increased synthesis by juxtaglomerular cells. Sodium restriction further augments this process. With increased renin activity, there is greatly enhanced angiotensin secretion. This is manifested not by a pressor effect but rather by aldosterone secretion. Sodium depletion will also result in this sequence. Aldosterone causes increased sodium reabsorption in the kidney tubules. About 850 mEq. of additional sodium (19.5 gm.) is retained during the course of normal pregnancy. In view of these needs and the ephemeral foundation upon which salt restriction is based, it is difficult to justify continuing this practice.

Weight control is likewise without basis in pregnancy as a means of preventing preeclampsia. Aside from its cosmetic advantage, there is no evidence whatsoever that restricting dietary intake of calories is beneficial. Indeed, there are data supporting the view that it may be potentially harmful to the fetus, producing smaller fetuses with greater likelihood of dying or acquiring some neurological or developmental defect (see Chapter 68).

Use of diuretics has been purported to be beneficial in preventing preeclampsia. It has become a very popular approach despite the fact that no effect can be demonstrated in properly conducted double-blind studies (Kraus et al.). Moreover, the hazards of diuretics are too often ignored, including electrolyte imbalance, hemorrhagic pancreatitis, diabetogenic effects in both mother and fetus, neonatal hyponatremia and thrombocytopenia (Gray). Equally important is the fact that diuretics mask the appearance of the early warning signs of preeclampsia by preventing fluid retention, edema formation and acute weight gain, so that the disease is further advanced before it is detected.

Treatment

Because etiology and pathogenesis are undefined, treatment is entirely empirical. The objectives of therapy are embodied in the objectives of obstetrics as a discipline, namely, the preservation of the mother's health and life and the delivery of an optimally healthy infant atraumatically. For the former, it is necessary to make every effort to prevent convulsions, thereby averting the hazards of this complication for the mother; as to the fetus, certain constraints are imposed according to the severity of the preeclamptic or eclamptic process and the gestational age at which it occurs.

The process can be definitively terminated under most circumstances by effecting delivery; however, concluding the pregnancy prematurely may be quite detrimental to the fetus who is insufficiently developed to survive outside the uterus. Thus, one must try to strike a balance. On the one hand we desire to prolong the pregnancy for purposes of allowing the fetus to mature. Weighed against this are the possibilities of imposing risks on the mother due to progressive disease and jeopardizing the fetus as a consequence of the complications of progressive placental

insufficiency, abruptio placentae or eclampsia itself. The more severe the manifestations, the more urgent the need for termination of the pregnancy primarily in the interests of the mother. For the milder forms of preeclampsia fetal needs should be considered first.

If one recalls that all the prodromal manifestations of preeclampsia are essentially silent insofar as the patient is concerned, one begins to appreciate how very important astute periodic observations by the physician are in detecting the disease process in its earliest phases. Regular examinations for the development of hypertension, proteinuria and weight gain and for the appearance of edema, as described in Chapter 9, are imperative.

Once detected, hospitalization is advisable. The outline of a recommended program of management is shown in Figure 260. Whenever the disease is progressive

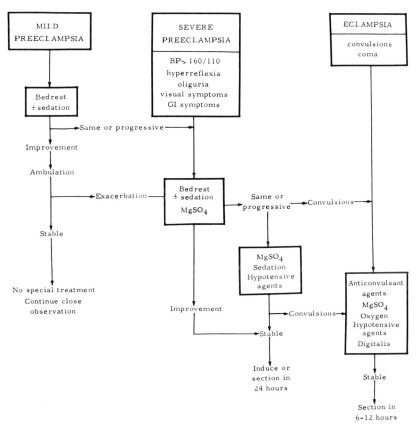

Figure 260 Schematic flow diagram illustrating program of management of patients with preeclampsia and eclampsia. For details see text.

or more than minimal in its manifestation, it is mandatory that the patient be hospitalized for purposes of intensive observation and care. Even patients with mild forms of this disease process may show rapid and unexpected progression over relatively short periods of time; thus, it is important to observe them carefully, if possible. Where hospitalization is not feasible for such mild cases, they should be examined no less often than twice weekly and carefully instructed concerning the development of such characteristic symptoms as visual disturbances, persistent headache, epigastric pain, nausea and vomiting, as well as puffiness of the hands and face and oliguria. When these symptoms arise, they must be reported at once so that hospitalization can be arranged.

Management of Mild Preeclampsia. The patient with mild preeclampsia need be treated with bed rest only. Dietary sodium restriction is universally practiced, albeit based on dubious evidence. Preeclamptic patients do not handle sodium well, however, and on this basis it is advisable to restrict sodium intake when manifestations of hypertensive states arise. The rationale for instituting salt restriction on a routine prophylactic basis in all pregnancies is not justified (see above). Moreover, few patients will realistically adhere to the unappetizing and tasteless diet which is prescribed for them.

Bed rest alone is usually sufficient for managing patients with mild manifestations of preeclampsia. With the patient at rest on her side, both renal and uterine blood flow is increased, diuresis is effected and blood pressure tends to return toward normal levels. The addition of a mild sedative or tranquilizing agent may be necessary in order to make it possible for the patient to remain restricted quietly at bed rest.

The hospitalized patient should be regularly evaluated so that the earliest indication of progressive changes will be detected. Blood pressure recordings every four hours are essential. Deep tendon reflexes should be tested at the same time and the ocular fundi examined for arteriolar vasospasm. Daily weighing, urinalysis for protein and microscopic search for red cells and casts are essential. Urinary output should be recorded and oliguria noted. Hematocrit should be followed periodically to detect the ominous sign of hemoconcentration. It is important that fluid intake not be restricted.

Most patients treated in this manner will show rapid subsidence of all manifestations and an associated diuresis. When this occurs, ambulation can be permitted. If the condition remains stable with normal blood pressure readings, minimal or no proteinuria and no evidence of vasospasm or active fluid retention, no further special therapy is necessary. The patient should be observed regularly in the clinic or office for exacerbations, however. Because it is likely that the underlying disease process has not completely subsided despite the absence of continuing manifestations, many physicians will attempt to terminate the pregnancies of such patients as soon as conditions are favorable for induction (see Chapter 24). This is an acceptable practice, but it must be remembered that the fetal risks of continuing the pregnancy may be counterbalanced by the risks inherent in attempting to induce labor under less than ideal circumstances.

Management of Severe Preeclampsia. The patient with manifestations of severe preeclampsia (see above) requires more aggressive management. This principle also applies to the patient with milder manifestations whose condition progresses, exacerbates after an interval of improvement, or remains essentially unchanged at bed rest. Here it is essential that maximum stabilization be pursued as shown in Figure 260. In addition to bed rest and sedation, there are a variety of agents that can be used effectively. Of all those available, perhaps magnesium sulfate is the most widely used.

Administered intramuscularly or intravenously, magnesium sulfate is effective because of its depressant action on the myoneural junction. It is very potent in this regard and will depress deep tendon reflexes at plasma levels exceeding 4 mEq. per liter and will completely obtund them in concentrations approaching 10 mEq. per liter. If this level is exceeded, respirations will cease and cardiac arrest will occur at still higher concentrations; the margin of safety is narrow so that great care must be taken not to exceed effective dosage. Since there is a delay in stabilizing of blood levels for 1.5 to 2 hours after intramuscular injection, intravenous administration is preferable for purposes of titrating to the appropriate therapeutic level.

While slowly administering 20 ml. of 10 per cent solution of magnesium sulfate, the knee jerks are tested and the respirations observed. Calcium gluconate is kept available for immediate use as an effective metabolic antagonist in the event of overdosage. The further administration of magnesium sulfate is discontinued immediately when the knee jerks become hypoactive. Since magnesium is eliminated by way of the kidneys, it is necessary to ensure good renal function before giving additional amounts of magnesium once an effective level has been reached. The intramuscular route requires injection of 50 per cent solutions with one per cent procaine introduced in 10 ml. amounts in each buttock. Because of the pain that results and the lack of close control on circulating levels, this approach is less preferable than the intravenous technique. Some have combined both approaches with satisfactory results (Pritchard).

Use of magnesium sulfate as described has several advantages. First, its depressant action on neuromuscular transmission will diminish hyperreflexia and result in some vasodilatation. The latter is seen in the acute skin flushing. Direct effect on the vasospastic component of the preeclamptic process does not occur to any great extent, however. Thus, the blood pressure is not affected directly in the usual therapeutic doses. Although larger doses may lower arterial pressure, more effective pharmacologic agents are available for this purpose when necessary. Magnesium also has a central effect, causing some degree of depression, but this action is less apparent than its effect on the myoneural junction.

When used in hyperosmolar concentrations intravenously, magnesium solutions also evoke osmotic diuresis and secondarily reduce intracranial pressure. In this latter regard 50 per cent glucose solution was once widely used, but its effect proved transitory. Today, 25 per cent mannitol is probably more effective when given intravenously in 12.5 gm. doses for purposes of effecting osmotic diuresis, particularly in the presence of oliguria. If this fructose derivative is used, care should be taken to avoid cardiac decompensation from circulatory overload by monitoring the central venous pressure.

In order to avoid masking or obtunding the signs and symptoms of progressively severe preeclampsia, it is advisable to withhold antihypertensive agents and sedation. Although it is common practice to give them, the administration of several powerful pharmacologic agents simultaneously tends to confuse evaluation and complicate management. Except for the fulminating varieties of preeclampsia and eclampsia, simplistic approaches tend to be more easily controlled and apparently just as effective.

If bed rest and magnesium sulfate are effective in reducing the overt manifestations of severe preeclampsia so that the patient's condition is stabilized, an appropriate course of action is to maintain control for 24 hours and then to consider means for terminating the pregnancy. This can entail induction of labor if conditions are favorable or cesarean section if they are not. The option to continue conservative management for prolonged periods of time under these circumstances is generally unwarranted. It might be undertaken only if the fetus were not viable and facilities for intensive, continuous monitoring of both mother and fetus were available. Most often, however, the wisest course is termination.

If bed rest and magnesium sulfate are insufficient to control the severe manifestations, additional measures should next be employed to achieve stabilization prior to terminating the pregnancy. For the patient whose blood pressure continues to increase and approaches levels at which one becomes concerned about the development of cerebrovascular accidents, hypotensive agents may be invoked. Pressure can be readily controlled with hydralazine hydrochloride administered by continuous intravenous infusion of a solution containing 20 mg. in 500 ml. The drug may also be given by intermittent intravenous injections of 10 to 20 mg. doses. By decreasing arteriolar resistance, hydralazine causes the blood pressure to fall. At the same time, it increases cardiac output and renal blood flow. Its effect on uterine blood flow and fetomaternal exchange is not yet well defined. The response of the blood pressure and the duration of effect will determine the initial and subsequent doses. Metaraminal bitartrate should be kept available as an effective antidote for hypotension produced by hydralazine (Apresoline) overdosage.

Usually, it is unnecessary to use reserpine, but it may be given in 2.5 to 5 mg. doses intramuscularly at intervals of 8 to 12 hours. Care should be taken to minimize the duration of reserpine administration because reversible parkinsonian rigidity may occur after five days and the newborn infant will have increased bronchial secretions as a consequence.

It is essential to bear in mind that use of hypotensive agents should be restricted to those patients only who are endangered by their rising blood pressures. The underlying preeclamptic process is unaffected, however, and blood flow to the uterus may be severely restricted as a result of the use of these agents, causing fetal demise. Urinary output will usually fall as well, but this effect tends to be transitory.

Sedation for purposes of allaying convulsions may be necessary for those patients with severe preeclampsia whose manifestations cannot be controlled as heretofore outlined. Morphine, although still widely used in 15 to 30 mg. doses, has the disadvantages of producing oliguria by reducing glomerular filtration and increasing intracranial pressure secondary to the carbon dioxide retention and acidosis caused by respiratory depression. Moreover, it invokes nausea and vomiting. Preferably, sedatives without these side effects, such as barbiturates or paraldehyde, should be used instead.

Phenobarbital, 300 mg., may be given subcutaneously at 12-hour intervals; amobarbital is likewise effective in 250 to 500 mg. doses; paraldehyde is also useful by rectal administration of 30 to 40 ml. diluted in mineral oil or olive oil. The disadvantages of paraldehyde include the fact that the profound sedation which results is difficult to distinguish from coma. Barbiturates enhance the increased cerebrovascular resistance and diminished oxygen consumption present in severe preeclampsia.

All effective sedative agents depress the fetus. Use of barbiturates for the preeclamptic patient in labor should be restricted in deference to the fetus, if fetal salvage is a matter of concern. The known depressant effect of these agents on the respiratory centers of the newborn will result in neonatal depression. This is not a consideration, however, if the fetus is dead or nonviable, or in those instances in which the hypertensive state does not extend into the intrapartum period. After stabilization has been achieved by these more aggressive means, an interval of 12 to 24 hours should be allowed to elapse before induction of labor or cesarean section is undertaken (see below).

Management of Eclampsia. The management of eclampsia requires efforts to stop the convulsions, to maintain ventilation, to avoid aspiration, to keep blood pressure within bounds, to avert cardiac decompensation and to effect termination of the pregnancy as soon as feasible with minimal maternal and fetal risk.

Hospitalization is mandatory, with the patient sequestered in a quiet room under constant observation. Nursing care is of utmost importance in the management of a patient with eclampsia. The patient is kept in bed on her side with padded siderails and the foot of the bed elevated to expedite tracheobronchial drainage. An intravenous line for administering drugs rapidly, central venous pressure and urinary catheter are essential.

During convulsions, injury to the tongue is avoided by placing a tongue blade covered with cotton and gauze between the patient's teeth. Any padded or rubber-covered piece of wood or rolled cloth will do for this purpose. Oxygen is given for cyanosis. Suction is used to prevent aspiration of vomitus, saliva and nasopharyngeal secretions. In some instances, a tracheostomy may be necessary to ensure adequate ventilation.

While the patient is unconscious, she must be given nothing by mouth. Observations of hourly urinary output, blood pressure, respiratory and pulse rates as well as rectal temperature are made and recorded, together with an accurate record of fluid balance. The patient must be watched for cyanosis and jaundice. Hyperreflexia progressing to clonus presages convulsions.

Convulsions can usually be readily controlled pharmacologically. Intravenous administration of a short-acting barbiturate is most effective. Thiopental (Pentothal Sodium) can be given intravenously in a 2.5 per cent solution in amounts sufficient to stop the convulsion; usually, no more than 2 ml. (500 mg.) is required. Sodium amobarbital (Sodium Amytal) 250 to 500 mg. intravenously is equally effective. Any of these may be combined with magnesium sulfate in the regimen described earlier. Diazepam (Valium) is also an effective anticonvulsive agent for use in controlling the eclamptic seizure. Intravenous titration to no more than a 20 mg. dose is used. If convulsions persist, muscle relaxants, such as succinylcholine 60 to 80 mg., may be given intravenously to produce complete muscular paralysis, but it is essential that this be done only if appropriate measures and skilled personnel are available to ventilate the patient properly.

Diuresis can be established by administering chlorothiazide or other diuretic agents. It is important to regulate dosage by means of serial electrolyte determinations. Supplemental potassium may have to be administered. These agents are relatively ineffectual in the presence of hemoconcentration. The patient may be resistant to hemodilution, but once it is achieved, diuresis generally occurs. Electrolyte disturbances and acute congestive heart failure may be initiated by injudicious administration of parenteral fluids. Strict attention to fluid balance and cardiovascular status is mandatory.

After stability is achieved and the patient's condition optimized, an interval of 6 to 12 hours should be allowed to elapse before pregnancy is terminated. Spontaneous onset of labor is common under these circumstances. If this does not take place, induction of labor may be attempted with intravenous oxytocin infusion. However, it is usually preferable to subject postictal patients to cesarean section in order to avoid exacerbating the disease process by the stimuli of labor.

The treatment of acute decompensation (see Chapter 41) requires rapid digitalization, the administration of oxygen and measures aimed at effecting diuresis and at decreasing central venous pressure. Cedilanid-D is an effective intravenous digitalis glycoside for use in congestive heart failure. Initially, an intravenous dose of 0.8 mg. is given slowly and followed at one- to two-hour intervals with additional intravenous doses of 0.2 to 0.4 mg. up to a maximum of 1.6 mg. per 24 hours. Digoxin can be used instead starting with 1.0 mg. intravenously, and 0.25 mg. every four to six hours to a maximum of 1.75 mg. in 24 hours. For rapid diuresis, furosemide (Lasix), 50 to 100 mg. intravenously, is very effective but may cause severe electrolyte imbalance. Precautions should be taken to make appropriate corrections in electrolyte requirements. Ethacrynic acid is a potent, effective diuretic for use in the presence of acute pulmonary edema. It can be given intravenously in 25 to 50 mg. doses. It is essential with the use of this agent to guard against electrolyte depletion.

Oxygen by intermittent positive pressure is helpful if the patient is cooperative, but it should not be forced on the patient who objects to its use. Rotating tourniquets on the extremities may be useful. Venesection for the purpose of reducing central venous pressure, however, is especially hazardous in severe preeclampsia and eclampsia because of the reduced volume of the total vascular circulation in these disorders. Evaluation of cardiac status and the management of relevant cardiac problems are detailed in Chapter 41.

Terminating the Pregnancy. Once the decision has been made to terminate the pregnancy according to the programs outlined above and schematically presented in Figure 260, it is imperative that this objective be pursued at an optimal time for both mother and fetus. Having delayed induction or section sufficiently long to allow one to correct fluid, electrolyte and acid-base problems and to make proper preparations for all eventualities, the physician is obligated to proceed forthwith with measures to terminate the pregnancy before the underlying hypertensive disorder exacerbates once again. The same principle generally applies to the fetus as well because delay may be associated with intrauterine demise in association with progressive placental insufficiency or abruptio placentae.

If conditions are particularly favorable for induction of labor, the membranes should be ruptured and oxytocin infusion begun. Constant observation of the mother for evidences of aggravation of her hypertensive state and surveillance of the fetus by heart rate monitoring (see Chapter 13) are essential. If the conditions of the mother and fetus remain stable and labor is progressive, vaginal delivery should be allowed.

On the other hand, if conditions for induction are unfavorable, if induction has failed, if labor progression is abnormally slow, if the manifestations of preeclampsia show any progression, or if the fetus demonstrates objective evidence of distress, cesarean section should be undertaken immediately. General inhalation anesthesia is usually most effective for delivery by either abdominal or vaginal routes.

CHRONIC HYPERTENSIVE CARDIOVASCULAR DISEASE

At least half the patients with hypertensive states of pregnancy have chronic hypertensive disease. In pregnancy the diagnosis is suggested by evidence of hypertension preceding pregnancy, hypertension during the first 20 weeks of gestation, hypertensive and arteriosclerotic retinopathy, hypertension in a multipara or hypertension in previous pregnancies. The differentiation from chronic renal disease is difficult. McCartney showed that 25 per cent of patients fulfilling the clinical criteria for chronic hypertensive cardiovascular disease have evidences of chronic renal disease in renal biopsy specimens. This distinction notwithstanding, the clinical manifestations and courses of chronic hypertensive vascular and renal diseases tend to be parallel in the pregnancy. Management is also similar.

Although by far the most commonly encountered form of hypertensive disease is that called *essential hypertension,* other varieties are encountered, including renal vascular disease, aortic coarctation, primary aldosteronism and pheochromocytoma. Hypertension based on renal disease extends from glomerulonephritis and pyelonephritis to diabetic nephropathy, collagen diseases and polycystic renal disease.

Retinal changes tend to be quite characteristic in long-standing chronic hypertensive vascular or renal disease. Arteriolar tortuosity is seen, together with variations in caliber and arteriovenous compression. In advanced stages of active disease, retinal hemorrhages and exudates are seen.

Superimposed preeclampsia refers to the appearance of the manifestations of preeclampsia (dealt with in detail in the previous sections of this chapter) in a pregnant woman with some form of preexisting chronic hypertensive disease. Usually, there is significant aggravation of the hypertension with or without the appearance of proteinuria and edema. The clinical picture may be quite rapidly progressive to extreme levels of hypertension with oliguria and azotemia. Rapid advancement of retinal changes are seen, including marked vasospasm, hemorrhages and cotton-wool exudates. Infrequently, progression to convulsions and coma occurs.

There is a high fetal loss that can be correlated with the severity of the disease. About one-third of infants are lost in association with severe forms, manifested by high levels of blood pressure exceeding 170/100, proteinuria exceeding 1 gm. in 24 hours or with coassociated arteriosclerotic retinopathy or impaired cardiac or renal function. Moreover, in patients with chronic hypertensive vascular or renal disease, there is a high incidence of late abortions and stillbirths. Frequently, infants are small for their gestational age because of intrauterine inanition due to placental insufficiency. Abruptio placentae is not uncommon in these patients, but congestive failure, azotemia and cerebrovascular accidents are seen infrequently. Abruptio placentae occurs much more frequently among patients with chronic hypertensive vascular disease, the incidence being eight times that of the normal gravid population; moreover, it tends to be more complicated when it does occur, particularly when seen with coassociated coagulopathy and renal cortical necrosis.

The definitive management of pregnant patients with chronic hypertensive vascular or renal disease is entirely empirical.

Maternal complications can usually be prevented and some of the fetuses can be salvaged by terminating the pregnancy at the most opportune time. Other measures are entirely palliative or temporizing and are used with the hope of retarding the progression of the disease until the fetus is sufficiently viable to survive. Unfortunately, it is the inherent severity of the disease rather than the type of therapy that determines whether these objectives can be achieved. Treatment consists of bed rest, sodium restriction, diuretic agents, sedatives and hypotensive drugs. Among these, bed rest is perhaps the most effective in enhancing renal and uterine blood flow. Evidence for its benefit is seen in the improvement in estriol excretion (see Chapter 13) when patients with signs of placental insufficiency are placed at bed rest.

It is not uncommon for blood pressure to return to the prepregnancy level with use of diuretic agents and low-salt diet alone. If the desired response is not achieved by this regimen, however, reserpine or hydralazine can be used. Such hypotensive agents are more particularly useful for the management of hypertensive crises and for the prevention of cerebrovascular accidents (see above).

Therapeutic abortion may be indicated for some patients with chronic hypertensive disease. Therefore, it is advisable that all such patients be evaluated as early as possible in the pregnancy. Cardiac, renal and retinal status should be studied. Termination is advisable if there is significant impairment of function, evidence of damage in any of these organ systems or indication of progression aggravated by the pregnancy.

If the decision is made to continue pregnancy, the patient should be examined biweekly during the first six months and weekly thereafter. At each visit, blood pressure, weight and urinary protein excretion are determined. Hospitalization should be advised for more thorough evaluation if there is any increase in hypertension, proteinuria or edema, or if there is evidence of impaired cardiac or renal function. Every effort should be made to prolong the gestation to 34 weeks or longer. However, sustained increases in systolic blood pressure of 30 mm. Hg or in diastolic of 15 mm. Hg, increase in proteinuria, progression of retinopathy, appearance of oliguria or azotemia are ominous signs. Such high risk pregnancies should be followed periodically with tests of fetal well-being as outlined in Chapter 13, including serial urinary excretion of estriol and ultrasound cephalometry.

When it is clear that the condition is progressive or that the fetus is in imminent jeopardy, the physician must decide whether it is better to deliver a premature infant who has some opportunity to survive or to accept the risk of death *in utero* by abruptio placentae.

It must be borne in mind that lowering the blood pressure through use of hypotensive agents does not necessarily have a favorable influence on the course of the disease. A false sense of security should not be derived from the relatively normal pressure levels that can be achieved. Increasing proteinuria and other manifestations of progression of the disease process must not be ignored under these circumstances.

The principles of terminating these pregnancies are essentially the same as those outlined for severe preeclampsia and eclampsia (see above). Appropriate delay to permit stabilization and optimization of the mother's condition is essential. Induction under favorable circumstances with close monitoring of mother and fetus is permissible; otherwise, cesarean section should be the method of choice. Following delivery, hypotensive drugs, barbiturates, sodium restriction and diuretic agents are used.

The prognosis is fairly good in that most patients with chronic hypertensive cardiovascular or renal disease survive and are delivered of living infants. There is no clear evidence that pregnancy accelerates the course of the hypertensive disease. There is a tendency for the clinical picture to exacerbate in more severe form with succeeding pregnancies. Therefore, such patients may with justification be advised against assuming the risks inherent in subsequent pregnancies. Sterilization is indicated for them.

REFERENCES

Altchek, A.: Electron microscopy of renal biopsies in toxemia of pregnancy. J.A.M.A. *175*:791, 1961.

Assali, N., Douglas, R. A., Jr., Baird, W. W., and Nicholson, D. B.: Measurement of uterine blood flow and uterine metabolism with the N₂O method in normotensive and toxemic pregnancies. Clin. Res. Proc. *2*:102, 1954.

Baird, D.: Combined Textbook of Obstetrics and Gynaecology for Students and Practitioners. Edinburgh, E. & S. Livingstone, 1969.

Bartholomew, R. A., Colvin, E. D., Grimes, W. H., Jr., Fish, J. S., Lester, W. M., and Galloway, W. H.: Criteria by which toxemia of pregnancy may be diagnosed from unlabelled formalin-fixed placentas. Amer. J. Obstet. Gynec. *82*:277, 1961.

Browne, J. C. M., and Veall, N.: The maternal placental blood flow in normotensive and hypertensive women. J. Obstet. Gynaec. Brit. Emp. *60*:141, 1953.

Carter, F. B., Cherny, W. B., and Crenshaw, C.: Serotonin studies in abnormal pregnancies: A preliminary report. Amer. J. Obstet. Gynec. *84*:913, 1962.

Chesley, L. C.: The renal excretion of sodium in women with preeclampsia. Clin. Obstet. Gynec. *1*:317, 1958.

Chesley, L. C., and Williams, L. O.: Renal glomerular and tubular function in relation to the hyperuricemia of pre-eclampsia and eclampsia. Amer. J. Obstet. Gynec. *50*:367, 1945.

Chesley, L. C., Annito, J. E., and Cosgrove, R. A.: Long-term follow-up study of eclamptic women. Amer. J. Obstet. Gynec. *101*:886, 1968.

Davies, M.: The Jerusalem toxemia study: III. Diet and toxemia in pregnancy. Washington, National Research Council, 1968.

Dieckmann, W. J.: The Toxemias of Pregnancy, ed. 2. St. Louis, C. V. Mosby Company, 1952.

Dieckmann, W. J., Smitter, R. C., and Pottinger, R. E.: Liver function studies in normal and toxemic pregnancy. Surg. Gynec. Obstet. *92*:588, 1951.

Eden, T. W.: Eclampsia: A commentary. J. Obstet. Gynaec. Brit. Emp. *29*:386, 1922.

Fahr, T.: Die Pathologisch Anatomischen Veränderungen der Niere und Leber bei der Eklampsie. *In* Hinselmann, H., ed.: Die Eklampsie. Bonn, F. Cohen, 1924.

Finnerty, F. A., Jr.: Toxemia of pregnancy as seen by an internist: An analysis of 1,081 patients. Ann. Intern. Med. *44*:358, 1956.

Freis, E. D., and Kenny, J. F.: Plasma volume, total circulating proteins and available fluid abnormalities in preeclampsia and eclampsia. J. Clin. Invest. *27*:283, 1948.

Friedberg, V.: Der Wasseraushalt und die Nierenfunction in der Normalen und Pathologischen Schwangerschaft. Leipzig, Georg Thieme Verlag, 1957.

Friedman, E. A.: Effect of blood pressure on perinatal mortality. *In* Vollman, R., ed.: International Workshop on the Clinical Criteria of Toxemia. Springfield, Ill., Charles C Thomas, in press.

Gray, M. J.: Use and abuse of thiazides in pregnancy. Clin. Obstet. Gynec. *11*:568, 1968.

Gray, M. J., and Plentl, A. A.: The variations of the sodium space and total exchangeable sodium during pregnancy. J. Clin. Invest. *33*:347, 1954.

Hughes, E. C., ed.: Obstetric-Gynecologic Terminology. Philadelphia, F. A. Davis Company, 1972.

Hunter, C. A., Jr., and Howard, W. F.: A pressor substance (hysteronin) occurring in toxemias. Amer. J. Obstet. Gynec. *79*:838, 1960.

Hutchinson, D. L., Plentl, A. A., and Taylor, H. C., Jr.: The total body water and the water turnover in pregnancy studied with deuterium oxide as isotopic tracer. J. Clin. Invest. *33*:235, 1954.

Hytten, F. E., and Leitch, I.: The Physiology of Human Pregnancy. Philadelphia, F. A. Davis Company, 1963.

Kraus, G. W., Marchese, J. R., and Yen, S. S. C.: Prophylactic use of hydrochlorothiazide in pregnancy. J.A.M.A. *198*:1150, 1966.

Kumar, D., Feltham, L. A. W., and Gornall, A. G.: Aldosterone excretion and tissue electrolytes in normal pregnancy and pre-eclampsia. Lancet *1*:541, 1959.

McCall, M. L.: Circulation of the brain in toxemia. Clin. Obstet. Gynec. *1*:333, 1958.

McCartney, C. P.: Pathological anatomy of acute hypertension of pregnancy. Circulation *30*(Suppl. 2):37, 1964.

McCartney, C. P., and Spargo, B.: An Evaluation of Renal Factors in the Toxemias of Pregnancy (in Edema). Philadelphia, W. B. Saunders Company, 1960.

McCartney, C. P., Pottinger, R. E., and Harrod, J. P., Jr.: Alterations in body composition during pregnancy. Amer. J. Obstet. Gynec. *77*:1038, 1959.

McKay, D. G.: Hematologic evidence of disseminated intravascular coagulation in eclampsia. Obstet. Gynec. Survey *27*:399, 1972.

McKay, D. G., Merrill, S. J., Weiner, A. E., Hertig, A. T., and Reid, D. C.: The pathologic anatomy of eclampsia, bilateral renal cortical necrosis, pituitary necrosis and other acute fatal complications of pregnancy and its possible relationship to the generalized Schwartzman phenomenon. Amer. J. Obstet. Gynec. *66*:507, 1953.

Page, E. W.: The Hypertensive Disorders of Pregnancy. Springfield, Ill., Charles C Thomas, 1953.

Palomaki, J. F., and Lindheimer, M. D.: Sodium depletion simulating deterioration in toxemic pregnancy. New Eng. J. Med. *282*:88, 1970.

Pollack, V. E., and Nettles, J. B.: The kidney in toxemia of pregnancy: A clinical and pathologic study based on renal biopsies. Medicine *39*:469, 1960.

Pritchard, J. A.: Use of magnesium ion in the management of eclamptogenic toxemia. Surg. Gynec. Obstet. *100*:131, 1955.

Robinson, M.: Salt in pregnancy. Lancet *1*:178, 1958.

Schmorl, G.: Pathologisch-Anatomische Untersuchungen über Puerperal-Eklampsie. Leipzig, F. C. W. Vogel, 1893.

Spargo, B., McCartney, C. P., and Winemiller, R.: Glomerular capillary endotheliosis in toxemia of pregnancy. Arch. Path. *68*:593, 1959.

Tillman, A. J. B.: The effect of normal and toxemic pregnancy on blood pressure. Amer. J. Obstet. Gynec. *70*:589, 1955.

Vollman, R., ed.: International Workshop on the Clinical Criteria of Toxemia. Springfield, Ill., Charles C Thomas, in press.

Chapter 37

Placenta Previa

Hemorrhage is a serious threat to the life of the pregnant woman. Its importance as a cause of maternal mortality cannot be overestimated. Most significantly, the majority, if not all, of deaths due to hemorrhage are probably preventable. Improved hospital facilities, advancement in technical skills, readily available bank blood and blood substitutes, measures to counteract shock, and the skilled use of anesthesia have created a milieu in which relative safety could exist for all obstetric patients. Unfortunately, standards of obstetric care are not uniform everywhere and patients are still lost because of inappropriate or inadequate measures taken to diagnose and treat bleeding in the third trimester of pregnancy. Among the leading causes of this serious problem are placenta previa and abruptio placentae. The latter will be dealt with in the next chapter.

The development of the placenta in part of or entirely in the lower uterine segment is *placenta previa*. Placenta previa is clinically divisible into two groups: *total placenta previa,* in which the internal os is entirely covered by the placenta (Figs. 261–263), and *partial placenta previa,* in which the internal os is only partially covered by the placenta (Fig. 263).

The term *low implantation of the placenta* is used when the placenta is located so that its edge can be palpated with a finger introduced through the cervix, but the placenta barely extends to the margin of the internal os (Fig. 263). The frequency of placenta previa is about 0.79 per cent (Davis and Campbell). Three of four women with placenta previa are multiparas.

ETIOLOGY

How the placenta comes to lie over the internal os is not fully understood. It is likely that the ovum must be implanted low in the uterus. The ovum burrows into the mucosa. As the ovum grows, the decidua vera and capsularis are carried across the narrow cervical slit and come to lie apposed to the vera of the opposite side, where fusion may or may not occur.

Hofmeier believed that many placenta previas are due to the development of the villi in the capsularis (Fig. 264). In general the nutritional power of the lower uterine segment is not great, and a placenta situated here spreads out to cover a large surface area, thus forming a *placenta membranacea*. In placenta previa not only is the placenta usually larger and thinner than normal but also, as emphasized by Macafee, there is frequently an eccentric insertion of the cord.

SYMPTOMS

Hemorrhage is the first and most constant symptom. It occurs in the last three months of pregnancy, most frequently in the eighth. Bleeding may actually begin much earlier, even before the twenty-eighth week. The patient may see silent vaginal bleeding with no forewarning; she may on awakening find a pool of blood, or she may notice fluid and clotted blood in the toilet bowl. A painless, apparently causeless, vaginal hemorrhage in the third trimester is often due to placenta previa,

415

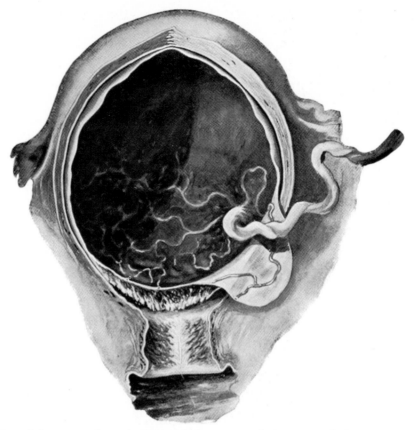

Figure 261 Frontal dissection of gravid uterus with fetus removed, showing total placenta previa; the placenta is implanted centrally over a partially dilated internal cervical os.

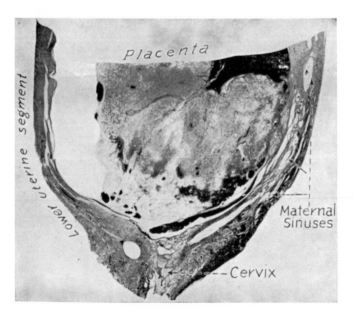

Figure 262 A section through the lower uterine segment and cervix in total placenta previa. Note the pathologic lower uterine segment. Extensive vascularization and increased thickness of the uterine wall are the result of the placental site in this abnormal locality. (Courtesy of M. E. Davis and R. Rubin.)

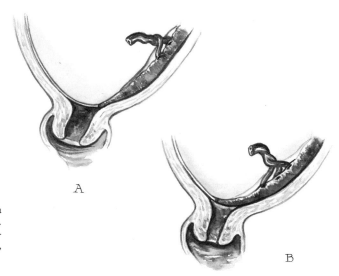

Figure 263 Different types of placenta previa. *A*, Low implantation of placenta. *B*, Partial placenta previa. *C*, Total placenta previa. (Courtesy of Bartholomew, R. A., et al.: Obstet. Gynec. *1*:41, 1953.)

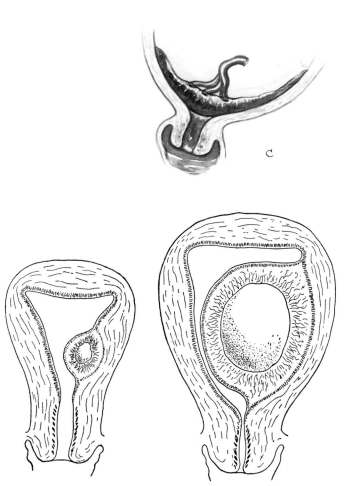

Figure 264 Diagrammatic representation of the probable mechanism by which placenta previa develops. The ovum implants in the lower segment and villi develop and persist in the decidua capsularis overlying the internal os. (After Hofmeier, M.: Störungen der Schwangerschaft durch vorzeitige Lösung der Placenta bei normalen Sitz. *In* von Winckel, F.: Handbuch der Geburtshülfe. Wiesbaden, J. F. Bergmann, 1904.)

but it is far from pathognomonic. The first hemorrhage may vary from a few drops to a profuse flooding; usually, the initial loss is a few ounces. Each succeeding hemorrhage is greater and, unless treated, anemia develops. An important sign is constant seepage of bloodstained serum, indicating that a large clot is forming in the lower uterine segment and vagina.

In total placenta previa the bleeding usually occurs earlier than in partial placenta previa and is more profuse. Partial placenta previa may not cause hemorrhage until labor begins or even toward the end of the first stage.

During the painless uterine contractions of pregnancy, the lower edge of the placenta is likely to be separated from the wall of the uterus, opening the placental sinuses and allowing blood to escape.

Bender found that 10 per cent of 444 multiparas with placenta previa had had a previous lower segment cesarean section. This suggests that uterine scars increase the chance of placenta previa in subsequent pregnancies threefold.

Placenta previa affects the course of pregnancy, labor and the puerperium. Many patients with placenta previa have had a history of threatened abortion in the early months. Both premature rupture of the membranes and premature labor are common.

Placenta previa causes malpositions, malpresentations and often delayed engagement. Air embolism is more common than usual because the uterine sinuses are exposed to the external air. Rupture of the uterus is frequent because the musculature is weakened by the ingrowth of the placenta and the presence of blood sinuses (Fig. 262).

Postpartum hemorrhage is frequent because the lower part of the uterine wall is thin and weak; the muscles contract tardily and imperfectly close the large venous sinuses at the placental site.

In the puerperium, placenta previa also causes trouble. Pieces of placenta may adhere and become infected because of the close proximity of the placental site to the vagina and cervix; subinvolution occurs and profound anemia results and further reduces resistance to infection.

DIAGNOSIS

Although an unexplained uterine hemorrhage in the third trimester is highly suggestive of placenta previa, the diagnosis must ultimately be verified by vaginal examination, ultrasonography, cystography, isotope placentography or arteriography.

When a vaginal examination is made in suspected placenta previa, the patient must be in the operating room with everything held in readiness for any treatment. The reason for this is that serious bleeding may result from such an examination even when performed gently. Because this examination must be made in a place where there are aseptic preparations for immediate termination of the pregnancy and for the treatment and the control of bleeding, it should be a universal rule to *hospitalize all pregnant women who bleed vaginally.* Vaginal examinations for bleeding should never be undertaken outside the hospital. Rectal examinations are of no value at all, in or out of the hospital, and should not be done if placenta previa is suspected. Profuse hemorrhage may result.

The patient should be transported to the hospital by ambulance at once. On arrival in the hospital, the patient's blood should immediately be typed, the Rh factor determined, and adequate amounts of blood cross-matched and made available. At least 1000 ml. of matched blood should be on hand.

In the differential diagnosis of placenta previa, bleeding from varicose veins of the vulva or vagina, cervical polyp, hemorrhoids, carcinoma of the cervix and hematuria are easily excluded, but rupture of the uterus, advanced ectopic gestation, abruptio placentae, bleeding from a vessel passing over the external os from a velamentous insertion of the cord (vasa previa) and placenta circumvallata require more careful study.

Placenta previa is the cause of bleeding near term in only about one-third of such hemorrhages. Nevertheless, all patients who present with vaginal bleeding in the third trimester should be considered to have placenta previa until it has been disproved.

Placentography

The objective of placentography is to locate the placenta in the course of conservative expectant management. If placenta previa can be excluded, a prolonged hospital stay can be avoided. The aim is to accomplish this accurately and with minimal hazard. Techniques include radiographic, radioisotopic, ultrasonographic and thermographic procedures.

Radiographic methods encompass soft-tissue exposures, use of contrast medium in bladder, rectum or amniotic fluid, and aortography. Ude et al. outlined the soft-tissue space between the fetal skull and bladder by instilling sodium iodide solution into the bladder. One injects 40 ml. of a 12.5 per cent aqueous solution of sodium iodide into the empty bladder and exposes an anteroposterior film centered on the midportion and lower part of the abdomen (Figs. 265 and 266).

Soft-tissue placentography, achieved by use of an aluminum wedge filter, is used widely. By the soft-tissue x-ray technique, Brown and Dippel clearly visualized the placenta in 90 per cent of cases. The placental implantations were almost equally divided between the anterior and the posterior walls of the corpus except with low insertions. Among these, there were about eight times as many placentas found on the anterior as on the posterior wall of the lower uterine segment. Only 12 per cent of women with vaginal bleeding were discovered roentgenographically to have true placenta previa. However, Moir pointed out that serious errors of interpretation are likely when soft-tissue placentography is used.

Another roentgen sign described by Ball and Golden is that a fetal head will normally dip into the pelvic inlet and occupy the midcoronal and midsagittal planes of the superior strait when the mother is standing. This sign rules out placenta previa but is applicable only with a single fetus in cephalic presentation.

Hartley advises a search for calcification

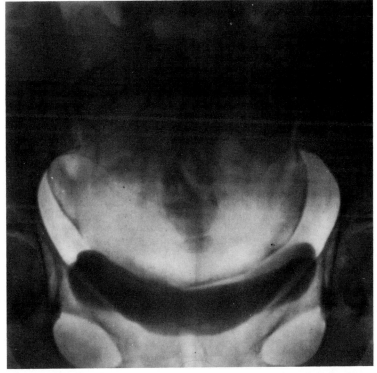

Figure 265 Cystogram of normally implanted placenta. The fetal head is directly above the bladder indicating the absence of forelying placenta. Compare with Figure 266. (Courtesy of J. Jarcho.)

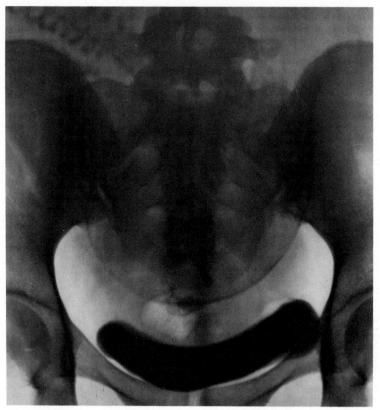

Figure 266   Cystogram of patient with total placenta previa. The fetal head is considerably above the bladder which was filled with sodium iodide solution. The placenta lies between the head and bladder. (Courtesy of J. Jarcho.)

in localizing the placenta. Calcification was demonstrated in 40 per cent of 80 cases. The technique uses low kilovoltage x-ray without filters.

Another diagnostic procedure for the detection of placenta previa is *arteriography*, first reported by Coutts et al. It is accomplished by the injection of contrast medium into the descending aorta either by translumbar approach or via a catheter in the femoral artery. Borell et al. used arteriography, improved by applying external pressure to the femoral arteries to occlude outflow, in 160 cases of placenta previa. They found that this procedure defines the placental site irrespective of the type of presentation, length of pregnancy or the presence of hydramnios. Arteriographic diagnosis was correct in 97 per cent of their cases.

Arteriography, although very accurate, carries significant risks to the patient: The injected artery may be injured; hematomas may form at the site; arterial spasm may occur in both femoral and uterine vessels;

tetanic uterine contractions have been reported occasionally as a consequence; premature labor may ensue; radiation dosage is relatively high. Where less hazardous techniques, such as ultrasonography, are available, such risks must be considered unacceptable.

Arteriography should not be done during uterine contractions because contractions may prevent satisfactory filling of the intervillous space and result in incorrect interpretation. Demonstration of both the ovarian and uterine arteries is of utmost importance when arteriography is done for placenta previa because the ovarian arteries may provide much of the uterine blood supply during pregnancy.

Radioisotopic methods are popular today. They entail intravenous injection of a radioactive isotope which is distributed uniformly in the maternal circulation. The amount of blood in a given organ will affect its distribution. A highly vascular structure such as the placental bed will be detectable by means of an external counter or an autoscan device as an area in which radioactivity is concentrated. Albumin is the most convenient carrier material used for labeling with an isotope. Although it does not cross the placenta to any significant degree, free isotope does readily. Free isotope is usually present in albumin preparations and more is freed by metabolic degradation. Iodine isotopes (I^{131}, I^{125} and, less availably, I^{132}) are used extensively as tracers. Technetium (Tc^{99m}) is especially useful because of its short half-life of six hours and good scanning properties. Red cells labeled with chromium (Cr^{51}) have also been used effectively for placental localization.

Weinberg et al. report that isotope placentography is highly accurate in localization of the placental site. Conditions such as prematurity, malpresentation, hydramnios, multiple pregnancy and pelvic tumors, which may lead to error or difficulties in roentgen placentography, do not affect isotope placentography. No operative procedures, such as are used in retrograde femoral arteriography, are necessary.

Whole body and gonadal radiation to mother and fetus is minimal in comparison to that received by the exposure needed for roentgen placentography. With a thyroid blocking agent, such as iodine, used preceding injection of isotopically labeled iodinated albumin (RISA), the absorbed dose delivered to the fetal thyroid will be well within the safe range listed by the Federal Radiation Council and constitutes about one per cent of the dose delivered by conventional roentgenographic techniques. Localization of the placental site in suspected placenta previa is often of such obstetric importance that the exposure of the fetus to some radiation is justified.

In localities where B-scan *ultrasonography* is available (see Chapter 13), the placenta can be localized with a fair degree of accuracy, and with no radiation hazard at all. This technique has much to recommend it in diagnosing placenta previa. Similarly, *thermography* is safe and probably just as reliable (but this is yet to be verified). It depends on the detection of areas of relative warmth over highly vascularized organs. Special facilities are needed to permit sensitive equipment to detect minute temperature changes based

in infrared emanations. These are plotted to yield a graphic display showing the concentrated sites of heat. The kind of sophisticated display equipment and special room needed for this study make it unlikely to become applicable everywhere.

PROGNOSIS

Maternal death rates as high as 1.5 per cent have been reported with placenta previa (Paalman and Hunt). Total placenta previa is more dangerous than the partial type.

Most deaths from placenta previa, in order of frequency, result from hemorrhage, infection, traumatic rupture of the uterus and air embolism. Usually, death occurs because an injury was inflicted during delivery. Infection is invited by the proximity of the susceptible placental site to the field of operation and because many hasty procedures are carried out. Rupture of the uterus is usually the result of excessively vigorous manipulations by the physician. Air embolism is rare. Thrombophlebitis is a common complication, occurring in about five per cent.

Fetuses fare poorly. They die from asphyxia secondary to hemorrhage (about 10 per cent of the blood lost vaginally is fetal in origin) or from dislocation, tearing or compression of the placenta. Prematurity is common. Many fetuses have developed anomalously.

PREVENTION

The principles of good antepartum care ensure that any medical disorders that place the patient at risk, either as a result of hemorrhage or because of a tendency toward hemorrhage, will be uncovered. Medical and obstetric diseases and bleeding tendencies are of obvious importance. Detecting and correcting anemia, with particular attention to those patients unresponsive to treatment, so as to provide adequate reserves in the event of hemorrhage, is equally noteworthy.

Perhaps the most meaningful measure to prevent the serious consequences of hemorrhage involves informing the patient what she should do in the event vaginal bleeding occurs. Under these circumstances, she should be told to notify her physician and to proceed immediately to the hospital by ambulance. She should be clearly advised as to the significance of bleeding, whether or not it is associated with pain and regardless of amount. Procrastination must be avoided.

TREATMENT

The factors that will determine when definitive diagnosis must be made and aggressive action taken include (1) the amount of bleeding because our prime goal in therapy is to arrest further blood loss before the mother's life is threatened; (2) the patient's cardiovascular and coagulation status; (3) the maturity of the fetus, our secondary goal being to attempt to salvage the fetus, if possible; and (4) whether or not the fetus is alive. The proper approach to management becomes clear once a correct diagnosis has been established. However, diagnostic evaluation, particularly by means of vaginal examination, must frequently be postponed. The decision to proceed must balance the benefits of postponement (usually to allow the fetus to mature further) against the dangers of delay (in terms of maternal risk from hemorrhage).

Every woman with profuse bleeding should be sent to a hospital in an ambulance without any internal examination or packing. Disturbing the placental site by means of rectal or vaginal examination or by anachronistic vaginal packing—a technique which can only be condemned in this situation—may produce torrential hemorrhage. When vaginal examination is withheld, maternal survival improves (Macafee; Johnson). It is important to reemphasize that a rectal examination should never be done in a patient who bleeds during pregnancy.

Immediate Evaluation

When first seen, patients should be assigned to one of two groups, namely, those few with profuse bleeding or shock and those with minimal or moderate bleeding. Patients who are bleeding heavily with increasing pulse rate and falling blood pressure present a serious problem that must be handled expeditiously and expertly. Although these cases are in the minority, immediate action is necessary to control further blood loss, thereby averting catastrophe.

Supportive measures for blood replacement, blood volume expansion, maintenance of blood pressure, cardiac output and tissue perfusion, as well as ventilation and oxygen exchange, must be instituted promptly. The indicated surgical procedures must be undertaken simultaneously. Under these exigent circumstances, only the most cursory attempts to establish diagnosis need be made by means of quick vaginal examination to ensure that the bleeding originates from within the uterus.

We should be mindful that only a small proportion of patients presenting with bleeding will require such emergency measures. The great majority can be evaluated carefully and handled with deliberation. Every patient, nevertheless, should be observed and handled as if she were about to begin to bleed profusely. Thus, suitably cross-matched blood should be made available and an intravenous infusion begun with a large bore needle to permit immediate access to a vein should it become necessary for purposes of transfusion.

Besides blood typing and cross-matching, it is important to obtain hemoglobin or hematocrit, urine analysis, bleeding and clotting time and a fibrinogen level (or clot observation, if unavailable). The urinary output should be recorded on a periodic basis (hourly, if blood loss is more than minimal) as a guide to the adequacy of renal perfusion. A more delicate index of cardiovascular instability is the central venous pressure catheter, which provides ongoing observations and can be used to indicate impending shock. During replacement it can serve to demonstrate approaching congestive failure.

Physical examination initially must include a survey of vital signs, checked repeatedly; the condition of the abdomen, particularly with reference to pain; guarding, tenderness and rebound should be noted. The uterus should be evaluated for size, contour, irritability, relaxation, fetal presentation and heart tones. Finding a malpresentation, an unengaged fetal presenting part or a placental souffle just above the symphysis pubis may be particularly significant.

Vaginal examination should be deferred until such time as a definitive diagnosis is to be made. No vaginal examination should ever be done until compatible blood is on hand, the clotting situation has been evaluated and all preparations have been made for both abdominal and pelvic surgery ("double setup"), including anesthesia, instrument trays and personnel ready to proceed without a moment's delay.

Although intracervical examination is contraindicated, it is wise to ascertain, by means of gentle speculum examination under a good light, the presence or absence of some vaginal or cervical condition that might be causing the bleeding. Cervical polyp, ruptured vaginal varix, laceration, chemical burn, erosion and cancer may be detected in this manner. Furthermore, digital palpation of the lower uterine segment, performed extracervically with the presenting fetal part impressed into the pelvis from above, may yield evidence supporting a tentative diagnosis of placenta previa by the palpation of a boggy interposed mass. Failure of the fetal presenting part to enter the pelvis also tends to authenticate the suspicion of placenta previa. On the other hand, if one is able to palpate the fetal parts readily in the lower uterine segment through the vaginal fornices in a full circle around the cervix, the diagnosis becomes tenuous.

Under most circumstances, expectant management is in order. The patient is put at rest and observed for progression or recurrence of bleeding. While awaiting stabilization or progression, certain diagnostic aids to help rule out placenta previa are available (see above).

The marked improvement in fetal survival from placenta previa in recent decades has been based almost exclusively on the principle of expectancy in vogue. If bleeding is not excessive and labor has not begun, it is clearly preferable to institute a program of observation and support, awaiting the onset either of another episode of hemorrhage or of labor. Proceeding to definitive examination to establish diagnosis will precipitate hemorrhage, thereby forcing intervention prematurely. The infant born under these circumstances has less opportunity to survive than one that has been permitted to mature further. It should be stressed, nevertheless, that this conservative approach is justified in the interest of the fetus only if maternal risks are minimized. Accordingly, this program includes detailed attention to patient care, especially with regard to evaluation of blood loss, replacement as necessary and adequacy and availability of all necessary facilities. If, while awaiting viability, profuse hemorrhage should occur, intervention becomes essential.

Active Treatment

The basic active approach to patients who have documented placenta previa is delivery by cesarean section. This applies to those with total placenta previa as well as to those with partial placenta previa. Only rarely is it feasible and safe to permit a patient with partial placenta previa to labor with the presenting fetal part tamponading the bleeding maternal uterine vessels. This approach should perhaps be reserved for the occasional multipara in active labor with negligible or no bleeding whose abnormal placental insertion is discovered fortuitously. Rupture of the membranes under these circumstances is usually quite effective. In the presence of active bleeding, however, unless labor is well advanced, abdominal delivery is preferable. Potentially dangerous and outmoded techniques to effect vaginal delivery, including bags, version and scalp traction, carry major risks to the mother and, therefore, are best avoided.

Definitive digital exploration within the cervix should be undertaken immediately prior to cesarean section, with everything in readiness, as previously stated. Under sterile conditions, the internal os is palpated for the characteristic spongy, gritty placenta. If it is not encountered, the fingers are advanced to palpate the lower uterine segment. Once the placenta is palpated, one must proceed immediately to perform the indicated cesarean section. The decision will usually be obvious, since manipulation may stimulate marked hemorrhage. Encountering this, one is impressed with the need for and the benefits of the "double setup" preparation previously described and how important it is that informal examinations never be done.

The choice of operative technique (that is, classic versus low cervical segment cesarean section) is debatable. Proponents of the classic section voice objection to an incision through the placental site because it increases fetal blood loss (it has been estimated that about 10 per cent of blood lost vaginally is fetal in origin). Those advocating the low cervical procedure purport advantage in having access to the placental site for purposes of providing hemostasis by means of well-placed sutures. In general, the classic operation is perhaps preferable, particularly since the lower segment is rarely thinned out well, tends to be rather vascular and is easily traumatized. Moreover, the fetus may be relatively inaccessible in an abnormal presentation high in the uterus.

Some obstetricians clamp the umbilical cord immediately after incising the placenta to prevent loss of blood from the fetus. However, the danger of initiating respiration of the fetus before an airway can be established by clamping the cord is greater than the loss of blood, which can nearly always be controlled by rapid delivery.

Wiener called attention to severe anemia of the newborn caused by unrecognized loss of blood from the fetal circulation via the placenta. Wickster emphasized the role of hemorrhagic shock in the death of the newborn associated, in placenta previa and abruptio placentae, with asphyxia, interference with nutrition and excretion, toxicity and prematurity and also with anemia from rupture of the capillaries in the cotyledons. Every infant born of a patient with placenta previa or abruptio placentae should have repeated hematocrit determinations. When anemia and shock are severe, appropriate replacement of compatible whole blood by transfusion is essential.

Novak showed that occult or manifest fetal bleeding during delivery is not rare. Among 879 cesarean sections there were 28 placentas which were cut or torn during operation; 11 of the babies had hemorrhagic shock. Some died at once; the mild shock state in others was aggravated if proper transfusion therapy was not given. In 643 cases of placenta previa 66 babies were anemic and 41 died before the mothers left the hospital. Most of these babies were premature.

In selected cases of partial placenta previa, where conditions are particularly favorable, one may proceed to rupture the membranes and permit the fetal head to descend and compress the bleeding edge of the placenta. This is excellent treatment in some instances of partial placenta previa if the bleeding ceases or is considerably reduced. As the cervix dilates after labor has begun, bleeding may recur or be aggravated, but it is usually not profuse enough to be alarming. Transfusion may be necessary. In most of these patients, spontaneous delivery may be permitted or outlet forceps may be used after the head has descended to the perineum.

For rupturing the membranes a small portion of membrane should be grasped with long dressing forceps or Allis forceps. This is safer than pushing the membranes upward to rupture them. This practice may lift the placental edge from its attachment to the uterine wall.

In the course of labor, the fetal heart tones must be carefully noted. The placental reserve is diminished by the tamponade of the fetal head. Fetal asphyxia may occur and be demonstrated by means of fetal heart rate monitoring (see Chapter 13). If hypoxic changes are encountered, delivery should be expedited. However, the fetus cannot be extracted vaginally until the cervix is fully dilated. If delivery must be effected before the cervix is sufficiently dilated, it is preferable to proceed with cesarean section.

One must be wary of attempting to extract the fetus through an incompletely dilated cervix. Laceration of the highly vascularized cervix is one of the most formidable accidents the physician can encounter. Use of oxytocin should be avoided and the slowest possible delivery must be practiced. If the head is restrained by a tight cervix, force must not be used to extract it.

With little or no hemorrhage there is no

reason to hurry. The patient will recover from the shock of the hemorrhage provided the lost blood is promptly and adequately replaced. While waiting for the cervix to dilate, the time should be employed in supplying the woman with sufficient blood, fluids and electrolytes as necessary, and preparing for the delivery. Everything must be ready and rehearsed beforehand so that, when the delivery occurs, there is no delay. Provision should be made for combating hemorrhage and for resuscitating the child.

Many women have died during the third stage after being skillfully carried through labor and vaginal delivery. It is necessary to conserve blood. The child is handed to an assistant as soon as it is delivered. The physician should devote all of his attention to the mother. The placenta is immediately removed manually, and 0.2 mg. of ergonovine is given intravenously. As soon

as the placenta is removed, the uterus usually contracts strongly and bleeding should cease. Sometimes the lower uterine segment remains atonic and bleeding from the placental site becomes profuse. Bleeding occurs from open sinuses in the lower uterine segment because the sinuses were uncovered when the placenta separated and remain open because of inefficient contraction.

No time should be wasted on uncertain methods of hemostasis. Packing the uterus, recommended by many in these circumstances, may be ineffectual and wasteful of time, and may contribute to the delay in providing adequate hemostasis. The uterus is held securely in forced anteflexion or the entire corpus is pushed up so as to stretch the uterine arteries (see Chapter 66). If hemorrhage persists or recurs, internal iliac ligation should be done.

REFERENCES

Ball, R. P., and Golden, R.: Roentgenologic sign for detection of placenta previa. Amer. J. Obstet. Gynec. *42*:530, 1941.

Bender, S.: Placenta previa and previous lower segment cesarean section. Surg. Gynec. Obstet. 98:625, 1954.

Borell, U., Fernström, I., and Ohlson, L.: Diagnostic value of arteriography in cases of placenta previa. Amer. J. Obstet. Gynec. 86:535, 1963.

Brown, W. H., and Dippel, A. L.: Uses and limitations of soft tissue roentgenography in placenta praevia and in certain other obstetrical conditions. Bull. Johns Hopkins Hosp. 66:90, 1940.

Coutts, W. E., Opazo, L., Banderas Bianchi, T., and Sanhueza Donoso, O.: Abdominal circulation during late pregnancy as shown in aortograms. Amer. J. Obstet. Gynec. 29:566, 1935.

Davis, M. E., and Campbell, A.: The management of placenta praevia in the Chicago Lying-in Hospital. Surg. Gynec. Obstet. 83:777, 1946.

Davis, M. E., and Rubin, R.: DeLee's Obstetrics for Nurses, ed. 18. Philadelphia, W. B. Saunders Company, 1966.

Hartley, J. B.: Incidence and significance of placental calcification. Brit. J. Radiol. 27:365, 1954.

Hofmeier, M.: Störungen der Schwangerschaft durch vorzeitige Lösung der Placenta bei normalen Sitz. *In* von Winckel, F.: Handbuch der Geburtshülfe. Wiesbaden, J. F. Bergmann, 1904.

Johnson, H. W.: The conservative management of some varieties of placenta previa. Amer. J. Obstet. Gynec. 50:248, 1945.

Macafee, C. H. G.: Placenta praevia: Study of 174 cases. J. Obstet. Gynaec. Brit. Emp. 52:313, 1945.

Moir, J. C.: Fallacies in soft tissue placentography. Amer. J. Obstet. Gynec. 47:198, 1944.

Moir, J. C., and Myerscough, R. P.: Munro Kerr's Operative Obstetrics, ed. 8. London, Ballière, Tindall & Cox, 1971.

Novak, R.: Posthemorrhagic shock in newborns during labor and after delivery. Acta Med. Iugosl. 7:280, 1953.

Paalman, R. J., and Hunt, A. B.: The selective management of placenta previa. Amer. J. Obstet. Gynec. 57:900, 1949.

Ude, W. H., Weum, T. W., and Urner, J. A.: Roentgenologic diagnosis of placenta praevia: Report of case. Amer. J. Roentgen. *31*:230, 1934.

Weinberg, A., Shapiro, G., and Bruhn, D. C.: Isotopic placentography: An evaluation of its accuracy and safety. Amer. J. Obstet. Gynec. 87:203, 1963.

Wickster, G. Z.: Posthemorrhagic shock in the newborn caused by occult placental hemorrhage. Amer. J. Obstet. Gynec. 63:524, 1952.

Wiener, A. S.: Diagnosis and treatment of anemia of the newborn caused by occult placental hemorrhage. Amer. J. Obstet. Gynec. 56:717, 1948.

Chapter 38

Abruptio Placentae

Abruptio placentae or premature separation of the normally implanted placenta may represent a catastrophic complication of pregnancy for both mother and fetus. The term *accidental hemorrhage* is still used by British authors to designate premature separation of the normally implanted placenta, whereas the term *unavoidable hemorrhage,* seldom used, means placenta previa. *Abruptio placentae* was suggested by DeLee for premature separation of the placenta and Holmes suggested *ablatio placentae,* both of which are today used interchangeably.

Clinically, it is usually easy to differentiate between placenta previa and abruptio placentae, but many times abruptio placentae is due to detachment low in the uterus. Indeed, abruption of a placenta previa may occur and probably takes place to some extent in nearly all cases of placenta previa with bleeding. Hence, the definition of abruptio placentae as "separation of a normally implanted placenta" is not always entirely correct, but in clinical practice, we refer specifically to separation of the placenta that is not implanted in the lower segment.

Abruptio placentae, including the mildest forms, occurs more often than is generally believed. Complete separation of the placenta is rare, occurring probably less often than once in 500 gestations. Major degrees of abruption are encountered in frequencies ranging from 1:139 to 1:85.

ETIOLOGY

The causes are largely unknown. Although recent evidence indicates the possibility that folic acid deficiency may produce this condition, there is neither confirmation of this relationship nor verification that the expected corollary is true, namely, that administering folic acid will prevent this disorder. The frequent coassociation of hypertensive states of pregnancy is also to be noted, although here, too, causal relationships are difficult to establish.

The association of preeclampsia with placental, retroplacental and myometrial hemorrhages is frequent. In one series of patients with abruptio placentae 69 per cent had preeclampsia (Dieckmann). Sexton et al. found that 42 per cent had a hypertensive state and, among 3654 women having some degree of albuminuria and/or hypertension, abruptio placentae occurred in one in 18.3. As the severity of the preeclampsia increases so does the chance of abruptio placentae.

The essential lesion of the placental site, apparently responsible for the separation, was first described by Williams and reemphasized by Hertig as an acute, degenerative arteriolitis. In the early stages a collection of phagocytes appears beneath the intima of the spiral arterioles. This phase is followed by a fibrinoid degeneration of the media which is in turn superseded by a fibroblastic proliferation of the intima that almost obliterates the lumen. Since the branches of the spiral arterioles nourish the endometrium and supply the placenta with blood, this leads to necrosis of the decidua beneath the placenta. Hemorrhage follows and the placenta becomes detached.

The time when abruptio placentae occurs differs in single and twin pregnancies. In singleton pregnancies, about two-thirds occur before the onset of labor; in multiple births, the onset is usually during the second stage of labor, when the first twin is delivered or soon afterward. The cause in twin gestations is a mechanical one due to the shearing effects that result from the sudden reduction in the uterine volume as the first baby is born and the uterus contracts. In single pregnancies the frequency of abruptio placentae during the second stage is only four to five per cent.

Trauma may cause a separation of the placenta. A hemorrhage having once begun may wend its way between the layers of decidua and complete the abruption. A jar, coitus, a blow or kick on the abdomen and severe coughing have been given as causes, although documented cases are rare (Davis and McGee).

During labor, several accidents may cause detachment of the placenta: sudden emptying of a large hydramnios; shearing of the placenta that sometimes follows the delivery of the first twin; manual manipulation during version; or traction on the placenta by a cord that is actually or relatively too short.

Experimental abruptio placentae was produced by Howard and Goodson in dogs by ligation of the left ovarian vein and the vena cava below the renal veins. Nesbitt et al. did the same in dogs by ligating the inferior vena cava just below the renal veins, but above the right ovarian veins. Examination revealed a characteristic picture of acute tubular degeneration in the maternal kidneys. These experiments would seem to incriminate elevated venous pressure as one possible factor in the pathogenesis of placental abruption. When this pressure is reduced by autonomic blockade, the chain of pathologic events, both local and systemic, is favorably modified. Mengert et al. caused abruptio placentae in two women near term during cesarean hysterectomy by the simple expedient of digital compression of the vena cava below the renal veins for five minutes.

PATHOLOGY

Separation of the placenta is always accompanied by profuse hemorrhage unless the fetus has been dead long enough for

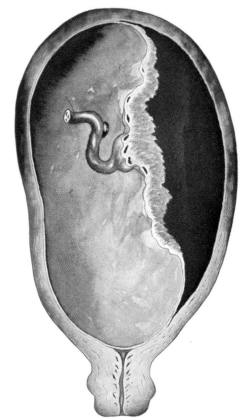

Figure 267   Abruptio placentae showing internal or concealed hemorrhage with formation of a large retroplacental hematoma sequestrated by the persisting attachment of the membranes to the uterine wall. The fetus has been removed.

thrombosis to have occurred in the uterine sinuses. The blood escapes under the decidua basalis and pursues one of four courses. First (Fig. 267), and most rarely, it may distend the uterine wall toward the abdominal cavity and encroach on the cavity of the conceptus, the placental edges remaining attached to the uterus. Second, it may dissect all the membranes around it, severing almost all the connections of the conceptus to the uterine wall. Third, it may break into the amniotic fluid. Fourth, it may seek a direct passage outward from the edge of the placenta under the membranes through the cervix into the vagina (Fig. 268). The first three types result in *concealed hemorrhage* and usually are the most serious. In all instances the blood may not reach the vagina because it is blocked by the fetal head or a firm clot in

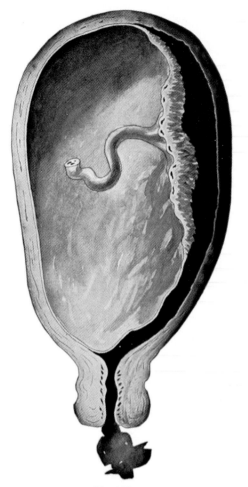

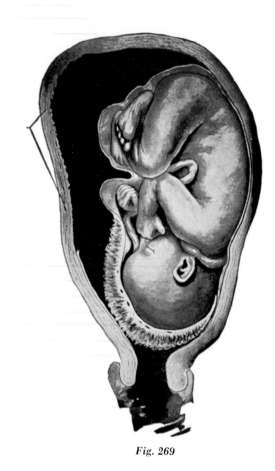

Fig. 269

Fig. 268

Figure 268   Abruptio placentae with combined internal and external hemorrhage, illustrating dissection of some of the retroplacental blood extraovularly until it reaches the cervix and escapes into the vagina.

Figure 269   Prolapse of the placenta in association with total separation of the placenta accompanying its dislocation from its original site in the upper uterine segment.

the cervix. The uterus may be so im-mensely distended by the blood that a fatal, exsanguinating intrauterine hemorrhage may occur without any blood appearing externally.

Rarely, the placenta drops from its site and lies over the internal os, a condition called *prolapse of the placenta* (Fig. 269). Most of these cases probably represent placenta previa, but true prolapse of the placenta can occur in association with abruptio placentae. This complication occurs most frequently in multiparas and in premature labor.

In most patients, external hemorrhage follows the internal so that, in general, the bleeding in abruptio placentae is first in-ternal or concealed and then combined, external and internal. The mildest cases are, fortunately, the most common. They are usually associated with purely external hemorrhages. Blood may also escape into the peritoneal cavity through the tubes.

Without doubt, small hemorrhages under the placenta may often occur during the later weeks of pregnancy and become organized without producing alarming symptoms. They can be disclosed from ev-idence on the delivered placenta; hard and almost completely fibrinous clots, ad-herent to or incorporated in the mem-branes or decidua, are found. The placenta in abruptio placentae may show evidences of hemorrhages or red infarcts of varying

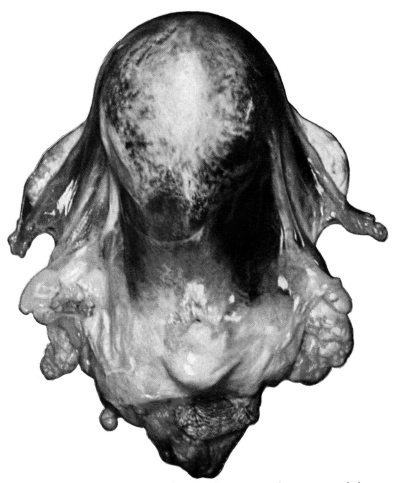

Figure 270   Anterior view of gross specimen of a Couvelaire uterus showing typical characteristics of utero-placental apoplexy. Note the purple discoloration of the ecchymotic areas extending over the uterine corpus and the broad ligaments, especially on the left side where blood has extensively infiltrated the myometrium and nearby connective areolar tissue.

degrees of organization; it may be torn or compressed by blood clots or it may show only a large retroplacental hematoma.

Couvelaire called attention to a special condition, which he called *apoplexie uteroplacentaire*. He likened the appearance of the uterus to an ovarian cyst with a twisted pedicle, because the uterus has a purplish, coppery color (Fig. 270). The uterine muscle is degenerated and infiltrated with blood, and various sized petechiae are found under the peritoneum covering the uterus and extending into the broad ligaments and culdesac. The most profuse bleeding in the uterine wall occurs near the placental site, but most of the muscular dissociation is in the middle and outer muscular layers. The serosa over the uterus may split in places and thus allow blood to escape into the abdominal cavity. The bloody extravasations between the muscle fibers disrupt their integrity and explain the atony of such uteri post partum.

SYMPTOMS

During pregnancy, slight, repeated hemorrhages from the uterus indicate the likelihood that there is some disturbance of placentation. The coassociation with evidence of preeclampsia is very suggestive of this complication.

Characteristically, the patient with abruptio placentae presents with vaginal bleeding and a painful, tender uterus that is quite irritable. In the mild varieties, the patient's cardiovascular status is good, the fetus presents no evidence of distress, and there is no coagulation defect. The moderately severe variety may exhibit uterine tetany and the fetus may or may not be dead; the patient is not in shock and the coagulation defect, if any, is minimal. The most severe form presents with uterine tetany of a boardlike quality, maternal shock, fetal death and a coagulation defect due to fibrinogen depletion. The severity of the disorder will dictate the program of management, modified according to the presence of toxemia, anemia and continuing hemorrhage.

Fortunately, most patients with abruptio placentae present with the mildest form and tend to be unrecognized as such until they deliver. At this time, a depressed organized scar on the maternal surface of the placenta indicates the site of separation which may have occurred weeks or months earlier. The patient may have exhibited a picture of uterine pain, irritability, focal uterine tenderness and vaginal bleeding, all of which subsided under expectant observation. Clearly, this patient and her fetus would have been unnecessarily jeopardized by a more aggressive attack.

The severity of the symptoms depends on the blood loss and shock. These vary widely. In severe cases, the usual first symptom is sudden, severe pain in the abdomen, often at the site of the placenta, sometimes described as knifelike or tearing, and later a dull tense ache, interrupted by colicky pains. Occasionally, nausea or vomiting occurs. Acute anemia and shock supervene. The blood pressure varies with the degree of shock and may be paradoxically high with complicating toxemia.

Soon blood or serum expressed from the intrauterine clots appears externally, but its amount is entirely disproportionate to the gravity of the symptoms. Examination of the abdomen will show that the uterus is larger than that which would correspond to the duration of the pregnancy. It enlarges every hour in response to enlarging collection of retroplacental blood. It often is boardlike in consistency, making it impossible to outline the fetus. A ligneous

consistency of the uterus is observed in more than 60 per cent of patients. Exceptionally, the uterus is relaxed and dilated. Of great diagnostic importance is a tender uterus. The patient may report that the fetus is no longer felt, but that it moved violently at the onset of severe pains. Very seldom can the fetal heart be heard in severe abruptio placentae.

Labor is usually sudden in onset and rapid in progression. The contractions of the uterus are strong and may be superimposed on an already hypertonically or tetanically contracted uterus. This event can be demonstrated objectively by using an amniotic fluid catheter attached to a strain gauge. The external cervical os may dilate quickly to effect delivery. The undelivered woman may die of shock and hemorrhage unless medical aid is given.

Fibrinogenopenia is a commonly associated disorder in severe abruptio placentae. It is the result of consumption of fibrinogen by disseminated intravascular coagulation caused by absorption of thromboplastin-like material from the placental site. Hypocoagulable states are discussed in Chapter 42.

DIAGNOSIS

Severe cases are recognized by the characteristic pattern of symptoms: acute abdominal pain, referred usually to one area of the uterus; sudden increase in the size and hardness of the uterus, with a tense abdominal wall; external hemorrhage and disappearance of fetal heart tones; and increasing anemia and deepening shock. If the membranes are ruptured, the amniotic fluid may be found admixed with blood. Its characteristic burgundy color was once thought to be pathognomonic of abruptio placentae, although it is now appreciated that any blood in the amniotic fluid will yield that sign. Differential diagnosis must consider placenta previa, rupture of the uterus and abdominal pregnancy, as well as torsion of the uterus, ruptured uterine varix and nonobstetric acute surgical conditions, such as cholecystitis with cholelithiasis, acute appendicitis with rupture and intraabdominal injuries. With a history of violent injury, laparotomy may be necessary for both diagnosis and treatment.

Distinguishing abruptio placentae from placenta previa is usually apparent, but difficulties may arise. The very mild abruption may mimic the silent vaginal bleeding of placenta previa. Contrariwise, some patients with placenta previa may present with uterine irritability and tenderness. As a general rule, whenever doubt exists, it must be assumed that there is a placenta previa and the program of management outlined in Chapter 37 should be followed until this diagnosis is ruled out definitively.

PROGNOSIS

Abruptio placentae is one of the gravest accidents with which the obstetrician has to deal. Overall maternal mortality can be as high as six per cent (Kellogg). With mild varieties of separation there is no mortality, whereas with the moderate and severe types the mortality ranges up to 15 to 20 per cent. Separations without hypertension have the lowest fetal death rate of only one per cent. The fetal mortality is 34 per cent in conjunction with hypertensive manifestations. Premature separation of the placenta occurring together with preeclampsia increases the fetal loss nearly five times over that associated with the hypertensive state alone.

TREATMENT

In addition to the basic problems previously enunciated in our discussion of placenta previa (Chapter 37) with regard to immediate evaluation and management of the patient with profuse hemorrhage, abruptio placentae adds the hazards of preeclampsia and hypofibrinogenemia as well as renal and pituitary damage. In general, occurrence of these complications can be related to a time factor: The longer the disease process persists prior to evacuation of the uterus, the more likely they are to be seen.

The basic premise underlying management of the patient with abruptio placentae (other than the minimal variety) is to effect delivery as quickly and as atraumatically as possible. We must consider the immediate status of the patient to determine whether delay — for the purpose of attempting to induce labor and effect vaginal delivery — is safe. We must further be aware of the likelihood that the situation will change with time, so that continual observation of cardiovascular status, blood loss (including that which is concealed within the uterus but is, nevertheless, no longer part of the circulating volume) and coagulation picture is necessary. The longer the delay before delivery, the greater the likelihood of increasing placental separation, enhancement of bleeding and risk of hypofibrinogenemia.

Severe cases of abruptio placentae require prompt diagnosis and treatment. Four objectives must be accomplished: Shock must be overcome; hemorrhage must be stopped; the anemia must be relieved; and the uterus must be emptied in due course after the diagnosis is made. The time factor is important because of the possibility of increased separation of the placenta with more alarming hemorrhage, increased danger of uteroplacental apoplexy and aggravation of preeclampsia, if it is present. Also the danger of hypofibrinogenemia is increased and renal failure may occur.

Accordingly, amniotomy and induction or stimulation of labor with oxytocin infusion should be undertaken only in those instances in which the patient is in good condition, blood is on hand, fibrinogen is available, coagulation status is known and coagulation studies can be done frequently thereafter. Moreover, it is essential that the ensuing labor progress rapidly and uninterruptedly. This approach can be modified at any time should the need arise. Fetal distress, falling fibrinogen, increasing bleeding, increasing tachycardia or falling blood pressure would militate toward more aggressive action in the form of immediate cesarean section. It is current practice to limit such attempts to stimulate labor to eight hours or less. This time limit may be increased if current investigations indicating that heparin prevents fibrinogen depletion prove this to be an effective approach.

Because many infants are still lost under these circumstances, it is probably reasonable to be more aggressive and proceed more perfunctorily to cesarean section if one is dealing with a viable fetus in the presence of a moderately severe abruption. Delay under these circumstances may well lead to fetal death or damage. On the other hand, if the fetus is already dead, greater conservatism may occasionally avert the need for cesarean section with its attendant greater morbidity and adverse influence on future obstetric experience.

In the presence of a severe abruption in which the fetus is already dead and the mother's life is in jeopardy, prompt, intensive action is necessary to empty the uterus. One should proceed with a laparotomy even in the presence of shock so as to control hemorrhage. Simultaneously, of course, blood replacement is essential, together with measures to maintain cardiovascular status.

Fortunately, very few patients present with a clinical picture demanding such immediate intervention. Most can be managed with a reasonable degree of conservatism by amniotomy and uterotonic stimulation. The rapidity of the labor that usually ensues is often quite surprising. Very rarely, following delivery the uterine muscle has been so inspissated by blood (Couvelaire uterus) that it cannot contract. Under these circumstances, hysterectomy may be necessary. It must be ascertained first, however, that the uncontrolled postpartum bleeding is not due to coagulation defect or laceration of the lower birth canal.

Hypofibrinogenemia presents a special problem. When plasma levels are not readily obtainable, the simple "clot observation test" gives a rough idea of the ability of a clot to form and subsequently lyse. A stable clot forming in less than six minutes indicates that the fibrinogen level is probably greater than 150 mg. per 100 ml. If it fails to form within 30 minutes, the level is probably less than 100 mg. per 100 ml. Quick semiquantitative tests, such as the Fibrindex test, will indicate a level above or below 100 mg. per 100 ml. Although these are of value in indicating the proba-

bility of fibrinogen depletion, they do not provide the quantitation necessary to measure serial changes in concentration during observation of patients. One can certainly be more secure in electing to handle a patient conservatively if quantitative fibrinogen and fibrinolysin determinations are available.

Replacement of fibrinogen only temporarily corrects the situation, while the cause, in the form of continuing autoinfusion of thromboplastin from disrupted placenta, decidua, myometrium and retroplacental clot, depletes fibrinogen stores by producing intravascular coagulation. The latter in turn is acted upon by the rapidly mobilized fibrinolysis mechanism, further complicating the coagulation picture.

The process terminates abruptly as soon as the uterus is emptied. Accordingly, it is imperative to end the pregnancy before the coagulation problem gets out of hand, if possible before the fibrinogen falls below the critical 100 mg. per 100 ml. level. Widespread hemorrhagic tendencies will be observed frequently in association with hypofibrinogenemia, requiring fibrinogen replacement (in amounts as high as 10 gm.), with its attendant risk of hepatitis. Furthermore, since fibrinogen replacement is only temporarily effective, it becomes mandatory to proceed more definitively forthwith.

If a woman who is apparently in normal labor suddenly has a hemorrhage, one must proceed to attempt to differentiate possible causes. An internal examination (with all operating facilities prepared for immediate intervention, as in the "double setup" described in Chapter 37) will disclose whether or not the hemorrhage is from a placenta previa. If the placenta is out of reach of the fingers, one is presumably dealing with abruptio placentae. The membranes should be ruptured and diluted oxytocin infusion begun to stimulate contractility. This is good temporizing treatment for detachment of the placenta because the labor may be much facilitated. If the hemorrhage continues, and especially if the fetal heart tones indicate hypoxia, diagnosis is definite and more aggressive intervention becomes essential. If the placenta separates after a twin is born, rapid delivery of the second twin is indicated.

At least 1000 ml. of grouped and matched blood should always be at hand, even if none of it is used. If much blood has been lost, it must be replaced, preferably before any operative procedure is undertaken.

Cesarean section is definitely indicated in many instances of abruptio placentae, especially when the abruption is associated with severe toxemia, when external or internal bleeding is profuse and when the cervix has not dilated or has dilated only slightly. A cesarean section should also be done when rupture of the membranes and oxytocin intravenously do not lead to delivery within eight hours. This rule applies even if the patient is not entirely out of shock, because it is necessary to stop the profuse bleeding. A conservative operation can be done in nearly all patients who require a cesarean section.

However, the uterus may have to be removed when it does not maintain its contractility. Fortunately, the necessity for this is rare, even in the presence of uteroplacental apoplexy (see above).

All danger is not over when the baby and placenta have been delivered. Because of the risk of late postpartum bleeding, a physician should carefully watch the patient for at least four hours after delivery. Postpartum atony may further complicate the situation as a consequence of uterine overdistention and myometrial injury or disturbance from blood inspissation. Management of this serious problem is dealt with in Chapter 66. Usually, the fibrinogenopenia is rapidly corrected in a spontaneous manner after the uterus is emptied, provided the liver is functionally intact and capable of replenishing the fibrinogen stores by synthesizing it.

REFERENCES

Couvelaire, A.: Deux nouvelles observations d'apoplexie utero-placentaire (hemorrhagies retroplacentaires avec infiltration sanguine de la paroi musculaire de l'uterus). Ann. Gynéc. Obstét. 9:486, 1912.

Davis, M. E., and McGee, W. B.: Abruptio placentae. Surg. Gynec. Obstet. 53:768, 1931.

DeLee, J. B.: A case of fatal hemorrhagic diathesis, with premature detachment of the placenta. Amer. J. Obstet. 44:785, 1901.

DeLee, J. B.: The Principles and Practice of Obstetrics, ed. 7. Philadelphia, W. B. Saunders Company, 1937.

Dieckmann, W. J.: Blood chemistry and renal function in abruptio placentae. Amer. J. Obstet. Gynec. 31:734, 1936.

Hertig, A. T.: Vascular pathology in albuminuric toxemias of pregnancy. Clinics 4:602, 1945.

Holmes, R. W.: Ablatio placentae: A study based upon two hundred cases in the literature. Amer. J. Obstet. 44:753, 1901.

Howard, B. K., and Goodson, J. H.: Experimental placental abruption. Obstet. Gynec. 2:442, 1953.

Kellogg, F. S.: Toxemias of pregnancy. Clinics 4:585, 1945.

Kellogg, F. S.: Hemorrhagic tendencies in toxemia of pregnancy (practical evaluation and management). Obstet. Gynec. Surv. 3:746, 1948.

Mengert, W. F., Goodson, J. H., Campbell, R. G., and Haynes, D. M.: Observations on the pathogenesis of premature separation of the normally implanted placenta. Amer. J. Obstet. Gynec. 66:1104, 1953.

Nesbitt, R. E. L., Jr., Powers, S. R., Jr., Boba, A., and Stein, A.: Experimental abruptio placentae: Histologic and physiologic studies. Obstet. Gynec. 12:359, 1958.

Sexton, L. I., Hertig, A. T., Reid, D. E., Kellogg, F. S., and Patterson, W. S.: Premature separation of the normally implanted placenta. Amer. J. Obstet. Gynec. 59:13, 1950.

Williams, J. W.: Premature separation of the normally implanted placenta. Surg. Gynec. Obstet. 21:541, 1915.

Chapter 39

Multiple Pregnancy

Because of the associated maternal and infant morbidity and the substantial fetal wastage, it is distinctly abnormal for the human female to bear more than one offspring at a time.

In 1895, Hellin propounded his "law" describing the incidence of multiple pregnancies as follows: twins occur once in every 89 births, triplets in 89^2 and quadruplets in 89^3. Greulich tested Hellin's statement in over 121 million births of 21 nations. He found 1:85.2 twin births, $1:87.3^2$ triplet births and $1:87.5^3$ quadruplet births. Guttmacher analyzed the plural birth data of more than 57,000,000 deliveries in the United States, concluding that the Hellin law is merely a mathematical approximation. Guttmacher showed a marked and consistent difference in the frequency of human multiple births among different racial groups. Multiple gestations occur with greatest frequency among blacks, least often among orientals. The difference in the twinning rates is almost entirely due to the relative frequencies of dizygotic twins. The incidence of monozygotic twins born to women of the black, white and yellow races is approximately the same. There is a significant correlation between maternal age and twinning frequency, the incidence rising progressively until the age of 39, then falling abruptly.

The incidence of quintuplets and sextuplets is very rare, estimated by Berbos et al. as once in every 15 to 20 million births. In recent years, the numbers have increased somewhat, perhaps related to use of agents, such as clomiphene, which can stimulate simultaneous maturation of many oocytes when administered in excessive dosages.

The marriage of twins increases the hereditary tendency. Twins and triplets are likely to be repeated in the same family. This refers to the incidence of multiple ovum pregnancies only (see below).

The sex ratio is markedly altered in multiple pregnancy. The ratio of females to males increases as the number of children born in one confinement increases. In single births there are 94 females born for every 100 males. In twins the ratio is 97 females to 100 males. In the higher order of multiple births, the sex ratio is reversed and females are in the majority. The ratio for triplets is 101 females for every 100 males and for quadruplets it is as high as 156 to 100 (Metropolitan Life Insurance Company). This observation is unexplained.

ETIOLOGY

Generally, two kinds of twin gestations are distinguished: those from separate and distinct ova (dizygotic or fraternal) and those arising from one ovum (monozygotic or identical). Two ova escaping from an ovary at the same time may be fertilized and develop synchronously. These ova may come out of the same graafian follicle or they may develop in separate graafian follicles in the same or opposite ovaries. When two or more separate ova implant in the uterus, several patterns of development are possible (Fig. 271): Two distinct placentas may develop or, if their implantation sites are near each other, the two placentas may fuse, but their circulations do not. Since each of the dizygous fetuses has its own amnion and chorion, a septum made up of four layers will be found intervening between

434

them, composed of an amnion and a chorion for each fetus. Occasionally, decidual remnants will be found in the septum, the residua of the decidua capsularis of the early stages of the development of the ova. Theoretically, six layers in the septum of dizygotic twins may be found, comprising two deciduas, two chorions and two amnions (Newman).

The identical variety of twins (Fig. 272) is not influenced by heredity, parity or age. There is comparative embryologic evidence suggesting that deleterious influences exerted on fertilized ova increase the incidence of twinning and other forms of pathologic doubling. Dizygotic twinning is an entirely different phenomenon; it obviously results from a double simultaneous ovulation. It is definitely influenced by heredity, parity and age.

Greulich's studies showed that the tendency to twinning is evident not only in both parents of fraternal twins but also in other members of the parents' families. He found no such predisposition to twinning in the families of identical twins. Both Greulich and Guttmacher's studies showed that monozygotic twinning occurs

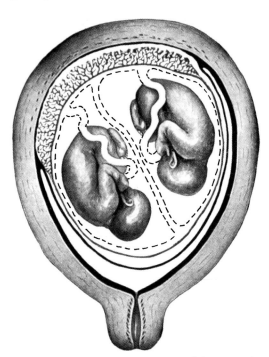

Figure 272 Monozygotic or single-ovum twins with two amnions but only one chorion. Here the intervening membrane has only the two amnions present.

most frequently in women between the ages of 20 and 35; this is the age group in which the greatest number of total births occur. On the other hand, dizygotic twinning is fundamentally a characteristic of older women. Guttmacher also found that dizygotic twinning is relatively infrequent in nulliparas and primiparas but common in grand multiparas. No such difference in the incidence of identical twins is encountered among women of different parity.

Tompkins determined that women with anomalous uteri have twins several times more often than the average for all women. For example, in all women there is one twin for every 84 obstetric cases, whereas in women with abnormal uteri the incidence is one in 20. It was possible to establish the zygosity in 80 per cent of 293 pairs of twins in a series reported by Potter: 23 per cent were identified as monozygotic on the basis of the finding of placentas with single chorions; dizygosity was clear in 57 per cent because of differences in sex and in blood groups of infants with the same sex. The remaining 20 per cent were probably monozygotic, but

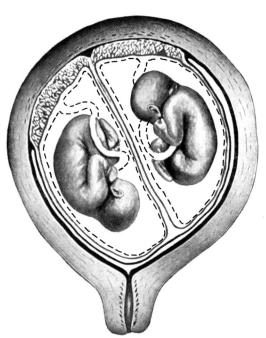

Figure 271 Double-ovum twins showing two chorions and two amnions in the intervening membrane.

Weinberg's rule

this could not be verified. These data corroborate Weinberg's rule which states that the total number of dizygotic twins in any population should be twice the number of twin siblings of different sex; this figure subtracted from the total should give the number of twins who are monozygotic.

CHARACTERISTICS

The placentas of twins are shown in Figures 273 and 274. The placenta in uniovular twins is single and the fetal blood vessels may anastomose with each other on the surface of the placenta and also within the villi themselves. The septum of the placenta never shows traces of decidua and only two layers, the two amnions, can be found in it. In the rarest of cases, two chorions or even separate placentas have been found. The children are very much alike in size and in mental and physical characteristics, including finger, palm and sole prints, and often may show identical physical deformities and mental malfunctions. Bak says their fingerprints, though similar, are not truly identical and can be used for police identification.

If there are two amnions and no chorion in the septum, the fetuses are uniovular. If fission occurred in the morula stage, however, there may be one placenta with two chorions or even two separate placentas (Newman). Wenner said the number of layers in the walls between twins is not a reliable indication of whether twins are monozygotic or dizygotic. He relied more on physical comparison made after the age of two years when most identical twins appear alike. The best estimate is that monoamniotic twins, in which no intervening septum exists and both fetuses occupy one sac, occur once in 60,000 births.

Macklin summarized the approach to distinguishing identical and fraternal twins: (1) If the babies' sexes are different, they are fraternal, whereas if they are alike, the situation is unclear. (2) Conjoined twins or those occupying the same sac must be identical. (3) If the intervening partition consists of only two amnions, the infants are identical; if there are two chorions as well, they may be either identical or fraternal. (4) A single placenta is associated with identical twins, but two placentas are found in both identical and fraternal twins. However, it must be emphasized that the placentas of fraternal

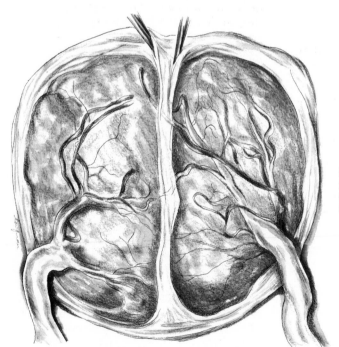

Figure 273 Placenta of single-ovum twins showing two layers of amnion composing the intervening membrane. The absence of chorion here establishes this as monozygotic twins.

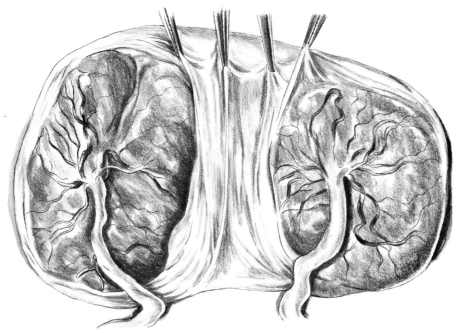

Figure 274 Placenta of double-ovum twins showing four separate membranes dissected from the intervening membranes: two chorions interleaved between the two amnions.

twins may fuse *in utero* and appear as if they were one.

Triplets and quadruplets may all come from one ovum, but usually two or three ova are concerned. One of these may further split to result in two fetuses. Twins usually differ in weight and length from each other and sometimes the differences are considerable. Twins are usually smaller than single children, but their combined weight may be greater. The largest combined weight of twins was reported by Warren as 16,102 gm. (35.5 lbs.). Leonard reported the delivery of twins weighing 9255 gm. (20.4 lbs.) in aggregate by cesarean section. More often, however, twins are small at birth, 54 per cent weighing less than 2500 gm., based on the greater likelihood of premature delivery among multiple pregnancies (Friedman and Little).

Twins of multiparas tend to be somewhat heavier than those of nulliparas. This is not caused by a greater length of pregnancy. Guttmacher ascribed it to a more rapid growth of the fetuses per unit of time of intrauterine existence. Twins derived from one ovum are smaller than those from two and the difference in weight between them is not as great. Also, the mortality among monozygotic twins is higher and they are more often deformed. Preeclampsia is said to be more common, too.

The two circulations frequently anastomose in the common placenta of monozygotic twins: artery to artery, vein to vein and artery to vein through the intercommunicating villous tree. Because of the anastomosis of the two blood systems, the cord of the first child delivered must be tied or clamped to prevent the other from bleeding through the open vessels.

As a result of this anastomosis there may be unequal distribution and size of the placental vessels, unequal circulation and unequal nutritional conditions. Anomalies may result. The heart of one fetus, because of better circulatory advantage and nourishment, may overpower that of the other via the anastomotic vessels. If this occurs at an early period, the weaker heart dilates into a tortuous vessel and the fetus remains undeveloped as an *acardius* or *acardiacus* monster. An *acardius acephalus* (Fig. 275) consists essentially of a pelvis and lower extremities, and an *acardius amorphus* has only a rudimentary head, extremities and heart.

If the imbalance occurs later, a condition known as the *fetal transfusion syndrome* may occur. It is seen only in monozygotic twins and is associated with good development, hydramnios, polycythemia and sometimes cardiac hypertrophy and edema in the "recipient" fetus. This is contrasted sharply with the small size, oligohydramnios, anemia, dehydration and microcardia seen in the "donor" fetus.

Hydramnios is so common with twins that, when it is discovered, multiple pregnancy should be suspected. If the twins lie in one amniotic cavity, a rare occurrence, the two umbilical cords may be twisted, causing the death of one or both fetuses. The high fetal mortality among monozygotic, monoamniotic twins is due chiefly to tangling and knotting of the cords. Raphael found reports of 183 monoamniotic twins in the world literature.

Dizygotic twins are also subject to abnormalities. One fetus may die and be retained or expelled, while the other develops normally to term. If one twin dies after nearly full development and is long

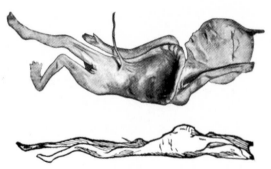

Figure 276 Two views of a fetus papyraceus or compressus. The head of the well-developed twin lay in the hollowed-out chest of the fetus compressus.

retained *in utero*, it is changed into a *fetus papyraceus* or *compressus* (Fig. 276). It may present before the normal fetus, giving rise to diagnostic errors, or it may be left in the uterus after delivery of the placenta and cause bleeding and infection. The placenta of the compressed fetus is white, hard, fibrous, infarcted and demarcated sharply; this finding should suggest an undiagnosed, retained second fetus.

Superfetation is the occurrence of a second fertilization and implantation in the uterus already occupied by a conceptus in the process of development. It occurs in animals (Fleming). Its occurrence in the human being seems most unlikely because ovulation is inhibited during pregnancy. Although a double uterus may carry a fetus in each side, this is not superfetation but rather the result of simultaneous fertilization of the separate ova as occurs with any dizygotic twinning in a single uterus.

Superfecundation is the impregnation of two different ova, at about the same time, by sperm from different fathers. Its occurrence in animals is demonstrated. Though doubted for the human being, it is possible but has never been proved.

CLINICAL COURSE

Plural pregnancy frequently gives rise to maternal and fetal disturbances. Anemia, toxemia, hydramnios, varices and edema are common. Hypertensive disorders occur in 21 per cent in comparison to eight per cent expected for all deliveries (Potter and Fuller). The abdominal distention associated with multiple pregnancy interferes with bowel function and respiration,

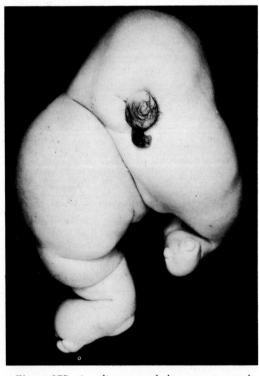

Figure 275 Acardiacus acephalus monster resulting from maldistribution of circulation between twins. (Courtesy of O. Agüero.)

especially in the presence of hydramnios. Softening and relaxation of the pelvic joints are sometimes extreme and, in association with the abdominal overdistention, make locomotion difficult.

About 80 per cent of twin pregnancies terminate before term and so do practically all triplet and quadruplet gestations. In Guttmacher's series, labor occurred on an average of 22.2 days before the calculated date.

Guttmacher and Kohl found the median birth weight for a twin to be 2377 gm. (5.25 lbs.). By the end of the thirty-fifth week of pregnancy, twins weigh approximately 650 gm. less than comparably aged singletons, a difference that is maintained thereafter. The birth weight of a twin is affected by the length of the pregnancy, sex and zygosity. Male twins weigh more than females and twins from two ova weigh more than twins from one ovum. Also, the second twin tends to be smaller than the firstborn.

Labor with twins is often abnormal. Due to the overstretching of the uterine muscle, the contractions may be ineffectual in dilating the cervix during the active phase of labor. Friedman and Sachtleben showed that some degree of cervical dilatation often precedes labor in these cases, giving rise to foreshortened latent phases. This is usually followed by slow dilatation in the active phase of the first stage, frequently in a dysfunctional pattern.

Since the fetuses are small and there is usually much amniotic fluid, frequent changes of presentation and position occur; the lie of the second twin may be affected by delivery of the first. For example, as the first is born, the second may change from shoulder to breech presentation. Various combinations of presentations are possible (Fig. 277). Most often both are vertex (45 per cent) or one is vertex and the other breech (38 per cent); infrequently, both are breech (9 per cent) or one is transverse (7 per cent) (Guttmacher and Kohl; Portes and Granjon). The incidence of cephalic presentation for all the twins is 66 per cent. For the first twin it is 75 per cent and for the second twin it is 58 per cent.

The fetuses usually lie parallel to each

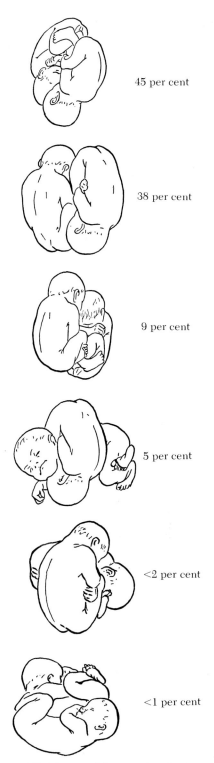

45 per cent

38 per cent

9 per cent

5 per cent

<2 per cent

<1 per cent

Figure 277 Types and frequencies of twin presentations based on the data of Guttmacher and Kohl and of Portes and Granjon.

other, one on each side of the spinal column, but one may lie anteriorly and the other be entirely beyond the reach of manual palpation. Occasionally, when the amount of amniotic fluid is scant, the fetuses are dovetailed into each other.

If one placenta lies in juxtaposition to the other, it is not unusual to find the lower edge of the placenta near or over the internal os. Breech and shoulder presentations are favored by low implantations and placenta previa. Abruptio placentae may follow delivery of the first twin because the uterine wall shears off the placental site as it contracts to accommodate the reduced intrauterine volume.

After delivery of twins, the uterus usually contracts firmly. However, hemorrhage due to uterine atony, the result of overstretching, is more common than after single births.

DIAGNOSIS OF TWINS

Twins may almost always be diagnosed during pregnancy without the aid of a roentgenogram if one's index of suspicion is high. A large and globular abdomen, especially if larger than expected for the gestational age, associated with rapid uterine growth, pronounced edema, proteinuria and fetal motion over the entire abdomen suggests twins. The diagnostic points are:

1. A sulcus or longitudinal indentation is felt in the fundus or down the front of the uterus. However, this may occur in uterus arcuatus or a distorted uterus with a single fetus, and it may be absent in twins.

2. An unusually large and globular uterus is present. However, the possibility of hydramnios with a single large fetus must be considered.

3. Palpation reveals three or more large parts, two heads and one breech or two breeches and one head. One should not make a diagnosis on the multiplicity of small parts because the fetus can place these in many locations.

4. When the distance from one pole of the fetus to the other is too great to be the length of one fetus, for example, more than 30 cm., twins may be present.

5. Auscultation will show two sets of fetal heart tones. Characteristically, (a) both are asynchronous with the maternal pulse, (b) both are asynchronous with each other, and (c) a free zone exists between the two areas of greatest intensity. The use of an ultrasound device (Doppler effect) is most helpful (see Chapter 13). It is sometimes best for two observers to listen at the same time. If one fetus is dead, the auscultatory method leaves one in doubt. It is also possible for two living fetuses to have their hearts beating synchronously for a time. In such cases irritation of one fetus until it moves will accelerate the heart beat or compressing its head manually may reduce its heart rate. A singleton fetus with a straightened spine may have heart tones audible on both sides of the uterus, or the placenta may divide the area of audibility.

6. Twins and triplets are readily seen on roentgenograms and B-scan ultrasonography (see Chapter 13). Even quadruplets and quintuplets have been diagnosed in this way. However, the techniques are not infallible because, if one of the fetuses moves during the procedure, it may not be distinguishable by x-ray. Roentgenography or sonography is most valuable for differentiation between one large and two small fetuses. It is not always easy to rule out a double monster unless repeated studies reveal that the relation of the fetuses to each other is always the same.

7. During labor, twins are suspected by palpation of an intact amniotic sac after one sac has ruptured. This sign may be misleading if the chorion alone ruptures but the amnion remains intact in a singleton fetus.

Diagnosis of twins is made at the time of delivery in about half the cases. After the delivery of one child, the diagnosis that another fetus remains in the uterus is easily made by palpating the corpus, but leiomyomas may be mistaken for a fetus. It may be necessary to explore the uterus manually to be sure. When the delivered baby is considerably smaller than expected according to uterine size and dates, twins are likely to be present.

DIFFERENTIAL DIAGNOSIS

In the early months of pregnancy, the presence of twins may suggest hydatidiform mole because of the rapid uterine growth. Chorionic gonadotropin titers and B-scan will help to make the distinction.

The differential diagnosis of simultaneous extrauterine and intrauterine pregnancy from twins is possible only to a keen and experienced obstetrician and, even under the most favorable circumstances, it is rarely made before operation. However, unless symptoms are manifest, the problem does not arise.

Leiomyomas or ovarian neoplasms complicating pregnancy may simulate plural gestations. The absence of two heart beats on repeated examinations, the immobility of large and small masses, their constancy of location, the history of leiomyomas or ovarian cysts and roentgen or ultrasonographic study allow prompt differentiation.

PROGNOSIS

Both maternal and infant mortality rates are higher in multiple than in single pregnancy. The chief cause of maternal deaths is hemorrhage. Because of longer labors and the more frequent necessity for operative deliveries, infection is also more apt to occur. Granjon found prolapse of the cord or fetal small parts in 8.5 per cent of 1000 twins.

For the fetus the prognosis is serious. Prematurity is quite common, occurring in 54 per cent of twins as compared with about nine per cent of singletons (Friedman and Little). Since the majority of twin births are premature, many infants die of respiratory distress, infection or general debility. Record et al. studied the data concerning 23,206 single, 666 twin, 786 triplet and 108 quadruplet births. The perinatal mortality rates expressed as the number of stillbirths and neonatal deaths per 1000 total births of single, twin, triplet and quadruplet gestations were, respectively, 39, 152, 309 and 509. Review of a dozen large reported series by Little and Friedman showed a range of twin perinatal mortality rates from 9 to 31 per cent or from 3 to 10 times that expected for singletons.

Camilleri analyzed the results in 3455 twin deliveries reported in the literature and found that the perinatal mortality rate of the second twin is 50 per cent higher than that of the first twin. Little and Friedman found second twin mortality nearly twice as high as that of first twins. This relationship held for comparably sized first and second twins. Nixon found the death rate to be three times as high in the second twin. The incidence of malpresentations in second twins is as high as 43 per cent. Transverse lie occurs in about 12 per cent.

Twins from one ovum have a higher perinatal mortality rate and are exposed to certain vicissitudes which twins from two ova are spared. Salvage is maximum in twins born spontaneously in vertex presentations or by elective outlet forceps, regardless of birth weight. Twins delivered by version and extraction do relatively poorly. Congenital malformations are twice as common in twins as in singletons.

TREATMENT

During pregnancy a patient with plural pregnancy requires more care than one with a singleton pregnancy. Premature twin births may possibly be reduced by having gravidas rest a good deal after the thirty-second week. Excellent results were obtained by the following regimen: early diagnosis of twins, a high caloric and mineral diet, good general hygiene and preadmission to a hospital for bed rest. Brown and Dixon were able to reduce the incidence of small babies under 2500 gm. from 51 to 37 per cent (under 2000 gm. from 21 to 13 per cent) merely by means of putting the patients with twins to bed for up to four weeks from the thirtieth to the thirty-sixth week. Their perinatal losses fell from 6.1 to 4.0 per cent, a significant improvement in salvage.

During labor "intelligent expectancy" should be practiced. Preparations for operative delivery and for the treatment of a pathologic third stage must be made well in advance of the delivery. Multiple preg-

nancy *per se* is not an indication for cesarean section, but complicating features
that may demand operative interference
do occur (most often prolapsed cord) and
must be acted upon when they take place.

Delivery of the second twin is critical.
Friedman and Little showed excessive
second twin losses in association with all
forms of delivery, the worst rates occurring
with midforceps and breech deliveries,
especially those following internal podalic
version. The smaller the baby, the worse
the result, most particularly after version
and breech extraction. Second twins who
are delivered following delays between
2½ and 15 minutes after birth of the first
twin fared best of all. Mortality rates three
times as high occurred if delivery took
place sooner or later. The earlier ones
were associated with trauma as a result of
undue haste; the later ones with a variety
of complicating features involving cord
and placental problems.

On the basis of the high incidence of
prematurity, it is wise to allow the mother
to labor with a minimum of analgesic medication. Delivery of the first twin is probably best accomplished spontaneously or
by prophylactic outlet forceps over an
ample episiotomy, utilizing local infiltration, pudendal or paracervical block or
light inhalation anesthesia.

Following delivery of the first twin, the
subsequent course will depend on prevailing conditions. In order to evaluate these,
immediate vaginal examination is essential. Without rupturing the second amniotic sac, one must determine the fetal lie
and the presence of any complicating feature, such as a forward-lying loop of cord.

If it is clear that the vertex is presenting
and fits easily into the pelvis, the membranes may be safely ruptured and labor
allowed to progress. If the breech is presenting without a prolapsed loop of cord, it
is probably wise to desist and await further
developments. This conservative approach is particularly appropriate with
very small infants, in the face of their very
high mortality in traumatic deliveries.

On the other hand, if the fetus is in a
transverse or oblique lie, it is necessary to
turn it to the longitudinal axis internally,
so as to allow the normal mechanisms of
labor to evolve if at all possible. Version

(cephalic or podalic) thus performed will
require and should be carried out under
general anesthesia sufficiently deep to relax the uterus during the manipulations.
Whether it is necessary to continue with
the delivery once version to a longitudinal
presentation has been accomplished will
depend on the situation at that moment. In
the absence of the compelling urgency of
evidence of fetal distress, prolapsed cord
or placental complication, one may safely
allow the patient to awaken. Continuous
fetal heart monitoring (Chapter 13) is most
helpful, if available. The patient may then
resume labor and deliver at a later time by
less traumatic means than, for example,
breech extraction or a midforceps procedure, the latter so often done in association
with considerable fundal pressure.

It must be strongly urged that when this
conservative policy is followed, ideal conditions of observation must be in force,
particularly with as nearly continuous auscultation of the fetal heart tones as possible. Here electronic fetal monitoring, as
stated above, may provide the earliest evidence of fetal hypoxia. If detected, delivery should be effected as indicated.

The interval-delay between delivery of
the first and second twin must depend on
the considerations mentioned. It is imperative that undue haste be avoided, particularly in the performance of any operative
procedures which may be carried out, because of the increased risk of traumatizing
the fetus as well as the mother. It is essential that one pursue early detection and expeditious handling of cord or placental
complications which may jeopardize the
life of the fetus. In this conservative approach the principles of watchful expectancy and prompt action in the event of
mishap are of paramount importance, and
may help to reduce the deplorable loss of
second twins.

Because of overdistention of the uterus,
contractions are poor and the tendency to
postpartum hemorrhage is definitely augmented. Gentle massage of the corpus is
indicated and removal of the placenta is
usually needed earlier than in single pregnancies. As soon as the second baby is
born and the placenta delivered (either
spontaneously or manually), 0.2 mg.
ergonovine is given intravenously. The pa-

tient must be watched for several hours to be certain that the uterus does not relax again.

Treatment of Anomalies of Plural Births

1. Pathologic presentations, such as breech and shoulder, occur frequently and are treated as usual.

2. The presenting part may change several times before one is finally engaged and is delivered. Intervention is indicated only when delay in engagement is abnormal.

3. The membranes of the second twin may rupture before that of the first. Treatment is not necessary unless the cord of the second twin prolapses before its presenting part is delivered. If conditions for vaginal delivery are present, both fetuses should be delivered, if possible. Otherwise, a cesarean section should be done if both fetuses are alive.

4. Rarely is the placenta of the first twin delivered before the second one is born. If the placenta is independent of that of the other fetus, no harm results. If the two placentas are united, the associated abruption of the placenta of the second fetus will result in its death unless it is delivered at once. The signs of asphyxia and external hemorrhage apprise the physician of what is taking place. Rapid but careful delivery of the second fetus will save it and the mother from mishap.

5. The transit of the first fetus may alter the position of the second. Treatment depends on the conditions present after the first twin has been delivered.

6. Interlocking, impaction or collision may rarely occur as a cause of dystocia. The first twin is more vulnerable under such circumstances (Nissen); two-thirds of the twins die.

Collision is the contact of any fetal parts of one twin with those of its co-twin, thereby preventing engagement of either.

Impaction is the indentation of any fetal parts of one twin onto the surface of the other, thereby permitting partial engagement of both simultaneously.

Compaction is the simultaneous full engagement of the leading fetal poles of both twins, thus filling the true pelvic cavity and thereby preventing further descent or disengagement of either one.

Interlocking refers to a rare situation in which the first twin presents as a breech and, as it descends, its chin impinges on the forelying neck and chin of the second twin above the pelvic inlet, preventing any further progress. Delay in the delivery of the first twin should suggest interlocking. Usually there is no time for roentgenography, but it is helpful to know if a monster exists. An examination with the whole hand in the uterus is necessary to determine this. If interlocking is diagnosed, a deep episiotomy is done to avoid laceration of the perineum. The whole hand is inserted under sterile operative conditions with deep general anesthesia and the second head is pushed up and out of the pelvis. If the heads are small, such a procedure is possible. If not, and the first twin is dead (as is usually the case by this time), the first twin may be decapitated and the head pushed up into the uterine cavity. Then the second twin can be delivered readily by any appropriately atraumatic method. Subsequently, the severed head must be delivered, a procedure that is sometimes quite difficult. Because of the trauma involved in this procedure, cesarean section is much safer for both mother and second twin; it is therefore recommended.

REFERENCES

Bak, M.: Dactyloscopy of twins. Orv. Hetil. 78:946, 1934.

Berbos, J. N., King, B. F., and Janusz, A.: Quintuple pregnancy: Report of a case. J.A.M.A. *188*:813, 1964.

Brown, E. J., and Dixon, H. G.: Twin pregnancy. J. Obstet. Gynaec. Brit. Comm. 70:251, 1963.

Camilleri, A. P.; In defense of the second twin. J. Obstet. Gynaec. Brit. Comm. 70:258, 1963.

Craig, I. T.: Monoamniotic twins with double survival. Amer. J. Obstet. Gynec. 73:202, 1957.

Fleming, G.: Fleming's Veterinary Obstetrics. London, Baillière, Tindall & Cox, 1930.

Friedman, E. A., and Little, W. A.: An evaluation of

the management of the twin delivery. Bull. Sloane Hosp. *4*:39, 1958.

Friedman, E. A., and Sachtleben, M. R.: The effect of uterine overdistention on labor: I. Multiple pregnancy. Obstet. Gynec. *23*:164, 1964.

Granjon, A.: Les procidences au cours des accouchements gémellaires. Gynéc. Obstét. *44*:421, 1944–1945.

Greulich, W. W.: The incidence of human multiple births. The American Naturalist *64*:142, 1930.

Greulich, W. W.: Heredity in human twinning. Amer. J. Phys. Anthrop. *19*:391, 1934.

Guttmacher, A. F.: An analysis of 521 cases of twin pregnancy. Amer. J. Obstet. Gynec. *34*:76, 1937.

Guttmacher, A. F.: Analysis of 573 cases of twin pregnancy: Hazards of pregnancy itself. Amer. J. Obstet. Gynec. *38*:277, 1939.

Guttmacher, A. F.: Clinical aspects of twin pregnancy. Med. Clin. N. Amer. *23*:427, 1939.

Guttmacher, A. F.: The incidence of multiple births in man and some of the other unipara. Obstet. Gynec. *2*:22, 1953.

Guttmacher, A. F., and Kohl, S. G.: The fetus of multiple gestations. Obstet. Gynec. *12*:528, 1958.

Guttmacher, A. F., and Kohl, S. G.: Cesarean section in twin pregnancy. Amer. J. Obstet. Gynec. *83*:1, 1962.

Hellin, D.: Die Ursache der Multiparität der uniparen Tiere überhaupt und der Zwillingsschwangerschaft beim Menschen. München, Seitz and Schnauer, 1895.

Leonard, M. W. E.: Large twins: Report of a case. Obstet. Gynec. *9*:219, 1957.

Little, W. A., and Friedman, E. A.: The twin delivery: Factors influencing second twin mortality. Obstet. Gynec. Survey *13*:611, 1958.

Macklin, M. T.: The use of monozygous and dizygous twins in the study of human heredity. Amer. J. Obstet. Gynec. *59*:359, 1950.

Metropolitan Life Insurance Company: Statistical Bull. May, 1944.

Newman, H. H.: The Physiology of Twinning. Chicago, University of Chicago Press, 1923.

Newman, H. H.: Multiple Human Births: Twins, Triplets, Quadruplets and Quintuplets. New York, Doubleday, Doran and Company, 1940.

Newman, H. H.: Aspects of twin research. Sci. Month. *52*:99, 1941.

Nissen, E. D.: Twins: Collision, impaction, compaction, and interlocking. Obstet. Gynec. *11*:514, 1958.

Nixon, W. C. W.: Perinatal mortality: The challenge. J. Internat. Fed. Gynaec. *1*:16, 1963.

Portes, L., and Granjon, A.: Les présentations au cours des accouchements gémellaires. Gynéc. Obstét. *45*:159, 1946.

Potter, E. L.: Twin zygosity and placental form in relation to the outcome of pregnancy. Amer. J. Obstet. Gynec. *87*:566, 1963.

Potter, E. L., and Fuller, H.: Multiple pregnancies at the Chicago Lying-in Hospital 1941–1947. Amer. J. Obstet. Gynec. *58*:139, 1949.

Raphael, S. I.: Monoamniotic twin pregnancy: A review of the literature and a report of 5 new cases. Amer. J. Obstet. Gynec. *81*:323, 1961.

Record, R. G., Gibson, J. R., and McKeown, T.: Foetal and infant mortality in multiple pregnancy. J. Obstet. Gynaec. Brit. Emp. *59*:471, 1952.

Tompkins, P.: Comments on the bicornuate uterus and twinning. Surg. Clin. N. Amer. *42*:1049, 1962.

Warren, E. C.: A new-born infant of extraordinary size (Correspondence). Lancet *2*:1029, 1884.

Wenner, R.: Les examens vasculaires des placentas gémellaires et le diagnostic des jumeaux homozygotes. Bull. Soc. Roy. Belge Gynéc. Obstét. *26*: 773, 1956.

Chapter 40

Infectious Diseases

Acute infections in pregnancy, labor and the puerperium tend to have more deleterious consequences than in nonpregnant individuals. Both maternal and fetal mortality are high. Part of the increased maternal death rate results from the superimposed stress and strain of abortion or labor which often decrease the patient's natural defenses against the infection. Furthermore, some diseases result in secondary uterine infection and the full-blown entity of puerperal sepsis which will be dealt with in detail in Chapter 70.

Labor is not disturbed in most acute infections and the third stage is usually normal. Generally, the puerperium is also unaffected. Only when the pyogenic bacteria in the genital tract are stimulated to produce secondary infections is the susceptibility to puerperal complications increased. Involution is usually normal.

Not only may acute infections disturb pregnancy, labor and the puerperium but the course of these infections is also adversely affected in turn so that they are much more serious during pregnancy than otherwise. Their severity may be increased if pregnancy is interrupted while the infection is active. Therefore, artificial interruption of pregnancy is contraindicated in the presence of an acute infectious process. Some resistant intrauterine infections may be exceptions to this rule (see Chapter 70).

Abortions occur frequently. The high fever or perhaps the bacterial toxins associated with acute infections may be responsible for the abortions. Transfer of immunity from the mother to the fetus has long been recognized. Various antibodies have been demonstrated in the umbilical cord blood. Active immunity in the mother may be attempted to protect her against a specific disease or to protect the newborn infant. Cohen et al. showed that multiple immunization of pregnant women in the last trimester provided a high titer of antibodies to diphtheria, pertussis, tetanus and influenza in more than 80 per cent of the mothers and infants.

After exposure or during epidemics, it is wise to immunize actively against diphtheria, pertussis, tetanus, typhoid, influenza or poliomyelitis; there are no deleterious effects to the mother or the fetus. Ordinary precautions must be taken against possible allergic reactions and when known contraindications exist. Materials containing live viruses should not be administered indiscriminately to pregnant women until it can be conclusively proved that the fetus will not be adversely affected by the resulting viremia. These include rubella, smallpox and live attenuated Sabin polio vaccines. In the presence of epidemics, however, it is prudent to immunize against smallpox or poliomyelitis because the risks of the disease are much greater than the theoretical hazard to the fetus. The fetal risks of rubella vaccine are uncertain and do not justify use of this material in pregnancy. Following vaccination, Vaheri et al. recovered rubella virus from fetal tissues.

In general, pregnant women are no more susceptible to acute infectious disease than others, except for poliomyelitis and Asiatic varieties of influenza (see below), which appear to have an increased morbidity and mortality. The discovery by Gregg that rubella in pregnancy caused deleterious effects in the fetus has stimulated extensive studies for parallels in other diseases. The incidence of anomalies occurring after many infectious diseases confirms the importance of protecting expectant mothers from any infection,

445

especially during the first eight weeks. Kaye and Reaney collected 1915 case reports of virus disease in pregnancy. The incidence of fetal abnormality overall was 4.5 per cent; in association with mumps, 13 per cent; measles, 7 per cent; varicella, 5.7 per cent; poliomyelitis, 1.6 per cent; infectious hepatitis, 4.3 per cent; and influenza, 4.1 per cent.

Transplacental transmission of the viruses of several different disorders has been demonstrated, including all of the above plus cytomegalovirus, Western equine encephalitis, herpesvirus hominis types 1 and 2 and the Coxsackie B group. Those with demonstrated teratogenicity are rubella, cytomegalovirus and herpes virus (Sever; Monif).

INFLUENZA

Pregnant women seem predisposed to influenza, probably because this disease especially attacks young, healthy individuals. Characteristic of the epidemic in 1918 were severe pulmonary complications, especially pneumonia. Recent epidemics of Asian influenza have reconfirmed this tendency, especially among infants, debilitated people and pregnant women. Both the incidence and the mortality are higher in gravidas than among others (Freeman and Barno).

Harris showed that about half of 1350 cases of influenza among pregnant women developed pneumonia; about 50 per cent of these patients died, giving a gross mortality of 27 per cent (before use of antibiotics). Gestation was interrupted spontaneously in from 35 to 60 per cent of such patients. When influenza was complicated by pneumonia, termination of pregnancy was much more frequent than otherwise, and then the maternal mortality was distinctly higher than when the gestation was unmolested.

Labor is usually rapid in association with influenza. There are generally no disturbances in the third stage, but bleeding may occur in the puerperium. During the delivery, it is hazardous to use an inhalation anesthetic; therefore, local or regional block anesthesia should be employed when necessary.

After labor, any existing pulmonary complication becomes worse. If influenza develops during the puerperium, the results are no worse than for nonpregnant women. The fetal mortality varies between 20 and 45 per cent and is due almost entirely to the early interruption of pregnancy.

The treatment of influenza during pregnancy is the same as that in nonpregnant individuals. Antibiotics are usually effective against the bacterial pneumonias that follow. Pregnancy should never be interrupted deliberately during the course of the infection. All patients should be isolated.

Baer and Reis found that mammary infections showed a direct increase in phase with the waves of influenza. Hence, special care should be taken of the nipples and breasts. However, such prophylaxis will prevent only a small number of mammary infections because most are hematogenous in origin.

DIPHTHERIA

Diphtheria of the throat is rare among pregnant women just as it is extremely uncommon among adults in general. However, if it does occur and it is not treated adequately, abortion results in about one-third of cases. Diphtheria of the genitals of pregnant women is likewise rare and it is also uncommon during the puerperium. The first symptoms usually appear three to four days after infection. It is usually transmitted by direct contact with an individual who has in turn been in contact with the disease.

Isolation is imperative. The most important step in therapy is prompt administration of sufficient amounts of diphtheria antitoxin. For mild cases, the dose is 10,000 to 20,000 units; for moderate ones, 25,000 to 50,000 units; and for severe ones, 50,000 to 100,000 units. The total dose should be given at one time, either intramuscularly or intravenously. The former route is preferable for doses up to 20,000 units and the intravenous route for larger doses. In addition, the patient should be given aqueous procaine penicillin G, 2 million units daily for 7 to 10 days. Erythromycin is useful for patients who are sensitive to penicillin; dosage is 40 mg. per kilogram per day in four divided doses. Precautions should be taken against anaphylactic reactions because diphtheria antitoxin is a foreign protein.

RUBELLA

Most congenital defects from rubella occur during the first eight weeks of gestation. The defects include congenital cataract, heart disease, deafness and central nervous system damage. Other reported eye lesions include glaucoma and microphthalmia. Patent ductus arteriosus, pulmonary stenosis and a variety of septal defects are found. Meningoencephalitis and intrauterine growth retardation are also encountered. Even if the fetus is grossly unaffected, however, it may still harbor the virus in active culture and continue to discharge virus-laden secretions for many months after it is born. Thus, the neonate may serve as a source of the virus for infecting other infants as well as susceptible personnel.

Siegel and Greenberg studied 294 pregnant women who had German measles and who did not have therapeutic abortions. Fetal deaths occurred in 14.3 per cent. Half of these took place during the first eight weeks and 20 per cent during the third month of gestation. Prematurity, determined by birth weight, was observed in 25 per cent of the newborn infants exposed to rubella in the first weeks of fetal life. Exposure in the second month of pregnancy was associated with a sharp drop in prematurity to 11 per cent in the third month and to below 10 per cent in the second and third trimesters.

Ingalls reviewed the reports of more than 1000 rubella-complicated pregnancies. The total infant death and deformity rate was 30.7 per cent if the rubella infection occurred during the first trimester, 6.8 per cent during the second and 5.3 per cent during the third trimester. He also noted that between one-third and one-half of the mothers lost their babies or gave birth to babies with significant defects when they had rubella during the first two months of pregnancy.

Lundström et al. have shown that administration of convalescent gamma globulin to mothers with rubella did not prevent fetal damage. Although use of gamma globulin may modify or even nullify the clinical manifestations of rubella in the mother, the viremia may still occur and the fetus be injured (Brody et al.).

Whitehouse reported a case to illustrate the danger of rubella in the period preceding conception. It is known that a virus may persist for a long time in the tissues of the host. The rubella virus may persist until fertilization takes place and then possibly damage the developing embryo, or the ovum may be damaged during maturation. If it can be proved that rubella before pregnancy can harm the fetus, it is possible that delaying conception after infection will prevent calamities and avoid the problems raised by therapeutic abortions.

Therapeutic abortion is indicated when rubella occurs during the first trimester because of the great probability of irrevocable damage. Errors in clinical diagnosis are very common, however. Serologic verification of the infection requires two blood specimens to be examined, one at the appearance of the rash and the second two to three weeks later. A significant increase in titer is serodiagnostic.

It has been suggested that all girls be exposed to German measles before the childbearing period. With the introduction of an effective means for immunization, it becomes essential to ensure that every female is provided this protection before adulthood and well before pregnancy is undertaken. Use of rubella vaccine is not entirely innocuous, arthralgias and arthritis having been reported, nor is the immunity that results absolute or necessarily permanent. It must not be used during pregnancy because the viremia may affect the fetus. In many places routine serologic testing for rubella antibody is carried out on all pregnant women to ascertain those that are not immune and are, therefore, at risk. It is even wiser to consider undertaking such tests as part of the premarital examinations so that appropriate preventive measures can be taken at that time.

RUBEOLA

Measles is frequently severe in adults. Pregnancy is often interrupted spontaneously; the incidence reported varies from 45 to 76 per cent. The uterus usually empties itself in the exanthematous stage. While labor is usually normal, the puerperium may be complicated by respiratory disease. Complicating infections are due to secondary invaders and can be treated with antibodies.

The prognosis for the baby is grave when pregnancy is interrupted. Since most adults have had measles in childhood, they have circulating antibodies which readily cross the placenta so that most newborn infants are immune for three to five months. However, infants of mothers ill with measles have been born with the disease. Measles of the mother in the first trimester, as other viral disease, may cause fetal defects. There is no specific treatment for measles. Bed rest is important. The disease is self-limited.

CYTOMEGALOVIRUS

This is a rare cause of congenital defects which may affect the fetus of an otherwise perfectly normal mother. Usually, the infection in the gravida is entirely silent and, therefore, is unrecognized, but the result to the fetus may be catastrophic. It is born with hydrocephalus or microcephalus and microphthalmia. It is subject to seizures and blindness. Encephalitis is common with blood changes such as hemolytic anemia, thrombocytopenia and hepatosplenomegaly. There is no known effective treatment.

HERPESVIRUS HOMINIS

Another mild clinical disease in the adult with potentially serious consequences to the fetus is herpes. It is possible that the virus is transmitted both by direct contact, as in herpes genitalis, or hematogenously. Although it has been recommended that babies be delivered by cesarean section in the presence of genital herpes, no proof is yet available to show that this aggressive approach is effective or even necessary. The rare neonatal death associated with generalized herpesvirus infection contrasts sharply with the rather frequent occurrence of herpetic lesions on the vulva or in the vagina. Available treatment is ineffectual.

COXSACKIE VIREMIA

Infection of the gravida with Coxsackie virus will produce only minor symptoms in the gravida. It can be fatal to the fetus, however, producing encephalomyelitis and myocarditis. Detection in the mother is very difficult and the disease is usually unsuspected. No treatment is available.

VARICELLA

Chickenpox in pregnant or puerperal women is an extreme rarity. It may be transmitted to the fetus. The disease is seldom serious, though sometimes it produces permanent scars. Varicella pneumonia, however, can occur rarely and may be fatal. There is no evidence of any harmful effects to the fetus from maternal chickenpox during pregnancy. There is no specific therapy; treatment is symptomatic.

MUMPS

Mumps in the adult may be of major import. While the testes are involved in about 28 per cent of adult males, the ovaries are much less frequently involved in females. Oophoritis may occur more often than is recognized because it is usually asymptomatic. Hyatt reviewed the literature and found that mumps during gestation can cause maternal morbidity and mortality. Abortions, stillbirths and congenital defects usually occurred when the mother had mumps in the first trimester. Congenital defects were present in slightly less than 16 per cent of 95 infants;

15 per cent of the pregnancies ended in abortion or stillbirth. There is no specific treatment, but rest in bed and symptomatic relief of pain are helpful.

SCARLET FEVER

Scarlet fever is rare among pregnant women since it is an uncommon disease in adult life. When it does occur, pregnancy is frequently interrupted during the acute eruptive process. The causative organism, *Streptococcus haemolyticus,* is extremely sensitive to antibiotics, especially penicillin, and is readily controlled. Adequate therapy will ensure a negative throat culture and an uneventful pregnancy and delivery. The scarlatinal form of puerperal sepsis is caused by the same streptococcus entering the puerperal wounds. Treatment is the same as for other streptococcal infections, namely, the use of antibiotics, such as penicillin, to which the responsible organism is usually quite sensitive.

ERYSIPELAS

Erysipelas during pregnancy is rare. The gestation proceeds unmolested when the disease is localized. However, when the infection is generalized, the uterus usually empties itself. It is exceptional for the fetus to be infected via the placenta. The umbilicus of the fetus may serve as the portal of entry of the infection during delivery. Puerperal infection of the mother may also occur by way of the birth canal.

The treatment of gravidas or puerperas is the same as that of nonpregnant persons and the same as for other hemolytic streptococcal infections. Penicillin is the preferred treatment. The neonate should not be permitted to nurse at the breast because of the danger of infection and also because the mother is frequently extremely ill.

TYPHOID FEVER

Typhoid fever in pregnant women is rare in the United States, but has a higher mortality than among the nonpregnant. The death rate among puerperal patients is still higher. Pregnancy is interrupted spontaneously in 60 to 80 per cent of gravidas with typhoid fever. The earlier in pregnancy that typhoid fever sets in, the more certainly will the gestation be interrupted. Termination of gestation does not shorten its course. Treatment consists of chloramphenicol. Better results may be obtained by giving adrenal corticosteroids at the same time.

The fetus is infected in about half the cases. In contrast to infections in the mother, it is generalized in the fetus and not merely confined to the intestines.

During epidemics of typhoid fever, many mothers were vaccinated. They stood the vaccinations well, but the children derived no benefit from them. Typhoid bacilli do not reach the mother's milk, but occasionally agglutinins are found in the milk. However, since there are so many ways in which such a mother can transmit the infection to her baby and since she is usually too ill to stand the strain of nursing, the baby should be separated from her immediately after birth. Treatment does not differ from the customary therapy for this infection. Artificial interruption of pregnancy is never indicated.

SMALLPOX

Smallpox is rare and seldom occurs in pregnant women. However, when it does, the danger is greater than it is among nonpregnant individuals. Pregnancy is spontaneously terminated in from 30 to 69 per cent of the patients and this may occur in any stage of the illness, but most frequently during the stage of eruption. The further advanced the pregnancy, the greater is the likelihood of interruption. The average fetal mortality is 45 per cent. In most instances in which the child is born healthy it remains so. Intrauterine infection is common and a child may be born pockmarked. Some fetuses acquire the disease during labor and show signs of it two weeks after birth. A few babies are born with smallpox even though the mothers had no signs of the disease. When the disease is mild, labor is usually uneventful. When it is severe, hemorrhage occurs frequently. Likewise, excessive bleeding during the puerperium is not uncommon.

During epidemics, pregnant women and their newborn babies should be vaccinated; whatever the theoretical fetal risks of the cowpox viremia secondary to the administration of the vaccine (Tucker and Sibson), they are smaller than the risks of smallpox to someone who is unprotected. Vaccination of the mother during pregnancy resulting in a positive reaction does not convey any specific immunity to the fetus. There is no specific treatment. The most frequent complications are bacterial infections that require specific antibiotic therapy.

TOXOPLASMOSIS

An asymptomatic adult disease that is transmissible to the fetus is toxoplasmosis. This protozoan disorder may seriously damage the fetus or result in abortion or premature birth. The fetus may die or be born with granulomatous lesions in the central nervous system. There are calcifications in the cerebrum, chorioretinitis, hydrocephalus or anencephaly. Surviving infants are prone to seizure disorders and mental retardation.

VIRAL HEPATITIS

Hepatitis in pregnancy may be very serious for the mother regardless of the nature of the etiologic virus. High maternal mortality has been reported from abroad; twice the number with hepatitis in pregnancy die than with hepatitis unassociated with gestation (D'Cruz et al.). Treatment in pregnancy is essentially the same as in nonpregnant patients, namely, bed rest, fluid and diet. Transmission of the virus to the fetus is uncertain, but likely because isolated cases of hepatitis in the fetus have been described.

MALARIA

Pregnancy and malaria frequently coexist in the parts of the world where malaria is endemic. Its deleterious influence on pregnancy is shown by the fact that about 40 per cent of the pregnancies are interrupted. Pregnancy may cause latent infections to relapse. This is more common late in pregnancy, during labor and the puerperium. Most women with a recent infection will go to term under proper treatment, but when the malaria is severe the prognosis is bad for both the mother and the fetus.

Labor may be difficult because it is prolonged in exhausted women, and postpartum hemorrhage is common owing to atony of the uterus. The maternal and infant mortality is high. Chloroquine, amodiaquine and primaquine may be administered with safety to pregnant women.

TETANUS

Tetanus is one of the most serious complications, and perhaps postabortal and puerperal tetanus is the most dangerous form. During pregnancy, the period of *Clostridium tetani* incubation is shorter than in nonpregnant individuals; it varies from 4 to 21 days with an average of 9 days. This is due to the favorable absorptive processes in the puerperal uterus. The shorter the period of incubation, the more dangerous is the disease. Puerperal tetanus is especially serious because muscle spasms frequently affect the respiratory muscles and cause death from asphyxia. Tetanus occurs more often after abortion, particularly after induced abortion, than after full-term labor.

Treatment is aimed at neutralizing nonfixed toxin and preventing the elaboration of more toxin. The wound is debrided and antibiotics administered. Tetanus antitoxin must be given without delay. The usual dose is 100,000 units, half of which is given intravenously and half intramuscularly. However, a preliminary test must be made to determine whether the patient is hypersensitive to horse serum. Muscle spasm and hypertonicity must be controlled with tranquilizers, sedatives or even curariform drugs. Adequate ventilation should be maintained by tracheostomy, if necessary.

SYPHILIS

Obstetricians should constantly be on the alert for this protean disease. The actual effects on pregnancy vary with the duration of the syphilis and the success of treatment. If the patient has been successfully treated, she will bear healthy children. If the syphilis is not treated, the fetus may die and abortion occur.

Premature labor in the seventh to eighth month is characteristic of untreated syphilis. If the syphilis was contracted during the early months of pregnancy, premature labor is the rule, but if it was acquired in the later months, the fetus may escape infection as the placenta offers a relative barrier to the spirochete. Effective treatment prior to the eighteenth week of pregnancy will prevent fetal infection because the organism does not appear to cross the placenta before this time.

It is imperative to use the opportunity of antepartum care programs to detect this serious disease and to institute treatment. All obstetric patients should be screened by a sensitive serologic test when first seen. This is a legal requirement in some areas. The test becomes positive within four to six weeks after infection. Repetition of the serologic test in the third trimester is a good routine practice because it will detect infections which have occurred later. Any suspicious lesion should be studied by darkfield examination to detect the presence of *Treponema pallidum* in the primary chancre even before the blood test becomes positive.

Syphilis must be treated adequately as soon as discovered, regardless of the period of pregnancy. If treatment is instituted early, nearly all babies are born alive and healthy because early intensive therapy renders the mother noninfectious and penicillin reaches the fetus readily and in adequate amounts.

On the basis of published reports, penicillin should be universally used. Adequate dosage consists of 2.4 million units of benzathine penicillin G intramuscularly, half in each buttock, or procaine penicillin G (PAM) 4.8 million units, divided into two or three parts given intramuscularly three days apart. Penicillin treatment is seldom followed by serious reactions, but allergies must be recognized. If the patient is known to be sensitive to penicillin, either erythromycin or tetracycline can be used (erythromycin 500 mg. or tetracycline 1 gm. 4 times daily for 10 to 15 days).

The most significant advantage of penicillin therapy is that, regardless of the duration of the pregnancy, the drug is delivered to the fetus in effective amounts. Only a single course is required to protect the fetus, although cases of persistent fetal infection have been reported.

The serologic test is not a good guide to the effectiveness of treatment. The average time required for a seronegative reaction in the adequately treated mother is 245 days. Many women treated in the last half of pregnancy are still seropositive at delivery, but deliver a healthy, nonsyphilitic infant.

Penicillin must be given in full dosage as soon as the diagnosis is made. Abortions or stillbirths occurring during or soon after treatment result from failure to treat the mother soon enough rather than from ineffective or faulty therapy. It was once believed that a pregnant woman with syphilis had to be treated in every pregnancy. It is now recognized that a woman successfully treated in one pregnancy need not be treated again in subsequent pregnancies, unless reinfected.

For early congenital syphilis in the neonate the following treatment is recommended: (1) a total dose of 100,000 units of PAM or aqueous penicillin per kilogram of body weight (PAM may be given in divided doses at intervals of two to three days), or (2) a single intramuscular injection of 50,000 units of benzathine penicillin G per kilogram of body weight.

GONORRHEA

Gonococcal infections in pregnancy may be entirely silent. Routine culturing of the cervix in pregnancy will uncover these potentially serious but dormant infections. Unlike the usual form of acute gonorrhea, in which the inflammation is most pronounced in the urethra, the vulvar glands and the cervix, in the pregnant patient the gonococcus may cause an acute inflammatory process that attacks the vaginal and vulvar epithelium in addition. Profuse secretion of greenish-yellow pus results; the vulva is red and is sometimes covered with a grayish exudate or it is ulcerated or covered with pointed condylomas. The vagina is thick and granular, like a nutmeg grater, and bleeds even on light touch. The cervix is swollen, vascular and eroded, and emits a foul mucopus in which the gonococci are readily found.

Chronic infection is the form generally encountered and it is usually localized in the urethra, Skene's tubules, the Bartholin ducts and glands and the cervix. As a rule the gonorrheal infection remains latent until after delivery, when gonorrheal endometritis, salpingitis, oophoritis and pelvic peritonitis may occur. Gonococcal ophthalmia of the neonate will occur if appropriate prophylactic measures are not used (see Chapter 67).

In acute cases smears are dependable, but in chronic cases smears alone are of little value. The diagnosis usually requires culture. The history is valuable. An obstinately inflamed single distal extremity joint is strongly suggestive. Ophthalmia in the infant does not prove the existence of gonorrhea in the mother unless the gonococcus is found in the pus, and other sources of infection of the child's eyes are eliminated.

In acute cases rest in bed is important.

Sexual intercourse must be forbidden. The drug of choice for the treatment of gonorrhea is penicillin. Aqueous procaine penicillin G, 4.8 million units intramuscularly, is divided into two doses of 2.4 million units and given in each buttock. This is effective against all but the most resistant strains. If sensitive to penicillin, the patient should be given tetracycline 1.5 gm. orally and then 0.5 gm. every four to six hours for four days to a total of 9.0 gm. Since tetracycline may affect bone growth and discolor the teeth anlage of the fetus in late pregnancy, it should not be used unless essential. Cephaloridine, kanamycin and erythromycin have also been shown to be effective.

Retreatment is indicated if the discharge in uncomplicated gonorrhea persists for three days or more after initial adequate therapy or if smears or cultures are still positive. The retreatment dose is twice that of the initial dose. This double total dose may be given as a single injection or as equally divided injections over a period of three to five days, or until signs and symptoms have subsided and smears and cultures are negative.

Smears and cultures should be taken at intervals of 28 days to be certain that a cure persists. If gonococci reappear, treatment must be repeated. During labor, in cases of known, untreated or resistant gonorrhea, vaginal explorations and operations should be limited to an irreducible minimum. Immediately after the baby is born, silver nitrate must be instilled into its eyes, and repeated on the second and third days. Subsequently, the baby should be given penicillin.

REFERENCES

Baer, J. L., and Reis, R. A.: Breast infections. Surg. Gynec. Obstet. 32:353, 1921.

Brody, J. A., Sever, J. L., and Schiff, G. M.: Prevention of rubella by gamma globulin during an epidemic in Barrow, Alaska, in 1964. New Eng. J. Med. 272:127, 1965.

Cohen, P., Schneck, H., and Dubow, E.: Prenatal multiple immunization. J. Pediat. 38:696, 1951.

D'Cruz, I. A., Balani, S. G., and Iyer, L. S.: Infectious hepatitis in pregnancy. Obstet. Gynec. 31:449, 1968.

Freeman, D. W., and Barno, A.: Deaths from Asian influenza associated with pregnancy. Amer. J. Obstet. Gynec. 78:1172, 1959.

Gregg, N. M.: Congenital cataract following German measles in mother. Trans. Ophthal. Soc. Aust. 3:35, 1942.

Harris, J. W.: Influenza occurring in pregnant

women: A statistical study of thirteen hundred and fifty cases. J.A.M.A. 72:978, 1919.

Hyatt, H. W., Sr.: Relationship of maternal mumps to congenital defects and fetal deaths, and to maternal morbidity and mortality. Amer. Pract. Digest Treat. 12:359, 1961.

Ingalls, T. H.: German measles (1900–1960): Risks for the fetus. Arch. Environ. Health 5:576, 1962.

Kaye, B. M., and Reaney, B. V.: Virus diseases in pregnancy: Prevention and fetal effects. Obstet. Gynec. 19:618, 1962.

Lundström, R., Thoren, C., and Blomquist, B.: Gamma globulin against rubella in pregnancy II. Manifest maternal rubella in early pregnancy treated with convalescent gamma globulin: A follow-up study. Acta Paediat. 50:453, 1961.

Monif, G. R. G.: Viral Infections of the Human Fetus.

New York, The Macmillan Company, 1969.

Sever, J. L.: Viral teratogens: A status report. Hosp. Pract. 75, 1970.

Siegel, M., and Greenberg, M.: Fetal death, malformation and prematurity after maternal rubella: Results of prospective study, 1949–1958. New Eng. J. Med. 262:389, 1960.

Tucker, S. M., and Sibson, D. E.: Foetal complication of vaccination in pregnancy. Brit. Med. J. 2:237, 1962.

Vaheri, A., Vesikari, T., Oker-Blom, N., Seppala, M., Parkman, P. D., Veronelli, J., and Robbins, F. C.: Isolation of attenuated rubella-vaccine virus from human products of conception and uterine cervix. New Eng. J. Med. 286:1071, 1972.

Whitehouse, W. L.: Rubella before conception as a cause of foetal abnormality. Lancet 1:139, 1963.

Chapter 41

Cardiovascular Disorders

PREGNANCY CHANGES

Normal pregnancy is accompanied by significant alterations in circulatory physiology. A knowledge of these changes is essential for management of pregnancy complicated by heart disease.

The heart rate begins to rise between the eighth and tenth week, gradually increases to a maximal level of about 10 beats per minute more than prepregnancy rates during the thirty-fourth to thirty-sixth week, and subsequently returns toward normal at term.

Oxygen consumption begins to rise about the second month and increases progressively, reaching a value between 10 and 20 per cent above normal at term. The rise is due primarily to fetal metabolic demands superimposed on the increased needs inherent in increased maternal tissue masses, including uterus and breasts.

The arteriovenous oxygen difference begins to decrease about the eighth week, falls to an average of 3.4 volumes per cent during the fourteenth to thirtieth weeks, and increases subsequently to normal at term.

The mean blood pressure tends to decrease, especially in the second trimester. It rises back to prepregnancy levels in the third trimester. It is not at all unusual for patients with hypertension to become essentially normotensive during the midtrimester. There is a disproportionate fall in the diastolic level, which may produce capillary pulsation. The peripheral resistance begins to fall in the first trimester, reaches its lowest value between the fourteenth and the twenty-fourth week, and rises progressively to normal levels at term.

Venous pressure in the upper extremities remains fairly constant, although there is a tendency for a slight decrease in the second half of pregnancy. Venous pressure in the lower extremities rises progressively, beginning about the twelfth week, and the term value may reach a level as high as 10 to 20 cm. of water above normal when measured while the patient is in the supine position. This rise is due primarily to pressure of the gravid uterus on the vena cava and on adjacent pelvic veins. Obstruction to venous return frequently produces hemorrhoids and varicose veins of the legs. If the pregnant patient lies on her side, the obstruction is relieved and femoral venous pressure falls.

In some otherwise normal pregnant women, the assumption of a supine position produces hypotension, tachycardia and syncope. These symptoms of the *supine hypotensive syndrome* are relieved promptly by changing to the lateral position, by sitting or standing erect, or displacing the uterus to the left off the vena cava. The syndrome is attributed to a decrease in venous return to the heart. It is encountered during the last trimester and in labor, and disappears following delivery.

Total blood volume increases during pregnancy. The rise begins about the tenth week and reaches a maximum up to 45 per cent (Pritchard) above normal during the thirty-second to thirty-fourth week, where it remains to term. The rise is due to increments in both plasma volume and red cell mass. Most investigators heretofore noted a decline in blood volume during the last four to six weeks of pregnancy; these observations are probably specious because recent evidence with measurements taken while the patients were lying on their side rather than supine showed persistence of the increased blood volume to term.

The increase in plasma volume exceeds the increase in red cell mass during pregnancy. As a consequence, there is a corresponding reduction in the erythrocyte count and in hemoglobin and hematocrit concentrations. The mean corpuscular volume, corpuscular hemoglobin and corpuscular hemoglobin concentration, color index, and appearance of erythrocytes remain unaltered during pregnancy unless coassociated with iron deficiency or other disorder.

Starting about the tenth week, the uncorrected sedimentation rate increases progressively to term. However, when correction is made for hemodilution, the rate does not begin to rise until about the twenty-fourth week. The rise is associated with changes in blood protein, especially fibrinogen and globulin. The average normal corrected sedimentation rate at term is 30 mm. per hour.

Starting about the eighth week of pregnancy, the leukocyte count increases progressively to term. A leukocytosis of 10,000 to 15,000 per cubic mm. is common during the second and third trimesters. The increase is largely due to a relative increment in neutrophiles.

The blood viscosity and circulation time decrease during pregnancy. These decreases are caused by and bear a reciprocal relation to the increase of plasma volume.

The cardiac output begins to rise about the tenth week of gestation and reaches a peak somewhere between the twenty-fifth and twenty-eighth week. Although believed to return gradually to normal at term, as indicated above when venous return is normalized by relieving the caval obstruction by the gravid uterus, cardiac output remains increased. The maximal reported values average between 30 and 40 per cent above the normal nonpregnant level. Since the rise in output is proportionately greater than the rise in pulse rate, it follows that the stroke volume is increased.

The alterations in cardiac output have been attributed to (1) increased metabolic demands of pregnancy, (2) hemodynamic effects of hypervolemia and (3) circulatory adjustments accompanying an arterio-

venous shuntlike mechanism of the placenta.

However, the increase in oxygen consumption is proportionately less than the increase in cardiac output, and the arteriovenous oxygen difference falls as the cardiac output rises. Hypervolemia undoubtedly contributes to augmented cardiac output, but plasma volume reaches a maximal level about the thirty-second week, whereas there is an earlier peak in cardiac output.

The hypothesis that the placenta functions as a modified arteriovenous fistula is supported by increased heart rate, decreased systemic diastolic pressure, decreased arteriovenous oxygen difference, presence of a continuous bruit with systolic accentuation over the placental site and higher oxygen content of venous blood leaving the uterus as compared with other mixed venous blood. The concept is supported further by the finding of decreased total peripheral vascular resistance during the second trimester.

As pregnancy advances the heart is displaced upward, forward and laterally. Roentgenograms may show the transverse diameter to be increased as much as 1 cm., and the cardiothoracic ratio may exceed 50 per cent. The apex impulse moves upward to the fourth intercostal space and laterally to or beyond the midclavicular line. Lateral and oblique x-rays may reveal the barium-filled esophagus to be encroached upon by the left atrium. Frequently, anteroposterior roentgenograms show straightening of the left border. There is, however, no conclusive evidence that the heart actually hypertrophies during pregnancy.

Auscultatory changes are common in pregnancy. There is accentuation of the first apical and second pulmonic sounds. Systolic murmurs are heard commonly over the entire precordium and split sounds may develop. Pregnancy appears to predispose to extrasystoles and to supraventricular tachycardia.

Electrocardiographic changes may be seen. As pregnancy progresses, a large Q wave may develop in Lead III and the T wave may become negative. The axis shifts to the left with advancing pregnancy, corresponding to rotation of the heart around its anteroposterior axis. There are no electrocardiographic manifestations of ventricular hypertrophy. The cardiorespiratory responses to exercise during pregnancy remain fairly constant. This has been established in normal subjects as well as in compensated cardiac patients through catheterization studies and through observations of the pulse and respiratory rates, oxygen debt and subjective symptoms.

CHANGES IN LABOR

Adams and Alexander employed the dye dilution technique to study hemodynamic changes associated with labor and found cardiac output rose 20 per cent during each uterine contraction. This increase in labor was cumulative to a moderate degree (Ueland and Hansen). During contractions pulse rate, blood pressure and left ventricular work also increased. Stroke volume, circulation time and total peripheral resistance were not altered appreciably. Changes were not seen after saddle block or caudal anesthesia, suggesting that response to pain, anxiety and muscular activity played a more important role in raising the cardiac output than any autotransfusion from the uterine sinuses into the systemic circulation with the contraction. Moreover, it is likely that the changes seen resulted from increased venous return by way of the inferior vena cava when partial obstruction is relieved as the uterus rotates forward in the abdomen during a contraction (see Chapter 14).

Sequential determinations performed in labor showed no cumulative hemodynamic effect. The cardiac output, heart rate, stroke volume and left ventricular work between contractions were unchanged by a normal first stage labor. Hendricks, using the blood pressure method to calculate cardiac output, showed that the output rose about 30 per cent during each uterine contraction. Blood pressure rose quite consistently during contractions, the systolic 10 to 20 mm. Hg and diastolic somewhat less. The heart rate and stroke volume maintained a reciprocal relationship throughout each contraction cycle. The heart rate rose during the initial phase, fell below base level at the peak of contraction and then returned to its original value. The stroke volume dropped slightly in the early phase of contraction and then rose significantly above base level before returning to its original value. Central and femoral venous pressures rose during contractions, but brachial venous pressure did not change.

Volume redistribution or the amount of uterine blood extruded during each contraction was estimated at between 250 and 300 ml. Both spontaneous and oxytocin-induced uterine contractions produced identical hemodynamic responses. Anxiety, pain and physical effort altered the findings significantly. When consistent changes were obtained with the patient supine, variable alterations ensued after shifting to the lateral position. The latter indicates the unreliability of any studies based on observations made on gravidas in the supine position. Until these investigations are verified in parturients lying on their side, theories concerning hemodynamic changes in labor should be considered at best conjectural.

When bearing down begins at the time of full cervical dilatation, these efforts reproduce the Valsalva maneuver. Normally, straining efforts should impede venous return to the heart but this may be countered somewhat by the increased venous return associated with effective uterine contractions.

The pulse and respiratory rates between contractions remain unchanged or increase (Pardee and Mendelson). Seldom does the pulse increase more than 20 beats per minute, but tachycardia is sometimes seen. Seldom do the respirations increase more than eight per minute.

Prolonged labor and a prolonged second stage enhance the possibility of increasing pulse and respiration rates. During actual delivery there is a variable increase in cardiac output and pulse rate.

McCausland and Holmes found that cerebrospinal fluid pressure increases during uterine contractions. This is undoubtedly a reflection of increased venous pressure in the azygous and vertebral venous system. Bearing-down efforts markedly increased cerebrospinal fluid pressures during uterine contractions. The highest values (more than 700 mm. water) were observed with patients in the supine position.

PUERPERAL CHANGES

In the third stage the pulse rate falls. Typically, bradycardia is encountered, sometimes to a marked degree. Pain and anxiety are alleviated and the patient is at rest. Augmented venous return is undoubtedly the primary factor involved. The rise in cardiac output that results is accompanied by an increase in left ventricular work. There is an increase in stroke volume as well (Adams).

The augmented venous return derives from expansion of plasma volume and from release of caval obstruction. A brief but significant rise in plasma volume coincides with the initial uterine contraction after the birth of the baby. Third stage blood loss is reflected over the next few hours by a decrease in plasma volume. However, the plasma volume then returns to higher than normal levels by hemodilution due to mobilization of accumulated interstitial fluids. This elevation persists for about two weeks.

Routine oxytocic agents administered at childbirth, especially ergot preparations, raise venous pressure markedly during the first 24 hours after delivery (Brown et al.). They are best avoided on a prophylactic basis.

The leukocyte count rises to an average of 14,000 to 15,000 per cubic mm. on the second postpartum day and gradually returns to normal in the next two to four weeks.

The corrected erythrocyte sedimentation rate reaches a peak averaging 37 mm. per hour the day after delivery and returns to normal within two to three weeks.

CESAREAN SECTION

Scant laboratory data are available concerning the hemodynamic changes that accompany abdominal delivery. Tatum was unable to demonstrate any immediate rise in plasma volume after emptying the uterus. There was a later rise as seen following vaginal delivery. It is possible there is no immediate rise because the uterine autotransfusion is counterbalanced by the relatively large volume of blood lost during cesarean section.

Infusions and transfusions, commonly administered during cesarean section, increase volume to the right side of the heart. Central venous pressure monitoring is important whenever this is or may be an issue in management. Postoperative complications, such as fever and abdominal distention, augment the cardiac burden associated with cesarean section.

CARDIAC BURDEN IN PREGNANCY

Pregnancy imposes a significant and predictable circulatory burden which is due mainly to increases in oxygen consumption, cardiac output and blood volume. This burden starts in the first trimester, increases progressively throughout the second trimester and persists to term. Transient rises occur during labor and immediately after delivery. A return to the normal nonpregnant hemodynamic state is achieved by the second postpartum week.

The normal pregnant woman manifests physiologic deviations which easily can be misinterpreted to indicate organic heart disease. These include changes in cardiac contour and electrocardiographic pattern, systolic murmurs, accentuated and split heart sounds, dyspnea, edema, capillary pulsation, transient basilar rales and increased venous pressure in the lower extremities.

CARDIAC DISEASE IN PREGNANCY

Heart disease is encountered in two to four per cent of pregnant women. Although at one time most heart disease in pregnant women was of rheumatic origin, the incidence of congenital heart disorders has increased over the past decade. This appears to be the result of two phenomena: First, there has been a worldwide reduction in the occurrence of rheumatic fever with widespread use of effective antistreptococcal therapy. Second, more children with congenital heart disease are being subjected to corrective surgery and are surviving to reproductive age. Thus, it becomes progressively more important for physicians to appreciate the subtle nuances of care required for gravidas with cardiac conditions heretofore rarely encountered in obstetric practices.

Functional Classification

The four classes of functional capacity, according to the criteria of the New York Heart Association, are:

Class I. Patients with cardiac disease, but without resulting limitation of physical activity. Ordinary physical activity does not cause undue fatigue, palpitation, dyspnea or anginal pain.

Class II. Patients with cardiac disease resulting in a slight limitation of physical activity. They are comfortable at rest. Ordinary physical activity results in fatigue, palpitation, dyspnea or anginal pain.

Class III. Patients with cardiac disease resulting in marked limitation of physical activity. They are comfortable at rest. Less than ordinary activity causes fatigue, palpitation, dyspnea or anginal pain.

Class IV. Patients with cardiac disease resulting in inability to carry on any physical activity without discomfort. Symptoms of cardiac insufficiency or of the anginal syndrome may be present even at rest. Discomfort is increased by any physical activity.

Therapeutic Classification

The functional capacity of the patient does not in all instances determine the amount of physical activity which should be permitted. The following therapeutic classifications are, therefore, useful:

Class A. Patients with cardiac disease whose physical activity need not be restricted. This is seldom the case in pregnancy because of the added burdens involved.

Class B. Patients with cardiac disease whose ordinary physical activity need not be restricted, but they should be advised against severe or competitive physical efforts.

Class C. Patients with cardiac disease whose ordinary physical activity should be restricted moderately and whose more strenuous effort should be discontinued.

Class D. Patients with cardiac disease whose ordinary physical activity should be restricted markedly.

Class E. Patients with cardiac disease who should be at complete rest or confined to bed or chair.

Prognosis

The mortality rate associated with heart disease in pregnancy ranges from one to five per cent. Experiences at most obstetric clinics throughout the country indicate that decompensation is the major cause of maternal death in cardiac patients, and that onset of severe failure and time of death coincide with the periods of greatest hemodynamic burden of pregnancy. The mortality in severe congestive failure is 15 per cent. There is no evidence to indicate that normal childbearing causes permanent deterioration of the cardiac status, or that childbearing shortens life expectancy, provided the patient survives each pregnancy. Outcome depends on preventing severe heart failure, the major cause of death.

Death also may result from other cardiovascular complications. These special problems include postpartum venoarterial shunt and vascular collapse, vascular accident, bacterial endocarditis and coronary occlusion.

A pregnant woman with congenital heart disease runs a risk of giving birth to a congenitally deformed infant. Antepartum maternal cyanosis is associated with small babies and with premature labor. Fetal deaths have been attributed to hypoxia associated with maternal cyanosis and with maternal paroxysmal tachycardia. Maternal heart disease by itself in the absence of congestive failure or chronic cyanosis does not affect the fetal morbidity or mortality. The incidence of spontaneous abortion and of premature labor is the same in cardiac patients as in the general gravid population. Fetal losses result primarily from antepartum death of the mother, other underlying medical conditions in the mother or from coincidental obstetric complications.

Clinical Appraisal

The functional classification of the New York Heart Association is the most important clinical guide to prognosis. Most Class I and Class II patients tolerate the hemodynamic burden of pregnancy without serious cardiac difficulty. Although only 10 to 12 per cent of the cardiac patients are in Class III and IV, this small group accounts for most of the maternal deaths.

As far as death from heart failure is concerned, less prognostic significance is attached to such factors as age, parity, multiplicity of valvular lesions, heart size and cardiac mechanism than to functional classification. Similarly, in patients with adequate cardiac reserve, chronic atrial fibrillation in rheumatic heart disease, cyanosis and polycythemia in congenital heart disease, previous coronary occlusion in hypertensive disease, and previous bacterial endocarditis in rheumatic or congenital heart disease are not by themselves necessarily incompatible with childbearing. However, these complicating features suggest a more serious problem deserving our close attention.

Experience in prior pregnancies aids in appraising cardiac reserve. Antepartum heart failure due to mitral stenosis is likely to recur in successive pregnancies. On the other hand, absence of serious cardiac insufficiency in one pregnancy does not guarantee a similar course in the ensuing one. The current functional classification is of primary significance, and due allowances must be made both for improvement (for example, following cardiac surgery) and for deterioration after the last delivery.

The value of functional classification in pregnant women has been questioned because of possible shifts in class that normally might accompany the antepartum circulatory burden. However, the responses to exercise remain fairly constant throughout pregnancy. In fact, reactions to exercise tests provide a reliable guide to functional classification, especially when the history is equivocal.

A simple test requires the patient to climb 20 stairs at a normal pace. The pulse and respiratory rates are recorded prior to the exercise, immediately after its completion and one, two and three minutes later. In normal patients and in Class I and II cardiac patients, the rates return to original levels by the last observation. Such tests should not be performed in the presence of serious incapacity, as they may precipitate pulmonary edema.

Laboratory Appraisal

Routine studies for the gravid cardiac patient include anteroposterior and lateral chest x-ray films, electrocardiogram and vital capacity test. In addition circulation time, venous pressure, exercise tolerance tests, cardiac catheterization, angiography and response to Valsalva maneuver may be required. Cardiac catheterization and angiography should be reserved for those serious problems in pregnancy that urgently require classification to ensure proper management. The procedures are not innocuous. Uterine shielding is essential to minimize radiation to the fetus.

Cardiac Catheterization. Cardiac catheterization in patients with obscure rheumatic or congenital heart disease provides a direct method of evaluating the underlying anatomic lesions and their hemodynamic significance. Except in the presence of atrial fibrillation or a history of embolism, this laboratory procedure may be performed during pregnancy if essential.

The Valsalva Maneuver. Pulmonary congestion due to alteration in mitral valvular hydraulics or left ventricular hemodynamics produces characteristic abnormal responses to the Valsalva maneuver. The initial rise in systolic blood pressure that accompanies a forced expiration persists throughout the period of straining, and the characteristic poststraining overshoot does not occur. These deviations from the normal response do not occur in dyspnea associated with obesity, in the hyperventilation syndrome or in psychogenic dyspnea.

MANAGEMENT

Heart Failure

Cardiac insufficiency manifests itself at first only when circulatory demands are increased, as with exercise. It may be absent in the resting state. As insufficiency progresses, there is further diminution in the ability of the heart to meet increased circulatory burdens. The different degrees of this ability are expressed by the cardiac functional classification (see above).

With the onset of congestive failure, there is diminishing cardiac output, circulation time is prolonged and functional changes occur in the various organs. Retention of salt and water due to impaired renal function produces hypervolemia that aggravates the congestive state. Cardiac output is normal or increased in cardiac failure associated with hyperthyroidism, beriberi, pulmonary disease and anemia.

The heart fails because of diminished efficiency of myocardial contractility. This may be caused by a defective coronary blood supply or by fatigue of the energy system due to unphysiologic volume or pressure loads. Volume loads pertain to high stroke volumes against low vascular resistance or pressure gradients. Pressure loads are created when normal or reduced stroke volumes are ejected against high resistance. The left side of the heart fails more rapidly than the right under volume loads; the right side fails more rapidly under hydrostatic pressure stress.

The clinical picture in the early stages of cardiac insufficiency may be predominantly that of left-sided or of right-sided failure, but generally, the late clinical picture is that of bilateral failure.

Primary left-sided failure is more common and occurs in mitral and in aortic valvular disease, hypertension, coronary artery disease and left-to-right intracardiac shunts due to patent ductus arteriosus or ventricular septal defect. The clinical

manifestations result from pulmonary congestion and increased pulmonary capillary pressure. Symptoms include dyspnea, orthopnea, cough and hemoptysis; there usually are pulmonary rales, accentuated pulmonary second sound and decreased vital capacity. The venous pressure is normal. Acute left-sided failure produces paroxysmal dyspnea and paroxysmal pulmonary edema.

Usually, right-sided failure follows upon left-sided failure. It occurs in pulmonary hypertension, pulmonic stenosis, cor pulmonale, myocarditis, tricuspid stenosis and constrictive pericarditis. The manifestations are due largely to engorgement and elevation of pressure in the systemic venous circuit. Signs include engorgement of the superficial veins, subcutaneous edema, enlargement and tenderness of the liver, cyanosis, ascites, hydrothorax, hydropericardium and disturbances of the gastrointestinal, urinary and nervous systems.

Heart failure, when it occurs during pregnancy, is usually left-sided and is manifested by reduced vital capacity, persistent basilar rales, prolonged circulation time, cough, hemoptysis, paroxysmal dyspnea and paroxysmal pulmonary edema.

Severe heart failure in pregnancy may be manifested by acute, fulminating pulmonary edema. The intractable nature of this complication has been responsible for many maternal deaths. It is due to sudden intensification of pulmonary congestion and a rise of pulmonary capillary pressure. The process may be initiated by a definite increase in resistance to outflow from the left cardiac chambers, sudden decrease in left ventricular or left atrial outflow or by an excessively rapid increase in venous return and right ventricular output. The hypervolemia of advancing pregnancy, coupled with increased heart rate and cardiac output predispose to pulmonary edema. Paroxysmal dyspnea and hemoptysis warn of impending pulmonary edema; these manifestations may occur suddenly.

Acute cardiac failure may develop in a pregnant patient with a previously normal heart. Augmentation of the physiologic antepartum hypervolemia beyond the capacity of the heart to handle may lead to high output failure and pulmonary edema. Acute cor pulmonale may develop with massive intraluminal or extraluminal pulmonary vascular obstruction, particularly in association with air embolism, fibrin emboli and gastric acid aspiration.

General Treatment

The general treatment of severe heart failure is the same as in the nongravid patient. It includes a regimen of digitalis, oxygen, rest, sedative, diuretic and a restricted intake of sodium and fluids. Mercurial diuretics, including mercaptomerin (Thiomerin) and meralluride (Mercuhydrin), thiazides, such as chlorothiazide (Diruil) and hydrochlorothiazide (Hydro-Diuril), as well as furosemide (Lasix) and ethacrynic acid, have proved to be effective. Continued administration may produce severe electrolyte imbalances and hyperuricemia.

Once severe heart failure has occurred during pregnancy it is advisable, in most cases, for the patient to remain under close continuous observation and treatment in the hospital until after delivery. This is important and should be stressed, even if complete recovery from the current episode of failure occurs or facilities for home supervision and care appear adequate.

Treatment of Pulmonary Edema

In pulmonary edema morphine 10 to 15 mg. is given to allay anxiety and to quiet the respiration. Aminophylline 250 to 500 mg. is administered slowly intravenously to maintain the cardiac output and to lower the venous pressure. This is especially useful if bronchospasm is present. If needed, it may be repeated at hourly intervals. To avoid cardiac arrest, it should be given slowly over a period of minutes, and injection should be discontinued immediately if the patient experiences any distress.

In undigitalized patients, rapid digitalization is induced to maintain cardiac output. Cedilanid-D may be given slowly over a one- to two-minute period starting with an initial intravenous dose of 0.8 mg.

(4 ml.); this can be followed at hourly or two-hourly intervals with additional doses of 0.2 to 0.4 mg. intravenously up to a maximum of 1.6 mg. in 24 hours. Oral digoxin maintenance therapy can be started 12 hours after the course of Cedilanid-D is completed. Antifoaming agents reduce pulmonary obstruction due to frothing of the edema fluid. The desired effect is achieved by bubbling pressurized oxygen through ethyl alcohol before the oxygen enters the tent or mask. Ethacrynic acid 25 to 50 mg. intravenously or furosemide (Lasix) 50 to 100 mg. intravenously will produce prompt and rapid diuresis in the presence of pulmonary edema, especially when there is coassociated hypervolemia. Diuresis may begin within 15 minutes after giving one of these agents and reach a maximum in one to two hours. Furosemide can then be given orally in 40 to 80 mg. amounts three to four times daily as needed. However, it is essential that electrolyte balance be strictly observed and maintained.

Venous tourniquets may be applied serially to the extremities to remove a volume of blood from the overloaded circulation. This procedure is preferable to phlebotomy, especially when anemia might aggravate the patient's condition. Occasionally, phlebotomy may be necessary if tourniquets do not achieve the desired results. Obstetric intervention has absolutely no place in the treatment of pulmonary edema.

When pulmonary edema develops as a result of hypervolemic congestion or when acute cor pulmonale develops as a result of embolism or gastric acid aspiration, the circulatory emergency is handled according to the same principles. However, recognition of the basic pathologic process is a prerequisite for definitive management. The accompanying hypotensive state may confuse the clinical picture.

This is true especially in acute cor pulmonale due to fibrin emboli complicating abruptio placentae, amniotic fluid infusion or retention of a dead fetus. In these patients excessive bleeding may result from an associated coagulation defect. Care should be exercised not to increase the cardiac embarrassment by overloading the circulation with infusions or transfusions.

The central venous pressure may be a useful guide here. Packed red cells are used for replacement, when needed, instead of whole blood.

Prevention

The prevention of severe heart failure during pregnancy requires attempts to: reduce the predictable or contributory burdens; improve the ability of the heart to withstand the expected increase in load by digitalization and, when appropriate, cardiovascular surgery; remove the cause of the predictable burden by therapeutic abortion, if desired and acceptable; and prevent future comparable or greater problems by sterilization or contraception.

Infection. Patients are carefully and repeatedly instructed to report at once any infection. Hospitalization is advised, cultures are taken as indicated and appropriate therapy is rendered. Infections of the upper respiratory tract command the greatest respect since their complications, especially bronchitis and pneumonia, are the most important contributory causes of severe heart failure in pregnancy. If difficulties arise in distinguishing signs and symptoms of pulmonary infection from those of severe heart failure, such patients should be treated for both conditions simultaneously. Infections also create special hazards of bacterial endocarditis in patients with valvulopathies. Prophylactic administration of broad spectrum antibiotics is, therefore, recommended during labor and after delivery or abortion.

Vascular Congestion. Vascular congestion is the second most common contributory cause of severe heart failure in pregnant women. It may result from excessive retention of fluids. Infusions and transfusions are avoided, if at all possible, since the augmented hypervolemia produced may lead to pulmonary edema.

It is also extremely important to limit the sodium intake. In order to supply the basic nutritional needs of pregnancy and still maintain the desired restriction of sodium, the patient should use low-sodium products. Dietary instructions should be given in detail.

Overactivity. Physical exertion is an important cause of severe heart failure. Patients whose cardiac reserve is limited should compensate for the burden of pregnancy by resting and by avoiding undue physical and emotional stresses. The therapeutic classification of the New York Heart Association (see above) is a useful guide to the amount of physical activity to be permitted.

It is advisable to hospitalize some patients in functional Class III as they approach the peak antepartum circulatory burden toward the end of the second trimester or whenever they show evidence of beginning decompensation. Complete bed rest may mobilize fluid from the lower extremities and actually precipitate failure in the presence of significant dependent edema. Care should be taken in this regard.

Arrhythmias. Tachycardia, atrial fibrillation or atrial flutter may precipitate severe failure in the presence of structural heart damage. These disorders should be diagnosed correctly and treated properly. The management of the underlying cardiac disease is the same as outlined above.

Anemia. In order to supply tissue oxygen demands in anemia, the cardiac output increases and the circulation time decreases. The resultant burden imposed on a damaged heart may lead to severe failure of the high output variety. Heart disease caused primarily by anemia is rarely encountered in pregnancy, but cardiovascular complications do occur in patients with sickle cell anemia and sickle cell–hemoglobin C disease (see Chapter 42). Decompensation may also occur when anemia aggravates other etiologic types of heart disease.

Severe failure can readily be precipitated by whole blood transfusions to pregnant cardiac patients. When profound anemia necessitates transfusions, it is prudent in severe heart disease to use packed erythrocytes rather than whole blood and to give them very slowly, watching the central venous pressure.

Obesity. Overweight may sometimes be a contributory cause of severe heart failure. Great care is necessary whenever weight reduction is considered or undertaken in pregnancy (see Chapter 10). It is usually not advisable.

Hyperthyroidism. The combined hemodynamic burdens of pregnancy and thyrotoxicosis may cause severe heart failure. Medical or combined surgical and medical regimens are available for adequate control during pregnancy. Fetal hazards of agents used should be kept in mind. Heart failure is treated in the customary fashion. Digitalis is continued if arrhythmia is present. Attempts to reestablish normal rhythm by cardioversion are deferred until the euthyroid state is reestablished.

Pulmonary Embolism. Pulmonary embolism may precipitate severe heart failure. Thromboembolic phenomena are associated with thrombophlebitis, coronary occlusion, sickle cell anemia, sickle cell–hemoglobin C disease, polycythemia, myocarditis, endocardial fibroelastosis, heart block, atrial fibrillation and bacterial endocarditis. Anticoagulant drugs are essential for prevention and treatment of thromboembolic complications (see Chapter 27).

Cardiovascular Surgery. Supportive care as outlined above suffices to carry most Class III patients safely through pregnancy. Recent experiences have demonstrated that cardiovascular surgery prior to or during pregnancy may render childbearing safer for those patients in whom the risk of severe heart failure or of vascular accident is prohibitively high. Operations can be performed during pregnancy with little more than expected risk from the surgery provided adequate oxygenation is maintained. Whenever possible, however, indicated cardiovascular surgery should be undertaken prior to childbearing.

Mitral valvotomy during pregnancy can be performed successfully (Schenker and Polishuk), although pregnancy and delivery complications can occur and puerperal deaths are reported. Similarly, patients who have valvotomy done prior to pregnancy may develop signs of congestive failure during the course of the ensuing pregnancy. The surgical procedure, therefore, cannot be considered a panacea.

Therapeutic Abortion. Supportive measures generally improve the ability of the heart to function and enable most cardiac patients to carry through pregnancy. There are patients whose cardiac status is compromised so severely that the burden of pregnancy may be excessive. One cannot expect the heart to tolerate the added gestatory burden. There are reports of deaths associated with congestive failure in such patients, even though they were managed optimally at absolute bed rest. Therapeutic abortion is, therefore, indicated for serious impairment of cardiac reserve.

Therapeutic abortion, if undertaken, should be done as early in pregnancy as possible, preferably by vacuum curage (see Chapter 35). For patients whose gestation is too far advanced to permit simple transcervical evacuation, the risks of hysterotomy may be as great, if not greater, than the risk of managing the pregnancy with supportive measures. Intrauterine hypertonic saline, on the other hand, while not innocuous, carries much less risk than hysterotomy and may be undertaken where indicated for interruption of midtrimester pregnancies.

Management of Labor and Delivery

Ideally, the cardiac patient should be hospitalized for at least a week before labor commences. This allows the physician ample time to evaluate the patient and to optimize the cardiac status. The practice of inducing labor prematurely in patients with severe heart disease is no longer acceptable. Frequently, such premature induction produces a prolonged and difficult labor. This imposes an unnecessarily great burden on the patient while at the same time imposing the risk of prematurity on the baby. Still worse results can be expected in cesarean sections done for the purpose of terminating the pregnancy of a cardiac patient prematurely. Although cesarean section may have to be done for clear-cut obstetric indications, it cannot be considered a valid procedure to do strictly for cardiac reasons (Mendelson).

Most cardiac patients will tolerate spontaneous, unstimulated term labor. The circulatory burden of labor and vaginal delivery is discontinuous and noncumulative.

There is a popular misconception that

women with severe cardiac disease have short, easy labors. Based on careful study of dilatation patterns (Friedman), it has been shown that cardiac patients actually undergo the labor progression expected for them according to conditions prevailing. Their heart condition does not appear to influence the course of labor.

Meticulous observation is mandatory during labor. One should follow pulse, blood pressure and respiratory rate, as well as maternal electrocardiogram, central venous pressure and blood gases. Periodic measurement of cardiac output and blood volume can be very helpful. Fetal monitoring is important also. Pulse rate during labor provides a valuable measure of cardiac status. In the absence of fever, a pulse rate of 110 per minute or higher between uterine contractions is very suggestive of approaching cardiac failure (Mendelson and Pardee). There is usually ample warning of impending failure so that adequate anticipatory measures can be taken to correct the problem before it becomes serious. At the same time, the likelihood of intrapartum failure is remote when the pulse rate remains below 110 per minute.

Tachycardia may or may not be associated with tachypnea, with respiratory rates exceeding 24 per minute. When tachypnea is seen alone, however, it does not necessarily signify the approach of heart failure, unless coassociated with dyspnea or moist rales in the lung fields. Cardiac patients with tachycardia in labor who have not been previously digitalized should have complete digitalis effect induced as rapidly as possible.

Such patients are allowed to labor in a comfortable position, either semirecumbent on their side or kept upright in bed. They are given oxygen by nasal catheter or face mask as indicated. As a general rule, they are delivered as soon as feasible after full cervical dilatation in order to shorten the period of bearing down in the second stage. With use of regional conduction anesthesia (see below), reflex bearing down is obtunded. Under these circumstances, it is preferable to allow descent to take place in the second stage by the forces of uterine contraction only, rather than to substitute a potentially traumatic midforceps proce-

dure ill-advisedly in an effort to shorten the second stage electively.

Of course, if there is evidence that allowing the labor to continue will jeopardize the mother or that no further progressive descent can occur without expulsive effort, midforceps procedures may have to be undertaken to effect delivery expeditiously. However, it is imperative for the obstetrician to weigh the hazards of midforceps operation under these conditions against its ostensible benefits. Prolonged straining to achieve natural childbirth is contraindicated in patients with serious heart disease.

Analgesia. The principles and practices relating to analgesia described in Chapter 21 pertain equally to cardiac patients in labor. It is important to try to reduce anxiety, reduce discomfort and maintain the patient's confidence and composure. This can be accomplished by giving adequate combinations of a narcotic-analgesic agent and a synergistic tranquilizer. Depression should be avoided. Scopolamine may cause restlessness, agitation and tachycardia; therefore, it should not be given for its amnesic effects.

Anesthesia. Inhalation agents afford a safe anesthetic technique for the delivery of cardiac patients when administered properly after adequate preanesthetic medication and in the absence of respiratory disease or a full stomach. Inhalation has the advantage of reversibility, short induction and recovery periods, predictable and constantly controllable depth and duration, feasibility of maintaining an oxygen-enriched atmosphere and adaptability to a wide range of obstetric procedures. Among its disadvantages are the possibilities of hypoxia, aspiration, acid-base imbalance and postoperative nausea or vomiting.

It is most important that anesthesia for the delivery of cardiac patients be administered by a fully competent, skilled anesthesiologist (see Chapter 22). The inherent risks and associated cardiovascular and pulmonary pathophysiology must be completely understood and he must have full knowledge of the recognition and management of all complications that may arise.

High oxygen flows should precede induction of anesthesia. Smooth and rapid induction can be accomplished with intravenous thiopental, followed by a balanced maintenance anesthesia of succinylcholine and nitrous oxide.

Regional anesthesia, particularly continuous peridural (see Chapter 22), is recommended for the total relief of pain during labor as well as for the delivery of cardiac patients. When properly given, there are no adverse effects. It can serve effectively as a substitute for all narcotic agents in labor, providing relief of pain, apprehension and anxiety. Its advantages also include elimination of the bearing-down reflex in the second stage. Hemodynamic changes are minimal (Ueland and Hansen) unless inappropriately given so as to produce hypotension.

Where even transient hypotension may be life-threatening, as in patients with severe aortic stenosis, this form of anesthesia should be avoided. Hypotension should be combated quickly as it develops by turning the patient on her side or displacing the uterus to the left off the inferior vena cava and elevating the patient's legs. Vasopressors may have to be used, although they may be harmful in patients whose cardiac function cannot accept increasing the output to any great degree. This latter is particularly the case in association with severe mitral stenosis.

Third Stage. It is advisable to ensure that blood loss is minimized in order to avoid hypovolemia and secondary circulatory strain of anemia. Ergonovine maleate as a uterotonic prophylaxis should be omitted because of its tendency to raise the venous pressure. Synthetic oxytocin can be given instead intramuscularly. Direct intravenous injection of undiluted oxytocin is dangerous in cardiac patients because it may produce hypotension.

Intravenous therapy should be limited and no large volumes administered because infusions of glucose or saline solution or plasma expanders may aggravate the cardiac burden. Packed erythrocytes are used rather than whole blood in the event of massive hemorrhage requiring transfusion. Because of the dangers of bacterial endocarditis from puerperal infection and mastitis, patients with valvular damage should be given broad spectrum antibiotics during labor and the puerperium, provided there is no known idiosyncrasy.

Intensive observation and continued care must be extended post partum, especially during the first day. Fowler's position may have to be maintained. Oxygen is administered as needed. Early ambulation is encouraged as tolerated to prevent thromboembolic complications. Routine use of anticoagulants is not advocated, but these drugs are prescribed when specifically indicated. When fully recovered, these patients should be offered sterilization.

Vascular Collapse Syndrome

In patients having anomalous communications between the two circulations, the development of pulmonic-systemic pressure imbalance associated with parturition may cause reversal of an arteriovenous shunt or augmentation of a venoarterial shunt. The volume of shunted blood is determined mainly by the size of the communicating defect and the relative pressure changes on either side of the defect. Extensive shunting produces a critical hypoxic state characterized by hypotension, tachycardia and the appearance or intensification of cyanosis. This potentially catastrophic clinical picture develops most often immediately post partum as a result of hemorrhage, but may be encountered intrapartum if systemic hypotension occurs.

In order to avoid this serious complication, hypotension must be stringently guarded against. Spinal and epidural anesthetics are withheld. Major obstetric operations are avoided whenever possible and blood loss kept at a minimum. Hemorrhage is treated quickly by replacement with transfusion of whole blood or packed erythrocytes. Rapid shifts in blood pressure levels in patients with hypertensive states are prevented or combated. Precautions are instituted to prevent the development of a right-to-left shunt through abrupt rise in venous pressure. Thus, uterotonic agents, such as ergot preparation, should not be used post partum unless there is uterine atony with hemorrhage.

Bacterial Endocarditis

Pregnancy does not specifically predispose patients with heart disease to bacterial endocarditis. Moreover, the occurrence of bacterial endocarditis during pregnancy does not alter accepted medical treatment of the infection or obstetric management of the underlying heart disease. However, the incidence of severe cardiac failure is significantly greater than that ordinarily encountered in heart disease complicating pregnancy. There is corresponding increase in maternal and fetal mortality. The indications for therapeutic abortion may be liberalized under these circumstances. This is particularly the case if the cardiac status is not stabilized after appropriately aggressive antibiotic therapy.

The prophylactic use of antibiotics during labor and for several days after delivery or abortion may prevent the development or recurrence of bacterial endocarditis in patients with valvular damage. It is appropriate to obtain blood cultures on all gravidas with heart disease who develop fever prior to instituting such an antibiotic regimen.

Coronary Artery Disease

Coronary artery disease is an extremely rare but very serious complication of pregnancy. It occurs most often in older gravidas who have hypertension, cardiovascular syphilis or diabetes. However, it may sometimes be encountered in younger, apparently normal women. The advisability of pregnancy in patients with coronary artery disease depends mainly on cardiac functional classification (see above). Pregnancy can be undertaken successfully after previous myocardial infarction, provided the patient has recovered without residual manifestations. Significant functional incapacity justifies therapeutic abortion.

Myocardial infarction can be recognized during pregnancy, and must be differentiated from dissecting aneurysm of the aorta, pulmonary infarction and myocarditis. The treatment of coronary occlusion in pregnancy is the same as in nonpreg-

nant patients. Anticoagulants may be given and heart failure is treated in the usual manner. Neither coronary artery disease nor myocardial infarction is a valid indication for operative obstetric intervention. Any form of surgery is undertaken with considerable risk, but these conditions are not absolute contraindications to surgery when it is clearly required for obstetric complications. Elective procedures should be postponed as long as possible after an acute myocardial infarction.

Uncomplicated labor does not appear to create special risks. Appropriate shortening of second stage bearing-down efforts is advocated. Conduction anesthesia is especially useful for managing labor and delivery, but hypotension must be prevented. Hypoxia is avoided if general anesthesia is employed.

Precordial pain is frequent during the antepartum period and may be due to a variety of extracardiac causes. Gastric hyperacidity, pylorospasm and hiatus hernia are common sources of angina-like discomfort, especially in the last trimester. Electrocardiographic studies are recommended to establish the correct diagnosis. Due consideration should be given to physiologic Q waves and T-wave inversions that accompany normal gestation.

Cor Pulmonale

Acute cor pulmonale in pregnancy is due most often to overloading of the circulation and to massive pulmonary vascular obstruction. Hypervolemia is usually the result of giving large amounts of fluids intravenously to patients suffering from water retention. Pulmonary vascular obstruction may result from embolism originating in a thrombus of the systemic veins or the right side of the heart, or from intravascular coagulation secondary to amniotic fluid or fibrin embolism. Aspiration of liquid gastric contents results in extraluminal pulmonary vascular obstruction from an intense peribronchiolar congestive and exudative reaction.

Chronic cor pulmonale is due primarily to ventilatory or pulmonary vascular defects. Dyspnea, accentuation of the pulmonic second sound, changes in cardiac contour, hypervolemia and increased cardiac output may all be seen in otherwise normal gravidas. They are sometimes so severe that they can simulate chronic cor pulmonale. Cardiac catheterization may be required for verification.

Limitation of functional reserve does not necessarily imply that heart disease is present, because dyspnea and impaired vital capacity may be due to pulmonary disease rather than to actual cardiac insufficiency. Patients who exhibit severe heart failure, marked pulmonary hypertension or arterial oxygen desaturation should be advised against childbearing. Therapeutic abortion is recommended in early pregnancy.

Kyphoscoliotic Heart Disease

Kyphoscoliotic gravidas with good cardiorespiratory reserve tolerate the hemodynamic burden of pregnancy without difficulty. However, kyphoscoliosis can be associated with severe cardiopulmonary embarrassment. Maternal prognosis cannot be determined strictly on the basis of functional capacity. Moderate dyspnea, impaired vital capacity and persistent basilar rales may result from pulmonary restriction alone due to rib cage distortion. They do not signify that the heart is involved or that a dire outcome is inevitable.

If dyspnea is marked and the vital capacity falls below 1000 ml., especially when accompanied by cyanosis, polycythemia or pulmonary hypertension, there is a significant risk of severe heart failure and death. This risk is aggravated as pregnancy progresses because the expanding uterus encroaches progressively on the thorax. The initial episode of decompensation may develop with peak circulatory loads at term or in labor.

Therefore, patients with impairment of cardiac reserve are advised against childbearing. Therapeutic abortion is recommended early in pregnancy. Intervention may be considered at any time if the cardiac status deteriorates progressively in spite of a strict supportive regimen. However, operative interference cannot be undertaken in severe heart failure.

Labor and delivery present other spe-cific problems in kyphoscoliosis. Lesions of the upper part of the spine cause compensatory lordosis, but do not affect the pelvis. However, involvement of the lower part of the lumbar spine produces distortions or anthropoid changes in pelvic architecture (see Chapter 62).

During the latter part of pregnancy, limited space in the abdominal cavity causes the expanding gravid uterus to be displaced anteriorly, creating a pendulous abdomen in which the fundal contents may lie at a lower level than the presenting part. Angulation of the uterine axis impairs the efficiency of contractions. Use of an abdominal binder may help to correct this faulty alignment. However, the resulting constriction may aggravate intrapartum cardiorespiratory distress.

Usually, dystocia can be predicted at term or at the onset of labor if the abdomen is markedly pendulous and the presenting part is unengaged. Cardiac strain and obstetric difficulty accompanying parturition may cause maternal decompensation and compromise the fetus. Fetal mortality in kyphoscoliotic dystocia is 12 per cent in association with hypoxia, acidosis and birth trauma. Therefore, cesarean section should be considered for delivery in the presence of pelvic distortion sufficient to cause dystocia.

If allowed to labor, the patient should be managed carefully to prevent decompensation. Maintenance of a high Fowler's position may be necessary throughout labor, delivery and the immediate postpartum period. Oxygen is indicated for relief of maternal hypoxia, but prolonged oxygen therapy and sedatives require great caution because kyphoscoliotic patients may have carbon dioxide retention and secondary depression of the respiratory center. Heart failure is treated with conventional measures. The second stage of labor is shortened appropriately. Regional block is advocated for delivery to avoid the respiratory complications which are more likely to occur with inhalation anesthesia.

Compatible blood is kept available to be used in the event of hemorrhage. Care is exercised not to overload the circulation if transfusion becomes necessary. Packed erythrocytes are used rather than whole blood if chronic cor pulmonale exists. Patients with evidence of severe heart failure during pregnancy should be advised against future childbearing. The uterine tubes can be ligated at the time of cesarean section, if section is done. If the patient is delivered vaginally, interval sterilization or effective long-term contraception is advisable.

Myocarditis

Idiopathic myocarditis is a serious complication of pregnancy because it can cause congestive heart failure, embolism and death. It should be suspected whenever cardiac decompensation, especially the right-sided variety, cannot be accounted for on the basis of other documented heart disease. Shock and chest pain may confuse the diagnosis with that of coronary occlusion, pulmonary infarction or dissecting aneurysm of the aorta. If hypotension is dominant, the clinical picture may suggest concealed hemorrhage. The majority of cases have been reported in southern black puerperas.

Acute myocarditis superimposed on the circulatory burden of pregnancy may lead to intractable cardiac failure. Right-sided congestive manifestations may dominate the picture in contrast to most other types of heart disease which tend to produce left-sided failure in pregnancy. The prognosis is more favorable with puerperal onset of the disease because congestive failure is not aggravated by pregnancy changes. It tends to be less severe and to disappear gradually. Complete recovery is usual in the absence of thromboembolic complications.

In early pregnancy complicated by active myocarditis, therapeutic abortion is justified. It is contraindicated in the presence of severe heart failure, however. Treatment of myocarditis in pregnancy or post partum is largely supportive with specific measures aimed at combating the complications of congestive failure and thromboembolism.

Cardiac Arrest

Cardiac arrest refers to sudden ventricular standstill or ventricular fibrillation. In neither of these does the heart expel blood; thus, the circulation is completely arrested. Cardiac arrest may occur (1) in Adams-Stokes disease, (2) during reflex vagal stimulation, (3) during treatment with cardioactive drugs, (4) after myocardial infarction and (5) during various diagnostic and therapeutic procedures.

Cardiac arrest occurs most often in association with anesthesia. The complication is estimated to develop in one of every 2000 anesthetized patients. The incidence is highest in older patients, those in poor physical condition and in those with underlying heart disease. The pathogenesis of cardiac arrest is not always clear, but the major contributory factors include hypoxia, hypercapnia, hyperkalemia, deepening and mismanagement of anesthesia and reflex phenomena.

The actual incidence of cardiac arrest in obstetric patients is not known. The pregnant woman has a predisposition to certain disorders of the heartbeat perhaps with increased myocardial irritability; she is also subject to reflex phenomena associated with pregnancy, labor and delivery. Anesthetic complications may arise, such as hypoxia and aspiration with inhalation methods, hypotension with regional blocks and accidental intravenous injection of local agents. Postpartum hemorrhage and fibrin embolization create additional hazards related to cardiac arrest.

Most general anesthetics are capable of producing some degree of hypoxia or coronary ischemia. Cyclopropane, chloroform and trichloroethylene may increase cardiac irritability and sensitize the heart to epinephrine. Arrhythmias and cardiac arrest with anesthesia tend to be especially associated with hypoxia and hypercarbia. The recovery rate in cardiac arrest has risen considerably over the years. Immediate diagnosis is a prerequisite for survival since irreversible brain damage begins to develop in four to six minutes unless treatment is begun promptly.

Patients with cardiac arrest may be resuscitated by external cardiac massage combined with artificial ventilation. Compression of the heart between the sternum and thoracic vertebral column is safe and simple. Open thoracotomy and direct heart massage restore circulation, but this method requires special expertise and equipment. Artificial respiration is given simultaneously with cardiac massage to assure adequate ventilation. Two individuals are needed as a minimum. An electrocardiogram should be obtained as soon as possible to determine the type and progress of arrest.

As soon as the diagnosis of cardiac arrest is made, the physician should strike the sternal region with a sharp blow. This often starts the heart beating again immediately. If unsuccessful, there should be no delay in proceeding as follows: The time of arrest is noted and help is summoned. The patient is ventilated by any means available. This usually consists of mouth-to-mouth resuscitation at a rate of 12 inflations per minute (once every five seconds). The patient is placed on a firm surface for cardiac massage. The physician places the heel of one hand on the sternum just above the xiphoid, with the fingers extended at right angles to the sternum. The other hand is placed atop the first. Then, using body weight, he thrusts the sternum vertically downward with a pressure of 80 to 100 pounds using only the heel of the hand. The sternum can easily be depressed 4 to 5 cm., and the resulting compression of the heart forces blood into the systemic and pulmonary circulations. Then the pressure is relaxed completely, the thoracic cage expands and the heart refills. With a compression rate of about 60 to 80 per minute, a systolic pressure of more than 200 mm. Hg is frequently obtained. Peripheral diastolic pressure is always low, 30 to 50 mm. Hg. One should not stop for more than five seconds for other procedures. Ventilation should be synchronized so that there is one deep breath for every five cardiac compressions.

If cardiac action is not restored within two minutes, 0.5 mg. epinephrine is given by the intracardiac route into the left ventricle and repeated, if needed, every five minutes. A metaraminol (Aramine) drip is started in a large-bore venous cutdown. Endotracheal intubation is done and pure oxygen ventilation assistance begun. Calcium chloride 0.5 to 1 gm. is administered into the heart and repeated intravenously at intervals of 5 to 10 minutes. Sodium bicarbonate is given to correct metabolic acidosis in 50 ml. (3.75 gm. or 44.6 mEq.) doses every 5 to 10 minutes. Decompression of the stomach with a nasogastric tube is useful to relieve distention resulting from the artificial ventilation.

External defibrillation is done if the heartbeat does not begin within five to six minutes of massage and drug therapy. Defibrillation is safe even if electrocardiographic evidence of fibrillation is lacking. Electrode plates are placed inferior to the medial third of the right clavicle and over the apex of the heart. The plates and skin sites are lubricated with electrode jelly and firm pressure is applied. Electrical countershock (100 to 400 watt seconds) is given and external massage resumed. Two or three shocks may be needed. Intracardiac procaine 250 mg. may reduce irritability and aid in defibrillation.

Postresuscitation measures consist of appropriate supportive therapy and close monitoring of the electrocardiogram, central venous and arterial blood pressures for at least 72 hours. An intensive care facility is essential, if available. Arterial blood gases should be followed as well as electrolytes and urea nitrogen. Urinary output is monitored as a measure of tissue perfusion. Central nervous system damage may be combated by hypothermia, and convulsions controlled with intravenous amobarbitol. Care must be instituted for cardiovascular decompensation as needed.

REFERENCES

Adams, J. Q.: Cardiovascular physiology in normal pregnancy: Studies with the dye dilution technique. Amer. J. Obstet. Gynec. 67:741, 1954.

Adams, J. Q., and Alexander, A. M.: Alterations in cardiovascular physiology during labor. Obstet. Gynec. 12:542, 1958.

Brown, E., Sampson, J. J., Wheeler, E. O., Gundelfinger, B. F., and Giansiracusa, J. E.: Physiologic changes in the circulation during and after obstetric labor. Amer. Heart J. 34:311, 1947.

Friedman, E. A.: Labor: Clinical Evaluation and Management. New York, Appleton-Century-Crofts, 1967.

Hendricks, C. H.: The hemodynamics of a uterine contraction. Amer. J. Obstet. Gynec. 76:969, 1958.

McCausland, A. M., and Holmes, F.: Spinal fluid

pressure during labor: Preliminary report. West. J. Surg. *65*:220, 1957.

Mendelson, C. L.: Cardiac Disease in Pregnancy: Medical Care, Cardiovascular Surgery, and Obstetric Management as Related to Maternal and Fetal Welfare. Philadelphia, F. A. Davis Company, 1960.

Mendelson C. L., and Pardee, H. E. B.: The pulse and respiratory variations during labor as a guide to the onset of cardiac failure in women with rheumatic heart disease. Amer. J. Obstet. Gynec. *44*:370, 1942.

New York Heart Association: Nomenclature and Criteria for Diagnosis of Diseases of the Heart and Blood Vessels, ed. 5. New York, Peter F. Mallon, Inc., 1953.

Pardee, H. E. B., and Mendelson, C. L.: The pulse and respiratory variations in normal women during labor Amer. J. Obstet. Gynec. *41*:36, 1941.

Pritchard, J. A.: Changes in blood volume during pregnancy and delivery. Anesthesiology *26*:393, 1965.

Schenker, K. G., and Polishuk, W. Z.: Pregnancy following mitral valvotomy. Obstet. Gynec. *32*:214, 1968.

Tatum, H. J.: Blood volume variation during labor and the early puerperium. Amer. J. Obstet. Gynec. *66*:27, 1953.

Ueland, K., and Hansen, J. M.: Maternal cardiovascular dynamics: II. Posture and uterine contractions. Amer. J. Obstet. Gynec. *103*:1, 1969.

Ueland, K., and Hansen, J. M.: Maternal cardiovascular dynamics: III. Labor and delivery under local and caudal analgesia. Amer. J. Obstet. Gynec. *103*:8, 1969.

Chapter 42

Diseases of the Blood

ANEMIAS

The anemia most frequently encountered during pregnancy is iron deficiency anemia. Much less often one finds megaloblastic anemia and sickle cell anemia. Anemia is rarely a serious complication of pregnancy but its recognition, diagnosis and treatment are important to the well-being of the pregnant woman. The incidence of anemia in pregnancy ranges from 10 to 75 per cent, depending on the criteria used for diagnosis and the nutritional and socioeconomic status of the patients (Holly). The incidence is greatest among gravidas who are poorly nourished and who do not receive adequate prenatal care.

Iron Deficiency Anemia

At least 95 per cent of pregnancy anemia is caused by a deficiency of iron. The responsible constellation of factors generally precedes the pregnancy, including a diet poor in iron content coupled with menstrual losses and a rapid succession of pregnancies in which supplemental iron was not provided. Nutritional aspects of iron deficiency are discussed in Chapter 10. Most women begin their pregnancy with partially or completely depleted iron reserves. This is the case even though the hemoglobin concentration and hematocrit may be normal. The demand for iron created by the fetus and the maternal needs of pregnancy is sufficient to produce anemia. The severity of the anemia is inversely related to the amount of iron reserves.

The total quantity of body iron in the normal adult is 3500 to 4000 mg. Approximately 70 per cent of this is contained in the mass of circulating hemoglobin. About 25 per cent is stored as ferritin in the bone marrow, spleen and liver. The remainder is contained in myoglobin and oxidative enzymes. Regulation of body iron is a function of the absorptive process. Usually, the amount absorbed from the ingested food equals the amount excreted. This totals about 1 mg. each day to provide a balance. More iron can be absorbed in pregnancy and in the presence of iron deficiency, but this amount probably cannot exceed 5 to 10 mg. daily.

Iron is transported in the plasma bound to a β_1-globulin known as transferrin. Between 25 and 40 mg. of iron are involved daily in the synthesis and degradation of hemoglobin. Storage iron can be mobilized for hemoglobin synthesis or cellular metabolism if needed. Iron is stored only when intake is greater than metabolic requirements.

Hematologic values for nonpregnant women apply equally to pregnant women. A hemoglobin concentration of 10 gm. per 100 ml. and a hematocrit of 30 per cent or less are generally accepted as indicative of the presence of anemia significant enough to warrant evaluation and treatment. Diagnosis of iron deficiency can be established by determination of serum level and the study of a blood smear. There will be evidence of hypochromia and microcytosis. A serum iron concentration below 60 μg. per 100 ml. is indicative of iron deficiency. Confirmation will be seen by the patient's response to iron. A more complete diagnostic survey is required if the anemia is severe, if the serum iron is in the normal range or if the anemia fails to respond to iron medication.

Rx:

The treatment of iron deficiency anemia consists of administration of iron. Because it is simple and inexpensive, oral administration of a ferrous salt is preferred. It should be given three times a day to reduce the incidence of gastrointestinal symptoms and to provide 100 to 150 mg. of elemental iron daily. Ferrous sulfate or ferrous gluconate is equally effective.

6-12 mos.

The duration of oral iron therapy should be calculated to provide sufficient iron for hemoglobin regeneration and for storage. This usually means continuous treatment during pregnancy and for 6 to 12 months after delivery. It is not enough to treat only until the hemoglobin concentration returns to normal because, as stated above, iron is not stored until the normal metabolic requirements are fulfilled.

Parenterally administered iron is indicated when iron deficiency exists in a patient who does not tolerate medication orally or when the anemia is diagnosed too near term for orally administered iron to be effective. In general it is stated that 250 mg. of iron-dextran is needed for each gram per 100 ml. of hemoglobin deficiency recorded. Actually, a parenteral dose of about 100 mg. will raise hemoglobin 1 gm. per 100 ml. in the average sized female, but an additional 500 mg. is needed to replenish storage iron.

Iron-dextran (Imferon) can be safely given in 5 ml. doses (250 mg.) into each buttock. A Z-track method of injection should be employed to prevent staining. This consists of drawing the skin laterally before injecting so that the needle track through the skin does not override the injection site in the muscle. Repeated injections may be used at intervals of two to four weeks until the total required dose has been administered. If iron-dextran is to be administered intravenously, a small gauge needle limits the speed of injection and reduces the incidence of side effects, such as facial flushing, substernal pain or headache. If side effects do appear, the injection should be discontinued at once.

A gradual and progressive response should be anticipated to oral iron. On the other hand, hemoglobin regeneration is more rapid after parenteral iron.

Use of whole blood transfusions for the treatment of iron deficiency in the course of pregnancy cannot be condoned. It is a dangerous practice because of the risks of hepatitis and provides relatively little iron to the pool of body iron. The one exception is to correct a severe anemia during labor in anticipation of possible acute blood loss at the time of delivery.

Megaloblastic Anemia

Megaloblastic anemia is a rare complication of pregnancy in the United States. It is more common in association with poor nutrition (see Chapter 10) and sepsis. The usual causes include folic acid deficiencies in the diet or a defect in the metabolism of nucleic acid which in turn can be produced by any condition that interferes with the normal conversion of folic acid to folinic acid. The bone marrow pattern is changed from normoblastic to megaloblastic development.

Megaloblastic anemia may develop rapidly late in pregnancy or in the puerperium. Extreme hemoglobin deficiencies may occur with levels of 3 to 5 gm. per 100 ml. Diagnosis can be verified by examining the bone marrow to show the abnormal megaloblasts. Erythrocytosis depends on the duration of the anemia and the extent to which megaloblastic change has occurred in the bone marrow. Other significant laboratory findings include leukopenia and thrombocytopenia. There may be a concomitant increase in the plasma iron concentration.

The treatment of megaloblastic anemia consists of administration of folic acid. The usual dose is 1 mg. daily by mouth. Response is often dramatic and reticulocytosis should be seen in four to five days. Whole blood transfusions are seldom required unless the anemia is first uncovered in labor. Iron is given simultaneously to ensure maximal hematopoietic regeneration because the synthesis of hemoglobin is rapid and there is often a coexistent iron deficiency.

Acquired Hemolytic Anemia

Patients with Coombs-positive idiopathic hemolytic anemia in pregnancy are characterized by rapid red cell destruction due to foreshortening of the life span of circulating erythrocytes by autoimmune hemolysins. They can be treated effectively with corticosteroids; these agents are equally effective in the nonpregnant and the pregnant states. Splenectomy may be required for those unresponsive to treatment. These patients should be advised against undergoing additional pregnancies.

Deficiency of glucose-6-phosphate dehydrogenase is an inherited enzymatic defect which is seen in severe form in about two per cent of black women and in a milder form in an additional 10 to 15 per cent. This disorder is inherited as an X-linked trait. It becomes manifest by hemolytic episodes precipitated by infections and various oxidative drugs, including aspirin, phenacetin or other analgesics and antipyretics, as well as sulfonamides, nitrofurantoin, quinine and primaquine. Correcting the infection or discontinuing the offensive agent will allow the resulting anemia to correct itself, provided there is no concomitant iron deficiency or toxic marrow depression.

Sickle Cell Anemia

Sickle cell anemia and related hemoglobinopathies result from genetically determined abnormal hemoglobins. Erythrocytes containing these hemoglobins have markedly foreshortened life spans. With decreased oxygen tension, sickling deformity of the red cell occurs. This in turn increases blood viscosity and leads to stasis, agglutination, thrombosis, tissue hypoxia, perivascular hemorrhage and even necrosis.

Abnormal variants of the hemoglobin molecule include hemoglobins S and C. Hemoglobin S is found in sickle cell trait (SA), sickle cell anemia (SS) and sickle thalassemia. Hemoglobin C is found in sickle cell–hemoglobin C disease (SC) and homozygous hemoglobin C disease (CC).

These various types of hemoglobin can be identified by plasma electrophoresis. All of the hemoglobin types are inherited as mendelian dominant traits; S and C types are inherited as alleles. Hemoglobins S and C occur predominantly in black patients; about 8 to 10 per cent of black gravidas have the trait (SA). Hemoglobin S can be detected with a sickle cell preparation using sodium metabisulfite. The characteristic sickle deformation of the red blood cells is demonstrated *in vitro* by this method. Recently instituted programs for routine screening will undoubtedly uncover many affected patients and benefit them substantially.

Persons with the sickle cell trait (SA) only have no clinical manifestations and often are unrecognized. Sickle cell disease (SS), hemoglobin SC disease, sickle thalassemia and homozygous hemoglobin C disease (CC) all produce anemia, sometimes of profound significance. Sickle thalassemia and homozygous hemoglobin C disease resemble sickle cell anemia in their manifestations, but are usually milder. Hemoglobin SC disease tends to be much more severe; it is characterized by anemia and recurrent bouts of pulmonary infarction and bone pain. Sickle cell anemia is characterized by chronic anemia, frequent infections and abdominal crises. Both SC and SS diseases are associated with as many as 50 per cent fetal losses. It is also possible that fetuses of mothers with sickle cell trait only may be at risk from hypoxic stress (Platt).

Treatment during pregnancy should consist of whole blood or packed red cell transfusions at term or in labor to protect the patient during labor and delivery. Supportive measures should be used during a hemolytic crisis. Oxygen therapy may alleviate symptoms during crises. Rapidly falling hemoglobin is an indication of acute sequestration of sickled cells in liver, spleen and bone marrow. This results in enlarging liver and spleen and the appearance of bone pain in these patients.

There is little justification for raising the

patient's hemoglobin concentration above the level that she normally maintains (which is usually at or above 7 gm. per 100 ml.) except at the time of the delivery. Partial exchange transfusions (Ricks) may prove a valuable therapeutic measure in due course. They avoid circulatory overload, provide nonsickling circulating donor cells with normal life span and diminish the possibility of transfusion hemosiderosis.

Folic acid needs are increased during crises and recovery, so that supplementation is essential. However, these patients tend to have adequate iron stores. Although iron deficiency anemia can occur, iron should not be given unless clearly needed so as to avoid hemosiderosis.

Sterilization is advisable in patients with severe forms of sickle cell disease so that they may avoid the hazards of subsequent pregnancies and possibly prolong their lives.

Anemia of Infection

Although anemia of infection resembles iron deficiency anemia, treatment with iron is ineffectual. Storage iron is not depleted. The anemia is chronic and refractory to treatment. It appears to result from decreased erythropoiesis primarily; infection somehow interferes with hemoglobin synthesis. Any chronic infection may produce the anemia, but urinary tract infection is the most frequently encountered problem (and simultaneously the most common infection occurring in pregnancy).

Hemoglobin, hematocrit and plasma iron concentration are decreased. The erythrocytes are microcytic and hypochromic. The diagnosis requires recognition of a chronic infection in a patient with an anemia resistant to iron medication. Iron stores can be demonstrated to be present in the bone marrow.

Treatment should be directed primarily at eliminating the infection by the use of appropriate antibiotics. Iron should be administered at the same time to ensure an adequate supply for hemoglobin regeneration.

COAGULOPATHY

During normal pregnancy the concentration of plasma fibrinogen rises and preconvertin activity may increase slightly. Neither of these changes is significant insofar as the well-being of the pregnant patient is concerned.

The most important clinical aids in suggesting the presence of defects in coagulation are bleeding problems manifested by easy bruising, epistaxis or menorrhagia. Any coagulation defect may complicate pregnancy, but thrombocytopenic purpura and fibrinogenopenia are the most important.

Thrombocytopenic Purpura

Thrombocytopenic purpura may be idiopathic or secondary to drugs or sensitization. It may also be associated with acquired hemolytic anemias (see above) or fibrinogenopenic states (see below). The idiopathic variety results from the development of platelet agglutinins in the blood. The criteria for the diagnosis of thrombocytopenic purpura include (1) purpuric skin lesions, (2) positive tourniquet test showing increased capillary fragility, (3) platelet count below 100,000 per cubic ml., (4) prolongation of bleeding, clot retraction and prothrombin consumption times and (5) increased numbers of megakaryocytes in the bone marrow.

The plasma agglutinin readily passes the placental barrier so that the fetus acquires a transient thrombocytopenia. The process in the infant may persist for periods up to two months, though it is rarely a serious clinical problem. However, circumcision should be postponed until platelet counts return to normal. Steroid therapy should be considered for the infant if clinical manifestations of the disease are severe.

Idiopathic thrombocytopenic purpura should be treated with a steroid. Either prednisone or prednisolone generally suffices. Splenectomy should be reserved for patients in whom this treatment is not effective. Transfusion of platelets is of limited value, but may be used if bleeding cannot be controlled or when operative bleeding is anticipated. Uterine bleeding is not seen characteristically, but hemorrhage from lacerations and perineal or abdominal wall incisions is common.

Fibrinogenopenia

The obstetric conditions commonly associated with depletion of fibrinogen are amniotic fluid embolism, abruptio placentae and retention of a dead fetus (Pritchard; Pritchard and Wright). Less often bacteremia, profuse hemorrhage or a transfusion of mismatched blood may initiate the process. The mechanisms by which fibrinogenopenia develop vary. Gradual liberation of thromboplastic substances during necrosis of the decidual or the fetal products is the mechanism in the dead fetus syndrome. With abruptio placentae most of the depletion of fibrinogen occurs as fibrin is formed in the retroplacental clot. In amniotic fluid embolism thromboplastic material in the amniotic fluid triggers widespread intravascular clotting and rapidly depletes the plasma fibrinogen. Fibrinolytic mechanisms may be activated secondarily by any of these mechanisms.

The detection and recognition of fibrinogenopenia is of utmost importance to the obstetrician. Some simple tests are available for diagnosis. Clot observation is easiest and gives important information. Carefully drawn blood is placed in a clean Pyrex tube. The blood should clot within a short period; the clot formed should be firm and retract well; there should be no evidence of clot lysis. This test can be repeated hourly or as often as the condition warrants it.

Plasma fibrinogen levels can be measured more accurately in sophisticated laboratories. Normal levels in pregnancy exceed 300 mg. per 100 ml.; when the levels fall below 100 mg. per 100 ml., abnormal clotting mechanisms exist. Although not every patient with such low levels will necessarily bleed, one can anticipate that hemorrhage may occur at any time. Aggressive treatment becomes essential under such circumstances.

Management of the fibrinogenopenia involves prompt management of the obstetric complication. Excessive bleeding requires adequate replacement of the blood. Treatment consists of blocking the consumptive process by use of heparin (Waxman and Gambrill) or replacing the lost fibrinogen. If the causative process (e.g., retained dead fetus) is ongoing, heparin may be very effective in arresting the intravascular coagulation and allowing the liver to replenish the fibrinogen. Levels may return to normal in a day or two. If the obstetric process is completed (the fetus is delivered) and the patient is bleeding copiously, fibrinogen should be given to replenish this clotting factor quickly. Usually, about 4 gm. are needed, but sometimes much more will be necessary. Use of epsilon-aminocaproic acid to combat fibrinolysis is no longer felt to be necessary unless there is clear evidence of massive plasmin formation in a patient whose bleeding is uncontrollable by other means.

LEUKEMIA

Leukemia is a rare complication of pregnancy. Acute or chronic myelogenous and lymphatic types may occur in about the same frequencies as in nongravid populations. Chronic myelogenous leukemia is the type most often encountered. The average survival time in acute leukemia from the onset of symptoms is approximately six months. Pregnancy does not alter the course of the disease (Lee et al.).

Acute leukemia does not constitute a specific indication for therapeutic abortion, although pregnancy may unnecessarily complicate the terminal course of the disease. If the patient desires to continue the pregnancy, all efforts should be directed toward continuing the pregnancy to term or as near to term as possible. Vaginal delivery should be permitted unless cesarean section is indicated for obstetric reasons.

The incidence of premature labor is increased. Postpartum hemorrhage may result because of increased fibrinolytic activity and decreased serum fibrinogen concentrations.

Chronic forms of leukemia are also unaffected by pregnancy and the disease does not alter the normal course of a pregnancy. The average survival time is three to four years. The disease has not been shown to develop in infants born to mothers with leukemia; thus, transplacental transmission does not occur.

Chemotherapeutic agents, because of their possible teratogenic effect, should be limited to the second and third trimesters. Whole blood transfusions should be given as needed. Patients with chronic leukemia should be advised against pregnancy because of the poor prognosis for survival and not because the disease will be aggravated or the pregnancy endangered.

HODGKIN'S DISEASE

Hodgkin's disease is a form of lymphoma closely related to leukemia and lymphosarcoma and characterized by Reed-Sternberg cells in the lymph nodes. Pregnancy is not uncommon because fertility is usually not impaired. The disease does not alter the normal course of a pregnancy but may be transmitted to the fetus. Equally important, the pregnancy does not adversely affect the natural course of the disease (Barry et al.).

Radiation therapy can be directed to the involved nodes if satisfactory shielding of the fetus is provided. Nitrogen mustard or related compounds may be administered, preferably during the second and third trimesters after the critical period of fetal development, without adversely affecting the fetus.

Therapeutic abortion is not indicated specifically for this disease. Women with active and progressive disease should be advised against pregnancy because of the poor prognosis. Women desirous of pregnancy should be urged to wait until their disease has been quiescent for at least two years.

POLYCYTHEMIA

Abnormally active hematopoiesis will result in polycythemia. It is seen in chronic hypoxic states associated with congenital heart disorders or pulmonary diseases. It will result in thromboses. It can be manifested clinically by paresthesias and skin and mucosal hemorrhages; headaches, malaise and myalgias are common. Patients have high red blood cell counts and increased blood volume. Blood viscosity is augmented.

The rare reported pregnancies with this condition are associated with high perinatal mortality. Aside from management problems related to the underlying heart or lung process, these patients can be treated with repeated phlebotomies to reduce red cell mass. Serial hematocrit determinations are useful in this regard. Myelosuppressive therapy is reserved for those unrelieved by this approach and, if possible, withheld during pregnancy because of the known fetal effects of alkylating agents. Radiation and radioisotopes should not be used at all during pregnancy.

PORPHYRIA

Porphyria is a disease caused by an inborn error of metabolism in which the urinary excretion of coproporphyrin and uroporphyrin is increased. The acute intermittent form (Tricomi and Baum), which is the most common variety, can be identified by the excretion of porphobilinogen in the urine. Porphyria is a rare complication of pregnancy.

Gastrointestinal and neurologic symptoms are common and often mimic other abdominal or neurologic disorders. Patients may be erroneously considered to be psychoneurotic until the true nature of their disease is recognized. Pregnancy has no adverse effect on the course of the disease nor does porphyria affect pregnancy. Treatment is supportive and nonspecific. Barbiturates, alcohol, sulfonamides and ergonovine have caused exacerbations of porphyria; their use should be avoided in susceptible patients.

REFERENCES

Barry, R. M., Diamond, H. D., and Craver, L. F.: Influence of pregnancy on the course of Hodgkin's disease. Amer. J. Obstet. Gynec. *84*:445, 1962.

Holly, R. G.: Anemia in pregnancy. Clin. Obstet. Gynec. *1*:15, 1958.

Holly, R. G.: Refractory anemia in pregnancy. Amer. J. Obstet. Gynec. *80*:946, 1960.

Lee, R. A., Johnson, C. E., and Hanlon, D. G.: Leukemia during pregnancy. Amer. J. Obstet. Gynec. *84*:455, 1962.

Platt, H. S.: Effect of maternal sickle cell trait on perinatal mortality. Brit. Med. J. *4*:334, 1971.

Pritchard, J. A.: Fetal death in utero. Obstet. Gynec. *14*:573, 1959.

Pritchard, J. A., and Wright, M. R.: Pathogenesis of hypofibrinogenemia in placental abruption. New Eng. J. Med. *261*:218, 1959.

Ricks, P., Jr : Exchange transfusion in sickle cell anemia and pregnancy. Obstet. Gynec. *25*:117, 1965.

Ricks, P., Jr : Further experience with exchange transfusion in sickle cell anemia and pregnancy. Amer. J. Obstet. Gynec. *100*:1087, 1968.

Tricomi, V., and Baum, H.: Acute intermittent porphyria and pregnancy. Obstet. Gynec. Survey *13*:307, 1958.

Waxman, B., and Gambrill, R.: Use of heparin in disseminated intravascular coagulation. Amer. J. Obstet. Gynec. *112*:434, 1972.

Chapter 43

Gastrointestinal Disorders

MINOR GASTROINTESTINAL SYMPTOMS

Gastrointestinal function may be altered in many different ways during normal pregnancy. Usually, these changes are of no major significance or importance, but they may cause annoying symptoms. Patients complain, for example, that their sense of taste or smell is distorted or is characterized by heightened sensitivity. Certain odors become disagreeable and may evoke nausea and vomiting. Appetite may fail as a consequence. The problem is generally not serious. Treatment includes avoidance of the source of odor, whenever possible, together with reassurance and mild sedation, if necessary. Occasionally, the pregnant woman craves unusual substances, such as chalk, ice, mud, starch, salt or clay. This craving, called *pica,* is discussed in Chapter 27.

Normal pregnancy frequently is accompanied by an increase in salivary secretion, called *ptyalism* or *sialorrhea.* True ptyalism is rare; it usually is associated with nausea and vomiting, beginning during the second month and often persisting until quickening, though the symptoms may continue throughout pregnancy into the postpartum period. The cause is not known, although neurogenic, reflex or psychologic etiology has been proposed. It is commonly seen in association with pica, especially with starch ingestion.

Adequate doses of anticholinergic compounds, such as belladonna alkaloids (e.g., atropine) or any of several good pharmaceutical preparations (e.g., methscopolamine or Pamine, propantheline bromide or Pro-Banthine), are useful. In addition to lowering the gastric secretion, they tend to suppress salivary secretion. The response to such medication varies considerably; dosages must be adapted to individual tolerance and requirements.

As the uterus enlarges during pregnancy, the abdominal organs are displaced. Late in pregnancy, the stomach is pushed up to the left dome of the diaphragm and its axis is rotated 45 degrees towards the right (Hansen). Gastric emptying may or may not be prolonged, a factor implicated in the development of heartburn, flatulence and vomiting (Hunt and Murray).

Nausea and vomiting occur frequently in most pregnant women. These symptoms may appear as early as the second week of gestation, but more often develop at about the fifth week; they may continue for several weeks to three months or longer. The patient is nauseated on arising or after breakfast, and vomits this meal or the overnight accumulation of mucus and gastric secretion. The nausea seldom recurs during the remainder of the day.

The cause is not known. Various unproved theories include psychologic and emotional disturbances, temporary adrenal depression, duodenal spasm, hormone imbalance involving estrogen and progesterone, allergies and pyridoxine deficiency (Wager). It is usually self-limited, disappearing at about 12 weeks.

In relatively mild cases, therapy includes frequent feedings, liquids in small amounts, sufficient sleep, rest after meals, avoidance of unpleasant odors, mild sedation and reassurance. More severe cases require tranquilizers and antiemetic compounds. Antihistamines, such as meclizine (Bonine) and buclizine, are effective.

Patients with intractable vomiting not

478

responding to these simple measures and with nutritional and electrolyte imbalance, perhaps with evidence of hepatic or renal damage and ketosis, should be hospitalized. The term *hyperemesis gravidarum* or *pernicious vomiting of pregnancy* is applied to this serious condition. Its treatment is outlined in Chapter 31.

Heartburn and eructation are common during pregnancy. Regurgitation of gastric contents as a result of relaxation of the cardioesophageal area and the increasing intraabdominal pressure caused by the enlarging uterus contribute to gastroesophageal reflux. Esophagitis, sometimes with ulceration, has been found in most patients with symptoms of heartburn, belching and epigastric distress (McCall et al.). Similarly, it has been shown by transducer pressure recordings that the resting pressures of the inferior esophageal sphincter, which normally prevents reflux, progressively weaken with advancing pregnancy in more than half the pregnant women with heartburn (Nagler and Spiro).

In many gravidas the heartburn and eructation disappear spontaneously near term as the uterus descends. Symptomatic relief may be obtained with a diet of small, bland meals. Antacids combining aluminum hydroxide, magnesium trisilicate and magnesium hydroxide may be effective. Other helpful measures include avoiding the recumbent position after eating and eliminating highly sweetened drinks and foods.

Constipation is common during pregnancy. Pressure of the enlarging uterus on the descending colon and rectum may be a contributory factor. The constipation is rarely caused by decreased bowel tone. Normal bowel function usually can be restored without irritating laxatives or enemas. An abundant intake of water is helpful. A glycerin suppository may be inserted rectally to initiate defecation when the fecal mass is not readily expelled.

The diet should contain substantial amounts of cooked or canned fruits and vegetables. Bulk producers, such as Metamucil, and laxatives, such as milk of magnesia or fluid extract of cascara, may be prescribed when indicated for severe constipation; usually, they are not necessary.

For hard and dry fecal collections in the rectum, several ounces of warm saline solution or mineral oil may be helpful. However, enemas are not desirable and their use should be limited.

Rest and a mild antispasmodic, such as tincture of belladonna (10 drops in half a glass of water before meals), help to relieve bowel irritability. The addition of a mild sedative, such as phenobarbital 15 mg. three or four times daily, is valuable. Perhaps the most important principle in management is the avoidance of unnecessary manipulation or drastic medication.

HIATUS HERNIA

Hiatus hernia is four times more common in women than in men (Quinlan) and is not uncommon in pregnancy. Siegel et al. diagnosed hiatus hernia in 17 per cent of women examined in pregnancy. The hernia was not demonstrated again in any of them during the early postpartum period. Sutherland et al. reported a 22 per cent incidence during the last trimester. The incidence of hiatus hernia accompanying pregnancy is greater in multiparas than in nulliparas and is more common in the older pregnant patient. The most frequent symptoms are heartburn and vomiting, especially during the latter half of pregnancy. Occasionally, there are no symptoms. No therapy is required except for symptomatic relief of heartburn.

PEPTIC ULCER

Approximately 10 to 20 per cent of peptic ulcers during adult life occur in women (Kirsner). Although accurate incidence figures are difficult to obtain because of the infrequency of gastrointestinal roentgen studies during gestation, active peptic ulcer appears to be infrequent during pregnancy. Recurrences of preexisting peptic ulcers during pregnancy are more frequent in the final trimester than during the rest of pregnancy. Bleeding and perforation are not uncommon and the course of the disease may be severe. The postpartum period seems especially hazardous.

The occasional tendency for active peptic ulcer to heal early in pregnancy and for it to relapse later in gestation appears to be correlated with trends in gastric secretion. Various observers (Murray et al.; Hunt and Murray) have reported a decrease in gastric secretion during the first six months of pregnancy and a rise in the gastric output of hydrochloric acid and pepsin during the last trimester, with a maximum during the early postpartum period. Lactation seems to be associated with a significant rise in gastric secretion. This rise is not seen, however, in mothers who are not breast feeding their infants. Of related interest are studies of gastric secretion in dogs with gastric pouches. Although pregnancy appeared not to influence acid secretion consistently (McCarthy et al.), hypersecretion of gastric juice occurred during lactation.

The treatment of peptic ulcer in pregnancy is conservative, where possible. Medical management with a bland diet is recommended unless hemorrhage makes it imperative that surgery be undertaken.

ULCERATIVE COLITIS

Ulcerative colitis is encountered in pregnancy among patients with a long history of the disorder or it may develop *de novo* during gestation or the postpartum period. The symptoms include rectal bleeding, diarrhea, abdominal cramps, fever, anorexia and weight loss. The disease is characterized by numerous local and systemic complications. Its course during pregnancy may be unchanged, improved or aggravated. The factors involved in its genesis are not entirely known, though emotional disturbances have been emphasized.

Crohn et al. studied 110 women with ulcerative colitis who had had 150 pregnancies. In 40 of 74 pregnancies there was a recrudescence, although the colitis was quiescent at the time of conception. Most of the exacerbations occurred during the first trimester. In 29 of 38 pregnancies the colitis, active at inception of pregnancy, was aggravated. Nineteen women had their first onset during pregnancy; in another 19 onset occurred post partum.

Mild or moderate ulcerative colitis has no significant effect on fertility or the viability of the fetus. It does not increase the hazard of spontaneous abortion. However, the nutritional depletion and poor general health of gravidas with severe colitis undoubtedly have a deleterious influence. Numerous or rapidly successive pregnancies tend to decrease the patient's resistance and perhaps thereby increase her vulnerability to the disease and its complications.

Patients with ulcerative colitis should be advised definitely to avoid pregnancy until the disease has been quiescent for at least two years, perhaps three to five years. Factors requiring consideration are not only the patient's general health and the severity of the disease but also her desire for the pregnancy and the availability of household help to care for the new infant. Sterilization to prevent future pregnancies should be given serious consideration in selected patients, especially those who already have several children, those with continuously severe and complicated ulcerative colitis and those with little likelihood that the disease will improve.

Ulcerative colitis rarely threatens life during pregnancy, and the usual procedure is to continue the treatment already in progress. Adrenal corticosteroids during pregnancy as adjunctive treatment have resulted in the delivery of healthy normal babies (Kirsner). Similar observations have been made with the continued use of antibiotic agents, sedatives, antispasmodics and antidiarrheal agents.

Colectomy and ileostomy no longer constitute contraindications to successful pregnancy. There may be an increased tendency to prolapse of the stoma, bleeding, cracking of the skin at the margin or temporary partial obstruction. However, these do not seem to constitute major problems (Bargen). The increased scar tissue in the perineum in patients who have had abdominoperineal resections may create problems in effecting descent in the second stage, but these are usually not serious. The scarred perineum apparently does not offer an obstacle to outlet forceps delivery with an episiotomy.

Scudamore et al. reported 13 viable births in 18 pregnancies among 12 women with ileostomies for ulcerative colitis. All patients had vaginal deliveries. The determining factor in the successful outcome undoubtedly was the patients' excellent general health. Similarly good results have been reported by Priest et al.

According to Crohn et al., pregnancy usually has a deleterious effect on the course of *regional enteritis*. However, the harmful effects are less pronounced than in ulcerative colitis. Evaluation of the effect of gestation on such chronic diseases as regional enteritis or ulcerative colitis is difficult because their courses are variable and unpredictable. The many physiologic, metabolic and endocrinologic phenomena associated with pregnancy do not appear to have any direct influence on the disease. The emotional factors associated with pregnancy and with both ulcerative colitis and regional enteritis undoubtedly play an important role.

APPENDICITIS

Although appendicitis is no more frequent during pregnancy than in nongravid women, ruptured appendix occurs 1.5 to 3.5 times more frequently during pregnancy than in the nonpregnant state (Warfield). Perforation is particularly serious during pregnancy because it is not likely to be walled off by inflammatory adhesions. The omentum and intestines are displaced by the enlarging uterus. The inflammation is intensified because of the increased vascularity of the uterus. Thrombophlebitis is more common. Obstructive symptoms arise earlier.

Appendicitis offers a better outlook the earlier in pregnancy it occurs. Of greater importance, the sooner it is recognized and treated, the better the prognosis. During labor, the contracting uterus may cause an abscess to rupture. An adherent or perforating appendix may tear with resulting general peritonitis. This danger is greatest during the third stage and the first few days of the puerperium when the uterine corpus makes its greatest involutionary excursions. Acute appendicitis in the puerperium is easily mistaken for puerperal infection. Moreover, the two conditions may coexist.

If the cecum is mobile, the appendix may be displaced upward by the growing uterus. It generally reaches the level of the iliac crest at the end of the fifth month. The long axis of the appendix undergoes a counterclockwise rotation, first becoming horizontal and pointing medially and finally pointing vertically in 60 per cent of women at the end of the eighth month. If the cecal attachments are such as to fix its location, the appendix will not be displaced during pregnancy. By the end of the tenth day post partum, the appendix has returned to its normal position (Fig. 278).

Diagnosis should present no special difficulties if one approaches the pregnant patient who has abdominal pain with a high index of suspicion. Ectopic gestation and twisted ovarian tumor should be considered, but most often it is confused with ureteritis and ureteral stone. All possible causes of acute peritonitis must be ruled out. During labor, abruptio placentae, torsion of an ovarian cyst or of a pedunculated leiomyoma, pyelonephritis and acute uterine infection must be differentiated.

Prognosis is no worse than in nonpregnant individuals. The use of the antibiotics has considerably reduced the mortality. The longer the delay in operating, the higher the death rate. Likewise, the mortality rate rises if labor should begin during an attack of acute appendicitis. The incidence of premature labor after perforation of the appendix is variously quoted as 40 to 80 per cent.

Treatment of appendicitis in the pregnant woman calls for immediate operation. Appendectomy is mandatory. Even in cases of doubt, operation is the safer course. The incision is made higher than ordinarily. A right paramedian incision overlapping the upper third of the uterine corpus is preferable to the usual McBurney type incision in providing easy access to the diseased appendix without disturbing the gravid uterus. Uterine manipulation should be restricted to the very minimum. Drainage is usually not done unless there has been abscess formation.

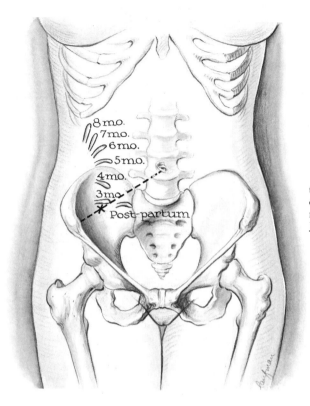

Figure 278 Diagrammatic representation of the probable location of the appendix at the different months of pregnancy and the puerperium. X marks McBurney's point. (From Baer, J. L., et al.: J.A.M.A. 98:1359, 1932.)

If abortion or labor should occur after the appendectomy, it should be allowed to run as natural a course as possible. Because of the high mortality from peritonitis at or near term, the issue of removing the appendix and doing a cesarean hysterectomy at the same time has been raised. The question is not clearly answered, but cesarean section is certainly contraindicated in the presence of acute appendicitis. It is not advisable to empty the uterus, because the uterus is easily infected and it is very possible that pregnancy may continue without further trouble. If a walled-off abscess has formed, it is dangerous to attempt to induce labor or to empty the uterus. If labor begins spontaneously, it should be allowed to progress into the second stage. An episiotomy should be made and an outlet forceps operation done as soon as the head reaches the perineum. Intrauterine manipulation should be avoided. Labor does not usually interfere with healing of the abdominal wound.

ILEUS

Ileus due to intestinal obstruction is a rare complication in pregnancy. It may be caused by compression or torsion of the intestines by the enlarging uterus, especially in association with adhesions secondary to previous abdominal operations. Other etiologic factors are volvulus, intussusception and hernias.

In general, treatment consists of intestinal decompression and restoration of fluid and electrolyte balance, followed by immediate surgery. Before viability, laparotomy should be performed and the cause of the obstruction corrected. After viability, cesarean section should be done and the ileus treated. Ileus after delivery may be due to the trauma of labor, to obstruction of the intestines by adhesions, to the large uterus incarcerated in the pelvis or to peritonitis. Ileus in pregnancy, especially when accompanied by signs of peritonitis, must always be considered to be an acute emergency and one must not temporize before operating.

HERNIA

Various hernias are encountered in pregnancy, although they tend not to be symptomatic. In fact, unless the bowel is adherent, the enlarging uterus pushes the contents of the sac away from the hernial opening and makes incarceration unlikely. The same situation also usually applies during labor. Even strong bearing-down efforts do not enlarge the hernial ring in inguinal, femoral or umbilical hernias. However, during the puerperium, the ring may be enlarged and bowel enter the sac, though incarceration is rare. Adherent intestines may be incarcerated, twisted or stretched at any time during pregnancy or the puerperium to produce ileus. Hiatus hernia was discussed earlier (see above).

Treatment is the same as at any other time when threatening symptoms occur. During labor, it is wise not to allow the patient to bear down too strongly if the hernial sac is enlarging. Forceps should be applied soon after cervical dilatation is complete, provided this will not be a traumatic obstetric procedure. It is not safe to hold the intestines back manually during strong expulsive efforts. Umbilical and postoperative ventral hernias are usually permanently enlarged by pregnancy. Traction on adherent omentum, when present in these cases, often causes pain.

LIVER DISEASE

The liver is not significantly affected functionally or anatomically by normal pregnancy (Schiff). Aspiration biopsies in normal pregnant women demonstrate no abnormality (Ingerslev and Teilum). The only changes in hepatic function tests during pregnancy have been a slight rise in the alkaline phosphatase during the ninth month and occasional slight impairment of the bromsulphalein test (Bodansky). These are temporary and apparently of no consequence. It is important to remember that such changes occur, however, when evaluating liver function in the pregnant female.

The liver may be affected during such special pregnancy problems as hyperemesis gravidarum and preeclampsia. These conditions are discussed elsewhere (Chapters 31 and 36). The hepatic lesion noted most often in preeclampsia is peripheral hemorrhagic necrosis of the lobules. Histological study of fatal cases of hyperemesis gravidarum complicated by jaundice demonstrates accumulation of fat, especially in the central zones of the lobules. This probably results from severe malnutrition.

Sheehan described a condition he called "obstetric acute yellow atrophy." It resembles severe viral hepatitis. It begins usually in the last month of pregnancy, with severe vomiting and epigastric pain, followed by jaundice. Maternal and fetal mortality are high. The symptoms rapidly increase in severity. There may be hypertension, edema and convulsions.

Grossly, the liver is small in size. The microscopic appearance of the liver differs somewhat from that of acute yellow atrophy secondary to viral hepatitis. It is characterized by severe fatty infiltration without inflammation or hepatic cell necrosis.

The etiology of this disease is unknown. The usual therapeutic measures for hepatitis in the nonpregnant patient should be followed (see below).

Idiopathic or *recurrent jaundice of pregnancy* is characterized by jaundice occurring in the last trimester, usually preceded by generalized pruritus. Both of these findings disappear after delivery, but frequently reappear during subsequent pregnancies. *Pruritus gravidarum* most likely reflects a milder form of idiopathic jaundice of pregnancy. Usually, the serum bilirubin, alkaline phosphatase and bromsulphalein tests are abnormal and return rapidly to normal levels after delivery. Intrahepatic cholestasis is observed on liver biopsy. Treatment is entirely symptomatic. The prognosis for both mother and infant is excellent.

Infectious and serum hepatitis develop occasionally during pregnancy. The course is the same as in the nonpregnant patient. The symptoms include anorexia, nausea, vomiting, fever, pain and tenderness over the liver, followed by jaundice. The prognosis of viral hepatitis in the first two trimesters is about what is expected in nonpregnant women. However, the mortality rate increases in the third trimester and during the postpartum period. There appears to be a greater tendency to acute yellow atrophy and chronic residual liver damage than in nonpregnant patients (Glotzer; Long et al.).

Serum hepatitis is transmissible to the fetus. The overall fetal mortality is 15 per cent. Abortion and premature labor are common in severely ill patients. Congenital abnormalities appear to occur no more frequently among children of mothers who had viral hepatitis during pregnancy than in the children of other pregnant women (Sherlock; Millen).

Treatment is the same as in the nonpregnant patient. Interruption of pregnancy is to be avoided, if possible, because of the added hazard of the procedure to the already jeopardized liver and the risk that severe hepatic necrosis may occur. Moreover, the outcome of hepatitis has not been shown to be improved when pregnancy has been interrupted. When labor begins spontaneously, analgesics and anesthetics having the least potential for hepatic toxicity should be selected (see Chapter 22). Vaginal delivery is appropriate, unless there are overriding obstetric reasons against it.

Pregnancy does not appear to alter the course of cirrhosis of the liver significantly (Moore and Hughes). Patients with cirrhosis of the liver can undergo pregnancy under careful supervision, with normal delivery and without deterioration of hepatic function as a result of the pregnancy. Cirrhosis cannot be considered an especially urgent indication for the termination of pregnancy. Successful full-term pregnancies have been reported in a patient with severe portal cirrhosis and a portacaval shunt (Abrams).

CHOLELITHIASIS

Gallstones are up to three times more common in women than in men. Although it is generally thought that the incidence is increased during pregnancy, Robertson and Dochat showed this not to be true. Pregnancy elevates both serum and biliary cholesterol levels and delays gallbladder emptying. These conditions favor the formation of gallstones.

Acute cholecystitis and biliary colic may develop at any time, but usually occur during the latter half of pregnancy and the postpartum period. They become increasingly frequent in subsequent pregnancies. Surgery should be postponed until after delivery, whenever possible, because premature labor may occur (Greene et al.). Cholecystectomy is technically more difficult during pregnancy because of the large uterus. Conservative medical treatment, including antibiotics parenterally, usually suffices unless there is associated bile duct obstruction or other complicating factors. When medical management is ineffective, the pregnancy must be disregarded and surgery performed. Pregnant patients who recover from acute cholecystitis or biliary colic with nonsurgical measures should undergo cholecystectomy at an appropriate time after delivery because recurrent attacks are likely.

ACUTE PANCREATITIS

No etiologic relationship between pregnancy and pancreatitis has been demonstrated. Its apparent rarity during pregnancy is probably due to the fact that the diagnosis is not considered or is obscured by the usual expected nausea and vomiting. It is likely that many cases are unrecognized. Deaths have been reported in association with this condition. Present evidence showing its production in rats by the administration of thiazide diuretics suggests both caution in the use of diuretics in pregnancy and the need for closer surveillance for pancreatitis in the gravid population. Acute pancreatitis should be considered in all instances of abdominal pain and vomiting in any trimester of pregnancy, and appropriate diagnostic tests undertaken. The treatment is the same as in the nonpregnant state.

REFERENCES

Abrams, F. R.: Cirrhosis of the liver in pregnancy: A review of the literature and a report of a case with electrophoretic studies. Obstet. Gynec. *10*:451, 1957.

Baer, J. L., Reis, R. A., and Arens, R. A.: Appendicitis in pregnancy with changes in position and areas of normal appendix in pregnancy. J.A.M.A. *98*:1359, 1932.

Bargen, J. A.: Chronic Ulcerative Colitis. Springfield, Ill., Charles C Thomas, 1951.

Bodansky, M.: Changes in serum calcium, inorganic phosphate and phosphatase activity in the pregnant woman. Amer. J. Clin. Path. 9:36, 1939.

Crohn, B. B., Yarnis, H., and Korelitz, B. I.: Regional ileitis complicating pregnancy. Gastroenterology *31*:615, 1956.

Crohn, B. B., Yarnis, H., Crohn, E. C., Walter, R. I., and Gabrilov, L.: Ulcerative colitis and pregnancy. Gastroenterology *30*:391, 1956.

Glotzer, S.: Hepatitis in pregnancy. New York J. Med. 57:3185, 1957.

Greene, J., Rogers, A., and Rubin, L.: Fetal loss after cholecystectomy during pregnancy. Canad. Med. Ass. J. 88:576, 1963.

Hansen, R.: Zur Physiologie des Magens in der Schwangerschaft. Zbl. Gynäk. *61*:2306, 1937.

Hunt, J. N., and Murray, F. A.: Gastric function in pregnancy. J. Obstet. Gynaec. Brit. Emp. 65:78, 1958.

Ingerslev, M., and Teilum, G.: Biopsy studies on the liver in pregnancy: II. Liver biopsy on normal pregnant women. Acta Obstet. Gynec. Scand. *25*:352, 1946.

Ingerslev, M., and Teilum, G.: Biopsy studies on the liver in pregnancy: III. Liver biopsy in albuminuria of pregnancy, eclampsism, and eclampsia. Acta Obstet. Gynec. Scand. *25*:361, 1946.

Kirsner, J. B.: Hormones and peptic ulcer. Bull. N.Y. Acad. Med. 29:477, 1953.

Long, J. S., Boyson, H., and Priest, F. O.: Infectious hepatitis and pregnancy. Amer. J. Obstet. Gynec. 70:282, 1955.

Mansell, R. V.: Infectious hepatitis in the first trimester of pregnancy and its effect on the fetus. Amer. J. Obstet. Gynec. 69:1136, 1955.

McCall, M. L., Wechsler, R. L., Anzalone, J. T., and Brougher, D. E.: Endoscopic studies of the esophagus and stomach during pregnancy. Amer. J. Obstet. Gynec. *82*:1125, 1961.

McCarthy, J. D., Evans, S. O., and Dragstedt, L. R.: Gastric secretion in dogs during pregnancy and lactation. Gastroenterology *27*:275, 1954.

Millen, R. M.: Jaundice during pregnancy. Brit. J. Clin. Pract. *11*:341, 1957.

Moore, R. M., and Hughes, P. K.: Cirrhosis of the liver in pregnancy. Obstet. Gynec. *14*:753, 1960.

Murray, F. A., Erskine, J. P., and Fielding, J.: Gastric secretion in pregnancy. J. Obstet. Gynaec. Brit. Emp. *64*:373, 1957.

Nagler, R., and Spiro, H. M.: Heartburn in late pregnancy: Manometric studies of esophageal motor function. J. Clin. Invest. *40*:954, 1961.

Nagler, R., and Spiro, H. M.: Heartburn in pregnancy. Amer. J. Dig. Dis. 7:648, 1962.

Priest, F. O., Gilchrist, R. K., and Long, J. S.: Pregnancy in the patient with ileostomy and colectomy. J.A.M.A. *169*:213, 1959.

Quinlan, D. K.: Heartburn in pregnancy. S. Afr. Med. J. 35:628, 1961.

Robertson, H. E., and Dochat, G. R.: Pregnancy and gallstones: Collective review. Internat. Abstr. Surg. 78:193, 1944.

Schiff, L., ed.: Diseases of the Liver. Philadelphia, J. B. Lippincott Company, 1956.

Scudamore, H. H., Rogers, A. G., Bargen, J. A., and Banner, E. A.: Pregnancy after ileostomy for chronic ulcerative colitis. Gastroenterology 32:295, 1957.

Sheehan, H. L.: Pathology of acute atrophy and delayed chloroform poisoning. J. Obstet. Gynaec. Brit. Emp. *47*:49, 1940.

Sherlock, S.: Diseases of the Liver and Biliary System. Springfield, Ill., Charles C Thomas, 1955.

Siegel, L. H., Greenfield, H., and Kogan, E.: The relationship between hiatus hernia and pregnancy: A clinical study. Gastroenterology 32:479, 1957.

Sutherland, C. G., Atkinson, J. C., Brogdon, B. G., Crow, N. E., and Brown, W. E.: Esophageal hiatus hernia in pregnancy. Obstet. Gynec. 8:261, 1956.

Wager, H. P.: Emesis gravidarum: Mechanism and control with a review of the literature. Obstet. Gynec. 6:99, 1955.

Warfield, C. I.: Acute appendicitis complicating pregnancy. Postgrad. Med. 8:10, 1950.

Chapter 44

Renal Disorders

FUNCTIONAL CHANGES IN PREGNANCY

Glomerular Filtration Rate

Renal blood flow and the effective renal plasma flow are elevated significantly above nonpregnant levels by the tenth to twelfth week (Bucht; Sims and Krantz). The para-amino hippurate clearance averages 750 to 850 ml. per minute in pregnancy compared with nonpregnant values of 550 to 600 ml. per minute. Only a small part of this increase can be accounted for by the increased cardiac output. Prior to term the renal plasma flow progressively returns to normal. Post partum it may be well below normal nonpregnant levels for as long as 25 weeks.

Glomerular filtration rate is also increased to about 30 to 50 per cent above normal. The mean inulin clearance values may be 150 to 170 ml. per minute compared to 100 to 130 ml. per minute in the nonpregnant subject. The glomerular filtration rate is increased from as early as the tenth week and remains elevated to the thirty-eighth week. It may fall to the normal nonpregnant rate in the last two weeks of pregnancy and post partum.

The filtration fraction (glomerular filtration rate divided by effective renal plasma flow) is elevated throughout pregnancy. Because the glomerular filtration rate is maintained at elevated levels while the plasma flow returns to normal, the filtration fraction increases further as term approaches.

Urea Nitrogen and Creatinine

As a result of the greatly increased glomerular filtration rate, the level of nitrogenous breakdown products in the serum is diminished during pregnancy. From the fifteenth week to term, the plasma urea nitrogen level averages 6 to 12 mg. per 100 ml. (Sims and Krantz), which is considerably less than nonpregnant levels. After delivery, the levels return rapidly to the nonpregnant range. Plasma creatinine level is lowered to 0.2 to 0.7 mg. per 100 ml. in pregnancy and returns to the normal nonpregnant range after delivery. These physiologic changes must be kept in mind when the functional state of the kidneys is assessed in pregnancy.

Urinary Tract Changes

After the third month of pregnancy the ureters, renal pelves and calices usually become dilated. Dilatation is more frequent and of greater magnitude in nulliparas than in multiparas (Baird). The urinary tract on the right is dilated in 85 per cent and on the left in 72 per cent. These changes are present as early as the sixth week of pregnancy in nulliparas and the tenth week in multiparas, and may persist 10 to 16 weeks into the puerperium. Intravenous pyelography shows the renal calices to be enlarged, with rounded rather than sharp outlines. The renal pelvis is enlarged and the narrowing at the ureteropelvic junction, which is normally present in the nonpregnant state, is lost (Fig. 279).

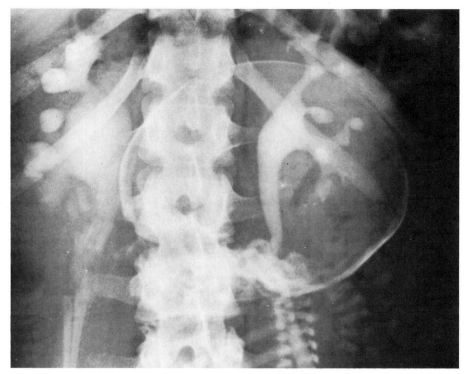

Figure 279 Intravenous pyelogram in late pregnancy showing dilatation and blunting of the renal calices and dilatation of renal pelves. The changes are more prominent on the right side.

The cause of this dilatation and atony is not known. It may be associated with the hormone changes of pregnancy. There is hyperplasia of the muscle of the calices and ureter and an increase in the elastic connective tissue of the wall of the ureter. As the uterus enlarges, it may compress the ureters at the pelvic brim. The tendency of the uterus to tilt somewhat to the right may lead to greater compression of the right than the left ureter.

Orthostatic Proteinuria

Orthostatic proteinuria occurs most frequently in young adults. Its incidence varies from 5 to 20 per cent. The incidence in pregnancy is not well documented, and the range of normal protein excretion in pregnancy is unknown. The mechanism of this condition is poorly understood. The rotation of the liver which occurs in the lordotic position and is exaggerated in pregnancy may be contributory by compressing the inferior vena cava, causing a slight rise in venous pressure in both renal veins and consequent proteinuria. The left renal vein may be compressed by the gravid uterus as it crosses the midline and this may have the same effect. If orthostatic proteinuria is suspected, specimens of clean voided urine should be collected when the patient is up and about and also when she is recumbent.

Glucosuria and Lactosuria

The urine of most gravidas contains reducing substances. It is important to differentiate between the physiologic glucosuria and lactosuria of pregnancy and the pathologic glucosuria of diabetes mellitus in pregnancy (see Chapter 49). Using Benedict's qualitative reagent, Flynn et al. found reducing substances in the urine of 73 per cent of healthy gravidas and in 88 per cent of puerperas. With paper chromatography, lactosuria was more common both during pregnancy and post partum. Glucosuria disappeared rapidly after delivery, but the incidence and amount of lactosuria increased.

Welsh and Sims have shown that the glucosuria of pregnancy is probably the result of the increased minute volume of glomerular filtrate which exceeds the maximal tubular capacity to reabsorb glucose. The lactosuria is probably caused by high levels of lactose of mammary origin in the maternal blood. Lactose is excreted by glomerular filtration and is not reabsorbed by the tubules so that all the filtered lactose appears in the urine. Lactosuria and glucosuria can be differentiated simply by using a dip stick or test tape impregnated with glucose oxidase. A positive test identifies the reducing substance as glucose.

DIAGNOSIS IN PREGNANCY

The problem of clinical differentiation of the several hypertensive states in pregnancy has been discussed in Chapter 36. A dilemma is posed when hypertension, edema and proteinuria are present late in pregnancy. They may be manifestations of preeclampsia, hypertensive disease or primary renal disease. The diagnosis is somewhat simplified if there is an antecedent history or the objective evidence of renal disease is recognized and confirmed before pregnancy begins. Hypertensive retinopathy with narrowing and tortuosity of the retinal arterioles suggests long-standing vascular or renal disease. Its differentiation from the retinal arteriolar spasm and the retinal sheen of preeclampsia may be difficult, however.

The amount of protein excreted in 24 hours should be measured quantitatively. There is no direct relationship between the underlying renal disease and the degree of proteinuria, except in broad terms. Persistent massive proteinuria of greater than 10 mg. in 24 hours is suggestive of the nephrotic syndrome. There may be a daily urinary protein excretion of between 4 and 10 gm. in various types of glomerulonephritis and in preeclampsia with severe glomerular lesions. Proteinuria in pyelonephritis and in hypertensive disease may be minimal or absent and rarely exceeds 2 gm. daily.

Microscopic examination of early morning urine may provide valuable information. The presence of many erythrocytes, red cell casts and crenated erythrocytes strongly suggests acute or active glomerulonephritis. Many pus cells with leukocyte casts suggest pyelonephritis. This may be confirmed clinically by a Gram stain of the urine sediment and quantitative culture showing a colony count of 100,000 or more organisms per milliliter. Occasionally, however, both red and white cells may be found in large numbers in the urine of patients with severe preeclampsia or with the nephritis of systemic lupus erythematosus.

Fatty casts and doubly refractile fat bodies appear in the urine in the nephrotic syndrome and in diabetic nephropathy. Occasionally, they may also be found when there is tubular degeneration from some other cause. The number of hyaline, granular and epithelial casts varies considerably. Their number is influenced by the rate of urine flow, urinary pH and other factors. Large broad casts are characteristic of advanced renal disease.

The demonstration by percutaneous renal biopsy of a characteristic renal lesion in preeclampsia has permitted recognition of the nature of the underlying disease process. This technique has also brought clearly to light the clinical difficulties in distinguishing between preeclampsia, hypertensive vascular disease and renal disease, and has broadened our understanding of the range of renal abnormalities occurring in pregnancy (see Chapter 36).

Bacteriuria

Kass is responsible for drawing attention to the importance of asymptomatic bacteriuria in pregnancy. Between 5 and 10 per cent of pregnant women have significant bacteriuria. Significant bacteriuria is defined as the finding on two successive occasions of more than 100,000 microorganisms per milliliter of urine when a clean voided midstream specimen is collected and cultured immediately. Bacteriuria is frequently present without pyuria. *Escherichia coli* is the most common organism found. Other organisms are infrequent except in association with previous instrumentation or urinary tract disease.

The significance of bacteriuria lies in the fact that about 25 per cent of gravidas with it will develop acute pyelonephritis or other symptomatic urinary infection in the course of the pregnancy. Although ostensibly associated with an increased incidence of small babies, this relationship has not been confirmed.

Acute Pyelonephritis

Acute pyelonephritis is one of the most common complications of pregnancy, occurring in at least two per cent of all pregnancies. The disease usually begins at or after the fifth month. The infection is frequently bilateral; when unilateral, it occurs more often on the right side. Stasis and obstruction in the urinary tract is contributory. When the uterus rises out of the pelvis, partial compression of the ureters occurs, particularly on the right side where the ureter crosses the pelvic brim (Fig. 280).

The route by which organisms reach the kidney is not known. Kass claimed that most cases of acute pyelonephritis of pregnancy occur in patients previously shown to have asymptomatic bacteriuria. Not all are agreed that this is so. In a carefully controlled study, Bryant et al. found no significant increase in the incidence of later symptomatic infection of the urinary tract in women who had asymptomatic bacteriuria early in pregnancy.

Acute pyelonephritis may also develop during the postpartum period. Difficulty in initiating micturition is common. It occurs particularly after prolonged anesthesia, prolonged labor and difficult delivery. Overdistention of the bladder results, and there may be incomplete emptying with

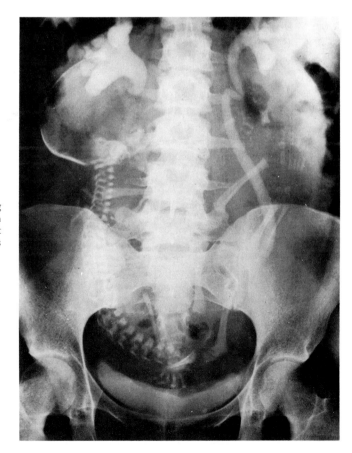

Figure 280 Pyelogram demonstrating hydroureter and hydronephrosis with kinking of ureter clearly seen on the left side. Obstruction at the pelvic brim is likely.

residual urine. Every effort should be made to prevent overdistention of the bladder, but catheterization should be used only as a last resort.

The use of an indwelling catheter before or after delivery may serve to initiate or augment urinary and renal infection. Although a full bladder may interfere with or be traumatized by delivery procedures, it is not a good practice to subject every patient to routine bladder catheterization at the time of delivery. This time-honored practice deserves to be reconsidered in light of its recognized risks. Catheterization to obtain urine specimens for microscopic or bacteriologic analysis should be avoided; a clean voided midstream urine specimen, properly obtained, gives equally satisfactory results.

One other factor may play a part in the development of acute pyelonephritis, namely, underlying renal damage. Patients with renal diseases, such as chronic glomerulonephritis or chronic pyelonephritis, are particularly susceptible to acute pyelonephritis. The only symptoms in mild cases may be backache, slight fever, urinary frequency and dysuria. In more severe attacks there may be shaking chills, high fever and pain and tenderness in the costovertebral angles. Leukocytes and organisms are found on microscopic examination of the urine, and the urine culture is positive. Because of the high incidence of asymptomatic bacilluria in pregnancy, the finding of leukocytes in the urine is more important than a positive urine culture.

Acute pyelonephritis should be treated vigorously with appropriate antibiotics. Treatment should be continued for at least one month because there is a great tendency to relapse in pregnancy. It may be necessary to continue treatment throughout pregnancy. If the infection cannot be controlled and renal function is deteriorating, therapeutic abortion may be lifesaving.

Acute pyelonephritis in pregnancy leads to a significant incidence of chronic pyelonephritis later in life (Pinkerton et al.). Thus, effective treatment with antibiotics is important and should be controlled by serial bacteriologic cultures.

Preeclampsia

The renal histological and functional changes associated with preeclampsia are detailed in Chapter 36. The glomeruli are involved uniformly with characteristic lesions. They are enlarged and may distend Bowman's capsule. The glomerular capillary wall is swollen, the swelling affecting both endothelial and epithelial cells. The glomerular tuft is ischemic, very few erythrocytes being seen in the capillaries. The capillary basement membrane is not thickened. There are some degenerative changes in the tubules, and patchy edema of the interstitial tissue in severely involved kidneys. These changes return to normal after delivery.

With essential hypertension in late pregnancy, the kidneys show only thickening of the walls of the small arteries and arterioles. The glomeruli are normal. Except for the rare patient with preeclampsia in whom acute renal failure develops from tubular necrosis or renal cortical necrosis, there is little relation between the severity of the renal lesions and the clinical picture.

Acute Renal Failure

Renal failure is the most serious renal complication of pregnancy. It is usually caused by acute tubular necrosis. This may result from or be associated with eclampsia or severe preeclampsia, septic abortion and abruptio placentae. Less commonly, it may complicate severe postpartum hemorrhage or transfusion reactions. The direst situation arises from bilateral renal cortical necrosis, a complication of severe abruptio placentae. Acute renal failure is manifested by oliguria of less than 400 ml. of urine per day or by anuria.

Acute renal failure can usually be avoided. In abruptio placentae commonly the magnitude of blood loss is underestimated because bleeding may be occult. When hemorrhage occurs, the blood volume should be maintained by immediate and adequate whole blood transfusion. In severe preeclampsia and eclampsia, profound vasoconstriction may lead to tubular necrosis. Treatment should be directed at decreasing renal vasoconstriction and thereby preventing tubular damage.

With regard to treatment, acute renal failure may be so mild as to go unrecognized unless the urine volume is carefully measured hourly. Patients with transient oliguria require little specific treatment. If oliguria lasts longer than a few hours, however, treatment must be initiated. Adequate transfusion may be needed to ensure replacement of blood loss. If there is concern about overhydration, central venous pressure determinations are helpful to monitor this problem. The principles of treatment in the oliguric phase (Parsons) include (1) giving sufficient fluid to replace the insensible loss plus urinary output, (2) supplying sufficient calories to reduce endogenous protein breakdown and thereby minimize formation of nitrogenous wastes and the accumulation of potassium, and (3) instituting dialysis if potassium or urea nitrogen levels are rising rapidly.

Acute Glomerulonephritis

Acute glomerulonephritis in pregnancy is rare. It is usually associated with respiratory or other infection with type A beta-hemolytic streptococci. Hematuria, proteinuria, oliguria, edema and hypertension are frequently present. Occasionally, severe oliguria or anuria may occur. Cardiovascular and cerebral manifestations may be present. Death is uncommon, but may result from cardiac failure, cerebral vascular complications, anuria or uremia. The history of healed glomerulonephritis is not a contraindication to subsequent pregnancy.

Treatment is the same as for nonpregnant patients with attention to rest, sodium restriction, fluid and electrolyte balance, control of hypertension and antibiotics to combat the infection. Interruption of pregnancy is usually not required unless the disease persists or renal function degenerates.

Chronic Glomerulonephritis

Since chronic glomerulonephritis usually antedates pregnancy by years, proteinuria or abnormal urinary sediment is generally encountered early in pregnancy when the patient is first examined. The clinical patterns include patients with proteinuria only, those with impaired renal function and those with the nephrotic syndrome.

Young gravidas in whom persistent proteinuria is found during routine examinations may have a mild form of glomerulonephritis. Renal function should be tested in these patients. If the serum urea nitrogen and creatinine are not elevated and urea and creatinine clearances are minimally diminished, then the outcome for both mother and child is probably good (Werkö and Bucht).

Women with chronic glomerulonephritis advanced to the point of renal failure tend to be sterile or they abort early in pregnancy. Some with chronic renal disease and severe azotemia may carry the pregnancy further, but hypertension increases the chances of abortion. Renal function, if severely compromised, may deteriorate rapidly during pregnancy. Whether this is due to the effects of the pregnancy or merely to the natural history of the underlying disease cannot be determined.

The fetal prognosis is usually poor. Many pregnancies terminate spontaneously by abortion or premature labor. Placental infarction and abruptio placentae are common and account partly for the high perinatal losses. Even when the pregnancy is carried successfully to full term, placental dysfunction (see Chapter 54) is seen.

In managing pregnant women with chronic glomerulonephritis, renal function should be measured frequently. The clinical condition and urinary findings should be periodically checked for functional deterioration and superimposed acute pyelonephritis. Maternal outlook makes it desirable to consider therapeutic abortion and sterilization.

The *nephrotic syndrome* may be caused by many underlying diseases, such as glomeruconephritis (most commonly), lupus nephritis, diabetic nephropathy and amyloidosis. The clinical findings are edema, massive proteinuria, hypoalbuminemia and increased levels of blood cholesterol. The immediate maternal prognosis is good unless there is some concomitant hypertension or the underlying disease is rapidly progressive (Schewitz and Seftel; Wilson). The fetal prognosis is also good provided hypertension is not also present.

Chronic Pyelonephritis

Chronic pyelonephritis may be present with no symptoms. The only abnormality may be an elevated blood pressure or transient, inconstant proteinuria. Microscopic examination of the urine may be negative. If there is no evidence of active renal infection, the outcome of the pregnancy depends on the state of renal function and the level of the blood pressure. The urine should be examined microscopically and bacteriologically at frequent intervals. Any evidence suggesting active infection requires that the patient be treated aggressively for the acute exacerbation (see above).

Lupus Nephritis

Systemic lupus erythematosus occurs in women of childbearing age. The kidney is involved in 70 per cent. With advanced lesions, especially when coassociated with lupus glomerulonephritis, progression to renal failure and death may occur rapidly. Many red and white cells and various casts are seen in the urinary sediment. Evidence of renal functional impairment is ominous.

The renal disease is probably not significantly affected by the pregnancy. Acute exacerbations may result in additional damage to the kidney and consequent progression to death from renal failure. Acute exacerbations of systemic lupus erythematosus are particularly liable to occur post partum or following abortion

(Friedman and Rutherford; Garsenstein et al.). Use of corticosteroids may be effective in controlling such exacerbations.

Polycystic Kidneys

The finding of polycystic kidneys is not a contraindication to pregnancy unless associated with impaired renal function. The good maternal and fetal prognosis seen with this condition has been attributed to the fact that the pregnancies usually occur comparatively early in the course of the disease before damage has progressed to the point where function is affected (Dalgaard).

Diabetic Nephropathy

The pregnant diabetic with proteinuria should be suspected of having diabetic nephropathy. The kidneys are likely to be involved in long-standing diabetes mellitus. They are surely involved when microaneurysms are found in the optic fundi. When the diabetic nephropathy is severe, pregnancy is contraindicated and therapeutic abortion should be advised. In addition to the severely compromised renal function, preeclampsia frequently occurs in the pregnant diabetic subject and may lead to further deterioration of renal function.

Urinary Tract Malformations

If a patient has only one kidney, its functional state should be carefully assessed before pregnancy is advised. Malformations, such as horseshoe kidneys and double ureters, are not contraindications to pregnancy provided renal function is not severely compromised. If a pelvic kidney is found, the type of delivery should be carefully weighed. It may serve to obstruct descent during labor, necessitating cesarean section. Structural abnormalities of the kidney and urinary tract increase susceptibility to infection.

REFERENCES

Baird, D.: The upper urinary tract in pregnancy and puerperium with special reference to pyelitis of pregnancy. J. Obstet. Gynaec. Brit. Emp. *43*:1, 435, 1936.

Bryant, R. E., Windom, R. E., Vineyard, J. P., Jr., and Sanford, J. P.: Asymptomatic bacteriuria in pregnancy and its association with prematurity. J. Lab. Clin. Med. *63*:224, 1964.

Bucht, H.: Studies on renal function in man with special reference to glomerular filtration and renal plasma flow in pregnancy. Scand. J. Clin. Invest. 3(Suppl. 3):1, 1951.

Dalgaard, O.: Bilateral polycystic disease of the kidney: A follow-up of 284 patients and their families. Acta Med. Scand. Suppl. *328*:1, 1958.

Flynn, F. V., Harper, C., and de Mayo, P.: Lactosuria and glycosuria in pregnancy and the puerperium. Lancet 2:698, 1953.

Friedman, E. A., and Rutherford, J. W.: Pregnancy and lupus erythematosus. Obstet. Gynec. 8:601, 1956.

Garsenstein, M., Pollak, V. E., and Kark, R. M.: Systemic lupus erythematosus and pregnancy. New Eng. J. Med. *267*:165, 1962.

Kass, E. H.: Symposium on the newer aspects of antibiotics: Chemotherapeutic and antibiotic drugs in the management of infections of the urinary tract. Amer. J. Med. *18*:764, 1955.

Parsons, R. M.: Obstetric anuria and the artificial kidney. Mod. Trends Obstet. 3:115, 1963.

Pinkerton, J. H. M., Wood, C., Williams, E. H., and Calman, R. M.: Sequelae of urinary infection in pregnancy: A five-year follow-up. Brit. Med. J. 2:539, 1961.

Schewitz, L. J., and Seftel, H. C.: The nephrotic syndrome in pregnancy: A review of 20 cases. M. Proc. South Africa 4:304, 1958.

Sims, E. A. H., and Krantz, K. E.: Serial studies of renal function during pregnancy and the puerperium in normal women. J. Clin. Invest. *37*:1764, 1958.

Welsh, G. W., and Sims, E. A. H.: The mechanisms of renal glucosuria in pregnancy. Diabetes 9:363, 1960.

Werkö, L., and Bucht, H.: Glomerular filtration rate and renal blood flow in patients with chronic diffuse glomerulonephritis during pregnancy. Acta Med. Scand. *153*:177, 1956.

Wilson, C.: Renal hypertension and pregnancy. *In* Morris, N. F., and Brown, J. C. M., eds.: Symposium on Non-Toxaemic Hypertension in Pregnancy. London, J. & A. Churchill, Ltd., 1958.

Chapter 45

Pulmonary Disease

PULMONARY FUNCTION IN PREGNANCY

In the course of normal pregnancy, the oxygen consumption rises in response to metabolic demands. The respiratory rate increases. This reduces plasma CO_2 content. Residual lung volume is reduced as the diaphragm is elevated by the growing uterus. Dyspnea occurs in more than 60 per cent of women in the course of pregnancy. The cause is incompletely understood. No correlation has been found between the intensity of this symptom and the various measures of pulmonary function (Cugell et al.). Bader et al. demonstrated an increase in the oxygen cost of breathing in dyspneic gravidas, but only near term. This observation does not explain the dyspnea of early pregnancy.

Vital capacity, maximal ventilatory capacity and total pulmonary resistance to airflow are essentially the same in pregnancy as in the nonpregnant state. Dyspnea may occur before there is any increase in abdominal girth or impingement of the growing uterus on the diaphragm. Normal women do not become increasingly dyspneic when the circulatory load is greatest and diaphragmatic movement is most constricted in the third trimester. Orthopnea may occasionally be seen, however, based on the difficulty encountered in breathing, especially if the uterus is greatly overdistended, as in association with multiple pregnancy or hydramnios. Dyspnea may be the result of subjective response related to an unfamiliar low level of CO_2 partial pressure during exercise (Gilbert et al.) which is seen in pregnancy.

remain stable

Pulmonary Function Tests

The patient who has chronic pulmonary disease or who has had major thoracic surgery should be evaluated carefully before conception or during pregnancy in order to determine her pulmonary reserve. This will help to define her ability to go through pregnancy and labor. It will also ascertain whether or not pulmonary complications are likely to develop as a consequence of the pregnancy.

Several simple and quick tests are available for this purpose (Meneely and Ferguson). They include (1) vital capacity, (2) timed vital capacity and (3) maximal breathing capacity tests. Vital capacity alone is capable of detecting only about one-third of patients with pulmonary impairment. Maximal breathing capacity, on the other hand, detects two-thirds or more. It has some major drawbacks, however, in that it requires considerable exertion on the part of the patient; its proper performance is dependent on the free use of abdominal and thoracic musculature and these, of course, may be impinged upon by the large uterus in advanced pregnancy. Timed vital capacity is probably the best procedure for preoperative evaluation of pulmonary function expressed as the volume of air expelled in the first half second by a maximal forced expiration beginning at full inspiration. The combination of total vital capacity with timed vital capacity is still better (Miller et al.): vital capacity of less than 85 per cent of predicted value provides evidence of some restrictive ventilatory defect; timed vital capacity of less than 60 per cent of the observed vital capacity suggests some airway obstruction.

494

TUBERCULOSIS

Serious consequences may arise from pulmonary disorders during pregnancy, labor or post partum if they are not recognized and treated appropriately. Therefore, it is essential that every obstetric patient be evaluated for lung pathology. In many areas routine posteroanterior chest x-ray is still done in a search for evidence of tuberculosis. The yield is low and the risks of fetal radiation are present. Therefore, this is being replaced by skin testing by Mantoux reaction (intracutaneous injection of 0.1 ml. or 5 units of purified protein derivative, PPD). If positive, a standard 14 × 17-inch chest film is obtained. Photofluorography is avoided because of the increased radiation associated with its use.

Pulmonary tuberculosis remains a frequently encountered major pulmonary infection. It is estimated that active disease exists in at least one per cent of the gravid population (Schaefer). The reported incidence depends in large part on the intensity of the effort made to diagnose it.

There have been many significant and dramatic changes in the treatment of tuberculosis in recent years. Effective chemotherapy has essentially replaced traditional forms of therapy such as pneumothorax, pneumoperitoneum and phrenic nerve operations. Thoracoplasty has been replaced by resection as the most effective surgical method. Complete bed rest has given way to modified bed rest. These changes are reflected in the obstetric management of the tuberculous gravida.

Medical Management

The management of the pregnant woman with active pulmonary tuberculosis must be individualized. Basic principles of accurate diagnosis must be carried out, including chest x-rays, sputum and gastric analyses. The patient known to have active disease before conception is continued on the same course of therapy through pregnancy without interruption. The antituberculosis drugs used are isoniazid, streptomycin and para-aminosalicylic acid (PAS). Initial therapy should include isoniazid and at least one of the other agents. Current practice is to use 300 mg. oral isoniazid daily, and 12 gm. oral PAS daily. If the disease is advanced, 1 gm. of streptomycin is given intramuscularly daily for several weeks and then the schedule is reduced to 1 gm. twice a week. These drugs are continued throughout the entire pregnancy and for at least six months post partum or until the disease is considered to be arrested. Very few deleterious effects on the pregnant patient or her offspring have been observed with this program. Isolated reports indicate the possibility of eighth nerve damage to the fetus. In balance, the drug is of such vital importance to the mother that it should be given whenever indicated.

If active tuberculosis is first discovered during pregnancy, the patient should be hospitalized immediately. The type and extent of the disease should be delineated and drug therapy promptly instituted. The patient with inactive tuberculosis should have at least three sputum or gastric analyses done. Adequate diet must be ensured and vitamin and iron supplements prescribed, if indicated. Daily rest periods should be advised.

Pulmonary tuberculosis is almost never an indication for therapeutic abortion unless pulmonary function is markedly impaired. Thoracic surgery may sometimes come up for consideration during pregnancy. Generally, it should not be undertaken until the patient has had the benefit of at least six months of antimicrobial therapy. Subsequent reevaluation will show whether there has been substantial improvement with no residual cavitations. If so, chemotherapy should be continued; if not, surgery may indeed be indicated, but it is preferably undertaken in the nonpregnant state.

Obstetric Management

The principles of care outlined for the cardiac gravidas (see Chapter 41) apply equally here. Labor and delivery should be made as easy as possible for the tuberculous patient. Heavy sedation should be avoided because it may diminish the cough reflex. Combinations of small doses of a narcotic analgesic and a synergistic tranquilizer are effective. Continuous peridural anesthesia (see Chapter 22) will provide suitable pain relief for labor as well as for delivery and is highly recommended. Local infiltration or pudendal block is also appropriate for delivery procedures. If general anesthesia should be necessary, one may effectively use balanced anesthesia consisting of thiopental induction, succinylcholine muscle relaxation and nitrous oxide maintenance. Ether tends to be too irritating for use in these patients.

If labor is progressing satisfactorily, the descent should be allowed to continue without interruption or stimulation. To preclude excessive bearing down in the second stage, forceps procedures are frequently undertaken. Cesarean section is not indicated for pulmonary tuberculosis, but may have to be done for clear-cut obstetric reasons.

The prognosis for the infant is good. Perinatal mortality is not increased in association with pulmonary tuberculosis in the mother and there is also no elevation of the prematurity rate. Congenital tuberculosis is extremely uncommon, although some cases have been described. The danger of neonatal infection of an infant does exist, however, if he is exposed to the mother with a positive sputum. For this reason, mothers with active tuberculosis should not be permitted to take care of their infants. Breast feeding should be prohibited.

Rest is essential for tuberculous patients post partum. Even with previously inactive disease, extended hospitalization for rest and evaluation is very important. Gastric analysis should be done in search of tubercle bacilli and chest x-rays obtained. Reexaminations are carried out again at six weeks and at three months after delivery.

UPPER RESPIRATORY INFECTIONS

The significance of upper respiratory infections in a patient undergoing labor and delivery should not be underestimated. They are so common, unfortunately, that there is a tendency to ignore or overlook them. The risks of postpartum or postabortal complications may be significantly increased by them. Pneumonia is often preceded by common colds or other forms of upper respiratory infection. The hazards of surgery, anesthesia and delivery are multiplied by the presence of such active infections. Half of the patients who develop pulmonary atelectasis postoperatively have had recent respiratory infections (Goodwin); it is a rare event in others. Furthermore, hemolytic streptococcal puerperal infections are most common among patients who have had precedent acute infection of the upper respiratory tract at delivery.

Acute respiratory infection may be developing during labor, but may be undetectable. Patients should be questioned about such respiratory symptoms as pharyngitis, rhinorrhea, cough, sputum, chest pain and malaise. A thorough physical examination is essential.

These infections should not be regarded lightly, but should be treated vigorously when they occur near term. Supportive measures include bed rest, steam inhalations, codeine for cough and antihistamines when indicated. It is now generally considered inappropriate to use antibiotics prior to delivery as prophylaxis against pneumonia. Antibiotics should be reserved for treatment of specific bacterial infections, if they should develop (see below). General anesthesia should not be used for either vaginal or abdominal delivery, if possible, in the presence of an active upper respiratory infection.

BRONCHITIS

Acute bronchitis is commonly associated with pulmonary and upper respiratory infections. It may also result from physical or chemical irritants, aspiration and acute exanthemata. Bronchitis is manifested clinically by a cough that may or may not be productive. The cough may cause pain or substernal rawness. It is usually associated with low grade fever, chills, hoarseness and headache. It tends to be a mild and self-limiting disease. Symptoms are worse in the winter months and are especially troublesome in the morning on awakening. Deep breathing may result in intense episodic coughing and breathlessness.

The danger of bronchitis to the pregnant patient is that it may extend to the parenchyma of the lung and give rise to pneumonia. Early treatment is essential with the usual supportive measures, including bed rest, codeine, expectorants, steam inhalation and bronchial vasodilators, such as ephedrine. If bronchitis is present during labor or when operative intervention is expected, inhalation anesthesia should be avoided.

PNEUMONIA

Bacterial Pneumonia

Although viruses and mycoplasmas are probably the most common causes of pneumonia today, bacterial pneumonias are still seen frequently. In pregnancy, pneumonia may embarrass ventilation sufficiently to produce hypoxia. This has a potentially serious effect on the fetus. It is important to define the cause quickly so that early effective treatment can be instituted. Diagnosis is made easier by the prevailing epidemiologic picture, clinical pattern of the disease, coassociated or precedent infections, x-ray findings and bacteriologic studies.

Pneumonococcal pneumonia may occur in isolated cases or in small epidemics. It is frequently secondary to an acute respiratory infection. Consolidation is usually confined to one or more lobes. When the infection extends to the bloodstream, the prognosis is grave. Complications include pleural inflammation with effusion, empyema, pericarditis or endocarditis. The prognosis may be adversely influenced by pregnancy, particularly in the third trimester (Hinshaw).

Hemolytic streptococcal pneumonia is usually secondary to acute epidemic infectious diseases, such as influenza and measles. Staphylococcal pneumonia may be secondary to a staphylococcal infection elsewhere in the body. Its onset is insidious, but its symptoms may be severe.

Klebsiella (Friedländer's bacillus) pneumonia is uncommon and is manifested by multiple foci of consolidation in the lungs. Other bacteria may also cause pneumonia. These include hemophilus, pseudomonas and mixed coliform organisms. They tend to occur in debilitated patients and are difficult therapeutic problems.

It is important to distinguish the causative agent and its antibiotic sensitivities so that appropriate specific treatment may be initiated as early as possible. This requires a bacteriologic diagnosis and precise *in vitro* determination of sensitivity of the organisms to various antibiotic agents. Sputum and blood cultures should be obtained before instituting therapy. Pending definite identification of the organism, a simple Gram stain of the sputum will indicate the probable nature of the infection and its treatment. If the stain shows large numbers of Gram-positive cocci, the infection is probably responsive to penicillin or a broad spectrum antibiotic. If Gram-negative bacilli predominate, agents effective against these organisms should be given instead, including kanamycin, gentamycin or chloramphenicol.

Prompt treatment may prevent premature labor and increase the chances of fetal survival. When bacteriologic identification of the etiologic organism is made and its sensitivities known, one may then consider changing the antibiotic regimen. If the patient's response has been good, there is no need to do so even if this contradicts the laboratory findings. For pneumococcal pneumonia, 200,000 units of crystalline penicillin G intramuscularly, followed by 100,000 unit doses every 12 hours, is usually very effective. Dosage levels should be increased or may be given intravenously in the presence of bacteremia or multilobar involvement. If the patient is allergic to penicillin, erythromycin or lincomycin may be given instead in 500 mg. oral doses every six hours.

Hemolytic streptococcal pneumonia can be treated in the same manner, but with larger doses of antibiotics. Ampicillin tends to be effective also. Staphylococcal pneumonia is often penicillin resistant and should be combated with agents to which the organism may be sensitive, such as cephalothin, ampicillin, methicillin or naf-cillin. If not resistant, staphylococcal pneumonia is preferably treated with penicillin G, 1 million units intravenously every six hours. Klebsiella pneumonia requires streptomycin 2 gm. daily by intramuscular route combined with equivalent amounts of chloramphenicol or tetracyclines. Combinations of sulfadiazine (2 to 4 gm. daily) and streptomycin or tetracycline are recommended for hemophilus pneumonia; ampicillin only may also be used with good results.

Supportive therapy for the pneumonias includes treatment of dehydration and anemia when present. Edema may require salt restriction and diuretics. Oxygen therapy may be necessary for dyspnea and cyanosis. Bed rest is essential. Analgesics are given to relieve pain and antitussives to suppress coughing.

Pneumonia is a serious complication of pregnancy, particularly when it develops near term. At one time it resulted in many maternal deaths, but this is fortunately no longer true. However, premature labor may occur and if the patient goes into labor while suffering from pneumonia, the problem is compounded. Narcotic-analgesic drugs that depress respiration should be avoided. General inhalation anesthesia should not be used. Continuous peridural anesthesia is preferable; if unavailable, paracervical and pudendal blocks are effective. The patient should receive oxygen throughout labor and delivery. Expulsive efforts should be averted in the second stage and delivery effected by means of an atraumatic forceps procedure. Antibiotics should be continued for several days after the temperature becomes normal.

Viral Pneumonia

A large variety of viruses can cause pneumonitis, including Coxsackie viruses and the viruses of chickenpox and measles. Characteristically, viral pneumonia begins insidiously with low grade fever and cough. Chest x-ray shows patchy infiltrates contradicting the negligible findings on physical examination of the lungs. There tends to be neither consolidation nor pleural effusion. In contrast to the leukocytosis expected with bacterial pneumonias, the white count is usually normal. Diagnosis is generally made by ruling out a bacterial etiology, although techniques are available for isolating the virus or verifying the infection by demonstrating a specific antibody response.

Treatment is nonspecific. It consists of bed rest in a hospital with oxygen available as needed plus fluid and electrolyte replacement. Codeine is useful as an antitussive agent to control the distressing and sometimes exhausting cough. The patient should be carefully watched for the possible development of secondary bacterial pneumonia. If it should develop, appropriate antibiotics must be given (see above) after cultures are obtained.

Pregnant women are particularly susceptible to influenza and suffer a greater than expected mortality from this disease (see Chapter 40). Moreover, many undergo abortion or premature labor. Because the hazards are so great, it is important that pregnant women be immunized against specific influenza viruses during epidemics and sheltered from exposure if possible.

Mycoplasma Pneumonia

The so-called atypical pneumonia is now known to be caused by *Mycoplasma pneumoniae*, a pathogen of animals and fowl. The disease is probably often subclinical and unrecognized in its usual form. Manifestations tend to be relatively mild with moderate fever, cough and patchy infiltrates on x-rays of the chest similar to those in viral pneumonias. There is usually no leukocytosis, but nonspecific cold hemagglutinins are often detectable. The disease is particularly prevalent in adolescents and young adults. When the clinical pattern is severe enough to warrant treatment, response to erythromycin or tetracycline is generally very good. Treatment should be continued for at least two to three days after the temperature has returned to normal so as to avoid the common problem of recrudescence by viable organisms still present in the patient. General principles of supportive care are the same as those outlined above for viral pneumonia.

Aspiration Pneumonia

Mendelson described a severe chemical pneumonia in obstetric patients caused by the aspiration of stomach contents into the lungs during anesthesia (see Chapter 22). It usually occurs in association with aspiration under deep general inhalation anesthesia, especially during induction and as the patient awakens, but may even be encountered in patients under high spinal anesthesia, during eclamptic convulsions or while preeclamptic patients are under heavy sedation.

Two different syndromes may follow the aspiration of stomach contents. Laryngeal or tracheal obstruction may occur and cause suffocation if solid food is aspirated. Death will occur if obstruction is not relieved immediately. Incomplete obstruction of one or more mainstem bronchi produces massive atelectasis with cyanosis, tachycardia, dyspnea, mediastinal shift and signs of consolidation. Prompt bronchoscopy may be helpful in relieving some of this problem, but secondary pneumonia and abscess formation is common.

Aspiration of gastric liquid material containing hydrochloric acid results in a serious problem called *Mendelson's syndrome*, associated with ventilatory obstruction due to severe bronchial and bronchiolar spasm. Cyanosis, tachycardia and dyspnea develop, but there is neither mediastinal shift nor massive atelectasis. Patients demonstrate tachypnea with many rales and rhonchi in the affected lobes. Therapy for this asthmatoid syndrome should be directed against bronchiolar spasm and cardiac enlargement. Treatment should be started promptly and pursued aggressively because of the potentially serious consequences of the disorder. In addition to the mechanical measures outlined in Chapter 22 for effecting drainage by positioning and suction, patients who have aspirated gastric fluid should be given (1) corticosteroids in large doses (e.g., hydrocortisone 1 gm. or equivalent intravenously); (2) broncholytic agents, such as aminophylline (500 mg. by slow intravenous injection), isoproterenol (0.5 ml. of 0.5 per cent solution) or epinephrine (0.1 to 0.5 ml. of 1:1000 solution); (3) antibiotics to combat secondary infection; and (4) oxygen, especially under intermittent positive pressure, to reduce pulmonary edema and correct hypoxia. Such patients deserve the special expertise and facilities of a surgical intensive care unit, if available. Shock may occur and require all measures needed for support of the cardiovascular system (see Chapter 51).

BRONCHIECTASIS

Dilatation of the bronchial tree may be initiated by prolonged bronchial obstruction and infection with bronchospasm to produce bronchiectasis. The symptoms include those of chronic suppurative bronchitis, such as productive cough and hemoptysis. Recurrences are common. If the disease is prolonged and extensive, the patient shows progressively developing weakness, loss of appetite, dyspnea, palpitation and clubbing of the fingers and toes.

Treatment during pregnancy should be directed toward controlling symptoms by postural drainage and by the administration of expectorants and antibiotics for the specific bacterial invaders. Aerosols may be useful. After delivery, resection of affected areas may be considered if medical treatment has not been successful.

As a rule, pregnancy has no particular effect on the course of bronchiectasis. Aggravation of cough and dyspnea depend on the extent of the disease and the occurrence of active infection. General inhalation anesthesia should be avoided at delivery, if possible.

SARCOIDOSIS

The typical granulomatous lesions of sarcoidosis may involve lymph nodes, lungs, liver, spleen, skin and eyes primarily. The roentgen finding of symmetrically enlarged hilar mediastinal lymph nodes is highly suspicious; Hodgkin's disease, tuberculosis, lymphoma, berylliosis and other granulomatous diseases must be excluded. A characteristic of sarcoidosis is the disparity between the extent of the disease and its clinical manifestations. The symptoms are mild despite extensive lymph node and organ involvement. The natural history of this disease is its unpredictable remissions and exacerbations.

Laboratory findings are not consistent or pathognomonic. A negative tuberculin test is of value in ruling out active tuberculosis; tuberculin anergy is encountered in two-thirds of patients with sarcoidosis. A specific skin test, the Kveim test, is positive in 80 per cent of patients. This requires intradermal injection of a suspension of lymphoid tissue obtained from patients with sarcoidosis and biopsy of the papule which develops six weeks to one year later to show the characteristic granuloma formation. The albumin-globulin ratio is frequently reversed owing to hypergammaglobulinemia. Leukopenia, eosinophilia and slight monocytosis are common. Erythrocyte sedimentation rate is usually rapid. Alkaline phosphatase and serum and urine calcium levels are generally increased. Many patients with sarcoidosis have a mild hypochromic, microcytic anemia.

Pregnancy appears to have no special effect on the course of sarcoidosis (O'Leary). Steroid therapy may have to be given during pregnancy because of a progression of the pulmonary lesion or eye involvement. Patients receiving steroids for sarcoidosis and those with a positive tuberculin test should receive isoniazid concomitantly.

Other than avoidance of heavy sedation and general inhalation anesthesia, pregnant patients with sarcoidosis require no special management of their labors and deliveries. Therapeutic abortion or cesarean section is not especially indicated for sarcoidosis. Complications such as pneumonia may result in pulmonary insufficiency. This rare occurrence should be treated, preferably well before labor begins. Delivery should be carried out under conduction anesthesia. A nontraumatic forceps procedure may be used, if necessary, to effect delivery without requiring the patient to bear down in the second stage.

ASTHMA

The incidence of bronchial asthma in antepartum patients is about one per cent.

It is manifested by breathing difficulties, wheezing and cough, as well as by orthopnea and chest tightness occasionally. Some asthmatics complain that they are unable to take in sufficient air, especially during the acute phase. In general, asthma seems unaffected by pregnancy, most patients experiencing no severe exacerbations (Schaefer and Silverman).

Medical Management

The gravida can be reassured that her asthma will have essentially no bearing on her pregnancy or on the outcome of her delivery. However, certain precautions should be observed. Needless to say, she should avoid conditions that might precipitate an acute exacerbation. Known responsible agents or contributory factors that produce attacks, such as dust, fumes, smoke or cold air, should be shunned. Similarly, since exertion may also precipitate an attack, particularly during the last trimester when the respiratory excursions are limited by the enlarging uterus, physical activities should be curtailed. Respiratory infection, which plays an important role as either a primary or precipitating factor in asthma, should be treated promptly and aggressively. If possible, emotional stresses should be avoided.

Treatment is the same as in the nonpregnant asthmatic patient. Iodides should not be used in large doses over long periods because they may cause fetal goiter. Some patients with chronic asthma are able to control their symptoms by the rectal administration of aminophylline at bedtime. An imminent attack may be aborted by inhalation of a fine spray of ephedrine by nebulizer. Antihistamines may give relief when used during periods of seasonal allergy.

When an asthmatic attack occurs during pregnancy or labor, the obstetrician must provide emergency treatment. The basic principles of care include (1) relieving anxiety, (2) administering a bronchodilator, (3) providing sedation and (4) maintaining oxygenation. The physician's calm, confident and sympathetic attitude is most important in providing warmth and reassurance to the asthmatic. Effective bronchodilators include self-administered aerosols of 2.25 per cent epinephrine or 1:200 isoproterenol. If these are ineffectual, one should give a subcutaneous injection of epinephrine 0.2 to 0.3 ml. of a 1:1000 solution. Caution is necessary when such vasopressor agents are used in the presence of a hypertensive state of pregnancy. Mild sedation is useful in the form of phenobarbital 30 mg., pentobarbital sodium 100 mg. or chloral hydrate 0.5 to 2.0 gm. One should avoid the respiratory depressant effects of narcotics.

It is well to remember that, in seriously ill patients with anoxia and hypercapnia, sedation in any form may depress ventilation and lead to even greater respiratory insufficiency and carbon dioxide retention. For a mild attack aminophylline should be given as a 500 mg. suppository, or 500 mg. may be administered rectally in 15 ml. of water. For a more severe attack 500 mg. of aminophylline in 20 ml. of solution may be given intravenously.

The patient should be hospitalized if relief is not obtained promptly by these measures. Hospital treatment should start with an intravenous infusion of 1000 ml. of 5 per cent dextrose in water containing 500 mg. of aminophylline. A total of 3 liters may be given within 24 hours.

When oxygen is necessary because of hypoxia, it should be given by intermittent positive pressure. Maternal arterial pO_2 should be determined, if possible, as an indirect measure of possible fetal hypoxia. Bronchoscopic aspiration may sometimes result in spectacular improvement in the very ill patient whose bronchial tree contains inspissated, tenacious secretions. The reestablishment of the airway by this means may be lifesaving.

For patients who are more than mildly ill, frequent nebulization with bronchodilators and wetting agents with an intermittent positive pressure breathing device is advised. Steam inhalations of Superinone (Alevaire) and postural drainage may be of some value in ridding the patient of accumulated secretions.

Bronchial infection should be vigorously treated with antibiotics. Corticosteroids may be used for their antiinflammatory and antiallergic effects when conventional methods prove ineffective.

Obstetric Management

Patients should be closely questioned concerning sensitivity to medications commonly used in the management of labor and delivery, including analgesic, hypnotic, ataractic, anesthetic and antibiotic agents. It is essential for the physician to avoid using any to which the parturient may be allergic.

Analgesia for labor should be minimized to prevent respiratory depression. Small doses of Demerol and promethazine or other antihistaminic tranquilizer are useful. Morphine is contraindicated in the asthmatic patient. Neither atropine nor scopolamine should be used because their drying action may lead to mucus inspissation.

The principles outlined in Chapter 22 with reference to anesthesia practices are especially applicable here. Irritation of the bronchial mucosa and respiratory depression must be guarded against. Local or regional blocks are preferable to inhalation anesthesia, but nitrous oxide and trichloroethylene are acceptable for short periods. Ether may be used for deep anesthesia, but it is contraindicated for light anesthesia because it is very irritating to the mucous membrane. As a consequence, ether may cause bronchospasm and increase bronchial secretions. Spinal or peridural anesthesia is recommended for cesarean section or for operative vaginal delivery, although sensitivity to local anesthetic solutions may preclude their use. Oxygenation must be assured at all times. If corticosteroids have been used, it is essential to maintain the cardiovascular state and avoid hypotension. Maintenance or supplemental doses of steroids should be given during the course of labor as required.

FUNGAL INFECTIONS

Coccidioidomycosis

Coccidioidomycosis is a fungal disease confined to endemic areas in the southwestern United States. It is caused by the fungus *Coccidioides immitis* and is spread by inhalation of the spores from the soil. Manifestations vary widely. The disease is usually a benign infectious process from which recovery is the rule; it is commonly unrecognized. At the other extreme, it could be an overwhelming infection that causes death within a few weeks. Chills, fever, substernal chest pain, generalized muscular aches, backache, pharyngitis, headache, weakness and night sweats occur together with cervical adenopathy.

The disease may simulate pulmonary tuberculosis. Treatment consists of rest and supportive measures to enable adequate focalization. Permanent immunity results after recovery.

Active coccidioidal infection during pregnancy is serious because of the tendency of the disease to disseminate, especially during the last trimester. When infection occurs in the first trimester, abortion is frequent; in the third trimester, premature labor can be expected (Vaughn and Ramirez).

Dissemination may be catastrophic. Surgical therapy by lobectomy is recommended for excision of large residual cavities of more than 5 cm. in diameter or for recurrent hemorrhage (Melick). Medical therapy consists of the administration of amphotericin B, which is highly toxic. It is given intravenously, by dilute infusion, starting with 0.25 mg. per kilogram of body weight and increasing to 1.0 mg. per kilogram over three to four days. Daily infusions up to a 1 gm. limit usually suffice, but patients with progressive disease may require as much as 2 gm. The renal toxicity increases at this dosage. Hospitalization is necessary because of the severe side effects of the treatment, including fever, anorexia, emesis, phlebitis, thrombocytopenia, hypokalemia and azotemia. It is clear that therapy is given only for the most severe cases in which the risk of the disease exceeds that of the treatment.

Histoplasmosis

Histoplasmosis is also frequently unrecognized because the symptoms are so mild. In endemic regions the disease is contracted and recovery occurs without any awareness of the infection. It appears to be universal in distribution, transmitted by way of the feces of domesticated fowl and wild birds.

It may be detected on routine chest x-ray examinations of pregnant patients. The lungs show extensive involvement by numerous spherical nodules, and the hilar nodes may be enlarged. There may be x-ray evidence of healed primary histoplasmosis with calcification. In addition, fibrocaseous lesions resembling pulmonary tuberculosis occur. This condition is indistinguishable from chronic pulmonary tuberculosis on clinical and roentgenographic grounds alone. Moreover, tuberculosis and histoplasmosis may coexist.

A differential diagnosis is made from the absence of tubercle bacilli and the presence of *Histoplasma capsulatum* in the sputum, with a negative tuberculin test. A positive histoplasmin skin test is diagnostic provided that coccidioidomycosis and blastomycosis have been eliminated.

The treatment of histoplasmosis is reserved for symptomatic patients with progressive or generalized disease, especially those with hepatosplenomegaly, emaciation, recurrent fever, leukopenia and anemia. Amphotericin B may be helpful. It must be used with all due care because of its great toxicity (see above) and stopped if renal damage is encountered.

REFERENCES

Bader, R. W., Bader, M. E., and Rose, D. J.: Oxygen cost of breathing in dyspneic subjects as studied in normal pregnant women. Clin. Sci. *18*:223, 1959.

Cugell, D. W., Frank, N. R., Gaensler, E. A., and Badger, T. L.: Pulmonary function in pregnancy. Amer. Rev. Tuberc. 67:568, 1953.

Gilbert, R., Epifano, L., and Auchincloss, J. H., Jr.:

Dyspnea of pregnancy: A syndrome of altered respiratory control. J.A.M.A. *182*:1073, 1962.

Goodwin, J. F.: Study of post-operative pulmonary atelectasis. Brit. J. Surg. 36:256, 1949.

Hinshaw, H. C.: Diseases of the Chest. Philadelphia, W. B. Saunders Company, 1969.

Melick, D. W.: The surgical treatment of pulmonary

coccidioidomycosis with a comprehensive summary of the complications following this type of therapy. Amer. Rev. Tuberc. 77:17, 1958.

Mendelson, C. L.: Aspiration of stomach contents into the lungs during obstetric anesthesia. Amer. J. Obstet. Gynec. 52:191, 1946.

Meneely, G. R., and Ferguson, J. L.: Pulmonary evaluation and risk in patient preparation for anesthesia and surgery. J.A.M.A. 175:1074, 1961.

Miller, W. F., Wu, N., and Johnson, R. L., Jr.: Convenient method of evaluating pulmonary ventilatory function with a single breath test. Anesthesiology 17:480, 1956.

O'Leary, J. A.: Ten year study of sarcoidosis and pregnancy. Amer. J. Obstet. Gynec. 84:462, 1962.

Schaefer, G.: Tuberculosis in Obstetrics and Gynecology. Boston, Little, Brown & Company, 1956.

Schaefer, G., and Silverman, F.: Pregnancy complicated by asthma. Amer. J. Obstet. Gynec. 82:182, 1961.

Vaughan, J. E., and Ramirez, H.: Coccidioidomycosis as a complication of pregnancy. Calif. Med. 74:121, 1951.

Chapter 46

Skin Diseases

During pregnancy and the puerperium, the *skin* and its appendages undergo many changes. The hair may be altered significantly. In particular, postpartum hair loss may be acute and when it occurs, it evokes anxiety. Actually, hair loss usually decreases during pregnancy and increases again after delivery (Lynfield; Schiff and Kern). The onset of significant hair loss is reported to start between 8 and 16 weeks post partum. The degree of alopecia varies considerably and lasts from 1 to 15 months after onset. In most instances alopecia repeats after successive pregnancies. It is believed that direct hormone stimulation on the hair metabolism controls hair loss and regrowth. The prognosis for regrowth without specific therapy is excellent. Reassurance is most important.

Vascular changes are common. Spider nevi or angiomas, varicose veins, hemorrhoids and palmar erythema are found in most pregnant women. These are primarily the result of increased intravascular pressure and endocrine changes, especially increased estrogens in the blood. After pregnancy, most vascular changes return to their prepregnant state. Purpuric lesions and edema may accompany circulatory changes, but more important pathologic causes should not be overlooked.

Pigmentary changes include darkening of the nipples and the appearance of the linea nigra in the lower abdominal midline. *Melasma* is characteristically seen in pregnancy as localized patchy hyperpigmentation of the face. It is also known as *chloasma* or *pregnancy mask*. The skin color tends to revert to normal after delivery.

PREGNANCY-ASSOCIATED DERMATOSES

Herpes gestationis is a rare but important skin disease associated with pregnancy. It is a herpetiform lesion by virtue of the grouped, pruritic and vesicular lesions. Sensitivity to iodides may be present. Peripheral eosinophilia, occasionally as high as 30 to 40 per cent, is common. The incidence is about 1:3000 deliveries.

Onset may be as early as the first trimester, but is most often in the second and third trimesters or in the first week or two of the puerperium. Once it occurs, the condition recurs in all subsequent pregnancies. It is associated with a high incidence of congenital abnormalities (Keaty et al.; Downing and Jillson). The eruption clears in 4 to 16 weeks after delivery (Russell and Thorne). Persistence of the eruption for as long as eight months after delivery has been observed.

The rash may range from erythematous macules through vesicobullous lesions; one type usually predominates. Pruritus and burning are the primary symptoms and there may be diagnostic confusion with tinea corporis, drug reactions, erythema multiforme and pemphigus.

Treatment tends to be ineffectual, although corticosteroids may control the disease. Supportive measures, such as antipruritic creams and lotions, analgesics and sedatives, are of value.

Papular dermatitis of pregnancy is a generalized, widely scattered, pruritic eruption (Spangler et al.). Associated with the eruption are increased urinary chorionic gonadotropin in the last trimester, lowered plasma hydrocortisone levels and shortened hydrocortisone half-life. Corticosteroid therapy is generally effective. Perhaps this condition is a variant of herpes gestationis.

Impetigo herpetiformis is a rare pustular disease affecting the skin and mucous membranes and accompanying serious systemic disease. It probably represents a manifestation of bacteremia and sepsis. Treatment should be directed at the underlying infection.

Adventitious changes of the gingiva represent a spectrum of conditions called stomatitis gravidarum, gingivitis gravidarum, proliferative gingivitis of pregnancy, hypertrophic gingivitis of pregnancy, epulis gravidarum and pregnancy tumor. The gingiva tends to become hypertrophic and proliferative in varying degrees. The changes last throughout pregnancy and may persist for several months after delivery. Local surgical removal gives temporary relief, but the proliferative changes usually continue to progress until spontaneous recession after delivery.

Prurigo of pregnancy and pruritus probably represent variations or subclinical cases of herpes gestationis. However, search for other causes of the pruritus, such as renal and liver disease, drug reactions, xerotic skin and contactants, should be undertaken. Local antipruritic measures and oral antihistamines usually control those cases in which no specific underlying cause can be found.

Molluscum fibrosum gravidarum consists of pinhead to pea-sized pedunculated tags usually present on the neck, chest, axillary and mammary areas. They develop during the later months of pregnancy and may partially or completely disappear after delivery. Electrodesiccation is the best treatment.

COINCIDENTAL DERMATOSES

Alopecia areata and *alopecia totalis* may rarely appear during pregnancy (Fig. 281). Treatment is ineffectual. Psychologic support is needed. The use of wigs is recom-

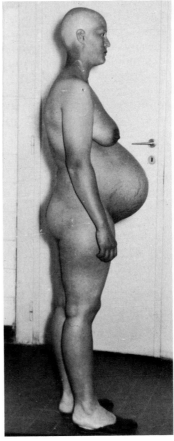

Figure 281 Patient showing spontaneous alopecia totalis occurring in pregnancy. (Courtesy of B. Beric.)

mended. In general, the prognosis for regrowth is good, but no specific time can be predicted.

New *pigmented nevi* may appear during pregnancy; those present may change in size, shape and color. The usual clinical signs of growth and change, suggesting neoplastic disease, should be the basic reason for removal and laboratory examination of a pigmented tumor. Prophylactic removal of pigmented nevi is not recommended as a routine procedure.

Melanosarcoma may occur rarely during pregnancy. There is no increased incidence of melanosarcoma during pregnancy (Pillsbury et al.). Radical surgical treatment, if feasible and indicated, should not be altered out of consideration for the pregnancy. Abortion or castration does not affect the course of metastases. Pregnancy does not change the survival rate.

Pemphigus vulgaris and *erythema mul-*

tiforme bullosum affect skin and mucous membranes with the development of bullae. Acantholysis in the epidermis is histologically diagnostic for pemphigus. This is seen as degeneration of the epidermal intercellular bridges. Both of these potentially fatal diseases can be controlled with corticosteroids. Abortion is not generally indicated. Drugs are frequently the cause of erythema multiforme; the cause of pemphigus is unknown.

Verruca or *condyloma acuminata* are soft, fungating warts usually found about the vulva and anus. They usually increase in size and number in pregnancy, especially during warm weather. They are easily distinguished from the highly infectious, flattened *condyloma lata* of syphilis. Topical treatment with 25 per cent podophyllin in compound benzoin tincture tends to control these warts, but recurrences are usual. Treatment with this caustic agent may be accompanied by discomfort and should not be pursued too vigorously during pregnancy. Moreover, podophyllin may be absorbed systemically, cross the placenta and adversely affect the fetus, even causing death (Gorthey and Krembs). Cryosurgical techniques with liquid nitrogen are rapidly replacing this older approach.

The course of *acne vulgaris* during pregnancy is unpredictable. Some cases become worse, especially during the first three months, while improvement generally is evident during the last two trimesters.

Atopic dermatitis (disseminated neurodermatitis) frequently improves during pregnancy. Emotional undulations, sweating and intertriginous friction frequently precipitate exacerbations and increase itching. Local neurodermatitis *(lichen simplex chronicus)* is worse in the anxious patient. Active treatment of hand involvement is important so the mother can adequately care for her newborn baby and her home.

Miliaria or prickly heat is best prevented by frequent cleansing, liberal use of dusting powder and minimized friction. Treatment with shake lotions, aerosol preparations, powders and compresses gives the best results.

Both discoid and systemic *lupus erythematosus* is usually well tolerated in pregnancy. Pregnancy does not seem to affect the course of the disease adversely, although exacerbations are common post partum. Exposure to sunlight and other ultraviolet light sources is to be avoided. Treatment is indicated with active and progressive disease. Corticosteroids are effective in progressive, serious disease. The prognosis of systemic lupus erythematosus depends on the degree of involvement of the kidney (see Chapter 44) and the heart. Suspicion of lupus erythematosus should be aroused by a weakly positive serologic test for syphilis.

Psoriasis generally remains static during pregnancy. It is advisable to use topical therapy for control. Systemic therapy with steroids is best avoided. Aminopterin sodium and related drugs are contraindicated.

Morbilliform eruptions, especially during the first trimester of pregnancy, should be investigated thoroughly. German measles (see Chapter 40) or other exanthematous viral diseases may be present, and drug reactions may mimic these diseases.

REFERENCES

Bean, W. B., Cogswell, R. C., Dexter, M., and Embick, J. F.: Vascular changes of the skin in pregnancy: Vascular spiders and palmar erythema. Surg. Gynec. Obstet. 88:739, 1949.

Downing, J. G., and Jillson, O. F.: Herpes gestationis. New Eng. J. Med. 241:906, 1949.

Gorthey, R. L., and Krembs, M. A.: Vulvar condyloma acuminata complicating labor. Obstet. Gynec. 4:67, 1954.

Keaty, C., Jones, P. E., and Lamb, J. H.: Progesterone therapy in dermatoses of pregnancy (herpes gestationis). Arch. Derm. Syph. 63:675, 1951.

Lynfield, Y. L.: Effect of pregnancy on the human hair cycle. J. Invest. Derm. 35:323, 1960.

Pillsbury, D. M., Shelley, W. B., and Kligman, A. M.: A Manual of Cutaneous Medicine. Philadelphia, W. B. Saunders Company, 1961.

Russell, B., and Thorne, N. A.: Herpes gestationis. Brit. J. Derm. 69:339, 1957.

Schiff, B. L., and Kern, A. B.: A study of postpartum alopecia. Arch. Derm. 87:609, 1963.

Spangler, A. S., Reddy, W., Bardawil, W. A., Roby, C. C., and Emerson, K.: Papular dermatitis of pregnancy: A new clinical entity? J.A.M.A. 181:577, 1962.

Chapter 47

Orthopedic Problems

The pregnant woman is subject to a variety of problems of a musculoskeletal nature. Orthopedic disorders relating to obstetric mechanisms, particularly those associated with pelvic deformities that may obstruct labor, are discussed in Chapter 62. Similarly, back pain due to postural factors and unrelated to organic disease is dealt with in Chapter 7. We shall review here other problems encountered in pregnancy that are important to the practitioner.

RELAXATION OF PELVIC JOINTS

Pregnancy is associated with relaxation of the pubic joint as evidenced by a separation of the pubic bones. The amount of separation varies considerably and may be pathologic in some cases (Fig. 282). This process begins during the first half of pregnancy and reaches a maximum at the seventh month. It does not increase during labor. The amount of relaxation diminishes after delivery and generally returns to the nonpregnant state within six months. Similar changes involve the sacroiliac and sacrococcygeal joints. They are probably a consequence of hormonal activity, although the exact mechanism by which these changes arise is unknown.

Signs and Symptoms

The presence and extent of symptoms depend on the amount of relaxation. Small

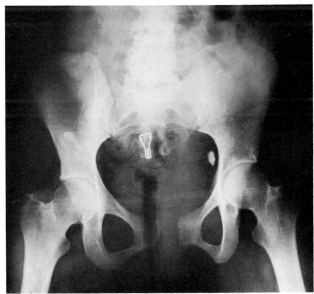

Figure 282 Anteroposterior x-ray view of a patient taken after a spontaneous delivery, showing abnormally wide separation of the symphysis pubis.

symphysial separations of less than 1 to 2 cm. usually present no discomfort. To determine the movability of the pubic joint, the patient is placed on her back. The examiner's forefinger is inserted in the vagina and the thumb of the same hand is placed over the pubis. Then an assistant pulls on one ankle while pushing on the other foot. The fingers on either side of the pubic joint can readily feel the amount of movability during these manipulations. Roentgenograms will reveal the condition more accurately if taken while the patient first stands on one foot and then on the other.

The chief symptoms of excess pelvic mobility are pain and tenderness in the pubic and sacroiliac joints. The symptoms appear about the sixth or seventh month of pregnancy. At first, the patient experiences pain only on walking and during exertion. The pain may appear suddenly and be so severe that walking or standing is impossible. The pain is excruciating even when turning in bed. The gait is usually affected. When the pain is mild, there is a limp on one side; when severe there is a characteristic broad-based, side-to-side waddle.

The most characteristic sign is tenderness on pressure over the pubic joint and the affected sacroiliac joint. Symptoms may first appear after labor as a result of loosening of the sacroiliac joint or diastasis of the pubic joint, but this is a rare event. Prognosis is guarded because half the women with this problem continue to have symptoms subsequently (Young), sometimes quite severe and crippling.

Treatment

In mild cases, relief can be obtained by wearing a properly fitted girdle. Some restriction of activities is helpful. The girdle should be worn for a few months after delivery. For severe cases complete rest in bed may be necessary. After 7 to 10 days, patients may get up but must wear strong supports. A few patients require use of slings similar to those used for fractured pelves while confined to bed. This treatment may have to be continued throughout pregnancy and for a few weeks after delivery.

The management of patients during labor is important because they cannot protect themselves by voluntary muscular control while under general inhalation or spinal or peridural anesthesia. Therefore, movements of the pelvis or limbs may damage softened or vulnerable joints. The lithotomy position is particularly harmful in this regard and delivery in the lateral Sims position (see Chapter 59) is recommended.

ARTHRITIS

Various arthropathies, including those of infectious origin (gonococcal and tuberculous), those of a traumatic or degenerative nature (osteoarthritis) and those related to systemic disorders (rheumatoid, sickle cell, gouty and syphilitic), may be encountered in women of childbearing age. The musculoskeletal involvement in rheumatoid disease is well recognized when associated with polyarthritis, fever and prostration. The joints of the hands, wrists, feet and knees are primarily involved and demonstrate characteristic warm, red, painful, tender swelling of the joints, generally in a symmetric pattern. Anemia is commonly coassociated; it is usually hypochromic and microcytic, and unresponsive to iron therapy. The erythrocyte sedimentation rate is high while the disease is active. The C-reactive protein test is not helpful because the protein may be present normally in pregnancy. Abnormal gamma globulin, the rheumatoid factor, is often found.

Differentiation from other arthropathic problems is sometimes difficult. If acute rheumatic fever does not present with clinical evidence of myocarditis, it may be readily confused. Precedent pharyngitis, erythematous rash or choreiform symptoms may help to distinguish it, together with the findings of β-hemolytic streptococcal organisms in the throat, immunologic response and electrocardiographic changes. Patients with rheumatoid arthritis generally, but not invariably, undergo significant remission during pregnancy (Hench).

Therapy depends on etiology; it is directed against causative factors and the underlying systemic disease. Management is not usually altered because of the coexistent pregnancy, but one should bear in mind potential effects on the fetus of the measures used for specific or symptomatic relief. This applies especially to the use of cytotoxic agents which are still sometimes given to patients with rheumatoid arthritis for purposes of immunosuppression; they are best avoided in pregnancy.

TRAUMA

The pregnant woman can be expected to experience some minor trauma as pregnancy advances because of her progressive clumsiness, awkwardness (see Chapter 7) and shifting body balance. Falls are common. She will instinctively try to protect her uterus and its contents so that she will be subject to all varieties of minor injuries, such as bruises, lacerations, sprains and even fractures (Dyer and Barclay). Severe injuries may also occur, particularly in automobile accidents. The patient may find it difficult to maneuver quickly and comfortably behind the wheel of her car in late pregnancy. Seatbelts may be uncomfortable and even somewhat hazardous in terms of potential direct injury they might cause to the uterus (Rubovits), but they are essential, nevertheless, for the overall safety of the gravida. Lap belts should never be worn over the fundus (Crosby et al.). Shoulder harnesses are particularly recommended (Keller).

The fetus within the gravid uterus is fairly well protected against injury and tends to do well in noncatastrophic maternal trauma (Fort and Harlin). Such injuries include direct blows to or falls on the abdomen, other falls and minor automobile accidents. However, it is quite possible that direct trauma may damage the fetus and/or the placenta, causing irreparable damage or death, or initiating abortion or labor. The uterus may also be damaged or ruptured and produce a catastrophic maternal condition based on internal hemorrhage demanding immediate and aggressive management. *Contrecoup* type of fetal injury has been reported in which the fetus is thrust against the mother's sacral promontory. Both uterine rupture and placental separation can occur; depressed fetal skull fractures have also been reported. Moreover, fetal death may occur on impact without discernible maternal injury.

Fractures

Fractures continue to be the most common type of severe injury occurring during pregnancy. Aside from long bone and skull fractures, most relevant to obstetrics are pelvic fractures. Commonly, these involve the anterior half of the pelvic ring, usually the anterior rami of the symphysis pubis (Fig. 283). Since the relaxation of the sacroiliac joints and the junction of the pubic bones reach their maximum in the last trimester of pregnancy (see above), if the traumatic force is severe enough, displacement of the pubic rami and disruption of the sacroiliac joint may be observed as well. Fractures of the pubic rami may be single or multiple and with or without comminution (Dyer).

As a rule, the pregnancy is unaffected by severe pelvic fractures, although they may interfere with labor mechanisms (see Chapter 62). Of course, concomitant uterine injuries may have occurred to affect continuation of the pregnancy. Treatment consists of attempts to correct any deformity, particularly if the pelvic cavity is impinged upon extensively, and any concurrent damage to other pelvic structures, most especially the bladder. Most patients with pelvic fractures can deliver vaginally without difficulty. This is so because the nature of the fracture of the pelvic ring usually does not affect the available diameters for fetal descent to any great degree.

Abdominal Trauma

Visceral trauma is most serious. Automobile accidents (see above) are responsible for about half the nonpenetrating abdominal wounds; the remainder result from falls, blows, kicks and other mishaps. If there is evidence of internal bleeding or the likelihood of bowel damage, aggressive management is essential. Immediate

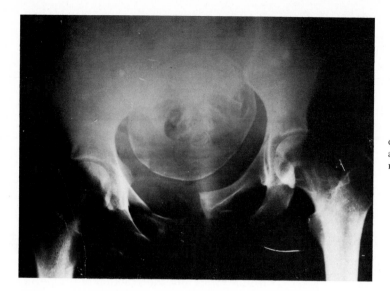

Figure 283 X-ray showing comminuted fracture of both the anterior and the posterior pubic rami. (Courtesy of I. Dyer.)

laparotomy for control of the hemorrhage and repair of the injured viscus should be done.

With penetrating gunshot or stab wounds of the abdomen, the intestines are usually uninvolved, especially in advanced pregnancy, because they are displaced superiorly and posteriorly. However, for a penetrating abdominal wound it is almost always necessary to perform a laparotomy to search for and repair any ancillary injury. As to uterine wounds, simple suture of the entrance wound is usually sufficient. If premature labor or abortion ensues, the uterus can be allowed to empty itself normally. Many patients go into labor within 72 hours and deliver uneventfully. If the fetus is alive, it is possible for the pregnancy to continue without interruption all the way to term, but this is not the usual course.

Stab wounds may produce lacerations of the uterus which can bleed a great deal. The hemorrhage is sometimes so difficult to control that hysterotomy is necessary for evacuation and hemostasis.

Abdominal injury that involves the viscera, the uterus or its adnexa warrants immediate surgical investigation. This may have to be preceded by appropriate measures to maintain cardiopulmonary status, blood replacement, nasogastric intubation and bladder catheterization. X-ray evaluations should be carried out as needed, weighing potential fetal hazards against the critical importance of such studies to the welfare of the mother.

The surgical approach should not be altered just because a pregnancy is present. The uterus need not be disturbed during surgical exploration unless necessary for exposure or to repair direct uterine injuries. The uterus should be handled minimally if pregnancy is to be preserved. The fetus need not be removed unless uterine damage is extensive. Near term, one might make an attempt to salvage a living, viable fetus who may be compromised by direct injury or placental damage. Intrauterine fetal wounds do heal slowly if the fetus does not die as a result of the trauma sustained (Buchsbaum).

REFERENCES

Buchsbaum, H. J.: Accidental injury complicating pregnancy. Amer. J. Obstet. Gynec. *102*:752, 1968.

Crosby, W. M., Snyder, R. G., Snow, C. C., and Hanson, P. G.: Impact injuries in pregnancy: I. Experimental studies. Amer. J. Obstet. Gynec. *101*:100, 1968.

Dyer, I.: Discussion of paper by Crosby et al.

Dyer, I., and Barclay, D. L.: Accidental trauma complicating pregnancy and delivery. Amer. J. Obstet. Gynec. *83*:907, 1962.

Fort, A. T., and Harlin, R. S.: Pregnancy outcome after noncatastrophic maternal trauma during pregnancy. Obstet. Gynec. 35:912, 1970.

Hench, P. G.: Ameliorating effect of pregnancy in chronic atrophic (infectious rheumatoid) arthritis, fibrositis and intermittent hydrarthrosis. Proc. Mayo Clin. *13*:161, 1938.

Keller, W. K.: Automobile safety belts during pregnancy: A.M.A. Committee on Medical Aspects of Automotive Safety. J.A.M.A. *221*:20, 1972.

Rubovits, F. E.: Traumatic rupture of the pregnant uterus from "seat belt" injury. Amer. J. Obstet. Gynec. *90*:828, 1964.

Young, J.: Relaxation of pelvic joints in pregnancy: Pelvic arthropathy of pregnancy. J. Obstet. Gynaec. Brit. Emp. *47*:493, 1940.

Chapter 48

Neurologic Disease

The neurologic aspects of eclampsia have been detailed in Chapter 36. Beginning with early visual disturbances, headache and hyperreflexia of preeclampsia and progressing to the convulsions of eclampsia, the clinical manifestations result from the generalized central nervous hyperirritability. The latter is probably a consequence of vasospastic reduction of blood flow to the brain combined with edema. Generally, one can readily distinguish this condition in pregnancy from other seizure disorders on the basis of coassociated hypertension, albuminuria and the progressive nature of the clinical picture. However, it is not always clear-cut and the obstetrician must be familiar with other neurologic problems which have similar manifestations. Differential diagnosis is especially problematic when one is faced with a convulsing patient who has not been previously seen or recently followed. Both proteinuria and hypertension may follow as a result of seizures caused by other conditions, thus confusing the issue still further.

Aside from epilepsy (see below), hyperventilation is quite common and may be etiologic. It is most often associated with an acute anxiety reaction, although it is seen in labors conducted with the breathing exercises of psychoprophylactic techniques (see Chapter 11). The typical hyperventilation syndrome begins with quivering tremulousness in the extremities, usually with subjective feelings of numbness in the fingers and around the mouth. Carpopedal spasm occurs as a result of hypocapnia. The patient may ultimately lose consciousness and develop generalized jerky muscular movements that are similar to those of a clonic seizure.

Other causes of seizures in pregnancy include organic brain disease (tumors, trauma or infection) and a variety of systemic disorders leading to cerebral ischemia, anoxia, hypoglycemia or uremia. As drug abuse becomes more widespread (see Chapter 50), physicians may expect to see more patients manifesting fits due to acute withdrawal from such agents as barbiturates, meprobamate, anticonvulsants and even alcohol. Seizures have also been reported to occur on an hysterical basis.

HEMIPLEGIC STATES

Puerperal hemiplegias, when seen, tend to be subclinical and minimal. They may be easily missed. One may encounter only a slight flattening of the side of the face, a widened palpebral fissure and an altered nasolabial fold. These subtle changes are difficult to document but are very important because they may set the stage for subsequent hemiplegias or even epileptic seizures later in life.

Hemiplegic states, whether transient or permanent, result from impairment of blood flow in a significant cerebral vessel by mechanisms of spasm or thrombosis. Embolization or rupture may occur, but only rarely. Venous and dural sinus thrombosis may be the cause, especially if the sequence of events includes severe postdelivery headache and convulsions followed by hemiplegia and signs of increasing intracranial pressure (Stevens; Hyland). It may progress to disturbances of consciousness and coma. Papilledema occurs and spinal fluid pressure is elevated. Since the symptoms tend to disappear spontaneously in this condition, treatment is expectant and symptomatic.

Anticonvulsants should be used as needed. The use of anticoagulants does not seem to be justified.

SUBARACHNOID HEMORRHAGE

Subarachnoid hemorrhage is a rare complication that demands early diagnosis. It is a particularly treacherous problem with a high mortality in pregnancy. It occurs most frequently before labor or after delivery, and least often during labor when cerebral intraarterial pressures are highest (Conley and Rand). Suboccipital headache and nuchal rigidity are seen, together with nausea, vomiting, syncope and neurologic manifestations such as coma, convulsions or hemiplegia. Diagnostic spinal puncture may reveal many erythrocytes. Angiography may locate the source of the bleeding in an aneurysm or angiomatous tumor.

Treatment is not satisfactory. Surgical intervention may sometimes be indicated and feasible, although results have not been uniformly favorable. Some believe that labor is contraindicated in these patients because of the fear of rupture of the aneurysm or angioma with increased intracranial pressure, but there is no proof of this contention. Vaginal delivery may be successfully accomplished, although it is advisable to conduct the labor under peridural anesthesia (see Chapter 22) and interdict expulsive efforts in the second stage. Cesarean section should be done for obstetric indications only.

MIGRAINE

Migraine is a common disturbance usually manifested by an aura of scintillating scotomas followed by severe unilateral pulsatile headache, nausea and vomiting. It may be associated with paresthesias or aphasia. It is often ameliorated during pregnancy. Rarely, it becomes worse or begins during gestation with more unusual auras, hemiparesis, hemianopsia, scotomas or amaurosis.

That such disturbances may be the pre-

monitors of the hypertensive states of pregnancy or impending cerebrovascular accident has been conjectured on the basis of certain similarities between migraine and eclampsia (Rotton et al.). For example, migraine diathesis is a widespread disorder involving many organ systems. Water and sodium balance may be disturbed, with increasing serum sodium levels and hemodilution, interstitial fluid retention, facial and dependent edema and diuresis following the attack. It is the spasm of the pial and cerebral arterioles, and their subsequent dilatation, that result in the localized cortical edema of migraine. This is analogous to the more extensive vasospastic changes of preeclampsia.

In both conditions there is a suggestive correlation with epileptoid tendencies. It is conceivable that seizures are more likely to occur in patients who are seizure-prone, that is, who have an "epileptogenic terrain," such as is seen in patients with rheumatic fever who convulse. Cerebral dysrhythmias are seen on electroencephalography characteristically in migraine patients, as well as among many patients who develop eclampsia. Thus, it is possible that the predisposition to convulsions may exist in many patients; this predisposition becomes manifest when triggered by such metabolic disorders as preeclampsia. Migraine diathesis in pregnancy should alert the obstetrician that he may be dealing with a patient prone to develop rapidly fulminating eclampsia. The exacerbation of migraine is thus an ominous sign.

Treatment of migraine includes rest, sedation and dehydration. Caffeine is sometimes effective if given during the prodromal phase. Ergonovine may also be useful, but there is an expected reluctance to employ this uterotonic agent during pregnancy. However, in usual dosages of 2 mg. orally or 0.25 to 0.5 mg. intramuscularly, it does not seem to have any observable adverse effect on intact gestations (Robb).

EPILEPSY

Epilepsy of either grand mal or psychomotor varieties commonly coexists in pregnancy. Nearly two million Americans are affected by this condition. Although hereditary relationships are not clear, epilepsy appears to be more frequent in the relatives of epileptics than in the relatives of those who are free of the disease. A woman suffering from idiopathic epilepsy has a 1:40 chance of bearing an epileptic child (Lennox), compared to 1:200 in the general population. By contrast, epilepsy which follows infection, trauma, tumor or malformation is transmitted at about the same rate as in the normal population. A recent study by Speidel and Meadow, however, showed twice the incidence of other major congenital anomalies among offspring, including most often congenital heart disease, cleft lip and microcephaly. Subnormal mentality was seen in 1.5 per cent (0.2 per cent in a control group). Perinatal mortality overall was 38.6 per 1000 births among epileptics or twice the regional rate and did not seem to be related to the use of anticonvulsant agents.

About 70 per cent of epileptic patients can be well controlled medically and another 15 to 20 per cent can be partially controlled. Seizures in the remainder are resistant to control. Most are effectively treated with sodium diphenylhydantoin (Dilantin) in doses of 100 mg. two to three times daily. Dosages may have to be increased to a tolerance of 400 to 500 mg. daily or supplemented with phenobarbital 100 to 200 mg. per day in divided increments. Other agents may have to be substituted, such as primidone (Mysoline) or methylethylphenylhydantoin (Mesantoin), but they cause drowsiness or have toxic effects.

The disease is generally unaltered in terms of control during pregnancy. Sometimes patients may experience some difficulty during the first trimester when troubled by hyperemesis because they are unable to take or to retain their regular oral anticonvulsant medication. The same situation may also arise in labor when oral intake is often automatically and thoughtlessly omitted. When this occurs, convulsions may develop. Parenteral medication, such as intramuscular Dilantin, is essential to ensure against convulsions.

Epilepsy does not usually affect pregnancy or delivery. Folate deficiencies may be aggravated by some anticonvulsants (Chanarin) and supplementation is indicated. Sodium and water retention is encountered among epileptic gravidas (Suter and Klingman) and should be watched for carefully. Diuretics are effective in correcting this when needed for acute fluid retention.

Status epilepticus is a serious life-threatening emergency crisis. It should be treated as in the nonpregnant state with amobarbital (Amytal sodium) intravenously in a 2.5 per cent solution injected slowly until the convulsions cease. An airway is vital. Hypoxia should be guarded against by avoiding overdosage. Artificial ventilation and even tracheotomy may become necessary to maintain oxygenation. With expert anesthesia available one may consider curarizing and ventilating the unresponsive patient in status epilepticus (James and Whitty). Diazepam (Valium) is also very effective when given slowly intravenously in the dose necessary to stop the seizures, up to 20 mg. Intractable status epilepticus may require interruption of pregnancy. This is especially recommended where the epilepsy is caused by a progressive degenerative or neoplastic disease process.

MULTIPLE SCLEROSIS

Pregnancy is unaffected by concurrent multiple sclerosis, and the course of the disease is apparently unaltered by pregnancy (Hirschmann). Multiple sclerosis undergoes remissions and exacerbations unpredictably during pregnancy just as it does at other times. Whether or not pregnancy is advisable depends on the extent of the disability and the patient's willingness to accept the burden of bearing and caring for a child in the face of possible progression of disability in the future. Both therapeutic abortion and sterilization are issues that may have to be faced on this basis. The answers are not arrived at easily unless the patient is already severely handicapped.

Generally, vaginal delivery is readily accomplished. The uterus is unaffected even if there is severe paraplegia, so that labor progresses normally up to the second stage. Expulsive efforts may be impeded because of abdominal wall involvement, and a forceps operation may become necessary. Traumatic delivery procedures should be avoided. Cesarean section should be undertaken for obstetric indications only. Spinal anesthesia is best avoided.

MYASTHENIA GRAVIS

The relationship between pregnancy and myasthenia gravis is also unpredictable (Osserman). Cholinergic drugs are usually very effective in controlling manifestations so that pregnancy, labor and delivery will be uneventful. Prostigmin (neostigmine) methylsulfate 1.5 mg. subcutaneously or 0.5 mg. intravenously will reverse the symptoms promptly; prostigmin bromide 15 mg. is effective orally for three to four hours. Both the dosage and the interval between doses must be adjusted according to the patient's specific needs. Overdosage is hazardous. Maintenance dosage is titrated carefully. One must be watchful for signs of respiratory embarrassment, however. Artificial ventilation may become necessary and long term use of a mechanical respirator required.

It is wise to keep the mother in the hospital for two to three weeks after delivery to observe for flare-up and to watch the baby, who may be born myasthenic (McKeever). If overlooked, death, hypoxic damage or aspiration may result. The child usually responds well to small doses of cholinergic drugs. Most often neonatal myasthenia clears up completely in two to four weeks. A rare, permanent congenital myasthenia is also reported to occur in neonates.

OTOSCLEROSIS

Otosclerosis is a disorder with a familial tendency associated with progressive deafness. It is said to be aggravated by pregnancy. Hearing loss becomes worse. Bony changes are believed to be augmented on the basis of the altered calcium metabolism of gestation.

Therefore, therapeutic abortion is generally advocated when this condition preexists. However, the evidence for this recommendation is not irrefutable. The actual effect of pregnancy on otosclerosis is variable and unpredictable. Moreover, the effect of previous pregnancies on the disease cannot be used as an accurate index of the expected effect during any subsequent pregnancy. Abortion is not necessarily associated with a favorable effect on otosclerosis. The progression of hearing loss encountered during pregnancy may or may not be arrested by abortion.

Other causes of hearing loss during pregnancy and the puerperium include the deafness that results rarely from severe preeclampsia or the toxic effects of drugs such as streptomycin, which may also affect the hearing of the fetus. Syphilis and rubella viremia may play a role as well.

REFERENCES

Chanarin, I.: The Megaloblastic Anaemias. Oxford, Blackwell Scientific Publications Ltd., 1969.

Conley, J. W., and Rand, C. W.: Spontaneous subarachnoid hemorrhage occurring in noneclamptic pregnancy. Arch. Neurol. Psychiat. 66:443, 1951.

Hirschmann, J.: Gestationsprozesse und multiple Sklerose. Arch. Psychiat. 181:530, 1949.

Hyland, H. H.: Intracranial venous thrombosis in the puerperium. J.A.M.A. 142:707, 1950.

James, J. L., and Whitty, C. W. M.: The electroencephalogram as a monitor of status epilepticus suppressed peripherally by curarisation. Lancet 2:239, 1961.

Lennox, W. G.: The genetics of epilepsy. Amer. J. Psychiat. 103:457, 1947.

McKeever, G. E.: Myasthenia gravis in a mother and her newborn son. J.A.M.A. 147:320, 1951.

Osserman, K. E.: Myasthenia Gravis. New York, Grune and Stratton, 1958.

Robb, J. P.: Neurologic complications of pregnancy. Neurology 5:679, 1955.

Rotton, W. N., Sachtleben, M. R., and Friedman, E. A.: Migraine and eclampsia. Obstet. Gynec. 14:322, 1959.

Speidel, B. D., and Meadow, S. R.: Maternal epilepsy and abnormalities of the fetus and newborn. Lancet 2:839, 1972.

Stevens, H.: Puerperal hemiplegia. Neurology 4:723, 1954.

Suter, C., and Klingman, W. O.: Seizure states and pregnancy. Neurology 7:105, 1957.

Chapter 49

Metabolic and Endocrine Disturbances

DIABETES MELLITUS

Disordered carbohydrate metabolism is an important complication in pregnancy because it is associated with high fetal losses. It is most important that diabetes mellitus be detected in its earliest stages prior to or early in pregnancy in order to avert its serious consequences. If undetected, patients with inherent defects in pancreatic function will manifest clinical symptoms due to the diabetogenic effects of the pregnancy itself. This is not to imply that pregnancy causes diabetes, but rather that it may either uncover underlying tendencies or aggravate the overt disease.

The impact of pregnancy on carbohydrate metabolism is profound. It is evidenced by elevated serum levels of lactate and pyruvate. Fasting blood sugar levels are not increased, however, nor is carbohydrate tolerance impaired (see below). Plasma insulin levels rise progressively in the last trimester, both in the fasting state and in response to intravenous glucose load (Spellacy). There is a diminished hypoglycemic response to administered insulin indicating either an altered metabolism of insulin during pregnancy or the presence of some form of anti-insulin factor. Both of these possibilities may exist because the half-life of insulin is reduced, and increased levels of synalbumin antagonist to insulin have been found in pregnancy (Ginsburg). An attractive hypothesis to explain the paradoxical increase in circulating insulin unassociated with hyperglycemic stimuli is the possible regulatory role of chorionic somato-mammotropin (see Chapter 4) which is known to decrease insulin sensitivity while at the same time stimulating its production and diminishing its capability to produce hypoglycemia. The role of the placenta in insulin degradation is incompletely understood, but enzymatic destruction has been shown *in vitro* (Freinkel and Goodner).

Classification

In its full-blown clinical form, frank diabetes occurs in about 0.7 per cent of all pregnancies (Niswander and Gordon). However, the actual number of patients with latent or subclinical forms of diabetes is probably more than twice this figure. Patients with the greatest risk of having such underlying proclivity include those with a family history of the disease (hereditary transmission as an autosomic recessive trait seems likely), those who have delivered infants of excessive weight or have had unexplained perinatal deaths or repeated abortions and those who are obese or demonstrate glucosuria. The disease process has a spectrum of patterns ranging from minimally disturbed carbohydrate metabolism as evidenced by a somewhat abnormal glucose tolerance test at one extreme to a clinical picture of juvenile onset and brittle control in a patient who is prone to develop ketoacidosis. Paralleling this gamut is the range of potentially deleterious effects on both mother and fetus.

In order to take advantage of the prognostic value of the clinical pattern, several descriptive classifications have evolved. Although each tends to be somewhat arbitrary, they afford means for standardization of diagnosis and therapy. Perhaps the most widely used is that of Priscilla White, which takes into account age of onset, duration, severity and complications:

Class A, with abnormal glucose tolerance test only; also variously called latent, chemical, subclinical or gestational diabetes.

Class B, clinically overt or frank diabetes beginning in adulthood after age 20 years and of less than 10 years' duration with no evidence of vascular involvement.

Class C, overt diabetes present for 10 to 19 years or beginning in adolescence between ages 10 and 19 years and without vascular disease.

Class D, disease of long duration (20 years or more) or onset in childhood before age 10 or with evidence of vascular involvement, including arteriosclerotic changes in retinal and leg vessels, and retinitis.

Class E, with radiographic evidence of pelvic vascular disease.

Class F, with nephropathy, including intracapillary glomerulosclerosis (Kimmelstiel-Wilson syndrome), pyelonephritis or papillary necrosis.

In addition, she includes a *Class G* to denote patients with adverse obstetric history and a *Class R* for the seriously complicating features of retinitis proliferans or vitreous hemorrhage.

Because of the artificiality of this and other classifications, albeit useful in investigative situations, many merely categorize patients according to whether or not the diabetes is clinically manifested and whether or not it is insulin dependent. The subdivision into juvenile and maturity onset is useful in indicating relative severity for prognostic purposes. Dichotomy into ketoacidosis-resistant and ketoacidosis-prone is also helpful for therapeutic reasons. In general these several factors are closely interrelated. The juvenile diabetic, for example, usually has a more severe variety of disease and is ketoacidosis-prone; her disease is insulin dependent and difficult to control; she is likely to develop renal, retinal, vascular and neural complications.

Prediabetes is the term used to identify people who are in a dynamic phase with regard to the sequence of pathogenesis, and who have the proclivity to develop clinical diabetes under certain kinds of stresses. They have underlying anatomic and metabolic derangements present from conception which do not become evident in terms of abnormal carbohydrate metabolism until some transitory stress acts to uncover the problem. Such stresses include infections, trauma, vascular crises, impaired nutrition, endocrine disorders, starvation, neoplastic processes, obesity, emotional problems and exogenous medications, including adrenal corticosteroids, diphenylhydantoin, beta-adrenergic blocking agents and certain thiazides.

Steroids have been used diagnostically in conjunction with a glucose load to aid in the identification of predisposed patients. It is clear that pregnancy serves this same role in the form of a stressful situation that is capable of disclosing prediabetes. It has been shown that 60 per cent of gestational diabetics will develop overt diabetes in 5.5 years (O'Sullivan and Mahan).

Diagnosis

Gestational or Class A diabetes is diagnosed on the basis of abnormal response to glucose tolerance testing. Standards are variable based on acceptable ranges of normal values, differences between oral and intravenous glucose load administration and differences in the methods for obtaining blood specimens and testing for the presence of reducing substances. Blood sugar values in capillary blood are known to be 10 to 20 mg. per 100 ml. higher than in venous blood; tests for total reducing substances yield values about 20 mg. per 100 ml. greater than those which measure glucose only. There are about one-fourth fewer false negative determinations with the oral glucose tolerance test than with the intravenous test (Benjamin and Casper).

The current standard oral glucose tolerance test is performed after the patient has fasted overnight. In order to ensure that no starvation effects are present, at least 300 gm. of carbohydrate per day must have been taken for three days prior to the test. Specimens of blood and urine are obtained and a glucose load of 100 gm. is administered. Subsequent blood and urine specimens are obtained at intervals of one-half, one, two and three hours. Levels indicating the presence of diabetes have been standardized by the American College of Obstetricians and Gynecologists (Hughes) as follows:

Fasting: Normal or less than 100 mg. per 100 ml.

One-half hour: More than 150 mg. per 100 ml.

One hour: More than 160 mg. per 100 ml.

Two hours: 120 mg. per 100 ml. or more.

Three hours: Normal or more than 120 mg. per 100 ml.

Much more conservative diagnostic values have been recommended by White and by O'Sullivan and Mahan for both peak values (170 and 165 mg. per 100 ml., respectively) and subsequent points at two hours (130 and 145 mg. per 100 ml.) and three hours (120 and 125 mg. per 100 ml.). The oral test is generally considered more physiologic but has the disadvantage of being adversely affected by impaired gastric function and the occasional intolerance of the gravida to ingestion of hypertonic glucose. Intravenous glucose is well tolerated and the response is more consistent, although false negatives are common and the test requires more frequent and more accurately obtained blood samples.

Every pregnant patient should have her urine studied for the presence of reducing substances at each antenatal visit by such simple, practical means as a glucose oxidase test strip (Tes-Tape or Clinistix). This easy dip technique, using an enzymatic method, is specific for glucose and, therefore, preferable to the use of Benedict's reagent or Clinitest tablets, both of which will react nonspecifically to other sugars present in the urine, such as lactose and fructose. Every patient showing glucosuria is studied further with regard to both fasting blood sugar determination and either the full oral glucose tolerance test as described or a more simple screening procedure. The latter consists of administering 100 gm. of glucose orally after an overnight fast and obtaining blood and urine specimens two hours later. Blood glucose levels in excess of 130 mg. are highly suggestive of diabetes. Fasting blood sugar levels are seldom useful for screening purposes. Consistently elevated fasting levels above 130 mg. per 100 ml. are encountered only in association with clinically overt diabetes.

Even in the absence of glucosuria, screening procedures are carried out for all gravidas with a familial history of diabetes, for those who have delivered babies weighing in excess of 4000 gm., for those who are obese or those who have had prior adverse obstetric experiences, including anomalous or dead babies and habitual abortion.

The manifestations of overt diabetes include the range of classic symptoms such as polyuria, polydipsia, polyphagia, pruritus, excessive thirst and hunger with associated weakness and weight loss. Untreated, it may progress to ketoacidosis with lassitude, malaise, anorexia, nausea, vomiting and vertigo, leading to coma and death.

Effects on Pregnancy

Before insulin was available and widely used, amenorrhea and infertility were common among diabetic women. Today this does not constitute a major problem, particularly if the diabetes is well controlled by proper insulin dosage and dietary management. Similarly, there does not seem to be any increase in the incidence of spontaneous abortion among diabetic women, contrary to what has been taught in the past. In the more severe cases, however, particularly in the presence of vascular complications, the frequency of abortion may be increased (White).

Pregnancy in the diabetic female tends to be complicated in many ways. The gravida may be more prone to infection; if infections arise, they will in turn make diabetic control more difficult. Hospitalization may be necessary for purposes of aggressive evaluation and treatment. This holds especially for urinary tract infections, which tend to be common in diabetic gravidas. Respiratory and skin infections must likewise be treated as potentially serious disorders.

Hypertensive states of pregnancy occur

three to six times as commonly among diabetic women as in nondiabetics. Although some of the typical manifestations of edema, proteinuria and hypertension may be on the basis of intracapillary glomerulosclerosis accompanying the diabetic state, most arise without concomitant underlying vascular disease. The course and management of the preeclamptic diathesis in association with diabetes is essentially the same as in the nondiabetic (see Chapter 36), except for the use of thiazides. Thiazides appear to alter carbohydrate metabolism (Shapiro et al.); therefore, if diuretic agents are needed, other forms should be used. Even though the management of the hypertensive state is not made more complicated by the presence of diabetes, the reverse is not true; control of the diabetes is made much more difficult by the superimposed hypertensive state.

Hydramnios is common in the gravid diabetic. Incidence figures as high as 50 per cent have been reported. It may arise very rapidly, causing great discomfort and respiratory embarrassment by impinging on the diaphragm; it may even adversely affect renal function. Intrauterine pressure may be increased so high as to interfere with uterine blood flow and fetomaternal exchange of vital substances.

The incidence of congenital malformations is high among infants of diabetic mothers, including cardiac and skeletal abnormalities most often. Macrosomia is seen among the milder forms of diabetes with the delivery of very large infants. The babies are longer and heavier and have correspondingly larger visceral organs, except for the brain. This may occur as a result of the stimulus for hyperinsulinism and growth secondary to long-standing maternal and fetal hyperglycemia. These babies tend to do poorly owing to their propensity to develop respiratory distress. Despite their large size, the physiologic function of various organs, such as the lungs, may be incompletely developed.

Increased birth weight is partly due to acceleration of true skeletal growth, but there is also excessive deposition of fat in the subcutaneous tissues. Water retention is also evident in the pitting edema found in newborn infants, and in the postnatal diuresis and weight loss which occur subsequently. The large fetuses complicate labor and delivery to the extent that they may contribute to cephalopelvic disproportion.

Fetuses die rather commonly in the course of diabetic pregnancies. Aside from congenital anomalies, maternal ketoacidosis and placental insufficiency are the most common causes. Hypoglycemia due to insulin shock is rarely a factor because this condition is so readily detectable and correctable in the mother. Ketoacidosis, on the other hand, may be present for some time in the poorly controlled diabetic gravida and cause serious damage to the fetus owing to the effects of altered pH on the placental enzymatic transfer mechanisms. Severely damaging ketoacidosis may thus exist in the mother without clinical manifestations, but with major adverse effects on the fetus.

Placental insufficiency may develop insidiously late in the diabetic pregnancy. Methods for its detection have been described in Chapter 13, particularly with regard to use of serial urinary estriol determinations and oxytocin stress testing. The specific mechanism by which placental insufficiency comes about in diabetes is not completely understood, but it is undoubtedly the result of microvascular changes occurring in the placental vascular tree (see Chapter 3). The placenta of diabetics shows characteristic microangiopathic changes with microcapillary aneurysms and endarteritis. There are reduplications of the basement membrane, endothelial proliferation and polysaccharide deposition in the vessels. The same typical alterations are also encountered in the lesions of diabetic glomerulosclerosis and retinopathy; they are seen as well in other small arteries, arterioles and capillaries of skin, skeletal muscle, nerves and myocardium.

Management

The primary objectives of management include optimal control of the maternal diabetes, prevention of progression of the disease, detection and control of complicating features and the delivery of a healthy infant who will survive. It is clear that the better the control, the better the outcome for both mother and baby (Pedersen). Such control consists of dietary measures and insulin. The caloric intake should be idealized according to the patient's weight, height and activities. Strict adherence to diet is essential so as to provide appropriate daily requirements of protein and carbohydrates to satisfy nutritional needs for fetal development (see Chapter 10). A total of 200 gm. of carbohydrate and 100 gm of protein per day is generally necessary, together with enough fat content to total the ideal daily caloric intake.

If dietary management alone is insufficient to correct the metabolic disturbance, insulin is indicated. One must be on guard because insulin requirements may change rapidly and unpredictably during pregnancy. Oral hypoglycemic therapy tends not to be satisfactory for use during pregnancy. In determining the type and dosage schedule of insulin, closest cooperation is necessary between obstetrician and internist. Attempts to maintain blood sugar levels entirely within the physiologic range may result in hypoglycemic episodes which threaten the fetus. Careful attention must be given to the specific needs of individual patients. In this regard no guidelines can be given as to whether crystalline zinc insulin or the more intermediate or longer acting NPH, globin or lente insulins will be required alone or in combination. Even after a dosage schedule has been established, it is imperative that it be carefully checked and modified to take into account changing insulin requirements based on pregnancy effects, altered physical activity and the appearance of complicating features such as infection.

Patients are usually begun on protamine insulin 15 units on arising in the morning. This provides relatively long term control, but may require supplementation with crystalline zinc insulin to satisfy the morning needs. Such combinations are commonly used early in pregnancy. As insulin needs increase in the second trimester, an additional nighttime dose of intermediate-type insulin may be required; in the third trimester, combinations of insulins may be needed before breakfast and before dinner for purposes of adequate control. Dose

levels are adjusted according to the degree of glucosuria encountered before meals, increasing the insulin dosages until the urine is almost free of sugar.

The patient should be instructed carefully concerning the great importance of her cooperation and stringent attention to details of diet, exercise, evaluation of her diabetic status and insulin dosage. She must be informed about complications of diabetes, pregnancy, intercurrent disease and the treatment she is receiving. She must be seen frequently by both obstetrician and internist, perhaps alternating visits to each. The patient should test her urine daily for glucose and ketone. In order to ensure that hypoglycemia will not occur, it is generally acceptable to adjust insulin dosage so that the gravida will have some glucosuria at all times. Tighter control to eliminate glucosuria entirely might lead to episodic hypoglycemia. Acetonuria, on the other hand, requires that additional insulin be given and the subsequent regimen adjusted accordingly.

Routine sodium restriction and use of diuretic agents are decried. Even though diabetic gravidas are more prone to develop preeclamptic diatheses, such prophylactic measures are without foundation. Similarly, the use of hormones, heretofore given ostensibly to correct demonstrated hormonal deficiencies in diabetic pregnancies (White et al.), is no longer defensible and cannot be recommended. Use of stilbestrol in pregnancy is specifically contraindicated because of the apparent hazard of the female fetus subsequently developing vaginal adenocarcinoma as a result (Herbst et al.).

It is most important to hospitalize the patient for at least one week before delivery is anticipated. This is necessary in order to ensure ideal control of carbohydrate metabolism and to correct any underlying concurrent disorder, if possible, thereby optimizing maternal and fetal outcome. Hospitalization is required also for the patient who develops ketoacidosis, sudden alteration in insulin requirements, infection, preeclampsia or acute hydramnios. These represent potentially ominous events for the diabetic patient in the course of pregnancy.

Timing of Delivery. Determining the

optimal time for delivery is difficult. There is general agreement that patients with frank diabetes are best delivered at around the thirty-seventh week of pregnancy. Mortality data (Hagbard; Gellis and Hsia) show high risk of death from prematurity if delivery is carried out prior to the thirty-sixth week and comparably high risks of intrauterine death if the pregnancy is allowed to progress beyond the thirty-seventh week. One quarter of fetuses can be expected to die *in utero* during the last three weeks of the diabetic pregnancy and this has given rise to a fixed policy with regard to timing of delivery in many areas.

This practice is most unfortunate because many fetuses are lost as a consequence of premature delivery undertaken too early by virtue of errors in determining the duration of pregnancy; others die before the time assigned for delivery as a result of diabetic complications or inadequate means for assessing fetal well-being objectively (see Chapter 13). If it were possible to individualize each case so that pregnancy will be allowed to continue as long as possible, provided the fetus is not in jeopardy and delivery is undertaken only when it can be objectively demonstrated to be necessary, it is theoretically possible to improve overall salvage rates.

The question of whether or not periodic urinary estriol is a reliable means for determining when delivery should be done has yet to be answered definitively, although several studies have been very encouraging in this regard (Greene et al.; Schwarz et al.). However, estriol assay is of little use prior to the thirty-fourth week of pregnancy (Klopper). Weekly estriol excretion levels may be helpful in identifying fetuses at serious risk and requiring prompt delivery; those not at risk whose delivery can be delayed further are likewise identified. When used in conjunction with periodic oxytocin stress tests as described in Chapter 13, diagnostic acumen may be increased considerably in this regard. At the same time it is important to ascertain fetal maturity so that one has relevant information dealing with both the intrauterine risks of placental insufficiency and the hazards of extrauterine life.

In regions where tests of fetal status are not available, it is advisable that gravidas with overt diabetes be delivered at 36 to 38 weeks' gestational age. An earlier time may be selected if urgency is suggested by a clinical indication in the form of sudden alteration in insulin requirements, the appearance of preeclampsia or hydramnios, decreased fetal activity or a history of intrauterine death earlier in pregnancy. Great care must be taken, however, to avoid excessive prematurity if at all possible.

Similar principles apply with reference to timing the delivery of Class A or gestational diabetics. The hazards for the fetus are substantially smaller and one is usually justified in allowing the pregnancy to continue closer to term before intervening. Given the advantages of testing for fetal status, one may safely carry the unaffected fetus to term. Intervention is justified only if periodic examinations show clear evidence of placental insufficiency. Without these measures, induction is appropriate as soon as the cervix is favorable at about 38 to 39 weeks. This conservative approach yields good results.

Method of Delivery. The method chosen for delivery will depend on the situation prevailing. In Chapter 24 we have extensively discussed methods of induction of labor. Usually, the optimal criteria do not apply, and failure of induction under these circumstances occurs commonly. Nevertheless, it should be tried in the patient under good diabetic control with no contraindicating medical or obstetric complications. Fetal monitoring for intrapartum hypoxia, as evidenced by alterations in fetal heart rate pattern, is strongly recommended.

Cesarean section should not be considered the routine method for delivery in diabetes. Cesarean section may be undertaken for delivery if the attempt at induction fails. Similarly, abdominal delivery is indicated without prior attempt at induction (1) for those patients in whom difficult vaginal delivery is anticipated, as with cephalopelvic disproportion associated with the excessively large fetuses of diabetic mothers; (2) for those with documented placental insufficiency when the uterine contractions of labor can be expected to affect fetoplacental exchange adversely; (3)

for those with bad prior obstetric experience, particularly previous traumatic vaginal delivery or intrapartum fetal death; (4) for patients previously delivered by cesarean section; and (5) for those problems that may arise in the course of labor, whether or not related to diabetes, that demand prompt termination of the pregnancy in the interests of mother or fetus. As to the last group, the gamut of acceptable indications is detailed in Chapter 76.

The hazards of induction under suboptimal circumstances and the probability of failure are significantly and progressively reduced the closer the patient is to term. Analogously, the need for cesarean section is also related to the proximity to term. It is, therefore, easy to understand the importance of the practice of periodic testing for fetal well-being with the objective of allowing those fetuses not yet at risk to remain *in utero* and continue to mature (see above).

In preparation for induction and vaginal delivery or for cesarean section, insulin dosage should be altered. The daily dose should be halved on the morning of delivery. Subsequent regulation by means of small doses of crystalline zinc insulin are given as needed. This regimen should be continued after the delivery for several days until the patient is at full activity again and daily insulin needs can be more precisely determined. Generally, the patient's requirements return to the levels of control in existence prior to the time she became pregnant. Care must be taken in providing adequate fluid intake and glucose supply, by the intravenous route if necessary, during labor and in the immediate puerperium. Careful control is ensured by frequent determinations of blood sugar and observations for urinary ketones.

Prognosis

A maternal death from diabetes is very rare, particularly if the patient has had good medical and obstetric care during her pregnancy. When it occurs, it is usually associated with the major complications of long-standing, severe diabetes, including especially vascular or renal involvement. For most diabetic women, however, pregnancy should not pose a serious threat (White).

The fetus, on the other hand, is in jeopardy. The more severe the diabetes, the greater the risk. There is a wide range in reported perinatal mortality rates based on the admixture of subclinical, mild and severe forms as well as on the intensity of the medical supervision patients received. In general 10 to 15 per cent of infants can be expected to die in association with maternal diabetes. The rate for gestational diabetics is about one-tenth that of overt diabetics (Schwarz et al.). The greatest risk to the fetus exists in pregnancies associated with diabetes of Class D, E and F (see above).

Not only are mortality rates increased but there may be long-term neurological and developmental effects as well. Churchill et al. studied neuropsychologic deficits in children born of diabetic mothers and found lower intelligence quotients if the diabetes was associated with ketoacidosis manifested by acetonuria. Offspring of diabetic gravidas who were in good control and, therefore, without acetonuria were essentially unaffected. The relationship between acetonuria and subsequent outcome of the infant applied equally in mild and severe forms of diabetes. Moreover, offspring appeared to have been unaffected by maternal insulin reactions during pregnancy.

Second in importance only to the special attention required during pregnancy for proper maternal control is the care of the newborn infant. Infants of diabetic mothers, although large and apparently healthy at first, are subject to a wide variety of potentially lethal complications. Physiologic immaturity of various organ systems occurs. The gross appearance is deceiving and the infant may behave much like a premature neonate, developing characteristic respiratory distress. Between one-fifth and one-third will have major manifestations of respiratory distress evident within the first 12 hours of life, including tachypnea, increasing cyanosis, intercostal and infrasternal retraction, high-pitched cry, lethargy and expiratory grunt. The babies tend to be hyperirritable and jittery at first, becoming depressed and sluggish later as a result of progressive hypoxia. This picture may progress to respiratory failure. Chest x-ray shows finely reticular granular infiltrates throughout the lung field. Pulmonary hyaline membranes are commonly found on autopsy examination (Winter and Gellis). This is undoubtedly the primary cause of death among infants born alive.

Hypoglycemia is encountered frequently and may persist for long periods of time. This is especially true in premature infants. Such transient severe hypoglycemia may be due to intrinsic hyperinsulinism acquired *in utero* as a consequence of exposure to the maternal hyperglycemic environment. Active therapy is essential to avoid the neurologic sequelae of prolonged, severe hypoglycemia. There is poor correlation between the blood sugar level and clinical manifestations in the newborn infant. Major fluid and electrolyte imbalance is also common, particularly with respiratory acidosis and hyperkalemia. Electrocardiographic abnormalities reflect the increased blood potassium levels, including prolongation of the P-R and QRS intervals (Usher).

It is patently clear that skilled and knowledgeable pediatric consultation must be available at the time of birth so that appropriately aggressive evaluation and management may be instituted immediately. The baby should be transferred at once to a neonatal intensive care unit if such a facility is available for use. Regardless of the infant's healthy general appearance and large size, it should be considered for evaluation and appropriate treatment as if it were a sick, premature infant. It requires humidified incubator atmosphere with supplemental oxygen according to demonstrated needs, together with close supervision and correction of acid-base balance and hypoglycemia. Even digitalization may be necessary for evidences of progressive congestive failure with the appearance of bilateral rales and enlarging liver, although this practice is of questionable value. It is important to ensure that congenital anomalies, such as tracheoesophageal fistula, imperforate anus and diaphragmatic hernia, be disclosed if present so that timely measures may be taken to correct them.

DIABETES INSIPIDUS

Diabetes insipidus may result from any lesion producing damage of the neurohypophysis or the supraoptic and paraventricular nuclei of the hypothalamus. It is characterized by polyuria and polydipsia. The effect of pregnancy on the clinical course of diabetes insipidus is unpredictable (Chau et al.). Although one might expect to encounter problems during labor and the puerperium as a result of diminished or absent production of oxytocin, such is not usually the case. Severe atony and missed labor have been reported, but they are seen only rarely. Similarly, lactation is usually undisturbed. These paradoxical phenomena are explained by the probability that oxytocin is actually being produced in hypothalamic nuclei and released in the posterior pituitary gland by a mechanism separate from that of antidiuretic hormone.

Diagnosis is established by use of a therapeutic test of vasopressin (Pitressin). The manifestations are readily controlled with this agent, given intranasally as a powder or intramuscularly in oil, but care should be taken during pregnancy. The uterotonic effects of Pitressin are likely to become increasingly manifest near term. In order to avoid missed labor and the possibility of an intrauterine death, elective induction of labor (see Chapter 24) with oxytocin infusion is indicated at term provided conditions are optimal. One must ensure that fluid and electrolyte balance is maintained during labor and the puerperium by means of intravenous infusions.

THYROID DYSFUNCTION

Physiologic changes in thyroid activity during pregnancy may produce clinical and laboratory patterns that can be easily confused with hyperthyroidism. The basal metabolic rate increases slowly from the fourth month to term, reflecting the increasing oxygen demands of the fetus, uterus and other organs augmented by pregnancy. Basal metabolic rates not uncommonly increase 15 to 25 per cent during pregnancy. During the first 12 weeks of pregnancy, measurable thyroid hormone increases to about double the nonpregnant values, where it remains until delivery. This is shown in determinations of protein-bound iodine as well as butanol-extractable iodine. Thyroxine levels are similarly affected. The metabolically active fraction of thyroxine, the free or unbound moiety, is not increased, however; it may actually be slightly decreased in euthyroid pregnancies (Burrow). Thyroxine-binding proteins dramatically increase in gestation as a response to estrogenic stimulation. Simultaneously, the I^{131}-T_3 red cell or resin uptake test (Visscher) will be considerably decreased into the hypothyroid range.

Thus, we have the paradoxical situation in pregnancy of thyroxine levels in the hyperthyroid range and thyroxine-binding proteins and T_3 uptake suggesting hypothyroidism, while clinically the patient is euthyroid. The former reflect the increased amounts of circulating bound and, therefore, inactive thyroxine; the latter, the increased amount of thyroxine-binding globulin and its available unsaturated binding sites.

The diagnosis of thyroid dysfunction in pregnancy is also made difficult by virtue of the clinical manifestations sometimes exhibited by euthyroid gravidas. Thus, diffuse enlargement of the thyroid gland may occur together with tachycardia, palpitation, dyspnea, fatigue, nervousness, diaphoresis and altered appetite, all mimicking hyperthyroidism. Comparable confusion with hypothyroidism is encountered if the pregnant woman complains of constipation, irritability, cold intolerance, coarsening of the hair and drying of the skin.

Hyperthyroidism

Hyperthyroidism is rare in pregnancy, occurring in about 0.2 per cent of the gravid population (Niswander and Gordon). Menstrual aberrations are common and, therefore, fertility may be diminished. Fetal wastage has been shown to be increased if pregnancy occurs, and the prematurity rate is significantly elevated. Clinical experience suggests, however, that the fetus of a well-managed patient

with hyperthyroidism is not in jeopardy. The incidence of preeclampsia is also reported to be increased somewhat.

Diagnosis of thyrotoxicosis in pregnancy is based on clinical manifestations, such as exophthalmos, lid lag, hyperkinesis, tachycardia at rest and tremor. Laboratory confirmation in markedly elevated levels of circulating thyroid hormone is necessary. Radioactive iodine must not be given to the gravida for purposes of measuring uptake in the thyroid gland because of its disastrous effect on the fetus. The fetal thyroid gland concentrates iodine beginning about the twelfth week of intrauterine life and has much greater affinity for circulating iodine than the maternal thyroid. Since placental transfer is very rapid, radioactive iodine given to the mother is quickly concentrated in the fetal thyroid, where it causes serious radiation damage. In addition to the general fetal effects of radiation, the baby is likely to be born with diminished or absent thyroid function.

There is no unanimity of opinion with regard to therapy. Medical management with antithyroid drugs can be effective for the mother but may adversely affect the fetus. Thiourea compounds, such as propylthiouracil and methimazole, block thyroid hormone synthesis. They can be given to control maternal hyperthyroidism, but fetal goiter may be anticipated because they cross the placenta readily. Fetal goiter can sometimes be avoided by minimizing dosage and by giving the mother desiccated thyroid simultaneously to suppress fetal production of thyroid stimulating hormone (Herbst and Selenkow).

Subtotal thyroidectomy is another form of treatment effective in correcting maternal hyperthyroidism. It is necessary to ensure that the thyrotoxicosis is under control before undertaking surgery. This can be accomplished by administering iodine in the form of Lugol's solution, five drops twice daily for two weeks, to block secretion of thyroid hormone and decrease the glandular vascularity. If iodine treatment is continued unduly long, the fetus may develop massive goiter. In this regard it is important to bear in mind the possibility that fetal goiter may develop if the gravida is taking large doses of iodides for other medical problems, such as respiratory disturbances. Thyroidectomy is best performed, when indicated, in the midtrimester (Talbert et al.), but can be done earlier if necessary (Werner). The risks of abortion and fetal damage are minimized if proper cardiopulmonary support and oxygenation are provided during surgery.

Hypothyroidism

The rare concurrence of hypothyroidism and pregnancy is based on the fact that hypothyroid women tend to be anovulatory and, therefore, infertile. There is also increased risk of abortion, congenital anomalies and cretinism of the fetus. Diagnosis is based on finding low levels of circulating thyroxine, protein-bound iodine or butanol-extractable iodine, or normal levels at a time in pregnancy when a rise is expected. Clinical manifestations of gross myxedema, with hoarse voice, large tongue and periorbital edema, are rare. More often, the patient may merely be fatigued and have dry skin and coarse hair. Paresthesias and asymmetrically distributed delayed deep tendon reflexes may be found.

Treatment consists of administering full replacement doses of desiccated thyroid, 200 mg. or its equivalent in L-thyroxine or L-triiodothyronine. Desiccated thyroid is preferable; dosage levels can be adjusted according to serum protein-bound iodine determinations. Beginning with 60 mg. daily, dosage can be increased at weekly intervals by 60 mg. daily until the optimal euthyroid level is reached.

PARATHYROID DYSFUNCTION

Abnormalities of parathyroid activity are very rare in pregnancy. Most often primary hyperparathyroidism is due to an adenoma. In a review of patients afflicted by this condition, Ludwig found a very high incidence of spontaneous abortions and stillbirths; in addition, neonatal tetany and permanent hypoparathyroidism in the infant were encountered. In fact, tetany occurring during the neonatal period often led to the retrospective diagnosis of maternal hyperparathyroidism and surgical exploration for removal of the parathyroid adenoma. In view of the high incidence of fetal loss and morbidity, it is recommended that definitive surgical treatment for hyperparathyroidism be undertaken when diagnosed rather than after delivery.

Hypercalcemia may be associated with anorexia, easy fatigability, difficulty in swallowing, nausea and vomiting, constipation and muscular hypotonicity. In addition, hypercalciuria may result in stone formation in the urinary tract with associated progressive renal damage and infection.

Hypoparathyroidism most frequently occurs following thyroid surgery, owing to removal of parathyroid tissue. Typically, one finds elevated serum phosphorus and diminished serum and urinary calcium levels. This results in increased neural excitability leading to tetany. Laryngeal stridor, dyspnea and cyanosis occur, together with tonic muscular contractions, gastric pain, nausea and vomiting. Generalized convulsions may occur and are difficult to distinguish from eclamptic or epileptic seizures.

Intravenous calcium is the specific treatment for acute hypocalcemic tetany. It can be given as 10 per cent calcium lactate, 10 to 30 ml. as needed. Maintenance therapy in the form of oral calcium lactate (4 gm. 6 times daily) and vitamin D in large doses (50,000 units daily) will be needed. The urine calcium level serves as a useful index of the adequacy of therapy. Dihydrotachysterol (AT 10) may be used as an effective substitute for vitamin D.

REFERENCES

Benjamin, F., and Casper, D. J.: Comparative validity of oral and intravenous glucose tolerance tests in pregnancy. Amer. J. Obstet. Gynec. 97:488, 1967.

Burrow, G. N.: The Thyroid Gland in Pregnancy. Philadelphia, W. B. Saunders Company, 1972.

Chau, S. S., Fitzpatrick, R. J., and Jamieson, B.:

Diabetes insipidus and parturition. J. Obstet. Gynaec. Brit. Comm. 76:444, 1969.

Churchill, J. A., Berendes, H. W., and Nemore, J.: Neuropsychological deficits in children of diabetic mothers. Amer. J. Obstet. Gynec. 105:257, 1969.

Freinkel, N., and Goodner, C. J.: Insulin metabolism and pregnancy. Arch. Intern. Med. 109:235, 1962.

Gellis, S. S., and Hsia, D. Y.: The infant of the diabetic mother. Amer. J. Dis. Child. 97:1, 1959.

Ginsburg, J.: Carbohydrate metabolism. In Philipp, E. E., Barnes, J., and Newton, M., eds.: Scientific Foundation of Obstetrics and Gynaecology. Philadelphia, F. A. Davis Company, 1970.

Greene, J. W., Jr., Smith, K., Kyle, G. C., Touchstone, J. C., and Duhring, J. L.: The use of estriol excretion in the management of pregnancies complicated by diabetes mellitus. Amer. J. Obstet. Gynec. 91:684, 1965.

Hagbard, L.: Pregnancy and Diabetes Mellitus. Springfield, Ill., Charles C Thomas, 1961.

Herbst, A. L., and Selenkow, H. A.: Hyperthyroidism during pregnancy. New Eng. J. Med. 273:627, 1965.

Herbst, A. L., Kurman, R. J., Scully, R. E., and Proskanzer, D. C.: Clear-cell adenocarcinoma of the genital tract in young females: Registry report. New Eng. J. Med. 287:1259, 1972.

Hughes, E. C., ed.: Obstetric-Gynecologic Terminology. Philadelphia, F. A. Davis Company, 1972.

Klopper, A.: The assessment of feto-placental function by estriol assay. Obstet. Gynec. Survey 23:813, 1968.

Ludwig, G. D.: Hyperparathyroidism in relation to pregnancy. New Eng. J. Med. 267:637, 1962.

Niswander, K. R., and Gordon, M., eds.: The Collaborative Perinatal Study of the National Institute of Neurological Diseases and Stroke: The Women and Their Pregnancies. Philadelphia, W. B. Saunders Company, 1972.

O'Sullivan, J. B., and Mahan, C.: Criteria for the oral glucose tolerance test in pregnancy. Diabetes 13:278, 1964.

Pedersen, J.: Foetal mortality in diabetes in relation to management during the latter part of pregnancy. Acta Endocr. 15:282, 1954.

Schwarz, R. H., Fields, G. A., and Kyle, G. C.: Timing of delivery in the pregnant diabetic patient. Obstet. Gynec. 34:787, 1969.

Shapiro, A. P., Benedek, T. G., and Small, J. L.: Effects of thiazides on carbohydrate metabolism in patients with hypertension. New Eng. J. Med. 265:1028, 1961.

Spellacy, W.: Plasma insulin measurements. In Wynn, R., ed.: Fetal Homeostasis, Vol. IV. New York, Appleton-Century-Crofts, 1969.

Talbert, L. M., Thomas, C. G., Jr., Holt, W. A., and Rankin, P.: Hyperthyroidism during pregnancy. Obstet. Gynec. 36:779, 1970.

Usher, R.: Respiratory distress syndrome of prematurity: I. Changes in potassium in serum and electrocardiogram and effects of therapy. Pediatrics 24:562, 1959.

Visscher, R. D.: T_3-^{131}I binding capacity of serum proteins. Amer. J. Obstet. Gynec. 86:829, 1963.

Werner, S. C.: Hyperthyroidism in the pregnant woman and neonate. J. Clin. Endocr. 27:1637, 1967.

White, P.: Pregnancy and diabetes: Medical aspects. Med. Clin. N. Amer. 49:1015, 1965.

White, P., Gillespie, L., and Sexton, L.: Use of female sex hormone therapy in pregnant diabetic patients. Amer. J. Obstet. Gynec. 71:57, 1956.

Winter, W. D., and Gellis, S. S.: Pulmonary hyaline membranes in infants of diabetic mothers. Amer. J. Dis. Child. 87:702, 1954.

Chapter 50

The Drug Problem[*]

In the United States today clinicians are increasingly confronted with patients who have been exposed to or are chronic users of psychotropic drugs of various kinds. This problem is rapidly becoming widespread around the world. The use of illicit drugs cuts across all socioeconomic and geographic barriers. The problem exists on a vast scale and involves many young individuals, including teenage and adult women. Few obstetricians have had any meaningful experience with management of pregnancy in addicted women, even though the issue has expanded to major proportions. The problem of caring for the pregnant addict and the addicted newborn infant is a relatively new one for physicians. Principles of prenatal care and both recognition and treatment of the withdrawal syndrome in the neonate demand our attention.

HEROIN

Heroin is a chemical congener of morphine with marked addicting potentialities. Its use in the United States was declared illegal in 1923 on this basis. It is manufactured directly from raw opium and generally adulterated for commercial use with lactose, glucose or quinine to one to three per cent concentrations (Louria et al.), although as much as 10 per cent may be present, each "bag" containing 10 to 30 mg. (Blinick et al.). Heroin can be absorbed from almost any body surface and is effective if taken orally, nasally by sniffing, subcutaneously, intravenously or intramuscularly.

The pregnant addict tends to be immature and relatively unstable. Her moods characteristically change abruptly and frequently, reflecting cyclic variations in drug levels. She may be quite euphoric soon after she has taken the drug, appearing sedated, tranquilized and absorbed in herself. A brief normal interval follows during which she appears alert and well. If no additional drug is administered, the abstinent state ensues with craving for narcotics together with malaise, nausea and perspiration, as well as other early manifestations of withdrawal (Blinick). These latter may include thirst, anxiety, restlessness, rhinorrhea, gooseflesh, hot and cold flashes, yawning and dilatation of the pupils. Late manifestation of the withdrawal syndrome in the heroin addict includes severe aching in bones and muscles, abdominal pain, vomiting and diarrhea; one may find tachycardia, tachypnea, hypertension and temperature elevation as well.

After the patient has been on the drug for some time, her system adjusts to the drug intake and the fluctuations in mood decrease markedly. In order for her to continue to reach the euphoric state, the addict finds she must take more and more heroin. Thus, higher doses and more frequent usage become common (Graham).

Menstrual aberrations are seen commonly among patients who use large doses of heroin. After one to four months on heroin, menstruation usually ceases altogether (Claman and Strang). About two-thirds of female addicts have oligomenorrhea or amenorrhea (Gaulden et al.). The mechanism by which this comes about is unknown, although it is postulated that ovulatory suppression is mediated by the

---

[*]Written with Johanna F. Perlmutter, M.D.

527

direct depressing effect of the narcotic on the pituitary or the hypothalamus or by the effecting of a neural block between hypothalamus and pituitary which results in decreased gonadotropin output. The latter is supported by observations that morphine, which is chemically related to heroin, decreases ACTH and affects adrenal function (McDonald et al.; Eisenman et al.). The fact that heroin addicts do become pregnant about as often as nonaddicts (Blinick; Stoffer) suggests that many may actually be receiving only small amounts of the drug which are insufficient to affect their pituitary-ovarian axis.

The physician can recognize the addict if he is alert to certain telltale features. Besides the patient's general demeanor and behavior, pinpoint pupils that are nonreactive to light are characteristic. Needle track marks along the arms and the backs of the legs, if found, are confirmatory.

Prenatal Care

Several options are available to physicians who provide care to the pregnant woman, including (1) provision of optimal support without altering the addiction pattern, (2) acute detoxification by withdrawal, (3) slow detoxification using methadone substitution and subsequent withdrawal of the methadone and (4) methadone maintenance (Blinick; Neuberg; Wallach et al.). There is still much controversy as to which of these approaches is optimal.

The results are not very good if one merely encourages the patient to come for prenatal care while permitting her to support her habit through usual channels. Heroin has low molecular weight and, therefore, readily crosses the placenta. It is found in fetal tissues within an hour after its administration to the mother. Thus, the unaltered maternal heroin addiction will lead commonly to intrauterine addiction of the fetus which will become manifest in withdrawal during the neonatal period (see below). Moreover, prenatal care of such patients tends to be spotty and erratic because the patient is primarily motivated to pursuing the time-consuming activity of supporting the habit. Since addiction is

not always disclosed by the patient, the physician may find himself following this program unwittingly by default.

Acute detoxification without use of any other supportive agent tends to be unacceptable to the addict and is not without complications. The fetus, if addicted also, may simultaneously undergo detoxification during this time. The incidence of fetal loss is high. Whether this results from the addiction *per se* or other factors, such as poor maternal nutrition, is unknown.

Slower means of detoxification by administering large doses of tranquilizers or methadone and then slowly withdrawing the substitute medication is another difficult approach. The effect is to convert the heroin addict first into a methadone addict and then gradually diminish the methadone dose over a long period of time. This usually requires prolonged hospital stay. Methadone withdrawal is not accomplished easily and indeed may be more difficult than heroin withdrawal in some patients. Moreover, at least 40 per cent of detoxified patients are back on heroin by the time they return for delivery (Blinick).

The approach currently most widely recommended is methadone maintenance. This requires that the gravida be hospitalized for purposes of substituting high doses of methadone for her heroin. The patient is then maintained on a daily controlled dose of the drug, between 80 and 120 mg. a day. The ostensible advantages of the methadone maintenance program include (1) better participation by addicts in their own prenatal care, (2) shorter hospital stay for the neonate, (3) improved attention by the mother to the health care needs of her child and (4) creation of a more stable social environment for both mother and baby (Sullivan et al.).

Preliminary reports of methadone maintenance programs for gravidas have been very encouraging. Most women in the programs resume their regular menstrual cycles. The pregnant women have no ill effects from the methadone; they lead a more normal life; they feel better and eat well; they are considerably more cooperative and easier to take care of; their babies are larger, less premature and, although addicted to the methadone at birth, the neonates do better and need active therapy less often (Blinick; Wallach et al.). With the high doses of methadone used, the patient is less apt to want to (or have to) supplement with heroin.

Within the constraints of availability and legality, it is the patient who tends to choose the program of care for her own pregnancy. Whichever she selects, it is important for the physician to avoid moralization. To do so will often cause the patient to go elsewhere or to avoid further care until she is in labor. These patients deserve the best in prenatal care and it should not be denied to them. Although they are difficult to manage, they warrant our close attention.

Complications of Pregnancy

Many of the medical problems encountered among pregnant addicts occur as a result of their life style and habits (Blinick et al.). Hepatitis and multiple peripheral abscesses are common because they use unsterile technique for injections. Similarly, thrombophlebitis and pulmonary embolism may result from local vein injury or irritation. Tetanus from use of unsterile needles has also occurred in addicts, although no gravid or neonatal tetanus has yet been reported. Venereal disease is frequent because women commonly support their addiction primarily by prostitution. The rapidly spiraling expense of heroin addiction usually leaves the addict in poverty so that nutrition is poor and anemia a common consequence. Chronic constipation and loss of libido occur, and the addict becomes progressively debilitated.

Death may occur almost instantaneously during intravenous heroin injection. It may be an acute allergic reaction associated with severe, rapidly developing pulmonary edema. Drug overdosage may also be a fatal factor, particularly if drug concentration administered exceeds 20 per cent (Louria et al.). Treatment should be directed at establishing cardiorespiratory function. Artificial ventilation, together with vasopressors and gastric lavage, is essential.

There are no specific obstetric problems that are peculiar to pregnant addicts. Prenatal care, as indicated earlier, is rather poor in general. They rarely see a physician prior to delivery (Krause et al.; Stone et al.); only one in four ever registers for care prior to labor. Most who do seek care wait until the last trimester of pregnancy. They often have a poor obstetric history with increased numbers of prior abortions and late fetal wastage.

Premature labor is common, occurring in at least half the cases (Perlmutter; Stern). As a result, pregnancies among addicts are associated with increased numbers of stillbirths and neonatal deaths. Perinatal mortality is reported to be about 17 per cent (Perlmutter). There are larger numbers of breech deliveries consistent with the incidence of prematurity. Placental abnormalities, as well as preeclampsia and abruptio placentae, are reported to be frequent (Neuberg; Stern). Retained placenta and postpartum hemorrhage are also said to be increased among these patients.

The management of labor and delivery must be individualized as with any other gravida. The amount of analgesia required is usually the same as or less than that needed by other women (Blinick et al.). The amount will depend upon how recently the patient took her drug before being admitted to the hospital. Usually, because of her fear that she will not be able to maintain her habit in the hospital, she deliberately remains at home during most of the labor, taking the last dose of heroin and coming to the hospital only when the delivery is imminent. She generally feels she can thereby shorten the hospital stay and minimize her need for drugs. Caution should be used whenever employing any drug or anesthetic agent that is known to be hepatotoxic because addicts are particularly likely to develop impairment of liver function as a result of repeated attacks of overt and subclinical hepatitis.

Meconium staining of the amniotic fluid is frequently seen at delivery. This may be unrelated to intrapartum fetal hypoxia. It is more likely due to repeated insults to the fetus prior to labor resulting from periodic narcotic overdosage, withdrawal or other maternal stresses. Addicts frequently report that the fetus becomes quiescent after they have taken the drug and hyperactive during withdrawal. Northrup et al. have recently shown that estriol urinary excretion levels in gravidas on methadone maintenance are consistently very low, negating the value of this test for monitoring fetoplacental function (see Chapter 13) in these patients.

Care of the Infant

Objective evidence of withdrawal is seen in infants delivered of addicts (Neuberg; Perlmutter), with reports ranging from 58 to 91 per cent incidence. However, perhaps only one-third of these will require treatment (Statzer and Wardell). The first signs will be manifest within 24 hours of the delivery in 50 to 63 per cent of these infants, but it can take as long as seven days before the problem becomes evident.

Attempts have been made to correlate severity, onset and duration of symptoms to the amount of heroin the mother has taken, when she took it and the length of her addiction. Although one would expect a short interval between drug and delivery to be associated with long delays in neonatal manifestations of withdrawal, this is not the case (Perlmutter). As to drug dosage, there does seem to be a good correlation; when a critical limit is exceeded (and this is estimated to be six "bags" daily), there is a 75 per cent probability that the infant will show signs of withdrawal. A similar correlation exists for the duration of the addiction, particularly if the mother is addicted for more than one year. With smaller drug dosages, withdrawal occurs in 63 per cent, and with shorter durations, 55 per cent (Zelson et al.).

The signs of neonatal withdrawal are not pathognomonic. The typical addicted neonate is usually described as an irritable baby with a high-pitched cry who does not feed well (Stone et al.). His characteristic irritability is manifested by hyperactivity, hypertonus, trembling, twitching, scratching of the face and convulsions. He may show vomiting, diarrhea, sneezing, yawning and sucking of the fingers. Mucus secretion is increased and respiratory distress may occur with tachypnea, grunting, rib retraction, intermittent cyanosis and periods of apnea. Hyperpyrexia with perspiration is seen. The baby loses weight excessively and may have an incomplete Moro reflex.

If left untreated, convulsions and death may occur in 93 per cent (Stone et al.). The diagnosis is difficult and the condition must be differentiated from hypocalcemic tetany, hypoglycemic reaction, central nervous system damage and pyridoxine deficiency. Neonatal mortality may be as high as 34 per cent, even with aggressive treatment.

About half the infants of addicted mothers weigh less than 2500 gm. (Perlmutter); half of these are small for gestational age (Stone et al.; Zelson et al.). Growth retardation has not been explained but may be related to the effects of the heroin or the adulterating quinine on the fetus or on placental function. It is possibly a consequence of pervading maternal nutritional deprivation. High perinatal mortality is primarily attributable to prematurity and may also be related to respiratory distress in association with undiagnosed withdrawal.

The incidence of congenital anomalies is not increased, although inguinal hernias are seen somewhat more often than expected (Perlmutter). When present, hernias become manifest fairly early, perhaps as a result of excessive straining and hypertonic activity of the newborn during withdrawal.

Still unresolved is the question of whether or not permanent brain damage will occur in these infants. It has been suggested that heroin causes histological changes in the brain during fetal life (Courville). These may be due to the direct action of the narcotic on the nerve cell or to indirect vasomotor action. Abnormal sleep patterns are seen in all addicted neonates that have been tested. None has quiet sleep patterns or the normal fluctuations in patterns from active to quiet sleep; periods of rapid eye movement are often disorganized (Schulman).

The incidence of physiologic jaundice is lower than expected among neonates, occurring in six per cent only. It is possible that intrauterine exposure to heroin or quinine has prematurely induced microsomal enzymes of the liver, thereby maturing the glucuronyl transferase. This possibility is supported by the observed ability of addicted infants to tolerate chlorpromazine treatment. Other neonates are usually unable to metabolize chlorpromazine, excreting it intact in the urine. Infants delivered of addicts, however, are able to metabolize this agent through the glucuronyl transferase system of the liver and excrete it in the urine as chlorpromazine-*o*-glucuronide. Moreover, one does not see the extrapyramidal effects of chlorpromazine in these infants (Zelson et al.).

When treatment is indicated for the addicted neonate, the infant is first sedated and then slowly withdrawn from all drugs. The most commonly used agents are paregoric, phenobarbital and chlorpromazine (Reddy et al.). Each works well alone, but combinations have been used effectively. None has been found to be especially superior to the others. Diazepam has also been used recently with good results (Nathenson et al.), although some feel it should be held in reserve for the babies with severe withdrawal symptoms (Blinick). Neither methadone nor morphine is generally administered to newborn infants because difficulties have occasionally been encountered in withdrawal.

The usual regimen of therapy for the infant known to be addicted is one of the following: (1) elixir paregoric, 4 to 6 drops with each feeding, (2) phenobarbital, 5 to 15 mg. every four to six hours, or (3) chlorpromazine, 0.7 to 1.1 mg. per kilogram every four to six hours. Doses are then slowly reduced and the time intervals lengthened until the infant is completely withdrawn. The total duration of this course averages one month and may vary from 10 to 60 days. The speed of withdrawal must be titrated against the infant's response. If too rapid, signs of acute withdrawal arise and necessitate return to the previous level. There is a delicate balance that must be maintained between withdrawal manifestations and the signs of oversedation, such as shallow respirations. The latter is especially important and is reflected in the large number of neonatal deaths associated with respiratory failure in the absence of hyaline membrane disease. Breast feeding is not encouraged because both heroin and methadone are secreted in the milk.

AMPHETAMINES

Long-term usage of amphetamines may lead to significant psychiatric disturbances (Lemere). Physical problems are generally not related to the drug itself, but are secondary to the resulting poor eating habits and undernutrition. The diagnosis of amphetamine abuse cannot be made by physical examination alone. The manifestations of fear, anxiety and excitement so commonly seen in amphetamine users cannot be distinguished from comparable manifestations in frightened gravidas who are nonusers.

Patients who use amphetamines may be unreliable with regard to antepartum care. They may miss appointments and neglect important instructions. It is essential that dietary deficiencies be detected and corrected for the sake of the fetus. However, there are no known specific adverse effects of amphetamine usage on the fetus or neonate. Neonatal withdrawal was considered to be responsible for marked drowsiness in one newborn infant whose electroencephalogram was reported to be normal (Neuberg). Acute withdrawal can be accomplished with no apparent reactions. However, some amphetamine users may become depressed as a result (Neuberg).

LYSERGIC ACID DIETHYLAMIDE (LSD)

Patients who take LSD exhibit none of the characteristics of psychological or physical dependence. One of the serious risks of its use, however, is periodic spontaneous recall of its previous effects long after the drug has been discontinued. There is conflicting evidence concerning the teratogenicity of LSD in human beings. In mice and rats LSD causes abortion, stillbirth, stunted growth and gross anomaly when given in early pregnancy; if given late in pregnancy, no fetal effects are found (Alexander et al.; Auerbach and Rugowski).

Although chromosomal abnormalities were found to be increased in human leukocytes (Cohen et al.; Irwin and Egozcue), this could not be substantiated (Tjio et al.). There is an increase in the frequency of spontaneous abortions among women who acknowledge using LSD prior to or early in pregnancy, and their aborted fetuses have a high incidence of abnormalities. Fetal abnormalities have also been reported when only the father has used LSD, presumably based on the chromosomal defects in the fertilizing spermatozoon. There have also been isolated reports of grossly deformed infants born to LSD users, but the actual incidence of this occurrence is unknown. Whether or not LSD is actually teratogenic in the human fetus is conjectural at this time (Zellweger et al.).

CANNABIS (MARIJUANA)

The use of marijuana is very widespread, analogous to the more prevalent use of alcohol. Only after long and heavy intake does any overt effect occur in the user. Mood and personality changes, including severe depression, may then be seen. Although there have thus far been no documented ill effects in the human fetus, marijuana has been shown to be teratogenic in lower animals (Persaud and Ellington). In mice, for example, it results in fetal resorption and stunting of growth. Despite its extensive use among people of childbearing age, little is actually known about its immediate and long-term effects on either the adult user or the fetus exposed to it by transplacental absorption from its mother (Hecht et al.).

REFERENCES

Alexander, G. J., Miles, B. E., Gold, G. M., and Alexander, R. B.: LSD: Injection early in pregnancy produces abnormalities in offspring of rats. Science *157*:459, 1967.

Auerbach, R., and Rugowski, J. A.: Lysergic acid diethylamide: Effect on embryos. Science *157*:1325, 1967.

Blinick, G.: Fertility of narcotic addicts and effects of addiction on the offspring. Soc. Biol. *18*:S34, 1971.

Blinick, G.: Babies seem better off when mothers are on methadone. Med. World News, July 21, 1972, p. 16.

Blinick, G., Wallach, R. C., and Jerez, E.: Pregnancy in narcotics addicts treated by medical withdrawal: The methadone detoxification program. Amer. J. Obstet. Gynec. *105*:997, 1969.

Claman, A., and Strang, C.: Obstetric and gynecologic aspects of heroin addiction. Amer. J. Obstet. Gynec. *83*:252, 1962.

Cohen, M. M., Marinello, M. J., and Back, N.: Chromosomal damage in human leukocytes induced by lysergic acid diethylamide. Science *155*:1417, 1967.

Courville, C. B.: Contributions to the study of cerebral anoxia. Bull. Los Angeles Neurol. Soc. *15*:99, 1950.

Eisenman, A. J., Fraser, H. F., Sloan, J., and Isbell, H.: Urinary 17-ketosteroid excretion during a cycle of addiction to morphine. J. Pharmacol. Exp. Ther. *124*:305, 1958.

Gaulden, E. C., Littlefield, D. C., Putoff, O. E., and Seivert, A. L.: Menstrual abnormalities associated with heroin addiction. Amer. J. Obstet. Gynec. *90*:155, 1964.

Graham, J.: The nature and properties of drugs which give rise to dependence. Community Health *1*:84, 1969.

Hecht, F., Beals, R. K., Lees, M. H., Jolly, H., and Roberts, P.: Lysergic-acid-diethylamide and cannabis as possible teratogens in man. Lancet *2*:1087, 1968.

Irwin, S., and Egozcue, J.: Chromosomal abnormalities in leukocytes from LSD-25 users. Science *157*:313, 1967.

Krause, S., Murray, P., Holmes, J., and Lurch, R.: Heroin addiction among pregnant women and their newborn babies. Amer. J. Obstet. Gynec. *75*:754, 1958.

Lemere, F.: The danger of amphetamine dependency. Amer. J. Psychiat. *123*:569, 1966.

Louria, D., Hensle, T., and Rose, J.: The major medical complications of heroin addiction. Ann. Intern. Med. *67*:1, 1967.

McDonald, R. K., Evans, F. T., Weise, V. K., and Patrick, R. W.: Effect of morphine and nalorphine on plasma hydrocortisone levels in man. J. Pharmacol. Exp. Ther. *125*:241, 1959.

Nathenson, G., Golden, G., and Litt, I.: Diazepam in the management of the neonatal narcotic withdrawal syndrome. Pediatrics *48*:523, 1971.

Neuberg, R.: Drug dependence and pregnancy: A review of the problems and their management. J. Obstet. Gynaec. Brit. Comm. *77*:1117, 1970.

Northrup, G., Ditzler, J., Ryan, W. G., and Wilbanks, G. D.: Estriol excretion profile in narcotic-addicted pregnant women. Amer. J. Obstet. Gynec. *112*:704, 1972.

Perlmutter, J. F.: Drug addiction in pregnant women. Amer. J. Obstet. Gynec. *99*:569, 1967.

Persaud, T. V. N., and Ellington, A. C.: Cannabis in early pregnancy. Lancet *2*:1306, 1967.

Reddy, A. M., Harper, R. G., and Stern, G.: Observations on heroin and methadone withdrawal in the newborn. Pediatrics *48*:353, 1971.

Schulman, L.: Alterations of the sleep cycles in heroin addicted and "suspected" newborns. Neuropediatrics *1*:89, 1969.

Statzer, D. E., and Wardell, J. N.: Heroin addiction during pregnancy. Amer. J. Obstet. Gynec. *113*:273, 1972.

Stern, R.: The pregnant addict: A study of 66 case histories, 1950–1959. Amer. J. Obstet. Gynec. *94*:253, 1966.

Stoffer, S.: A gynecologic study of addicts. Amer. J. Obstet. Gynec. *101*:779, 1968.

Stone, M. L., Salerno, L. J., Green, M., and Zelson, C.: Narcotic addiction in pregnancy. Amer. J. Obstet. Gynec. *109*:716, 1971.

Sullivan, R., Fischbach, A., and Hornick, F.: Treatment of a pregnant opiate addict with oral methadone. Arizona Med. *29*:129, 1972.

Tjio, J.-H., Pahnke, W. N., and Kurland, A. A.: LSD and chromosomes: A controlled experiment. J.A.M.A. *210*:849, 1969.

Wallach, R. C., Jerez, E., and Blinick, G.: Pregnancy and menstrual function in narcotics addicts treated with methadone: The methadone maintenance program. Amer. J. Obstet. Gynec. *105*:1226, 1969.

Zellweger, H., McDonald, J. S., and Abbo, G.: Is lysergic-acid diethylamide a teratogen? Lancet *2*:1066, 1967.

Zelson, C., Rubio, E., and Wasserman, E.: Neonatal narcotic addiction: Ten year observation. Pediatrics *48*:178, 1971.

Chapter 51

Intensive Care of the Gravida

There is no special immunity bestowed upon the pregnant woman with regard to major life-threatening illnesses. She is subject to all the ills that may befall any woman plus those that are peculiar to pregnancy itself. Thus, almost any condition for which females require intensive care may be complicated by the presence of coincidental pregnancy. The pregnancy in turn may affect the presenting condition and, further, may require modification of management.

Aside from the obvious factors involving simultaneous care of two individuals (the patient and the fetus), critical questions invariably arise and demand attention: What is the effect of the disorder on maintenance of the pregnancy; is there potential risk of the disorder producing fetal injury or death; how may treatment affect continuation of the pregnancy and the well-being of the fetus; in what way may the pregnancy affect the course of the disorder; what are the hazards of allowing the pregnancy to continue; what are the comparable risks of interrupting the pregnancy?

To further complicate the situation we find the need to consider that pregnancy may alter physiologic mechanisms and pharmacologic actions in diverse and sometimes unpredictable ways. The complex interrelationships between these various aspects require a nicety of judgment for the intelligent, discriminating management of each individual case. All facets must be taken into account so that appropriate decisions can be made.

Death in pregnancy may occur from factors relating to hemorrhage, infection and hypertensive states of pregnancy most commonly. These three complications alone account for three-quarters of all reported maternal deaths. Detailed explora-tions of the etiologic factors, measures essential for prevention and programs of management are presented elsewhere (see relevant chapters).

It is imperative to appreciate that obstetric hemorrhage may occur suddenly, essentially without warning, and proceed unremittingly to exsanguination if unchecked in association with abortion, especially in conjunction with Gram-negative septicemia, ectopic pregnancy, abnormal placentation (placenta previa and abruptio placentae), trauma or uterine rupture. Preeclampsia may progress with lightning rapidity to convulsions, coma and death if not managed aggressively in its premonitory phases.

Similarly, infection of the pregnant or recently pregnant uterus spreads rapidly and widely to produce septic thrombophlebitis, peritonitis and disseminating bacteremia. Particularly treacherous is the problem of sepsis in association with abortion, most especially in the middle trimester, where the picture of endotoxin shock may arise, characterized by cardiovascular instability, oliguria as a manifestation of renal failure and concomitant coagulopathy. Septic abortion is probably the single most commonly encountered phenomenon associated with maternal mortality.

Some essential principles pertaining to the intensive care of the pregnant patient must be reviewed. A basic general objective involves the necessity to maintain fetal oxygenation. Embryogenesis may be adversely affected by diminished oxygenation during the first eight weeks of gestation. At any time during the course of pregnancy, anoxia may lead to irreversible tissue damage, especially involving the central nervous system, or death *in utero*. Although the fetus is somewhat less susceptible to hypoxemia than the adult, he is nevertheless vulnerable. Adequate fetal oxygenation requires smooth functioning and integration of a chain of phenomena: (1) pulmonary ventilation and oxygenation of maternal blood, (2) suitable blood flow to the uterus and the placenta, (3) prompt, efficient placental exchange, and (4) adequate fetal circulation.

Ventilation and oxygenation may be deleteriously affected by many conditions, including an assortment of acute and chronic pulmonary disorders, obstructive and inflammatory processes, severe anemia and states characterized by altered oxygen carrying capacity, such as methemoglobinemia. Blood flow reflects maternal cardiovascular status and is adversely altered by failure or shock. Placental exchange is influenced primarily by metabolic factors, renal and hypertensive diseases, febrile disorders and toxins. Fetal blood flow appears to be diminished during the drug-induced uterine hypercontractile states. One can see how important it is to maintain pulmonary ventilation and support adequate blood flow to the brain as well as to the uterus.

DRUGS AND UTERINE ACTIVITY

With regard to uterine contractility as influenced by various drugs, obstetric and pharmacologic literature is often contradictory. Basically, this is a result of inherent difficulties in attaining objectivity. Of prime importance here are drugs with documented uterine effects, including those that stimulate as well as those that inhibit contractility. The former are important because uterine hypercontractility may reduce intrauterine fetoplacental circulation; the latter, because they reduce efficiency of contractions in the course of labor, thereby either permitting significant delays where indicated or producing unwanted protraction of labor. Thus, agents used for management of the concurrent condition may be undesirably inhibitory.

Less well known for their oxytocic effects than posterior pituitary extracts, synthetic oxytocin preparations and ergot alkaloids are a myriad of frequently used agents with valuable nonobstetric pharmacologic functions. Among these are adrenergic blocking agents, including imidazolines (Priscoline and Regitine) and benzodioxamines (piperoxan and prosympal); ganglionic blocking agents, such as nicotine and tetraethylammonium ion; and parasympathomimetic agents, acetylcholine in large doses and the synthetic choline derivative, carbachol. The cholinesterase inhibitor, physostigmine, also stimulates the uterus in high concentrations. Neostigmine, on the other hand, does not affect the pregnant uterus, except at term. Among cholinergic alkaloids, pilocarpine will stimulate the uterus that has been primed by estrogens. Sympathomimetic agents have paradoxical effects: epinephrine inhibits contractility, while norepinephrine stimulates it. Histamine acts directly on the uterine muscle as a stimulant; interestingly, antihistamines are generally mildly spasmogenic as well. The cardiac glycosides, digoxin, ouabain and strophanthin G, have all been demonstrated to increase contractility.

Inhibition of uterine muscle activity, generated either spontaneously or by therapeutic stimulation, occurs with the use of many analgesic, sedative and hypnotic agents, including morphine, methadone, barbiturates, tribromoethanol and paraldehyde. Similarly, anesthetic gases, such as diethyl and divinyl ether, chloroform, cyclopropane and especially halothane, are strongly inhibitory. Variably depressant effects are seen following use of antispasmodic agents, such as isoxsuprine, adiphenine, dicyclomine and others. Suppression has also been encountered with magnesium sulphate, proportional to the level of magnesium ion in circulation, and with ethyl alcohol.

DRUGS AND THE FETUS

Aside from the direct effect of uterotonic agents upon the uterus (and therefore potentially on the fetus) as indicated above, many drugs are known to influence the fetus. As discussed in Chapter 4, any substance found in the maternal circulation can be expected to cross into the fetal circulation. Some traverse slowly or are altered in transit so that they exert little pharmacologic or toxicologic effects on the fetus. Others, however, are transferred freely and exert readily demonstrable actions. One must weigh this consideration before administering any drug to the pregnant female.

Examples of drugs that may endanger the fetus cover the entire spectrum of our pharmacopoeia. Anomalies, death or damage may result from use of antimetabolites (aminopterin and related drugs), anticoagulants (Dicumarol, but not heparin), antihistamines, antithyroid drugs (propylthiouracil), hypoglycemic agents (sulfonylurea derivatives), tranquilizers (phenothiazines, thalidomide) and antibiotics. The adverse effects of this last group are well documented and growing. They include: eighth nerve and cochlear damage and possible teratogenicity from streptomycin; aplastic anemia and circulatory collapse from chloramphenicol; liver and pancreatic dysfunction, bone growth inhibition, and discoloration of teeth from tetracycline; interference with bilirubin conjugation leading to kernicterus from sulfonamides and novobiocin; liver damage from erythromycin; and hemolysis from nitrofurantoin. Cortisone and its analogues have been suspected of causing cleft palate, but this is unproved in humans. Hepatic toxicity has been encountered from anticonvulsants, and hemorrhagic manifestations have followed use of barbiturates and reserpine. Reserpine administered to the mother has also been implicated in producing respiratory distress of the newborn. Masculinization of the female fetus may occur following administration of progestins and androgens. Even salicylates may predispose the infant to hemorrhagic crises in the newborn period. The development of clear cell adenocarcinoma in the vagina of adolescents whose mothers were given stilbestrol during pregnancy has recently been reported also.

Even more here than in other medical disciplines, the overriding rule prevails that the relative hazards of a disorder must be balanced against the potential risks of the treatment used. Clearly, no lifesaving measures should be avoided, regardless of danger to fetus, providing there is no available alternative choice of regimen equally suitable for care of the mother but less hazardous to the fetus. Theologic considerations aside, it would be unthinkable to withhold such measures, thereby jeopardizing maternal well-being and survival, particularly if it is done to preserve the life of a fetus that is not likely to survive independently. Fortunately, the dilemma does not arise often.

In this regard, one's approach may perforce have to be modified according to whether or not the fetus is viable. Dating the duration of pregnancy on the basis of last menstrual period is notoriously inaccurate. Other, more accurate means for determining fetal age and the likelihood of survival if the fetus is delivered are reviewed in Chapter 13. In most instances, the fetus delivered at or before 28 weeks' gestational age cannot be expected to live. The further along the pregnancy has advanced beyond this point in time, the more optimistic the outlook for the infant. Survival rates are quite high for infants born after 36 weeks. Accordingly, where casuistic considerations are not limiting, the fetus is essentially ignored in handling critical situations prior to the twenty-eighth week; beyond this time, his welfare should be considered in developing suitable programs of management.

ACUTE PROBLEMS

Nearly every medical disorder somehow affects pregnancy, or in turn is affected by the concurrent gravid state. In general, the programs of care acceptable in the nonpregnant state for conditions requiring intensive care should prevail. Nevertheless, it is important to stress briefly areas of special importance, most particularly those critical conditions peculiar to pregnancy that demand our attention. Reference should be made to the more detailed discussions in the chapters dealing with the specific disorders. Physicians who are called upon to deal with such serious, critical issues should always bear in mind the importance of seeking expert consultative aid for the management of special medical problems.

Cardiac Disorders

Heart disease remains a major obstetric problem (see Chapter 41). Fortunately, very few afflicted obstetric patients have valvular lesions that interfere sufficiently to impair cardiopulmonary function. Despite increased cardiac output, blood volume and heart rate associated with pregnancy, most of these patients do very well. It is in the remaining group, comprising those with major functional deficiency, that problems arise. Patients with functional Class IV disability may be in serious jeopardy in pregnancy. These patients should be advised against pregnancy; if pregnant, they should be evaluated for therapeutic abortion in the first trimester. If pregnancy is advanced to a later stage or if therapeutic abortion is contraindicated on theologic grounds, the patient with severe mitral stenosis, especially if already manifesting decompensation, may be considered a candidate for mitral valvotomy. For terminating the late pregnancy, vaginal delivery is a more reasonable and less taxing modality than cesarean section. Unless cesarean section is indicated for obstetric reasons, these women can endure properly conducted labor and delivery much better than the major surgical assault of cesarean section.

In general, treatment of cardiac complications, including congestive failure, pulmonary edema and arrhythmias, should be exactly as in the nonpregnant state. This tenet applies despite the fact, previously noted, that cardiac glycosides are mildly uterotonic. Special obstetric measures refer primarily to management of labor and delivery. If possible, labor should be short and uncomplicated; delivery should be smooth and assisted. The labor should be conducted with sufficient analgesics to allay discomfort and anxiety. The delivery should be accomplished under regional block anesthesia preferably, with timely intervention by low forceps early in the second stage to minimize the bearing-down efforts. Induction of labor is generally not indicated and may be ill-advised if the labor that results is long and trying. Under no circumstances should any attempt be made to induce labor until after functional compensation has been reestablished and the cardiovascular status stabilized. The additional cardiac burden of labor and delivery may prove fatal.

The immediate postpartum period is particularly dangerous. Acute hemodynamic changes, including autotransfusion from the suddenly emptied, contracting uterus, splanchnic pooling or acute blood loss due to uterine atony or tissue laceration, may produce failure or shock following delivery. It is essential, therefore, that the patient be observed most carefully during this critical period of circulatory readjustment.

Labor has been shown to exert an intermittent burden on the heart, increasing oxygen consumption and accelerating pulse and respiratory rates, as well as augmenting venous return, venous pressure and cardiac output. Uterotonic agents, unless clearly indicated for obstetric reasons, should probably be avoided because, by stimulating the uterus to contract more forcefully, they may enhance the cardiac work load. Similarly, in the postpartum period, although it is important to ensure that the uterus contracts to prevent hemorrhage from open maternal sinuses at the placental site, overstimulation is best avoided.

Shock States

Shock in the obstetric patient is one of the leading causes of obstetric death and is undoubtedly the overriding factor in nearly all preventable maternal deaths. Always serious, its treatment requires the greatest measures of skill in diagnostic acumen and therapeutic judgment. Urgency is necessary in handling this disorder; yet it usually occurs under the worst possible conditions insofar as personnel and facilities are concerned. Thus, where possible, even though the obstetric factors may be paramount, these patients are often best handled in intensive care units specifically created for these purposes.

There are obviously many causes of shock, but in obstetrics we tend naturally to think first of hemorrhage and trauma. Nevertheless, among the many possible pathogenic mechanisms, six major categories exist and are pertinent to obstetric patients: (1) hypovolemia in association with hemorrhage primarily, and also with dehydration and protein loss; (2) neurogenic reaction in conjunction with vasomotor paralysis, spinal shock, ganglionic blockade, trauma, pain, uterine inversion, toxemia and other conditions; (3) circulatory block resulting from pulmonary embolism (catastrophically in association with amniotic fluid infusion, and also from thrombi or air) or the supine hypotensive syndrome; (4) bacteremia with endotoxin shock; (5) hypersensitivity phenomena with anaphylaxis in response to exogenous agents including blood or oxytocin preparations; (6) cardiac failure with myocardial infarction, or cardiac dysrhythmia.

Because of the variety of disorders that can produce shock pictures and because of their serious nature, it is essential that every precaution possible be taken to avoid situations potentially leading to shock. One should be prepared to handle the problem expeditiously when it does arise and take extra precautions with patients who are high-risk candidates for the development of shock. Pertinent prophylactic measures should include such accepted principles of good patient care as correction of malnutrition, anemia, fear, infection, debilitation and exhaustion, while avoiding trauma, ill-advised manipulation, excessive blood loss, prolonged anesthesia, electrolyte imbalance and dehydration.

Successful treatment of shock is based upon the following essential requirements: a comprehensive grasp of the physiopathologic derangements; careful clinical evaluation; accurate diagnosis; prompt initiation of treatment; determination of the course of treatment based on diagnosis and physiologic abnormalities prevailing; and appreciation of the dynamic nature of the condition that usually requires continuous observation, repeated reevaluation and timely modification of treatment wherever necessary.

One must appreciate that the basic underlying mechanisms of shock, all causes considered, include hypovolemia to some degree, decreased cardiac output, decreased capillary perfusion, vasoconstriction, hypoxia and acidosis. In most instances the hypovolemia is the stimulus resulting in decreased cardiac output and capillary perfusion, which in turn result in tissue hypoxia. As a consequence, tissue acidosis may occur on the basis of anaerobic oxidative mechanisms. Hypoxia and acidosis in turn stimulate an adrenergic response that results in vasoconstriction. This additionally decreases capillary perfusion by increasing peripheral vascular resistance, contributing still more to the hypoxia and acidosis. Unfortunately, vasoconstrictive compensatory mechanisms may maintain arterial blood pressure at relatively normal levels so that the clinical picture may be masked. One must be aware that blood pressure measurement is a very unreliable index of blood flow or cardiac output.

The prime requisite in handling the obstetric patient in shock is making an accurate diagnosis. Starting with essentials of knowledge and logic, the physician must integrate data obtained by careful and extensive history, where time permits, as well as appropriate, detailed physical examination and probing laboratory and x-ray investigations. Thus, one might establish the presence of shock, its cause and the existence of concomitant physiologic derangements which may result from, complicate or mask the prevailing picture. Ordinarily, however, one does not have the luxury of time to pursue exhaustive study, but it is often critical that measures along these lines be undertaken simultaneously with the institution of active treatment of the shock state.

The fundamental measures indicated include the following: (1) make an accurate diagnosis; (2) establish an airway, provide for pulmonary ventilation and oxygenation of blood and tissues; (3) staunch the hemorrhage; (4) replace blood loss, restoring blood volume and maintaining circulation, cardiac output, capillary perfusion and renal function; (5) watch for and correct coagulation defects; (6) treat concomitant injuries; (7) continue to evaluate at intervals, weighing the need for altered or additional therapy as demanded by the course of the disorder.

The basic approach to establishing an

airway and providing adequate pulmonary ventilation includes: proper positioning of the head, neck and tongue; clearing the oropharynx and bronchial tree of secretions or aspirate; endotracheal intubation by laryngoscopic technique under direct vision or tracheotomy, if necessary; and artificial ventilation with oxygen administration, perhaps even under intermittent positive pressure if suitable equipment is available.

Uterine hemorrhage may be controlled by manual compression of the uterus (see Chapter 66). This temporizing measure is effective in cases of uterine atony and even rupture. Search for and repair of lacerations is, of course, mandatory. Adjunctive aids should also be used, such as oxytocin and ergot preparations to maintain uterine contractility, where indicated. There seems no longer to be any good indication for the use of uterine or vaginal packing in these situations. Packing merely delays definitive treatment unnecessarily and may convert a difficult problem into an irreversible one. Discussion of the use of hypothermia and adrenolytic agents to reduce tissue metabolic requirements is beyond our purview here, and there is considerable doubt as to their efficacy in the acute clinical situations with which we must deal in obstetrics.

Exploratory laparotomy may be indicated where intraperitoneal or retroperitoneal bleeding is occurring. Ligation of the internal iliac arteries may be highly advantageous in critical situations resulting from otherwise uncontrollable pelvic hemorrhage. Although stabilization of the clinical picture is a sound fundamental principle in managing the patient with shock, it is imperative to remember that there are extenuating circumstances when surgical intervention is a necessary means for correcting a situation which cannot be stabilized in any other way. This aggressive approach should be entertained when it is clear that the need exists and conservative measures, such as rapid blood transfusions, are inadequate.

One of our first concerns after ensuring adequate pulmonary ventilation and while taking measures to control hemorrhage is the restoration of adequate blood volume, cardiac output and peripheral circulation. Whole blood transfusion of properly cross-matched donor bank blood may be administered rapidly intravenously to compensate for blood loss. Much has been written about the superiority of intraarterial transfusion, but this can apparently be reserved only for the most extreme situations. In the interim, until the blood has been properly prepared, type O, stored bank blood (preferably with the proper Rh factor, where this is known, or Rh negative, if unknown) may be used. In preparation for unexpected situations that are so common in obstetrics, type O, Rh negative blood should be kept available in the delivery unit at all times. Where this is impossible or impractical, plasma volume expanders, such as dextran, plasma or serum albumin, should always be on hand for emergency administration.

With regard to the amount of blood to be administered in patients with massive hemorrhage, it is imperative that rapid replacement be given, provided that the circulatory capacity is not overloaded. Here central venous pressure monitoring, by way of a catheter inserted into the jugular, subclavian or brachial vein, may be very useful. Equally important with large blood losses is the occurrence of compensatory shifts of fluid from the interstitial space to the intravascular space. This fluid requires replacement by solutions such as lactated Ringer's solution. Isotonic saline apparently is less effective and dextran is actually detrimental.

The use of vasopressor agents seems in general to be contraindicated in hypovolemic hypotension since they tend to complicate the physiopathologic changes, causing intensified vasoconstriction and elevated peripheral vascular resistance, further diminishing tissue perfusion and aggravating hypoxia and tissue acidosis. On both theoretical and practical grounds, some vasopressors, such as epinephrine, should not be used. Other sympathomimetic agents, including Aramine (metaraminol), effectively raise blood pressure and increase renal blood flow and glomerular filtration rates (see below).

Shock in the patient with septic abortion (see Chapter 34) is a very serious problem, especially when associated with enterobacillary septicemia and intravascular hemolysis. The pathogenesis of *endotoxin shock* is incompletely understood, but circulatory failure in conjunction with overwhelming bacterial infection, especially by Gram-negative organisms, is now well documented. Therapy in these cases consists of the administration of antibiotics, whole blood transfusion, oxygen, Aramine, corticosteroids, early evacuation of the uterus and laparotomy, if indicated. Attention to acid-base balance and fluid requirement is important, since acidosis enhances the shock picture and reduces response to therapy.

The choice of antibiotic will depend upon the organism, but it is imperative to begin therapy empirically before accurate identification can be made and sensitivities determined. It is important to treat this condition aggressively with large doses of bactericidal antibiotics. In *Clostridium welchii* septicemia, further complicated by jaundice, oliguria and hemoglobinuria, treatment may also include administration of antitoxin, although its value is rather dubious. If oliguria or anuria becomes a significant problem, dialysis by extracorporeal exchange using the artificial kidney may be required.

Aramine may be very effective in preventing irreparable damage that may result from prolonged hypotension. It acts to prevent pooling in the splanchnic bed, by peripheral vasoconstriction, and to increase cardiac output and venous return. It may be administered in doses of 200 mg. per liter, the rate of drip and dosage level being adjusted to the patient's response. The minimum amount necessary to maintain the arterial pressure at or somewhat below normal levels is given. Again, central venous pressure monitoring is a much more sensitive indicator of adequate response. Pressures should be maintained at levels sufficient to provide urinary flow of 30 to 50 ml. per hour. Dosage should be reduced as the general condition of the patient improves. Risks implicit in the use of vasopressors, including vasoconstriction leading to permanent organ or tissue damage, must be accepted in these very seriously ill patients.

Blood replacement is obviously essential here, too, in the presence of blood loss superimposed on hypovolemic shock. It should be emphasized that pressor amines may produce a false sense of security in the presence of shock due to blood loss. The use of corticosteroids in endotoxin shock has been very encouraging. They must be given early and in large doses, but should be reserved for the treatment of the shock state and not used prophylactically. Their modality of action is not yet completely defined. Responses when corticosteroids are given late in the course of the disease, after other measures have been shown to be inadequate, are relatively poor. Since the prognosis in these cases is very grave, it is recommended that all measures be used early. Preliminary investigations have indicated that the use of vasodilators may be very promising.

Timely surgical intervention is an unresolved problem in these cases. Superimposition of anesthesia and a surgical procedure on an already jeopardized patient with an unstable cardiovascular system may be fatal. However, it is sometimes critical to empty the uterus of its infected contents so that there will no longer remain a source for bacterial showers and the production of more endotoxin. Furthermore, in the presence of hemorrhage, bowel injury or other intraabdominal complication, surgical intervention may actually be lifesaving. Above all, in every instance of shock in obstetric patients, astuteness, aggressiveness, expediency and individualization must prevail.

Pulmonary Embolism

Acute catastrophic crises may arise in pregnant patients in association with pulmonary embolization. Aside from those originating from thrombosed veins in the pelvis or legs, both of which are common sites in conjunction with abortal or puerperal infection, air and amniotic fluid may be much more serious sources of embolization. Air embolism in pregnant women following self-administered douches, vaginal insufflation or abortion attempts or occurring in the course of sex play (air blown into the vagina) has been implicated as an infrequent cause of sudden death in pregnancy.

Amniotic fluid infusion syndrome

(variously called *obstetric shock* or *amniotic fluid embolism*) is characterized by sudden chest pain, acute dyspnea, cyanosis, pulmonary edema, shock and coassociated uncontrollable hemorrhage, leading quickly to death (see Chapter 42). Its pathogenesis appears to be the infusion of amniotic fluid containing thromboplastin-like material into the circulation, there causing widespread intravascular coagulation and defibrination of the blood. With exhaustion of circulating fibrinogen and simultaneous mobilization of the fibrinolytic mechanism, hemorrhagic diatheses result. Tumultuous labor, whether spontaneous or due to overstimulation with uterotonic agents in conjunction with rupture of the membranes, is predisposing. The site of entry of amniotic fluid into maternal circulation may be by way of an open venous sinus at the placental site or a laceration opening onto the endometrial surface.

Although almost uniformly fatal, it is probable that some patients survive, especially if the infusion of amniotic fluid has been minimal and treatment has been aggressive. Therapy includes administration of oxygen under intermittent positive pressure to combat pulmonary edema and to provide for ventilation, fibrinogen to replace acutely depleted reserves and digitalis for failing cardiac function.

The diagnosis in the surviving patient is suspect, however. The typical picture is catastrophic, with instantaneous collapse and death. Under these circumstances, supportive measures, regardless of the degree of aggressiveness, are usually ineffective. Despite this, treatment is occasionally (and surprisingly) beneficial. As much as 8 to 12 gm. of fibrinogen may be necessary in these patients, complete defibrinogenation having occurred. Use of heparin may be advantageous in preventing further defibrination from occurring by arresting the intravascular coagulation phenomenon. Papaverine may be useful against reflex vasospasm and atropine may combat cardiac depressor reflexes. It has also been suggested on the basis of animal experimentation, but unconfirmed in man, that isoproterenol may counter the pulmonary effects which are seen, including pulmonary hypertension, rapid fall in lung compliance and arterial hypoxemia.

Eclampsia

An uncommon but nevertheless significant differential diagnostic dilemma may face the physician in the general medical or intensive care milieu. This concerns itself with the acute disorder of eclampsia (see Chapter 36) occurring in the third trimester of gestation, characterized by variable prodromal symptoms, including cephalgia, disorientation, visual disturbances, somnolence, nausea, emesis, epigastric pain and hyperreflexia. It is usually associated with progressive anasarca and may rapidly develop full-blown focal and generalized convulsions leading to coma and death. Death in eclampsia is usually due to congestive heart failure, cerebral hemorrhage or a variety of hemorrhagic, hepatic, respiratory or renal complications. This idiopathic condition is best treated in its prodromal phase when signs of water retention, rising blood pressure and proteinuria become manifest. If unchecked, the disease is rapidly progressive and carries with it a high fetal and maternal mortality. The differential diagnosis requires an appropriate index of suspicion based on recognizing the existence of the pregnancy. Among the various disorders manifested by convulsions, eclampsia has the worst prognosis if not promptly treated.

The essential feature of therapy involves termination of the pregnancy. However, in the acute phase, the superimposition of induced labor or the major operative procedure of cesarean section to effect delivery may seriously jeopardize an already unstable, tenuously balanced situation. Therefore, it is most important to stabilize the process while simultaneously maintaining ventilation and cardiovascular support.

Eclampsia must ultimately be distinguished from such conditions as hypertensive encephalopathy, epilepsy, various encephalitides, cerebrovascular accidents, drug toxicities, trauma and uremia. Most often it is confused with chronic hypertensive cardiovascular disease with encephalopathy. Except for renal biopsy studies, attempts to make this differentiation by laboratory means have been largely unsuccessful. Nevertheless, the course of events will help to define the problem more clearly. Thus, the surviving patient with persistent hypertension is likely one with precedent hypertensive disease, whether idiopathic or due to underlying renal disease. On the other hand, the patient who survives uncomplicated eclampsia is usually completely devoid of residua.

Treatment of the preconvulsive state, marked by severe and progressive hypertension, edema, albuminuria and hyperreflexia, consists empirically of magnesium sulfate, heavy sedation, diuretics and perhaps antihypertensive agents. Magnesium sulfate is given in an initial dose of 20 ml. of 10 per cent solution slowly intravenously, watching the deep tendon reflexes; an equivalent dose of calcium gluconate should be available for intravenous use to combat potential magnesium overdosage, manifested by areflexia and respiratory depression. Additional magnesium is given in the same manner until reflexes are obtunded. Often no other form of therapy is needed. Sedation with barbiturates is probably preferable to sedation with opiates, since the latter (especially morphine) tend to depress glomerular function. Diuresis may be effected with either mercurials (Mercuhydrin) or carbonic anhydrase inhibitors (Diamox or Diuril). Use of anticonvulsants, such as Dilantin, has been suggested because they do not sedate the fetus, but they have limited usefulness during the acute phase because of the long intervals needed before the desired clinical effect can be achieved.

The question of the use of hypotensive agents in preeclampsia or eclampsia is essentially unresolved. These drugs tend not to affect the course of the disease except that, in association with severe hypertension, they are potentially useful in preventing cerebrovascular accidents. Good results have been obtained with Apresoline, Unitensen and protoveratrine in lowering blood pressure. It is important that the pressure not be diminished to a point where tissue perfusion is adversely affected. Observations of urinary output become important under these circumstances as a significant measure of tissue (renal) perfusion.

For the patient who is convulsing or in postictal coma, the problem is far more critical. Convulsions must be controlled while attempts are made simultaneously to ameliorate the underlying eclamptic process by the measures indicated earlier. Additionally, oxygenation should be maintained, a mouth gag inserted and, if needed, a tracheotomy performed. Large doses of a rapidly acting barbiturate (sodium pentobarbital) or tranquilizer (Valium) are valuable in controlling the acute convulsion, but should be used with caution since the depressive effects may augment the postictal coma. Thus, only that amount necessary to control the convulsion should be given. Neuromuscular blocking agents, such as succinylcholine, are much more effective in controlling convulsions, but of course require artificial ventilation because of the concomitant diaphragmatic paralysis.

It is also essential that hydration, urinary output, blood pressure and cardiopulmonary function be observed carefully. The decision to evacuate the uterus at some subsequent time after stabilization (6 to 12 hours) must be made in these patients. If the cervix is favorable, induction of labor by the use of intravenous oxytocin infusion should be attempted. If not, cesarean section is indicated. Active treatment must be maintained throughout labor and during the immediate postpartum period. Uterotonic agents, such as ergot preparations, should be avoided because of their vasopressor effects. Stringent nursing care is mandatory.

please note

Chapter 52

Rh Isoimmunization

The last thirty years have seen the evolution of the etiology, pathogenesis, therapy and prophylaxis of Rh isoimmunization. It is gratifying to know that the tragic consequences of fetomaternal blood group incompatibility are now almost completely preventable. Nevertheless, despite the availability of adequate means for prevention (see below), it is likely that we will continue to be confronted with sensitized women and affected babies for some time to come. This is so because we cannot be assured that every pregnant woman at risk will receive proper preventive treatment, because prevention is not necessarily completely effective in every instance and because there is no known practical means for desensitizing those women who are already affected.

Erythroblastosis fetalis is an especially treacherous hemolytic disease of fetuses and newborn infants. It affects less than one per cent of all pregnancies. It is characterized by excessively rapid destruction of red blood cells. This in turn produces profound anemia, toxic hyperbilirubinemia and severe generalized edema in the fetus. Red cell destruction is the result of hemolysis caused by specific antibodies entering the fetal circulation during pregnancy. These antibodies are produced by the mother in response to the antigenic stimulus of fetal red cells entering the maternal circulation by way of the placenta. These fetal erythrocytes are coated with antigenic factors not present in the mother, namely, the D factor or Rh_0. Fetal red cells containing this factor are capable of initiating or augmenting antibody production in the mother who does not possess this factor when these cells enter her circulation.

Fetomaternal incompatibility may involve any one of the many different genic blood characteristics. The most common and most important instances of erythroblastosis fetalis are those associated with the more potent antigens, the Rh and the ABO factors. The ABO system is involved in two-thirds of all cases of isoimmunization. This tends to result in a rather mild form of erythroblastosis fetalis, often occurring with the first pregnancy and clinically mild. It is as yet not detectable before birth. The Rh system, although less frequently the cause of isoimmunization, is the most significant cause of severe erythroblastosis fetalis and will be dealt with here exclusively.

The incidence of Rh incompatibility between mother and fetus, in which an Rh-negative mother is carrying an Rh-positive fetus, is about 10 per cent of all pregnancies. Sensitization, however, occurs in only about five per cent of the fetuses. The overall incidence of erythroblastosis is between 0.4 and 1.0 per cent of all births.

The discrepancy between the incidence of Rh incompatibility and the occurrence of Rh isoimmunization is apparent when one appreciates that only 1 in 20 of such pregnancies becomes sensitized. This has been explained on the basis of variations in immunization potential or the ability of the mother to respond to the antigenic stimulus by antibody production; it is also explained by differences in the intensity of antigenic stimulus in terms of the quantity of fetal red cells crossing the placenta into the maternal circulation. Additionally, first pregnancies are rarely affected and, as a rule, the degree of sensitization increases with subsequent pregnancies. In these instances, it appears that small antigenic stimuli may be cumulative and mitigate toward more intensive sensitization. The incidence of sensitization increases with parity, illustrating that isoimmunization is

543

a variable phenomenon and that the mere presence of fetomaternal Rh incompatibility does not necessarily mean that erythroblastosis will occur.

The D factor is found in 85 per cent of whites, 92 to 95 per cent of black Americans and nearly 99 per cent of Orientals. More than 90 per cent of cases of erythroblastosis are caused by this factor. In the small remaining number unassociated with D isoimmunization, other Rh factors may be responsible, including c (hr'), C (rh'), E (rh") and e (hr").

In perspective we see that the probability of any individual Rh-negative woman becoming sensitized during pregnancy is relatively small, at about five per cent or less. The risk mounts if she has received a prior transfusion of Rh-positive blood, if her husband is Rh positive and especially if he is homozygous for the Rh factor, if she has delivered Rh-positive infants previously and if fetomaternal ABO compatibility is also present. In general, there is a relatively good outlook for the unsensitized Rh-negative woman contemplating pregnancy. Her chances of marrying an Rh-positive male are 85:15 or 5.6:1. If she should, her chances of becoming sensitized during any subsequent pregnancy should be no greater than about 10 per cent overall. Furthermore, it is quite likely that neither the first nor the second child will be affected. Taking into account all children of such incompatible matings, one finds that only one in 20 to 30 infants exhibits hemolytic disease.

The optimistic outlook does not apply, unfortunately, once sensitization has occurred. Because of the rapid changes in clinical and laboratory approaches to evaluation and treatment of this disorder, it is difficult to determine precise morbidity and mortality frequencies. The disease process may take any one of a wide range of forms, all the way from mild jaundice in the neonatal period to severe hydrops fetalis with massive anasarca, cardiac failure and anemic anoxia. The combination of these latter proves almost invariably fatal. The approximate perinatal loss due to erythroblastosis is 25 to 30 per cent. The more severe the sensitization, the graver the prognosis.

Introduction of techniques of amniocentesis and spectrophotometric analysis of the amniotic fluid, in combination with realistic and meaningful programs for termination of pregnancy, when indicated, have effectively reduced the overall mortality of affected infants to 5 to 10 per cent. The more recent introduction of intrauterine transfusion has effectively halved the figure again (Freda).

DIAGNOSIS AND TREATMENT

Determining the existence of sensitization and assessing its intensity in a given pregnancy are based upon evidence accumulated from several areas (Table 8). The past obstetric history of the patient is quite important, particularly if the patient has delivered affected infants previously. Information on the Rh factors of children born earlier, the severity of their disease, the gestational age at time of intrauterine death, when this has occurred, and pertinent findings on autopsy can be very helpful. Since progression of the disease can be

TABLE 8 CLINICAL CRITERIA FOR EVALUATION OF Rh ISOIMMUNIZATION

I. Past History
1. Transfusion of incompatible blood.
2. Outcome of previous pregnancies.
   a. Rh factor of infants.
   b. Severity of hemolytic disease.
   c. Gestational age at intrauterine death.
   d. Autopsy confirmation of erythroblastosis.

II. Determination of Husband's Rh Genotype
1. Homozygous: All infants Rh positive.
2. Heterozygous: 50 per cent chance for Rh-negative infant.

III. Estimated Fetal Weight and Gestational Age
Timing of delivery may be critical (see Chapter 13).

IV. Maternal Anti-D Antibody Titers
Limited value in interpretation of levels and changes.
Variable and unpredictable reliability.

V. Spectrophotometric Analysis of Amniotic Fluid
Begin at 28–32 weeks; earlier according to history.
Repeat every 2–3 weeks, as needed.

expected with successive pregnancies, one can easily understand how important such detailed information is. Determination of the husband's Rh genotype is also important, as this may give information on heterozygosity. In much the same way, previous delivery of an Rh-negative infant will give important data provided, of course, the biologic father of both infants is the same.

Once a gravida is known to be Rh negative, certain elementary precautions should be taken to uncover developing sensitization. Figure 284 outlines a recommended program of evaluation and management for these patients. Initial anti-D antibody titers should be determined as soon as possible. This initial titer will serve as a base line for all future studies. Even if antibodies are not detectable at first, blood should be subsequently drawn at regular four-week intervals throughout the pregnancy. In the absence of any circulating antibodies, one may be reasonably confident that the infant will be unaffected. The importance of periodic examination for antibodies should not be underestimated.

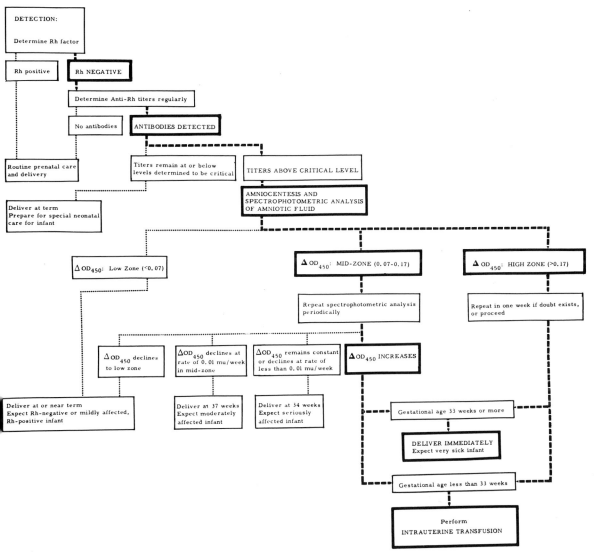

Figure 284 Systematic outline of programmatic plan for detection, evaluation and management of the gravida with potential Rh isoimmunization. (From Charles, A. G., and Friedman, E. A., eds.: Rh Isoimmunization and Erythroblastosis Fetalis. New York, Appleton-Century-Crofts, 1969.)

The limitations of maternal anti-D antibody titers, however, must be borne in mind. At one extreme, antibodies may appear anamnestically in the absence of sensitization or, at the other extreme, they may not rise significantly in some severe cases. Thus, although high or rising titers are strongly suggestive of the presence of Rh sensitization or of increasing sensitization, they cannot be entirely relied upon. Although anti-D antibody titer levels and increments of rise clearly reflect the overall prognosis (Allen et al.), it is not possible in the individual case to predict the severity of hemolytic disease of the infant. This is the chief drawback to the use of antibody titers as guides for prognostication and therapy. They serve only to inform us that the mother is sensitized. They are insufficiently accurate in predicting fetal outcome, thus precluding use for anything but for determining the presence or absence of isoimmunization. In two-thirds of cases in which fetal death will occur, the antibody titer may actually be fixed (Freda).

The history of a stillborn infant is very significant because, once it has occurred, the chances are less than 30 per cent that the patient will ever be able to deliver a living child. All available records should be checked to verify the cause of the previous stillbirth because, occasionally, death may have been unrelated to isoimmunization. Thus, critical review of prior autopsy findings is very important.

The pathologic diagnosis of erythroblastosis fetalis is important in terms of future care of the mother (see above). One may expect to find excessive extramedullary erythropoiesis and abnormal deposits of iron in the liver, spleen and kidneys. These changes are nonspecific, occurring in any condition which will cause excessive hemolysis *in utero*. Histological study is unfortunately difficult because of the autolysis which is usually present. In addition to severe anemia, one may find marked anasarca together with lymphatoid hypoplasia, whitening and necrosis of the fetal adrenal cortex and hyperplasia of the islets of Langerhans. It is of importance to note that infants who survive for several days may show no evidence of extramedullary hematopoiesis, but may have jaundice and kernicterus. Some adequately treated neonates, particularly after intrauterine transfusion, may have no residual evidence of erythroblastosis at all.

Examination of the placenta will show characteristic but not pathognomonic changes (Figs. 285 and 286). Grossly, the placenta is edematous and porky. Microscopically, there are hydropic villi with many erythroblasts in the fetal blood vessels.

History of the previous course of the isoimmunization phenomenon is important. It is generally agreed, as stated above, that there is a tendency for the clinical picture to become increasingly severe with each subsequent Rh-positive fetus delivered.

If the husband is blood type A and the wife type O, the possibility of an ABO incompatibility must be anticipated. The

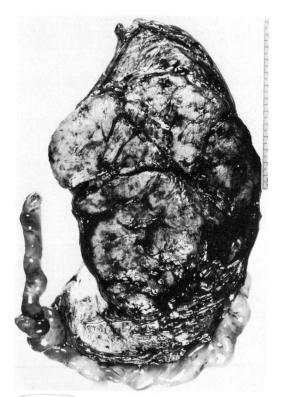

Figure 285 Gross view of maternal surface of the enlarged, edematous placenta in severe erythroblastosis fetalis. The cotyledons are broad, sharply demarcated and gray-white. The cord is thick and edematous. (From Charles, A. G., and Friedman, E. A., eds.: Rh Isoimmunization and Erythroblastosis Fetalis. New York, Appleton-Century-Crofts, 1969.)

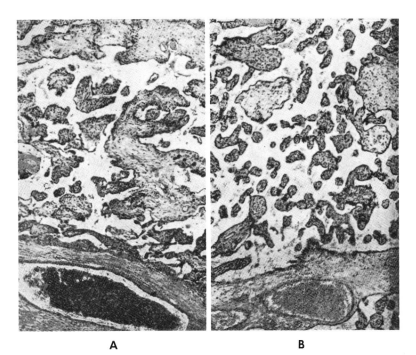

A   **B**

Figure 286 Histological appearance of the placenta in erythroblastosis fetalis, showing different severity. *A*, Changes include large, immature, edematous villi typical of hydrops, as well as the presence of large numbers of nucleated red blood cells in the fetal vessel. *B*, Villi more mature in a less severe case. Some edema is still present. The fetal vessel contains fewer nucleated erythrocytes. (Magnification × 60.) (From Javert, C. T.: Surg. Gynec. Obstet. 74:1, 1942.)

inhibiting effect of ABO incompatibility on Rh isoimmunization is well documented. However, Rh isoimmunization can and does occur even in the presence of ABO incompatibility.

The importance of correctly dating the duration of an Rh-sensitized pregnancy cannot be overestimated. Errors in either direction may be fatal to the infant, allowing death from progressive disease *in utero* if timely action is not taken or from prematurity if delivered too early. Unfortunately, timing of the duration of pregnancy tends to be rather uncritical. Available methods are detailed in Chapter 13.

Amniocentesis

When antibody titers in the mother indicate the presence of Rh isoimmunization, it is important to attempt to determine the precise extent to which the fetus is involved. This can be accomplished by studying the amniotic fluid for its content of bilirubin and other pigments of blood breakdown resulting from the hemolysis

inherent in the sensitization phenomenon (Bevis). Critical diagnostic accuracy is obtained by this means. The procedure is generally carried out in an outpatient surgical suite, but it may also be done in a clinic or an office if facilities are comparable.

The presence of blood pigments in the amniotic fluid is closely related to the severity of the hemolytic process (Liley). Amniotic fluid readily obtained by transabdominal amniocentesis can be analyzed for its blood pigment content by chemical determination or by means of a spectrophotometer. In the latter, the characteristic absorption curve is produced by plotting optical density against the wavelength of visible light spectrum. As the destruction of fetal red blood cells progresses, there is an increase in the concentration of the various breakdown products of hemoglobin in the amniotic fluid. These pigments absorb monochromatic light between wavelength range 400 to 500 mμ, and the cumulative peak is seen at 450 mμ.

The initial amniocentesis and analysis of amniotic fluid should be done in sensitized patients between the twenty-eighth and the thirty-second weeks of pregnancy (Alpern et al.). For those patients who have lost infants from hemolytic disease at an earlier gestational age, the initial examination should be done prior to that time indicated by their histories because it can be anticipated that sensitization will occur earlier and be more severe in later pregnancies. If the initial analysis demonstrates no peak in the critical range or only an insignificant one, additional analyses tend to be unnecessary. In other cases, amniotic fluid should be reexamined at intervals of two to three weeks. With moderate to very abnormal peaks, repeat examination must be done more often.

The basic technique of amniocentesis requires only skin antiseptic solution, sterile towels, syringe and needle for local anesthetic infiltration and syringe and 22-gauge, 4-inch spinal needle for purposes of puncturing through the abdominal wall to enter the uterine cavity. The patient first empties her bladder and then is positioned on her back with her head slightly elevated. The uterus is palpated and the unobstructed area anterior to the fetal shoulder is located. The selected site is then prepared with antiseptic solution. Infiltration with local anesthetic agent is optional and tends not to be needed. The puncture needle is deftly introduced into the amniotic cavity and fluid is aspirated.

Fluid specimens are placed in clean test tubes and protected from the light to avoid deterioration of pigments. The fluid is cen-trifuged for 20 minutes at 3000 rpm and filtered. Analysis is carried out in a continuously recording spectrophotometer (such as Model 11 Cary) and the height of the 450 mμ peak is measured directly from the recorded spectral absorption curve in optical density units (Fig. 287).

The technique of amniocentesis has a wide margin of safety, but does present specific risks to both mother and fetus (Alpern et al.; Liley). Although complications tend to be very infrequent, there have been reports of augmented maternal antibody titer, maternal, fetal and placental hemorrhage, premature labor, infection and fetal damage. Thus, the procedure should not be undertaken lightly. The theoretical effect on maternal antibody titer is brought about by the hazard of increasing sensitization due to fetomaternal transfusion during the procedure.

The height and progression of the spectral absorption curve at 450 mμ is critically important for diagnosing severity of disease and predicting fetal survival. Two or more sequential analyses are needed in order to determine a valid prognosis because the findings in a single test may be misleading.

The smooth, undeviating, upward curving spectrophotometric absorption curve (Fig. 288) indicates the absence of detectable bilirubin and signifies that (1) the fetus is Rh negative, (2) it is an unaffected Rh-positive fetus, or (3) it is only so mildly affected by the hemolytic process that no immediate intervention is necessary. Simi-

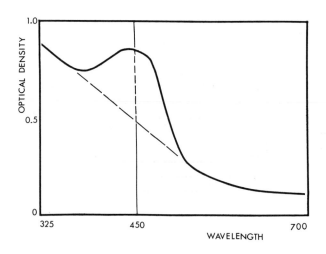

Figure 287 Spectral absorption curve obtained by continuously recording spectrophotometer, with optical density on vertical axis plotted against wavelength on abscissa. Pattern seen in amniotic fluid obtained in Rh-sensitized pregnancy is shown, measuring blood breakdown pigments at 450 mμ in optical density units above the interpolated base line.

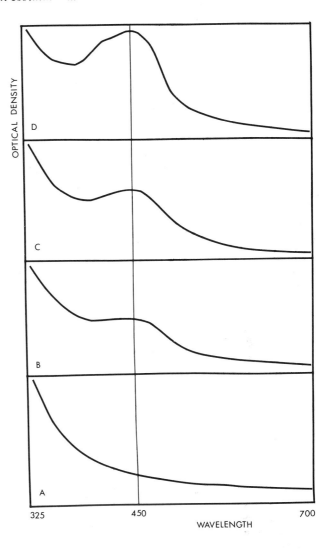

Figure 288 Representative spectrophotometric curves, showing progression of severity of erythroblastosis. *A*, Normal or negative curve with smooth progression over entire wavelength. *B*, Appearance of bile pigment peak of mild degree, 0.07 unit at 450 mμ, indicating mild disease requiring no immediate intervention. *C*, Moderate elevation in upper range of midzone, 0.17 unit peak, showing presence of active and potentially severe disease demanding close observation and preterm intervention. *D*, Marked elevation in high zone, 0.25 unit, requiring immediate delivery if beyond 34 weeks' gestational age or intrauterine transfusion if previable.

larly, 450 mμ peaks of less than 0.07 optical density unit appear to require only expectancy in our experience (Charles and Friedman). In the middle range, peaks between 0.07 and 0.17 unit indicate that an Rh isoimmunization phenomenon of moderate severity exists. Under these circumstances, if the level does not rise into the more severe range, early termination of pregnancy around the thirty-sixth week seems in order. Peaks greater than 0.17 unit forecast the severe nature of the condition and the urgent need for action. Here we face the dilemma of risking fetal death or damage from erythroblastosis fetalis if delay should occur or the equally real hazards of neonatal death from prematurity if pregnancy is interrupted too soon.

We thus have a delicate technique which enables us to make rather clear-cut diagnoses of the sensitization phenomenon, with regard to both its existence and its severity. These findings are based on the work of Liley who correlated the bilirubin peaks at various gestational ages with outcome. He was thus able to divide his material into three zones according to the height of the 450 mμ peak. Values in the low zone pointed to a good outcome, and delivery could be delayed to term or near term. The midzone values indicated a need for repeated analysis and early delivery. Fetuses with values falling into the upper zone before the thirty-second week required some form of intervention, such as intrauterine transfusion, in order to prevent a fatal outcome; after the thirty-second week, immediate delivery was required to prevent fetal death.

Thus, using this information, we can proceed to think in terms of early termination of pregnancy in those cases in which a significant compromise is necessary between urgent delivery and unavoidable prematurity. We still face the serious problem of the severely affected previable fetus who could not possibly survive outside the uterus. This problem results from a pregnancy in which fetal involvement has become so severe at such an early stage that extrauterine survival is unlikely because of marked immaturity. In this case, if the fetus is left in the uterus without special attention to gaining valuable time to mature, the outcome will invariably be intrauterine death or irreversible neurologic damage.

Intrauterine Transfusion

Amniocentesis is invaluable in determining those cases of isoimmunization in which the fetus will not survive to viability undamaged. In this situation, the technique of intrauterine transfusion may allow us to leave the fetus *in utero* for additional intervals. The procedure consists of administering blood to the fetus by injecting it into the fetal peritoneal cavity. This approach is effective in combating the consequences of the marked hemolysis that results from severe isoimmunization and produces progressive anemia and even high output congestive heart failure with fetal ascites and anasarca, typical of *hydrops fetalis.*

The high degree of accuracy afforded by amniocentesis and spectrophotometric analysis of amniotic fluid for bile pigment has been pointed out for the severe cases of Rh isoimmunization in which it is obvious that intrauterine death will occur at or before 32 weeks' gestation, well before extrauterine fetal survival could possibly be considered reasonable. It is for these hopelessly involved fetuses that the technique of intrauterine transfusion described by Liley offers some hope for correcting anemia *in utero.* Intrauterine transfusion depends upon the proclivity

for whole donor blood to be absorbed intact from the fetal peritoneum and the practical capability to localize and gain access to the fetal peritoneal sac by way of the mother's abdominal wall.

The technique consists of inserting a needle through the maternal abdominal wall, the uterine wall, the amniotic sac, the fetal abdominal wall and into the fetal peritoneal cavity. It is simplified by the use of special x-ray monitoring devices. Radiopaque material is injected into the amniotic cavity for purposes of amniography. An aqueous solution of radiopaque dye is used, such as 10 to 15 ml. of Renografin or Conray. About five hours are allowed to elapse between this injection and the intrauterine transfusion to permit adequate concentration in the fetal bowel. Because the fetus actively swallows amniotic fluid, it will demonstrate the fetal intestinal tract (Fig. 289). In this way the site of the intestinal contents is located and serves as the target for puncture. When the needle has been inserted into the area of the fetal intestines, additional radiopaque dye is injected and the characteristic pattern of demilunes is seen around the loops of fetal bowel (Fig. 290). Freshly drawn type O, Rh-negative, packed red blood cells, compatible by cross-matching with the mother's serum, are then transfused. The amount given is determined by the estimated fetal blood volume based on 15 per cent of the fetal weight. The usual amount is 80 to 150 ml.

The technique results in significant elevations of the fetal hemoglobin (Charles et al.; Queenan). The injected cells enter the fetal circulation probably by way of the subdiaphragmatic lymphatics. The procedure can be repeated every week or two, depending upon the changing fetal needs owing to continued destruction of fetal Rh-positive erythrocytes and the additional expansion of fetal circulation with further growth. Benefit is strictly limited to those fetuses whose disease has not progressed to the extreme form of hydrops fetalis. This state prevents adequate absorption of infused blood from the peritoneal cavity and one cannot expect such a fetus to survive.

It should be emphasized that this technique is not without danger to the fetus.

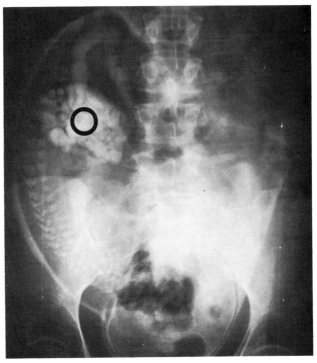

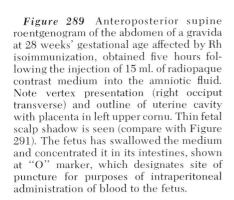

Figure 289 Anteroposterior supine roentgenogram of the abdomen of a gravida at 28 weeks' gestational age affected by Rh isoimmunization, obtained five hours following the injection of 15 ml. of radiopaque contrast medium into the amniotic fluid. Note vertex presentation (right occiput transverse) and outline of uterine cavity with placenta in left upper cornu. Thin fetal scalp shadow is seen (compare with Figure 291). The fetus has swallowed the medium and concentrated it in its intestines, shown at "O" marker, which designates site of puncture for purposes of intraperitoneal administration of blood to the fetus.

Perforation of various organs, including gastrointestinal tract, bladder and liver, has occurred. In consideration of the hopelessness of the situation for these fetuses,

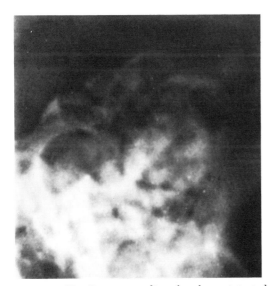

Figure 290 Contrast medium has been injected into the fetal peritoneal cavity to demonstrate that the transabdominal needle has been properly placed for transfusion. The characteristic demilune pattern appears as the dye coats the serosal surfaces of the fetal bowel.

whether delivered prematurely or allowed to remain *in utero* without therapy, these hazards are readily accepted in selected instances.

Once fetal transfusion has been performed, further amniocenteses for purposes of spectrophotometric analysis are useless. Contamination of the amniotic fluid by transfused blood makes interpretation impossible. Transfusions are repeated periodically until a total of about 350 ml. is given or until the thirty-second week is reached. When completed, delivery is accomplished by the most expeditious route approximately three weeks after the last transfusion.

Hydropic fetuses are easily recognized by means of amniography (Fig. 291). The presence of subcutaneous edema and a protuberant, distended abdomen, and absence of swallowing by the fetus facilitate the diagnosis. Heroic efforts to salvage these infants do not seem warranted, particularly if detected prior to 34 weeks' gestational age. Intrauterine transfusion is unrewarding. Vaginal delivery of these infants may be complicated by unexpected soft tissue dystocia due to a markedly distended fetal abdomen. Paracentesis may be needed.

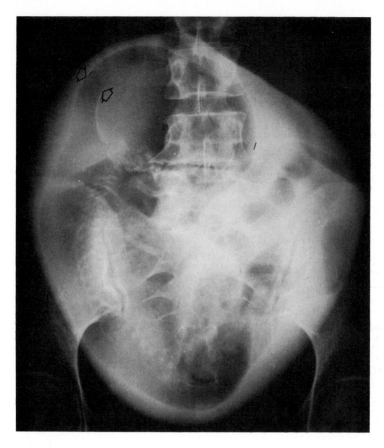

Figure 291 Amniogram showing characteristic findings of hydrops fetalis, with large radiolucent halo around fetal skull due to marked scalp edema (arrows). The absence of intestinal concentration of the contrast medium is evidence that the fetus is unable to swallow, suggesting it is seriously ill. (From Charles, A. G., and Friedman, E. A., eds.: Rh Isoimmunization and Erythroblastosis Fetalis. New York, Appleton-Century-Crofts, 1969.)

Exchange Transfusion

The infant born with erythroblastosis fetalis is generally pale, edematous and hypotonic. Severe edema has a serious prognosis as a sign of hydrops fetalis, accompanied by ascites, pleural effusion and pulmonary edema (Fig. 292). Edematous infants are generally in respiratory distress and suffering from congestive heart failure as well. Hepatosplenomegaly characteristically parallels the severity of the disease. Jaundice is usually absent at birth, but may develop rapidly in the first few hours of life. The rapidity of its appearance reflects the severity of the hemolytic process. Rapidly developing jaundice with anemia is one of the important criteria for exchange transfusion (Allen and Diamond).

It is essential to determine the newborn infant's cord blood hemoglobin, hematocrit, Coombs test, reticulocyte count and serum bilirubin. The Coombs antiglobulin test is very reliable for the detection of Rh antibodies. Hemoglobin and hematocrit will provide meaningful guides to the infant's condition. Abundance of reticulocytes and nucleated red cells is evidence of active erythropoiesis. Similarly, serum bilirubin will reflect both the severity of the hemolytic process and the degree of impairment of the liver in its ability to conjugate bilirubin. Serial bilirubin determination should be done every four to six hours.

No absolute level can be set at which exchange transfusion is required. Although 20 mg. per 100 ml. is frequently used to indicate a serious risk of kernicterus, today the rate of rise is used more often than the absolute level itself. The toxic effects of unconjugated or free bilirubin on nerve cells are well documented, particularly when they affect the globus pallidus and other cerebellar and subthalamic nuclei, although other regions of the brain and spinal cord may be affected as

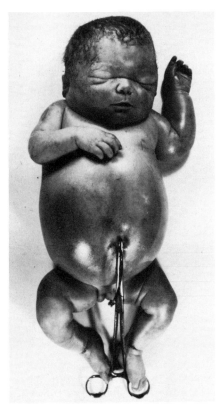

Figure 292 Stillborn infant with typical manifestations of hydrops fetalis, including anasarca and ascites.

well. However, the correlation between serum bilirubin levels and incidence of kernicterus is not clear-cut (Hsia et al.).

Kernicterus is manifested in the newborn infant by such nonspecific signs as diminished muscular activity and poor feeding. Opisthotonus may occur, with characteristic rigid extension of the arms associated with clenched fists and pronated forearms. Survival is infrequent, but survivors may be afflicted with an athetoid variety of cerebral palsy affecting motor function primarily.

The need for exchange transfusion is generally decided on an individual basis. If the infant is found to have a positive Coombs test with cord hemoglobin of 14 gm. per 100 ml. or less and cord unconjugated bilirubin level of 4.5 mg. per 100 ml. or more, exchange transfusion is clearly indicated. Moreover, serial bilirubin determinations indicating a rise of more than 0.5 mg. per 100 ml. per hour

during the first 48 hours of life or projected to exceed 20 mg. per 100 ml. warrant such treatment.

The techniques of exchange transfusion are beyond our scope, but it is important that this delicate procedure be carried out under optimal circumstances by individuals fully skilled in managing its complications. The proper preparation of the infant, careful selection and screening of blood to be used, employment of adequate equipment for the transfusion and monitoring of the infant's vital functions will minimize morbidity and mortality from the procedure. To this end it is strongly recommended that all mothers affected by Rh isoimmunization be referred to centers equipped for their evaluation and management and the care of their offspring.

The technique for exchange transfusion requires sterile, aseptic, surgical preparation (Allen and Diamond). Continuous monitoring of the heart rate, respiratory rate and body temperature is essential. Equipment for nasopharyngeal suction and resuscitation must be at hand. Blood previously cross-matched with maternal blood (or group O, Rh negative) is given. Thermal control for heat regulation is important, together with available oxygen and facilities for correction of acidosis and hypocalcemia. Digitalis may be needed for cardiac failure.

Blood is given in 10 to 20 ml. increments, withdrawing and discarding equivalent amounts after each injection. At least 500 ml. of blood should be used for each exchange transfusion so as to ensure removal of 90 per cent of the infant's red cells and Rh antibodies. The rate of exchange is limited by the infant's ability to withstand the changes in blood volume. If given or withdrawn too quickly, the infant will become restless and develop tachycardia.

Hemoglobin, hematocrit and bilirubin should be determined before and after the exchange transfusion. If anemia coexists, somewhat more blood should be given than withdrawn. Additional exchange transfusions may be given as needed, utilizing the same criteria (see above). The baby should be followed carefully over the next six to eight weeks in order to detect development of late anemia due to suppression of the infant's own bone marrow and the gradual destruction of the transfused erythrocytes.

Phototherapy has been used to advantage in reducing the effects of neonatal jaundice, although its efficacy is far better in combating the so-called physiologic jaundice of the newborn than that due to hemolytic disease. Exposing the infant to light reduces the level of circulating bilirubin (and the incidence of its neurologic sequelae) apparently by means of accelerating the breakdown or conjugation of bilirubin to products that are more readily excreted via the kidneys and liver. Recommended exposure is 200 to 400 footcandles of fluorescent daylight-type light (Behrman and Hsia). The question of retinal damage is as yet unanswered and, although it seems unlikely to occur, the baby's eyes should be shielded against the light. The overall need for exchange transfusion has been markedly reduced with the institution of this therapeutic regimen for the infant who is at risk and is demonstrated to have moderate or rising serum bilirubin levels.

PREVENTION

Much progress has been made in the prevention of Rh isoimmunization. Successful prevention of antibody formation is now a reality with the wide availability of anti-D antibody (commercially available as RhoGAM). Attention directed at protecting the placental barrier to avert the possibility of fetal cells entering the maternal circulation has been generally unsuccessful. Similarly, desensitization by neutralizing or inactivating circulating antibodies already present in maternal circulation has thus far been ineffective.

The basic tenet for preventing antibody formation is the administration of passive antibody as a means of suppressing the active immunization processes. The antigen stimulus in the mother for production of anti-D antibody is nearly always the fetal erythrocytes that have entered the maternal circulation by way of the placenta. It is conceivable that immediate injection of anti-D, either as plasma or as gamma glob-

ulin, blocks the antigen sites through a specific feedback inhibition mechanism to prevent antibody formation at an extracellular or intracellular site. Alternatively, perhaps the primary mechanism is the rapid clearance of the offending fetal cells from the maternal circulation before antibody production has had a chance to be initiated.

Initial isoimmunization of an Rh-negative mother by the D factor of fetal origin has been shown to be preventable almost without exception by passive administration of high titer Rh antibody in the form of either plasma or gamma globulin concentrate (Clarke; Finn et al.; Freda et al.). It is not known how long after a transplacental hemorrhage the administration of anti-D immunoglobulin can be delayed and still be effective in preventing immunization.

It is generally recommended that high titer anti-D gamma globulin be administered only in the postpartum period and only in the first 72 hours after the birth of an Rh-positive infant. This is a highly effective program; only rare failures have been reported. It has been shown that most Rh-negative women can be protected against immunization by the intramuscular injection of 1 ml. of high potency gamma globulin or the equivalent of about 150 μg. of anti-D. This dosage appears to be effective against all but the most severe transplacental hemorrhages.

All unsensitized Rh-negative patients with Rh-positive husbands must be protected. Passive antibody must be given after the first pregnancy and repeated with all subsequent pregnancies. The objective is to prevent sensitization from occurring. This includes abortions as well because they might serve to provoke isoimmunization by means of the passage of small numbers of Rh-positive fetal cells into the mother's bloodstream. Commercially prepared high titer anti-D gamma globulin, such as RhoGAM, is useful in this regard. Before administering this material, one should determine that the patient has delivered within 72 hours, is Rh-negative, is not already sensitized to the Rh factor, and her infant is Rh positive (or she has just had an abortion with unknown Rh factor) and has a negative Coombs test. Crossmatching is required to ensure compatibility of the anti-D preparation and the patient's own red cells. If all these factors are verified, the immunoglobulin is given intramuscularly to the postpartum mother. It must never be injected intravenously nor given to the infant. Each subsequent pregnancy should be followed carefully and managed in the same manner.

REFERENCES

Allen, F. H., Jr., and Diamond, L. K.: Erythroblastosis Fetalis, Including Exchange Transfusion Technique. Boston, Little, Brown & Company, 1957.

Allen, F. H., Jr., Diamond, L. K., and Vaughan, V. C., III: Erythroblastosis fetalis: II. Prognosis in relation to history, maternal titer and length of fetal gestation. Pediatrics 6:441, 1950.

Alpern, W. M., Charles, A. G., and Friedman, E. A.: Amniocentesis in the management of Rh-sensitized pregnancies: Technique, accuracy of results, and complications. Amer. J. Obstet. Gynec. 95:1123, 1966.

Behrman, R. E., and Hsia, D. Y. Y., eds.: Summary of a symposium on phototherapy for hyperbilirubinemia. J. Pediat. 75:718, 1969.

Bevis, D. C. A.: Composition of liquor amnii in haemolytic diseases of the newborn. Lancet 2:443, 1956.

Charles, A. G., and Friedman, E. A., eds.: Rh Isoimmunization and Erythroblastosis Fetalis. New York, Appleton-Century-Crofts, 1969.

Charles, A. G., Alpern, W. M., and Friedman, E. A.: Intrauterine transfusion. Obstet. Gynec. 28:182, 1966.

Clarke, C. A.: Prevention of Rh haemolytic disease: A method based on the post-delivery injection of the mother with anti-D antibody. Vox Sang. 11:641, 1966.

Clarke, C. A.: Prophylaxis of rhesus iso-immunization. Brit. Med. Bull. 24:3, 1968.

Finn, R., Clarke, C. A., Donohoe, W. T. A., McConnell, R. B., Sheppard, P. M., Lehane, D., and Kulke, W.: Experimental studies on the prevention of Rh haemolytic disease. Brit. Med. J. 1:1486, 1961.

Freda, V. J.: The Rh problem in obstetrics and a new concept of its management using amniocentesis and spectrophotometric scanning of amniotic fluid. Amer. J. Obstet. Gynec. 92:341, 1965.

Freda, V. J., Gorman, J. G., Pollack, W., Robertson, J. G., Jennings, E. R., and Sullivan, J. F.: Prevention of Rh isoimmunization: Progress report of the clinical trial in mothers. J.A.M.A. 199:390, 1967.

Hsia, D. Y., Allen, F. H., Jr., Gellis, S. S., and Diamond, L. K.: Erythroblastosis fetalis: VII. Studies of serum bilirubin in relation to kernicterus. New Eng. J. Med. 247:668, 1952.

Liley, A. W.: The technique and complications of amniocentesis. New Zeal. Med. J. 59:581, 1960.

Liley, A. W.: Liquor amnii analysis in the management of the pregnancy complicated by rhesus sensitization. Amer. J. Obstet. Gynec. 82:1359, 1961.

Liley, A. W.: Intrauterine transfusion of foetus in haemolytic disease. Brit. Med. J. 2:1107, 1963.

Queenan, J. T.: Intrauterine transfusion: A cooperative study. Amer. J. Obstet. Gynec. 104:397, 1969.

Chapter 53

Trophoblastic Disease

Proliferative changes may occur in the course of the development of the gestational trophoblast ranging from the mildest forms of hydropic degeneration of the benign hydatidiform mole to the overtly neoplastic alterations of choriocarcinoma. They produce tumors of fetal origin. They are usually found in the absence of a recognizable embryo, but may occur concomitantly or subsequently. Recent progress in chemotherapy has made the malignant varieties of these tumors amenable to treatment. Heretofore, they were considered particularly lethal, although very rare. The more common benign forms are of considerable abiding interest as potential forerunners or harbingers of malig-

nancy. The several variants are difficult to distinguish clinically because histological differentiation is not predictive of biological activity.

HYDATIDIFORM MOLE

Hydatidiform mole results from the deterioration of the villous circulation in a pathologic ovum. It is characterized histologically by proliferation of both the syncytiotrophoblastic and cytotrophoblastic layers covering the chorionic villi and edematous dissolution and cystic cavitation of the avascular stroma of the villi (Fig. 293). The villi are converted into

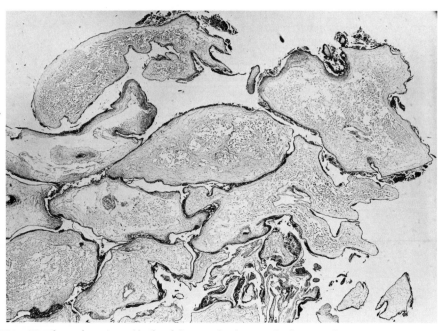

Figure 293 Histological pattern of hydatidiform mole showing hydropic, edematous swelling of the villous stroma, diminished number of blood vessels and proliferation of trophoblastic epithelium. (Magnification × 10.5.)

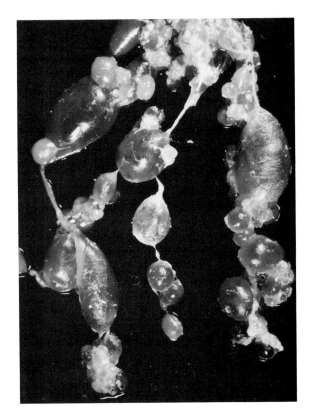

Figure 294 Gross appearance of the grape-like structures characteristic of hydatidiform mole. The isolated vesicles are submerged in water to demonstrate the hydropic distention of the interconnected villi.

molar cysts resembling grapes connected to one another by tenuous tissue (Fig. 294). The diameter of the hydropic villi is usually 0.5 to 1 cm., but may vary from 1 mm. to 3 cm.

Most blighted ova (see Chapter 33), if examined carefully, will show some hydropic degeneration of villi (Hertig and Edmonds). About one in ten or less of grossly diagnosed hydatidiform moles will be complicated by chorionic malignancy. However, choriocarcinomas are preceded or accompanied by hydatidiform mole in at least half of the cases.

Proliferative changes in a mole help to distinguish it from the so-called false or transitional mole (Alter and Cosgrove). Swollen, edematous villi are found in association with a blighted ovum, usually somewhat preserved, but the surrounding trophoblastic elements are flat and show no evidence of active proliferation. True moles often show considerable trophoblastic activity, but there may be very little cellular pleomorphism. There is variability in the histological appearance of

moles, even those seen in different parts of the same specimen.

Correlation is poor between the histological appearance and the malignant potential, although the more pronounced the anaplasia and exuberant the trophoblastic growth, the more likely that the lesion is malignant (Hertig and Sheldon). However, a benign appearance does not provide assurance that malignancy will not develop.

Hydatidiform mole secretes comparatively large amounts of chorionic gonadotropin which appears in the blood serum, urine and even in the spinal fluid. Urinary levels may be as high as 2 million international units, but may fall well within the range of levels expected for a normal pregnancy up to about 100 days after fertilization. At this time pregnancy levels become relatively low. Gonadotropin production by a mole may be quite variable, however (Hobson).

In many women with hydatidiform mole, one or both ovaries are enlarged by multiple theca lutein cysts (Fig. 295). The ovarian masses may become huge, but will

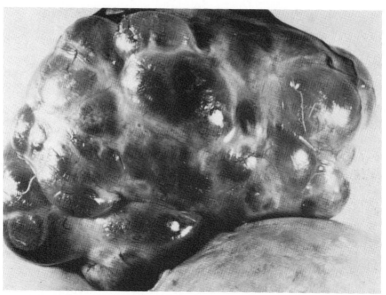

Figure 295   Multiple lutein cysts of ovary associated with hydatidiform mole. (Life size.) (Courtesy of A. J. Bret.)

regress spontaneously after the mole is evacuated. They do not require any form of surgical therapy unless they have undergone torsion. The cysts appear to result from chorionic gonadotropin stimulation of the lutein elements. They are particularly likely to be seen in benign moles of long duration. They occur in about one-quarter of women with hydatidiform mole (Hobson).

The incidence of hydatidiform mole appears to be geographically related. In the United States, about one in 2000 pregnancies is affected (Hertig and Sheldon), whereas in the Far East the disease is much more frequent: in Japan, 1:232 (Hasegawa); in Taiwan, 1:125 (Wei and Ouyang); in Hong Kong, 1:530 (King); and in the Philippines, 1:145 (Acosta-Sison and Baja-Panlilio).

There seems to be a greater tendency for moles to occur in older gravidas. Whereas the incidence in young Philippine gravidas under age 30 is 0.4 per cent, it increases sixfold to 2.4 per cent in those aged 40 to 49 years and 12.5 per cent in those still older (Acosta-Sison and Baja-Panlilio).

Clinical Course

Hydatidiform moles in most instances have a tendency to grow rapidly and en-large the uterus more quickly than a normal pregnancy. Thus, the uterine size is typically larger than expected for the gestational age. In some, however, the uterus is not unduly enlarged and may even be smaller than expected; this occurs in about one-third of cases.

As part of the mole becomes separated from its attachment, uterine bleeding occurs. This usually takes place at the third or fourth month of gestation, but may not occur until as late as the sixth month. The bleeding may be slight or profuse. Anemia may develop and the patient will become pallid and weak from blood loss. The patient may have severe morning nausea. Hypertension and other signs of pre-eclampsia may be seen. Whenever a hypertensive state of pregnancy arises before the twentieth week, a diagnosis of mole should be entertained. The patient may also have fever and tachycardia from secondary infection.

Some hydropic grapelike vesicles may be passed vaginally. A part of the mole may be expelled spontaneously after several episodes of bleeding, but its complete expulsion is seldom spontaneous. Continued or recurrent bleeding indicates incomplete evacuation. Severe hemorrhage may occur at the time of or immediately after the expulsion of the mole. Shock may result.

Diagnosis

The diagnosis of hydatidiform mole is most often made by hindsight after the tissue has been partially or completely evacuated from the uterus. A high degree of suspicion is needed to make the diagnosis prospectively, and accuracy is often lacking. A uterus enlarging at a rate in excess of that expected for normal pregnancy is suspicious, but may indicate multiple pregnancy instead. Chorionic gonadotropin levels may be supportive, but are usually not diagnostic unless they are very high or the pregnancy has advanced beyond 100 days (and the dates are accurate). Early preeclampsia is very suggestive.

Absence of fetal heart sounds, especially with use of ultrasound (Doppler) auscultation, is also helpful, but not truly diagnostic. X-ray search for a fetal skeleton is not useful prior to 20 weeks' gestation; moreover, a normal fetus may coexist with a mole. Ultrasonographic B-scanning (see Chapter 13) will yield the characteristic speckled pattern of a mole. Care must be taken to view the uterine contents both longitudinally and horizontally so as to ensure that one is not misled by the ultrasonic pattern of a transected normal placenta. Injection of a small amount of radiopaque dye into the uterus will give a typical amniographic honeycombed pattern as the dye coats the vesicles of the mole. Pelvic aortography has also been shown to be of some value (Borell et al.) for diagnosis.

Acosta-Sison recommended gently sounding the uterine cavity via the cervix; if a normal pregnancy is present the membranes will offer resistance to the sound, whereas a mole will not and the sound can be introduced to 10 cm. or more in the midline. She indicated that this very simple approach will establish the diagnosis readily in a uterus that is more than four months' gestational size, but it is not accurate earlier because the decidua capsularis in a normal pregnancy may not yet be firmly attached to the decidua vera and allow the sound to pass. Moreover, the sound may be introduced if the fetus is macerated and the membranes offer no resistance, as in missed abortion. The procedure is not without complications, especially bleeding, but this is usually not severe.

Treatment

Once diagnosed, hydatidiform mole must be evacuated from the uterus. Usually, spontaneous mechanisms are in progress when the diagnosis is made and the uterus is in the process of emptying itself. Management of molar abortion is the same as for incomplete abortion (see Chapter 33). Uterotonic stimulation with oxytocin infusion is given and instrumental evacuation accomplished under appropriate anesthesia and aseptic conditions using suction curage or ovum forceps. The uterus is particularly delicate and great care must be taken to prevent perforation. Hemorrhage may occur and whole blood should be made available in anticipation of its need for transfusion. For the uterus larger than 12 to 14 weeks' size, it is preferable to evacuate by way of a hysterotomy incision. In this way hemostasis can be secured, one can be assured that the mole is evacuated completely and specimens of myometrium can be obtained for the purpose of determining invasiveness.

Total hysterectomy leaving the mole *in situ* has been recommended as treatment for women aged 40 years or more, especially if they already have living children, because the potential for malignancy is so high in this group. It is also said to be useful in other situations in which the malignancy rate is found to be high, such as those with a history of previous mole, high parity or pulmonary tuberculosis. This approach is probably acceptable because it may prevent some malignancies, although hysterectomy is no guarantee against choriocarcinoma, and closely supervised follow-up is essential nevertheless. Since chemotherapy is equally effective with or without hysterectomy, one must question the wisdom of adding the risks of operative morbidity.

Use of chemotherapy has been advocated for prophylaxis (Acosta-Sison; Goldstein), especially where the incidence of malignant disease is high and follow-up is poor. There is no doubt about its effectiveness. However, since treatment is not innocuous, this cannot be recommended for general use. Severe and even fatal drug toxicity can develop. Closely following these patients to detect rising gonadotropin titers is a much more acceptable and rational program for choosing patients for chemotherapy. No treatment is given to the majority of patients whose titers fall quickly and do not rise again; the few who show evidence of persistently functioning trophoblastic tissue are treated aggressively (see below).

Search should be carried out for the presence of local or distant metastases, including examination of vulva, vagina, lungs and central nervous system. Negative findings serve as useful base line information for later comparisons; positive findings demand more aggressive study by biopsy, if feasible, and treatment.

Prognosis

The outlook for patients with hydatidiform mole will depend on the complications that may arise and how expeditiously they are handled. These include acute hemorrhage, secondary infection, preeclampsia, uterine perforation (by the mole itself or by the instrumentation used to evacuate it), pulmonary trophoblastic embolism and malignant progression. The risk of malignancy is variously considered to be about 8 to 10 per cent, but has been reported over a wide range up to 16 per cent, and is especially seen in older gravidas.

Since it is now possible to detect these neoplasms early on the basis of their biological hormonal activity by means of serial determinations of chorionic gonadotropin, particularly with the recent development of a sensitive radioimmunoassay (Taymor), every patient with a mole should be considered at risk and carefully monitored. The bioassay should become negative within two to four weeks after evacuation; the radioimmunoassay will fall to levels of luteinizing hormone (with which it cross-reacts) by four to six weeks. Careful periodic follow-up subsequently at weekly or biweekly intervals should quickly demonstrate any rising gonadotro-

pin activity of persistent or recurrent disease. After the level has been in normal range for three weeks, determinations are repeated monthly for at least six months; during this time it is essential that the patient avoid conception because the new pregnancy will interdict any possibility of following the gonadotropin levels meaningfully. About 90 per cent spontaneous cures should be expected in untreated cases of hydatidiform mole; with the addition of careful postevacuation surveillance and chemotherapy as indicated, the outlook is even brighter.

CHORIOADENOMA DESTRUENS

Chorioadenoma destruens, also called *malignant mole, invasive mole* or *destructive mole,* is a rare trophoblastic neoplasm showing both villous and trophoblastic elements. Masses of pleomorphic, hyperplastic syncytium and cytotrophoblastic cells locally invade deeply into myometrium and perforate blood vessels. Grossly, one finds hemorrhagic nodules in uterine muscle (Fig. 296). The finding of molar vesicles microscopically distinguishes this lesion from overt choriocarcinoma. It tends to remain localized, but infrequently it may metastasize widely, especially to the lung. Acute pulmonary hypertension may be seen as a consequence of embolic metastatic showers (Evans and Hendrickse). Invasion may extend to the vagina and parametrium (Fig. 297). Intraabdominal hemorrhage may occur due to penetration and perforation by the tumor (Fig. 298).

Invasive mole appears to arise invariably from or be closely associated with hydatidiform mole (Hertig); choriocarcinoma, on the other hand, may arise in conjunction with a normal pregnancy. About one in 6 to 10 patients with hydatidiform mole can be expected to have chorioadenoma destruens.

The clinical picture before evacuation may be indistinguishable from hydatidiform mole. Occasionally, the patient may present with manifestations of intraperitoneal bleeding. One may find hemor-

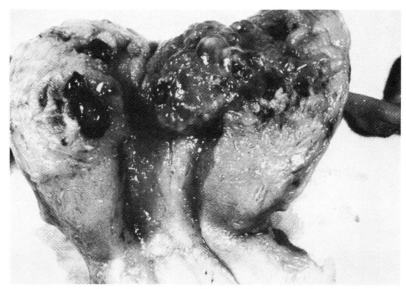

Figure 296 Uterus opened along the anterior midline to show chorioadenoma destruens occupying the uterine fundus with typical hemorrhagic nodules in the myometrium. (Courtesy of A. J. Bret.)

rhagic vaginal nodules. Diagnosis is established histologically at the time of evacuation by biopsy of the myometrial bed or a vaginal nodule.

Management is the same as for chorio-

carcinoma (see below). Good results are seen with aggressive chemotherapy. Hysterectomy is also advocated, especially if perforation has occurred or is anticipated, so as to prevent or correct sepsis and hem-

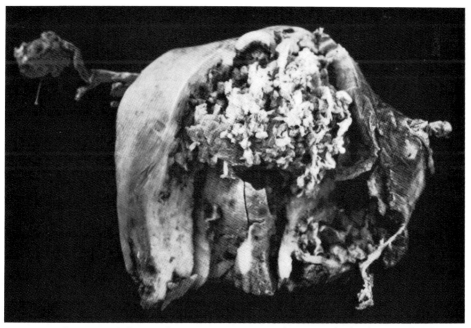

Figure 297 Fixed specimen of opened uterus containing a malignant mole that has invaded deeply into the myometrium and both parametria, seen especially well on the left (right side of the photograph).

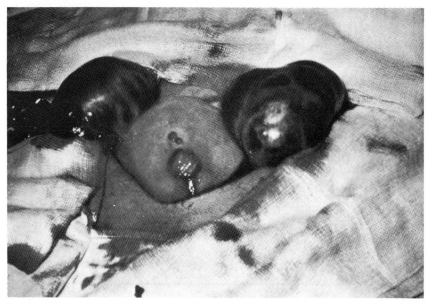

Figure 298 Photograph obtained at time of surgery with abdomen open, showing uterus and adnexa *in situ* with enlarged uterus containing a chorioadenoma destruens which is perforating the anterior wall in three sites. Note the ovaries enlarged bilaterally by multiple lutein cysts. (Courtesy of J. W. Lumsden and F. H. Tow.)

orrhage. However, hysterectomy is not an essential element in the chemotherapeutic regimen even if the disease is extensive, and the intact uterus may be preserved if future childbearing is an important consideration. There is no particular justification for removing the adnexal organs when doing a hysterectomy for this condition, although it is often advocated.

In prognostic terms chorioadenoma destruens occupies an intermediary position between benign mole and choriocarcinoma. In the uncomplicated case, cure can be expected with early, effective treatment. Although prognosis is generally favorable, it is not a benign lesion because death may result not only from perforation with its complications but also from distant metastases.

CHORIOCARCINOMA

One of the most malignant neoplasms affecting women is choriocarcinoma or chorionepithelioma. It is fortunately rare, varying in reported occurrence rate from 1:13,850 (Schumann and Voegelin) to 1:1382 (Acosta-Sison) pregnancies. Recent advances in its management by chemotherapy have been very gratifying. Choriocarcinoma arises most often from a hydatidiform mole, but may also follow an abortion, a normal pregnancy and even an ectopic pregnancy. It may make its appearance in the course of the pregnancy, more often relatively soon after it is terminated, or rarely years later.

It is characteristically made up only of trophoblastic elements with masses of both cellular and syncytial components (Fig. 299). No formed villi are found. The cell morphology of the tumor is similar to that of the early normal placenta in its anaplastic characteristics. It invades deeply into myometrium and into blood vessels. Mitotic activity, together with pleomorphism, is common in the cytotrophoblast, but these "malignant" findings are also seen in the trophoblast of the normally developing conceptus. Hemorrhage, necrosis and inflammatory reaction are usually present in the lesion and peripherally.

Grossly, the uterine mass is nodular in appearance; it is soft, friable and granular; it bleeds easily and is usually quite hemorrhagic (Fig. 300). The myometrium is occupied by the demarcated lesion which

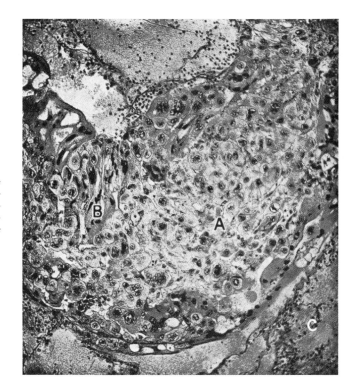

Figure 299 Histological appearance of choriocarcinoma demonstrating cytotrophoblastic cell mass (A), deeper staining syncytiotrophoblast (B) and characteristic surrounding blood and necrotic debris (C). (Magnification × 125.)

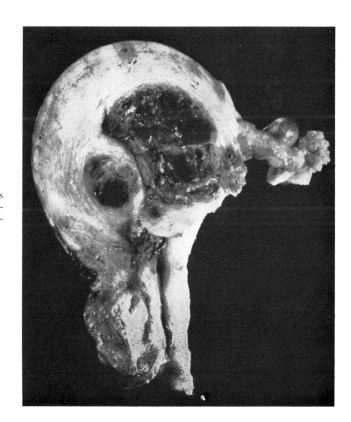

Figure 300 Gross appearance of uterus transected frontally to show large hemorrhagic and necrotic masses of a choriocarcinoma (Courtesy of M. E. Davis.)

may extend to either the luminal or the serosal surfaces or both. Growth is rapid and blood vessels are invaded early. Secondary infection may complicate lesions contiguous with the endometrial cavity; perforation and intraperitoneal hemorrhage may result from serosal penetration.

Clinical Course

Choriocarcinoma most often presents with vaginal bleeding. There may be no uterine bleeding when the growth is deep in the myometrium far from the endometrium or when it grows outward toward the serosa. The uterus is usually larger than normal and softened. Metastases are blood-borne and usually occur early in the course of this disease. The manifestations vary according to the organ involved. The most frequent site of metastases is the lung, occurring in at least two-thirds of cases. Cough with blood-tinged sputum or a sensation of chest oppression may be the earliest symptom. Hemoptysis is common. Early pulmonary metastases may not be revealed by x-ray.

Vaginal metastases are present in about half the patients with choriocarcinoma; they may be detected by palpation or by the typical appearance of a pink or purple mass under the vaginal mucosa. These growths may break through the mucosa and bleed. Cerebral metastases are less common, occurring probably via the azygos vein system. They may give rise to various neurologic signs. Brain metastases are usually fatal. Less common metastases may also be found in liver, kidney, ovaries, vulva and gastrointestinal tract. As in other locations, hemorrhagic sequelae are encountered in these sites also.

Diagnosis

Precise diagnosis requires histological verification, but that is not always available. The patient who has had a hydatidiform mole evacuated and is being followed may be discovered to have rising chorionic gonadotropin titers; she presents *prima facie* evidence of the existence of choriocarcinoma even though tissue confirmation is not provided. Similarly, the patient with hemoptysis and metastatic lung lesion on x-ray is considered to have choriocarcinoma even if the uterine curettings are negative. At the opposite extreme, the finding of typical anaplastic trophoblastic elements on curettage, unless massive, does not ensure the diagnosis because one may be dealing with a normal conceptus implanting deep in the myometrium. The negative curettage may have missed the tumor bed or the tumor may be inaccessible to sampling because of its location deep within myometrium.

Persistence of gonadotropin excretion after abortion or delivery, especially in high or rising amounts, is very suspicious of malignancy. A new pregnancy must be ruled out with certainty. It should be noted that some highly anaplastic or necrotic choriocarcinomas may produce very little gonadotropin and yield a negative or weakly positive test. Thus, it is often the clinical picture coupled with the strong suspicion of the physician which leads to the correct diagnosis.

Treatment

An encouraging milestone in oncological management was reached with the discovery of effective chemotherapy for choriocarcinoma (Hertz). A highly lethal tumor was found to be amenable to control by medical means in a significant number of instances. Originally, the cytotoxic agent, methotrexate, an antifolic acid derivative, was used. It is given in 10 to 30 mg. intramuscular doses daily for five days. This regimen is found to yield therapeutic response in about half the cases with metastatic disease, as evidenced by objective regression in tumor size by x-ray, visual or palpatory observations and suppression of gonadotropin excretion. Significant toxicity is encountered with hepatic, renal and bone marrow manifestations. Thrombocytopenia and leukopenia are common, along with stomatitis, nausea, vomiting, diarrhea and alopecia. Sepsis and death have been reported also. Careful surveillance is essential during treatment.

Remissions, when they occur, may be permanent. The course can be repeated at four- to six-week intervals as dictated by the persistent or rising level of chorionic gonadotropin. Experience with other forms of antimetabolites has shown some good results, especially with use of actinomycin D alone (10 μg. per kilogram per day for five days by intravenous infusion) or, in resistant cases, with combinations of methotrexate, chlorambucil and actinomycin D (Li). Actinomycin D appears to have less tendency to produce toxic side effects.

Close supervision for evaluation of response following treatment is essential. Chorionic gonadotropin excretion must be determined periodically as described after evacuation of hydatidiform mole (see above). The titer should continue to fall progressively to luteinizing hormone levels; if it does not, additional chemotherapy will be needed. Brewer et al. consider the treatment to have failed if there is no response to two courses of treatment and they recommend that another agent then be tried.

The current role of surgery in management of metastatic choriocarcinoma is in doubt (Brewer et al.; Lewis et al.). One can acknowledge its usefulness primarily for control of uterine bleeding due to tumor growth in the small number of cases in which this is a serious consideration. It does not augment the efficacy of chemotherapy in any way. Hysterectomy offers no special advantage, therefore, and is not recommended for the treatment of metastatic choriocarcinoma. Whereas hysterectomy was the primary form of treatment before chemotherapy, it is rarely considered justifiable today. Its use is limited to patients with intractable bleeding and to those few whose metastases regress with cytotoxic agents but whose gonadotropin levels remain elevated because of persistent uterine tumor. By preserving the uterus, subsequent reproductive function may be retained. Normal pregnancies have followed successful chemotherapy (Spellacy et al.), but the potential genetic effects are still undetermined.

Prognosis

Choriocarcinoma is highly malignant. Before effective chemotherapy was available, it was almost uniformly fatal unless the hysterectomy was done at a very early stage before metastases occurred. Even with the advent of chemotherapy about half the patients cannot be cured. Some cancers are or become resistant to one or more of the oncolytic agents; some will respond only to combination of drugs, and some patients are unable to tolerate adequate cancericidal dosages because of toxicity effects. Choriocarcinoma with brain or liver metastasis is especially difficult to treat; remissions are rare even when the tumor is responsive to the agent or to supplemental local radiotherapy. One can expect remission rates of more than 90 per cent in nonmetastatic disease and about 60 to 65 per cent with metastatic lesions (Brewer et al.).

Delays in diagnosis adversely affect cure rates. If treatment is begun within four months of onset of disease, Hertz reported 72 per cent cure; if delayed longer, only 26 per cent could be cured. Ross et al. confirmed this and also showed that the effectiveness of treatment was closely associated with the titer of chorionic gonadotropin, a reflection of the extent of disease. With the titers over 1 million mouse uterine units in 24 hours, there were 41 per cent remissions; with lower levels, 91 per cent. Early referral of patients to centers equipped for intensive observation, evaluation and therapy is important.

REFERENCES

Acosta-Sison, H.: Will the uterine sound go up the cervico-uterine canal unobstructed in all cases of hydatidiform mole? Philip. J. Surg. *16*:185, 1961.

Acosta-Sison, H.: Choriocarcinoma in the Philippines. Philip. J. Surg. *19*:27, 1964.

Acosta-Sison, H.: Changing attitudes in the management of hydatidiform mole. Amer. J. Obstet. Gynec. 88:634, 1964.

Acosta-Sison, H., and Baja-Panlilio, H.: Statistical study of 177 cases of hydatidiform mole in the Philippine General Hospital from April 6, 1946 to

December 31, 1950. J. Philip. M.A. 27:652, 1951.

Alter, N. M., and Cosgrove, S. A.: Hydatidiform mole: Practical considerations. Obstet. Gynec. 5:755, 1955.

Borell, U., Fernström, I., Moberger, G., and Ohlson, L.: The Diagnosis of Hydatidiform Mole, Malignant Hydatidiform Mole and Choriocarcinoma with Special Reference to the Diagnostic Value of Pelvic Arteriography. Springfield, Ill., Charles C Thomas, 1966.

Brewer, J. I., Torok, E. E., Webster, A., and Dolkart, R. E.: Hydatidiform mole. Amer. J. Obstet. Gynec. 101:557, 1968.

Brewer, J. I., Eckman, T. R., Dolkart, R. E., Torok, E. E., and Webster, A.: Gestational trophoblastic disease: A comparative study of therapy in patients with invasive mole and with choriocarcinoma. Amer. J. Obstet. Gynec. 109:335, 1971.

Brewer, J. I., Gerbie, A. B., Dolkart, R. E., Skom, J. H., Nagle, R. G., and Torok, E. E.: Chemotherapy in trophoblastic diseases. Amer. J. Obstet. Gynec. 90:566, 1964.

Evans, K. T., and Hendrickse, P. d. V.: Pulmonary changes in malignant trophoblastic disease. Brit. J. Radiol. 38:161, 1965.

Goldstein, D. P.: Prophylactic chemotherapy for patients with molar pregnancy. Obstet. Gynec. 38:817, 1971.

Hasegawa, T.: Statistical investigations on hydatidiform mole and choriocarcinoma in Japan. Tokyo, Japan, Proceedings of the First Asiatic Congress of Obstetrics and Gynecology, 1957.

Hertig, A. T.: The evolution of a research program. Amer. J. Obstet. Gynec. 76:252, 1958.

Hertig, A. T., and Edmonds, H. W.: Genesis of hydatidiform mole. Arch. Path. 30:260, 1940.

Hertig, A. T., and Sheldon, W. H.: Hydatidiform mole: A pathologico-clinical correlation of 200 cases. Amer. J. Obstet. Gynec. 53:1, 1947.

Hertz, R.: Chemotherapy of choriocarcinoma and related trophoblastic tumors in women. *In* Greenhill, J. P., ed.: The Year Book of Obstetrics and Gynecology. Chicago, Year Book Medical Publishers, 1961.

Hobson, B. M.: Further observations on the excretion of chorionic gonadotropin by women with hydatidiform mole. J. Obstet. Gynaec. Brit. Emp. 65:253, 1958.

King, G.: Hydatidiform mole and chorion-epithelioma: The problem of the borderline case. Proc. Roy. Soc. Med. 49:381, 1956.

Lewis, J., Jr., Ketcham, A. S., and Hertz, R.: Surgical intervention during chemotherapy of gestational trophoblastic neoplasms. Cancer 19:1517, 1966.

Li, M. C.: Management of choriocarcinoma and related tumors of uterus and testis. Med. Clin. N. Amer. 45:661, 1961.

Ross, G. T., Stolbach, L. L., and Hertz, R.: Actinomycin D in the treatment of methotrexate-resistant trophoblastic disease in women. Cancer Res. 22:1015, 1962.

Schumann, E. A., and Voegelin, A. W.: Chorioepithelioma with especial reference to its relative frequency. Amer. J. Obstet. Gynec. 33:473, 1937.

Spellacy, W. N., Meeker, H. C., and McKelvey, J. L.: Three successful pregnancies in a patient treated for choriocarcinoma with methotrexate: Report of a case and review of the literature. Obstet. Gynec. 25:607, 1965.

Taymor, M. L.: Bioassay and immunoassay of human chorionic gonadotropin (HCG). Clin. Obstet. Gynec. 10:303, 1967.

Wei, P.-Y., and Ouyang, P.-C.: Trophoblastic diseases in Taiwan. Amer. J. Obstet. Gynec. 85:844, 1963.

Chapter 54

Abnormalities of Placenta, Cord and Amnion

Variations in shape and size of the placenta have been described in Chapter 3. They are common and usually insignificant. Exceptions are *placenta succenturiata* and *placenta membranacea*, which are important because an accessory lobe may be left *in situ* at delivery and give rise to subsequent bleeding and possibly infection.

PLACENTAL DYSFUNCTION

The term *placental dysfunction* refers simply to a condition in which the placenta is incompetent anatomically and physiologically to nourish and oxygenate the fetus and to maintain its growth and development at a normal rate. It is clear that this can occur at any time during pregnancy in association with a variety of conditions. The fetus that is the product of a pregnancy complicated by placental dysfunction may not survive, but if it does survive, it has the characteristic manifestations of *fetal dysmaturity*, variously called a syndrome of *intrauterine inanition* or *growth retardation*, and the fetus is considered *small for dates* or *small for gestational age*.

Characteristic features described by Clifford include loss of vernix caseosa, leaving the baby with macerated, cracked, wrinkled, parchment-like skin and scanty subcutaneous tissue due to nutritional deficiency. Oxygen deprivation causes meconium to be passed, and golden staining of skin, cord and membranes results. At least half of these fetuses will die *in utero* or during the neonatal period.

It is too often diagnosed retrospectively when the sick baby is born or after it dies *in utero*. Improved salvage requires detection during pregnancy before the fetus is adversely affected. Objective means for uncovering this problem by investigating fetal well-being are detailed in Chapter 13, including serial urinary estriol determinations, ultrasonography and oxytocin stress testing. Designating certain patients to be in an especially high risk category in this respect is most helpful to ensure instituting surveillance measures early enough to benefit the fetus. Such patients should include those with diabetes mellitus, hypertensive states of pregnancy, cardiac and renal disease, syphilis, Rh isoimmunization, placenta previa, abruptio placentae and various debilitating diseases, as well as those with unexplained stillbirth in a previous pregnancy. Another group encompasses those whose pregnancies extend two or more weeks beyond term, the so-called postmature, prolonged, postterm or postdate gestation.

The relationship between *postmaturity* and placental dysfunction is highly controversial and not at all well established. Most fetuses carried beyond term do quite well. A few fare poorly; they fail to grow and will develop the stigmata of fetal dysmaturity described above. Typically, they have long nails and hair. They often develop severe respiratory distress as well as late neurologic sequelae.

In some areas, notably Great Britain, postmaturity is considered to be a great threat to the fetus and elective induction of labor is frequently undertaken or, failing this, cesarean section. The rationale for this approach is the work of Walker, unfortunately not satisfactorily verified, which purported to show rapidly diminishing fetal oxygen supply beyond the fortieth week, reaching critical levels at the forty-third week. At this time, the fetus is said to have no further reserve and cannot withstand labor contractions which have the effect of periodically cutting off fetoplacental exchange by obstructing uterine blood flow.

There does not seem to be ample justification for the practice of induction of labor or cesarean section for postmaturity unless one can demonstrate objectively that placental insufficiency actually exists and the fetus is truly at risk. In the absence of such documented need, one must weigh the risks of induction under conditions that may not be optimal (see Chapter 24) or the hazards of anesthesia and surgery inherent in cesarean section against the dubious benefits of these measures. Furthermore, once the fetal well-being has been shown to be in jeopardy, labor may carry considerable risk of hypoxic damage; under these circumstances, cesarean section is a more logical approach to management than induction. Thus, we recommend that the postterm patient be allowed to initiate labor spontaneously; in the interim, the fetus should be carefully monitored periodically to detect the earliest manifestations of placental dysfunction and the patient should be given appropriate reassurances. Nearly all will show no signs of failing placental function and will deliver uneventfully in due course. Monitoring during labor is also important; potentially traumatic procedures must be avoided. Clear evidence of fetal hypoxia in the form of characteristic heart rate patterns (see Chapter 13) warrants cesarean section unless the fetus is promptly deliverable *per vaginam* by atraumatic means.

PLACENTAL INFARCTS

Nearly every placenta can be found to contain whitish, nodular, hard areas on the fetal or the maternal surface or both. They vary in size from 2 mm. to several centimeters. These structures are called *infarcts* (Fig. 301). Several varieties are found. In order of frequency, they include (1) flat subchorial infarcts which form the

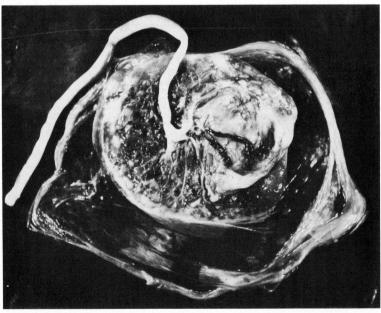

Figure 301 Fetal surface of a placenta with its attached membranes, showing a large white infarct on the right side involving 25 per cent of the placental substance.

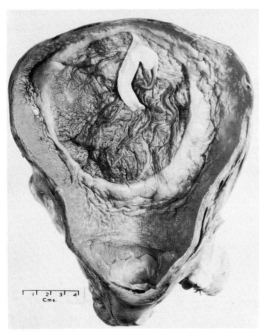

Figure 302 A puerperal uterus with placenta attached *in situ* on the posterior wall, illustrating characteristics of both placenta circumvallata (at the right lower aspect of the chorionic plate with raised fold) and placenta marginata (at left upper margin without a fold).

placenta marginata or *circumvallata;* (2) nodular infarcts on the fetal surface; and (3) extensive full-thickness infarcts of the cotyledon.

At the edge of the placenta, at the site of the subchorial decidua, a more or less complete white ring may be present. This ring varies in width from 2 to 16 mm. and in thickness from 1 to 4 mm. It is called *placenta marginata.* Sometimes the ring is raised from the surface and the attached membranes are doubled back over its edge, a condition called *placenta circumvallata* (Fig. 302). Both are variants of *placenta extrachorialis.* It is not clear how they arise.

In placenta marginata adhesion of the membranes may occur and the placenta may be delivered naked or decrowned of its membranes. The membranes may be retained. As the result of this retention, hemorrhage sometimes ensues. An abnormal mechanism in the third stage, with retention or adhesion of the placenta, requires manual exploration of the uterus more often than with normal placentas.

There is also an increased risk of abruptio placentae. It is possible that placental separation may be the result of the abnormal relationship of the placenta to the underlying degenerated decidua at its margins.

The incidence of occurrence of placenta circumvallata is reported to be as high as 18 per cent (Scott). It is associated with a high frequency of maternal and fetal complications, including abortion, hemorrhage, infection and third stage complications. Although premature labor may occur in this disorder, it is not found in increased numbers (Shanklin).

A diagnosis of circumvallate placenta cannot be made until the placenta is delivered and inspected. The common symptoms which suggest circumvallate placenta are intermittent vaginal bleeding and hydrorrhea. It is most often confused with placenta previa and abruptio placentae (see Chapters 37 and 38).

On the fetal surface of the placenta nodular infarcts are often seen, ranging in size from scarcely visible ones to 3 to 5 cm. in width and up to 1 cm. in thickness. The smaller ones predominate; they may be bunched or a thin, nodular layer of fibrin may cover a considerable portion of the fetal surface. Generally, these are of no great significance unless extensive.

Some infarcts involve the whole thickness of one or more cotyledons. Extensive infarct formation may compromise fetal oxygenation or nutrition. There may be fetal inanition of long duration, resulting in the birth of an infant that is small for dates, weak and in poor condition. If a substantial area is infarcted, the fetus will die. Such placentas are likely to be prematurely detached with manifestations of abruption.

Infarcts may be caused by obliterative periarteritis or endarteritis in villous vessels. This process obstructs the lumina and produces multiple infarcts on the fetal surface characterized by necrosis of the stroma and the walls of the villi with subsequent clotting of the blood in the adjoining intervillous spaces. Alternatively, endometritis may occur with decidual overgrowth and consequent necrosis of the villi and fibrin deposition yielding infarcts on the maternal side. Primary alteration or desquamation of the chorionic epithelium

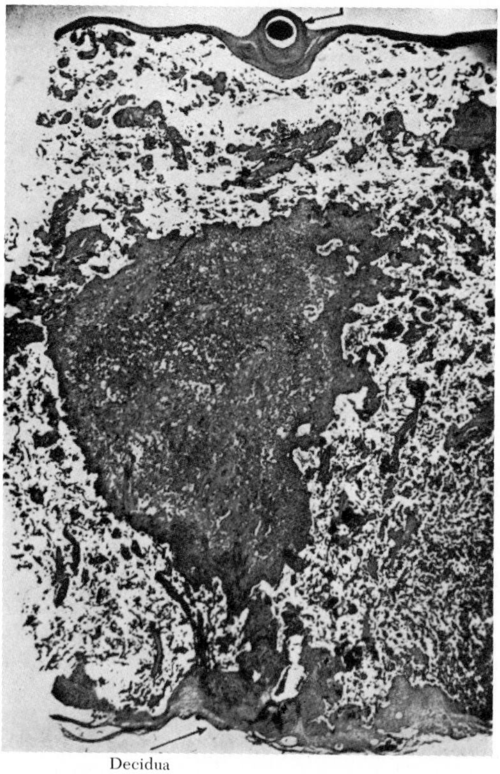

Figure 303 Low power photomicrograph of transected placenta showing an early placental infarct undergoing fibrinous degeneration and necrosis.

also causes deposition of fibrin and microscopic infarcts of necrotic ectodermal cells. These are almost a constant finding in term placentas.

Microscopically, circumscribed areas of placental tissue which have undergone necrosis are found (Fig. 303). In the advanced stages, the whole mass is changed into fibrin with only traces of the previously existing villi.

PLACENTAL EDEMA

An edematous placenta has villi that are club-shaped and irregularly swollen. It can be distinguished by its consistency from the fatlike syphilitic placenta. Fluid can be squeezed from the edematous placenta which is pale, thick, soft, shaggy and mushy, and often has a torn basalis. Edema of the placenta is caused by maternal and fetal heart disease, nephritis, diabetes, generalized anasarca and erythroblastosis. These conditions are all discussed in relevant chapters. Abortion or stillbirth generally results.

PLACENTAL CALCIFICATION

Frequently the basalis surface of the placenta is filled with white, sandy deposits. These may be discrete or, rarely, fused together into small plates of hard, brittle masses. They are composed of calcium carbonate, calcium phosphate and magnesium phosphate. They lie in the upper layers of the decidua basalis, especially around the anchoring villi. They result from the deposition of the calcium salts in areas which had previously undergone fibrinous degeneration and, therefore, are associated with white infarcts. They occur as a manifestation of the normal aging process of the placenta (Tindall and Scott). They have no clinical significance, but may aid in locating the placenta by x-ray study.

PLACENTAL CYSTS

Cysts are occasionally found on the fetal surface of mature placentas, underneath the amnion and just under the chorial membrane (Fig. 304). They vary in size from microscopic to about 6 cm. in diameter. Often a white infarct is found underneath the cyst. The lining may resemble decidua, but it is actually degenerated Langhans' cells. Occasionally, a cyst may contain a blighted twin.

PLACENTAL TUMORS

Various tumors are found in the placenta, including myxoma fibrosum, hemangioma (Fig. 305), hyperplasia of the chorionic villi and especially

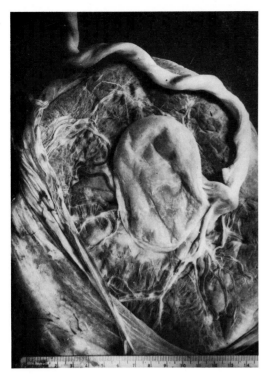

Figure 304 Large chorionic cyst of placenta on the fetal surface located under the chorion.

chorioangioma. DeCosta et al. indicate that hemangiomas of the placenta have clinical importance. About one-third of placental tumors are found in association

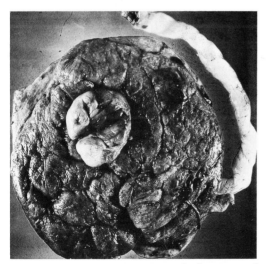

Figure 305 Maternal surface of placenta with chorioangioma evident. (Courtesy of E. J. DeCosta et al.)

with hydramnios and prematurity. The newborn infant may exhibit heart failure and be found to have an angioma as well. Perinatal loss is high and the incidence of antepartum and postpartum hemorrhage is also increased.

KNOTS IN THE CORD

Since the umbilical vein is longer than the arteries and the vessels are longer than the cord itself, twisting of the vessels occurs so that the vein is twisted around the arteries. This vein is especially prone to form loops with the arteries. The jelly of Wharton is thicker at such places, and nodes or *false knots* appear on the cord.

True knots in the cord are rare and occur as the result of the fetus passing through a loop. Such knots have no clinical importance unless they form early in pregnancy and active fetal movements draw the loop so tight that death results.

TORSION OF THE CORD

Torsion of the cord is often present with aborted fetuses, but usually it cannot be ascertained whether or not the torsion caused the fetus to die. Occasionally, the cord is almost twisted off at the umbilicus or at some point along its length; stenosis of the vessels follows with fetal death. It may be impossible to determine whether the death of a fetus resulted from stricture of the cord, whether torsion of the cord was produced by active agonal movements of the fetus before death or whether twisting occurred after fetal death.

COILING OF THE CORD

Coiling of the cord around parts of the fetus affects the fetus only when the cord is abnormally short or the coils are so tight that the umbilical circulation is compromised. Monoamniotic twins often have their cords intertwined.

Coiling of the cord around the baby's neck, sometimes called *nuchal cord,* is present in one-fifth of all deliveries. This may make the cord functionally short. It is probable that, in its active movements, the fetus twists so that the cord comes to lie entwined around its limbs, body or neck in a random manner. The condition probably exists for weeks before delivery. Coils of cord around the neck may interfere with the mechanism of labor, especially when the cord is so short that descent is impeded (see below).

The coiling of the cord around the neck, particularly with a loop alongside the head, has caused fetal death. Compression of the cord during labor or delivery may asphyxiate the fetus. This may be detected by noting the characteristic acute slowing of the fetal heart rate best detectable by electronic monitoring (see Chapter 13).

During labor, the funic souffle of the nuchal cord can sometimes be heard plainly at the fetal neck. Digital pressure will slow the fetal heart. During forceps operations, the fingers should be passed all around the head as far up as possible and a finger also passed behind the symphysis pubis up the nape of the fetal neck to the back so as to be able to detect a low-lying cord.

It is advisable to feel for the cord around the neck immediately after delivery of the fetal head and before attempting to deliver the shoulders. This is especially important when further descent seems to be obstructed. In such instances it may be necessary to doubly clamp and cut the cord before it is possible to deliver the body. In this way one can avoid excessive traction on the placenta.

SHORT CORD

Clinically, cords can be either absolutely or relatively short; the latter are those that have coiled around the fetal neck or extremities one or more times so that they become too short for the proper mechanism of labor. A cord must be long enough to reach from the placental site to the vulva. For the placenta located in the uterine fundus, a length of 32 cm. is necessary.

A cord that is too short sometimes leads to (1) delay in second stage descent, (2) characteristic cord pattern of fetal heart rate, (3) rupture of the cord with fetal hemorrhage and asphyxia, (4) tearing of the cord from the placenta, (5) tearing of the placenta from the uterus, causing abruptio placentae or a pathologic third stage, or (6) inversion of the uterus.

A short cord cannot always be diagnosed before delivery. The condition is rare. If diagnosed, the fetal status should be observed carefully, preferably by the sensitive techniques described in Chapter 13, and delivery effected at the first sign of hypoxia. As soon as the head is delivered, the cord is cut between two clamps.

RUPTURE OF THE CORD

Rupture of the cord is a serious accident because it will cause hemorrhage and hypoxic damage to the fetus. Intrauterine death may occur. The accident usually takes place in the course of the delivery, however, so that it is often possible to institute appropriate measures at once to save the infant.

NEOPLASMS OF THE CORD

Neoplasms in the cord are exceedingly rare. Myxoma, sarcoma and dermoid have been found. Rupture of a varix of the cord with hematoma formation, especially near the abdomen of the child, is occasionally observed. An immense increase of Wharton's jelly may change the cord to a heavy, thick, glassy rope. Cysts comprising remnants of the omphalomesenteric duct or of the allantois may rarely be found also.

ABNORMAL CORD INSERTION

Ordinarily, the cord is inserted at or near the center of the placenta. Eccentric inser-

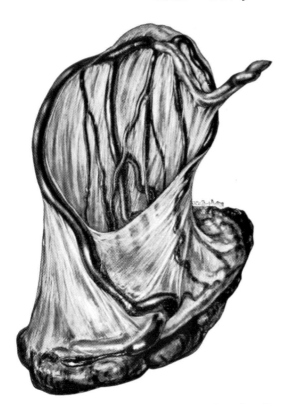

Figure 306 Velamentous insertion of cord with large umbilical vein on the left alongside the rent in the membranes through which the fetus passed. The infant was asphyxiated at birth, but was not anemic.

tion, even attachment at the margin, is not rare. *Battledore placenta* is the marginal insertion of the cord and has some clinical importance because sometimes it is associated with slight bleeding that may be confused with placenta previa. Brody and Frenkel found that 68 per cent of patients with battledore placenta had premature labor.

When the cord inserts into the membranes so that the umbilical vessels course between the amnion and the chorion to the placenta it is termed *velamentous insertion* (Fig. 306). This condition is often accompanied by other anomalies of the placenta, such as infarcts, placenta succenturiata, bilobata and previa. Velamentous insertion occurs nine times more often with twins than with single infants and is the rule with triplets. This insertion is dangerous to the fetus, especially when the vessels traverse the lower uterine seg-ment and cross over the internal os, a condition known as *vasa previa.*

VASA PREVIA

Vago and Caspi showed that trauma to the velamentous vessels may occur. They encountered an incidence of 1:2761 in nearly 20,000 deliveries. The most frequent presumptive diagnoses in cases of bleeding from velamentous vessels are the more common problems causing third trimester bleeding, namely, abruptio placentae and placenta previa. Velamentous vessels are usually torn at the time of rupture of the bag of waters, but this is not always true. In some cases the vessels are torn before the membranes rupture. It is presumed that bleeding stops because of thrombus formation. In contradistinction, bleeding can also begin long after the membranes rupture.

The diagnosis is based on identifying the blood as fetal in origin (see below). Treatment consists of delivery as quickly as feasible without causing additional fetal or maternal trauma. Vasa previa endangers the fetus by causing exsanguination from a torn fetal blood vessel or asphyxia from pressure on the velamentous vessels by the presenting part.

If the required high index of suspicion for vasa previa is maintained in all cases of antepartum hemorrhage, it would not be difficult to determine if the bleeding were fetal or maternal in origin. The Apt test is particularly suitable for this purpose (Israel). It is based on the resistance of fetal hemoglobin to alkali in contradistinction to maternal hemoglobin which changes to alkaline heme in an alkaline medium. About 2 to 3 ml. of bloody material is mixed with an equal amount of water. The distinct pink-red hemoglobin solution obtained is centrifuged for two minutes at 2000 r.p.m. The resultant supernatant fluid is decanted and one part of 0.25 N sodium hydroxide is added to five parts of the decanted solution. A color reaction appears within one or two minutes. Yellow-brown (alkaline heme) shows the blood to be of maternal origin. Red indicates fetal hemoglobin that has resisted conversion to alkaline heme. The extreme simplicity of the Apt test makes it readily applicable to every case of antepartum hemorrhage. Merely observing a stained smear of the blood under a microscope for nucleated fetal erythrocytes is also useful. Having demonstrated the bleeding to be of fetal origin, the obstetrician can then take immediate steps to effect delivery.

The high perinatal mortality associated with vasa previa might be significantly reduced in this way. The fetal mortality in vasa previa is almost 60 per cent, probably the highest single mortality rate for any of the so-called accidents of pregnancy. The baby may be born anemic and require blood, but there is no danger to the mother.

If the diagnosis is made before the membranes rupture, cesarean section is the proper treatment. This is appropriate even if the blood vessel is intact, unless vaginal delivery can be accomplished promptly and atraumatically.

HERNIAS INTO THE CORD

Herniation of fetal bowel into the cord at its abdominal insertion is not rare. A hernia must always be considered and carefully searched for while tying the cord. Occasionally, the skin of the abdomen extends up for a varying distance on the cord. This is called *skin umbilicus* and, after the stump has dropped off, retraction of the center causes the skin to invert and result in a deep, retracted umbilicus.

HYDRAMNIOS

Hydramnios (or polyhydramnios), a condition in which there are excessive amounts of amniotic fluid, occurs about once in 200 pregnancies. A volume of more than 2000 ml. of amniotic fluid should be considered as indicating hydramnios, although clinical estimates of amounts are inaccurate. Uterine overdistention is usually quite evident and the diagnosis is apparent,

especially when the accumulation of fluid has been rapid. The possible mechanisms by which this condition comes about have been detailed in Chapter 5. Coassociated phenomena include (1) fetal malformations, especially esophageal or pyloric occlusions, anencephaly and spina bifida, (2) vascular obstructive disorders, such as cord stenosis, fetal heart disease or cirrhosis, (3) multiple pregnancy, and (4) certain maternal diseases, including diabetes and Rh isoimmunization, as well as those disorders of the heart, lung, liver and kidney that may produce anasarca. About 26 per cent of patients with hydramnios will be found to have an anomalous fetus. Hydramnios occurs in seven per cent of twin pregnancies.

There are two recognized clinical types of hydramnios, based on differences in the rapidity with which they develop, their relative severity and prognostic significance. *Acute hydramnios* is a very serious problem, occurring only once in 12,000 deliveries. It may begin as early as the fourth or fifth month of pregnancy, rapidly expanding the uterus over an interval of just a few days.

The patient experiences pronounced pressure symptoms with pain in the abdomen, back and thighs. Dyspnea may occur with nausea and vomiting. Secondary edema of the abdominal walls, vulva and lower extremities develops. The abdomen is tightly distended and sensitive. The fetus cannot be palpated easily and it is difficult to hear the fetal heart tones. The cervix tends to efface early and undergo some prelabor dilatation. Premature labor or abortion is common. Ultrasonography (see Chapter 13) readily confirms the diagnosis, although it is usually obvious on clinical grounds. Acute hydramnios may have to be differentiated from a rapidly growing hydatidiform mole, an ovarian cyst or ascites.

Treatment consists of attempts to reduce the volume of amniotic fluid so as to provide relief of the discomfort. Diuretics tend to be ineffectual. Amniocentesis (see Chapter 52) can give temporary relief of the overdistention, but fluid tends to reaccumulate quickly and the procedure must be repeated often. Although spontaneous premature labor (or abortion) usually occurs in due course, pregnancy may have to be terminated by inducing labor. Usually, amniotomy suffices, but care must be taken to avert shock by withdrawing amniotic fluid slowly.

The outlook in acute hydramnios is generally good for the mother, although she is at risk with regard to possible cardiac and respiratory failure. Abruptio placentae may result from the sudden reduction in uterine volume when the fluid is released. Shock may develop from sudden diminution in intraabdominal pressure. Prognosis for the fetus is particularly poor; most die as a consequence of their prematurity, an anomaly, the maternal disease that caused the hydramnios, or the complications of the condition, including prolapsed cord and abruptio placentae.

Chronic hydramnios occurs about 10 times as often as the acute form, or once in 1200 pregnancies. Reported incidence varies according to the criteria used for diagnosis. Mild asymptomatic forms tend to be overlooked. The course is much less stormy than acute hydramnios. It does not lead so often to abortion, although premature labor is frequent.

Symptoms are the same as those of the acute form, but less pronounced and of longer duration. Enormous distention of the uterus may occur, with resulting cardiac or pulmonary distress. The patient may have episodic false labor contractions for weeks before delivery. The condition is most often confused with multiple pregnancy. It must be remembered that the two conditions may coexist. Roentgenograms or ultrasonograms help to distinguish multiple pregnancy or monsters.

The treatment program is essentially the same as for acute hydramnios, except that there is less urgency. When the symptoms become pronounced, labor should be induced by needle amniotomy. The fluid should be drained slowly to avoid the shock of sudden decrease of intraabdominal pressure and to prevent prolapse of the cord or fetal extremities. Delivery should also be slow so that the uterus may adapt itself to the diminishing volume without shearing the placenta. Oxytocin and ergonovine should be used prophylac-tically after the delivery to prevent the hemorrhage from uterine atony seen so commonly in association with uterine overdistention.

Overdistention of the uterus has been found to raise the tonus and reduce the intensity of contractions (Caldeyro-Barcia et al.). There may be increased uterine contractility leading to premature labor, but the intensity of contractions during labor may be reduced. However, progressive cervical dilatation patterns of labor (Friedman and Sachtleben) show that most patients with hydramnios experience entirely normal labors.

OLIGOHYDRAMNIOS

Oligohydramnios is a rare, ill-defined entity in which there is a paucity of amniotic fluid. Nothing is definitely known of its cause, but it has been reported present with renal agenesis of the fetus. It can affect one twin, with coassociated hydramnios in the other. There may be a few spoonfuls of thick, viscid or cloudy, yellowish-green fluid which is barely sufficient to fill the interstices between the fetus and the uterus. If the condition occurs early, some adhesion of the amnion to the fetus results or amniotic bands develop. Both conditions may cause deformities. The gamut of fetal consequences is reviewed by Torpin. If the amniotic fluid is absent in the later months, the fetal skin becomes dry and leathery and its body is cramped together. Clubfoot and clubhand are seen, as well as strangulation or amputation of digits or extremities. Shortening of muscles, such as in wryneck and talipes calcaneus, are also encountered. The same conditions may occur in extraamniotic development and in extrauterine pregnancy.

Labor often begins prematurely. Uterine contractions may be ineffectual or particularly painful. Progress in labor may be protracted. Fetal hypoxia may develop more often than in normal pregnancies, perhaps as a result of cord compression which is more likely to occur because of the diminished amniotic fluid.

REFERENCES

Brody, S., and Frenkel, D. A.: Marginal insertion of the cord and premature labor. Amer. J. Obstet. Gynec. 65:1305, 1953.

Caldeyro-Barcia, R., Pose, S. V., and Alvarez, H.: Uterine contractility and polyhydramnios and the effects of withdrawal of excess of amniotic fluid. Amer. J. Obstet. Gynec. 73:1238, 1957.

Clifford, S. H.: Postmaturity. Advances Pediat. 9:13, 1954.

DeCosta, E. J., Gerbie, A. B., Andersen, R. H., and Gallanis, T. C.: Placental tumors: Hemangiomas with special reference to an associated clinical syndrome. Obstet. Gynec. 7:249, 1956.

Friedman, E. A., and Sachtleben, M. R.: The effect of uterine overdistention on labor: II. Hydramnios. Obstet. Gynec. 23:401, 1964.

Israel, R.: Vasa previa in binovular twins: Report of a case. Obstet. Gynec. 17:691, 1961.

Scott, J. S.: Placenta extrachorialis (placenta margin-ata and placenta circumvallata): A factor in antepartum hemorrhage. J. Obstet. Gynaec. Brit. Comm. 67:904, 1960.

Shanklin, D. R.: The human placenta: A clinicopathologic study. Obstet. Gynec. 11:129, 1958.

Tindall, V. R., and Scott, J. S.: Placental calcification: A study of 3025 singleton and multiple pregnancies. J. Obstet. Gynaec. Brit. Comm. 72:356, 1965.

Torpin, R.: Fetal Malformations Caused by Amnion Rupture during Gestation. Springfield, Ill., Charles C Thomas, 1968.

Vago, T., and Caspi, E.: Antepartum bleeding due to injury of velamentous placental vessels. Obstet. Gynec. 20:671, 1962.

Walker, J.: Foetal anoxia. J. Obstet. Gynaec. Brit. Emp. 61:162, 1954.

Walker, J.: Prolonged pregnancy syndrome. Amer. J. Obstet. Gynec. 76:1231, 1958.

PATHOLOGY OF LABOR

Chapter 55

Dysfunctional Labor

Classically, abnormalities of labor may be considered under four headings: (1) dysfunction of the powers (uterus and abdominal muscles); (2) anomalies of the passengers (fetus and placenta); (3) disturbances of the passages (bony and soft tissues), and (4) complications threatening the mother, the fetus or the placenta. This is an artificial classification based on retrospective evaluation and provides little practical basis for early detection, diagnosis, evaluation and management.

In Chapter 15 we reviewed the functional aspects of normal labor with particular regard for an approach to objective evaluation of labors in progress. Based on studies of the pattern of progression of cervical dilatation and descent of the fetal presenting part (Friedman), we determined the component functional divisions of labor (preparatory, dilatational and pelvic) and what should be expected to occur during these intervals in terms of limits of normal activity.

Using this information, we may now define specific aberrant labor patterns. Each is characterized according to its location in the course of labor and by its significant temporal deviation from normal. Thus, we have three groups of labor abnormalities according to location in the functional subdivisions, namely, (1) those of the *preparatory division*, in which the latent phase of dilatation is prolonged; (2) those of the *dilatational division*, charac-

terized by abnormally slow rates of cervical dilatation and descent; and (3) those of the *pelvic division*, in which there is arrest of dilatation and descent or protraction of the deceleration phase of dilatation (Friedman).

As indicated in Chapter 15, the latent phase in most nulliparas terminates in less than 20 hours. The disorder of *prolonged latent phase*, therefore, exists when the latent phase exceeds 20 hours in nulliparas. Similarly, in multiparas it is present when the latent phase extends beyond 14 hours. *Protracted active-phase dilatation* is defined by a rate of cervical dilatation of less than 1.2 cm. per hour in nulliparas and 1.5 cm. per hour in multiparas. The related disorder of *protracted descent* occurs when there is a rate of descent under 1 cm. per hour in nulliparas and 2 cm. per hour in multiparas, based on station determinations in centimeters above or below the plane of the ischial spines (see Chapter 19). *Prolonged deceleration phase* exceeds three hours in nulliparas and one hour in multiparas. *Secondary arrest of dilatation* is apparent when the expected linear progression of cervical dilatation in the active phase ceases for at least two hours; *arrest of descent* is recognized by interrupted descent, usually in the second stage, for at least one hour. These patterns are displayed graphically in Figure 307 and will be discussed in detail below.

Some classifications of abnormal labor

577

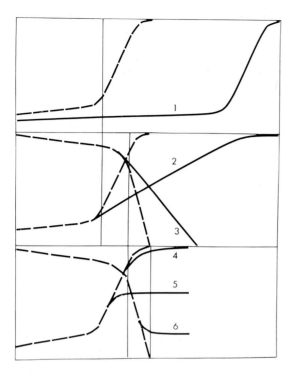

Figure 307 Representations of the six graphic disorders of the functional divisions of labor, with cervical dilatation and fetal station on the vertical axis and time on the horizontal. At the top, the normal dilatation curve (broken line) is compared with the preparatory division abnormality of *prolonged latent phase* (1). The middle group presents the protraction disorders of the dilatational division, namely *protracted active-phase dilatation* (2) and *protracted descent* (3). At the bottom are the pathologic states of the pelvic division, including *prolonged deceleration phase* (4), *secondary arrest of dilatation* (5) and *arrest of descent* (6).

are based on abnormal uterine activity as determined by clinical examination. Jeffcoate et al. divided cases into (1) hypotonic uterine action with weak ineffectual contractions, (2) cervical dystocia, in which there is rare mechanical obstruction at the external os, and (3) hypertonic states. Three varieties of hypertonic states were recognized, including (1) that with poor propagation of the contraction as well as poor upper segment contractility, (2) the dyskinetic or discoordinate contraction without gradient or propagation, and (3) constriction ring dystocia with formation of an obstructive annular ring in the lower segment as the end result of reversed polarity.

In clinical practice this classification, although reasonable, is difficult to apply and the distinctions are not always clear. Abnormal labor cannot be defined without a clearer understanding of the physiology of normal labor and its variants. Unless normal labor and its limits can be defined more critically by the methods described in Chapter 15, the diagnosis of an abnormality is at best nebulous. It is a rather difficult matter to study labor in detail and to analyze it critically because of the dynamic nature of the several changes that take place simultaneously. The simple, clinically applicable and objective method of graphic evaluation is useful in this regard.

With this approach a definition of average labor is possible in quantitative terms, and at the same time the limits of normal are described. It should be noted that the concept of *prolonged labor* has been eliminated. The maximal allowable total duration of labor has heretofore been variously and arbitrarily set at between 18 and 48 hours in centers throughout the world. Total duration by itself has relatively little significance.

Similarly, the ephemeral terms *uterine inertia* and *inert labor* are avoided because their meaning has never been fully elucidated or defined in a manner that permits clear understanding or application to clinical situations. It is recommended that these terms be discarded in favor of the descriptive terms for the six specific labor aberrations defined above.

Utilizing this method of approach to follow the individual patient and collectively to study pregnant patients in general, it is possible (1) to determine more eas-

TABLE 9   DYSFUNCTIONAL LABOR PATTERNS

	Prolonged Latent Phase	*Protraction Disorders*	*Arrest Disorders*
Diagnostic features	Nulliparas: >20 hr. Multiparas: >14 hr.	Nulliparas: <1.2 cm./hr. dilatation <1 cm./hr. descent Multiparas: <1.5 cm./hr. dilatation <2 cm./hr. descent	Dilatation: >2 hr. arrest Descent: >1 hr. arrest
Etiologic factors	Excessive sedation Unprepared cervix False labor Anesthesia Uterine dysfunction	Unknown CPD° 28 per cent Malposition Excessive sedation Anesthesia	CPD° 45 per cent Malposition Excessive sedation Anesthesia
Therapy	Rest	Support Avoid inhibitory factors	Section† for CPD° Oxytocin (only if no CPD°)
Expected response	85 per cent "cure" 10 per cent out of labor	90 per cent uninterrupted progression	94 per cent "cure"
Delivery prognosis	Vaginal delivery	Vaginal delivery usually Section† for CPD°	Delivery prognosis varies with response
Fetal prognosis	No risk	Slightly increased risk	Threefold risk

°Cephalopelvic disproportion.
†Cesarean section.

ily the progressive changes occurring in individual labors in progress; (2) to study the management of labor; (3) to investigate the effects of various factors that may potentially influence the course of labor; and (4) to examine aberrations critically as to diagnosis, etiology, treatment and prognosis.

These abnormalities are easily definable and detectable in individual labors merely by the expediency of plotting estimates of cervical dilatation against time. Abnormalities may occur individually or in any one of several combinations. All together they constitute about six per cent of labors. Their clinical features are shown in Table 9. A total of 63 possible combinations have all been found in nature, suggesting why there has been so much confusion in clinical recognition and characterization of abnormal labors in the past.

PROLONGED LATENT PHASE

Patients with prolonged latent phase lasting more than 20 hours in nulliparas or 14 hours in multiparas have frequently been subjected to the inhibitory effects of excessive sedation or anesthesia. These factors appear to have contributed to the development of prolonged latent phase in as many as 45 per cent of patients with this disorder. There can be little doubt that sedation and anesthesia given too early in labor (that is, before the latent phase is terminated) will prolong labor.

Second only to the influence of sedation and anesthesia is that of prelabor cervical preparation. Patients who begin labor with the cervix unprepared (that is, thick, uneffaced, undilated and unyielding) can be expected to have a long latent phase during which the cervix is being prepared for subsequent active dilatation. This is a factor in about 20 per cent.

Other patients with abnormally prolonged latent phase are later found to have been in false labor (about 10 per cent). When the contractions finally stop, the diagnosis is apparent in retrospect. In others (less than 10 per cent), investigation of the subsequent dilatation pattern reveals an abnormally slow rate of progression in the active phase, which is characteristic of the protraction disorders mentioned earlier. On this basis, we can assume that the latent phase was probably prolonged by a similar dysfunctional process which could not be diagnosed until later in the active phase.

Patients with prolonged latent phase are quite exhausted and emotionally discouraged. Such patients benefit from a significant period of rest, accomplished by use of a narcotic agent, such as morphine, given in sufficient amounts to suspend labor temporarily. The effectiveness of this treatment is equivalent to that of oxytocin stimulation for this disorder, 85 per cent responding with active dilatation subsequently. Rest, however, is preferable because of the frequency of unrecognized false labor in these patients and the consideration of their emotional and physical needs. Aside from rest or oxytocin, no other form of therapy has been consistently effective in correcting this disorder.

With this conservative treatment regimen for prolonged latent phase, the prognosis is very good with regard to delivery and fetal outcome. At least 85 per cent of patients thus treated respond later with normal, active dilatation and descent, followed in most instances by vaginal delivery. These patients do not progress to delivery during the interval in which the sedative drug is active; the depressant effects have abated long before the infant is born.

Following rest therapy, about 10 per cent of patients awaken out of labor. In these patients, the difficult differential diagnosis of false labor has been established in retrospect. In the remaining five per cent thus treated, the original condition recurs; contractions are ineffective in producing dilatation. Only in this residual group is further active therapy required. In the absence of any contraindication, oxytocin infusion is usually effective in stimulating labor to terminate the latent phase and produce normal active phase progression.

This program of management is most useful in treating patients with documented prolonged latent phase aberrations. The choice of therapeutic rest rather than oxytocin stimulation is based on a desire to make the diagnostic differentiation between false labor and the abnormal disorder of prolonged latent phase. In false labor, stimulation may unnecessarily increase fetal and maternal risks, particularly since many of these patients are not physiologically or functionally prepared for labor (see Chapter 24).

Amniotomy has not been consistently effective as a stimulatory device when the latent phase is prolonged. It is advisable, therefore, not to perform amniotomy in these cases if the membranes are still intact, because of the possibility that the labor may be false. Moreover, ultimate delivery may be delayed for many hours, raising the likelihood of infection.

Prolongation of the latent phase does not influence fetal or maternal morbidity or mortality adversely, provided that it is handled expeditiously when the diagnosis is made. There is no reason to resort to cesarean section as a primary therapy for prolonged latent phase. The prognosis for vaginal delivery is excellent. Patients who are delivered by cesarean section during the latent phase, particularly for such controversial reasons as inertia, lack of progress and cervical dystocia, are often subjected to operative delivery unnecessarily. On this basis, cesarean section merely for prolonged latent phase without a more definitive indication is unjustified.

PROTRACTION DISORDERS

Protracted active-phase dilatation and protracted descent patterns are analogous in many ways. Underlying pathogenesis is essentially unknown, but many common factors appear to be associated or perhaps contributory. These include minor malpositions, excessive sedation and improperly administered conduction anesthesia. By the last is meant an epidural or caudal anesthetic given too high (above the tenth thoracic dermatome), too early (before the onset of the active phase) or in conjunction with other inhibitory factors. Additionally, cephalopelvic disproportion is encountered in 28 per cent of these patients. Definitive evaluation of fetopelvic relationships by digital and x-ray examination is obviously needed.

The treatment of these aberrations is uniformly ineffectual. These rare disorders do not appear to be remediable by any of the stimulatory methods in our current clinical armamentarium. At the same time, however, it is quite easy to inhibit further progress or even to produce arrest of dilatation or of descent by such potentially deleterious measures as excessive sedation or regional block anesthesia.

If one finds insurmountable bony dystocia in these patients, one may justifiably elect cesarean section because it avoids subjecting the patient to a long, tedious labor with risk of ascending infection. Support is essential if labor is allowed to proceed in order to provide for emotional and physical needs, with special attention to fluid and electrolyte balance.

Continued progress should be expected if patients with protraction disorders are properly managed conservatively. The prognosis remains good as long as progress continues. The risk to mother or fetus from these conditions appears to be only slightly increased, provided that no ill-advised measures for stimulation or, even more important, for traumatic delivery are undertaken. Expectancy is very strongly recommended.

If the patient with a protraction disorder develops the further complication of an arrest pattern, in the form of either arrest of dilatation or arrest of descent, the prognostic outlook becomes considerably worse. Here cesarean section becomes a more likely possibility, and the fetal risks increase substantially. The risk to the fetus in protraction disorders is primarily related to the type of delivery utilized. Midforceps procedures, for example, are especially hazardous. Conservative management must be employed to optimum advantage in these cases, limiting delivery techniques to easy low forceps or spontaneous maneuvers.

It is important to recognize and accept the apparent facts that (1) the slow progressive dilatation and descent cannot be prodded even though occurring at abnormal rates; (2) provision should be made for support of these patients as required; (3) anything that even remotely impedes progress must be avoided; and (4) above all else, unnecessarily complicating the problem with factors that may increase the maternal, fetal and delivery hazards of labor must be prevented. Prognostically, about two-thirds of these patients will deliver normally if given the opportunity to do so.

ARREST PATTERNS

Perhaps the most ominous cause of arrest of dilatation or of descent is concomitant cephalopelvic disproportion. It occurs in about 45 per cent of patients. The potential for atraumatic vaginal delivery in the presence of disproportion is negligible. Other associated factors include minor malpositions, excessive sedation and conduction anesthesia.

Patients frequently present with a pattern of arrest as the first sign of disproportion. Under these circumstances, the pattern of dilatation or descent serves as a useful prognostic index. The association of bony dystocia and arrest of dilatation or descent constitutes a significant warning. Patients presenting with this combination warrant cesarean section as the safest and the most conservative approach.

Whenever arrest patterns are diagnosed, it is vital that an intensive search be undertaken to discover problems in fetopelvic relationships. Since disproportion carries the worst prognosis, accurate digital and x-ray pelvimetry should be performed promptly (see Chapter 12). It should be stressed that no form of therapy should be instituted for arrest before the pelvic relationships are adequately investigated. Any degree of disproportion in association with an arrest pattern does not deserve a further trial of labor, because vaginal delivery is most unlikely.

If one can rule out disproportion in the patient with arrest of dilatation or descent, subsequent therapy can then be chosen according to the condition of the patient. If arrest has resulted from excessive sedation or from improperly administered conduction anesthesia, expectancy alone may suffice, while the effects of the offending agent are allowed to dissipate. Therapeutic rest is in order for the patient who is thoroughly exhausted; during this time adequate support can be given.

In the remaining patients, as well as in those who have had adequate rest but who have failed to reinstitute labor spontaneously, stimulation with oxytocin infusion should be undertaken, barring contraindications. Most patients respond well to such uterotonic stimulation as primary therapy if it is administered cautiously and in sufficient doses to simulate strong, normal labor. The required optimal duration of stimulation with the infusion titrated so as to produce uterine contractions simulating good labor is between three and seven hours. Most patients will respond with additional progress in dilatation and descent in less than three hours.

The expected success rate of more than 90 per cent permits an optimistic forecast for most of these patients. Therefore, cesarean section should not be the primary means of therapy in the absence of documentable disproportion. It must be emphasized once again that no form of uterotonic stimulation should be instituted in these cases before the bony relationships have been investigated thoroughly and disproportion ruled out with certainty.

Arrest of dilatation or of descent is a serious abnormality with a particularly poor prognosis for vaginal delivery. Many patients with these patterns ultimately require cesarean section because of disproportion. If pelvic relationships are adequate, the prognostic outlook for vaginal delivery is better. One can determine the prognosis more carefully if one compares the rate of progression in the slope of dilatation or descent before arrest with the rate that occurs after therapy for the arrest. Delivery prognosis improves with the increment in slope. The more rapid the postarrest slope, the more likely that the delivery can be *per vaginam*. All patients whose postarrest slope is more than 2 cm. per hour greater than the prearrest slope should be expected to deliver vaginally. None should require cesarean section, unless indicated for some other reason (such as fetal distress).

The specific fetal risk factor for arrest patterns appears to be greater than that expected for comparable normal labor. This is true even when the delivery hazards, such as occur in midforceps procedures, are taken into account. On this basis, arrest of dilatation or of descent must be considered a labor pattern which is inherently deleterious to the fetus. Therefore, it requires early diagnosis, prompt evaluation for disproportion and careful definitive management.

Since most arrest patterns can be diagnosed readily within a short time after cessation of progression in dilatation or descent, it should be relatively easy to discover these high-risk situations expeditiously by graphing the progress of labor in an ongoing manner. If one waits for some arbitrary total labor duration to pass before becoming aware of the possible presence of labor abnormalities, the early diagnosis of arrest patterns will be missed.

FALSE LABOR

False labor consists of the intrinsic contractions of the uterus that, toward the end of gestation, become perceptible or even painful. They are often especially pronounced at the time of lightening. All the usual symptoms of actual labor, including pain, hardening of the uterus and regularity of the contractions, may be present. It may help in the diagnosis to point out that false labor contractions are usually not progressive, while true labor contractions tend to become stronger. False labor contractions usually cease after a few hours.

It is important to recognize false labor because, if a woman is considered to be in labor when actually she is not, unnecessary and harmful interference may be instituted. Treatment consists of rest in bed, narcotics and expectancy. An approach to help make this sometimes rather difficult differential diagnosis has been discussed in considering the management of the prolonged latent phase (see above).

PRECIPITATE LABOR

An abnormally fast, tumultuous labor in which cervical dilatation occurs quickly and descent of the presenting part is rapid is called *precipitate labor.* This is to be distinguished from "precipitate delivery," which refers to rapid delivery over an unsterile field.

Precipitate labor has been variously limited to labors of two to four hours. Objectively, the rate of cervical dilatation in the active phase is greater than 5 cm. per hour in nulliparas or 10 cm. per hour in multiparas. Since these represent very rapid changes in dilatation, it is easier to consider them in more realistic terms, such as 1 cm. every 12 minutes for nulliparas and 1 cm. every 6 minutes for multiparas. This is an objective clinical entity and can be detected graphically. Etiologic factors are not clearly defined, but precipitate labor may occur even in the presence of heavy sedation, relative bony disproportion and minor malpositions.

In general, this condition results from overactive uterine contractions, occurring too frequently and too intensely, in conjunction with negligible resistance of the maternal soft parts. Often there are concomitant powerful contractions of the abdominal muscles so that labor is enhanced and delivery effected quickly.

Precipitate labor may be injurious to both mother and baby. Perinatal mortality with precipitate labor is increased from both trauma and coassociated hypoxia. The hypercontractility of the uterine muscles may be diminished by ether or halothane anesthesia or with peridural anesthesia to levels up to T-6.

For precipitate delivery, abolition of the perineal reflex with local, pudendal or general inhalation anesthesia is sometimes effective in preventing the powerful abdominal muscle action from terminating the labor too rapidly. It is strongly emphasized that under no circumstances should a forcible attempt be made to hold the head back during a precipitate delivery. There can be no possible excuse for such unconscionable techniques as holding the legs together or other delaying tactics with a view toward awaiting the arrival of the obstetrician. Serious injury to mother and baby can occur.

Attempts to guide the head over the perineum with the modified Ritgen maneuver, as described in Chapter 20, are recommended for purposes of control in order to prevent traumatic, explosive damage to the perineum and the fetal head. After precipitate labors and deliveries, thorough exploration of the birth canal is essential to detect injuries to the uterus, cervix, vagina or perineum.

TETANIC UTERINE CONTRACTIONS

Any local irritant to the cervix or uterine wall may evoke tempestuous action. In abruptio placentae, the uterus is not infrequently in a tetanic state. Any uterotonic agent, especially if administered in excessive amounts, may produce tetanic contractions. By convention, any contraction lasting longer than 90 seconds is considered tetanic. The major danger is that the fetus may die from asphyxia, because the increased intrauterine pressure effectively impedes exchange across the placenta, diminishing or abolishing oxygenation of the fetal blood.

Treatment of uterine tetany due to oxytocic drugs has been detailed in Chapter 24. Tetanic contractions occurring during oxytocin infusion are effectively handled by stopping the intravenous drip immediately. Tetany occurring spontaneously or after an intramuscular injection of a uterotonic agent may respond to deep inhalation anesthesia. Open drop ether, chloroform and especially halothane are useful in this regard. In abruptio placentae, amniotomy and additional stimulation to augment labor should be used to effect prompt evacuation of the uterus (see Chapter 38).

CONSTRICTION RING DYSTOCIA

Dystocia due to constriction ring or contraction ring is a rare phenomenon. It is caused by an abnormally persistent contraction of an area of circular fibers in the myometrium. It should not be confused with the physiologic or pathologic retraction ring seen in parturient uteri at the junction of the upper and lower uterine segments. The constriction ring is usually localized to a thickened area of myometrium over a point of depression in the fetal body or at a level just below it (Fig. 308).

The diagnosis may be made in the course of a prolonged labor, when progress in dilatation and descent stops. A depression at the site of the ring may be seen and felt through the abdominal wall. The area below the ring is usually flaccid, even during contractions. In other words, the contraction of the upper segment is not transmitted beyond the ring to the lower uterine segment and cervix. The diagnosis is rarely made in the first stage of labor.

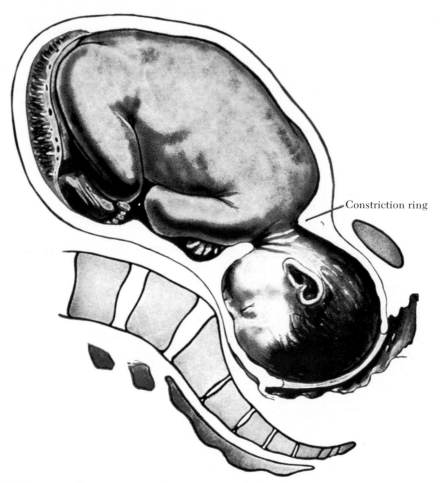

Constriction ring

Figure 308 Exaggerated representation of constriction ring formed around the fetal neck in the course of labor, indicating how further descent may be obstructed.

Definitive diagnosis requires vaginal and intrauterine examination. Characteristically, there is no advancement in the station or in the descent of the fetal presenting part during a uterine contraction. In some instances the head may even recede. The presenting part is loose in the pelvic cavity during and between uterine contractions, and there is no feeling of thrust downward during contractions.

A pathognomonic sign is the persistent relaxation of the cervix during a contraction. Normally, the cervix should become firm as it is pulled tight during contractions. During vaginal examination, the examining hand can easily pass upward into the uterine cavity to palpate the ring tightly constricted around some part of the fetus.

The ring is primarily a functional disturbance of the uterus. Etiologic factors are usually difficult to assign. Occasionally, it may follow intrauterine manipulation and premature rupture of the membranes. Cephalopelvic disproportion is neither an active nor a predisposing factor, but may coexist, of course.

Treatment for this condition may be expectant. Except when an indication arises for immediate delivery (for example, for fetal distress), temporization is usually in order. Hasty and potentially traumatic operative interference results in high maternal and infant morbidity and mortality. The patient should be supported and rested. Subsequently, attempts should be made to relax the ring if it has not relaxed spontaneously. Deep ether, chloroform or halothane anesthesia is usually effective. Many ancillary measures have been used in the past with varying degrees of success, including epinephrine, papaverine, amyl nitrite, magnesium sulfate and isoxsuprine.

Most constriction rings respond to time, drugs or anesthesia. Cesarean section through a classic incision may have to be done when a constriction ring cannot be overcome.

MISSED LABOR

Very rarely, labor begins at the proper time and some degree of cervical dilatation may be attained, but the contractions cease and gestation continues for weeks or months. The fetus dies. Oldham called this *missed labor.* In other varieties, no labor-like pattern of contractions occurs, and the pregnancy continues well beyond term. This condition is the same as missed abortion (see Chapter 33), except that it occurs later in pregnancy.

The reason for the failure of the uterus to expel the dead product of conception is unknown. Long after the fetus dies it mummifies and shrinks, the amniotic fluid is absorbed and the uterus applies itself closely to the body. A lithopedion may form as in extrauterine gestation (see Chapter 32), or infection may set in with purulent disintegration and extrusion of the bones through the cervix.

Examination shows a closed cervix and a nonresponsive uterus of relatively hard consistency, entirely lacking the spongy softness characteristic in normal pregnancy. The diagnosis is usually easy. Since the question of pregnancy is seldom uncertain, all that is needed is to prove that the symmetric mass is the uterus, that it is not enlarging and that the fetus is dead. Features for the determination of the life or death of the fetus are discussed in Chapter 8. One should strongly suspect abdominal pregnancy (see Chapter 32) and take appropriate measures to determine its presence.

It is advisable to wait to see if labor will begin spontaneously to empty the uterus.

The patient must be watched carefully while waiting. The uterine contents may become infected. More importantly, acquired afibrinogenemia with resultant hemorrhagic diathesis may occur from longstanding retention of a dead fetus (see Chapter 42). Acquired afibrinogenemia is a potential hazard for any patient whose dead fetus has been retained for several weeks. These patients deserve careful observation and periodic fibrinogen level determinations until delivery has been accomplished. It must be emphasized that defibrination may develop in the intervening weeks prior to labor. The use of heparin prophylactically for anticoagulation has been shown to prevent hypofibrinogenemia in these cases.

The patient should be hospitalized whenever alterations in the clotting mechanism are encountered or hemorrhagic manifestations appear. Diagnosis, evaluation and therapy are discussed in Chapter 42. During labor or any operative procedure, circulating blood volume should be maintained if necessary by transfusions, preferably of fresh whole blood to ensure adequate amounts of accelerator substances. Intrapartum or postpartum hemorrhage is not likely if clotting factors are restored.

PREMATURE RUPTURE OF MEMBRANES

At any time during pregnancy the membranes may rupture. Contractions almost always begin within a few hours or days, and the uterus empties itself. Premature rupture of the membranes is considered to exist when labor does not begin within one hour of rupture. The time between rupture of the membranes and the onset of labor is defined as the *latent period.*

The treatment of early rupture is expectancy. The dangers of rupture at or near term have been greatly exaggerated. In shoulder and breech presentations and in contracted pelves, however, it may lead to prolapse of the cord and other complications, particularly infection, especially if the labor is prolonged.

Premature rupture of the membranes is commonly associated with premature labor. It does not, however, increase the infant mortality of premature babies any more than that of mature babies. Babies are lost because the cord may prolapse or intraamniotic infection may develop.

Labor is shorter after premature spontaneous rupture of the membranes (Calkins). It does not follow, however, that rupturing the membranes artificially to induce labor will yield a labor that is foreshortened. There is agreement that labor induced by rupturing the membranes in normal patients in the presence of the proper conditions (see Chapter 24) is not prolonged nor necessarily fraught with danger. When conditions are not ideal, however, artificial rupture of the membranes may be hazardous. Labor may not ensue promptly, ascending infection may occur and labor may be dysfunctional.

The first essential of management of premature rupture of membranes is to discover any indication that may be present to justify immediate intervention. Intelligent expectancy should be followed in normal cases, but operation may be necessary for such indications as contracted pelvis, abnormal presentation or prolapsed cord. To reduce the danger of infection, as few vaginal or rectal examinations as possible should be made. There is no need to attempt induction of labor when the membranes rupture, unless the conditions are optimal for doing so on an elective basis (see Chapter 24). It is usually safe to wait without doing anything and without giving antibiotics prophylactically. This course may be pursued indefinitely or until some complication arises to demand intervention.

Prolonged rupture of the membranes may lead to infection in a small number of instances. When it occurs, very aggressive intervention is necessary, including antibiotics, induction or even cesarean section. It does not seem justified to employ such measures for the majority of patients in whom no infection will occur. Routine aggressive therapy merely substitutes potentially hazardous treatment (with the risks of induction under suboptimal conditions, of cesarean section and of fetal pre-maturity) for the real but limited chance of infection. The controversy over this matter is as yet unresolved.

DYSFUNCTION OF ABDOMINAL MUSCLES

In general, the second stage does not progress normally without active voluntary participation in expulsive bearing-down efforts by the patient. Descent may be delayed when the rectus muscles and diaphragm are ineffectual, attenuated or not brought to bear because of inherent weakness or fear. Multiparas with rectus diastases, pendulous abdomens and widely separated rectus muscles exhibit this phenomenon. The abdominal muscles do not contract reflexly when the perineal reflex has been abolished by narcosis or anesthesia. Similarly, patients may refuse to bear down, voluntarily inhibiting the reflex, if the discomfort is severe. The musculature may be weakened from exhaustion.

It is important to avoid having the patient bear down before the cervix is fully dilated and completely retracted and the second stage has begun because (1) expulsive force may prematurely dilate the cervix too rapidly, producing cervical lacerations; (2) expulsive force may cause the cervix to become impinged between the fetal head and bony pelvis so that it cannot dilate and becomes edematous; or (3) the patient may exhaust her strength in fruitless and harmful efforts in the first stage.

It should be borne in mind that, although the second stage may be prolonged in the absence of sufficient abdominal muscle action, delivery may sometimes be effected, especially in multiparas, when the reduced resistance of the soft tissues of the vagina and perineum is overcome by uterine contractility alone.

Women with cardiac and respiratory disorders should not be permitted to exert themselves in the second stage. In these patients conduction anesthesia is effective in abolishing the perineal reflex; elective midforceps procedures to shorten the second stage may be in order, but one must be certain that such procedures are carried out atraumatically.

As to treatment, most patients can be encouraged to bear down more efficiently. Relief of inhibiting pain by analgesics or light nitrous oxide anesthesia may help them to cooperate. Although the second stage may be prolonged, there is usually no indication for applying Kristeller expression (that is, pressure over the uterine fundus exerted in the axis of the inlet) nor for effecting forceps delivery before the forward leading portion of the presenting part is in the vulvar outlet.

REFERENCES

Calkins, L. A.: Premature spontaneous rupture of the membranes. Amer. J. Obstet. Gynec. *64*:871, 1952.

Friedman, E. A.: Labor: Clinical Evaluation and Management. New York, Appleton-Century-Crofts, 1967.

Friedman, E. A.: The functional divisions of labor. Amer. J. Obstet. Gynec. *109*:274, 1971.

Friedman, E. A.: High risk labor. J. Reprod. Med. 7:28, 1971.

Jeffcoate, T. N. A., Baker, K., and Martin, R. H.: Inefficient uterine action. Surg. Gynec. Obstet. 95:257, 1952.

Oldham, H.: A rare case of midwifery. Guy's Hosp. Rep. 5:108, 1847.

Chapter 56

Disordered Cephalic Mechanisms

The mechanisms of normal labor are detailed in Chapter 18. A thorough understanding of the material is essential before one attempts to grasp the nuances of the important irregularities in the mechanisms of labor that are found so commonly in clinical practice.

PERSISTENT OCCIPUT POSTERIOR POSITION

Clinical Course and Diagnosis

Occasionally during descent, the fetal head will not undergo normal internal rotation so that the occiput will come to lie beneath the symphysis pubis; rather, rotation will take place in such a way that the occiput will turn toward the sacrum. This condition may persist well into the second stage. The pathologic condition of *persistent occiput posterior* is distinguishable from the more common and usually innocuous occiput posterior position of early labor. The latter generally corrects itself during the course of labor, most often late in the active phase of dilatation, by internal rotation through a long arc to an occiput anterior position. The subsequent mechanism of labor is entirely normal after rotation has occurred.

The mechanisms of labor associated with persistent occiput posterior positions are depicted in Figure 309. Engagement may take place with the fetal head assuming any variant of posterior oblique or transverse occiput position, usually with some degree of deflexion. During subsequent descent, internal rotation takes place through the short arc, bringing the occiput to the sacrum. The head is brought under the symphysis by flexion along the curvature of the lower pelvis and is delivered over the distended perineum face up. After the head is delivered, restitution occurs as the head aligns with the shoulders once again. External rotation follows as the shoulders internally rotate. The mechanisms of delivery of the shoulders and the rest of the body are the same as for occiput anterior position.

In persistent occipitoposterior positions the progress of labor may be slowed toward the end of the first stage and during the second stage. Dilatation of the cervix proceeds well to the deceleration phase, but may be prolonged beyond that or even arrested. Descent may also be impeded because the head does not fit well into the pelvis. Spontaneous delivery requires more uterine and abdominal effort than for a comparable occiput anterior mechanism.

Perineal lacerations are common unless the fetus is small or the woman is a multipara. They occur because the head presents larger planes than usual and also because the perineum is forcibly dislocated downward. The presenting fetal diameter is the occipitofrontal rather than the suboccipitobregmatic of the occiput anterior (see Chapter 18), a difference of 2.5 to 3.0 cm.

In thin women, the diagnosis may sometimes be made abdominally because of the distinctive hollow over the pubis. Palpation reveals the shoulder far back from the midline, and probably the forehead and chin are found over the opposite pubic ramus. The heart tones are deep in the flank and distant from the ear unless, as often occurs, there is some deflexion of the fetal head and straightening of the spine which pushes the chest forward against

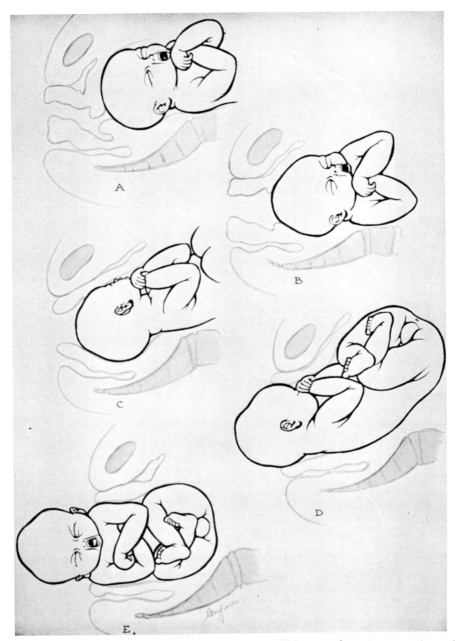

Figure 309 Diagrammatic representation of the mechanisms of labor in right occiput posterior position as it evolves into an occipitosacral or direct posterior position. *A*, Engagement of deflexed head in right oblique diameter with occiput posterior. *B*, Descent with partial internal rotation of the occiput to the posterior, but with little flexion. *C*, Internal rotation completed to the occipitosacral position. *D*, Flexion of head in the pelvic outlet under the symphysis and delivery over the perineum. *E*, Restitution and external rotation.

the abdominal wall and makes the heart tones loud and distinct. The heart tones are then on the same side as the forehead, that is, opposite to where the back is felt. This finding may give an erroneous diagnosis of face or of brow presentation be-

cause the physician may believe that the occiput is on the wrong side.

Vaginally, early in labor the head is felt up high. Usually, it is partly deflexed and the small posterior fontanel is higher or on the same level as the large one, which is nearer the center of the pelvis. The head is usually synclitic. If anterior rotation is going to occur, flexion takes place with descent. The tendency of the small fontanel to turn to the front during the contractions will be discovered on palpation, or it will be easy to push the occiput in this direction. If posterior rotation is to be the mechanism, the head descends in moderate extension. As the occiput turns into the hollow of the sacrum, the small fontanel is found deep on the rectovaginal septum and the large fontanel is behind the pubis. The sagittal suture occupies the midline. This variant of the occiput posterior position with the occiput in the midline, directed toward the sacrum, is called the *direct occiput posterior* or *occipitosacral position*. If extreme flexion occurs, the large fontanel is felt just under the pubis; if there is extension, the large fontanel lies in the center of the pelvis and the glabella will be felt behind the pubis.

Because of the usually large caput succedaneum which tends to develop here, it is not always easy to outline the sutures. Under these difficulties, a finger should be passed to the side until the ear is found; the direction of the tragus will reveal the diagnosis. The head is sometimes delivered with the occiput directed posteriorly over the perineum, when the reverse mechanism was anticipated.

Prognosis

Occiput posterior position *per se* does not produce a significant increase in either maternal morbidity or infant mortality (Calkins) unless it persists into the second stage and is associated with protraction or arrest of descent or an operative delivery. Since most occiput posterior positions rotate spontaneously to anterior positions and delivery is uneventful, the risks are small. The troublesome cases are those in which the occiput remains persistently posterior in spite of a long labor. In such cases delivery may sometimes be difficult and attended with extensive maternal lacerations and damage to the fetus. This is particularly true if the correct diagnosis is not made before instruments are applied for the delivery.

Treatment

When the fetal head is high, floating above the pelvis, a complete examination is made to determine the possibility of a contracted pelvis or other anomaly which may require specific treatment. Pelvimetric techniques are discussed in Chapter 12. During the first stage, the woman may be permitted to walk around until the head engages.

After the head has engaged, most cases undergo internal rotation to an anterior or obliquely anterior position, followed in due course by spontaneous delivery or easy forceps operation. The fetal head in the occipitosacral position often requires assistance. Techniques for manual rotation are described in Chapter 73; forceps rotation is detailed in Chapter 75. If the head is descending with good flexion, the perineum is not endangered as much as when the brow comes down and the head is partially extended. In either case a deep episiotomy is indicated unless the patient is a multipara with easily distended perineal tissues.

If the head is already on the perineum, forceps can be applied and delivery accomplished without rotating the occiput anteriorly. Forceps rotation through 180° for persistent occiput posterior position with the head on the perineum does not appear to be warranted because it will likely traumatize the mother or fetus. It is difficult to rationalize this result if the rotation is being done ostensibly to avert such trauma due to the aberrant position.

DEFLEXION ATTITUDES

Often during an examination early in labor, the deflexed head is found lying over the inlet with the large anterior fontanel lower than the small posterior one. The root of the nose and the eyes may even be palpable. After labor becomes established, the small fontanel will usually advance and a normal mechanism will ensue. Should the cause of the abnormal attitude of partial extension persist, the uterus will fix the trunk and body so that

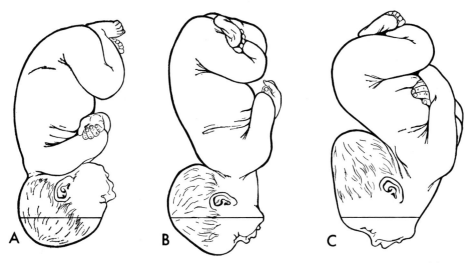

Figure 310 Gamut of deflexion attitudes from (*A*) sincipital and (*B*) brow presentations to (*C*) face presentation, showing altered presenting fetal diameter from occipitobregmatic to mentobregmatic to trachelobregmatic.

flexion cannot occur. A pathologic mechanism will result.

Three deflexion attitudes are recognized as distinct presentations. Each has a clearly defined course and mechanism. In the order of their degree of deflexion, they are *sincipital, brow* and *face* presentations (Fig. 310). The fetal trunk becomes extended to an S shape in these presentations instead of its normal flexed condition or C configuration.

Sincipital Presentation

With slight deflexion, labor is similar to that in occiput posterior positions. The occiput is still considered the point of reference. Sometimes in abnormal mechanisms, the forehead descends and becomes the point of reference, making it a brow presentation (see below), and potentially much more hazardous.

Labor may be long in association with sincipital presentations. Usually, however, after the head reaches the pelvic floor, the contractions improve, flexion takes place and the head is expelled without further difficulty.

Abdominally, the usual diagnostic points for determining presentation and position will reveal that the trunk of the fetus is straight and that the heart tones are near the midline. The shoulder is also in the midline, just above the pubis, and the occiput and chin are on about the same level. Internally, the two fontanels are found in the same plane, with the sagittal suture often transverse in the pelvis. Usually, the head is synclitic.

Treatment of labor with sincipital presentation is the same as for occiput posterior positions (see above).

Brow Presentation

Transitory presentation of the brow in the beginning of labor is occasionally observed. Descent of the occiput usually occurs as the head engages in the pelvis; the brow presentation is converted into a vertex presentation and a more normal mechanism results. Sometimes, further extension occurs and, as the deflexion is completed, a face presentation is produced.

Brow presentation occurs about twice as frequently in multiparas as in nulliparas. This may be because the decreased abdominal and pelvic muscular tone predisposes to an abnormal fetopelvic axis. Contracted pelves may partially explain the difficulties encountered when the fetus is above average in size. Prematurity is also common (Meltzer et al.), especially among nulliparas with brow presentations. Face and brow presentations may be due to ex-

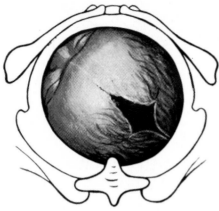

Figure 311 Details of palpatory findings in brow presentation, right bregma anterior position, showing large, centrally located anterior fontanel and root of nose within reach.

cessive tone in the extensor muscles of the fetal back and the neck (White).

Abdominally, the diagnostic findings are the same as in face presentations, with an elongated uterine ovoid and the cephalic prominence felt on the same side as the fetal back (see below). Vaginally (Fig. 311), the bregma is the lowest point and occupies the center of the pelvis. The large anterior fontanel is palpable on one side, and the root of the nose and orbital ridges are palpable on the other side. The nose, mouth and chin are up high and out

of reach unless the examination is being done with the patient anesthetized. The orbital ridges are on a level with the posterior border of the large fontanel.

Molding is characteristic. The head acquires a three-cornered outline. The face is flattened; the distance from the chin to the top of the forehead is great and this is exaggerated temporarily by the large caput succedaneum, as shown in Figure 312.

As to prognosis, brow presentation is especially dangerous to a large fetus because of operative intervention, prolonged and difficult labor and infection. The high fetal mortality is due to injuries sustained as a result of operative procedures or to the consequences of labor and delivery, including hypoxia, excessive cranial compression with tentorial or falx tears, and compression of the neck against the pubis with fracture of the trachea and larynx.

The treatment of brow presentation is intelligent expectancy because spontaneous extension to face presentation or flexion to vertex presentation will usually take place in the course of a normal, progressive labor. Subsequent vaginal delivery as an occiput or face presentation can be expected. This course of action should not be followed when the pelvis is contracted and the fetus is large. Cesarean section should be performed early in labor under these circumstances.

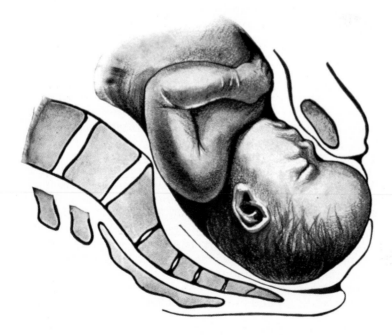

Figure 312 Schematic illustration of brow presentation, bregma anterior, demonstrating deflexion attitude and large caput succedaneum formation.

Those patients undergoing spontaneous conversion during labor cease to be a problem. The high success rate of attempted operative conversions in the remainder gives an optimistic outlook. The attempt should be made in all instances. Selection of proper timing is important. As long as labor is progressing normally in dilatation and descent, there seems to be no urgent reason to interfere. If arrest of dilatation in the active phase or of descent in the second stage should occur, action is indicated.

True cephalopelvic disproportion must first be ruled out. One should then attempt manual or, if unsuccessful, forceps conversion. Manual conversion is described in Chapter 73. Where conversion succeeds, further management will depend on the conditions prevailing. This includes allowing additional labor so as to permit the second stage to evolve fully and to avoid unnecessary, potentially traumatic operative delivery procedures.

Cesarean section is indicated for the ominous combination of secondary arrest and disproportion, as well as for failed conversion attempts following arrest. In all other instances, vaginal delivery should be anticipated. After conversion, second stage arrest of descent in the midpelvis without disproportion sometimes warrants trial midforceps. In the majority of cases, however, under a conservative regimen, delivery ought to be either spontaneous or by low forceps (Meltzer et al.).

Face Presentation

When the deflexion is carried to its greatest degree, the entire face comes to lie in the presenting plane (Fig. 313) so that it is bounded by the girdle of resistance and is felt on vaginal examination. This is face presentation, which occurs about three times as often in multiparas as in nulliparas. Monstrosities, especially anencephaly, account for about five per cent of face presentations. Cephalopelvic disproportion is commonly coassociated. Prematurity is also frequently encountered (Dede and Friedman). The chin or *mentum* is the point of reference. Mentum positions occur in the order of frequency of the occipital positions from which they develop; for example, since left occiput transverse is the usual position the head takes on entering the pelvis, the deflexion

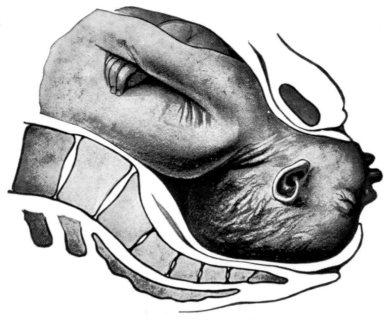

Figure 313   Face presentation with mentum anterior position, showing extreme extension of the fetal head under the symphysis and beginning flexion as the face is delivered over the perineum. Compare with Figure 317.

of the chin will bring the face down in a right mentum transverse position.

As a rule, face presentations are fully developed only after labor has been in progress for some time. Face presentations are commonly associated with normal progress in labor (Dede and Friedman). Delays or obstructed progress in labor are due to coassociated factors, such as sedation, anesthesia and disproportion, that will influence the course of labor regardless of presentation.

Diagnosis. Abdominally, the ovoid of the uterus is longitudinal, decidedly elongated, and the flanks are flat. The shape of the uterus alone may sometimes be sufficient for diagnosis. The head is felt over the inlet. The breech and the small parts are felt in the fundus. It is often difficult to outline the back.

A hard, round prominence, the occiput, is felt to one side and above the inlet on the same side as the back. It is separated from the back by a deep furrow. On the other side, the inlet is empty but, if the abdominal wall is relaxed, deep pressure with the fingers will elicit a horseshoe-shaped jaw. Great importance is attached to finding the feet, heart tones and chest on the same side. If a large, hard prominence with a sharp groove above it is felt over the inlet on the other side, face or at least brow presentation is certain. The heart tones may be unusually loud.

Vaginally, the pelvis is empty early in labor. The brow is felt up high, even in nulliparas, and it is generally movable. The anterior orbit, if not the root of the nose, is also felt. As soon as the membranes rupture, there is usually no difficulty in recognizing the eyes, nose, mouth and jaw (Fig. 314). Late in labor, when the caput succedaneum has obscured its characteristic features, the face becomes indistinguishable from the breech. When an irregular surface with prominences and depressions is felt with the finger, the examiner knows at once that the vertex is not the presenting part.

In differential diagnosis, breech presentation, brow presentation and anencephalic monsters must be considered. If the face is so swollen that the landmarks are obliterated, two points still remain: the saddle of the nose and the gums.

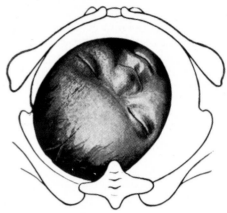

Figure 314   Findings on palpation of face presentation, left mentum anterior position, demonstrating the characteristic features of the brow, nose, ocular orbits, mouth and chin.

An important point in the diagnosis is the determination of the station. The head is engaged only when the biparietal diameter has passed the inlet. In occipital presentations, the parietal bosses are just below the plane of the inlet when the lowest part of the head, the vertex, is at or below the plane of the ischial spines. However, in face presentation, when the brow or the root of the nose (that is, the lowest portion of the presenting part) lies in this plane, the parietal bosses are still several centimeters above the plane of the inlet (Fig. 315). Only when the face is deep down on the pelvic floor and distending it may the head be considered to be engaged.

When internal examinations are made in face presentations, one must try to avoid the introduction of vaginal mucus and antiseptic solutions into the eyes of the fetus. Rectal examination may suffice for the diagnosis, but it is usually inadequate and a vaginal exploration is required. Roentgenograms should be taken early to disclose the presence of a fetal anomaly or cephalopelvic disproportion. Both are encountered in association with face presentations.

The head is usually engaged as a brow presentation first (Borell and Fernström). As the fetal head descends through the birth canal, it undergoes further extension, resulting in spontaneous conversion to a face presentation. Labor is generally un-

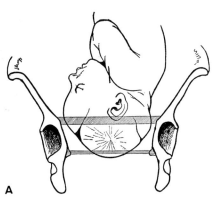
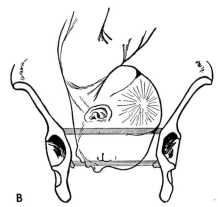

A   **B**

Figure 315   Diagrams showing relative degrees of engagement of vertex (*A*) and face (*B*) presentations when the forward leading edge has advanced to the plane of the ischial spines. The parietal bosses are at or below the inlet with the vertex presentation, but well above the inlet in the face presentation.

complicated in these cases because a comparatively favorable diameter of the fetal head, the trachelobregmatic, is presenting.

The molding of the fetal head in face presentations causes the parietal bones to be depressed, unlike vertex presentations in which the parietals are elevated. Molding generally starts when the fetal head is in the upper part of the birth canal. It is of major importance in labor, for it may result in a significant reduction in the dimensions of the presenting part. Internal rotation from the mentum transverse to the mentum anterior position (Fig. 313) takes place in the lower midpelvis at the same level as comparable rotation in vertex presentation.

The face is often disfigured (Fig. 316), especially if labor has been prolonged after the membranes have ruptured. Caput forms over the anterior cheek and eye and the whole face is involved; the eyes bulge out, the lids are swollen, a mucoserous discharge escapes from the eyes, the mouth is open because the lips are tumid and the tongue sometimes protrudes. Minute hemorrhages under the conjunctiva and the skin, intense venous congestion and cracks in the skin of the neck give the child a most discouraging appearance. The shape of the head is extremely dolichocephalic. The child lies on its side, with its head extended and its back straight; it may keep this attitude for two weeks. The mother should be reassured that the child's features will soon regain their proper appearance.

Prognosis.   Face presentation is pathologic in many cases. Maternal morbidity is higher than that of average deliveries because of the longer labor, the greater danger of infection, the increased frequency of contracted pelves and the operative intervention so often done. The infant mortality is also higher and is due to the same factors as in brow presentation (see above). Edema of the glottis and fracture of the larynx have been reported and should be carefully watched for in the neonate.

Diagnosis is not established until delivery in nearly half the cases, and few are discovered by abdominal examination

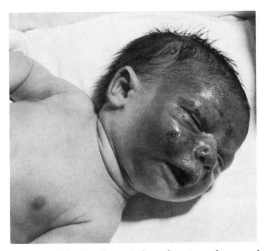

Figure 316   Newborn infant showing edema and suffusion of blood into subcutaneous tissue, especially over the anterior cheek and eye, as a result of face presentation. (Courtesy of E. L. Potter.)

(Dede and Friedman). Factors which affect the course of labor with vertex presentation act similarly in these cases. Progress is influenced not so much by the face presentation as by associated phenomena, particularly fetopelvic disproportion.

Delivery is spontaneous in two-thirds of cases and by cesarean section in about 20 per cent. There is a higher rate of operative intervention among mentum transverse and posterior presentations. This is especially true among patients with very large babies.

Treatment. Not all face presentations require special treatment. The majority can terminate spontaneously and without assistance, if allowed to do so. First, if possible, the cause of the face presentation must be determined. A contracted pelvis requires cesarean section. In the absence of special indications, intelligent expectancy should be pursued. Patience usually will be rewarded by either a spontaneous delivery or sufficient descent and anterior rotation so that forceps may be applied easily and safely.

More active conduct may be advisable if the chin is posterior to the transverse diameter of the pelvis, although in about half the cases the chin rotates to the anterior spontaneously. If the head remains high with the chin posterior, in spite of good contractions, a conversion procedure (Chapter 73) may be attempted; if unsuccessful, a cesarean section should be done.

When the head is engaged in the pelvis with the chin in the transverse diameter or even anterior to it, vaginal delivery may be feasible. After the fetal head has descended to the pelvic floor in the second stage, a forceps procedure may be undertaken. Before applying forceps, however, one should attempt to complete the rotation of the chin anteriorly by manipulation with the fingers. Purchase is obtained on the posterior malar and frontal bones and, during a contraction, gentle traction upward and forward is exerted with the fingers in an attempt to bring the chin under the pubis. This maneuver is aided by external abdominal pressure on the occiput over Poupart's ligament. If rotation can be completed in this way, the delivery may occur spontaneously or, at least, the forceps operation becomes easier, simpler and safer.

If the chin lies posteriorly to the transverse diameter or has turned toward the sacrum (Fig. 317), attempts to effect a vaginal delivery will almost certainly yield

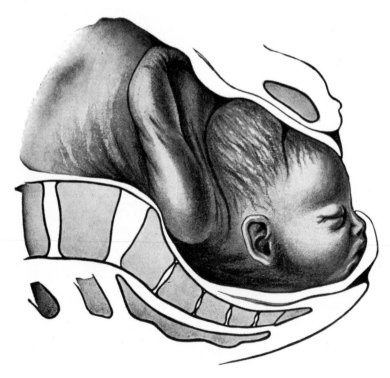

Figure 317 Face presentation with the particularly hazardous mentum posterior position. The fetal chin has rotated into the hollow of the sacrum and the head is fully extended. Vaginal delivery would require further extension and is, therefore, impossible unless rotation to mentum anterior position can be done.

a dead child. A cesarean section should be performed for the mentum posterior position when conversion cannot be accomplished or attempts at rotation to mentum anterior are unsuccessful.

In all spontaneous and operative face deliveries, the diameters and circumferences presented to the pelvic outlet are not as favorable as in vertex deliveries. The pelvic floor is pushed farther downward and may undergo damage. Deep episiotomy is almost always needed and is recommended to avert both maternal and fetal injuries.

REFERENCES

Borell, U., and Fernström, I.: The mechanism of labour in face and brow presentation: A radiological study. Acta Obstet. Gynec. Scand. 39:626, 1960.

Calkins, L. A.: Occiput posterior: A normal presentation. Amer. J. Obstet. Gynec. 43:277, 1942.

Calkins, L. A.: Occiput posterior presentation. Obstet. Gynec. 1:466, 1953.

Dede, J. A., and Friedman, E. A.: Face presentation. Amer. J. Obstet. Gynec. 87:515, 1963.

Meltzer, R. M., Sachtleben, M. R., and Friedman, E. A.: Brow presentation. Amer. J. Obstet. Gynec. 100:225, 1968.

White, T. G.: Deflexion attitudes of the foetus *in utero*, with special reference to the aetiology and diagnosis of face and brow presentation. J. Obstet. Gynaec. Brit. Emp. 61:302, 1954.

Chapter 57

Breech Presentation

About 3.5 per cent of deliveries are breech presentations. Since the consequent infant mortality is higher than in vertex presentations and the maternal morbidity is decidedly greater, breech presentations should be considered to be potentially abnormal. Their cause is unknown and subject to considerable conjecture. Coassociation with prematurity, placenta previa, multiple pregnancy and fetal malformations has been noted. Fetal hydrocephalus and anencephaly are especially incriminated (Potter and Adair). It is possible that extension of the fetal legs may somehow be etiologic also (Vartan).

NOMENCLATURE

There are several varieties of breech presentation according to the attitude or posture of the fetus: (1) *frank* or *single breech,* (2) *complete* or *double breech* and (3) *incomplete breech.* In frank breech presentations (Fig. 318), the legs are extended against the trunk and the feet lie against the face. This is by far the most frequent type. In the complete breech, the fetus maintains the same attitude as in vertex, but with reversed polarity. The thighs are flexed against the body and the forelegs flexed on the thighs so that the but-

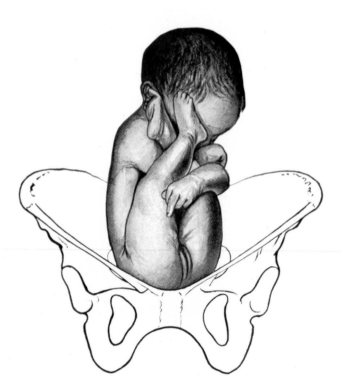

Figure 318 Fetus in frank or single breech presentation, right sacrum posterior position, with lower extremities extended fully across abdomen, chest and face.

598

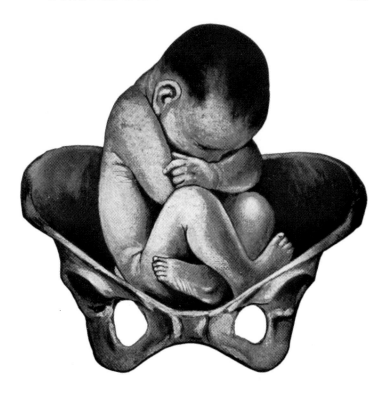

Figure 319 Fetus shown in complete or double breech presentation with buttocks and both feet presenting in the pelvic inlet, right sacrum posterior position. Compare with Figure 318.

tocks, with the feet alongside them, present at the internal os (Fig. 319). Incomplete breech is of two types: (1) one foot or both feet prolapse into the vagina producing single or double *footling presentation* and (2) one or both knees are prolapsed.

It is possible to distinguish six positions of breech presentation, analogous to those of other presentations. Two are most often seen, namely, left sacrum anterior and right sacrum posterior. The point of reference is the sacrum. In following the mechanism of labor, the genital crease is used for orientation in the same way as the sagittal suture or the facial line is used for occipital and face presentations, respectively.

MECHANISM OF LABOR

With very little variation, the mechanism of labor (Fig. 320) is the same whether the breech is frank, complete or incomplete. Let us consider what takes place in the left sacrum anterior position or

L.S.A. Even in nulliparas, the breech sometimes remains high in the pelvis until labor is well advanced and dilatation of the cervix is completed. *Descent* may be somewhat slow because the soft breech cannot wedge itself into the vagina as firmly as does the head, but normal rates of descent should be expected under normal conditions. *Lateral flexion* occurs as soon as the breech reaches the perineum. The posterior buttock is held back and the anterior buttock stems under the pubis. This movement is always associated with *internal anterior rotation*.

In L.S.A., the breech descends in the left oblique; that is, the bisiliac diameter lies in the left oblique diameter of the pelvis, the genital crease lies in the right and the anterior hip points to the right iliopubic tubercle and is a little deeper in the pelvis than the posterior hip. This is *anterior asynclitism* and it is analogous to the obliquity of Nägele (see Chapter 18). Anterior rotation occurs as the anterior hip rotates to the anterior midline from the right anterior quadrant of the pelvis and the sacrum points directly to the left side; the genital fissure now lies transversely.

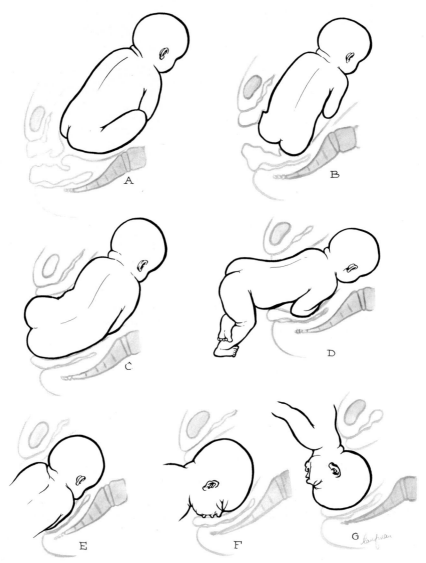

Figure 320   Diagrammatic sequence of steps in the mechanism of labor in the breech presentation, left sacrum anterior position. *A*, Engagement of the breech in the oblique diameter high in the pelvis, where it may remain until well into labor. *B*, Descent into the midplane with internal anterior rotation to left sacrum transverse position. *C*, Lateroflexion of the fetal pelvis until delivered over the perineum. *D*, Delivery of the legs and the body to the umbilicus with rotation of the back anteriorly. *E*, Delivery of the shoulders. *F*, Beginning delivery of the head with the occiput anterior under the symphysis pubis. *G*, Delivery of the head over the perineum with the body supported.

The causes of this movement are the same as in the other presentations.

Delivery involves continued *lateroflexion* as the anterior hip stems under the symphysis pubis; the posterior hip rolls over the perineum, and the whole fetal pelvis rises up over the pubis. *Restitution* and *external rotation* are not constant in breech presentation. Usually, the anterior hip turns again to the right side and the sacrum comes to lie directly anterior. Sometimes, the back remains in the transverse position and the shoulders are delivered in this position. Now the legs drop down and the back again lies in the oblique.

The movements of the shoulders are precisely the same as those of the breech. Descent occurs with the bisacromial diameter in the left oblique. If no attempt is made to aid delivery by traction from below, the arms lie folded closely against the chest. Strong contractions and good abdominal muscular exertion are needed for delivery of the shoulder girdle. The anterior shoulder rotates in the right anterior quadrant of the pelvis toward the pubis and stems behind it. By a process of lateroflexion, the posterior shoulder and arm are delivered. Then the anterior shoulder appears from behind the pubis and, if no assistance is given, the body drops down so that the neck is against the perineum and the nape of the neck is against the subpubic ligament. If the head is arrested high, restitution and external rotation take place and the back again rotates to the side. If the head follows the body closely and drops into the pelvis, the back may rotate to the front immediately.

Under normal circumstances, the head enters the inlet when the shoulders are passing the vulva. The head then undergoes the expected mechanisms. Descent, flexion and anterior rotation of the occiput occur in order. The sagittal suture enters in the right oblique as it does in left occiput anterior positions. When the chin has rotated to the hollow of the sacrum,

flexion occurs (Fig. 321). The nape of the neck stems centrally under the symphysis pubis, and the chin, face and forehead appear successively over the perineum. After this, the occiput escapes from behind the pubis. In sacrum posterior positions, the mechanism is nearly the same. The anterior buttock must rotate only 45° to reach the pubis.

UNUSUAL MECHANISMS

Occasionally, after the breech is delivered, the back overrotates beyond the pubis to the other side of the pelvis. Here the mechanism is similar to that of the shoulders in head presentations. The remainder of the fetus may appear with the back on the side opposite to that in which it started.

Even excessive internal anterior rotation of the breech may occur with the fetal abdomen facing toward the pubis. Subsequently, the shoulders enter in an oblique diameter and the proper mechanism is resumed. It is usually not possible to

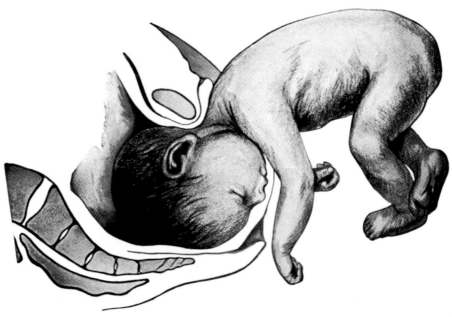

Figure 321   Lateral view showing best mechanism for delivering the well-flexed after-coming head. Note the occiput located anteriorly with the nape of the neck stemming just under the symphysis pubis. The face will be delivered over the perineum by further flexion as expulsive efforts are used and the body is elevated above the horizontal plane.

discover the cause of these irregular mechanisms.

Footling presentation undergoes the normal mechanisms unless the posterior foot has prolapsed. In all labors the tendency is for the lowest or leading portion of the presenting part to slip under the pubic arch. The construction of the front part of the pelvis and the arrangement of the sacrosciatic ligaments and the levator ani muscles are such that any movable body placed on these inclined planes and propelled from above tends to go in one direction. Thus, when the anterior leg has prolapsed, the breech glides along without difficulty. However, when the posterior leg has prolapsed, the breech is held higher, the anterior buttock impinges on the anterior ramus of the pubis and the posterior leg is prevented from reaching the anterior inclined plane. It finds a path of less resistance on the other side of the pelvis, and often the back rotates to face the sacrum. The posterior limb now becomes the anterior one and follows out the usual mechanism, but on the other side of the pelvis.

Abnormal rotation of the back is infrequent unless premature traction is made on the trunk. If the back does not rotate to the front, but to the sacrum instead, the fetus descends with its abdomen upward toward the mother's pubis. Usually, the uterine and abdominal muscle powers are insufficient to deliver the fetus in this position. Birth may be accomplished spontaneously with the shoulders being forced out in the transverse diameter, the elbows and arms falling from behind the pubis and anterior rotation of the trunk occurring late. As a rule, the head then causes the most trouble. If it turns so that the occiput is in the hollow of the sacrum and the chin faces the pubis, further progress may stop. Unless the physician intervenes, the fetus may die.

If left unattended, nature deals with the aftercoming posterior head in one of three ways: (1) If the head comes down well flexed with the chin applied to the sternum, anterior rotation of the occiput may occur. (2) If the head is relatively small and flexed (Fig. 322), delivery with the occiput posterior can occur. The root of the nose stems behind the pubis. The nape of the neck, occiput and vertex roll over or through the perineum, and then the face drops from behind the pubis. This mode of

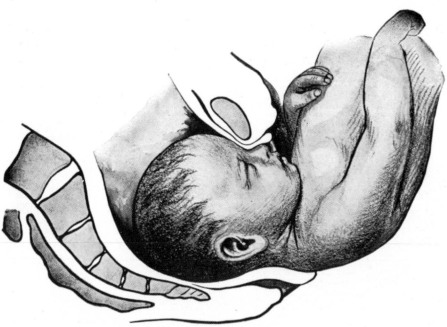

Figure 322   Less favorable mechanism for delivering the after-coming head in the occiput posterior position. The bridge of the nose stems under the symphysis pubis and delivery of the head will take place by the occiput crossing over or through the perineum. Compare with Figure 321.

delivery is facilitated by lifting the body of the child upward. (3) If the head is extended, the chin may be caught on the pubic ramus above the inlet. By lifting the child, one allows the occiput, vertex and forehead to pass over the perineum with the anterior neck forming the center of rotation. However, this cannot be accomplished without assistance.

In frank breech presentations, delivery is more difficult because the legs, extended against the body, act like a splint and interfere with the flexibility of the fetal cylinder. Therefore, descent and flexion are slow and difficult. To be considered also are the small size of the advancing wedge, which results in imperfect preparation of the soft parts, delay and danger in the passage of the shoulders and head, early rupture of the membranes and often weak labor contractions.

Labor is complicated when the fetal arms leave the chest and are stretched up over the head or even crossed behind the occiput in the nape of the neck. This so-called *nuchal arm* or *nuchal hitch* constitutes a serious obstetric problem. These cases require close, skilled attention (see Chapter 74).

CLINICAL COURSE

No consistent differences are found between labors associated with breech presentation and those associated with vertex presentation (Dunn et al.; Roth). The course of labor with breech presentation is essentially the same as in comparable vertex presentations insofar as cervical dilatation and descent are concerned (Friedman). Dysfunctional patterns can be expected with a large fetus and a relatively small pelvis. The appearance of an aberrant dilatation or descent pattern (see Chapter 55) is especially ominous and should serve to alert the obstetrician to the probability of fetopelvic disproportion.

Premature rupture of the membranes is common. Escaping meconium during breech deliveries has no significance. It is expressed for the same reason that the caput succedaneum forms; the meconium is pressed out in the direction of least resistance by the intrauterine pressure generated during labor contractions. Caput succedaneum is found on the anterior hip but may spread all over the buttocks. In boys, the penis and scrotum may be extremely edematous and ecchymotic. In girls, there may be a moderate vulvitis for a few days. If a leg has been down for any length of time, minute hemorrhages and severe congestion and swelling are present. All of these disappear within a week.

Ordinarily, the child's head, which is not molded, presents the round or square shape it had *in utero*. However, there may be distinct molding of the head. It may take the form of a dolichocephalus, the head having been pressed down by the fundus, or either side of the head may be flattened. This feature may reflect intrauterine hyperextension of the fetal head which is seen so commonly (Wilcox). Hyperextension may be of no great significance because most cases seem to correct themselves spontaneously in the course of labor; however, if uncorrected, spinal cord damage may be inflicted in the course of vaginal delivery (see below). Often the side of the head which was anterior against the abdominal wall will be flattened.

In oligohydramnios, the sternocleidomastoid and other neck muscles on the side opposite that showing the flattening may be shortened and atrophied and cause a wryneck. This congenital shortening is important because these muscles will tear or a hematoma or myositis will result if too much traction is applied to them during delivery. Wryneck may also result from faulty development, of course, but the same admonition applies.

DIAGNOSIS

Unless labor is advanced and the contractions are strong and frequent, making the uterus rigid, external abdominal examination should be sufficient for diagnosis. The ovoid is longitudinal, but the upper portion of the uterus is broader than the lower part. There is no hard, round body over the inlet; instead, one finds a soft yielding, irregular mass which slides upward from between the hands, allowing the hands almost to meet. Usually, the head is easily felt to one side of the fundus. If it is in the midline, it may be assumed that the body of the fetus has been straightened by the legs being stretched up toward the face. This indicates that there is a frank or single breech presentation.

The back is felt on one side and the shoulder is usually easily outlined above the umbilicus. Between the shoulders and the head, there is a deep sulcus. The heart tones are loudest on the side where the back lies and are always above the level of the umbilicus. This is an important diagnostic point. Often the head can be grasped between the hands or even measured with a cephalometer, but at other times it can be discerned only by ballottement (see Chapter 8).

The diagnosis of breech presentation can often be made on rectal examination, but a vaginal examination should be done for verification. The fingers may have to be inserted deep into the vagina before the presenting part can be touched, if the presenting part is high and the pelvis is empty. There is no convex hard mass in the vaginal vault; instead, a roundish, soft mass of prominences and depressions can be distinguished. This latter is the buttocks with a crease between them and at one end there is a pointed bone, the sacrum (Fig. 323).

The location of the sacrum indicates the

direction of the fetal pelvis, but for additional assurance the genital crease can be followed with the finger until the scrotum or vulva can be distinguished. If the finger is accidentally inserted into the anus, it may be covered with meconium. Higher up and to one side, one or both feet may be felt, although usually only the heels are within reach of the finger.

Mistakes are common in diagnosing the presence of breech presentation. The breech has been confused with a shoulder, a face and an anencephalus. Differentiating a foot from a hand is not easy (Fig. 324), but one can try to demonstrate the straight alignment of the toes contrasted with the curved line formed by the fingertips. Sometimes the heel can help distinguish the foot from the hand, but it is easy to be deluded when the fetal hand is folded back at the wrist. The closed axilla and the costal gridiron identify a shoulder presentation; the saddle of the nose, the orbital ridges, the nostrils and the gums identify a face presentation.

In frank or single breech, when the feet are extended up near the face, they may often be felt there abdominally. Vaginally, the feet cannot be felt. The anus is near the middle of the pelvis and the straightened thighs disclose the direction of the extremities. In footling presentation, the prolapsed extremity should be followed up to the pelvis of the fetus to make the diagnosis. The direction of the big toe and the flexure of the knee give added information. A hasty diagnosis of breech presentation should not be made if a foot is discovered because it may have prolapsed with the head in a compound presentation (see Chapter 59).

PROGNOSIS

The maternal morbidity is higher for breech than for occipital presentations. Perinatal loss associated with breech presentation is 12 to 15 per cent (Hall et al.). Much of the fetal loss is associated with prematurity, with a higher mortality occurring in premature breech births than in those at term (relative to premature and term vertex births). The aftercoming head is delivered through the unprepared pelvic floor and laceration of the perineum,

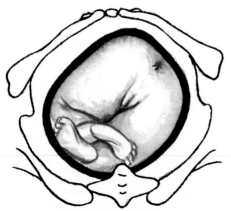

Figure 323 Composite tactile picture of the findings on vaginal examination in the complete breech presentation, left sacrum anterior position, with genital crease in the right oblique diameter, sacrum and anus in the left anterior quadrant and the feet palpable in the right posterior quadrant.

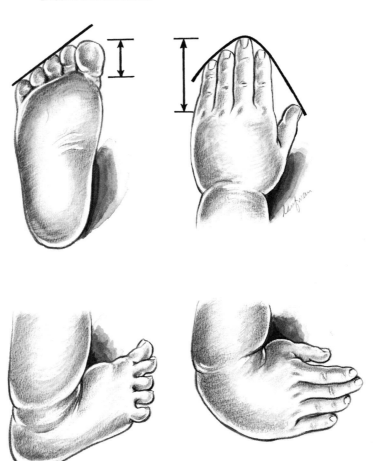

Figure 324 Features helpful in distinguishing the foot from the hand during vaginal examinations. The straight line formed by the toes is distinctive from the curve of the fingertips; the heel is sometimes recognizable as different from the wrist. (Redrawn from Beck and Rosenthal.)

often extending through the rectum, is frequent. Disturbances of the mechanism of labor often require operative measures. Most of these dangers can be eliminated by good obstetric judgment and use of skilled technique.

The chief causes of fetal death in breech presentations are prematurity, intracranial damage and asphyxia. Potter and Adair found intracranial hemorrhage in 43 per cent of autopsies on such babies. Cerebral hemorrhage and asphyxia result from difficulty in delivering the aftercoming head, usually because the cervix is not sufficiently dilated. Transection of the cervical spinal cord has been reported, especially in association with the hyperextended fetal head in breech delivery (Abroms et al.; Bhagwanani et al.). Asphyxia may also be caused by compression of the umbilical cord.

It is inevitable that there will be some cord compression in every breech birth. As the breech is delivered over the perineum, the fetal umbilicus enters the pelvic inlet, potentially compressing the cord at that point. Throughout the remainder of the delivery process, the cord is increasingly likely to be compressed between the fetal body and the maternal soft tissues or bones. Also, the cord may be compressed by its being stretched upward from between the fetal legs.

The progress of labor should not be too slow after the breech has passed the vulva, but undue haste must be avoided because of the danger of injury to the baby. The most frequent causes of infant death are rupture of the tentorium cerebelli and tears of the falx cerebri (see Chapter 68). These dangers are increased in parturients with rigid soft parts.

TREATMENT

If breech presentation is discovered during the last few weeks of pregnancy, it is not advisable to make any effort to bring the cephalic pole over the inlet by the procedure called *external cephalic version* (see Chapter 74). The maneuver is not without some intrinsic risk (Peel and Clayton) based on the possibility that it may cause a cord or placental accident or initiate premature labor. Moreover, many successfully turned babies will return to their previous presentation. Furthermore, spontaneous version from breech to vertex is very common (Vartan). The incidence of breech presentations in midpregnancy is about 25 per cent, most undergoing spontaneous version by the thirty-fourth week. Seldom do these fetuses return to the breech presentation.

Stevenson recommends that the implantation site of the placenta be determined in all cases of breech and shoulder presentation persisting after gestations of 30 to 32 weeks. The methods available for placental localization are discussed in Chapter 37. This knowledge is of great value because of the possibility of placenta previa in these cases.

Of utmost importance in the management of the breech delivery, especially in the nullipara, is thorough digital and x-ray evaluation of the pelvis (see Chapter 12). Accepting the limitation of x-ray pelvimetry, we are obligated to ensure that no fetopelvic disproportion exists. Cesarean section is indicated whenever any degree of disproportion can be documented in the patient in labor with a breech presentation. It is far better to err on the side of liberal indications for abdominal delivery than to risk serious fetal damage or even death from an overoptimistic interpretation of the fetopelvic relationships.

Zatuchni and Andros suggested a scoring system for purposes of recognizing potentially problematic cases. They considered the following features to indicate a poor outlook: large fetus over 8 pounds, high station of presenting part and little cervical dilatation in a nullipara at term. The smaller the fetus and the lower the station, the better the prognosis. No difficulty is anticipated with high score based on multiparity, prematurity and a history of previous term breech deliveries.

DELIVERY METHODS

There are three major variations in the techniques for vaginal delivery of the fetus in breech presentation. These include (1) *spontaneous breech delivery,* in which the entire fetus is expelled by uterine and abdominal muscle forces and no manipulation is done except for support of the infant (see the Bracht maneuver, Chapter 74); (2) *partial breech extraction* (often called *assisted breech delivery*), in which the fetus is extruded as far as the umbilicus by natural forces and the remainder of the body is extracted (see Chapter 74); and (3) *total breech extraction,* in which the entire body is extracted. When the term *breech extraction* is used without a qualifier, it is assumed to mean a total extraction.

Opinions differ as to whether or not spontaneous delivery should be permitted with breech presentations, or whether it is preferable to resort to partial breech extraction as a routine. In the hands of experienced obstetricians, it does not seem to matter which of these alternatives is used. However, there is complete agreement on one vital principle that must be fulfilled if one does intervene: There must be absolute certainty that the cervix is fully dilated before the fetus is extracted, or serious trouble will develop.

Spontaneous breech delivery is the safest procedure in the hands of general practitioners. With patience and the use of a deep episiotomy, breech presentations can be delivered spontaneously by most multiparas and by some nulliparas as well. This is especially true if the fetus is small and the pelvis ample.

Intelligent expectancy is the treatment of choice during labor. One must avoid hastening the processes of cervical dilatation and descent. The treatment of the first stage is as usual. When the second stage begins, everything should be made ready for an operative delivery.

When the breech reaches the perineum, the patient is placed on a delivery table and preparations made for vaginal deliv-

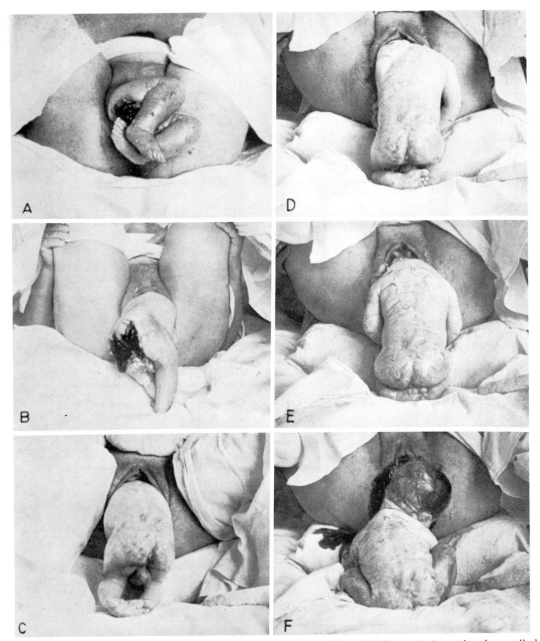

Figure 325 Sequence of photographs obtained at a spontaneous breech delivery. *A*, Legs already expelled and buttocks being delivered by lateroflexion with the breech in right sacrum transverse position. *B*, Body delivered to the umbilicus with external rotation to right sacrum anterior. *C*, Anterior rotation completed, fetal thorax delivered to the scapulas. *D*, Right shoulder and arm delivered, and left shoulder appearing. *E*, Baby delivered to the head. *F*, After-coming head in occiput anterior position expelled spontaneously over perineum by flexion. (Courtesy of H. Vermelin.)

ery. As the breech emerges, the physician should restrain from aiding by traction; instead, he should encourage the woman to bear down strongly. The breech or the foot, if it is down, is wrapped in a warm towel as it is delivered. Nothing more is done. The physician sits by and uses the head stethoscope to listen to the heart tones almost continuously. Continuous heart rate monitoring is preferable in order to detect and prevent asphyxia (Rovinsky et al.).

Local anesthesia is ideal here because the woman's fullest cooperation for further expulsion is required. A deep episiotomy is imperative before the breech is delivered. It saves delay in the delivery of the shoulders and the head. It may prevent severe perineal lacerations.

When the umbilicus appears, the rest of the birth should be enhanced by having the patient bear down with all her force. If the natural powers are successful, the baby is born as shown in the sequences in Figure 325. The physician may support the fetus as it emerges. He sponges the mucus out of the mouth when it first becomes visible in the vulva. He should gently restrain the head from passing through the pelvic floor too rapidly. The techniques used for aiding the delivery of the shoulders and the head when a delay occurs are detailed in Chapter 74. It is essential for every physician who is responsible for the delivery of breech presentations to become expert in these lifesaving maneuvers.

REFERENCES

Abroms, I. F., Bresnan, M. J., Zuckerman, J. E., Fischer, E. G., and Strand, R.: Cervical cord injuries secondary to hyperextension of the head in breech presentations. Obstet. Gynec. 41:369, 1973.

Bhagwanani, S. G., Price, H. V., Laurence, K. M., and Ginz, B.: Risks and prevention of cervical cord injury in the management of breech presentation with hyperextension of the fetal head. Amer. J. Obstet. Gynec. 115:1159, 1973.

Dunn, L., J., Van Voorhis, L., and Napier, J.: Term breech presentation: A report of 499 consecutive cases. Obstet. Gynec. 25:170, 1965.

Friedman, E. A.: Labor: Clinical Evaluation and Management. New York, Appleton-Century-Crofts, 1967.

Hall, J. E., Kohl, S. G., O'Brien, F., and Ginsburg, M.: Breech presentation and perinatal mortality: A study of 6,044 cases. Amer. J. Obstet. Gynec. 91:665, 1965.

Peel, J. H., and Clayton, S. G.: External version under anesthesia. J. Obstet. Gynaec. Brit. Emp. 55:614, 1948.

Potter, E. L., and Adair, F. L.: Clinical-pathological study of the infant and fetal mortality for a ten-year period at the Chicago Lying-in Hospital. Amer. J. Obstet. Gynec. 45:1054, 1943.

Roth, F.: Statistiche Auswertung von über 1,000 Beckenendlagen-Geburten. Schweiz. Med. Wschr. 91:1337, 1961.

Rovinsky, J. J., Miller, J. A., and Kaplan, S.: Management of breech presentation at term. Amer. J. Obstet. Gynec. 115:497, 1973.

Stevenson, C. S.: The principal causes of breech presentation in single term pregnancies. Amer. J. Obstet. Gynec. 60:41, 1950.

Stevenson, C. S.: Certain concepts in the handling of breech and transverse presentations in late pregnancy. Amer. J. Obstet. Gynec. 62:488, 1951.

Vartan, C. K.: The behavior of the foetus in utero, with special reference to the incidence of breech presentation at term. J. Obstet. Gynaec. Brit. Emp. 52:417, 1945.

Vartan, C. K.: Breech presentation and delivery. Clin. Obstet. Gynec. 2:390, 1959.

Wilcox, H. L.: The attitude of the fetus in breech presentation. Amer. J. Obstet. Gynec. 58:478, 1949.

Zatuchni, G. I., and Andros, G. J.: Prognostic index for vaginal delivery in breech presentation. Amer. J. Obstet. Gynec. 93:237, 1965.

Chapter 58

Transverse Lie

Another error of polarity of the fetus is *shoulder presentation* or *transverse lie* in which the long axis of the fetus crosses the long axis of the mother. The two terms are interchangeable, although the shoulder may not always be the presenting part over the pelvic inlet. The term *shoulder presentation* is used to correspond with vertex, face and breech presentation, and by analogy the point of reference is the acromial process of the shoulder. The use of the term *transverse lie* will avoid the confusion which frequently arises between the transverse presentation and the transverse position of the occiput in vertex presentations.

Rarely does the long axis of the fetus actually cross at a right angle; usually, the fetal cylinder is oblique to the mother's spine. This situation of an *oblique lie* is usually transitory in late pregnancy and is thus sometimes characterized as an *unstable lie*. Generally, the head is the lower pole, but the breech may be nearer the inlet.

ETIOLOGY

Shoulder presentation occurs about once in 300 to 400 deliveries (Johnson), much more often in multiparas than in nulliparas and more frequently in premature labor than at term. Anything that prevents engagement of the head in the pelvis and any condition that confers an extraordinary degree of mobility to the fetus may cause shoulder presentation.

The most important causes are contracted pelvis, placenta previa, obstructing pelvic tumor, multiple pregnancy, hydramnios and uterine and fetal anomalies.

Shoulder presentations occur twice as often with a contracted pelvis as with a normal pelvis. Anything in the pelvis which may prevent engagement, such as placenta previa, an ovarian tumor or leiomyoma, may result in a transverse lie. Placenta previa must especially be considered whenever a shoulder presentation is encountered. It was found to be present in 27 per cent of such patients studied by placentography (Stevenson). Hall et al. also found frequent coassociation of transverse lie with placenta previa and with contracted pelvis as well. They found prolapse of the umbilical cord to be common, but prematurity was the greatest single cause of perinatal loss, occurring in 32.2 per cent.

MECHANISM

Although either the back or the abdomen may lie across the inlet, the shoulder most often enters the pelvis first. On the shoulder, the following useful and diagnostic landmarks are distinguished: scapula, acromial process, axilla and clavicle. The acromial process is selected as the point of reference, as indicated above, for purposes of delineating the position relative to the pelvis. The left acromion anterior position is shown in Figure 326, with the head in the left lower uterine segment overlying the left iliac ala and the back facing anteriorly. One should note that it is the right arm that is presenting here; the nomenclature does not refer to the right or left shoulder, but rather to the direction of the acromial process in the pelvis.

The back-anterior positions, left and

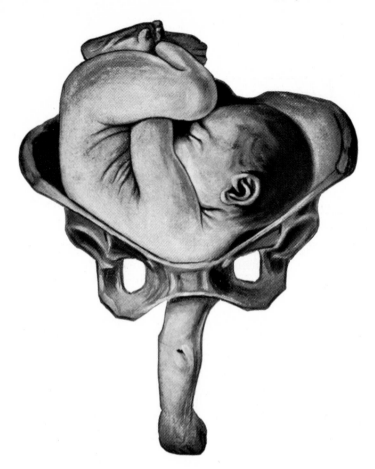

Figure 326 Schematic drawing of shoulder presentation, left acromion anterior position, in advanced labor with prolapsed right arm, head in the left iliac ala, back down and anteriorly located.

right acromion anterior, are common and are dealt with easily. The right and left acromion posterior positions, called back-posterior positions, are less common and there is much greater difficulty in dealing with them. The back may also lie with its convexity up so that the extremities and cord hang down; or the back may span the inlet with the extremities above in the upper uterine segment.

The attitude of the head and the limbs is characteristic. Early in labor the usual posture of flexion common to vertex presentations is present: the chin is on the sternum, the arms are crossed over the chest and the legs are crossed over the abdomen. Later, many changes may be observed. The most common of these is prolapse of the lower arm (Fig. 326) and the cord. When the uterus has contracted on the transversely placed fetal ovoid for any length of time, the fetus is compressed from side to side,

the head approaches the breech and the ovoid becomes more globular.

COURSE OF LABOR

Shoulder presentations are always pathologic and, therefore, may eventually demand aid. Early in pregnancy, transverse lie is the rule. Even in the last month, especially in multiparas, it is found occasionally, but it nearly always corrects itself before labor begins. This process is called *spontaneous rectification*.

In shoulder presentation, the uterine contractions are likely to be relatively infrequent and weak. The membranes often rupture early because they are exposed to the full force of the uterine contraction. After the membranes have ruptured, almost all the amniotic fluid escapes. As a result it is possible in due course for the uterus to become closely applied to the body of the fetus.

As labor progresses, uterine contractions become intensive. This may be brought about by manipulations. Such uterine activity forces the shoulder into the pelvis. The fetus is folded together, the breech approaches the head and the ovoid becomes still more globular. If the fetus is small or macerated and the pelvis is large enough, the uterus aided by powerful efforts on the part of the mother succeeds in expelling the fetus through the pelvis by a process called *spontaneous evolution* or *conduplicato corpore.* Spontaneous evolution is the least likely sequence of events under these circumstances and constitutes the most dangerous method nature has to overcome the malpresentation.

There are three types of spontaneous evolution, named for the men who described them: Roederer's, Douglas' and Denman's. Roederer's method usually occurs without prolapse of the arm. The fetus is folded like the letter V; the shoulder and back advance and the head is pressed deep into the chest and abdomen. Douglas' method occurs more often in back anterior positions with prolapse of the arm. The head is arrested above the inlet and rotates to the pubis. A greatly lengthened neck is applied to the pelvic brim. The chest, the abdomen and the breech roll down alongside the shoulder; the legs drop out; the other arm then delivers and finally the head appears. The rarest of the three mechanisms is Denman's, which is usually associated with back posterior positions. The head rotates behind and, as the breech descends, the shoulder ascends in the pelvis. This is actually a form of version taking place spontaneously in the pelvic cavity. The breech finally comes down and out. All three methods require exceptionally favorable conditions for success: a large pelvis, a small, soft molding fetus and strong uterine contractions. A full-term fetus cannot be delivered alive with any of them. These methods should never be relied on because the fetus is invariably lost and the mother is exposed to potentially fatal risks.

With obstructed labor, the contractions become irregular and tumultuous. The uterus may almost be in a state of constant contraction. The patient complains of constant pain and great tenderness over the lower part of the uterus. The pulse and temperature begin to rise. The uterus draws up over the fetus; the myometrium becomes thick in the upper segment and the lower segment is extremely thin. The uterus is likely to rupture under these circumstances (Fig. 327). This condition is called *neglected shoulder presentation.*

At the junction of the thick upper uterine segment and the thin lower uterine segment, there may be a groove or depression, the ominous *pathologic retraction ring.* Above this groove, no fetal parts can be distinguished by palpation; below it, the fetus is easily felt. Unless aid is given, the uterus ruptures and the mother may die of shock, hemorrhage or peritonitis. Fetal death usually occurs from interruption of placental circulation and cord compression before the uterus ruptures. If the fetus has not succumbed earlier, it dies after the rupture and it may be extruded in part or completely through the rent into the abdominal cavity. In order to avert such dire consequences, it is obvious that one must recognize when transverse lie exists and not allow it to evolve in this way.

DIAGNOSIS

Abdominally, there is no longitudinal ovoid, but a more or less transverse ovoid can be felt. There is nothing felt over the inlet. Likewise, nothing can be felt in the fundus. At best there are some small parts palpable or a deep furrow. The back is not in either flank. Since three of the four cardinal points for the diagnosis of presentation are negative, the diagnosis must rest on the observation of a transverse fetal ovoid. An x-ray or ultrasonogram will verify the diagnosis.

In left acromion anterior position (Fig. 326), the head will be on the left side, low in the flank. It is recognized as a large, hard, round mass, sometimes with ballottement. The breech is deep and up high to the right. The small parts are in the upper uterine segment to the right of the mid-

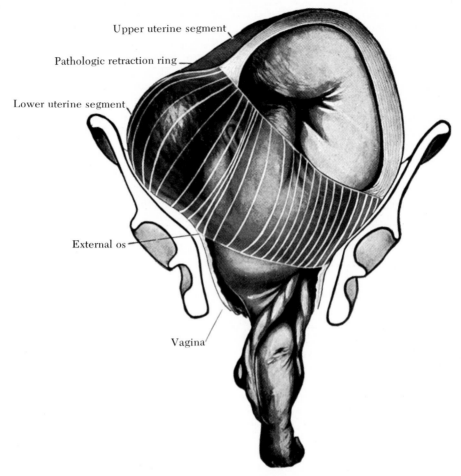

Upper uterine segment

Pathologic retraction ring

Lower uterine segment

External os

Vagina

Figure 327   The appearance of a neglected shoulder presentation, right acromion anterior position, with prolapsed cord and prolapsed left arm. The shoulder is tightly wedged into the pelvis and the uterus is shown at the point of rupturing. The thick upper uterine segment has retracted over the fetus and is separated from the greatly overdistended and thinned lower segment by the pathologic retraction ring.

line. The heart tones are loudest a little to the left and below the umbilicus.

In right acromion posterior position, the head is deep in the right flank. The breech is under the spleen. The back cannot be outlined; instead, the area under the umbilicus seems filled with small parts. The heart tones are to the right of the umbilicus and about on a level with it.

A vaginal examination is necessary for confirmation. An empty vaginal vault immediately suggests some abnormality. Sometimes, the forewaters hang down like a stocking, filling the pelvis. Any attempt to feel the fetus through the intact membranes may rupture them. This would be an unfortunate occurrence and should be

avoided, if possible. The cervix hangs down like the cuff of a sleeve. After labor has progressed for a while, the shoulder is more accessible and all the landmarks may be discernible.

The direction of the axilla (that is, its apex) points to the fetal head. By determining whether the hard edge of the fetal scapula points to the maternal pubis or to the sacrum, one is able to tell whether the back lies to the front or to the rear. In the left acromion anterior position, the apex of the axilla points to the left. The edge of the scapula lies to the front. The rib cage forms the costal gridiron to the rear (Fig. 328).

Prolapse of the arm or elbow will aid in diagnosis. When the hand is down, the di-

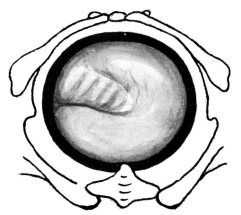

Figure 328 Tactile picture of vaginal examination findings in left acromion anterior position with apex of the axilla pointing to the head on the left and the costal gridiron facing posteriorly.

rection of the thumb and bend of the elbow will be toward the abdomen of the fetus. By attempting to "shake hands" with the fetus, one can decide which hand is prolapsed. In left acromion anterior position, the right or lower arm almost always comes down. Therefore, if the head is on the left side and the right arm is down, this position is likely to be present. One may follow the arm up to the thorax and try to outline the axilla, the ribs, the pipestem-like clavicle and the scapula. The spinal column also gives absolute information.

In right acromion posterior position, the axilla points to the right and rear. The costal gridiron and the clavicle face the pubis. The edge of the scapula is to the rear. The arm that will prolapse is the right one.

After labor has been in progress for a long time, the tissues become so swollen that diagnosis may be difficult. If the back or the abdomen is forced down into the pelvis, the difficulties may be great. In the differential diagnosis, breech, face, vertex and compound presentations have to be considered. Confusion will be avoided by carefully searching for the landmarks peculiar to each.

PROGNOSIS

If early diagnosis is made, the outlook for both the mother and the fetus is ex-

cellent. In neglected cases, infection and trauma from ill-conceived and poorly carried out intervention and from operative delivery make the situation grave. In such cases, the fetus almost always dies from the asphyxic or traumatic insults. Maternal prognosis is also guarded under these circumstances by virtue of the significant hazards of uterine rupture or the trauma inflicted by operative means. Prognosis is considerably improved by aggressive termination of the problem by cesarean section, as outlined below (Harris and Epperson).

TREATMENT

Before treatment is begun, search should be made for an overriding cause, such as a contracted pelvis or total placenta previa. If found, cesarean section is indicated as a fine and safe solution to the problem. With pelvic contraction, cesarean section should be the procedure of choice in all shoulder presentations of viable fetuses. Likewise, a cesarean section should be performed on every nullipara with a transverse lie in labor, whether or not it can be definitively demonstrated that the pelvis is contracted.

The operation should be performed early in labor. A longitudinal classic incision is preferable to a transverse uterine incision (see Chapter 76). This is recommended because intrauterine manipulation is usually necessary to effect delivery through the incision. The lower segment is generally not well developed except if the transverse lie has been long neglected. A vertical incision is also useful in the event that a large incision may become necessary because of impaction of the fetus in the pelvis.

External cephalic version may be tried if there is no pelvic contraction and the membranes are still intact. The fetus should be brought into a longitudinal position as a head presentation if possible. Wigand's method (Chapter 74) of external version consists of placing one hand over the breech, the other over the head and, with alternate pushing and stroking movements, manipulating the head down over the inlet. Each manipulation is executed between contractions. When the uterus contracts, the position gained is retained manually.

There are three conditions which govern external cephalic version: (1) There must be no immediate indication for the rapid termination of labor. (2) The fetus must possess a high degree of mobility; the contractions should not be strong and frequent and the membranes should be intact. (3) There must be no pelvic contraction. If external version fails, a cesarean section should be performed. Rupture of the membranes before the cervix is completely dilated is an unfortunate event in shoulder presentation. Serious consequences of this are prolapse of the cord and prolapse of an extremity. More than half the fetuses lost have a prolapsed extremity and more than one-third have a prolapsed cord.

Neglected shoulder presentations, especially those in which one of the modes of spontaneous expulsion (see above) is in progress, present intricate situations for the obstetrician to solve. These occur in the second stage of labor. The fetus may lie in the dilated lower uterine segment and cervix. The structures may be so thinned that the introduction of a hand may rupture them. No consideration need be given to the fetus in this type of case because it is usually dead. Decapitation and other destructive procedures are theoretically indicated, but the physician must understand that they are dangerous even for an expert obstetrician. After delivery, the uterus and vagina must be carefully and completely explored to determine the integrity of the parturient canal. In most neglected shoulder presentations, a cesarean section should be performed even if the fetus is dead.

REFERENCES

Denman, T.: Observations to prove that in cases where the upper extremities present at the time of birth the delivery may be effected by spontaneous evolution of the child. London Med. J. 5:64, 301, 1785.

Douglas, J. C.: An Explanation of the Real Process of the Spontaneous Evolution of the Fetus, ed. 2. Dublin, P. D. Hardy & Sons, 1844.

Hall, J. E., Kohl, S. G., and Kavaler, F.: Transverse lie and perinatal mortality. New York J. Med. 62:2186, 1962.

Harris, B. A., and Epperson, J. W. W.: An analysis of 131 cases of transverse presentation. Amer. J. Obstet. Gynec. 59:1105, 1950.

Johnson, C. E.: Transverse presentation of the fetus. J.A.M.A. 187:642, 1964.

Roederer, J. G.: Observationum medicarum de partu laborioso decades duae, prima et secunda. Göttingen, sumt. Bossiegelianis, 1756. Cited by Payer, A.: Zur Lehre von der Selbstentwicklung. Samml. klin. Vortr. 114:411, 1901 (Gynäk. vol. 314).

Stevenson, C. S.: Concepts in the handling of breech and transverse presentations in late pregnancy. Amer. J. Obstet. Gynec. 62:488, 1951.

Stevenson, C. S.: Transverse or oblique presentation of the fetus in the last ten weeks of pregnancy: Its causes, general nature and treatment. Amer. J. Obstet. Gynec. 58:432, 1949.

Wigand, J. H.: Von einigen äussern Handgriffen, wodurch man unter der Geburt die regelwidrigen Lagen der Frucht verbessern kann. Hamb. Mag. Geburtsh. 1:52, 1807.

Chapter 59

Funic and Compound Presentations

PROLAPSE OF THE CORD

Prolapse of the cord occurs approximately once in 200 cases (Myles). The terms *cord* and *funic presentation* refer to any situation in which the cord has prolapsed in front of or alongside the presenting part. Three degrees of prolapse may be distinguished: (1) *Occult* prolapse refers to the cord located at or near the pelvis, but not within reach of the fingers on vaginal examination. In such patients the condition is not suspected (Fig. 329). (2) The cord may be *forelying,* that is, palpable through the cervical os, but within the intact amniotic sac (Fig. 330). (3) The cord may be *prolapsed* into the vagina or even outside the vulva after the membranes have been ruptured (Fig. 331).

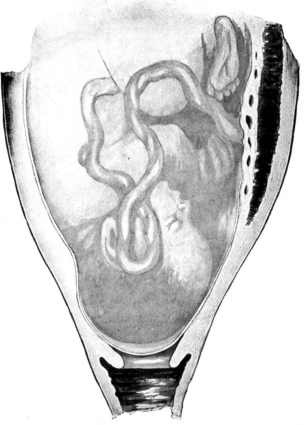

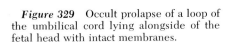
Figure 329 Occult prolapse of a loop of the umbilical cord lying alongside of the fetal head with intact membranes.

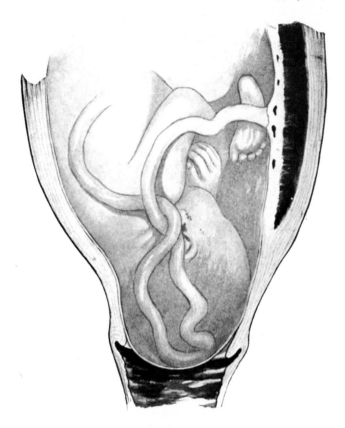

Figure 330 Forelying cord showing loop of umbilical cord lying in front of the fetal head within the intact amniotic sac. The funic presentation can be diagnosed by palpation through the membranes; compression of the cord may occur here.

Etiology

Anything which causes maladaptation of the presenting part to the lower uterine segment or prevents engagement of the head will favor prolapse of the cord. In normal presentations, the lower uterine segment is so evenly applied to the head that there is no room for the cord to slip down. Mechanical causes include the following: (1) Contracted pelvis with the head arrested high may allow the cord to prolapse. Indeed, the discovery of the cord should suggest a contracted pelvis. (2) Similarly, the cord may come down in association with malpositions and malpresentations. (3) Low attachment of the placenta with marginal insertion of the cord is commonly found with the presenting part held out of the pelvis, thereby favoring cord prolapse. (4) An unusually long cord may prolapse. (5) Displacement of the cord during obstetric operations may cause it to descend. (6) Prolapse of an arm in transverse lie, (7) twins and (8) hydramnios are all seen with funic presentations. As the membranes rupture, the cord may be washed down in these conditions and (9) in conjunction with any condition in which the head is unengaged.

Course and Prognosis

Prolapse of the cord does not affect the course of labor. Of course, some of the factors that cause prolapse, especially cephalopelvic disproportion, can and do influence labor adversely.

For the fetus there is great danger because the blood vessels in the cord may be compressed and cause asphyxia. Discounting very premature fetuses and those already dead before hospitalization, Savage et al. found that one-sixth of fetuses with prolapsed cord do not survive. Half of these or more might be salvaged by earlier detection of the funic presentation and cesarean section.

The cord is most readily compressed in cephalic presentations, especially when it lies behind the pubis. When it has slipped

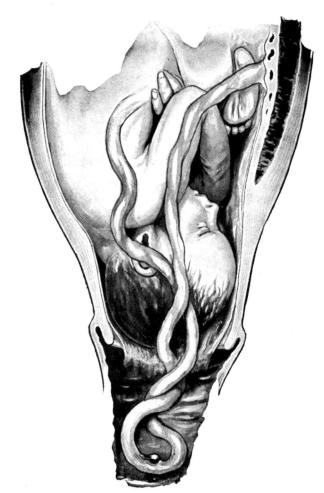

Figure 331 Cord prolapsed into the vagina after membranes have been ruptured. The danger of compression of the umbilical vessels is great under these circumstances.

down at the side, near the sacroiliac joints, the jutting sacral promontory affords some protection. However, compression by the soft parts alone can cause fatal obliteration of the umbilical blood vessels. Moreover, exposure of the cord to relatively cold room air causes reflex constriction of the umbilical vessels. The prognosis for the fetus is poor unless the situation is handled expeditiously and atraumatically (see below).

Diagnosis

Occult prolapse of the cord should be thought of when, in an otherwise normal labor, the fetal heart tones become irregular with sudden periodic episodes of bradycardia of variable duration and variably associated with contractions. The characteristic fetal heart rate pattern is seen when continuous, instantaneous monitoring is in progress (see Chapter 13). Prolapse should also be considered when, during forceps operations, auscultation reveals cardiac tumult during traction. By inserting the fingers deeply behind the pubis, one may sometimes discover a loop of the cord where it lies alongside the head.

A forelying cord in an intact amniotic sac should be apparent on vaginal examination. It should be easy to differentiate from velamentous umbilical vessels and from pulsating maternal arteries in the fornices.

After rupture of the membranes, there is no difficulty in diagnosing a prolapsed cord because it is often possible to see and feel it in the vagina. Pulsation in the cord may be absent or so slight that it is impalpable and yet the fetus may still be alive. The fetal heart must always be auscultated, particularly with a Doppler-type ultrasound device, before the death of the fetus is announced (see Chapter 8).

Treatment

All treatment must be preceded by a careful examination to discover the cause of the prolapse. A contracted pelvis may indicate cesarean section. As a prophylactic measure, an immediate vaginal examination should be made whenever the membranes rupture in the presence of an abnormal presentation, a high presenting part or a multiple pregnancy.

When the forelying cord is felt behind intact membranes or an occult prolapse is diagnosed by means of the fetal heart rate monitor, the physician should attempt its correction and replacement by posture. He should try to dislodge the head from the pelvis by raising the pelvis against gravity to a point higher than the uterine fundus using the Trendelenburg (Fig. 332), the elevated Sims' (Fig. 333) or the knee-chest (Fig. 334) position. To prevent rupture of the membranes before complete dilatation of the cervix, the patient is forbidden to bear down. All preparations are made for quick operative delivery. The physician must remain with the patient.

Spontaneous delivery is indicated immediately after the membranes rupture if

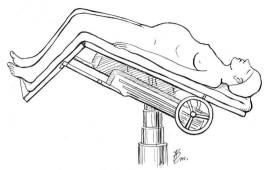

Figure 332 Method of managing the occult or forelying cord by placing the patient in the Trendelenburg position to try to ensure that the cord will not be compressed between the fetal head and the maternal pelvis. One can aid further by manually displacing the head out of the pelvis.

the cervix is completely dilated. The fetus should be delivered by forceps if its head is down on the perineum. However, if the membranes rupture and dilatation of the cervix is not complete, the patient must be treated differently (see below). Patients with early rupture of the membranes and a high presenting part have heretofore been kept in the prone position because it was believed that the upright position predisposes to prolapse of the umbilical cord. However, prolapse can occur while the patient is in the recumbent position (Fenton and D'Esopo). In the standing position, the presenting part actually dips further below the pelvic inlet than in the recumbent position, theoretically leaving less room for the cord to prolapse. Therefore, a more rational treatment of women with ruptured membranes and a high present-

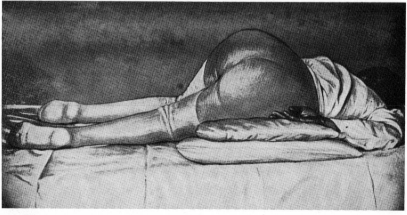

Figure 333 Another approach to managing the prolapsed cord is the elevated Sims' position, whereby the pelvis is raised on pillows above the level of the uterine fundus.

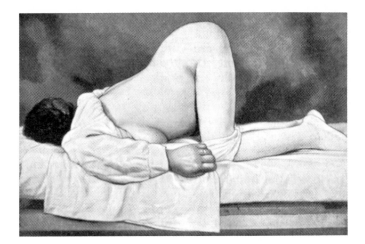

Figure 334 A useful method of displacing the head out of the pelvis to relieve cord compression by placing the patient in the knee-chest position.

ing part is to encourage ambulation, except for those with shoulder presentation and true cephalopelvic disproportion.

If the cord is prolapsed outside the vulva and the fetus is alive and viable, the fetal head should be held up out of the pelvis with a hand in the vagina. Delivery must then be effected. If conditions are right, immediate extraction is the most advisable procedure because it instantly extricates the fetus from its precarious position. However, for rapid extraction without doing damage to mother or fetus, the cervix must be effaced and completely dilated; unfortunately, these conditions are seldom present.

If the cervix is not completely dilated and the fetal heart tones are good, the best results will be obtained by immediate cesarean section. While waiting for the operation to be started, the patient should be placed in the Trendelenburg position, and an assistant should prevent the cord from being compressed between the bony pelvis and the head with his hand in the vagina until the operation is begun.

Any attempt to delay for the purpose of allowing vaginal delivery, such as in a multipara nearing second stage, requires that the cord be replaced. Usually, measures aimed at repositing the cord tend to be difficult and unsuccessful. Even when it is possible to replace the cord, it is likely to prolapse again. Moreover, handling the cord is hazardous in that it may cause spasm of the vessels. The wisest course of action with prolapsed cord, therefore, is immediate vaginal delivery or, if this is not possible, immediate cesarean section.

If the fetus is dead, it is best to leave the delivery to nature. Operative procedures, such as forceps or version, on a dead fetus are contraindicated. Of course, the fetus should have the benefit of the doubt if it is not known definitely whether it is alive. It is not easy to decide what to do when the cord is pulsating only feebly and there is reason to believe that the fetus may already have suffered irreparable hypoxic damage or that fetal death is not far distant. If delivery can be accomplished quickly without maternal injury, the fetus should be given the benefit of the doubt. However, if the operative delivery promises to be hard or dangerous, it is more than likely that the fetus will perish during or soon after the attempt to save it.

Prolapsed cord complicating breech presentation is slightly less dangerous than it is with a cephalic presentation. However, treatment is essentially the same. It is best to effect delivery as quickly and atraumatically as feasible. Cesarean section is indicated for prolapse of the cord with shoulder presentation.

COMPOUND PRESENTATION

When an extremity prolapses alongside the presenting part so that both enter the pelvic cavity at the same time, the condition is called *compound presentation*. The incidence of compound presentation is one in 1293 deliveries (Sweeney and Knapp). The main factors associated with this presentation are (1) twinning, (2) prematurity, alone or in combination with twins, and (3) an unengaged or a persistently high presenting part associated with ruptured membranes. Almost one-third of compound presentations occur in twin pregnancies and two-fifths involve premature infants. The frequency is still greater when twins and prematurity coexist.

Prolapse of the arm may influence the mechanism of labor. First, it may cause the fetal body to become rigid and prevent normal rotation and, second, it may prevent anterior rotation by occupying a portion of the pelvis which the occiput should traverse. An arm lying in the anterior half of the pelvis will obstruct labor more than if it is in the more spacious hollow of the sacrum. The anterior arm is the one usually found.

The diagnosis is simple. It must be remembered, however, that the prolapsed arm may be associated with a shoulder presentation or a second twin; sometimes a foot may be mistaken for a hand. Distinguishing characteristics are shown in Figure 324.

The best method of managing compound presentation without cord prolapse is watchful waiting with no manipulation. Generally, the hand will slip back as the cervix becomes completely dilated and the head descends. It is sometimes possible to induce the fetus to withdraw its own hand by gently pinching its fingers. In exceptional cases, however, when the forearm and the hand can be palpated vaginally, reposition may be indicated. With pelvic contraction or prolapse of the cord, a cesarean section should be performed.

After the head has engaged with the arm down, nothing need be done because there is clearly enough room in the pelvis for both structures. Forceps procedures are needed more often since labor is longer and abnormal mechanisms of rotation and descent are more common. Care must be used to see that the hand is not grasped with the blades of the forceps.

Prolapse of a foot alongside the head is rare. Since the fetal body is rigid, slow descent and delayed rotation are usual and, therefore, forceps operations are required commonly. If a foot prevents engagement of the head, the foot may be pushed away and the head led into the pelvis by combined manipulation. Watchful expectancy and forceps, if needed, are recommended if a foot and the head have engaged in the pelvis.

REFERENCES

Fenton, A. N., and D'Esopo, D. A.: Prolapse of the cord during labor. Amer. J. Obstet. Gynec. 62:52, 1951.

Myles, T. J. M.: Prolapse of the umbilical cord. J. Obstet. Gynaec. Brit. Emp. 66:301, 1959.

Savage, E. W., Kohl, S. G., and Wynn, R. M.: Prolapse of the umbilical cord. Obstet. Gynec. 36:502, 1970.

Sweeney, W. J., and Knapp, R. C.: Compound presentations. Obstet. Gynec. 17:333, 1961.

Chapter 60

Fetal Dystocia

FETAL GIGANTISM

The largest babies delivered vaginally weighed 11 kilograms or 24 lbs. (Belcher, Moss). These are exceedingly unusual because it is rare to see a baby born weighing more than 5 kilograms. Fetuses of excessive size can give rise to dystocic problems by virtue of their head dimensions as well as the coassociated phenomena of more rigid bony structure and limited ability to effect molding in the course of labor.

Etiology

(1) Prolonged or postterm pregnancy is a rare cause of overdevelopment of the child. (2) Women with adequate or abundant diets and indolent habits have larger babies than those who have inadequate diets during pregnancy; the latter group is more likely to have undersized babies instead. (3) Children of later pregnancies are usually larger than those of the first pregnancy. (4) Large parents usually have large children. (5) Women and some men with diabetes often procreate overweight babies. (6) Some infants with erythroblastosis, especially those with generalized edema, and (7) some with hypothyroidism are large.

Course

Overdistention of the abdomen may cause the same disturbances of pregnancy as are associated with twins. It is common for multiple pregnancy to be confused with an excessively large singleton pregnancy. Patients complain of a feeling of great weight, dyspnea and edema. If labor is postponed, intermittent false labor contractions may annoy the woman for several weeks.

Labor may be slow because the head may not engage in the pelvis or because it engages late. Cephalic presentations are the rule. In general, the course of labor resembles that seen in contracted pelves of the justominor type (see Chapter 63). The head molds into the pelvis if the cranial bones are not too hard. It is delivered with strong bearing-down efforts or by forceps.

The broad shoulders then cause delay (see below). After the head is delivered through the outlet, it characteristically snaps back against the perineum. Because of the elasticity of the fetal neck, the head presses the perineum inward. Unless the shoulders can be brought down quickly, the fetus dies. Rupture of the uterus from dystocia caused by delivery of the large shoulders may occur.

Postpartum hemorrhage and anomalies of placental separation are more frequent in association with excessively large fetuses because of uterine overdistention. The large uterus needs time to retract and it may not do so perfectly. Lacerations must also be expected, especially if manipulations are required.

Diagnosis

An excessively large, protuberant abdomen suggests a large fetus, twins or hydramnios. Absence of fluctuation will exclude hydramnios, and the recognized methods of diagnosis will determine the presence of twins (see Chapter 39). Ultrasonography is particularly valuable for diagnosis here (see Chapter 13).

Knowledge of the size of the fetus is just as important as information on the size of the pelvis. The principles and technique of cephalopelvimetry are discussed in Chapter 12. Of nearly equal significance is the hardness of the fetal head. This is determinable by bimanual palpation, from the size of the fontanels and by determining how well the bones of the head overlap as the head enters the pelvis during labor.

In a breech presentation, the size of the buttocks will give a good indication of the size of the fetus. If the foot is down, it will serve as a good indicator also. A large leg and foot usually mean a large fetus. X-ray or, preferably, ultrasound mensuration is helpful in determining the size of a fetus.

Prognosis

The prognosis for the mother depends on the degree of disproportion between the fetus and the pelvis. If this is great and unrecognized, the mother may suffer a ruptured uterus, infection, exhaustion or inflicted injuries. However, usually the mother may be delivered successfully if the fetus does not weigh more than 5000 gm., provided other conditions are favorable, especially with regard to pelvic capacity.

The prognosis for the fetus is not good. Many overlarge fetuses die in labor from asphyxia or from injuries occurring as a consequence of labor or inflicted during operative delivery. Intracranial hemorrhage, fracture of the skull, cephalhematoma, skull depressions and Erb's paralysis are frequent. The mortality rate is high and late neurological and developmental sequelae are unfortunately common (Sack).

Treatment

The issue of postdatism or postmaturity (see Chapter 54) is probably not relevant here because it is unlikely to contribute significantly to fetal overdevelopment. Prophylactic induction of labor in anticipation of this problem is practiced in some areas, but it does not seem to be warranted because the risks may outweigh the theoretical benefits, especially if the induction is done under suboptimal conditions. For the diabetic, induction is carried out as indicated according to the principles outlined in Chapter 49, based on fetal condition, placental status and maternal disease rather than on anticipated fetal size.

During labor, it is important to discover early that the fetus is large, because cesarean section may be easiest and safest for both patients. Management of labor and delivery will depend on prevailing conditions, particularly with reference to the evolution of the patterns of cervical dilatation and descent. Typical dysfunctional patterns of arrest (see Chapter 55) can be expected in the presence of insurmountable disproportion due to an excessively large fetus.

SHOULDER DYSTOCIA

Dystocia due to impaction of the baby's shoulder girdle occurs about once in every 60 deliveries of infants over 4000 gm. (Swartz). It carries with it a serious fetal prognosis with a mortality of 16 per cent.

The condition will usually be apparent immediately after the head has been delivered. The head will pull back tightly against the perineum. Traction serves only to stretch the neck. Many children have been lost at this stage of delivery and many uteri ruptured.

After delivery of the head, if the shoulders do not immediately follow with gentle traction, an examination should be made to determine the cause for the delay. There is great urgency in ascertaining the cause so that appropriate measures may be instituted promptly. One or more of the following will be found: (1) The shoulders are broad and firm. (2) The pelvis is contracted. (3) The shoulders have followed an unfavorable mechanism, the anterior shoulder being caught on the pubic ramus or having overrotated. When this is not recognized, the physician may try to bring the shoulder girdle down in the wrong diameter. (4) The chest of the fetus is too large, as in association with anasarca. (5) A double monster exists.

Treatment

Although it is important to deliver the infant quickly, excessive haste and overly aggressive manipulation and force are especially hazardous. Much skill is needed to effect the delivery of impacted shoulders without traumatizing mother and baby. If the woman is conscious, she should be asked to bear down strongly. Her legs are pressed firmly against her abdomen to aid her in expulsion.

With the fingers of one hand inside and the opposite hand outside, the shoulder girdle is rotated into the most favorable pelvic diameter, which is one of the oblique diameters, and the anterior shoulder is pressed down behind the symphysis pubis. Next, two fingers are inserted behind the pubis along the fetal back to gain a purchase on the scapula. By gentle pressure and slight traction in the axilla, the anterior shoulder is pushed to one side in the direction of the fetal chest so as to reduce the lateral dimension of the bisacromial diameter. This shoulder is then drawn down and out. The pressure slightly twists the body.

If this fails, the physician should try to dislodge the posterior shoulder from the sacral promontory and lead it down into the excavation of the sacrum by the following maneuver: Four fingers are passed up high into the vagina over the fetal back. The index finger is insinuated into the posterior axilla. Aided by gentle but firm suprapubic pressure from the outside on the anterior shoulder (Fig. 335), the shoulder girdle is turned into a favorable oblique diameter and at the same time drawn down into the pelvis. The torso is given a turbinal or corkscrew motion

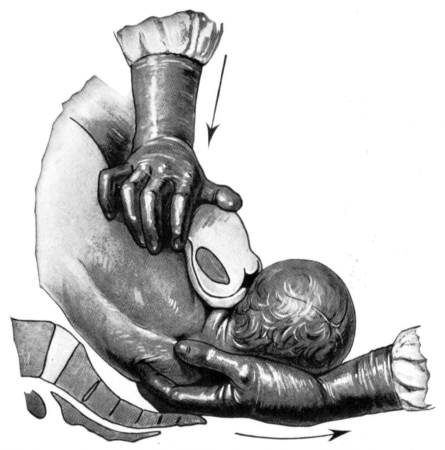

Figure 335 Demonstration of method for dislodging the posterior shoulder into the sacral excavation in a case of impacted shoulders. Note light suprapubic pressure exerted against the anterior shoulder, pressing it into the right anterior quadrant, while the posterior shoulder is being pulled downward and into the left posterior quadrant.

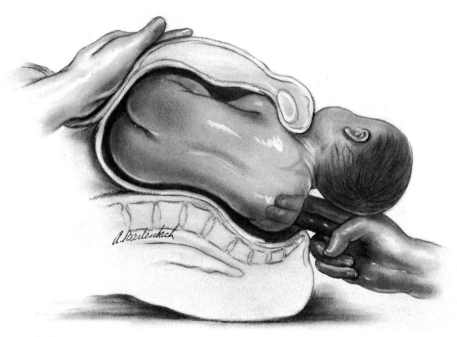

Figure 336 Corkscrew principle applied as an aid in the management of shoulder dystocia. The first step shown here involves lateral pressure on the posterior shoulder. Note Kristeller fundic pressure is also being applied.

which may carry the back over into the opposite side of the pelvis (Woods), as shown in Figures 336 and 337.

Caution is required because traumatic injury may be easily inflicted. The cervical plexus can be torn or pulled out of the spinal cord, the neck of the fetus may be broken or a hemorrhage can occur in the spinal canal. Purposeful fracture of the clavicle may sometimes be necessary to ac-

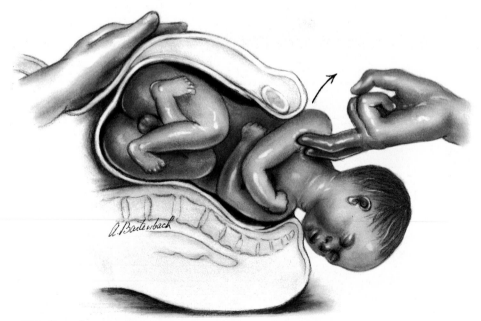

Figure 337 Second step in the maneuver begun in Figure 336, showing corkscrew rotation and delivery of the impacted shoulder by continued clockwise pressure against the shoulder.

complish delivery of impacted shoulders, although it is difficult to do in a large fetus with well-calcified bones. Some have advocated cutting the clavicle, but this is particularly risky for both mother and fetus. It is a good medicolegal practice to announce a deliberate fracture beforehand.

HYDROCEPHALUS

Hydrocephalus may cause severe dystocia. The skull may contain several liters of cerebrospinal fluid, although usually no more than 1000 to 1500 ml. is present in the ventricles. The association of hydrocephalus with spina bifida, clubfoot, ascites and other deformities is common. Fetal head size may be greatly increased as a consequence of hydrocephalus.

Course

Because of overdistention and thinning of the lower uterine segment and the me-

chanical obstruction to labor, rupture of the uterus may occur if the problem is neglected. Breech presentation is much more frequent than usual, occurring in nearly one-third (Feeney and Barry). A small hydrocephalic fetus may be delivered easily. A larger one always causes some degree of difficulty, but a large head that is not overly distended and with soft bones may mold its way through the pelvis.

Spontaneous delivery occurs in 40 per cent (Feeney and Barry). A dead and macerated fetus may pass easily through the pelvis, especially with strong contractions. Pressure necrosis and fistulas from prolonged labor and operative errors have occurred. The head often remains high for a long time.

Postpartum hemorrhage from uterine atony and lacerations is frequent. The mother is endangered by hydrocephalus unless it is recognized early. The disease is usually fatal to the fetus. Most of the babies who survive birth die within a few years after birth.

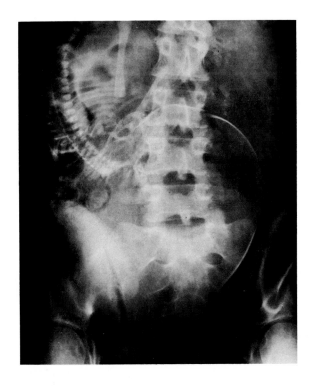

Figure 338 Anteroposterior roentgenogram illustrating characteristic features of hydrocephalus with thin cranial bones, globular distended head and relatively small facial features.

Diagnosis

If the possibility of this complication is kept in mind, the diagnosis is easy. Abdominally, the large uterine mass, the tense lower uterine segment, the rigidity of the abdomen, the broad head over the inlet or in the fundus, the lack of engagement and the tendency to dysfunctional labor all call attention to some anomaly. Vaginally, the vault of the pelvis is empty. The broad sutures, the large fontanels and the large flat elastic dome that remains high over the inlet will almost always confirm the diagnosis. By bimanual palpation the immense size of the head is easily distinguishable. Ultrasonography is diagnostic (see Chapter 13).

A thin-walled hydrocephalus may simulate the forewaters. A hydrocephalic fetus, presenting by the breech, is usually not discovered until after the baby's body is born and the aftercoming head is found to be arrested at the inlet. Occasionally, a spina bifida or other deformity will suggest an associated hydrocephalus.

Whenever a hydrocephalus is suspected, a roentgenogram (Fig. 338) or B-scan ultrasonogram should be obtained for verification. Hydrocephalus in head presentations is easily recognized, but errors are often made with breech presentations. Frequently, a roentgenogram of a breech presentation may show a large head that may be interpreted as a hydrocephalus, but in reality the head on the film has been magnified out of proportion because it was far from the film cassette when the picture was taken (see Chapter 12). The thickness of the skull bones and the size of the sutures and fontanels reveal the true state of affairs. The relatively small facial features and large, globular, thin-boned cranium of the hydrocephalic fetus are characteristic.

Treatment

In a vertex presentation the safest and simplest treatment is drainage of either the large or the small fontanel with a long 18- or 20-gauge needle through the vagina (O'Connor and Gorman). Only a minimal amount of dilatation of the cervix is necessary for this procedure. This treatment may be used in pregnancy or early in labor. It is entirely permissible to perform ventricular tap under these circumstances in Roman Catholic patients.

When it is technically not feasible to do the procedure because the head is high and not fixed over the inlet, or in a breech presentation, transabdominal ventriculocentesis may be done using the same approach as in amniocentesis (see Chapter 52). One must ensure that the urinary bladder has been emptied completely before undertaking either approach.

After the fluid is evacuated, the collapsed cranium offers little resistance to the soft parts and is usually delivered quickly and spontaneously. Traction may be exerted on the collapsed sac if a maternal indication for rapid delivery arises.

When a spina bifida is found with hydrocephalus in a breech presentation, the fluid in the brain may be removed easily by passing a ureteral catheter or narrow flexible metal catheter through the spina bifida into the brain. Even if a spina bifida is absent, the same technique may be used after making a lumbar puncture. This procedure is much simpler and safer than perforating the occipital bone of the aftercoming head. This latter technique can be used, if needed, for the trapped head in a breech birth, but the fetus cannot be expected to survive it. The mother may also be injured by this approach.

FETAL MALFORMATIONS

Single monsters are much more common than double ones. Because an enlargement of a part is often encountered, there is dystocia. Double monsters are frequently expelled spontaneously, especially when labor has evolved prematurely. When they give rise to dystocia, they are dangerous, and very complicated operations are often needed to effect delivery.

Malformed fetuses have a high frequency of abnormal presentations. The frequency of breech, shoulder, face and brow presentations in term-size malformed fetuses is seven times as great as in normal fetuses. Deflexion attitudes are also common.

Diagnosis

An abnormally formed fetus may be suspected before labor. Hydrocephalic and anencephalic monsters can be diagnosed by the alert examiner. Roentgenography readily confirms the findings. Since recurrence of monstrous children is common, the history is of aid in the diagnosis.

During labor, the possibility of a monster is to be considered when the vaginal examination reveals atypical findings. Before attempting cesarean section, it is wise in all instances of doubt to consider the shape of the fetus, its size and viability. It would be unfortunate to subject patients to a cesarean section for fetal indications, for example, and deliver a monster. On the other hand, cesarean section would be preferred to vaginal delivery if roentgenography proved the presence of a double monster that would be difficult to deliver *per vaginam*.

If anencephaly is associated with hydramnios, which is often the case, delivery usually is premature. If hydramnios is absent, the pregnancy tends to be prolonged. If an anencephalic monster is born alive, it dies quickly.

An anencephalic monster presenting by the head might easily cause confusion with breech presentation, placenta previa or face presentation. Grouping of deformities will help in diagnosis; for example, hydrocephalus may be expected when a spina bifida is found during a breech delivery. A single or double monster is suspected if the delivered head shows harelip and there is significant delay in delivery of the trunk. Hydramnios is so frequently present with fetal anomalies that one should always be alerted to look for anomalies whenever hydramnios exists.

If delay in delivery is not overcome by the usual manipulations, a vaginal examination should be made under anesthesia. The following must be searched for during such an exploration: enlargement of a part of the fetus, a tumor of the uterus or the fetus, a double monster and, if the last, the location and extent of fusion, the number of arms and legs and the movability of one fetus on the other.

In singleton pregnancies, various parts of the fetus are capable of being abnormally enlarged. Abdominal distention is associated with the ascites of erythroblastosis, a distended bladder and tumors of the liver or the kidneys. Goitrous enlargement of the thyroid may also cause obstruction. Conjoined twin monsters include those attached at the head (craniopagus), at the trunk (thoracopagus) and at the pelvis (ischiopagus or pygopagus), or with single fused lower parts (dicephalus).

Treatment

When double monsters are diagnosed, either clinically or roentgenographically, an elective cesarean section should be done. However, a monstrosity often is not discovered until labor is well established and obstruction is encountered. Breech presentation is most favorable for the mother. Single monsters with enlarged parts must be reduced in size. A hydrocephalus is punctured (see above) and a full abdomen is emptied.

It is best, if possible, to deliver the fetuses whole and not to amputate a head or trunk that has been expelled. It may be necessary to amputate the delivered portion in order to gain access to the rest or to render the balance of the mass movable, but such occasions are rare. Extremities should not be dismembered because they do not interfere with the manipulations; further, they may provide a means to grasp and pull on locked-in fetuses. Also, their removal destroys the relation of one twin to the other and complicates diagnosis and treatment.

Often the interconnection between double monsters is sufficiently flexible and elastic to permit one fetus to be delivered vaginally at a time, almost as if they were separated twins. Difficult and potentially traumatic manipulations should be avoided. Cesarean section is necessary if attempts at vaginal delivery fail, even though such patients may have become poor subjects for abdominal delivery.

REFERENCES

Barnes, A. C.: An obstetric record from *The Medical Record.* Obstet. Gynec. 9:237, 1957.

Belcher, D. P.: A child weighing 25 pounds at birth. J.A.M.A. 67:950, 1916.

Feeney, J. K., and Barry, A. P.: Hydrocephaly as a cause of maternal mortality and morbidity: A clinical study of 304 cases. J. Obstet. Gynaec. Brit. Emp. 61:652, 1954.

Moss, E. L.: Dystocia due to gigantic female foetus. Brit. Med. J. 2:643, 1922.

O'Connor, C. T., and Gorman, A. J.: The treatment of hydrocephalus in cephalic presentation. Amer. J. Obstet. Gynec. 43:521, 1942.

Sack, R. A.: The large infant: A study of maternal, obstetric and newborn characteristics, including a long-term pediatric follow-up. Amer. J. Obstet. Gynec. 104:195, 1969.

Swartz, D. P.: Shoulder girdle dystocia in vertex delivery: Clinical study and review. Obstet. Gynec. 15:194, 1960.

Woods, C. E.: A principle of physics as applicable to shoulder delivery. Amer. J. Obstet. Gynec. 45:796, 1943.

Chapter 61

Soft Tissue Dystocia

Anomalies of the soft parts are a more frequent cause of minor degrees of dystocia than anomalies of the bony pelvis. They are usually easy to manage, but require early recognition.

STENOSIS OF THE VULVA

Congenital closure of the vulva is usually complete and, if present, presents a barrier to menstruation, sexual intercourse and conception. Acquired closure may result from injury and inflammation with ulceration in childhood. Hymenal septums may offer a slight barrier to progress, but they usually break or can be easily snipped in two. Excessive edema of the vulva is sometimes encountered in preeclamptic and nutritional edema. Edema is also seen secondary to massive uterine overdistention in hydramnios. Varicosities do not delay labor, but they increase the dangers of hemorrhage and hematoma.

Obstructing vulvar tumors are occasionally encountered. Large condyloma acuminata have been reported to cause difficulty. Cesarean section may be necessary under these circumstances.

When it is obvious that the vulvar outlet is holding the presenting part back, the resisting ring of tissue must be stretched with the fingers or an episiotomy must be done. This usually allows vaginal delivery to occur and prevents extensive perineal lacerations.

STENOSIS OF THE VAGINA

The causative factors of a rigid or stenotic vagina are congenital deformities, atresia (which usually causes sterility), vaginal septums, tumors in and near the vagina, hematomas of adjacent tissue, cicatrices from previous ulcerative processes and injury or infection after labor.

Labor in women with vaginal constriction is not delayed until the head reaches the point of obstruction. Congenital septums are often pushed aside or torn by the presenting part; rarely is excision required.

Vaginal rigidity is usually overcome by natural powers. The vagina softens and dilates, although sometimes it splits longitudinally. The latter occurs more frequently during operative intervention. Scars often cause dystocia, but a scar may sometimes soften and dilate during pregnancy and labor.

Diagnosis is easy because a hard ring or narrow passage is felt with a finger; beyond it, the cervix is felt. Sometimes the vagina folds up before the oncoming head, and stricture is simulated. Such a fold is soft and easily pushed aside.

Cesarean section must be performed when an insuperable obstacle to delivery exists. A cicatricial septum may be split by one or more radial incisions; care must be exercised to avoid entering the rectum or the bladder. A narrow, tight vagina must be incised. A deep vaginoperineal incision will usually suffice, as the tears almost always occur in the lower half.

RIGIDITY OF THE CERVIX

M. Kolstad

Cervical stenosis is surprisingly rare. Among the etiologic factors are chronic cervicitis, deep cauterizations and surgical operations, such as trachelorrhaphy or cervical amputation (Fisher). Not every hard cervix is caused by anatomic disease. It is important to distinguish anatomic rigidity from functionally disordered labor (see Chapter 55). When it is evident that nature has accomplished as much as possible in terms of arrest of progression of effacement and dilatation, an effort must be made to overcome the rigidity by one of three methods: (1) digitally, (2) Dührssen's incisions or (3) abdominal cesarean section.

In mild rigidity in which the cervix is completely effaced and the os is almost completely dilated, the opening may be stretched slightly with the fingers to permit delivery. However, one must be aware of the likelihood that arrest of dilatation late in the first stage is most likely due to cephalopelvic disproportion rather than to any form of cervical rigidity. No treatment of the cervix should ever be instituted, therefore, unless the fetopelvic relationship has first been studied objectively. Almost invariably the cervix tears. If the ring is too tough to be stretched, clean incisions radiating to the fornices must be made or a cesarean section performed.

Dührssen's incisions are of limited use here and should be stringently avoided unless absolutely necessary because they are hazardous to both mother and fetus (Greenhill and Friedman). The patient should be given every opportunity to dilate the cervix with additional labor. The fetus that is unable to negotiate an inadequate birth canal should not be forced to do so by ill-advised vaginal operative manipulations. In the presence of disproportion, cesarean section is indicated; with an adequate pelvis, oxytocin infusion is preferable to overcome the arrest pattern.

CERVICAL INCISIONS

It is of greatest importance to distinguish between a cervix that is already effaced or obliterated and one that has not unfolded. During effacement and dilatation of the cervix, the pelvic connective tissue, the bladder and the lower uterine segment are drawn up; the pelvic peritoneum is elevated; the broad ligaments are unfolded and the large vessels at the sides of the uterus are raised up and retracted laterally. This means that these important structures are removed from the pelvis, where they could be subject to injury. Extensive unfolding of the cervix usually occurs in the last weeks of pregnancy and it is sometimes accompanied by false labor contractions. The more the cervix has been opened in the course of labor, the less the physician has to do.

Dührssen's incisions are seldom indicated any longer in obstetrics. Indications are complications which may prove haz-

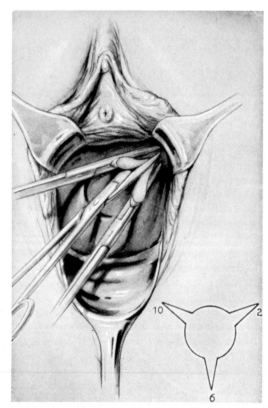

Figure 339 Dührssen's incisions. Under wide exposure of the field by broad specula the cervix is grasped and cut to the fornix between two 8-inch clamps or sponge forceps which are left on a few minutes to stop hemorrhage. Three incisions are made, corresponding to 2, 6 and 10 on the clock as shown in the inset.

ardous to the mother or the fetus, requiring rapid termination of labor at a time when the cervix is obliterated and there is only a thin partition between the dilated lower uterine segment and the vagina.

The conditions that must be fulfilled for Dührssen's incisions are that (1) there must be no cephalopelvic disproportion; (2) the fetal station must be at least at plus 1, although the risks to the mother and the fetus are considerably reduced if the fetal presenting part has reached the perineal floor; (3) there must be complete cervical effacement; (4) the dilatation must be at least 5 cm. and (5) there has been no progress for at least two hours after adequate sedation and maintenance of fluid balance. Placenta previa is a contraindication. Oxytocin stimulation in many of these cases will avert the need for this procedure and should be considered first unless the critical nature of the indication dictates urgent intervention. In most in-

stances in which there is urgency, cesarean section may be a far safer approach.

The usefulness of this operation is limited because the incisions are safe only after the cervix has been effaced completely. If the tissues are incised before effacement of the cervix is complete, the wounds are likely to tear further during the extraction and open up the broad ligaments and even the peritoneal cavity.

Three incisions are generally made, as shown in Figure 339, while holding the cervix carefully with sponge forceps. It is essential that the greatest deliberation be practiced in the subsequent extraction of the fetus to prevent extension of the incisions.

Suture of Dührssen's incisions is the same as for cervical lacerations (see Chapter 65), care being taken to ensure hemostasis and good apposition of cut surfaces. Dührssen's incisions do not seem to affect subsequent pregnancy and labor.

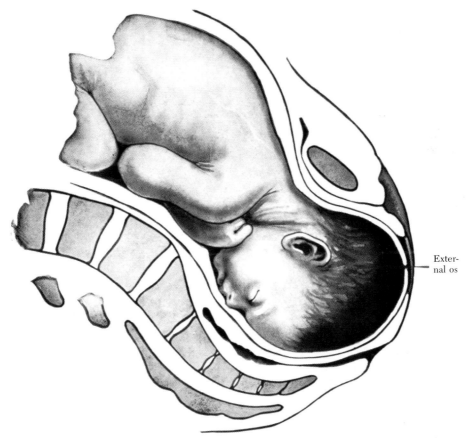

External os

Figure 340   Lateral diagrammatic view of the soft tissue relationships in conglutination of the external os with the markedly thinned out but closed cervix advanced to the introitus by the descending fetal head.

CONGLUTINATION OF THE EXTERNAL OS

This is a rare condition. The circular fibers around the external os do not dilate; as a result the cervix is not opened, but the lower uterine segment and cervical canal become progressively thinned. The cervix may protrude externally, completely ef- faced, but undilated and still covering the head (Fig. 340). The os cannot always be identified, but the opening, surrounded by a red ring, can be seen through a speculum as a tiny hole with some mucus in it. By pressure with a finger the resistance can be overcome and then dilatation usually progresses rapidly. Rarely will it ever be necessary to dilate the cervix further, digi- tally or with incisions.

REFERENCES

Dührssen, A.: Ueber vaginalen Kaiserschnitt. Samml. klin. Vortr. 232:1365, 1898.

Dührssen, A.: Eklampsie. *In* von Winckel, F.: Hand- book der Geburtshülfe. Wiesbaden, J. F. Berg- mann, 1905.

Fisher, J. J.: Effect of amputation of cervix uteri upon subsequent parturition: Preliminary report of seven cases. Amer. J. Obstet. Gynec. 62:644, 1951.

Greenhill, J. P., and Friedman, E. A.: Soft-tissue dys- tocia. Hosp. Med. 4:73, 1968.

Chapter 62

Abnormal Pelves

Clinical and x-ray pelvimetric techniques are described in Chapter 12. It must be made clear that the pelvis cannot in truth be evaluated accurately as an isolated entity without simultaneous consideration of the fetal head dimensions. This concept understood, we will deal here with the anatomic aspects of configurationally distorted and contracted pelves as they are encountered in clinical practice. Although such encounters are fortunately rare, it is essential for the physician to be able to recognize the basic features of abnormal pelves and understand how they may affect the mechanisms of labor.

Generally, a pelvis that shows a diminution of 1.5 to 2 cm. in an important diameter is considered to be contracted. Since contraction at the inlet is most common, the true conjugate is most often used as the determining diameter. A pelvis is contracted when the true conjugate is shortened; the degree of contraction is measured by the amount the true conjugate is shortened.

Litzmann proposed various grades of contracted pelves according to the length of the true conjugate; these grades still provide a reasonable guide to clinical estimation of pelvic capacity. (1) He considered 6.5 cm. as the shortest true conjugate that would permit the passage of a normal-sized fetus; pelves smaller than these were called *absolutely* contracted. (2) If the true conjugate was from 6.5 to 9 cm. long, the pelvis was called *relatively* contracted because a small living fetus could sometimes be forced through it and a macerated fetus always. (3) In a third grade were those with a true conjugate from 9 cm. to normal; labor complications in these were more often caused by errors of mechanism than by spatial disproportion between the fetal head and the pelvis. These measurements

apply to flat pelves primarily (see below). In *generally* contracted pelves, since there is diminution of all the diameters and the area of all planes is smaller, 0.5 cm. is added to the upper limit of each division.

Such classification is artificial, but serves a useful purpose in clinical pelvimetry. The size of the fetus, the hardness and moldability of its head, the presentation, position and attitude all make the pelvis more or less adequate insofar as spatial relationships are concerned. If the difficulty of precisely measuring the pelvis is appreciated, it becomes apparent why there is so much inaccuracy and variation in the evaluation of contracted pelves.

GENERALLY CONTRACTED PELVES

The small gynecoid or *justominor* pelvis is characterized by contraction in all diameters as shown in Figure 341. Its features are detailed in Chapter 12. It is actually a normal pelvis in miniature, found in short women and is in proportion to the rest of the skeleton. All its measurements are diminished. Often a slight flattening exists.

One may occasionally encounter a variant of the justominor pelvis of the infantile or juvenile type with typical anthropoid features. The inlet presents an anteroposterior oval and the sacrum is high and long. The pelvis is deep and the tuberosities are close together, giving the excavation a funnel shape.

The pelvic cavity may be encroached on if the bones are heavy and thick in the small pelvis with characteristics of the android pelvis. The sacrum is long and narrow; the arch of the pubis is high; the sides of the pelvis are close together and

633

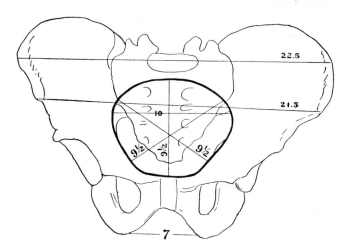

Figure 341   Typical justominor pelvis with diminished diameters in all dimensions, but with the good proportionality of a small gynecoid pelvis.

the inlet is heart-shaped with narrowing of the forepelvis.

Minor degrees of general pelvic contraction are common. Those with a true conjugate between 9 and 10 cm. are almost always associated with rickets and show pronounced flattening (see below). Only dwarf pelves have a true conjugate of 7 cm. or less.

PLATYPELLOID PELVES

Flat pelves are contracted in the anteroposterior diameters. They may be of two kinds: the *simple flat* and the *rachitic flat* (Figs. 342 and 343). However, the simple

flat pelvis is probably often rachitic in origin also. The sacrum has sunk downward and forward, causing the outline of the inlet to be broad and kidney-shaped, and the pelvic cavity to be slightly flattened.

Rachitic flat pelves are usually smaller than normal because the bones are smaller and thinner. The ilia flare outward and are flattened. The pelvic inclination is increased; the pubic arch is broad; the angle that the pubis makes with the inlet is obtuse; the ischial tuberosities are widely separated, and the direction of the acetabula is more anterior than normal. This peculiar insertion of the femurs gives the patient a distinctive gait; the feet are thrown outward.

The most characteristic changes are in

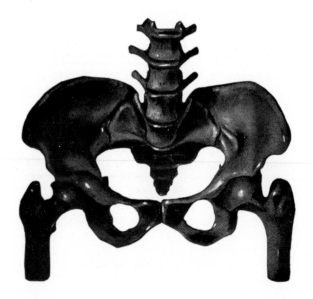

Figure 342   A rachitic flat pelvis with foreshortening of the anteroposterior diameter, forward displacement of the sacrum, anterior displacement of the acetabula and flaring ilia.

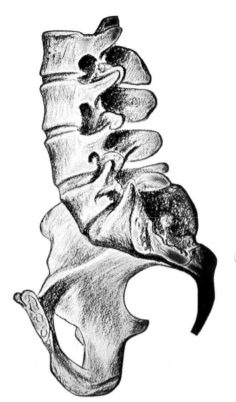

Figure 343 Sagittal section of a rachitic flat pelvis with forward protrusion of the sacrum to produce a false promontory.

the sacrum. This bone is forced downward into the pelvic cavity; the concavity of its anterior surface is changed in both directions so that it becomes flat. In advanced cases it is convex from side to side and straight from above downward; the bodies of the sacrum protrude from between the wings, and the sacrum is bent on itself. A second or false promontory is sometimes present below the true one (Fig. 343).

Important alterations result in the shape and size of the pelvic canal. Most prominent of these is the flattening of the inlet from anterior to posterior. The transverse and oblique diameters may be normal or even larger. The true pelvis is shallow; the outlet is usually much enlarged.

Thus, labor differs from that in generally contracted pelves. In the justominor pelvis, because the pelvis is usually uniformly contracted throughout the length of the canal, the head has to overcome resistance all the way down. In the flat pelvis, after the inlet has once been passed, the rest of the distance is usually traversed quickly and easily.

OBLIQUELY CONTRACTED PELVES

When rickets is severe and prolonged, the bony growth is so stunted that the pelvis does not attain normal size. Added to this are the deformities of the pelvic bones, the sinking down of the sacrum and other conditions; all of these combine to produce the generally contracted flat pelvis. The smallest pelves are of this class. When there is a major difference in the size of the two halves of the inlet, the pelvis is referred to as *obliquely contracted.*

The most common cause of obliquely contracted pelves is scoliosis of the vertebral column. Figure 344 shows such a pelvis due to fragilitas ossium. Much depends on the location of the spinal curvature because, if it is up high, compensation takes place lower down on the vertebral column and the effect on the pelvis is hardly noticeable. Another point is that the pelvic asymmetry may cause the scoliosis.

Asymmetry of the pelvic inlet is present in approximately 80 per cent of women who have had paralytic poliomyelitis. The distortion is usually slight so that dystocia is not produced. Hence, cesarean section is seldom necessary in these women.

Common to all obliquely contracted pelves are these features: (1) The inlet is smaller on the side to which the convexity of the lumbar scoliosis points. This is due to the fact that the sacrum is pushed over onto that side; because the pressure of the trunk is greater here, the sacrum sinks lower. (2) Since the pressure of the trunk is borne more on one wing of the sacrum than on the other, the part which bears the pressure is less well developed; the foramina are smaller and closer together and even the iliac portion of the sacroiliac joint is sometimes affected. (3) The pelvis is tilted so that the more contracted side is higher than the larger side; this is due to the fact that the line of direction of the body falls not through the midline of the sacrum but to the side away from the greatest convexity of the scoliosis. This throws the weight of the trunk almost entirely on one leg and, therefore, this femur is forced upward, inward and backward. (4) The sciatic notch is narrowed. (5) The pubic arch points to the contracted side. (6) The true conjugate

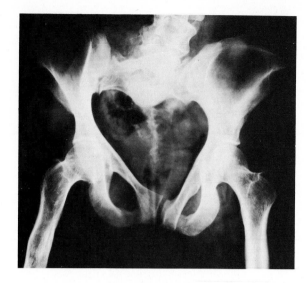

Figure 344 Anteroposterior roentgenogram of a contracted pelvis with fragilitas ossium, showing oblique contraction due to scoliosis.

runs obliquely backward. (7) The obstetric transverse diameter is always shortened. (8) The oblique diameters are decidedly unequal. (9) One ischial tuberosity is higher than the other.

Disease of the hip joint in infancy almost always leaves a pronounced pelvic deformity (Fig. 345), but rarely does sufficient encroachment on the lumen result to cause serious dystocia. In the typical *coxalgic pelvis* that results, the unaffected side is elevated. This tilts the pelvis up and the vertebral column away. Scoliosis here is a secondary phenomenon. There is diminished concavity on the sound side, with flattening and narrowing seen.

Another variety of the obliquely contracted pelvis is the *Nägele pelvis,* caused either by disease of the sacroiliac joint and the adjacent portions of the ilium and sacrum or by absent or undeveloped sacral ala on one side (Fig. 346). This type of pelvic deformity is perhaps somewhat more common than is usually believed (Chan et al.), although it is acknowledged to be relatively rare, nevertheless.

All the findings of oblique contraction and those caused by exaggerated pressure of one thigh are present in this type of pelvis. Moreover, since one wing of the sacrum is often atrophic, aplastic or even missing, in addition to the distortion, actual reduction in the size of half of the pelvis is present. What is important from a clinical point of view is that the narrowing of the pelvic lumen extends down to the outlet.

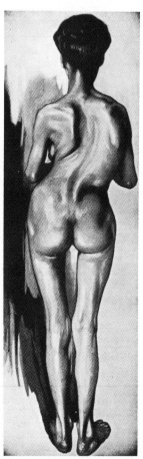

Figure 345 Standing back view of a patient with a coxalgic pelvis associated with ankylosed right hip joint. Note tilting and elevation of the left side of the pelvis, shown by the asymmetrical rhomboid of Michaëlis. Secondary scoliosis is also present.

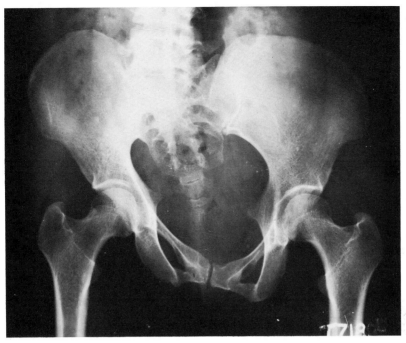

Figure 346 X-ray view of a Nägele pelvis showing oblique contraction associated with aplasia of the right sacral ala.

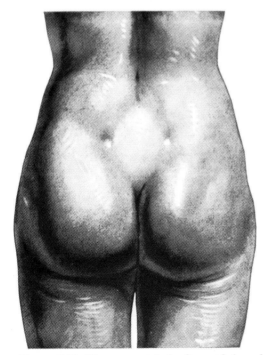

Figure 347 The symmetrical, diamond-shaped rhomboid of Michaëlis in a patient with a normal pelvis.

The diagnosis of an obliquely contracted pelvis is usually easy to make because of the uneven limping gait seen in association with scoliosis or unequal length of the legs. With oblique contraction, in addition to the scoliosis and the apparent shortening of the leg, the hip of one side will be higher and retroposed, the pubic region will be displaced to one side and the hair line will be oblique. The rhomboid of Michaëlis is asymmetric or tilted and the gluteal fold is lower on one side. The contrast between normal and asymmetric rhomboids is shown in Figures 347 and 348. Of course, a roentgenogram will clearly show the deformity. On vaginal examination, the corresponding half of the pelvis will be found to be very small and the encroachment of the ischium on the lumen persists even to the outlet.

TRANSVERSELY CONTRACTED PELVES

The classic transversely contracted pelvis, the *Robert pelvis*, is caused by os-

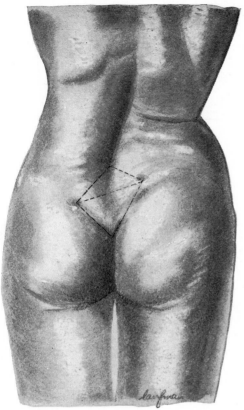

Figure 348 An asymmetrical rhomboid of Michaëlis encountered in a patient with an obliquely contracted pelvis. Compare with Figure 347.

teoarthritis affecting both sacroiliac joints. Both sides of the pelvic cavity are involved and the inlet assumes the form of a narrow wedge. The narrowing of the pelvis usually extends to the outlet.

The *kyphotic pelvis* is contracted in the transverse diameter and is seen in association with kyphoscoliosis. It also possesses some of the characteristics of the funnel-type pelvis (see below). The sacrum is drawn upward and out of the pelvis. At the same time, the sacrum rotates on a transverse axis so as to throw the promontory up and back and the coccyx forward and inward. As a result of this rotation, the innominate bones are rolled around the sacral articular surfaces so as to bring the ischia together and exaggerate the forward dip of the crests; this increases pelvic inclination.

The extreme pelvic inclination of these pelves is easily understood. The patient forces the lower part of the abdomen forward and holds her chest high and the shoulders back. Pendulous abdomens are more pronounced in these women than in all others.

Women with kyphoscoliosis compare favorably with those not so afflicted in their ability to conceive, deliver vaginally and withstand postpartum complications (Dugan and Black), although cardiopulmonary complications sometimes arise (see Chapter 41).

FUNNEL PELVES

When the capacity of the pelvis is progressively smaller from the inlet to the outlet, it is referred to as a *funnel pelvis*. Most pelves of the generally contracted type, as well as kyphotic, Nägele, Robert and some of the rachitic pelves, belong in this class.

Funnel pelves of the kyphotic type are easily recognized. The gibbus down low in the back will suggest it. Recognition of the android type pelvis is not as simple. The physician usually becomes aware of its existence only after labor progression ceases with the head down low in the pelvic canal. Such surprises will be infrequent if, in the routine pregnancy examination, the physician will palpate the descending rami of the pubis and measure the distance between the tuberosities (see Chapter 12). Palpation of the side walls of the parturient canal usually indicates narrowing and convergence.

ASSIMILATION PELVES

In the embryo, the iliac bones develop near the twenty-fifth to the twenty-ninth vertebras; later, these five vertebras fuse to form the sacrum. At first, the sacroiliac joint is usually made with the twenty-sixth spinal vertebra, but soon the twenty-fifth and twenty-seventh are involved. If the iliac bones are united with vertebras higher up in the spinal column, the sacrum is long and narrow and the first sacral vertebra presents the characteristics of a transitional stage from the last lumbar. The sacrum has six segments instead of five and five foramina instead of four. Therefore, the last lumbar vertebra appears *assimilated* with the sacrum; it has helped to make up this bone. Such a pelvis is called *high assimilation pelvis* because the union of the ilia with the spinal column is up higher than normal.

If this union omits the twenty-fifth vertebra, six lumbar vertebras instead of five are present; the last lumbar (sixth) has many of the characteristics of the first sacral. Such a pelvis is called a *low assimilation pelvis* because the union of the ilia with the spinal column is lower than normal and the sacrum is short, broad and has three or four foramina.

The characteristics of a high assimilation pelvis are an extremely high promontory and a long sacrum, usually with six vertebras and five sacral foramina (the first of which may lie above the plane of the inlet). The wings of the sacrum are thin and almost perpendicular. There is a deep pelvic canal and a lengthened true conjugate. Low assimilation pelves are characterized by foreshortening of the anteroposterior diameter and flattening of the inlet. Such problem pelves may cause dystocia.

SPONDYLOLISTHETIC PELVES

The essential feature of the spondylolisthetic pelvis is a sliding of the body of the last lumbar (rarely, the fourth or third) vertebra over the first sacral and into the pelvis; it carries the spinal column with it. The articular processes of the vertebra and sacrum are not dislocated; the slipping of the body of the vertebra is brought about by stretching or fracture of the interarticular processes. The lumbar vertebra is thus elongated from the front to the rear; it may even be bent over the sacrum so that the apposed portions of the two bones are compressed and often synostotic.

Spondylolisthesis exerts a deforming action on the pelvis: (1) The pelvic inclination is obliterated; in severe cases the inlet is almost horizontal. (2) The lower lumbar spine projects over and into the inlet, similar to the condition encountered with lumbosacral kyphosis, and the promontory becomes the fourth, third or even the second lumbar vertebra. (3) The available true conjugate may be reduced to as little as 5 cm., and the rest of the pelvis tends to become funnel shaped.

OSTEOMALACIC PELVES

Osteomalacia is an extremely rare disease consisting of failure of calcium and phosphorus to be deposited in newly formed bone matrix or osteoid tissue. It is attributable to inadequate availability of calcium and phosphorus concentrations in body fluids. The disease is not associated with failure of bone matrix production nor with increased bone destruction.

As a result of osteomalacia, the bones become much lighter in weight, softer and sometimes very flexible. If treated properly with high doses of calcium and vitamin D, calcium is again deposited in the osteoid substance and the skeleton becomes heavy, but the deformities remain. The pelvis, the vertebras, the ribs and the long bones are affected in the order named.

Osteomalacia resembles rickets pathologically, but rickets develops before the epiphyses close. Multiparas are affected much more frequently than nulliparas. Frequent childbearing seems to be a contributing factor. It occurs most often in women with poor nutrition. Dietary deficiency is clearly an underlying or aggravating cause, especially in those areas of the world where the problem is endemic, such as China and northern India.

The pressure of the trunk, the pressure of the heads of the femurs and the traction of the muscles and ligaments on the softened bones crowd the pelvis together (Fig. 349). The downward and forward sinking of the sacrum, the beaklike distortion of the horizontal pubic rami (from inward pressure of the femurs), the approach of the ischial tuberosities and the inward rolling of the iliac crests are characteristic. This invasion from three sides and

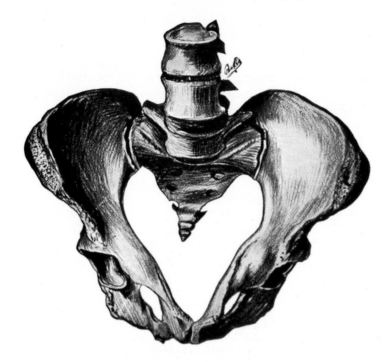

Figure 349 Osteomalacic pelvis with softening of the bones, resulting in downward displacement of the sacrum and inward distortion of the pubic rami and innominate bones.

from above produces marked effects on the pelvic lumen to the point that the cavity may be almost obliterated.

Vaginal delivery is impossible if the process is advanced, but if labor occurs when the osteomalacia is in the florid stage, the soft bones may give way to the head advancing under the influence of strong contractions and dilate enough to allow delivery; it is best not to depend on this, however. Cesarean section is usually indicated.

REFERENCES

Chan, D. P. C., Kan, P. S., and Chan, B. K. Y.: Nägele pelvis. J. Obstet. Gynaec. Brit. Comm. *71*:464, 1964.

Dugan, R. J., and Black, M. E.: Kyphoscoliosis in pregnancy. Amer. J. Obstet. Gynec. 73:89, 1957.

Litzmann, C. C. T.: Die Formen des Beckens, insbesondere des engen weiblichen Beckens, nach eigenen Beobachtungen und Untersuchungen. Berlin, B. Reimer, 1861.

Litzmann, C. C. T.: Die Geburt bei engem Becken. Leipzig, Breilkopf und Härtel, 1884.

Michaëlis, G. A.: Das enge Becken. Leipzig, G. Wigand, 1851.

Nägele, F. C.: Das schrägverengte Becken, nebst einem Anhange ueber die wichtigsten Fehler des weiblichen Beckens ueberhaupt. Mainz, V. von Zabern, 1839.

Robert, F.: Beschreibung eines in höchsten Grade querverengten Beckens. Karlsruhe u. Freiburg, 1842.

Robert, F.: Ein durch mechanische Verletzung und ihre Folgen querverengtes Becken, im Besitze von Herrn Paul Dubois zu Paris, beschrieben und zusammengestelt mit den drei übrigen bekannten querverengten Becken. Berlin, A. Hirschwald, 1853.

Chapter 63

Mechanisms of Dystocic Labor

CLINICAL CONSIDERATIONS

When labor begins at term in a woman with a severely contracted pelvis, it may soon become evident that something is wrong, based either on the high undescending presenting part or the evolution of a dysfunctional labor pattern (see Chapter 55). In these cases, a careful digital examination should be made and x-ray pelvimetry should be carried out. Such examinations are made to determine the type and location of the pelvic contraction, the degree of contraction and also the relative size of the fetal head. Too often pelvic contraction is not recognized until late in labor when both mother and fetus are in jeopardy (Jacobs).

Factors other than the spatial disproportion may cause the dystocia. These include abnormal presentation and position and irregular uterine action, discussed elsewhere. We will concern ourselves here primarily with dystocia in contracted pelves.

Abnormal presentations (breech, face, brow and shoulder) are four times as frequent with contracted pelves as with normal pelves. Prolapse of the arm, foot and cord are also common in all forms of pelvic contraction, particularly in the flat varieties, because the head is not firmly apposed to the lower uterine segment. It is held away by the jutting promontory of the sacrum, which leaves spaces through which the small parts slip easily.

A great deal depends on the size and moldability of the fetal head. If the bones are soft, they may lend themselves to the shape of the inlet and disproportion may thus be overcome. If the fetus is small,

there may actually be no disproportion relative to the pelvic contraction.

Of prime significance in all labors in contracted pelves is the action of the uterus. Generally, the force of the uterus is proportionate to the amount of work required of it. The recurring contractions adjust, compress, mold and propel the head through the narrowed canal in a fashion that the finest obstetric maneuvers fail to imitate. Furthermore, strong contractions dilate the cervix and prepare the soft parts for the passage of the fetus. Weak uterine action is an unwelcome complication of labor in contracted pelves. The majority of labors will terminate spontaneously by vaginal delivery if the passage is not too contracted, the fetus is of moderate size, the presentation and position are normal and the contractions are strong.

At the beginning of labor the head is usually high and not engaged. It does not fit the lower uterine segment accurately and the membranes over the os are exposed to the full force of the uterine contractions. The membranes may rupture and the amniotic fluid drain away. The possible consequences of early rupture of the membranes under these circumstances are (1) prolapse of the cord or an extremity and (2) ascending uterine infection.

Differences are observed in the way the cervix dilates in obstructed labor (see Chapter 55). Typically, one or more of the arrest patterns are encountered in the presence of insurmountable obstruction, including secondary arrest of dilatation, prolonged deceleration phase and arrest of descent.

Unless the head passes quickly into and through the pelvis, the expanded and overstretched lower uterine segment may rupture. Sometimes, the cervix is compressed between the bony surfaces of the head and the pelvis. The anterior lip is particularly likely to be caught between the head and the pubis and become enormously swollen, suggillated or even necrotic. Later, it may form a cervicovesical fistula.

If the head is arrested at the inlet, the contractions may become progressively and consistently stronger and the intervals between them become shorter, but no advancement is perceptible. A large caput succedaneum forms and the scalp may even be visible at the vulva when the head is actually not yet engaged. The fetus may die because the violent contractions reduce uterine blood flow and placental exchange. There may be cerebral injury or hemorrhage as a result of nature's attempt to crowd the head through a passage that is too small. If aid is not rendered, the woman will die from rupture of the uterus with intraperitoneal hemorrhage, shock or exhaustion. This should be an extremely rare occurrence today because, long before serious damage is done, a cesarean section should be performed.

If the disproportion is not absolute, nature may be able to accomplish the delivery. The course of such a labor is somewhat different from that just described. At first the head is high and is separated from the bony inlet by a pad made up of the thick cervix, the bases of the broad ligaments and the pelvic connective tissue. After the uterus has been active for a while, all these structures are drawn upward out of the pelvis with the retraction of the lower uterine segment and the head applies itself to the inlet.

The shape of the inlet determines the mechanism of engagement and also the subsequent mechanism. In the gynecoid pelvis, the head enters and proceeds normally unless the inlet is small or the fetus large. In the transversely contracted android or anthropoid types of pelves, the area of the inlet may be sufficient to allow the head to pass, but the occiput seeks the pelvic sagittal diameter and an occiput posterior position results. In obliquely contracted inlets, if the available area is adequate, the head usually comes down with the occiput facing into the larger half.

When the contractions grow stronger, molding begins and the intrauterine pres-sures gradually force the head through the narrowed superior strait. Because of the softness of the cranial bones and their mobility on each other at the sutures, the head is capable of being changed in form so that it accommodates itself to the shape of the inlet. The parietal bone that is first subjected to resistance is pressed under the other and the plate of the occipital bone lies under the two parietals. The overlapping may be so pronounced that the dura mater begins to strip off and a row of minute hemorrhages forms on either side of the longitudinal sinus.

The contractions become expulsive as soon as the head has been molded so that it is ready to pass through the inlet. The parturient bears down, the head drops into the excavation and the occiput begins to rotate to the front.

Three signs indicate that the head is descending: (1) the patient begins to bear down, (2) feces are discharged or the woman expresses a desire to defecate and (3) sometimes cramps occur in the legs. The first two signs are due to pressure of the head on the rectum and levator ani muscles; the last one is due to irritation of the sacral plexus by contact with the advancing head.

In flat pelves, in which the resistance is encountered only at the inlet, this part of the labor is completed with surprising rapidity. In multiparas, one or two powerful expulsive efforts produce anterior rotation and delivery of the head. In nulliparas, the soft parts have to be overcome and this requires time. If the pelvis is generally contracted, the resistance continues all the way to the outlet and labor is prolonged and tedious.

After the head is delivered, the main difficulty is overcome, but broad shoulders may cause trouble, especially in the generally and transversely contracted pelves. Many infants have been lost through repeated attempts to deliver impacted shoulders (see Chapter 60).

FETAL PROGNOSIS

In the highest degrees of pelvic contraction, the fetus' chances for life are best because the disproportion is recognized early and cesarean section is performed. With slight pelvic contractions, the fetal mortality is not much higher than expected because labor is usually not obstructed at all. However, many fetuses are lost with moderately contracted pelves because the physician has not carefully studied his patient. Too many women with this kind of problem are allowed to endure a prolonged, difficult labor before the spatial disproportion is discovered. This is particularly hazardous when the issue is brought to a head only after forceps delivery has failed. Such "failed forceps" cases are notably associated with high fetal morbidity and mortality.

Asphyxia causes many fetal deaths and is brought about by (1) interference with the placental circulation, the result of frequent and powerful uterine contractions, (2) compression of the brain and trauma to cranial supportive structures and vessels as the fetal head is jammed through the pelvis and (3) prolapse of the cord, a common occurrence in flat pelves.

The largest caput succedaneum occurs in contracted pelves. Of great clinical importance is the proper estimation of the caput because, even if the scalp is visible at the vulva, it may be wrongly concluded that the head is engaged with the biparietal plane well through the inlet. In reality the head may still be above the inlet. The caput also obscures the landmarks of the head and renders the diagnosis of position difficult.

The outlook for the fetus depends on the degree of pelvic contraction and the nature and difficulty of the operative delivery, as well as on the skill of the physician. Optimal outcome requires that problem labors be evaluated adequately and disproportion carefully determined. When the labor pattern verifies, by evolving into one of the characteristic arrest curves, that the pelvic contraction is indeed insurmountable, cesarean section should be done. In support of this recommendation is the observation (Friedman) that 98.8 per cent of patients who had arrest pattern in labor associated with documented disproportion ultimately required abdominal delivery; the remainder were all subjected to difficult, traumatic midforceps procedures, which in retrospect should not have been done (see Chapter 64).

LABOR IN FLAT PELVES

In flat pelves, abnormalities of position and presentation are common. Because of the forward jutting of the promontory, the head cannot enter the pelvis and, therefore, it overrides the pubis. The biparietal diameter is often too large to engage in the true conjugate, which is the diameter of greatest contraction. As a result, the head slides off to the side and the smaller bitemporal diameter comes to lie in the true conjugate, while the biparietal diameter occupies the larger space opposite the sacroiliac joint.

The forehead descends first because the resistance offered the occiput is greater. Thus, deflexion occurs instead of flexion. This results in a sincipital presentation. Owing to the long transverse and short sagittal diameters of the inlet, the head seeks the most accommodating position for its advance. The sagittal diameter of the head will be in the transverse diameter of the pelvis and the head will assume a deflexed occiput transverse position.

Since the jutting promontory forces the head forward, the available or obstetric transverse diameter of the inlet lies anterior to the true or anatomic transverse. Thus, the space actually available for the fetal head is quite small.

Anterior Asynclitism

A most important abnormality of the mechanism is the almost constant lateroflexion of the head. The parietal bone is inclined on one or the other shoulder. In other words, the head enters the pelvis in exaggerated synclitism (see Chapter 18). This lateroflexion of the head relative to the pelvic plane is called *parietal bone presentation* or *asynclitism*. It is designated anterior or posterior according to which parietal bone is lowermost in the pelvis.

In normal pelves, the head engages with the posterior parietal bone a little lower, that is, in slight posterior asynclitism. However, in flat contracted pelves, anterior asynclitism (Nägele's obliquity) is more common (Fig. 350). It may even be exaggerated to the extreme in which the anterior ear is palpable behind the pubis.

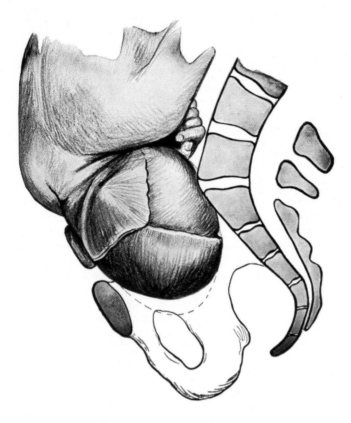

Figure 350 Anterior asynclitism in a flat pelvis with anterior parietal bone lowermost. Marked molding and overlapping of the cranial bones is evident. Caput succedaneum shown by dotted line. (Adapted from Smellie, W.: A Treatise on the Theory and Practice of Midwifery, ed. 2. London, D. Wilson and T. Durham, 1752.)

In the subsequent course of labor, the posterior parietal bone rolls over the promontory into the pelvis; the anterior parietal bone forms a sort of sliding fulcrum on the posterior wall of the pubis (Fig. 351).

The amount of molding of the cranial bones necessary for the head to descend depends on its size and hardness and the roominess of the inlet. The time required for its descent depends on these factors also and on the strength of the uterine contractions. The configuration of the head is sometimes remarkable.

As soon as the greatest periphery of the head has passed the area of the inlet, the occiput sinks, the large anterior fontanel ascends with associated flexion, the head descends and, as a rule, anterior rotation follows immediately (Fig. 352). The subsequent mechanisms are as usual: flexion, descent, extension, restitution and external rotation. Rapid progress to delivery should be expected.

Abdominally, one may suspect deflexion of the head by observing the straightening of the fetal spine and the lateroflexion at the neck. On vaginal examination (Fig. 353), the sagittal suture lies in the transverse diameter, but very close to the sacrum. The small posterior fontanel is on the same level as the large one or sometimes even higher, so that the brow comes down. The sutures are felt plainly at first because the cranial bones overlap, but later the caput succedaneum obliterates the landmarks.

Posterior Asynclitism

In the posterior parietal bone presentation (Fig. 354), the head is inclined on the anterior shoulder. The posterior parietal bone occupies the vault of the pelvis and, if lateroflexion is pronounced, the posterior ear may be palpable in front of the promontory. This mechanism is the reverse of that just considered. The posterior parietal bone stems on the promontory and the anterior one rolls down from behind the pubis.

In posterior asynclitism, the angle that the shoulder makes with the head can be felt just above the pubis. Often the

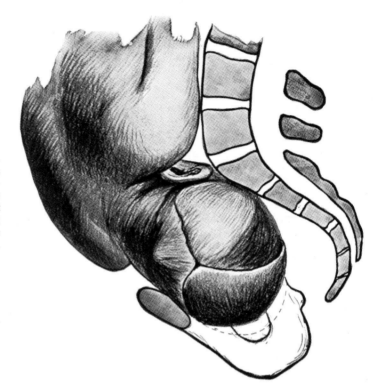

Figure 351 Progression of descent with anterior asynclitism in a flat pelvis, showing posterior parietal bone rolling downward over the sacral promontory so as to permit engagement of the head. Sagittal suture approaches closer to the midline. Compare with Figure 350.

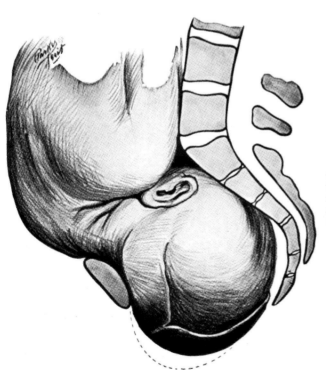

Figure 352 Further advancement with descent to the pelvic floor of a head with anterior asynclitism in a flat pelvis, showing rotation of the occiput nearly to the midline anteriorly. Dotted line is caput succedaneum. Compare with Figures 350 and 351.

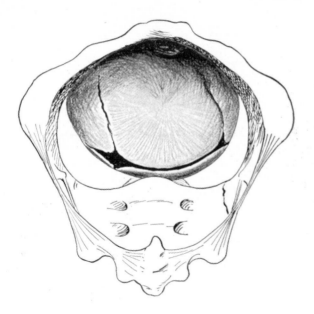

Figure 353 Palpatory findings in anterior parietal presentation, illustrating the location of the sagittal suture transversely near the sacrum and the ear up behind the symphysis pubis. Also shown is the way in which the jutting sacral promontory crowds the head anteriorly so that there is less available space for its descent in labor.

rounded parietal bone can be felt also. Vaginally, the sagittal suture is just behind the pubis, usually in the transverse or slightly oblique diameter. The small and large fontanels are on a level with each other, or the small posterior fontanel is high and out of reach.

As the head descends, the sagittal suture leaves the pubis and comes to lie nearer the sacrum. Later descent and anterior ro-

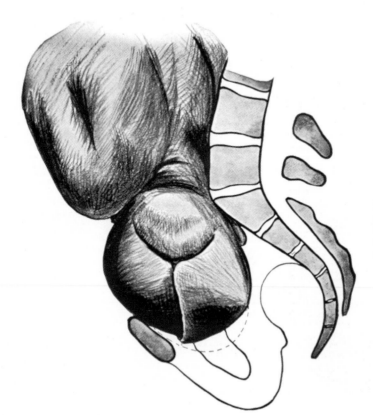

Figure 354 Posterior asynclitism in a flat pelvis represented by the posterior parietal bone leading into the pelvis in a markedly molded, unengaged fetal head. Caput succedaneum indicated by dotted line.

tation of the occiput bring this suture into an oblique diameter. The nape of the neck stems from behind one ramus of the pubis and the head is delivered in the oblique.

LABOR IN GENERALLY CONTRACTED PELVES

The fetal head usually fits well into the inlet of the small gynecoid or justominor pelvis. Abnormal attitudes, presentations and positions are not as frequent as in flat pelves. Prolapse of the cord is rare because the head fits the inlet accurately. Early in labor, the head lies in flexion and as soon as descent begins this flexion becomes extreme. The small posterior fontanel is the first that can be reached with a finger. The sagittal suture lies in an oblique diameter.

After labor has been in progress for some time and molding is advanced, the posterior fontanel lies almost in the center of the pelvis. It is usually covered by the caput succedaneum. The extreme flexion is caused by an exaggeration of the same mechanism which produces flexion in normal labor. The long sincipital end of the lever encounters greater resistance and rises higher.

Generally contracted pelves, unlike flat ones, are narrow all the way down and, therefore, progress is not rapid after the inlet has been passed, but the head has to make its way slowly through the birth canal.

Excessive length of the occipitofrontal diameter characterizes the molding seen in association with justominor pelves. The occiput is peaked, the forehead and face are flattened, the neck is almost in a line with the back of the head and the chin is buried in the chest. Extreme overlapping of the bones is common.

Labor is usually slow. The uterus acts poorly so that contractions are never very forceful; they may even diminish in intensity in advanced labor. Uterotonic stimulation is only occasionally effective. It should not be instituted here until it is certain that cephalopelvic disproportion is not present. Both stimulation and instrumental intervention are potentially dangerous to both the mother and the fetus because of the frequent injuries that result to the maternal soft parts and to the fetal brain.

The diagnosis is usually easy. Abdominally, the extreme flexion is indicated by the high forehead, easily palpable over one pubic ramus, and the deep occiput, usually not palpable. Vaginally, the small fontanel, almost in the axis of the pelvis, and the vertical position of the sagittal suture disclose the extreme characteristic flexion.

LABOR IN FUNNEL PELVES

In funnel pelves, the resistance increases to a maximum at the pelvic outlet and the head is arrested at or above this plane. Extreme flexion occurs and labor resembles that seen in generally contracted pelves.

Pelves contracted transversely at the outlet are sometimes encountered, albeit infrequently. Since the contraction lies between the descending pubic rami and ischial tuberosities, the broad occiput cannot utilize this space during its passage under the symphysis but is forced backward onto the perineum and against the sacrum and coccyx (Fig. 355).

As a result, the perineum and levator ani are often torn, the coccyx is fractured and, if the sacrum curves too far forward, vaginal delivery becomes impossible. Forceps delivery may result in deep injuries of the pelvic floor and tearing of the vagina.

When the head reaches the pelvic floor, it is arrested and impacted between the ischia, but usually anterior rotation of the occiput has been completed. Strong bearing-down efforts produce no advance, the perineum is not put on the stretch and bulging or crowning does not occur.

Vaginal examination will disclose the head in exaggerated flexion, squeezed between the spines of the ischia and covered with a large caput succedaneum. Rotation is usually complete, but sometimes the sagittal suture lies in the transverse diameter. This indicates that *deep transverse arrest* has occurred.

To determine whether the head will or

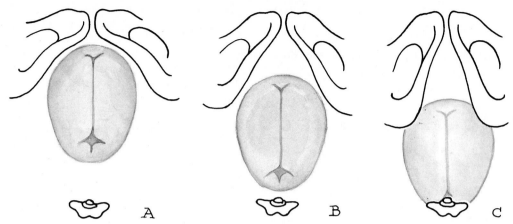

Figure 355 Interrelationships between bony outlet and fetal head, demonstrating the importance of the configuration of the subpubic arch and available posterior sagittal diameter. *A*, Normally shaped outlet with posterior sagittal ample to permit easy delivery. *B*, Somewhat contracted outlet with adequate room posteriorly to allow vaginal delivery. *C*, Narrow subpubic arch with insufficient posterior sagittal diameter, indicating cesarean section.

will not pass the outlet, the physician must know the measurement between the ischial tuberosities and the distance from the center of this diameter to the tip of the sacrum, the posterior sagittal diameter. Klien found that a normal outlet has a transverse diameter of 11 cm., an anterior sagittal of 6 cm. and a posterior sagittal of nearly 10 cm.

It is apparent that, if the sacrum does not curve forward too much, there will still be ample room for the passage of the hyperflexed head. The soft parts may be endangered considerably, however. If the bisischial (interspinous) diameter is less than 8 cm., difficulty with the delivery is the rule and a forceps procedure is often needed. In addition, if the posterior sagittal is less than 9 cm., vaginal delivery is difficult or impossible. A pelvis with a diameter of less than 7 cm. between the tuberosities and a posterior sagittal of less than 8 cm. with a normal fetus offers insuperable obstruction and demands cesarean section.

The smaller the transverse diameter of the outlet is, the larger must the posterior sagittal diameter be to permit the fetal head to escape from the pelvis. As a good guide, the two measurements added together should total at least 15.5 cm. (Williams). In all patients with known or suspected pelvic contraction, but especially in those with funnel and transversely contracted pelves, x-ray pelvimetry is imperative.

LABOR IN TRANSVERSELY CONTRACTED PELVES

Mild degrees of contraction in the transverse diameter will usually not be serious. A circular pelvis has the largest area for a given diameter and a small round inlet may have more available room than a large one which is rendered functionally inadequate by a jutting sacral promontory or compressed side walls. In android and anthropoid pelves, the head fits better when entering sagittally with the occiput posterior. When the posterior segment of the inlet is larger, the occiput tends to move in that direction. If the sacrum projects more forward, as in android types of pelves, the whole head is anteposed, but still the occiput favors the posterior or posterior oblique position after it is engaged.

The head descends until it is arrested between the prominent ischial spines. If the obstruction cannot be overcome, abdominal delivery is in order at this time. However, often it is possible for additional descent to take place if the head flexes well and undergoes rotation in the midplane either anteriorly or posteriorly. Rotation to the occiput posterior is most common. The subsequent mechanisms of delivery are those seen in persistent occiput posterior positions (see Chapter 18), with the occiput coming out over the perineum as the forehead stems between the pubic rami.

LABOR IN OBLIQUELY CONTRACTED PELVES

The obliquely contracted pelvis may present a serious impediment to delivery. Everything depends on the amount of contraction of the true conjugate and, of course, on the forward protrusion of the sacral promontory. If the latter projects low toward one iliopubic tubercle, it will essentially eliminate that half of the pelvis for use by the fetal head in its passage through the pelvis. In effect, this converts the large distorted pelvis into the equivalent of a generally contracted pelvis of the highest degree insofar as actual available space is concerned. Usually, it is most favorable for the occiput to come down in the large half of the pelvis. The mechanisms of labor that ensue will depend on the spatial configuration of the pelvis.

Obstruction in descent or arrest patterns of dilatation warrant cesarean section. Breech deliveries are difficult in obliquely contracted pelves; therefore, cesarean section is recommended when a breech presentation is encountered during the course of labor in a patient with this pelvic malformation.

REFERENCES

Friedman, E. A.: Trial of labor: Formulation, application, and retrospective clinical evaluation. Obstet. Gynec. *10*:1, 1957.

Jacobs, J. B.: Management and outcome of labor in 742 women with borderline pelves. Amer. J. Obstet. Gynec. *43*:267, 1942.

Klien, R.: Die geburtshilfliche Bedeutung der Verengerungen des Beckenausganges inbesondere des Trichterbeckens. Samml. klin. Vortr. *169*:687, 1896.

Smellie, W.: A Treatise on the Theory and Practice of Midwifery, ed. 2. London, D. Wilson & T. Durham, 1752.

Williams, J. W.: Frequency, etiology and practical significance of contractions of the pelvic outlet. Surg. Gynec. Obstet. 8:619, 1909.

Williams, J. W.: The funnel pelvis. Amer. J. Obstet. *64*:106, 1911.

Chapter 64

Conduct of Dystocic Labor

Many factors besides pelvic contraction enter into the course of labor. Success in the conduct of labor depends on the proper evaluation of each of the factors and their relations to each other. Some can be evaluated accurately before or during labor, including the presentation and position of the fetus, the size and hardness of its head, the shape of the pelvis, the height of the promontory, the inclination of the inlet, the state of the soft parts, the character of the uterine contractions and the general health of the parturient. Nature is usually able to overcome the difficulties inherent in many contracted pelves.

Diagnosis

The first thing to try to determine is whether or not it is likely that the fetus will go through the pelvis. The routine examination of the pelvis of every pregnant woman will have directed attention to pelvic contraction. The history of previous labors is of great value, but it must be weighed carefully. A woman may have had a serious dysfunctional labor and yet have a normal pelvis that will present no difficulty in the present labor. With experience and roentgenography, the actual size of the pelvic lumen may be determined with a reasonable degree of accuracy (see Chapter 12).

Not as much may be said with regard to evaluating the fetus. It is more difficult to form an opinion of its size and still more difficult to estimate the ossification and configuration of its head. The hardness of the fetal head is determined by the general impression of firmness of the bones conveyed to the fingers, the sharpness of the contour of the parietal bosses, the size of the fontanels, the extent to which the bones overlap during the uterine contractions and the width of the dome of the cranium.

The station of the fetal presenting part is important. Burke et al. found that engagement occurred at 38 weeks in 75 per cent of nulliparas with the vertex presenting, and in 95 per cent at the onset of labor. If the vertex is engaged at the onset of labor, pelvic delivery can be anticipated in 99 per cent, but if it is unengaged, the need for cesarean section can be anticipated in 36 per cent. Comparable data by Friedman and Sachtleben show a 39 per cent incidence of cephalopelvic disproportion if the fetal head is high at the onset of labor in nulliparas. There is an associated 30 per cent incidence of dysfunctional labor pattern in this group.

After as accurate an idea as possible is obtained of the size and station of the fetus, the physician tries to determine, by more direct means, if the head is likely to go through the pelvis. With the patient in active labor, the fetal head is applied closely to the inlet. This makes evaluation of the cephalopelvic relationship meaningful.

However, such conditions are not always present. Other characteristics can be evaluated. The head is forced down into the inlet by a uterine contraction and is steadied with the fingers (Fig. 356) in order to learn if the anterior parietal boss projects in front of the posterior surface of the pubis and how much overriding there is. The forehead will be prominent in front if the fetus presents with the occiput posterior.

Müller's procedure consists in having an assistant force the head down into the inlet. With the fingers inside the vagina, it

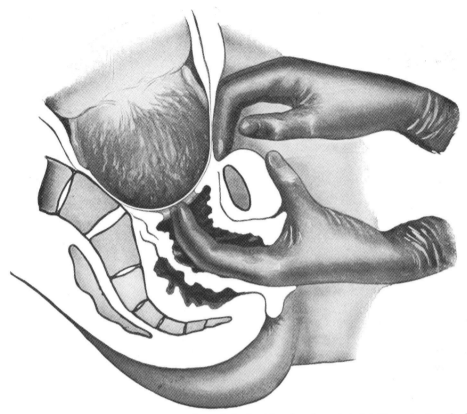

Figure 356 Method for determining overriding of the fetal head at the pelvic inlet by palpating the head in its relationship to the posterior surface of the symphysis pubis.

is determined how far the fetal head enters the pelvis. It has most value after the cervix is out of the way because the soft parts may prevent the head from engaging under the limited amount of downward pressure that it is possible to exert safely with both hands. This same information may also be obtained with the Müller-Hillis maneuver (Fig. 357), in which the fundic pressure is applied by the physician himself at the same time as he is evaluating descent. Still more information is obtainable by observing the "thrust" of the fetal head during a uterine contraction while simultaneously applying pressure to the uterine fundus.

When uncertainty exists, an anesthetic may be used to evaluate the situation carefully. The most valuable information is the determination of the degree of engagement or station (see Chapter 19). If the vault of the pelvis is empty and the head is high and floating in late active labor, the

pelvis is probably considerably contracted. If the head enters the inlet with a large segment projecting into the excavation, and if it seems to flex and rotate in the mechanisms best suited to the pelvis, it is reasonably certain that the contractions will succeed in molding it sufficiently for spontaneous delivery.

By passing the fingers around the head and alternately touching the walls of the pelvis, it is not difficult to form an accurate concept of the degree of disproportion. Engagement is usually certain if the lowest portion of the head has reached zero station at the interspinous plane (see Chapter 19), provided excessive molding has not taken place. Lengthening of the head from extreme molding may be misleading; therefore, it should be determined if the larger portion of the head is not still above the inlet even though the occiput has reached the midplane.

A diagnosis of presentation, position and

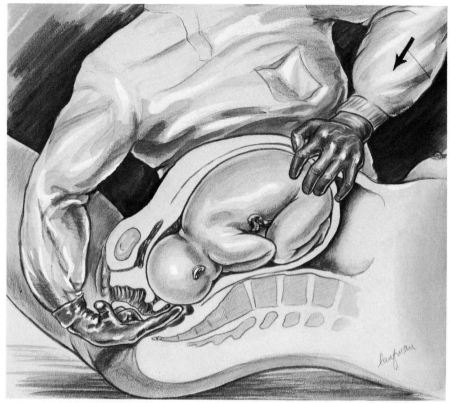

Figure 357 Demonstration of the Müller-Hillis maneuver for determining depth of descent of fetal head through the pelvic inlet by palpation through the vagina while simultaneously applying Kristeller fundic pressure during a uterine contraction.

attitude must be made, followed by a careful study of uterine action. Good regular contractions may overcome great resistances. One should accurately plot cervical dilatation and station against elapsed time in labor (see Chapters 15 and 55) so that aberrant patterns indicative of disordered labor will be detected promptly.

INLET CONTRACTION

The greatest difficulties arise in the management of patients with moderate degrees of pelvic inlet contraction. When it is discovered, one must decide whether to perform a cesarean section or to await a fair test of labor. In nulliparas whose fetuses do not seem overly large, when the pelvic contraction is near the upper limit with the true conjugate of 9 to 9.5 cm. or greater and when the contractions are strong, it is advisable to wait and see what

nature will accomplish. The contractions usually mold the head into the inlet and a disproportion that seemed insuperable is overcome. The head is generally advanced so low that it can be easily extracted by forceps. Such a termination is likely in most instances.

When the conditions are particularly unfavorable—that is, when the evaluation shows that the disproportion between the fetus and the pelvis is not likely to be overcome by the natural forces, when the presentation and position are abnormal, when the history of previous labors is unfavorable or the constitution of the woman is such that a prolonged, difficult labor and delivery cannot be accomplished—then cesarean section is the operation of choice.

Trial of Labor

In those situations in which disproportion may exist between the fetal head and the maternal pelvis, one may permit labor to evolve long enough to see if vaginal delivery is feasible. Definitions of *trial of labor* or *test of labor* vary widely because there are differences in philosophy among obstetricians as to which physiological or clinical criteria are most applicable in determining whether or not the fetopelvic relationships are adequate to permit a safe, atraumatic delivery. There are actually no specific clinical criteria that will define the adequacy of a trial of labor in association with disproportion.

Most formulations of such tests heretofore have been quite arbitrary in designating a specific number of hours in strong labor, with or without full cervical dilatation and ruptured membranes. We are not concerned here with other varieties of trial labors unassociated with cephalopelvic disproportion, such as labor after cesarean section (see Chapter 76), labor in association with prolonged latent phase (see Chapter 55) or labor induced for medical or obstetric complications (see Chapter 24). The principles are, nevertheless, the same. It is now felt that we can take advantage of the expected course of labor in terms of projected extrapolations of the cervical dilatation and descent patterns as detailed in Chapter 15.

Normal labors have been found to follow well-defined curves when cervical dilatation and station are plotted against time. Accordingly, it is felt that, in cases in which the lower limbs of these curves are established, a degree of predictability is present in that they may be projected in time (Fig. 358). In the phase of maximum slope, for example, in which dilatation proceeds essentially in a linear fashion, one can simply project the line upward to full dilatation. Thus, for a particular labor which has entered the active phase of dilatation, one may anticipate full dilatation after a period of time specified for the patient on the basis of earlier progress. The duration is dependent on the previously established rate of cervical dilatation.

For a labor which has entered the active phase under observation and in which the maximum slope is definable by two or more observations obtained within this phase, the slope line may be projected on the time axis as a straight-line extension to a point representing anticipated full dilatation. By adding to this a factor representing the maximum deceleration phase (3 hours in nulliparas, 1 hour in multiparas), one obtains the time when the second stage should be expected to begin. Furthermore, by adding a suitable interval for the duration of the second stage, one derives that time when delivery should theoretically be effected. The projected curve may be used effectively to define normal progress and to delimit what may be considered the proper sequence of an adequate trial of labor (Friedman).

In a group of 236 patients with documented disproportion who were allowed to labor, Friedman found 24 per cent fol-

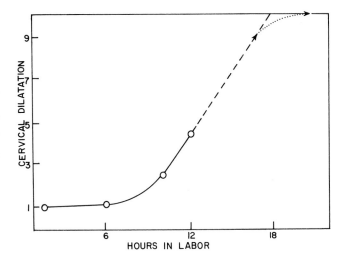

Figure 358 Plotting trial of labor using method for extrapolating dilatation curve in the active phase by projecting linear phase of maximum shape up to 9 cm. and adding an appropriate duration for the deceleration phase. (Modified from Friedman, E. A.: Obstet. Gynec. *10*:1, 1957.)

lowing the extrapolated curve precisely, 41 per cent developed prolonged deceleration and 35 per cent had arrest of dilatation or descent. Greater degrees of disproportion occurring more often at the inlet than the midplane were encountered in the last group. Only five per cent of those following the expected pattern required cesarean section, indicating the optimistic outlook for these patients. With prolonged deceleration, there were 36 per cent cesarean sections and 40 per cent midforceps. No patient with the combination of arrest and disproportion delivered normally. Fetal mortality was greatest in those babies subjected to midforceps procedures, especially after arrest of dilatation or descent or after prolonged deceleration. Thus, the labor pattern serves as an index of the feasibility of safe vaginal delivery.

Attention should be paid to the bowels, as a full rectum may prevent engagement. The same may be said of the bladder; occasionally, catheterization with a soft rubber catheter permits a head which is high and unengaged to sink into the pelvis. However, routine catheterization should be avoided so as to prevent infection. Bloody urine and the frequent desire to urinate indicate injurious pressure on the bladder. Psychic and physical exhaustion is to be avoided. The four dangers to be guarded against in labor are asphyxia of the fetus, exhaustion of the mother, infection and rupture of the uterus.

If spontaneous delivery does not occur, or if the head does not engage so that it may be delivered with relative ease by forceps, there is really no other option but cesarean section that will ensure delivery of a live, undamaged infant of a healthy, intact mother.

Version with extraction is mentioned here for completeness only. It is fraught with great danger to both the mother and the fetus. The fewer versions performed for any purpose the better, and most certainly this traumatic procedure should never be done when any degree of pelvic contraction is present.

Forceps is sometimes used inappropriately when the head has molded so that it appears to be deeply engaged. Here, the forward leading edge is at the perineal floor as the result of markedly exaggerated molding, but engagement and descent have not yet actually taken place and the contractions have ceased. This treacherous and highly hazardous practice must be stringently avoided. Both the mother and the fetus suffer seriously as a consequence. The procedure constitutes a *high forceps* operation and is categorically condemned because of the damage it does. It must never be done.

The concepts of *failed forceps* and *trial forceps* are, unfortunately, emotionally charged (see Chapter 75). The physician must not feel he is obligated to effect vaginal delivery just because he has applied forceps to the fetal head. It is far better to accept the fact that one has misjudged the cephalopelvic relationships, remove the forceps and proceed with cesarean section than to persist in a foolhardy attempt to force the fetus through the pelvis.

Aside from actual disproportion, the reasons for failed forceps include application before the cervix is fully dilated and undiagnosed malpositions with improper application. Both these latter situations are avoidable in the hands of experienced, competent obstetricians. It is imperative that forceps never be applied unless the cervix is fully dilated and fully retracted and the fetal position is accurately defined.

MIDPLANE CONTRACTION

The principles of trial labor based on cervical dilatation and descent patterns outlined above are equally applicable to labor in association with midplane contraction. Most patients with moderate to minimal degrees of midplane contraction go through perfectly normal labor progressions and deliver uneventfully.

Midplane diameters can be measured by clinical means (see Chapter 12), but accuracy tends to be suboptimal. Some reliance may be placed on roentgen pelvimetry whenever midpelvic obstruction is suspected, although it should be borne in mind that interpretation of the midplane measurements must be tempered according to available compensatory room. The fetal head is able to take better advantage of such available space in the midpelvis than in the inlet. The presence of the fetal head applied closely to midplane structures is helpful for providing a reasonable idea of the cephalopelvic relationships, especially if this information is considered in conjunction with the results of the Müller-Hillis maneuver (see above).

Midplane contraction is by no means uncommon as a cause of dystocia and operative delivery (Hanson). Midplane contraction such as is seen in android and anthropoid pelves may direct the occiput into the hollow of the sacrum and prevent anterior rotation of the occiput or only allow rotation to the transverse diameter. Deflexion attitudes are common in this type of contraction. If the spines of the ischia project too far, mechanical dystocia may render any attempt at rotation undesirable and vaginal delivery unlikely even in the occipitosacral position.

These are the women in whom the cervix, bladder and rectum may be torn from their fascial and bony anchorages by inept operating. Therefore, the utmost care in rotating the head must be observed if manual or forceps rotations (see Chapter 75) are undertaken. The head should be given time to mold itself in its new position. When the midplane transverse diameter is less than 10 cm. combined with anteroposterior shortening, the incidence of potentially traumatic operative delivery is unacceptably high. Hence, cesarean section should be performed for most combined transverse and anteroposterior contractions of the midplane.

OUTLET CONTRACTION

Serious outlet contractions are practically never present alone without concomitant midplane contractions. Usually, the obstruction offered by the narrow bony outlet is not recognized until the head has been arrested at this point for some time. Forceps may be applied in ignorance of the true condition. Engagement of the head is the rule unless there is a coexistent contracted inlet.

Before every forceps operation, it is wise to measure the distance between the tuberosities and to determine how far the sacrum and the coccyx encroach on the anteroposterior diameter of the outlet so as to avoid this kind of entrapment. Considerable damage can be done by trying to deliver a fetus through such a contracted outlet. Although the situation is rare, a pronounced outlet contraction with a large fetus justifies cesarean section. Usually, the prospect for a vaginal delivery is good if the outlet contraction is not great. If forceps must be used, extreme care is essential because severe damage can be inflicted on both mother and fetus under these circumstances.

REFERENCES

Burke, L., Rubin, H. W., and Berenberg, A. L.: The significance of the undiagnosed vertex in a nullipara at thirty-eight weeks' gestation. Amer. J. Obstet. Gynec. 76:132, 1958.

Friedman, E. A.: Trial of labor: Formulation, application and retrospective clinical evaluation. Obstet. Gynec. 10:1, 1957.

Friedman, E. A., and Sachtleben, M. R.: Station of the fetal presenting part: II. Effect on the course of labor. Amer. J. Obstet. Gynec. 93:530, 1965.

Hanson, S.: The transversely contracted midpelvis with particular reference to forceps delivery. Amer. J. Obstet. Gynec. 32:385, 1936.

Hanson, S.: Sagittal expansion in narrow midpelves. Amer. J. Obstet. Gynec. 63:1312, 1952.

Hanson, S.: The contracted upper midpelvis. Amer. J. Obstet. Gynec. 65:290, 1953.

Hillis, D. S.: Diagnosis of contracted pelvis. Illinois Med. J. 74:131, 1938.

Müller, P.: Über die Prognose der Geburt bei engem Becken. Arch. Gynäk. 27:311, 1886.

Chapter 65

Parturitional Trauma

VULVAR LACERATIONS

All nulliparas and many multiparas suffer injuries to the parturient canal. In nulliparas the most frequent lesions occur about the vulvar orifice and in the vagina. Figure 359 shows the most common vulvar lacerations. They are seldom deep. However, severe hemorrhage may occur if the tear extends through the clitoris and even through the vulva itself. Superficial wounds and simple splitting of the skin and mucosa seldom require suturing, as their edges are usually apposed when the

legs are brought together. Hemorrhage from tears is easily stopped by suture.

Paraurethral lacerations are particularly common. They result from excessive pressure of the fetal head against the anterior vestibule and urethra during expulsion, especially in the nullipara. A strong, well-preserved muscular perineum forces the head anteriorly as the occiput extends under the pubic arch. Overly vigorous pressure during the modified Ritgen maneuver will effect the same results by the posterior hand pushing upward against the fetal chin. Such damage can be largely

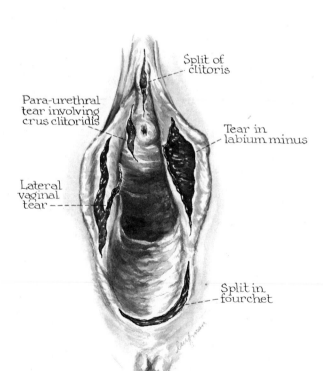

Split of clitoris

Para-urethral tear involving crus clitoridis

Tear in labium minus

Lateral vaginal tear

Split in fourchet

Figure 359 The vulvar structures showing the different varieties of lacerations that can be sustained during delivery.

avoided by use of a deep, timely episiotomy and a properly conducted, well-controlled, gentle Ritgen maneuver.

PERINEAL LACERATIONS

The perineal body is composed of fat, connective tissue of the *centrum tendineum* and rudimentary muscles. The sphincter ani and, at the sides, the strong rounded masses of the levator ani muscle coming down from the pubis are apparent. Lacerations of the perineal body occur in most first labors, but are less important than tears of the pelvic floor involving the levator ani and its fascia.

When the perineal body is torn and left unrepaired, the urogenital septum is destroyed, the anterior wall of the vagina sags, the posterior vaginal wall begins to roll out and the vulva is permanently open. If the tear is deeper, it may involve part or all of the sphincter ani or even extend up the rectal wall. Incontinence of feces results unless proper steps are taken to correct the damage (see below).

The levator ani muscle, with its superior and inferior fascia, is often damaged in labor at term. The muscle suffers less actual injury than the fascia. The following injuries are easily determined by a study of the conditions immediately after delivery and also years later when permanent results become more manifest.

Diastasis of the Levator Ani Pillars

As the head comes down it stretches the pelvic floor radially and axially. The portions in advance of the dilating wedge are forced downward as they are dilated. The fascia is stretched longitudinally from the cervix to the perineum. The two levator ani pillars are parted and the *intercolumnar fascia*, which holds them in their relations to the rectum, vagina, perineum and each other, is destroyed.

Abruption of the Levator Pillars

Tearing into the body of the levator ani muscle (Fig. 360) constitutes a continua-

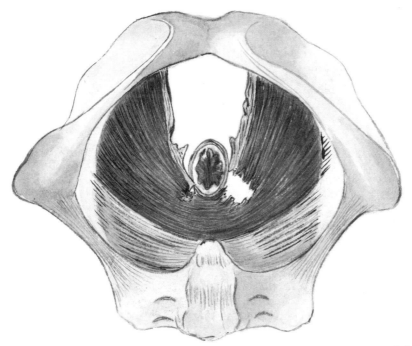

Figure 360 Diagrammatic representation of pelvic floor structures showing separation of the levator ani pillars with tearing of the overlying fascia and, posterolateral to the rectum, lacerations into the body of the levator ani muscle itself.

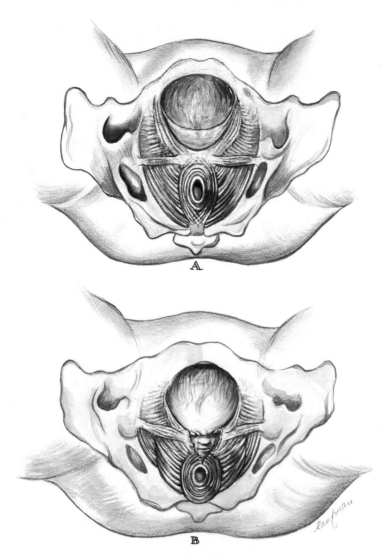

Figure 361 Pelvic floor structures during delivery, illustrating damage done by the fetal head to unyielding maternal soft tissues, (A) distending the urogenital diaphragm and (B) lacerating the perineal body through into the sphincter ani.

tion of the diastasis of the levator ani pillars. The two puborectal bundles are pushed far apart, leaving a wide breach. After healing has occurred, a thick muscle is found instead of a thin, flat, slinglike one; it forms two pillars at the sides of a gaping introitus with the rectum protruding between them.

Anatomically, in addition to the destruction of the intercolumnar fascia, the interlacing of the levator ani muscle with the sides of the rectum and sphincter ani is severed. The tear may extend deeply into the ischiorectal fossa. It may be bilateral and, usually, it is deeper on one side than the other. The vagina and the perineum are always torn and sometimes the sphincter ani, too (Fig. 361).

Subpubic Tears

Tears of the subpubic tissues are rarely seen. They are usually caused by rapid operative delivery. Parts of the levator ani may be cut between the anterior aspect of forceps blades and the descending pubic rami if the instrument is turned up too sharply as the head is delivered, or the levator ani may be twisted and severed from its attachment to the bone when the head is rotated with forceps. When such an injury is extensive, the bladder is denuded at the top of the wound, the vesicovaginal fascia is severed from its rootstock and the vagina is torn from the pubis.

Etiology

The most common cause of perineal lacerations is disproportion between the fetus and the soft parts. Either the head is too large or the canal is too small, as occurs with infantile genitals. The head may present unfavorable diameters to the passage, as in occiput posterior positions and brow presentations. Too rapid delivery causes many tears by not giving the parts time to dilate.

Therefore, the most extensive injuries occur during breech or forceps deliveries. Sometimes the perineum is crushed with forceps or torn by introducing the hand alongside the fetal body in breech deliveries. Other causes of laceration may be edema from prolonged labor, excessive rigidity in elderly nulliparas or scars from previous injury. Sometimes the perineum tears like wet blotting paper with no apparent reason.

An important and generally unrecognized cause of perineal tears is a narrow subpubic arch. Unless the head can occupy the space directly under the subpubic ligament, it is forced downward toward the coccyx to occupy the posterior aspect of the outlet (see Fig. 355), thus overstretching the levator ani muscles and the perineum. Extensive injuries thus occur in women with funnel pelves and in those with a narrow subpubic arch. In these patients, if the delivery is operative, the vagina may be caught between the head and the bones and be forced or dragged downward and outward. If rotatory movements are made with forceps at the same time, the vaginal walls may actually be torn off their pelvic attachments.

Sometimes the skin is intact but all the deeper structures down to the rectum are torn; in such instances superficial observation will not disclose the extent of the injury. It may even be thought that no lacerations exist. To repair such injuries it is necessary to incise the thin bridge of skin medially the whole length of the wound.

Perineal tears are classified in three degrees (see Chapter 20): *First degree* tears are those in which the skin and mucosa are torn, but not the fascia or muscle beneath. *Second degree* tears include all other tears except those in which the laceration is through the sphincter ani muscle (Fig. 362). A *third degree* or *complete laceration* is one in which the tear is through the sphincter muscle and/or mucous membrane of the rectum or anus (Fig. 363).

Treatment

Preventive. Protection of the perineum according to the principles stated in Chapter 20 will prevent many, but not all, injuries to the pelvic floor. Even episiotomy is not always sufficient to prevent lacerations, although in experienced hands they should seldom occur. Incision of the perineum should be done not only when it is rigid and inelastic but also in premature labors to prevent cranial compression and injury to the fetus, and in most nulliparas to prevent serious perineal trauma and preserve the sphincter ani from injury.

Slow delivery is the secret for preventing tears in spontaneous and operative deliveries. If very frequent auscultation of the heart tones or continuous monitoring of the rate shows that the fetus is in good condition, slow and persistent perineal dilatation can take place very effectively. Even with forceps deliveries, it is possible to mimic nature with intermittent traction during contractions over an interval of 20 minutes or more, and in this time the perineum can be dilated safely.

A deep episiotomy should be performed if danger to mother or fetus demands haste. A deep episiotomy is also indicated when the fetus is exceptionally large and when unfavorable diameters are presented for the passage of its head. A mediolateral episiotomy is preferable when space is expected to be a problem, but many obstetricians perform a midline episiotomy routinely and accept the fact that it may sometimes be necessary to cut the sphincter ani or even the rectal mucosa to provide more room. In favor of the latter approach are less postpartum pain and less bleeding. There is, of course, the risk of extension by laceration into the sphincter and rectum. This is most likely to occur in

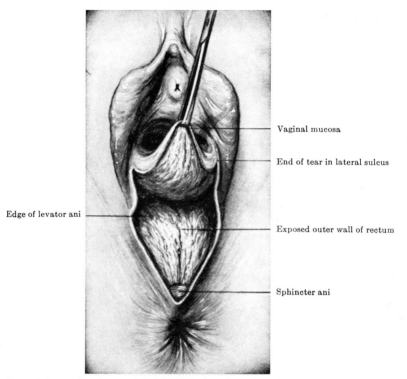

Vaginal mucosa

End of tear in lateral sulcus

Edge of levator ani

Exposed outer wall of rectum

Sphincter ani

Figure 362   Second degree laceration of the posterior fourchette, involving vaginal mucosa, levator fascia and the puborectal portion of the levator ani muscle, and exposing the anterior wall of the rectum and the sphincter ani.

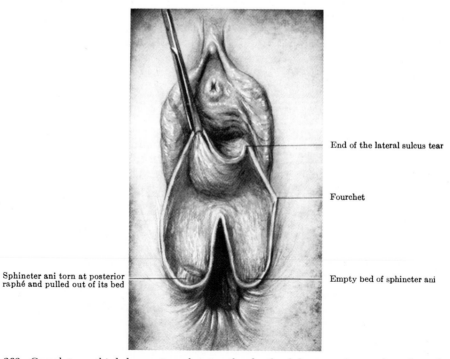

End of the lateral sulcus tear

Fourchet

Sphincter ani torn at posterior raphé and pulled out of its bed

Empty bed of sphincter ani

Figure 363   Complete or third degree tear showing the depth of the wound extending through the anal sphincter and the rectal mucosa. The flap of the vagina is raised.

unskilled hands, and is best avoided. Complete laceration occurs in about two per cent of patients. Repair of the complete laceration is usually satisfactory; repair of the incised sphincter is easier and heals better than one that has been lacerated.

Surgical Repair. Perineal tears seldom bleed profusely. Compression with a sponge will arrest bleeding until the tissue can be approximated by suture. Every tear of the perineum requires repair, but rarely it may not be advisable to do it immediately after labor. Although immediate hemostasis is essential, it may be best to postpone the full repair procedure if the woman is in collapse after delivery or is too exhausted for further operation. In the presence of infection and shock, it is preferable to put one or two chromic catgut sutures in the sphincter ani and one external stitch to support this muscle. The rest of the wound may be left open for drainage.

It is not advisable to place the sutures for completion of the repair before the placenta has been delivered because, if intrauterine manipulation should be required for exploration or control of hemorrhage, the perineal wound may be damaged or the sutures may have to be removed.

First, the wound and adjoining surfaces are cleansed. Care is taken not to touch the wound with anything unsterile. An assistant retracts the anterior vaginal wall with a speculum or right-angle retractors. The extent and depth of the anatomic structures involved are determined. If the fact that the muscles of the pelvic floor are torn escapes notice, one will risk repairing the skin only.

Perineorrhaphy is divided into four stages: (1) suturing the vagina, (2) uniting the torn puborectal portions of the levator ani, (3) suturing the urogenital septum and (4) closing the skin. Absorbable 00 chromic catgut is generally used for the levator ani and 000 gut for the vagina, the urogenital septum and the perineal skin. The sutures may be continuous or interrupted.

Suture of a third degree laceration is illustrated in Figures 364 to 366. Repair of

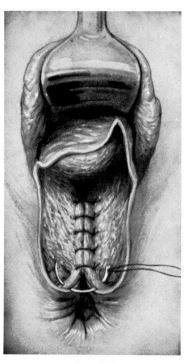

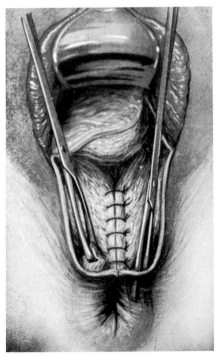

Fig. 364   *Fig. 365*

Figure 364 First step in repair of third degree laceration, showing suturing of rectal mucosa with interrupted atraumatic 000 or 0000 chromic catgut introduced submucosally. A second reinforcing layer of sutures may be placed if the tear is extensive.

Figure 365 Second step in repair, illustrating method for reaching into sphincter pit with Allis or tissue forceps to grasp and draw up the retracted ends of the sphincter ani muscle.

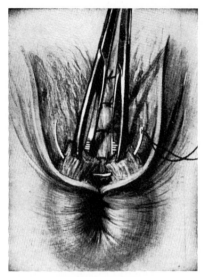

Figure 366 Third step in the repair, uniting the cut ends of the sphincter ani with figure-eight sutures of 0 chromic catgut. The remainder of the repair is the same as for second degree laceration or episiotomy (see Figs. 367 and 368).

a mediolateral episiotomy is illustrated in Figure 367, and suture of median episiotomy is shown in Figure 368. Tissues must be handled gently and carefully apposed with good hemostasis. Sutures should not strangulate tissues. Skin sutures should be placed loosely because edema can be expected. Deeply cutting sutures may have to be removed in a few days because of the pain they cause. Anesthetic spray, heat lamp or soaking in warm water is helpful in relieving discomfort, and may be given together with mild analgesic agents.

When the laceration has been complete, special instructions are necessary regarding the bowels. A low residue diet is given. After the third day, 15 ml. of mineral oil or milk of magnesia (or both) is given in the morning and evening. On the fifth day, an oil retention enema is given. If the bowels do not move spontaneously, it is followed a few hours later by a saline or other enema. With second degree tears, no special treatment of the bowels is necessary.

VAGINAL LACERATIONS

The vagina may tear during labor and certainly during operative delivery if it is congenitally small or strictured, or if it is rigid or scarred by previous lacerations or operations. Precipitate delivery, forceps and rapid breech extractions particularly cause vaginal tears. Difficult forceps rotation may split the whole length of the canal and open up the perivaginal spaces down to the bone. Hemorrhage in such patients is usually profuse and hemostasis may tax the physician's skill. Tears of the posterior vaginal wall are usually due to perforation by the tip or toe of the forceps blade and may go through into the rectum. Such lacerations are occasionally spontaneous; perforating tears may occur between the fetal head and prominent bony points, such as the ischial spines and the sacral promontory. During delivery after craniotomy, unprotected spicules of bone may penetrate the vaginal wall and even puncture the bladder.

Usually, the tears are longitudinal and occupy the vaginal sulci anteriorly or posteriorly. The bladder or the rectum is exposed. Anterior lacerations are often accompanied by tearing of the levator ani pillars from their pubic attachments.

The amount of hemorrhage depends on the location. Sometimes the tear extends more or less circularly around the vagina, near the cervix. It may even open into the peritoneal cavity. This serious accident is called *colporrhexis*. It is fortunately a great rarity because it may result in fatal hemorrhage if the uterine vessels are involved.

Repair requires good visualization, anesthesia and assistance. Sutures must be well placed to ensure hemostasis and good tissue apposition. Dead space should be avoided, if possible, so that hematomas or serous collections will not form. Vaginal packing may be necessary to tamponade the area, but usually this is not required.

LACERATIONS OF PELVIC FASCIA

Damage to the *retinaculum uteri* of the endopelvic fascia, in which the uterus is embedded, is an almost irreparable injury. Overstretching of the vagina and the underlying vesicovaginal fascia is responsible for most cystoceles. The retinaculum

A   **B**

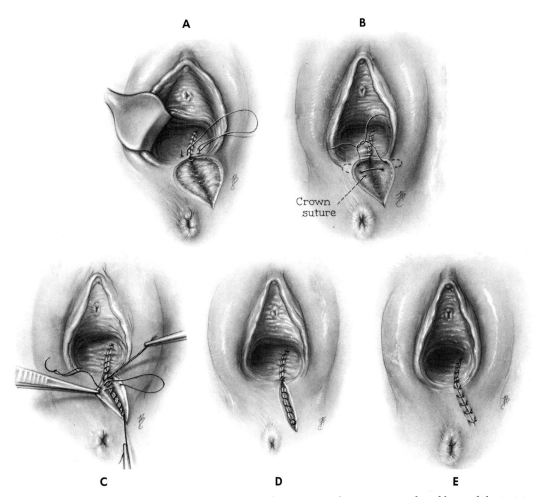

Crown
suture

C   **D**   **E**

Figure 367 *A,* Repair of a mediolateral episiotomy, beginning with a suture introduced beyond the incision of the vaginal mucosa to make certain bleeding will not occur in this area. *B,* The continuous surgical gut suture is tied only after it reaches the end of the vaginal mucosa. Then a "crown suture" is inserted as shown here. The needle takes a deep bite of tissue on each side and the suture is tied. *C,* The crown suture may be held by an assistant, while a continuous suture is begun at the bottom of the incision, making certain that all dead space is occluded by the suture. The suture is continued upward until it almost reaches the crown suture; it is then locked and continued downward. *D,* The continuous suture has been tied to the short end at the bottom of the episiotomy and cut. *E,* A few interrupted catgut sutures, usually four, are inserted to appose the edges of the skin, but they are tied very loosely to allow for tightening when postpartum edema follows.

uteri is destroyed if the parametria are overstretched radially and pulled down. The cervix slides down toward the hiatus genitalis, the corpus falls into the axis of the vagina and uterine prolapse may follow. The same sequelae may result if the sacrouterine ligaments are injured during traction. Destruction of the posterior endopelvic fascia causes high rectocele.

In some patients the urethra and the base of the bladder are detached from the posterior wall of the pubis. The vagina may actually be torn from its fascial moorings. This occurs whenever forceful traction is made before the cervix is fully dilated and fully retracted, as during a forceps delivery or a breech extraction. It is essential that such procedures never be undertaken unless the birth canal is completely prepared so that serious injuries will not occur.

While these injuries usually occur with operative delivery, they may result from the action of the natural forces alone. Pre-

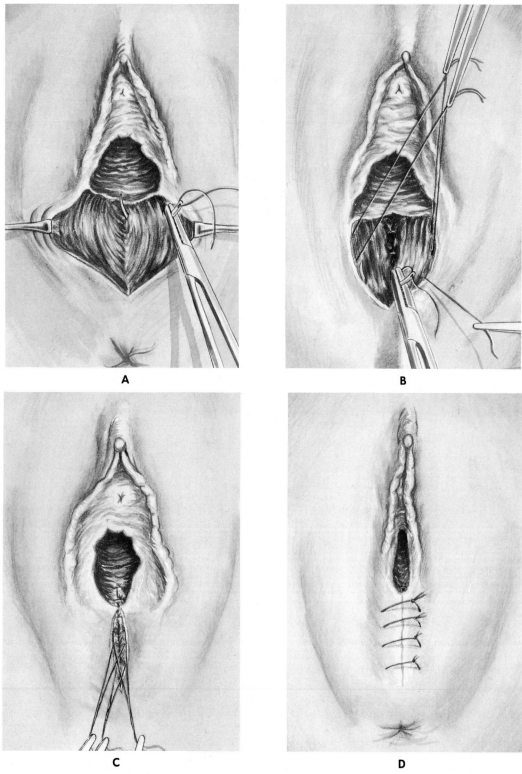

A

B

C

D

Figure 368 Repairing a median episiotomy. *A*, Interrupted suture being placed to bring the perineal body together. *B*, Additional sutures placed in Colles' fascia. *C*, Vaginal mucosa has been sutured; this may be done before the perineal body is sutured; perineal body sutures are being tied. *D*, Interrupted cutaneous or subcutaneous sutures in place and loosely tied.

mature bearing-down efforts have the same effect as forced traction from below. Expulsive efforts should never be encouraged before the cervix is completely dilated. If a patient should begin to bear down too early on a reflex basis, she should be instructed against continuing it or even anesthetized so as to ensure that she will stop.

Perineal and vaginal lacerations are not serious if properly treated. However, hemorrhage may be serious if large veins or arteries are involved. The invalidism following destruction of the pelvic connective tissue may not appear for many years.

Treatment

Physiologic evolution of a normally slow delivery best preserves the pelvic fascia. Manual dilatation and incisions are crude and destructive. Forceps delivery or breech extraction through an incompletely dilated cervix is especially hazardous and cannot be condoned. Oxytocin should be used with caution. A woman should not bear down until the head has passed through the cervix and the cervix is well retracted. If laceration of the vagina appears to be unavoidable and the levator ani muscles are endangered, it is certainly better to perform a deep episiotomy than to allow the vaginal walls and their attachments to the pubic rami to be jeopardized.

A few interrupted sutures usually stop the hemorrhage from tears in the upper third of the vagina, but sometimes the flow is so profuse that the wound cannot be seen. Anesthesia and adequate assistance for retraction and exposure are essential. Speed is required to staunch the blood loss. Transfusion with whole blood for replacement should be given if needed. If delay is anticipated before the laceration can be repaired, tight vaginal packing may be used, but it must be understood that this is a poor substitute and will hide active bleeding within the uterus, the cervix and even the upper vagina. After suturing, it may be necessary to use vaginal tamponade to prevent a hematoma in the loose paravaginal tissues. Tears around the base of the bladder require accurate repair and even then cystocele may not always be prevented.

HEMATOMAS OF VULVA AND VAGINA

Blood vessels, particularly the veins, may tear during pregnancy, labor, delivery or post partum and a hematoma may form in the loose pelvic connective tissue. Hematomas have been found under the skin of the vulva, around the vagina and in the broad ligaments. They tend to enlarge progressively and follow the lines of cleavage of the layers of fascia. If they are below the levator ani muscle and deep pelvic fascia, the hematomas distend the perineum and dislocate the rectum and anus. If they extend around the vagina, they may fill the pelvis and force the vagina to one side. If at the base of the broad ligaments, they may extend up anteriorly into the false pelvis under Poupart's ligament or, if they extend posteriorly, they may dissect up to the kidney retroperitoneally. Although a hematoma begins to form at once, a few hours may be required for it to become manifest.

Etiology

The bursting of a blood vessel may be caused by the trauma of spontaneous labor or forceps. Pressure necrosis explains the formation of hematomas late in the puerperium. Hematomas may form commonly above lacerations or episiotomies that have been repaired. Failure to start the suturing of the vaginal laceration or incision beyond the upper angle of the wound may leave open vessels unligated to result in a hematoma.

Rough uterine massage for postpartum hemorrhage may cause small hematomas in the subperitoneal connective tissue and in the broad ligaments. Large hematomas are rare, occurring about once in 4000 labors. Small hematomas are not uncommon, being seen in 1:742 (Pieri). Often they form when a vein is inadvertently pricked during perineal repair. It is likely that many are not diagnosed because they are not located where they can be readily seen or felt.

Symptoms

Intense pain is the most prominent symptom of hematomas, and the alert, unanesthetized and unsedated patient will describe the tearing open of the tissues and the intolerable pressure on the rectum and bladder. The skin over the hemorrhage is bluish or blue-black. This characteristic discoloration, along with intense local pain and swelling, is diagnostic. Signs of anemia from internal hemorrhage appear if blood loss into the hematoma is great.

Prognosis

If the hematoma does not become infected, recovery is the rule. However, secondary infection is common. It is wise to make a guarded prognosis until it is determined how far the hematoma has extended, whether bleeding has stopped or is under control and whether infection will occur. Delay in diagnosis means needless destruction of tissue and blood loss; hence, early recognition is crucial.

Treatment

If a hematoma begins to form during labor, it should be incised and a search made for the source of the bleeding. If bleeding vessels are seen, they should be ligated. The placenta is removed manually if the mass begins to form before the placenta is delivered; then the hematoma is treated. If the hematoma is found after labor, the usual time for its occurrence, the hemorrhagic cavity must be broadly opened through the vaginal mucosa, the clots and fluid blood removed and the bleeding vessels ligated. If no individual blood vessels are found, the wound should be carefully closed by suturing in layers to occlude any dead space and ensure hemostasis. The vaginal canal is then firmly packed. The pack is removed in about twelve hours. All patients in whom the amount of blood in the tissues was excessive should be given blood transfusions as needed. Antibiotics can be given if there is any evidence of beginning infection after appropriate cultures are obtained. Small hematomas may be left to be absorbed spontaneously, but all are to be opened and drained at the first sign of infection.

Whenever a woman who has delivered a baby complains of severe pain in the perineum, vagina or rectum, or down a leg a few hours after labor, the physician should inspect the perineum and buttocks carefully for a hematoma. He must not assume that the pain results from sutures.

CERVICAL LACERATIONS

Nearly every labor is attended by some injury to the cervix, especially at 3 and 9 o'clock, where separation is very common. Large tears result from (1) too rapid or too forceful dilatation by the powers of labor or by the physician during an operative delivery before the os is dilated completely, (2) disease of the cervix or healed scars from former deliveries or operations and (3) excessively large fetal diameters, as with malpositions or a large baby. Most of the tears are caused by violence. Every forced labor and every manual or instrumental dilatation of the cervix is attended by such lacerations.

The lesion may be a small nick in the mucosa or a deep rent extending through the cervix, the vaginal vault, the parametrium or even to the brim of the pelvis, up under the peritoneum of the broad ligaments or into the peritoneal cavity (see below under Uterine Rupture). Sometimes a portion of the cervix is pulled off the uterine body at the vaginouterine junction.

Rarely, the whole cervix may be amputated and cast off as a ring of tissue. At least 60 authentic cases of spontaneous amputation of the cervix have been reported, mostly in association with prolonged labor characterized by regular and forceful uterine contractions with the fetal head well down against the cervix. The picture is one of labor mechanically obstructed by the external os. Annular cervical detachment is, therefore, a complication of true cervical dystocia (see Chapter 61). The raw stump of the cervix practically never bleeds profusely, as the blood vessels are thrombosed. The recorded fetal mortality is high, stillbirth rates being approximately 30 per cent. This primarily reflects the very difficult labor rather than the ultimate delivery procedure.

Cervical tears are usually not discovered until after delivery, when bleeding begins. Bleeding is slight unless a large branch of the uterine artery or a vein is torn across. In placenta previa, cervical tears usually bleed profusely, as the immensely dilated veins are opened by even a superficial lesion.

Small tears of the cervix heal without trouble, but larger tears, unless repaired, leave deforming scars, leading to ectropion and other conditions. Perforating tears extending into the broad ligament may be fatal.

Treatment

An examination of the cervix should be routine after forceps and other operative deliveries or when injury is suspected. At the sides of the cervix, there is less muscular and fibrous tissue and the tears occur most often in this location, producing the usual bilateral split (Fig. 369). If only the fibromuscular part of the cervix tears, the external and internal mucosas remain intact and a thin bridge of tissue, uniting the anterior and posterior lips, is present.

In repairing such a laceration, the thin bridge should be cut open and the muscular tissue pulled out of the deep recesses at each side. If this is not done, the operation will only bring the edges of the mucosa together.

When bleeding is profuse, it is not easy to suture the cervix because it is hidden in a pool of blood. With vulsella or cervix forceps, the two lips of the uterus are drawn down to the vulva. Successive stitches may be passed through the most accessible portion of the cervical lips. By pulling on these, one may bring the higher regions into reach. Even the base of the broad ligament may be pulled into view in this way so that a spurting vessel that may have re-

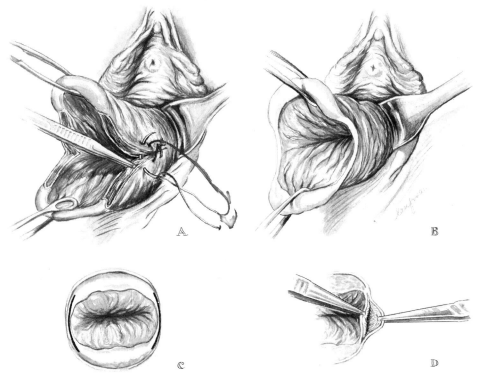

Figure 369 Cervical lacerations. *A,* The typical cervical tear is preferably sutured with a continuous suture of chromic catgut. It is important that the suturing be started *above* the apex of the wound. It is necessary to include a good bite of muscle which often retracts. *B, C* and *D,* An occult cervical laceration. The mucosa is intact, but the muscle has retracted deeply. The two edges of mucosa should be separated, the muscle drawn into view with Allis forceps and the wound sutured in the usual manner.

tracted can be ligated. The torn vessel must be encircled; otherwise, the bleeding continues retroperitoneally and a hematoma forms. Great care must be taken to avoid introducing a suture into the bladder or around the ureter.

The most important suture is the one near the fornix, since it is intended to stop the hemorrhage from the large vessels and from those that may have retracted somewhat. The highest suture in the cervical wound, analogous to the highest suture in a perineal laceration or episiotomy wound, must be placed beyond the uppermost part of the tear or incision in order to be certain that a retracted vessel will not bleed later. Continuous suturing is done more quickly than interrupted. Since the ureter is nearby, the needle for the first suture must be passed close to the uterus; the same principle applies for any suture placed in the lateral fornix.

UTERINE RUPTURE

The uterus may rupture during pregnancy or, more commonly, in labor. Ruptures of the uterus during labor are divided into three classes: *spontaneous, traumatic* and *postcesarean*.

Predisposing causes of spontaneous rupture include all the mechanical factors which obstruct the advance of the fetus through the birth canal, such as cephalopelvic disproportion, shoulder dystocia, malpresentations, malpositions, delayed rotation of the head and obstruction by maternal soft-tissue tumors or fetal enlargements, such as hydrocephalus. In addition, conditions that weaken the uterine wall may also cause rupture, including scars from myomectomies extending into the uterine cavity, pregnancy in an undeveloped horn of the uterus, interstitial pregnancy and grand multiparity.

The mechanism of spontaneous rupture often involves attenuation of the lower uterine segment as labor progresses, particularly in the presence of insurmountable obstruction to descent, so that it thins to the point of disintegration. Ruptures of the lower uterine segment are usually longitudinal or oblique; those in the

corpus and fundus are usually transverse. The normal contractions of the uterus alone may cause a rupture if the wall is diseased. In the presence of mechanical obstruction, even a normal muscle may rupture with strong pains. The hazardous effects of overstimulation with uterotonic agents, such as oxytocin, must be remembered.

Traumatic ruptures have no special mechanism but, as a rule, the upper uterine segment is already drawn up and the lower uterine segment is thinned out when the causative injury is inflicted. Because of this, the shape and location of the tear are similar to those in spontaneous ruptures. A forceps blade may be pushed through the uterine wall, or a portion of the musculature may be grasped with the instrument and crushed. Traction with forceps may pull the cervix down and a transverse split occurs in the lower uterine segment which is already stretched to the point of rupture. A hand introduced alongside the fetus in the maximally distended lower segment may cause the tear. Too rapid delivery through an unprepared cervix may also tear through the narrow canal. Such injuries take place in the overdistended lower uterine segment. At times the physician is completing the tear that was already in progress or just beginning.

The most common causes of traumatic rupture are podalic version and extraction, neglected obstructive labor, forceps delivery through an incompletely dilated cervix, great parity and the injudicious use of oxytocin, even when given by intravenous drip (Awais and Lebherz), especially in women of high gravidity.

With proper obstetric care, rupture of the uterus is almost unknown. Multiparas are affected eight or nine times as often as nulliparas and the danger increases with parity. This is due to weakness of the muscular fibers, scars and residues from previous labors. Obese women seem to be especially disposed to rupture of the uterus.

The incidence is about 1:1300 or 7.7 per 10,000 (Palerme and Friedman; Bak and Hayden). One-quarter occur after cesarean section and many of these are asymptomatic separations of the scar recognized only at a subsequent cesarean section. Most of the noncesarean ruptures are traumatic, including many caused by version and extraction. Pertinent primary causative factors include traumatic delivery procedures and prior uterine operation, most especially cesarean section.

Pathology

Ruptures are usually divided into two classes: *complete*, in which the peritoneal cavity is entered, and *incomplete*, in which the muscle is torn but the peritoneum remains intact.

The edges of the tear are suggillated and ragged. If the broad ligaments are opened, the veins and arteries may be felt traversing the spaces of the connective tissue, which are filled with blood. The bleeding may be slight if the tear is behind the broad ligaments. If it is through the bases of the broad ligaments or involves the site of the placenta, the woman may die in a few minutes from the sudden immense loss of blood. Meconium, lanugo, vernix caseosa and amniotic fluid may be present in the peritoneal cavity.

Usually, at the height of a contraction, the thinned portion of the uterus tears open, and is associated with intense, acute pain. Sometimes the separation of the fibers is gradual and the rupture is completed without producing alarming symptoms; this is the so-called silent rupture. The area which is most subjected to the strain gives way and then the uterine contractions force the fetus through the weak spot thus created. After the fetus is expelled through this new passage into the peritoneal cavity, the uterus contracts down beside it. Characteristically, no further contractions are felt by the patient or the bedside observer. Whenever contractions stop abruptly, one must assume rupture has occurred. Sometimes the rent is enlarged by an operative delivery. Intestines and omentum may protrude through the uterine opening into the vagina.

Incomplete ruptures occur under the same circumstances and from the same causes as the perforating ones. A hematoma develops as a rule. The tear is almost always located at a spot where the peritoneum is loosely attached to the uterus;

namely, at the sides and near the bladder. Cervical tears, if extensive, are usually of this type. Rupture of a varix in the broad ligament, with subperitoneal or intraperitoneal hemorrhage, and tearing of an artery in the broad ligament are rare events, but may cause death.

Symptoms

An alert physician will usually detect a dangerous thinning of the lower uterine segment. He should be especially watchful in contracted pelves, in mechanical obstruction and when the uterine wall is known to be weakened. However, the tear may sometimes occur so gradually that the symptoms will hardly attract notice, or the tissues will rupture suddenly without any apparent cause and without any warning. This may occur at the beginning of labor, with few contractions and intact membranes, or even during late pregnancy, especially after a classic cesarean section.

Fortunately, symptoms are usually present when a uterus ruptures. The parturient is restless; she is anxious about the labor because there is no progress in spite of strong contractions; she complains of constant soreness and almost continual pain over the hypogastrium, and unconsciously her hands support the lower uterine segment with every uterine contraction. Her face is reddened; her mouth and tongue are dry and red; there is a desire to urinate frequently, and she bears down with the contractions in a helpless sort of way. She begs for relief incessantly; the temperature is slightly elevated; the respiration is panting; the pulse is fast and usually of high tension. One can infer that slight tearing of the uterus has begun if she has syncopal attacks.

Suddenly, during the acme of a contraction or while the woman is tossing from side to side, she complains of a sharp, tearing pain in the lower part of the abdomen and she may exclaim that something burst within her. This symptom is not constant. Now the picture changes rapidly. As a result of the shock and internal hemorrhage, the face becomes pale; the lips turn white or cyanotic; the features sink in; a cold sweat appears on the nose and forehead; the temperature drops; the pulse becomes weak and rapid and the respirations sighing; the contractions cease and the patient is ominously quiet for a short time. She complains of shortness of breath, of precordial oppression, of a feeling of impending death and soon becomes restless again. The contractions almost always cease but, if the fetus has not been expelled into the abdominal cavity, they may continue, though weaker. They may even deliver the fetus through the vagina, although this is very rare.

Hemorrhage from the vagina appears, but usually it is not profuse. Pain is felt down one leg if the blood distends a broad ligament. If there is free blood in the abdominal cavity, it may seep under the diaphragm and cause pain in the shoulder. The fetal movements for the first few minutes are violent; then the fetus dies. This phenomenon may be observed with special distinctness when the fetus has escaped from the torn uterus under the abdominal wall.

If the rupture is untreated, the woman may die from hemorrhage, shock or peritonitis; rarely, she may recover unaided if the damage is not too great. The peritoneal edges of the tear adhere and, in the absence of infection, the wound heals. Occasionally, the rupture is symptomless as to pain, hemorrhage or shock, and it may not be discovered for days or weeks, until peritonitis and some other manifestation, such as foul vaginal discharge, pain, ileus or protrusion of bowel, draw attention to it.

Diagnosis

Threatened Rupture. It is vitally important that the diagnosis of dangerous thinning of the uterus be made before rupture occurs, because if anything can be done to save the woman, it must be done at this time. The findings on examination are: (1) a restless, excited, anxious patient with a rapid pulse and irregular respiration; (2) strong uterine contractions without a proportionate advance of the presenting part; (3) a uterus which is thick and hard and drawn up over the fetus, which lies in the dilated, thin, soft and ballooned-out lower uterine segment; (4) an oblique groove is sometimes visible and palpable across the abdomen; (5) the round ligaments are tender and wiry and are inserted high on the uterus; (6) the bladder is drawn up high, but the distended lower uterine segment may imitate a full bladder; (7) general abdominal tenderness is present, but the lower uterine segment is so sensitive that the woman will hardly allow it to be touched; (8) on vaginal examination, the cervix is stretched tautly around the presenting part and swollen or drawn up out of the pelvis with the vagina on the stretch. A caput succedaneum may reach the perineum with the head still at the inlet.

Acute Rupture. The symptoms of actual tearing of the uterus and the shock and anemia which follow will almost always be sufficient for diagnosis, but an examination of the patient must be made to confirm it. The findings in uterine rupture vary with the time in labor when it occurs and whether the fetus is in the uterus or in the abdomen when the examination is made. They are (1) a patient in collapse, with signs of anemia and shock; (2) uterine action stopped or weak; (3) external hemorrhage; (4) the fetus felt abdominally with distinctness, lying just under the abdominal wall, while the empty uterus is pushed to one side or posteriorly where it may not be palpable; (5) dullness in the flanks from free blood is rarely observed; (6) externally, a hematoma or emphysematous crackling may be felt; (7) internally, the ragged rent may be palpable and intestines or omentum may drop into the hand; (8) the presenting part disappears from the inlet or becomes freely movable.

It is a good rule to examine the uterus with the whole hand after every operative delivery to determine definitively if any injury is present. This practice cannot be too strongly recommended, especially after vaginal delivery in every woman who previously had a cesarean section. Care must be taken to avoid producing a rupture of the weakened scar with the hand during such an examination.

Differential Diagnosis

Little difficulty is experienced during labor in diagnosing uterine rupture, but sometimes abruptio placentae, placenta previa and extrauterine pregnancy must be considered. Collapse during or after labor may be caused by other conditions, but rupture of the uterus is to be thought of first. Threatened rupture of the uterus must be differentiated from tetanic uterine contraction because the dangers of the former are so much greater and treatment is quite different.

A point to determine is whether the rupture is complete or incomplete. Vaginally, fingers are passed gently through the uterine portion of the tear and come into a space filled with a soft clot. If the tear is complete, the fingers are passed directly into the peritoneal cavity which may be recognized by (1) the smooth, slippery surface of the adjacent uterus and the abdominal wall; (2) the presence of intestines and omentum; (3) the great freedom of motion for the fingers; (4) the edges of the wound may be outlined. If the peritoneum is so thin and stripped off the underlying structures that the intestines appear to be uncovered within the grasp of the fingers, differential diagnosis is merely academic. The thin veil of peritoneum will in all likelihood be torn through and treatment will be the same as for complete tears.

It is sometimes necessary to decide if organs other than the uterus, such as the bladder, rectum, intestine and omentum, have been injured. If there is the least suspicion of such an injury, the patient is to be treated as if such injury actually existed. The bladder may be examined with a cystoscope. A roentgenogram may show pneumoperitoneum. The rectum may be explored, but if any injury higher up is suspected, the abdomen should be opened.

Prognosis

The outlook for patients with ruptured uterus is always grave. Fortunately, improved modern obstetric practice, antibiotics, early recognition and timely operative treatment have effected a substantial reduction of the previous high mortality. Incomplete ruptures are perhaps a little less dangerous than complete ones.

The outlook for the fetus is very bad

unless delivery can be completed at once. The fetus may be delivered alive vaginally when the rupture occurs at the end of the second stage. If it is forced out into the abdomen, it usually dies in a few minutes. At least one-fifth of the fetuses die (Palerme and Friedman) and reports of up to 80 per cent mortality have appeared (Beacham and Beacham).

The incidence of ruptures of myomectomy scars that have encroached on or entered the uterine cavity is similar to that of previous classic cesarean section (Pedowitz and Perell). Predisposing factors include (1) the extent and depth of the incision in relation to the endometrial cavity and (2) postoperative infection of the scar. Postpartum exploration of the uterine cavity is advised after vaginal delivery of patients who have previously had a myomectomy. As a guide to future delivery, the record of a patient who has had a myomectomy should always indicate the extent and depth of the incision, particularly in relation to the uterine cavity. Elective cesarean section is the safest delivery for a patient who has had a previous myomectomy encroaching on or entering the endometrial cavity or who has had a febrile postoperative course.

Treatment

Prevention of uterine rupture is an important aspect of obstetric practice. The physician must constantly look for the first evidence of threatened rupture in every case of mechanical disproportion (contracted pelvis, malpresentation, hydrocephalus) or weakened uterus (previous cesarean section or deep myomectomy). If a diagnosis of threatened rupture is made, the uterus must be emptied as quickly as possible. Moreover, this must be done with the least possible increase in intrauterine tension. There must be no further distention of the already overstretched lower uterine segment, cervix and vagina.

If the head is well engaged but the cervix is imprisoned in the pelvis, the cervix must be pushed up first because traction on it from below would stretch it still further and produce the impending transverse tear. Usually, this cannot be accomplished, however. This is the operation of choice only if all the conditions for forceps delivery are fulfilled and it is feasible to dislodge the cervix upward. Version cannot and should not be done under any circumstances in these patients. A cesarean section must be done if the head is not engaged. In breech and shoulder presentations, cesarean section is indicated whenever rupture threatens. Cesarean section must also always be done with pelvic contraction or obstruction of the soft parts. To prevent a rupture while preparing for these operations, deep inhalation anesthesia can be used to stop the uterine contractions.

Treatment after Rupture. The conditions that govern management after rupture has taken place are the state of the patient (shock or anemia or both), the amount of bleeding present and the site of the tear. Traumatic ruptures are not uncommon during operative delivery; they bleed profusely. The tear is usually discovered during the removal of the placenta for hemorrhage. Immediate laparotomy is imperative. If, on opening the abdomen, the rent is smooth and the bleeding is easily stopped by sutures, simple repair may be made (Seth); otherwise, total hysterectomy is to be performed.

One must, however, weigh the patient's parity, reproductive desires and theological limitation before proceeding. However, one should never compromise the situation by using ill-advised, inadequate means to control the hemorrhage. Uterine packing, for example, is to be condemned here as wholly without merit. Such conservative measures are of no value in staunching hemorrhage. Maternal mortality has been essentially eradicated in this serious condition by early and aggressive management entailing hysterectomy or, in selected cases, repair of the laceration (Palerme and Friedman).

For severe hemorrhage, it may be necessary to ligate the hypogastric arteries. This is easily performed intraabdominally at the time of the operation for rupture of the uterus. Sterilization is indicated if the uterus is retained, because there is a definite risk of repeated ruptures in subsequent pregnancies. All bleeding must be controlled. Blood transfusion should be given during or immediately after operation according to the estimated amount of blood loss.

Incomplete rupture is usually an extension of a cervical tear and may sometimes be repaired from below if it is not too deep. It may be necessary to detach the bladder to reach the highest angle of the rupture, which must always be secured to prevent hematoma formation in the broad ligament. Usually, laparotomy will be necessary when the laceration extends so far into the parametrium.

A vaginal and cervical tear that extends high into the lower uterine segment is inaccessible to suture. A laparotomy should be performed. These cases are just as formidable as complete ruptures in terms of blood loss and threat to the mother's life.

Since the site of a healed rupture of the uterus is weak and the muscular fibers near it are usually atrophied, it is best to instruct the patient that in a subsequent pregnancy, about two weeks before term, a cesarean section should be performed, provided the fetus is large enough.

Uterine Rupture During Pregnancy

Ruptures of the uterus during pregnancy are rare events. They are classified in the same way as those in labor, namely, *spontaneous* and *traumatic*. The latter is further divided into those caused by direct uterine injury and those occurring indirectly, as from a fall. Spontaneous rupture may occur from yielding of the scar of a previous cesarean section, previous rupture of the uterus, deep myomectomy, thinning of the uterine wall from manual removal of the placenta, a malformed single or double horn uterus, interstitial pregnancy, carcinoma of the cervix, hydatidiform mole and from the same factors which predispose to rupture during labor. However, in labor, the lower uterine segment usually gives way; in pregnancy, it is usually the upper uterine segment that is involved.

Clinical Course. The symptoms resemble those of ruptured extrauterine pregnancy, but shock is usually more pronounced. This is especially so when external violence is the cause. Pain in the abdomen is the rule, and labor contractions may occur when the rupture is incomplete. These contractions complete the tear and expel the fetus from the uterus. Subsequently, the contractions subside.

The fetus usually dies and, if it is not removed, a lithopedion may later result. The hemorrhage may be internal or external or both; sometimes the fetus tamponades the rent and there is no hemorrhage, so that a diagnosis cannot be made until the abdomen is opened. Hematomas are rare because the tears are usually in the upper uterine segment. Delivery may take place through the vagina before the tear is completed.

Diagnosis. It is often difficult to make the diagnosis correctly. Since most of the conditions which simulate the accident require laparotomy anyway, it is not absolutely essential. To be considered in the diagnosis are torsion of a tumor near the uterus, rupture of the gallbladder or spleen, ileus, ruptured ectopic gestation, abruptio placentae and placenta previa, as well as a host of conditions that may give rise to an acute surgical abdomen.

Treatment. The treatment is laparotomy as soon as the diagnosis is made or seems likely. If a former cesarean scar ruptures and there is no infection, operation consists of removing the fetus and placenta, resecting the scar and suturing the wound. Sterilization by ligating the uterine tubes is indicated, if desired by the patient. The entire uterus should be amputated in infected cases, particularly if the patient has a number of living children.

BLADDER INJURIES

A full bladder may be mistaken for a dilated lower uterine segment, but catheterization will confirm the diagnosis. Varices of the bladder may rupture during pregnancy and labor. Cystocele may prolapse before the advancing head and delay the delivery. A protruding cystocele may be gently pushed back above the advancing head and an episiotomy performed to deflect the head from the posterior surface of the pubis and to relieve crowding.

Bladder injury is common during labor as shown by cystoscopy (Funnell et al.). The damage is directly proportional to the length and difficulty of labor and the trauma of operative delivery. Hence, prolonged or neglected labor and difficult forceps deliveries may produce permanent injury to the bladder in the form of pressure necrosis or direct traumatic laceration. The possibility of resulting fistula formation should be considered in weighing the indications for cesarean section in prolonged labor (see below).

Following prolonged labor or operative delivery, the bladder should always be catheterized. Gross blood in the urine denotes severe trauma and cystoscopy is indicated to determine the exact status of the bladder. If no irreversible trauma is present or there is only little blood in the catheterized urine, an indwelling catheter should be inserted and left in place until the hematuria disappears.

FISTULAS

Fistulas are becoming rare as a result of improved obstetric techniques. Pressure necrosis of the bladder results from prolonged compression between the head and the pelvis. Usually, the vesicovaginal septum is caught between the two hard objects and, as the result of prolonged ischemia, the area under compression becomes necrotic, is cast off as a slough in the first week of the puerperium and a fistula results. The patient notes urinary incontinence. If the cervix is not dilated but is caught in the zone of compression, the resulting fistula will involve the cervix or uterus as well. Various types of fistulas are encountered (Fig. 370).

Undoubtedly, infection with bacteria aids in causing the necrosis. Fistulas are also caused by direct trauma. An instrument may punch through the bladder or cut the ureter, or a wound of the uterus may extend into the bladder.

As soon as the danger of vesical fistula is recognized by the presence of bloody urine in labor, one must determine the optimal delivery approach. Although vaginal

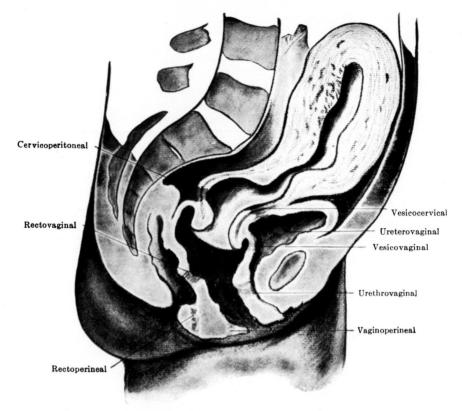

Cervicoperitoneal

Rectovaginal

Vesicocervical

Ureterovaginal

Vesicovaginal

Urethrovaginal

Vaginoperineal

Rectoperineal

Figure 370   The sites of the varieties of fistulas that may result from a difficult, obstructed labor.

delivery is often feasible, it may traumatize the bladder additionally; cesarean section may, therefore, be indicated. Each case must be individualized.

The bladder must be protected. After delivery, the bladder is catheterized. It is best to insert a Foley catheter open to gravity drainage and leave it in for at least 10 days if the urine contains blood or if there was prolonged pressure on the bladder. Suprapubic cystotomy with an indwelling catheter introduced for effective drainage may be very useful under these circumstances. An antibiotic should be given.

Infection often accompanies injury. The scars resulting from ulceration radiate to the sides of the pelvis, even to the bone, and by contracting pull open the fistula and may prevent it from closing. These scars also render curative operations difficult. If sloughing of the compressed area follows, a catheter must be left in the blad-

der until the fistula closes or until it becomes evident that spontaneous closure will not take place. Skin breakdown from continuous dribbling of urine may be prevented by proper nursing. Having the patient lie on her abdomen helps the fistula to heal.

Small fistulas, especially of the traumatic variety (that is, those perforations not attended by extensive necrosis and radiating scars), often heal spontaneously. Operation is not to be performed until the tissues are completely healed. At least three months should be allowed to elapse post partum. The repair procedure should not be undertaken in the presence of any residual infection.

A woman whose fistula has been successfully repaired should be delivered by elective cesarean section if she becomes pregnant again. Too often the trauma of another labor reopens the old wound and a new operation may not be successful.

JOINT AND BONE INJURIES

Rupture of the Pelvic Joints

Such ruptures during labor are not as uncommon as is generally believed. The symphysis pubis is the most common site for rupture, but sometimes the sacroiliac joints are involved. The rupture may be partial or complete. Trauma causes rupture of the joint but, since great force is required to disrupt the pelvic girdle, some inherent weakness of the joint must preexist. Contracted pelves predispose to rupture because the expansile force acts in the narrow transverse diameter. A large fetus or one with especially broad shoulders may act in the same way.

In three-fourths of these patients, the joint has been disrupted during operative delivery. Improperly directed forceps traction, such as pulling upward too soon or too strongly, will produce a rupture, perhaps even in the absence of pathologic softening.

Symptoms. The patient may have complained of pain in the symphysis pubis and sacroiliac joints with difficulty of locomotion for several weeks. During spontaneous labor, the rupture may be discovered at the moment that it occurs, being heard as a dull cracking sound, or the woman may say that something burst. Usually, the physician feels and hears the joint open during operative delivery and notices that the obstruction to the progress of the fetus has disappeared suddenly. Later, the patient complains of intense pain over the affected joint, radiating down to the thighs. She cannot move her legs, which lie everted and abducted. It is a sort of pseudoparalysis and may sometimes be mistaken for acute paraplegia caused by injury to the pelvic nerves. Overstretching of the joints without actual rupture sometimes occurs in difficult forceps deliveries and keeps the woman bedridden for months.

When spontaneous cure results, fibrous union takes place between the ends of the bones, but excessive play at the joint may make the patient an invalid for years. Suppuration may occur if the vagina communicates with the wound. Sometimes infection of the joint occurs hematogenously or by contiguity, especially if infection of the parturient canal exists. Chills and high fever indicate the advent of infection in the joints.

Diagnosis. The diagnosis is usually easy if the condition is considered. The history of difficult delivery, the position of the patient in bed, the pain and tenderness of the pubis and the palpation of a groove over the joint, with movability of the pubic bones on each other, contribute to the diagnosis on direct examination. In the differential diagnosis, paraplegia is excluded by finding the reflexes and muscle function normal and sensation unaffected, and a roentgenogram showing a normal symphysis pubis.

Even when recognized early, this accident is dangerous although recovery and restoration of function often occur in three to eight weeks. Permanent wide separation of the ends of the pubis may require wiring or nailing to restore function.

Loosening of the sacrum from the innominate bones, sacroiliac slip and hemorrhages in the joints may result from labor. These explain many of the backaches after normal and operative deliveries. Pain and tenderness over the joints and abnormal mobility are diagnostic. Treatment is orthopedic.

Injury to the Coccyx

During delivery the coccyx is often forced backward 2.5 cm. or more. This excursion is permitted by a healthy sacrococcygeal joint. If the joint is ankylotic, the bone itself may be fractured or the joint may break open and chronic arthritis may result. Dislocations of the bone onto the anterior or posterior surface of the sacrum occur and also chronic and painful pericoccygeal cellulitis. Many, if not most, cases of so-called *coccygodynia* are referable to these conditions. After injury, the ends may unite at a right angle, a deformity may occur at the joint or, because the bone is moved so frequently (during walking, defecation and sitting), pseudarthrosis may result.

Even while the woman is in bed, there are symptoms referable to the injury, such as tenderness and pain on defecation.

Usually, the first attempt to sit up attracts the attention of the physician. Inability to sit with comfort, pain radiating up the back and down the thighs and difficulty of locomotion are the main symptoms. The patient often rests the weight of her body on either trochanter.

The diagnosis is easy, since the history will draw attention to the location of the trouble. An examination with a finger in the rectum and the thumb over the coccyx will disclose dislocation, fracture (crepitus) or excessive tenderness. Roentgen study is helpful.

Spontaneous recovery is the rule, but sometimes many months are required for its accomplishment. At least six months should be allowed for spontaneous cure. Then, in the absence of improvement, the bone is excised. For coccygodynia, injections of a one per cent solution of procaine around the joint and the supplying nerves should be tried. Heat is helpful.

An ankylosed coccyx may obstruct labor. Occasionally, one can hear the joint crack during a forceps operation or a normal delivery. On rare occasions, the sacrococcygeal joint may have to be broken deliberately, but care must be taken not to injure the rectum. Rarely, the jutting bone may be so large and hard that a cesarean section must be done.

REFERENCES

Awais, G. M., and Lebherz, T. B.: Ruptured uterus: A complication of oxytocin induction and high parity. Obstet. Gynec. *36*:465, 1970.

Bak, T. F., and Hayden, G. E.: Rupture of the pregnant uterus. Amer. J. Obstet. Gynec. *70*:961, 1955.

Beacham, W. D., and Beacham, D. W.: Rupture of the uterus. Amer. J. Obstet. Gynec. *61*:824, 1951.

Funnell, J. W., Klawans, A. H., and Cottrell, T. L. C.: The postpartum bladder. Amer. J. Obstet. Gynec. *67*:1249, 1954.

Palerme, G. R., and Friedman, E. A.: Rupture of the gravid uterus in the third trimester. Amer. J. Obstet. Gynec. *94*:571, 1966.

Pedowitz, P., and Perell, A.: Rupture of the uterus. Amer. J. Obstet. Gynec. *76*:161, 1958.

Pieri, R. J.: Pelvic hematomas associated with pregnancy. Obstet. Gynec. *12*:249, 1958.

Seth, R. S.: Results of treatment of rupture of the uterus by suturing. J. Obstet. Gynaec. Brit. Comm. *75*:55, 1968.

Chapter 66

Third Stage Pathology

POSTPARTUM HEMORRHAGE

Postpartum hemorrhage refers primarily to bleeding which occurs immediately after the placenta is delivered. In practical terms, however, many consider under this heading all hemorrhages from the time the child is delivered until the puerperium is ended. Those occurring after the first 24 hours are *late postpartum* or *puerperal hemorrhages* and are considered separately (see below).

In healthy gravidas, a loss of blood up to 500 ml. is usually borne without any symptoms. Accepting the difficulty in estimating blood loss and the universal tendency to underestimate, most agree that a loss of more than 500 ml. should be considered abnormal. The average loss during labor and delivery should be less than 300 ml.; with laceration or episiotomy, an additional 150 ml. may be lost on average. Bloodless deliveries are rare and usually occur when the fetus has been dead a long time and placental thrombosis has occurred. Oozing should be slight, if any, before the expulsion of the placenta and membranes; after this, the puerpera should not lose more than 90 ml. in the first two hours. It is pathologic for blood to gush or ooze from the genitals in large amounts.

Etiology

During the separation and expulsion of the placenta, hemorrhage is prevented by uterine muscle contraction and later, by thrombosis of the uterine sinuses. The sinuses in the uterine wall are blood spaces which lie between the muscular bundles and are lined with a single layer of endothelium. As the uterus is emptied, the muscular layers and bundles crowd together so that the sinuses are twisted and occluded. The muscle effectively checks the flow of blood through these vessels.

Postpartum hemorrhage is caused primarily by absence of uterine contractions and lacerations of the parturient canal. Disorders of the blood or the blood vessels may also be contributory.

Lacerations of the genital tract play an important role in causing postpartum hemorrhage. The common sites are shown in Figure 371. Lacerations of the clitoris and the bulbocavernosus area of the vestibule may give rise to serious hemorrhage. Similarly, a ruptured varix of the vulva or vagina can bleed profusely. Perineal and vaginal tears usually do not result in major blood loss, but high vaginal tears extending into the sulci or the fornices may bleed profusely. They are usually combined with cervical tears and tend to be seen in operative vaginal deliveries.

A deep cervical tear gives rise to severe hemorrhage and usually occurs if a rapid delivery is effected before the cervix is effaced or dilated completely. Some postpartum hemorrhages with shock are associated with rupture of the uterus.

Special emphasis must be placed on lacerations of the cervix and lower uterine segment occurring in placenta previa. The increased frequency of postpartum hemorrhage in placenta previa is not usually from uterine atony but rather from open sinuses at the placental site and from lacerations. The extreme vascularization of the lower uterine segment and cervix, result-

677

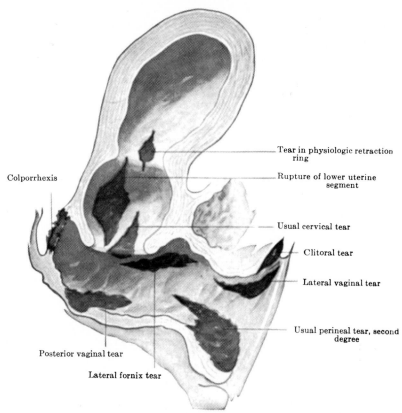

Colporrhexis

Tear in physiologic retraction ring

Rupture of lower uterine segment

Usual cervical tear

Clitoral tear

Lateral vaginal tear

Usual perineal tear, second degree

Posterior vaginal tear

Lateral fornix tear

Figure 371 Schematic drawing of uterus, vagina and introitus, illustrating sites of important lacerations occurring in the course of spontaneous or operative delivery.

ing from the low placental implantation, permits every tear to bleed profusely.

Atony of the uterus is a common cause of postpartum hemorrhage. It may be associated with lacerations. The causes of atonic hemorrhages include exhaustion from prolonged labor or inability of the uterus to contract on a pharmacologic basis, as occurs with certain types of anesthesia (see Chapter 22). Some women have atony in successive labors; therefore, any patient who has previously had a postpartum hemorrhage should have preparations made for a possible recurrence.

There are many local causes of uterine atony, such as overdistention of the uterus by twins, hydramnios, a large fetus or abruptio placentae. The elongated muscular fibers need time to accommodate themselves to the rapidly diminishing uterine volume at delivery; the sudden emptying of a distended uterus often predisposes to hemorrhage. Uterine anomalies, distortion

by tumors and scars from cesarean section and myomectomy interfere with uterine contraction and may allow the sinuses to remain open so that hemorrhage occurs.

A retained piece of placenta or membranes or a thick layer of decidua with clots prevents proper contraction of the uterus. These may cause the uterus to fill with blood; persistent oozing vaginally nay be sufficient to demand intervention. If the primary hemorrhage ceases, the foreign material may autolyze and come away in profuse and fetid lochia, or it may be discharged *en masse*. Cornual placentas separate poorly because of inadequate uterine action. Atony of the placental site is more frequent than is generally believed and may be a common site of postpartum hemorrhage from open maternal sinuses. It may be the beginning of inversion (see below).

Irregular action of the uterus itself or the formation of constriction rings, the best

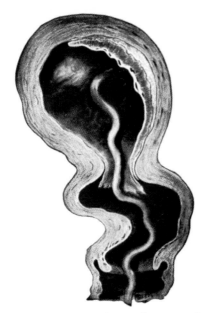

Figure 372 Drawing of sagittal section of uterus with placenta trapped *in situ* by an hour-glass contraction at the junction of the upper and lower segments of the uterus. Note the relaxed lower segment and cervix.

known of which is the *hour-glass contraction,* may be the cause of bleeding. The latter is a serious complication of the third stage. There is pronounced retraction of the upper uterine segment with formation of a constriction ring at the junction of the upper and lower uterine segments and retention of the placenta (Fig. 372). The lower uterine segment is flaccid and there is no bleeding unless the placenta separates. If the placenta should begin to separate, the upper uterine segment balloons out and there is usually considerable hemorrhage. The cause of hour-glass contraction is not known, but uterotonic agents play a role.

Conditions which disturb the normal mechanism of the third stage by producing abnormal uterine action which partially separates the placenta and favors retention of pieces of it, leading to hemorrhage, include: improper conduct of labor; too rapid delivery of the fetus, which does not permit time for the uterus to adapt its walls to its diminishing contents; premature attempts to expel the placenta by Credé expression; traction on the cord; and giving oxytocin or ergot preparations too soon.

Abnormal blood coagulation states, such as in afibrinogenemia or preexisting blood dyscrasias, or diseases of the blood vessels may cause severe and even fatal postpartum hemorrhage.

Symptoms

The symptoms are those of blood loss and vary in intensity with the rapidity and the amount of the loss and the condition of the patient. A sudden large loss is attended by shock. If this is corrected quickly and adequately (see Chapter 51), the patient improves rapidly. A slow, prolonged bleeding is more often fatal because it tends to be neglected.

The bleeding may be internal, external or both. If the cervix is occluded by a clot, membranes or the placenta, or if the vulva is closed by apposition of the thighs, an enormous amount of blood may be dammed back, distending the vagina and the uterus. Blood gushes out when a hand is pressed down on the abdomen or on the uterus. Sometimes a great rush of blood follows the child. Usually, there is a steady oozing or a more copious flow.

Bleeding is minimal or absent if the placenta is totally adherent (see Placenta Accreta below). The worst hemorrhages come from the sinuses opened by partial separation of the placenta; the attached portion of the placenta prevents the uterus from contracting to effect closure of the gaping vessels.

The local findings vary with the cause. If the bleeding is from lacerations, the uterus is well contracted and firm, although it may sometimes fill up with blood and become atonic. In severe uterine atony, it is difficult to locate the flabby corpus. If the placenta has separated but is incarcerated, the uterus is firm and globular but balloons out between contractions. With each contraction blood gushes from the vagina.

Diagnosis

Ideal obstetrics demands that blood loss at delivery be minimized so that anemia will not develop. If bleeding is excessive or symptoms of acute anemia are present, the physician must quickly determine the cause. Rupture of the uterus, inversion of the uterus and other acute conditions must be considered. Bleeding from a firm uterus results from lacerations, but atony (with or without coassociated lacerations) is the cause when the uterus is large, boggy or too soft to outline. The history of the labor will give valuable data; if the uterine action was sluggish in the first two stages, atony may be expected in the third stage and postpartum.

Lacerations must be looked for after forceps or other manipulative procedure. Before the placenta is out, it may be impossible to decide between atony and injury. Diagnosis and treatment go together. The uterus is massaged briskly. Then the vulva and introitus are sponged free of blood and inspected for tears. Atony is probably the cause if firm contraction of the uterus follows the massage and the hemorrhage ceases. Nothing further is done, except that the placenta is removed. If the bleeding continues and the uterus is firm, laceration is probably the cause.

A vaginal examination is done to explore the entire birth canal, palpating the uterine cavity and wiping it clean, and inspecting the cervix, vagina and introitus. It is best to explore the uterus with a hand, having the patient under anesthesia and using all necessary sterile precautions (see below). A large, elastic, globular uterus, with occasional gushes of blood, almost always contains some retained foreign material. Incarceration of the placenta is diagnosed when a tight constriction ring is felt with the placenta above it.

Prognosis

In hemorrhage, the prognosis as to life will depend on the amount of blood lost. Tachycardia, while a good guide, is not always a reliable one. Similarly, blood pressure is a relatively poor indicator. A blood pressure below 80 mm. Hg indicates great danger, and a pulse pressure less than 20 may constitute a fatal sign.

At the beginning, it is impossible to foretell how dangerous the bleeding will become. It is necessary to stop all bleeding as soon as possible and to replace the blood that has been lost in anticipation of additional hemorrhage.

There are remote dangers. Thrombosis and embolism are more common after severe blood losses. Infection also is more frequent because resistance has been lowered and because the physician, in his haste, may have been unable to adhere stringently to the principles of asepsis in the justifiable interest of saving the patient's life.

Management

Prevention. Prevention should begin during pregnancy. At least one hemoglobin or hematocrit should be obtained early in pregnancy and another about four weeks before term. All women should take iron during pregnancy and receive special treatment for anemia (see Chapter 42).

During labor, the possibility of postpartum hemorrhage must be borne in mind, particularly when the uterus is sluggish or overdistended with twins or hydramnios. At delivery, the uterus should be emptied slowly and the rules of the conduct of the third stage observed closely. If labor has continued for a long time, a prophylactic dose of ergonovine should be given as soon as the placenta is delivered. In cases of prolonged labor, great multiparity and other conditions that may be associated with postpartum hemorrhage, bleeding may be prevented by starting an intravenous drip of oxytocin shortly before the baby is born. Use of ergonovine at the time of delivery of the anterior shoulder in a routine manner is widely practiced, but it is a somewhat hazardous practice because of the risks of trapping a placenta or an unsuspected second twin.

Treatment During the Third Stage. When severe bleeding follows the delivery of a child, the uterus should be grasped and massaged evenly and gently. Ten units of oxytocin is given intramuscularly; it should not be administered intravenously because hypotension may result. As soon as the uterus contracts, the hemorrhage can be expected to cease. At the same time, the physician inspects the genitals to discover any laceration that may be bleeding. While doing this, he should continue to massage the uterus. If the uterus contracts but the hemorrhage continues, a vaginal examination should be made to see if there is a cervical or vaginal tear. It is necessary to remove the placenta in order to explore the uterus manually.

If the placenta is incarcerated by the uterine contraction resulting from the action of the oxytocin, in the absence of external and internal hemorrhage, one must wait for the effects of the drug to wear off.

Manual Removal of the Placenta. The patient should be anesthetized if she is not already under anesthesia. Before a hand is inserted into the vagina, the vulva should be sponged liberally with an antiseptic solution and the perineum draped as a sterile field. If there is time, the operator should scrub and regown. He inserts his hand, covered with fresh sterile gloves, into the vagina, avoiding the anus. The fingers are spread out in the cervix so that

the membranes and cord fall into their grasp; then the tips of the fingers are brought together to form a cone for insertion into the upper segment (Fig. 373). It is seldom necessary to use force, but if a tight constriction ring has formed, it may be helpful to exert steady but gentle conic pressure to gain entrance to the corpus. The edge of the placenta is sought with the fingers. With the hand on the abdomen, the uterus is forced down and over the fingers inside the vagina (Fig. 373). With a gentle combined movement, the placenta is usually easily separated from its bed by blunt digital dissection along the cleavage plane. One must be warned not to bore into or through the wall of the uterus; this is sometimes surprisingly easy to do.

After the placenta has been cleanly separated, and before the internal hand is removed, the uterus is briskly massaged

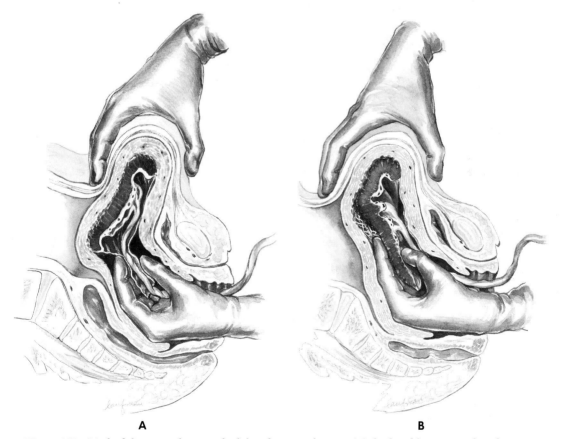

A   **B**

Figure 373 Method for manual removal of the placenta, showing (*A*) the hand being introduced in a cone shape into the uterus and (*B*) separating the placenta from its attachment to the uterus by gently dissecting in the cleavage plane.

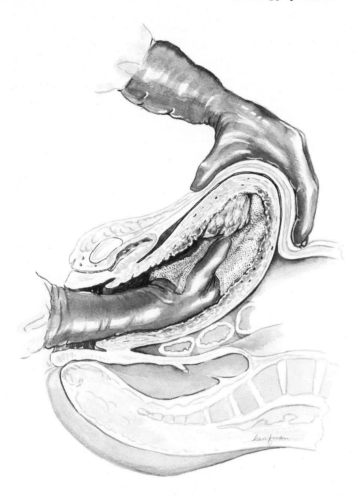

Figure 374 Method for removing adherent membranes left within the uterus after delivery of the placenta by wiping the endometrial surface with gauze-covered fingers of the intrauterine hand while supporting the uterine wall externally with the abdominal hand.

with both hands. A uterine contraction will expel the hand in which the placenta is held. It is essential to let the uterus expel the hand with the placenta rather than to pull the placenta out.

After the blood is washed off the glove and the perineum is again sponged with antiseptic solution, the hand is inserted once more. The whole interior of the uterus is palpated to ascertain that the uterus is completely empty. Care should be taken to remove all the membranes and adherent placental fragments or cotyledons. The rubber gloves are so slippery that shreds of membranes cannot be grasped. The fingers should be covered with gauze to aid in this process (Fig. 374). After this, oxytocin or ergonovine should be given intramuscularly.

A *placenta accreta* (see below), if total in extent, will resist any such measures to find a cleavage plane between the placenta and the uterine wall. It is discovered when the attempt at manual removal is made. With partial placenta accreta, the separation is begun and acute hemorrhage initiated. Hysterectomy must be performed as a lifesaving measure under these circumstances because the placenta cannot be removed completely, and persistent attempts may be fatal.

After the Placenta is Delivered. In all deliveries, the placenta should be inspected carefully as soon as it is delivered and before it is discarded because, if a cotyledon is missing, the uterus must be explored. It is recognized that gross examination of the placenta is imperfect and one may easily overlook a missing piece of placenta. Nevertheless, if the placenta is not intact, one can avert hemorrhage by exploring at once.

For all postpartum hemorrhages, *uterine massage* is the first step. The first motions should be slow and even. If the uterus does not respond promptly, the motions should be made more rapidly and spread over the entire corpus. If the hemorrhage is so profuse that it threatens the woman's life, the aorta should be compressed firmly against the spine with the fist on the abdomen. This will check the flow until the uterus can contract effectively or until the physician can put on sterile gloves and prepare for effective hemostasis.

Ten units of oxytocin is given intramuscularly and followed by 0.2 mg. of ergonovine intravenously. During hemorrhage and immediately after a patient has had a uterine hemorrhage, it is advisable to administer oxytocin intravenously by infusion (5 units in 500 ml. of 5 per cent aqueous glucose) and to permit the solution to run for at least four hours after delivery.

Usually, this medication stops the flow. If its action is not prompt enough or not satisfactory, fresh sterile gloves are put on quickly, a hand is inserted and the uterine cavity is cleared of clots, membranes, and placental and decidual debris. Search is carried out for lacerations. If any are found, they are managed as described below.

If severe uncontrollable atony is diagnosed, other measures must be instituted.

Time is an important element. To stop the hemorrhage, the uterus is compressed between the hand on the abdomen and a fist in the vagina, as in Figure 375. An essential part of this procedure is elevation of the uterus out of the pelvis and sharply anteflexing it as shown. One may feel the uterus gradually assuming its normal shape and consistency. After two to five minutes, the pressure is relaxed. If the flow has ceased, the hands may be removed.

Another helpful procedure (Dickinson) involves pulling the uterus up by seizing the corpus through the abdominal wall with the left hand (Fig. 376). The procedure is easiest to perform in a multipara with a relaxed abdominal wall or with diastasis recti. The right hand is arched (with the thumb spread away from the fingers) with the ulnar border resting against the symphysis. With the fingertips and the thumb of the right hand, the narrow and relaxed lower uterine segment and cervix are encircled as far as possible and massaged. With the left hand, in which the corpus is held, active massage and compression of the thick ball-shaped body of the uterus are carried out against the sacral promontory and the lumbar spine. Access is had to all parts of the uterus and the whole organ can be controlled completely between the two hands.

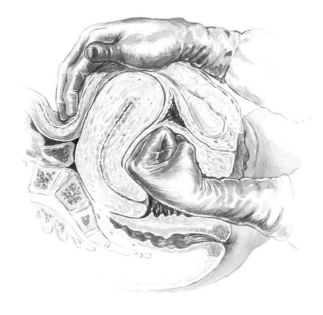

Figure 375 Technique for temporarily arresting acute postpartum hemorrhage from uterine atony by compressing the sharply anteflexed uterus between the closed intravaginal fist and the counterpressure of the suprapubic hand.

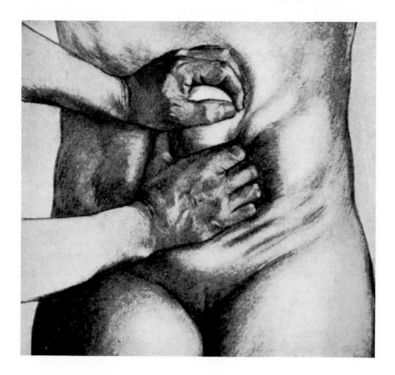

Figure 376 Emergency method for controlling postpartum hemorrhage, illustrating technique for lifting the entire uterus out of the pelvis by grasping it through the abdominal wall and compressing it firmly against the sacral promontory and lumbar spine with the left hand, while squeezing the lower segment in the encircling right hand. (After Dickinson, R. L.: Brooklyn Med. J. *13*:137, 1899.)

At intervals of a few minutes, the upper uterine segment should be pressed down into the pelvis and then lifted again. This movement expels any clots that have formed in the vagina. If the flow continues in spite of these maneuvers or recommences after the hands have been removed from the uterus, some obstetricians immediately resort to packing the uterus and vagina. This procedure tends to be ineffective and may cause loss of valuable time in correcting the problem definitively. It can no longer be condoned because it will not prevent intrauterine bleeding, but may hide it instead. It interferes with proper uterine contraction and it may lead to infection.

If aggressive conservative measures are ineffectual, one should resort to surgery. Bilateral internal iliac ligation is very useful in this situation and can be accomplished quickly, while preserving the uterus for future childbearing. If the latter is not an important consideration, hysterectomy is in order. Unfortunately, some physicians try desperately to avoid such surgery, only to realize too late that they have procrastinated too long and irreparable damage or death occurs.

Blood transfusion may be needed and should be given early, well before irreparable cerebral damage has occurred. Sufficient blood should be given to replace at least the amount lost.

Repair of Lacerations. Sometimes bleeding will cease if a clitoral, vulvar or lower vaginal tear is compressed for a few minutes; if not, well-placed sutures will suffice. High vaginal and cervical tears may cause serious hemorrhage. It is important to remove the placenta at once and try to secure contraction of the uterus. This part of the treatment is the same as for atony (see above), but the only way to stop hemorrhage from a laceration is to suture it (see Chapter 65).

Free bleeding may make suturing difficult. The following measures may be useful to expose the field: compression of the aorta with a fist by an assistant; wide retraction of the vaginal walls by two or more right-angle retractors; traction on the lips of the cervix with cervix forceps and compression of one side of the cervical tear while the other is being sutured.

Sometimes shock occurs during or after a he norrhage. One must ascertain (1) if the shock is due to postpartum hemorrhage or something else; (2) if there is internal bleeding from a ruptured uterus; (3) if the blood loss attending the required manipulations will turn the scale against the woman; and (4) if the patient can withstand an inhalation anesthetic.

Preparations for the operation should be begun while one is deliberating. Occasionally, the procedure has to be undertaken with the patient in shock or even *in extremis*, especially if there has been undue delay. Once the operation is begun, it should proceed quickly, carefully and thoroughly with no unessential frills in order to stop the hemorrhage immediately and minimize trauma, anesthesia and additional blood losses.

During the treatment program, the patient should be covered and kept warm. Morphine should be administered as needed. Blood transfusions must be given, but plasma or other volume expander may have to be given first if considerable time is required for blood typing and crossmatching. In acute exsanguinating hemorrhage, use of unmatched type O, Rh-negative blood is permissible and recommended.

There should be no hesitancy in giving sufficient amounts of whole blood as rapidly as feasible, using a large intravenous or intraarterial catheter, under pressure if needed. The dangers of incompatibility and hepatitis associated with use of whole blood must be accepted when transfusions are given as lifesaving measures, but they cannot be used indiscriminately. The management of patients in shock is dealt with extensively in Chapter 51.

PLACENTA ACCRETA

Placenta accreta is a rare but often tragically dangerous complication of pregnancy due to abnormal adherence of part or all of the placenta to the uterine wall. It is associated with partial or complete absence of the decidua basalis, especially the spongiosum layer, and defective decidua vera (Irving and Hertig), with chorionic villi in juxtaposition to or involving the myometrium.

There are three types: (1) *placenta accreta,* in which the placenta is pathologically adherent to myometrium with no in-

tervening decidua; (2) *placenta increta,* in which there is penetration of the uterine wall; and (3) *placenta percreta,* in which the uterine wall is invaded to its serosal layer. The invasion in placenta percreta may actually rupture the uterus. The condition is further subdivided into *partial* and *total* according to the amount of surface involvement. The incidence of placenta accreta is at least one in 2000 deliveries, and is perhaps more frequent because some cases of partial placenta accreta are overlooked.

The main factor involved in the etiology of placenta accreta is apparently some injury to the endometrium by trauma, infection, previous gynecologic surgery, associated gynecologic disorder or endocrine imbalance. Implantation may occur in areas of endometrial insufficiency, such as over leiomyomas or uterine scars, in the lower uterine segment with placenta previa, in the uterine cornu or in a congenitally anomalous uterus.

There are no symptoms in complete placenta accreta. There is no bleeding because there is no placental separation, and there is no shock unless rupture or uterine inversion is also present. On the other hand, in partial placenta accreta the classic symptoms are those of a partially separated or adherent placenta with acute hemorrhage.

Diagnosis is made definitively by microscopic examination, but clinical diagnosis is essential in order for proper therapy to be instituted promptly. The absence of a cleavage plane between the adherent placenta and the uterine wall makes the diagnosis during the course of an exploration for manual removal of the retained, unseparated placenta (see above). In partial placenta accreta, the cleavage plane may be started, but it cannot be followed completely across the maternal surface of the placenta because dense adhesion is encountered. Catastrophic hemorrhage results when partial separation is accomplished.

The treatment of choice in most patients is abdominal hysterectomy as soon as the diagnosis is made. To attempt to remove the adherent placenta carries a staggering maternal mortality due to massive hemorrhage, traumatic rupture or uterine inversion. Conservative measures, such as support and uterine tamponade, are rarely effective, although there are isolated reports of success in cases of total accreta when no attempts to remove the placenta have been made and there is no bleeding. These criteria appear to be essential for the nonoperative, expectant approach to management.

With partial accreta (or total accreta that has been manually undermined), bleeding demands hysterectomy; conservatism here may be fatal and packing must be condemned. Since the advent of treatment by hysterectomy immediately upon recognition of this condition, maternal mortality has fallen steadily (Rotton and Friedman). Considerable blood loss should be replaced by transfusion.

Placenta previa accreta is abnormal adherence of a placenta situated in the lower uterine segment. The coassociation of placenta accreta with placenta previa is seen in 18 per cent (Rotton and Friedman). The main etiologic factor here is the lack of decidual response at the site of the placental implantation. The preferred treatment of placenta previa accreta is the same as for placenta accreta, namely, total hysterectomy (Koren et al.).

UTERINE INVERSION

Complete inversion of the uterus is an exceedingly rare complication of the third stage (Fig. 377), in which the corpus vir-

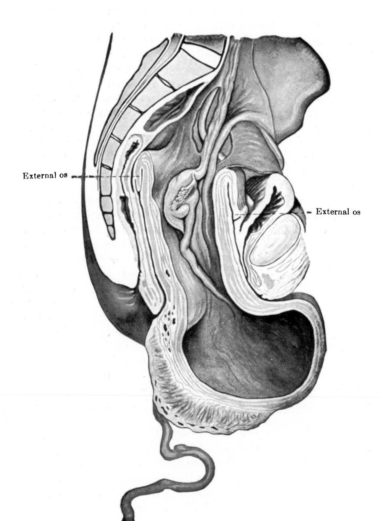

External os

External os

Figure 377 Diagrammatic illustration of a case of total uterine inversion with the placenta still attached to the posterior endometrial surface. Note the tube and ovary pulled down into the intra-abdominal inversion funnel. (From Halban, J., and Tandler, J.: Anatomie und Ätiologie der Genitalprolapse beim Weibe, Vienna, Wilhelm Braumüller, 1907.)

tually turns inside out. The most common form is that in which the inverted corpus lies in the vagina just within the introitus and feels like a soft, large, globular leiomyoma. The placenta may still be attached or only partially adherent. If the uterus lies outside the vagina, the open sinuses and tubal ostia may be visible. In the *inversion funnel* viewed from the abdominal side, the uterine tubes, the ovaries, the round and broad ligaments, and sometimes the intestines and omentum may be found.

Etiology

The conditions necessary for inversion are believed to be (1) sudden emptying of the uterus after distention of its cavity; (2) physiologic or pathologic thinning of its walls by the gradual development of some tumor within it; (3) a dilated cervix; and (4) usually some forceful pressure or traction on the fundus.

While atony of the uterus is the cause of most inversions, an inversion can be produced by focal contraction of the corpus with relaxation of the lower portion of the uterus. An atonic uterus may become inverted by a sudden contraction of the abdominal and diaphragmatic muscles increasing intraabdominal pressure (as from bearing down to express the placenta), changing position in bed and coughing. Inversions are described as spontaneous, as in these situations, in 40 per cent (Das); they follow cord traction in 21 per cent and improper placental expression in 19 per cent.

Symptoms

As a rule, inversion is gradual, beginning as a little depression and then suddenly the corpus drops into the vagina. If traction on the cord has been made, the movement is more abrupt. The patient cries out and bears down and this tends to increase the inversion.

Shock is often present and is certain to exist if the inversion was sudden. The shock tends to be disproportionate to the amount of blood loss.

Profuse hemorrhage is the rule, but it may be absent if the placenta still adheres to the inverted uterus. The placenta is completely or partially adherent at the fundus in nearly 75 per cent of the patients (Das). If the uterus contracts, especially if the cervix closes around the extruded corpus, the bleeding may be slight; but this is the exception. In rare instances, neither collapse nor severe bleeding is present; the condition is discovered only at a subsequent examination.

In the chronic cases, the corpus atrophies in the vagina and becomes covered with dry, slightly cornified epithelium. Menorrhagia, leukorrhea and irregular bleeding are often present with dragging pains in the back and a feeling of bearing down, but all of these symptoms may be remarkably absent.

Diagnosis

If the physician bears this accident in mind, there is no difficulty in diagnosis on direct examination. The uterine corpus is not in its proper place and there is a large, round mass in the vagina. The presence of shock and hemorrhage will suggest the diagnosis at once. It may be possible to feel the inverted funnel through the abdomen after the bladder is emptied.

Submucous leiomyoma, adherent placenta and uterine atony must be ruled out. A bimanual examination will easily decide the diagnosis. If the corpus is prolapsed, the bright red, rough, bleeding endometrium or the placenta discloses what has happened.

Prognosis

Immediate recognition offers the best chance of survival, irrespective of the treatment given. The mortality rises steadily as recognition is delayed up to 48 hours. The mortality decreases sharply if patients with unrecognized inversion survive beyond this time. Recurrence is common in subsequent pregnancies among survivors (Miller).

Treatment

Preventive. Although uterine inversion is rare, the physician's routine technique in handling labor should include means for its prevention. There should be no pressure on the corpus, particularly while it is relaxed. Traction on the cord must be stringently avoided. While drawing the membranes off the uterine wall, the hand outside must rest on the corpus to be sure that it is well contracted. Atony of the uterus post partum is to be overcome as soon as possible. In changing the newly delivered woman's position in bed, someone must place a hand on the uterus to be certain that it is firmly contracted. Inversion can always be detected if cervical inspection and immediate puerperal vaginal examinations are made routine procedures.

Active Management. Shock should be combated actively (see Chapter 51) and the uterus replaced immediately, if possible, under deep anesthesia by manual means. However, unless the patient is bleeding actively, correction may be delayed for days or even weeks if conditions interdict immediate intervention (McLennan and McKelvey).

Manual replacement of the uterus in acute cases is simple (Fig. 378). While the whole vaginal mass is in the grasp of a hand, the constricting portion of the uterus is spread out with the fingers and the inverted corpus is pushed up with the palm. All this is done in the direction of the axis of the pelvis, well forward, to avoid the sacrum. Great care should be exercised to avoid puncturing the soft atonic uterine wall.

For chronic inversion, a vaginal procedure is generally performed in which the constricted ring is incised in the midline anteriorly, the uterus is replaced and the incision is repaired as in a vaginal hysterotomy (Spinelli). Huntington's simple abdominal operation is also effective in pulling the inverted fundus up with vulsella from the depth of the inversion funnel by progressive traction as if unfolding it.

LATE PUERPERAL HEMORRHAGE

Even long after delivery there is danger of bleeding. It may occur as late as the fifth

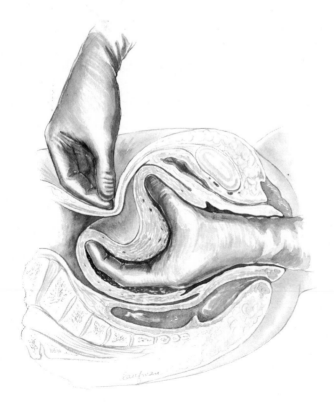

Figure 378 Mechanism for replacing the inverted uterus, showing the intravaginal hand grasping the inverted corpus, spreading the constricting cervical ring with the fingers and thumb and steadily forcing the fundus upward with the palm.

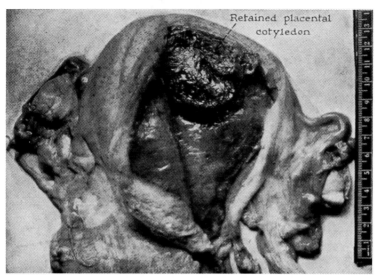

Retained placental cotyledon

Figure 379   Uterus removed from a patient who died of an exsanguinating postpartum hemorrhage, showing the source of the bleeding to have been retention of a placental cotyledon. (Courtesy of Davis, M. E., and Sheckler, C. E., 1957.)

month post partum. Bleeding from the genitals which begins after the first 24 hours post partum is called *late puerperal hemorrhage*.

The most common causes of late hemorrhage are thrombosed blood vessels at the placental site and subinvolution of the placental site. Only rarely is placental tissue the cause of late puerperal hemorrhage (Fig. 379). This is proved by the rarity of the finding of placental tissue when the uterus is curetted for late postpartum hemorrhage.

The important lesion that is usually causative is that associated with subinvolution of the uterus (Ober and Grady), consisting of thickening and hyalinization of the arterial walls at the site of implantation in the regenerating endometrium (Fig. 380). The lesion may be present whether or not placental tissue is present.

Other causes of late puerperal hemorrhage are withdrawal bleeding from estrogenic hormones used to suppress lactation, undiagnosed laceration, hematoma, local tumor, uterine inversion and systemic blood dyscrasias.

Even though severe, late hemorrhage is seldom fatal; it responds quickly to conservative treatment. In the puerperium,

ergonovine should be given orally (one tablet of 0.2 mg. four times a day). Rarely will it be necessary to give ergonovine hypodermically (0.2 mg. three times a day). Curettage should be performed at once if the bleeding is profuse; it should be done when convenient if the bleeding does not abate after uterotonic agents are given.

Other causes are treated as required by the prevailing circumstances. A hematoma, if found, is opened and the bleeding vessels are ligated. Degenerated leiomyomas usually require a hysterectomy. For malignancy, appropriate radical surgery or radiation therapy must be carried out. Hysterectomy is also indicated for uterine rupture if it is the cause of late hemorrhage. Inversion of the uterus is treated by vaginal or abdominal operation as described above.

ACUTE PUERPERAL CRISES

A patient may collapse and die suddenly, almost without warning. The cause of this catastrophe sometimes can be de-

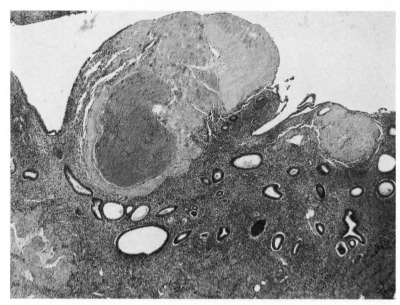

Figure 380   Photomicrograph of a section through the endometrium at hysterectomy, ten weeks post partum. A single spiral arteriole served as the source for copious vaginal bleeding. The endometrium has regenerated partially. The vessel is a gross caricature of an arteriole measuring about 12 times its normal size with part of its wall thickened and hyalinized; part is necrotic and opens upon the lumen which is filled with a coagulum of blood and necrotic material.

termined only at autopsy. Sudden collapse and death may be caused by hemorrhage and shock from obstetric accidents, such as postpartum hemorrhage, ruptured ectopic gestation, uterine perforation, rupture or inversion, placenta previa, abruptio placentae, lacerations, trauma and air or amniotic fluid embolism. Endotoxin shock is discussed in Chapter 34.

Eclampsia (see Chapter 36) may cause sudden death from cerebral hemorrhage, which may even occur without convulsions, or from acute pulmonary edema or vasomotor collapse. Rapid delivery or deep inhalation anesthesia may be a factor in the shock also.

Postural shock is most likely due to compression of the inferior vena cava and pelvic veins by the enlarged uterus with decrease in the amount of flow returning to the heart (see Chapter 41). The supine position is best avoided in treating the gravida or puerpera in shock because it may complicate the issue.

Sudden death may be caused by systemic conditions which complicate pregnancy and parturition, including cardiac disease, cerebrovascular accident and pulmonary insufficiency or embolism. Reactions to anesthetics and drugs may also be causative.

The most important factor in the treatment of shock is prevention. This consists of conscientious obstetric technique. Of the greatest importance are the prevention of blood loss and avoidance of any manipulation leading to undue bleeding. Harmful manipulations include Credé expression of the placenta, manual dilatation of the cervix, forceful instrumental extraction and version procedures.

Exhaustion should be prevented by ample sedation, parenteral replenishment of fluid and electrolytes, careful balance of the acid-base status and timely, gentle and atraumatic intervention. Appropriate anesthesia should be chosen according to the needs and expertly administered so as not to jeopardize the patient's health or life. The pathophysiology and management of the shock states, including hemorrhagic shock, endotoxin shock and amniotic fluid infusion syndrome are discussed in Chapter 51.

REFERENCES

Das, P.: Inversion of uterus. J. Obstet. Gynaec. Brit. Emp. *47*:525, 1940.

Davis, M. E., and Sheckler, C. E.: *In* DeLee's Obstetrics for Nurses, ed. 16. Philadelphia, W. B. Saunders Company, 1957.

Dickinson, R. L.: Lifting and manipulation of the uterus through abdominal wall to control postpartum hemorrhage. Brooklyn Med. J. *13*:137, 1899.

Halban, J., and Tandler, J.: Anatomie und Ätiologie der Genitalprolapse beim Weibe. Vienna, Wilhelm Braumüller, 1907.

Huntington, J. L.: Acute inversion of uterus. Boston Med. Surg. J. *184*:376, 1921.

Irving, F. C., and Hertig, A. T.: Study of placenta accreta. Surg. Gynec. Obstet. *64*:178, 1937.

Koren, Z., Zuckerman, H., and Brzezinski, A.: Placenta previa accreta with afibrinogenemia: Report on three cases. Obstet. Gynec. *18*:138, 1961.

McLennan, C. E., and McKelvey, J. L.: Conservative treatment of inversion of the uterus. J.A.M.A. *120*:679, 1942.

Miller, N. F.: Pregnancy following inversion of uterus. Amer. J. Obstet. Gynec. *13*:307, 1927.

Ober, W. B., and Grady, H. G.: Subinvolution of the placental site. Bull. N.Y. Acad. Med. *37*:713, 1961.

Rotton, W. N., and Friedman, E. A.: Placenta accreta: Review of the literature and report of four cases. Obstet. Gynec. *9*:580, 1957.

Spinelli, P. G.: Chirurgische konservirende Behandlung der chronischen Uterusinversion nach dem Verfahren von Kehrer. Centralbl. Gynäk. *23*:552, 1899.

Chapter 67

Care of the Neonate

A *liveborn infant* is defined by the American College of Obstetricians and Gynecologists (Hughes) as one that shows any sign of life, such as heart beat or respiration after it is delivered, regardless of its gestational age or size. A baby dying in the newborn period up to 28 days is called a *neonatal death*. *Fetal death* refers to cessation of fetal life before termination of pregnancy; subsequent to fetal death, a *stillborn infant* results when the pregnancy terminates. Delivery of a dead infant before the twentieth week of pregnancy or of one weighing less than 500 gm. is generally considered an *abortion* (the fetus is an *abortus*) and does not enter into the consideration of perinatal mortality rates.

Calculation of perinatal mortality is confused because standards vary widely. Some use the 20-week cutoff limit while others use 28 weeks, 500 gm. or even 1000 gm. Moreover, the denominator may be liveborn infants instead of total births. A plea is made for uniform standardization for purposes of clarity and comparison. Since there is little precision in timing the duration of pregnancy, birth weight tends to be more useful. Only fetuses weighing 500 gm. or more should be considered in the calculation, therefore.

Perinatal mortality rate is the number of stillborn infants plus neonatal deaths per 1000 total births. It consists of the summation of the *fetal death rate* (number of stillborn infants weighing 500 gm. or more per 1000 births) and the *neonatal death rate* (number of infants born alive weighing 500 gm. or more and dying before the twenty-eighth day per 1000 births). The perinatal period extends from the twentieth week of pregnancy to the twenty-eighth day of extrauterine life.

Principles of routine care of the healthy neonate, dealing with management of the umbilical cord and prophylactic treatment of the eyes against gonococcal infection, are dealt with in Chapter 20.

INFANT RESUSCITATION

Obstetricians, anesthesiologists, pediatricians and nurses must know how to (1) evaluate the infant's physical status, (2) establish and maintain an adequate airway, (3) deliver oxygen to the lung alveoli and provide proper artificial ventilation, (4) determine the presence and severity of acid-base imbalance and correct it, and (5) perform closed cardiac massage if the infant's heart is not beating. The extent to which such measures should be instituted depends on the degree of depression of the infant at birth.

Detailed instruction is essential for all personnel responsible for care of the pregnant woman and her baby. The most experienced person in attendance at a delivery should be delegated to assist in establishing respirations. Responsibility for resuscitation cannot be neglected or relegated lightly. Skill and experience are mandatory for endotracheal intubation and positive pressure ventilation.

The normal neonate usually breathes spontaneously within a few seconds after he is delivered, establishing respirations within a minute or so. Therefore, most newborn infants will need no special resuscitative measures. It is good practice to ensure nasopharyngeal drainage of amniotic fluid by keeping the baby's head down and his mouth open. During the delivery and immediately thereafter, one should gently clear the mouth and nose by aspirating with a rubber suction bulb or catheter. It is well to avoid vigorous or prolonged suction that will stimulate the pharyngeal area to inhibit respirations and cause bradycardia by a vagal mechanism.

After birth, the infant is held up by the feet and the cord is severed between clamps. The infant is placed in a heated bassinet in the Trendelenburg position with a slight lateral tilt, and the neck is extended to assure a patent airway (Moya).

There are a variety of good resuscitating units available today. Every delivery room should be equipped with at least one of these very useful devices. They provide a surface for access to the baby for intubation and other measures, oxygen (both for enriching the inspired atmosphere by face mask and for controlled positive pressure ventilation), heat, suction and space for needed ancillary resuscitative equipment. Minimally, a resuscitation tray should have a lighted infant laryngoscope, assorted sizes of endotracheal tubes, a plastic oral airway and a suction catheter. All equipment must be carefully checked to ensure good working condition before every delivery.

Evaluation of the Infant

The infant's condition requires continual evaluation from the moment of birth. The mother's general health, the course of labor and its complications, the amount and type of sedation and anesthesia she has received and the delivery procedures will all give advanced warning as to what may be expected in regard to the status of the neonate. A good guide is provided by the presence of pallor, cyanosis, bradycardia or flaccidity. Babies exhibiting these signs may be in difficulty. One should note the time to the first breath, the time to the initiation of spontaneous respirations and the time to the first cry. These are coarse measures of responsiveness and are prolonged beyond one minute in depressed infants. A better overall view of the infant's condition is given by the Apgar score.

The Apgar system considers the heart rate, respiratory effort, muscle tone, reflex irritability and color of the infant (Table 10). Each of the five signs is rated at 0, 1 or 2 and then totaled. Infants in excellent condition score 7 to 10. The moderately depressed infant scores 4 to 6. The severely depressed infant scores 3 or less.

The Apgar score should be determined and recorded formally at one minute and again at five minutes, preferably by the anesthetist or nurse. Some bias tends to be introduced by some obstetricians who overestimate scores consistently. The baby who is depressed at one minute of life has an Apgar score less than 7 and deserves active resuscitative measures. Five-minute Apgar scores are prognostic indicators of mortality and neurologic damage (Drage and Berendes). It was found, for example, that the incidence of neurologic abnormalities in infants weighing more than 2500 gm. was three times greater in babies scoring less than 7 as compared with those scoring 7 to 10.

Other systematic evaluation procedures have been described for use in determining the status of the newborn infant. Second in importance only to the Apgar scoring system is that of Silverman and Andersen, which weighs the features of respiratory obstruction, especially in premature babies. The infant is scored on the basis

TABLE 10 APGAR SCORING METHOD FOR EVALUATING THE INFANT

Sign	0	1	2
Heart rate	Absent	Slow (below 100)	Over 100
Respiratory effort	Absent	Weak cry; hypoventilation	Good; strong cry
Muscle tone	Limp	Some flexion of extremities	Active motion; extremities well flexed
Reflex irritability (response to stimulation of sole of foot)	No response	Grimace	Cry
Color	Blue; pale	Body pink; extremities blue	Completely pink

TABLE 11   SILVERMAN-ANDERSEN RETRACTION SCORING METHOD

Sign°	0	1	2
Synchrony of chest and abdomen	Synchronous	Lag	See-saw
Intercostal movement	None	Slight	Marked on inspiration
Xiphoid retraction	None	Slight	Marked
Chin excursion	No movement	Chin descends; lips closed	Chin descends; lips part
Expiratory grunt	None	Audible by stethoscope	Loud

°All refer to inspiration, except grunt.

of the appearance of one or more relevant signs, including (1) asynchronous inspiratory chest retraction, (2) lower intercostal retraction, (3) xiphoid retraction, (4) inspiratory chin tug and (5) expiratory grunt (Table 11). The higher the score, the greater the respiratory embarrassment and the worse the prognosis.

An essential feature inherent in the initial evaluation of the infant is the speed which enables vital resuscitative measures to be instituted as quickly as possible. Examination can be expedited by cooperative effort. For example, while the nurse is listening to the heart beat (or palpating it at the umbilicus) and indicating its rate by tapping or moving a finger, the physician can be aspirating the oropharynx and establishing an airway.

Resuscitation Measures

Most infants need no special care other than that described, namely, suctioning the mouth and nose, maintenance of warmth and gravity drainage (head down tilt). This applies to all vigorous babies with an Apgar score of 7 or greater who have breathed and cried spontaneously within a short time after being delivered. All others need supportive aid.

The moderately depressed baby will be found to deteriorate very quickly within one to two minutes if artificial ventilation is not initiated. Gentle slapping of the feet occasionally rouses such an infant, especially if the depression is the direct result of excessive sedation or anesthesia which the mother received late in labor. Any other, more vigorous method of stimulating the neonate is condemned, including such antiquated and potentially traumatic

methods as alternating hot and cold tubs, slapping the back or buttocks and dilating the anal sphincter.

Having cleared the oropharynx of amniotic fluid and mucus by gentle aspiration, the physician should *establish an airway* by inserting a small plastic oropharyngeal airway into the mouth to prevent obstruction by the tongue. He should then give *intermittent positive pressure ventilation* by administering oxygen in short puffs under pressure by means of a tightly fitting face mask equipped with some form of mechanical device for delivering oxygen under controlled positive pressure. A simple form of this useful equipment is shown in Figure 381. A rate of 30 to 40 puffs per minute is proper. The initial pressure should be no greater than 20 cm. of water and the interval of administration only one to two seconds. Although this is insufficient pressure to expand the alveoli, it does stimulate pulmonary stretch receptors and will often

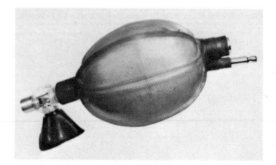

Figure 381   Ambu bag and mask for administration of air or oxygen. Bag is self-expandable. Oxygen or air under pressure is not required to expand the bag. Pressure above 35 to 40 cm. of water cannot be produced with the Ambu apparatus using one hand. (From Moya, F.: Conn. Med. 26:239, 1962.)

evoke an inspiratory gasp, thereby initiating respirations indirectly.

If spontaneous respirations are established, the ventilation is discontinued and the infant is carefully observed in an oxygen-enriched environment with 6 to 8 liters per minute of oxygen supplied by a face mask. Gentle suctioning of the mouth and nose may be needed from time to time as secretions accumulate.

If intermittent positive pressure oxygen by a face mask is ineffectual in maintaining adequate ventilation, postnatal acidosis will become increasingly aggravated, as evidenced by progressive cyanosis, flaccidity and bradycardia. Additional emergency measures must be taken promptly. Direct visualization of the larynx and *endotracheal intubation* should be done. Every delivery room physician should become proficient in this important, lifesaving technique. The requisite technical skills can be acquired easily by use of available models and practice on dead babies. The blind technique of introducing a tracheal catheter without visualization by a laryngoscope has been shown to be often traumatic and, although still widely practiced, it is no longer recommended.

The infant is placed with its head hyperextended facing the operator, and its shoulders elevated by a folded towel. The mouth is held open with fingers of the right hand and the laryngoscope is introduced by the left hand. The laryngoscope blade is advanced into the oropharynx along the right side of the tongue. The glottis is visualized in its anterior position. The tip of the laryngoscope blade is elevated to bring the glottis into view. The glottis is easily recognized as a dark vertical slit with the arytenoid cartilage identified posteriorly. Any foreign material should be quickly and gently aspirated. The endotracheal tube is then introduced through the glottis into the trachea.

It is important to ensure that one is not intubating the esophagus which lies posteriorly; direct visualization by way of the laryngoscope is the best way to ascertain the proper location. The endotracheal tube should fit snugly. Usually a No. 16 Cole-type tube is the proper size for an infant at term. Aspiration through the tube may dislodge additional foreign material, such as meconium, vernix and blood, from the trachea. This should always be done before proceeding.

With the endotracheal tube in place, the laryngoscope is withdrawn and positive pressure ventilation initiated unless the stimulus of intubation has started spontaneous respirations. Mouth-to-tube respiration may be given, using short puffs of breath to expand the lungs. This must not be done vigorously or damage may occur. The lower chest should rise if the lungs are expanding; if the tube is in the esophagus, the upper abdomen will rise instead. Aeration of the lungs should be checked periodically by means of a stethoscope. A face mask equipped with a bag or positive pressure device can accomplish the same objective.

Pressures of about 30 cm. of water (but no higher than 50 cm.) may be needed to expand the lungs and deliver oxygen, but these must not be sustained more than one to two seconds. Once expansion has occurred, lower pressure should be used. The dead space is reduced and the ventilation is made most efficient by attaching the endotracheal tube with a tightly fitting adaptor directly to the bag or device for delivering oxygen under controlled intermittent positive pressure. Ventilation is continued until the infant begins breathing spontaneously.

After sustained, spontaneous breathing has been established, the oropharynx should be cleansed of any fluid which has accumulated. When the baby's condition warrants it, the tube may be removed. Good muscle tone, heart rate and rhythm and skin color indicating satisfactory oxygenation should all be present before extubation.

For infants severely depressed at birth with Apgar scores 0 to 3, no time should be lost before proceeding to intubate the trachea, aspirate foreign material and administer positive-pressure ventilation. Cardiac arrest is managed by *external cardiac massage* done in conjunction with ventilatory measures. With one hand under the upper back and two fingers of the other hand on the midsternum, one compresses the chest wall $\frac{1}{2}$ to $\frac{3}{4}$ inch about 100 to 120 times a minute with periodic interruptions every five seconds to permit good expansion of the lungs. A 3:1 ratio of cardiac to respiratory rates should be maintained. Electrocardiographic monitoring is useful. These measures must be done gently because direct damage to heart, liver and rib cage may occur from overly vigorous massage.

Correction of Acid-Base Imbalance

Labor and the birth process are associated with progressive acidosis in the fetus. This appears to be the result of diminished fetomaternal exchange across the placenta and coassociated hypoxia. The situation is aggravated by maternal illness, labor dysfunction, cord and placental complications and difficult delivery. Babies, therefore, tend to be born in a relatively asphyxic state. Depressed infants are much more acidotic than alert babies and show substantially greater falls in blood pH; the drop is of longer duration and the recovery nuch slower (James). Asphyxia becomes rapidly and progressively more severe as long as the baby does not breathe. Very low arterial oxygen levels are associated with marked hypercapnia and falling pH to below 7.0. Recovery is hampered by analgesic and anesthetic agents given late in labor and by prematurity. Acidosis in turn causes high pulmonary vascular resistance and diminishes the effectiveness of resuscitative measures.

It is essential, therefore, that the acidosis be corrected promptly in the course of resuscitation. *Umbilical vein catheterization* should be done. Although this technique is not without its inherent risks of trauma, infection and thrombosis, it may be lifesaving for the severely depressed, acidotic neonate. A solution containing sufficient alkali to correct the problem partially should be given while awaiting the laboratory results of the blood sample taken for blood gas analysis. Sodium bicarbonate, 0.9 molar (7.5 per cent) solution, may be given slowly intravenously to the newborn infant in amounts of 3 to 5 mEq. per kilogram. In addition, 10 per cent glucose may also be helpful for the purpose of replenishing depleted glycogen reserves, especially for use by cardiac muscle.

Respiratory stimulants are of no demonstrable value in the asphyxic infant and should not be used. They include such agents as Metrazol, alpha-lobeline, Coramine and picrotoxin. These analeptic drugs may actually be harmful in that they increase the central nervous metabolism, making oxygen demands greater, and may cause hypertension and convulsions.

Narcotic antagonists may be quite useful if the depression is narcotic induced. They do not benefit the infant who is depressed from anoxia, trauma, inhalation anesthesia or barbiturates. Nalorphine (*N*-allylnormorphine, Nalline) and levallorphan (Lorfan) may reverse narcotic-induced respiratory depression, but can augment depression due to other causes. They especially synergize with general anesthetics, aggravating depression. Moreover, they should not be given unless adequate ventilation is being administered because of the risk of enhancing an existing asphyxic state. A newer agent, naloxone hydrochloride (Narcan), seems to be devoid of its own depressant properties and may, therefore, be particularly beneficial.

Narcotic antagonists may be given to the mother before delivery, to counteract large doses of narcotics given in labor, or to the baby at birth. The usual dosages of *nalorphine* are 5 to 10 mg. intravenously to the mother or 0.1 to 0.2 mg. to the infant; of levallorphan, 1 to 2 mg. to the mother or 0.05 to 0.1 mg. to the infant; of naloxone, 0.4 mg. to the mother. However, since their effectiveness is inconstant and cannot be relied on, and since they may enhance depression due to other causes, the use of both narcotics and narcotic antagonists in labor should be limited.

THE PREMATURE INFANT

Prematurity refers to the condition of the infant whose physiologic functions are not as sufficiently developed as those of the healthy baby at term. Because this condition is difficult to define accurately on a clinical basis, a premature infant is arbitrarily defined as any liveborn infant weighing 2500 gm. (5 lbs. 8 oz.) or less at birth. The duration of gestation as judged from the first day of the last menstrual period also varies rather widely, but in general infants born less than 37 weeks from this date are considered premature. These definitions are unsatisfactory.

To help distinguish those babies whose gestational age and birth weight are *discordant* from those delivered prematurely with appropriate weight for the gestational age, the terms *small for gestational age, small for dates* or *fetal dysmaturity* have been used (see Chapter 54). Birth weight, although providing a practical and objective index of the relative maturity of an infant, is influenced by many factors other than gestational age, including fetal disease, maternal nutritional status and socioeconomic, familial and probably racial factors. It stands to reason that ethnically small people have small babies and the same definition of prematurity by birth weight is inappropriate for them.

Prematurity occurs more often in women who are less than 20 years of age and this apparently holds true throughout the world. Whether this relationship is based on a nutritional factor (see Chapter 10) cannot be determined. There is little doubt that smaller babies are born among malnourished patients of all ages from lower socioeconomic strata. Prematurity, both by gestational age and by weight, even at term, occurs in multiple pregnancies (see Chapter 39). Similarly, any condition that affects placental function, including hypertensive states, renal disorders and diabetes, may yield a baby that is small for dates or actually premature.

Various other objective measurements, either singly or in combination, have been used as criteria of prematurity. Among these are a crown-heel length of 47 cm. or less, an occipitofrontal diameter of 11.5 cm. or less, an occipitofrontal circumference of less than 33 cm., a difference between the circumference of the head and that of the thorax of more than 3 cm., absence of centers of ossification in the distal femoral epiphyses and a high percentage of fetal hemoglobin in blood obtained from the umbilical cord (Brody). Although these provide objective data which are of some value in assessing the maturity of a newborn infant, they are subject to considerable variation.

Although premature infants comprise only 5 to 10 per cent of all live births, about two-thirds of all neonatal deaths occur in premature infants. The smaller the baby, the higher the mortality. Prematurity *per se* is seldom the sole cause of death, although it plays a major role in neonatal mortality. The premature infant, especially the extremely small one, has many functional and morphologic handicaps which make his life during the neonatal period a precarious one. He is particularly susceptible to infection, hypoxia, trauma and hemorrhage.

Incomplete differentiation of pulmonary alveoli (Farber and Wilson), inadequate vascularization of the lung and the relatively low reactivity of the respiratory center probably all contribute to the reduced ability of the premature infant to oxygenate its blood. This is further enhanced by less effective respiratory movements due to the softness and pliability of the bones of the thoracic cage, by weakness of the respiratory muscles and by a paucity of pulmonary elastic tissue. Diminished transfer of maternal antibodies with decreased amounts of serum gamma globulin, defective formation of granulocytes and diminished phagocytic ability (Gluck and Silverman) may all contribute to the increased susceptibility of the premature infant to infection.

Varying degrees of the following characteristics may be exhibited to help distinguish the premature infant: (1) The body is usually small and puny. (2) Weight of viable infants varies from 500 gm. to 2500 gm. (see Table 12). (3) The skin is soft and usually pinkish red in color; the epidermis is thin and the blood vessels are easily seen. (4) Adipose tissue is scant; the features are angular; the face looks old and the skin frequently hangs in folds. (5) Lanugo is abundant, especially on the extensor surfaces of the extremities, the forehead and the upper part of the back. (6) The skull is round or ovoid; the fontanels are large and the sutures are prominent. (7) Many small milia are visible on the nose and sometimes on the chin. (8) The ears are soft and small and hug the skull. (9) The nails have scarcely reached the ends of the fingers even in larger infants, while in smaller ones they may be poorly devel-

*TABLE 12   TABLE FOR CONVERTING NEONATAL WEIGHT FROM AVOIRDUPOIS TO METRIC SYSTEM**

Pounds Ounces	0	1	2	3	4	5	6	7	8	9	10	11	12	Pounds Ounces
0	0	454	907	1360	1815	2270	2720	3175	3630	4080	4535	4990	5445	0
1	28	482	936	1390	1845	2295	2750	3205	3655	4110	4565	5020	5470	1
2	57	510	964	1415	1870	2325	2780	3230	3685	4140	4595	5045	5500	2
3	85	539	992	1445	1900	2355	2805	3260	3715	4165	4620	5075	5530	3
4	113	567	1020	1475	1930	2380	2835	3290	3740	4195	4650	5105	5555	4
5	142	595	1050	1500	1955	2410	2865	3315	3770	4225	4680	5130	5585	5
6	170	624	1075	1530	1985	2440	2890	3345	3800	4255	4705	5160	5615	6
7	198	652	1105	1560	2015	2465	2920	3375	3825	4280	4735	5190	5640	7
8	227	680	1135	1590	2040	2495	2950	3400	3855	4310	4765	5215	5670	8
9	255	709	1160	1615	2070	2525	2975	3430	3885	4340	4790	5245	5700	9
10	283	737	1190	1645	2100	2550	3005	3460	3910	4365	4820	5275	5725	10
11	312	765	1220	1675	2125	2580	3035	3485	3940	4395	4850	5300	5755	11
12	340	794	1245	1700	2155	2610	3060	3515	3970	4425	4875	5330	5785	12
13	369	822	1275	1730	2185	2635	3090	3545	3995	4450	4905	5360	5810	13
14	397	850	1305	1760	2210	2665	3120	3570	4025	4480	4935	5385	5840	14
15	425	879	1330	1785	2240	2695	3145	3600	4055	4510	4960	5415	5870	15

*To change from pounds-ounces to grams, read across top line to find vertical column for the number of pounds and read down within that column for weight corresponding to the number of ounces. Weights over 1000 gm. rounded to nearest 5 gm. To convert to grams mathematically, multiply pounds by 453.6 and ounces by 28.4, and add the two products; to convert grams to pounds, multiply grams by 0.002205.

oped. (10) The cry is feeble, monotonous and whining. (11) The infant lies in a deep sleep and may have to be aroused for feedings; efforts at sucking may be weak or absent; all movements are slow; all functions are sluggish, and muscular inertia is pronounced. (12) The body temperature tends to be below normal and is inclined to be irregular. (13) Urine is scanty.

Management

Principles of care of the gravida in *premature labor* include attempts to arrest the process by inhibiting contractility. To date, such measures have been imperfectly successful, tending to work best when labor is early and not well established. The implication of this observation is that some of the patients in whom these approaches were successful in arresting labor may not have been in labor at all. Among agents reported to be useful in this regard are intravenous alcohol (Fuchs), pregnenolone (Bieniarz et al.) and a group of beta-adrenergic agents currently under investigation, such as isoxsuprine (Hendricks), ritodrine (Landesman et al.; Barden), diazoxide and orciprenaline (Baillie). The beta-mimetic effects of the latter group of drugs appear to inhibit uterine contractility effectively, but they have major cardiovascular side effects, including tachycardia and hypotension, that are unpleasant. Although promising, their clinical applicability has not yet been completely determined.

To date, a program of absolute bed rest, heavy sedation and abstinence from intravaginal examination or manipulation has proved to be fairly satisfactory. Zuspan warns against sedation by means of intravenous Demerol because of its potential uterotonic effect. When alcohol is used, it can be given by infusion according to the program described by Fuchs et al., with a loading dose of 7.5 ml. per kilogram of body weight per hour of a 9.5 per cent solution (made up by adding 100 ml. of 95 per cent ethanol to 900 ml. of 5 per cent dextrose in water). Maintenance requires 1.5 ml. per kilogram per hour for 10 hours or more.

A recent controlled study (Zlatnick and Fuchs) proved the effectiveness of alcohol in delaying or arresting threatened premature labor. Rapid infusion of large amounts of fluid may be effective alone by a reflex mechanism involving blood volume expansion, but the result is less impressive (Bieniarz et al.). It must be recalled that alcohol has been reported to produce fetal tachycardia, hypotension and acidosis in monkeys (Horiguchi et al.).

There are some situations in which inhibition of labor is contraindicated because it would be preferable if the fetus were out of its hostile intrauterine environment. Such conditions include intrauterine infection, premature rupture of the membranes, placental insufficiency, hypertensive states, erythroblastosis and diabetes.

The optimal management of the premature labor in progress involves (1) minimizing analgesic agents so that the very sensitive premature infant will not be depressed by them at birth, (2) utilizing conduction anesthesia and (3) employing a generous episiotomy to avoid compression of the soft, poorly calcified cranial bones and subsequent brain damage. Forceps as a prophylactic measure to protect the head against perineal compression is widely used for small premature infants, ostensibly to prevent intracranial injury. However, it is probably often abused when instruments are applied fairly early in the second stage before the fetal head has reached the pelvic floor; subsequent traction and compression by the forceps blades may actually do comparable or greater damage than is associated with spontaneous delivery. Gentleness is essential whenever forceps are applied, especially when used for delivery of the head of the premature baby.

The intensive care needed by many small premature infants at birth is beyond the scope of this book. The basic requisites include warmth, oxygen (not over 40 per cent concentration) and humidity in a protected environment safe from infection. The baby should be handled as little as is compatible with the requirements of resuscitation. Improvement in the organization of care of the premature infant has made a significant impact on perinatal salvage rates. The principles of resuscitation outlined earlier are completely applicable to premature infants, although their effectiveness is decidedly poorer in these babies. If real progress is to be made in this area, we must concentrate on prevention of prematurity.

CIRCUMCISION OF THE NEWBORN

Circumcision has been practiced for centuries by large groups of people irrespective of race or religion. Today it is routine among more than two hundred million people (Bryk), although there is a growing wave of opposition to the procedure based on ostensible risks of psychologic damage, blood loss, local penile damage, infection and hypesthesia. Against these arguments are the potential advantages of circumcision in preventing penile and cervical cancer, phimosis and infection. We have no wish to enter the debate, but merely to indicate that the procedure is widely performed and appears to carry small risk when well conducted.

Usually, circumcision is performed when a baby is two to four days old, but it may be done at birth or delayed for a week or longer, if desired. Circumcision at the time of birth is expedient, but may present some hazard if the neonate has an undetected coagulation defect. Prothrombin levels in the newborn begin to approach adult values at about one week of age.

There are numerous ways of performing circumcision but the following two procedures are the common ones. The baby is placed on a specially designed, well-padded wooden or plastic board (Figs. 382 and 383). It is wrapped on the board with towels to keep it from moving its arms and legs. The penis, scrotum and surrounding area are washed with soap and water and, if desired, covered with an antiseptic solution. A sterile towel with a hole in the center is placed over the baby so that the penis protrudes through the hole.

The penis is grasped in three fingers of the gloved left hand (for right-handed physicians) and a probe is inserted between the prepuce and the glans. The probe is moved all around the glans and down to the corona to break down adhesions. Then the dorsal edge of the prepuce is grasped with hemostats and a slit is made with scissors in the midline of the dorsal surface down to within 3 mm. of the corona (Fig. 384). The entire prepuce is pushed back of

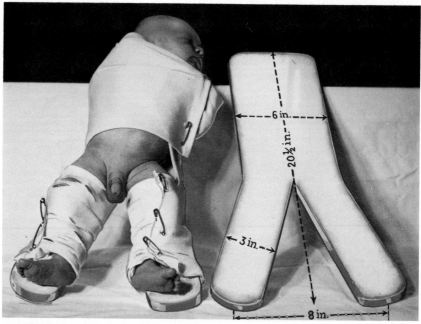

Figure 382 Padded wooden board for restraining the neonate for circumcision. Baby is attached to the board with towels and safety pins.

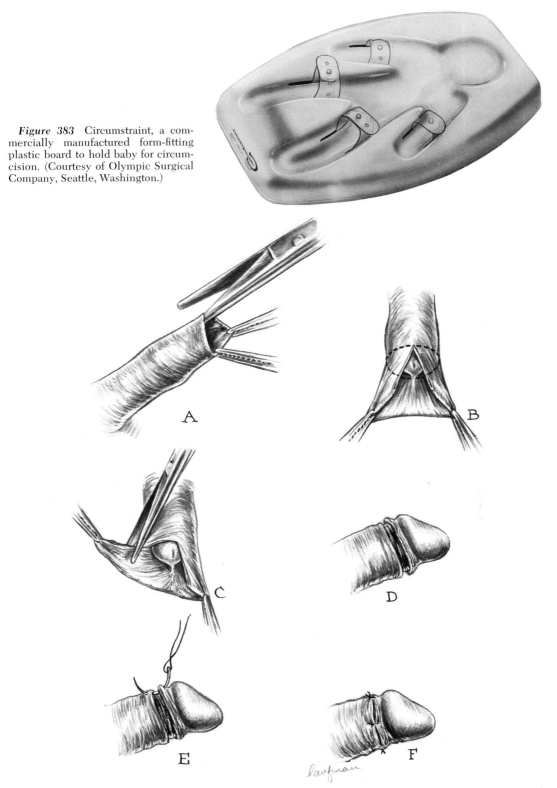

Figure 383 Circumstraint, a commercially manufactured form-fitting plastic board to hold baby for circumcision. (Courtesy of Olympic Surgical Company, Seattle, Washington.)

Figure 384 Free-hand method for performing circumcision. *A*, After the prepuce has been freed of its adhesions to the glans, the dorsal edge is grasped with hemostats and a slit is made in the dorsal midline. *B*, Slit completed to within 3 mm. of the corona; circumferential incision shown by broken line. *C*, Foreskin being cut away at 3 mm. from corona. *D*, Dissection complete. *E*, Interrupted 0000 catgut sutures being placed to approximate skin and mucosa. *F*, Hemostasis secured.

the glans and beyond the corona. The prepuce and mucous membrane must be free from the corona all around, especially at the frenulum on the ventral surface.

Then most of the foreskin is cut away with scissors, leaving about 3 mm. of mucous membrane attached all around the corona. The skin and the mucous membrane are approximated by inserting four interrupted sutures of 0000 chromic catgut with a curved cutting-edge needle. One suture is placed at the frenulum, one at the dorsal edge and one on either side of the dorsal surface. Any bleeding vessels are clamped and ligated.

After ensuring that there is no bleeding, one places a small piece of gauze covered with petrolatum gently around the penis. A cotton or gauze dressing is placed over this without compression.

No special after-care is necessary. When the dressings become soiled they are changed. Petrolatum or Alboline should be placed on the penis or on the dressing to prevent the dressing from adhering to the wound.

Circumcision with the Gomco clamp (Fig. 385) or Plastibell is popular because of the safeguards against trauma and bleeding which these devices provide. Cleansing, draping and preparing the prepuce are the same as in the free-hand method described above. A partial dorsal slit, just long enough to allow the cone to be applied easily, will facilitate the procedure. The cone is placed over the penis, permitting just enough of the mucous membrane to fit below it to ensure that not too much of this tissue is removed (Fig.

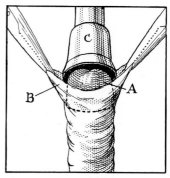

Figure 386 The prepuce (*B*) has been cleaned and detached from the glans (*A*) and is being held by hemostats. A dorsal slit has been made and the cone (*C*) of the Gomco clamp is applied to the glans.

386). The prepuce is then pulled through and above the bevel hole in the platform and is clamped in place (Fig. 387). In this way the prepuce is crushed against the cone, causing hemostasis. This pressure is maintained for five minutes. The excess of the prepuce is then cut with a sharp knife. There is no danger of cutting the glans, because it is protected by the cone portion of the instrument. A very fine ribbon-like membrane (¼ inch, 0.6 cm.) is formed between the new union of the skin and the mucous membrane. The pressure is then released. Suturing is very rarely needed. The circumcision is completed and the penis is covered with petrolatum gauze.

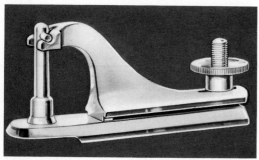

Figure 385 Gomco circumcision clamp in four parts: cone, plate, wedge and nut.

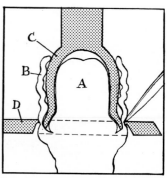

Figure 387 Schematic cross section showing cone (*C*) of Gomco clamp applied between glans (*A*) and prepuce (*B*). Plate (*D*) crushes prepuce against cone at circumcision line and excision is begun as shown at the right.

REFERENCES

Apgar, V., Holaday, D. A., James, L. S., Weisbrot, I. M., and Berrien, C.: Evaluation of the newborn infant: Second report. J.A.M.A. *168*:1985, 1958.

Baillie, P.: Treatment of premature labor with orciprenaline. Brit. Med. J. *4*:154, 1970.

Barden, T. P.: Effect of ritodrine on human uterine motility and cardiovascular responses in term labor and early postpartum state. Amer. J. Obstet. Gynec. *112*:645, 1972.

Bieniarz, J., Burd, L., Motew, M., and Scommegna, A.: Inhibition of uterine contractility. Amer. J. Obstet. Gynec. *111*:874, 1971.

Brody, S.: The intra-uterine age of the foetus at birth. Acta Obstet. Gynec. Scand. *37*:374, 1958.

Bryk, F.: Circumcision in Man and Woman. Translated by D. Berger. New York, American Ethnological Press, 1934.

Drage, J. S., and Berendes, H.: Apgar scores and outcome of the newborn. Pediat. Clin. N. Amer. *13*:635, 1966.

Farber, S., and Wilson, J. L.: Atelectasis of the newborn. Amer. J. Dis. Child. *46*:572, 1933.

Fuchs, F.: Treatment of threatened premature labour with alcohol. J. Obstet. Gynaec. Brit. Comm. *72*:1011, 1965.

Fuchs, F., Fuchs, A.-R., Poblete, V. F., Jr., and Risk, A.: Effect of alcohol on threatened premature labor. Amer. J. Obstet. Gynec. *99*:627, 1967.

Gluck, L., and Silverman, W. A.: Phagocytosis in premature infants. Pediatrics *20*:951, 1957.

Hendricks, C. H.: Use of isoxsuprine for the arrest of premature labor. Clin. Obstet. Gynec. *7*:687, 1964.

Horiguchi, T., Suzuki, K., Comas-Urrutia, A. C., Mueller-Huebach, E., Boyer-Milic, A. M., Baratz, R. A., Morishima, H. O., James, L. S., and Adamsons, K.: Effect of ethanol upon uterine activity and fetal acid-base state of the rhesus monkey. Amer. J. Obstet. Gynec. *109*:910, 1971.

Hughes, E. C., ed.: Obstetric-Gynecologic Terminology. Philadelphia, F. A. Davis Company, 1972.

James, L. S.: Onset of breathing and resuscitation. Pediat. Clin. N. Amer. *13*:621, 1966.

Landesman, R., Wilson, K. H., Coutinho, E. M., Klima, I. M., and Marcous, R. S.: The relaxant action of ritodrine, a sympathomimetic amine, on the uterus during term labor. Amer. J. Obstet. Gynec. *110*:111, 1971.

Moya, F.: Resuscitation of the newborn. Conn. Med. *26*:239, 1962.

Silverman, W., and Andersen, D.: A controlled trial of effects of water mist on obstructive respiratory signs, death rate and necropsy findings among premature infants. Pediatrics *17*:1, 1956.

Zlatnick, F. J., and Fuchs, F.: A controlled study of ethanol in threatened premature labor. Amer. J. Obstet. Gynec. *112*:610, 1972.

Zuspan, F. P.: Premature labor: Its management and therapy (Symposium). J. Reprod. Med. *9*:93, 1972.

Chapter 68

Neonatal Damage

For infants born alive, the first 28 days of extrauterine life are the most hazardous period of life. More than two-thirds of all deaths during the first year occur during this interval, and more than half the neonatal deaths occur during the first 24 hours of extrauterine life. The most common causes are hypoxic and traumatic damage with which we will deal here.

FETAL HYPOXIA

Fetal hypoxia is directly responsible for approximately 10 to 20 per cent of neonatal deaths and for an even higher percentage of intrauterine deaths. It may be the result of any of a variety of lesions of the placenta or the umbilical cord and other complications of pregnancy, labor and delivery.

There is ample evidence that the newborn animal tolerates anoxia better than the adult. This is probably related to the enhanced capacity of the fetal brain to function by utilizing anaerobic glycolysis (Himwich). Evidence from animal studies (Windle) indicates that sublethal anoxia during the fetal or neonatal period may lead to permanent neurologic defects. It is likely that the same is true in man.

When death from anoxia occurs suddenly, there may be no discernible morphologic changes seen on pathological examination. The diagnosis of fetal anoxia here is dependent on clinical data. With more prolonged fetal anoxia preceding death, one sees nonspecific morphologic changes. These consist of visceral congestion, scattered petechiae involving especially the serous surfaces of the pleural and pericardial cavities and ill-defined areas of hemorrhage in the subarachnoid

space over the cerebral hemispheres. When the anoxia is severe and prolonged, there may be pulmonary and adrenal hemorrhages, subcapsular hemorrhages and focal necrosis in the liver as well as in the centrum semiovale of the cerebral hemispheres and in the coronary arteries.

The amniotic fluid surrounding the fetus normally contains squamous epithelial cells, vernix caseosa and lanugo derived from the skin of the fetus; meconium may be present in the amniotic fluid of anoxic fetuses. Any of these solid constituents may be aspirated *in utero* into lung alveolar spaces as a result of deep intrauterine respirations accompanying fetal anoxia (Macgregor). The epithelial cells appear as blue, elongated, wavy, nonnucleated structures or as flattened, pink, squamous cells. Vernix caseosa consists of cellular debris embedded in fat and fatty acids. Lanugo is present infrequently and appears as long, highly refractile bodies. Meconium is recognizable as golden brown, spheric or ovoid bodies or as an amorphous, yellowish brown, granular precipitate.

Roentgenographically, the lungs of liveborn infants who have aspirated large amounts of amniotic debris *in utero* may reveal coarse, irregular densities indistinguishable from those associated with postnatal aspiration of feedings (Peterson and Pendleton). These densities are transient and probably result from focal areas of atelectasis secondary to obstruction of small bronchi by amniotic debris.

Although the most characteristic morphologic findings in fetal anoxia are located in the lungs, most deaths are probably the result of cerebral damage with subsequent depression of respiratory activity. Cerebral congestion, scattered subarachnoid hemorrhages and perivascular petechiae may be visualized in the central nervous system, but more specific changes are usually lacking in infants dying as a direct result of fetal anoxia, since death usually occurs before morphologic changes become manifest.

The clinical measures needed to combat neonatal hypoxia and to correct its sequelae are detailed in Chapter 67. Still more relevant to obstetric practice are the principles of good antenatal and intrapartum care of the gravida so that hypoxic states will be avoided, if possible, or detected early and treated aggressively when they arise.

RESPIRATORY DISTRESS SYNDROME

Pulmonary hyaline membranes (Fig. 388) are encountered in nearly half the neonates who die. This condition is the leading cause of death of premature infants (Smith; Bruns and Shields). The clinical pattern associated with pulmonary hyaline membranes and the commonly coassociated atelectasis is called *respiratory distress syndrome*. Although used interchangeably, *hyaline membrane disease* requires pathological identification in the fatal cases and is, therefore, inappropriate to use in the surviving infants.

Although more frequent in premature infants, especially those with a birth weight of under 1500 gm. (Claireaux; Landing), hyaline membrane disease may also occur in babies born at term, especially in infants born by cesarean section, in those of diabetic mothers or of gravidas with third trimester bleeding, and in twins. It is not seen in stillborn infants (Tran-Dinh-De and Anderson) or in babies surviving less than one hour after birth.

Clinical manifestations may be present at birth, but usually do not appear for several hours after delivery. Classically, the infants exhibit increasing dyspnea with retraction of the suprasternal and infracostal regions, increasing respiratory rate, cyanosis and apnea. Auscultation of the chest reveals poor exchange of air.

Roentgen examination (Fig. 389) reveals a uniform miliary mottling or reticulogranular appearance throughout both lungs. This picture is apparent within a

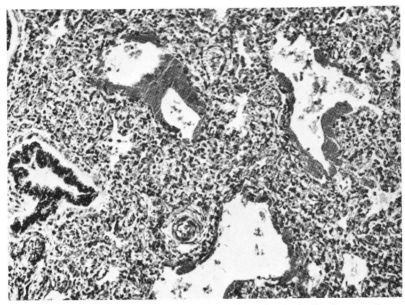

Figure 388 Photomicrograph of the lung in a premature infant who died of hyaline membrane disease in the neonatal period. Acidophilic membranes are shown lining the expanded alveolar spaces. The interalveolar septums appear to be widened, but this is due to atelectasis. (Magnification × 200.) (From Nelson, W. E., Vaughan, V. C., III, and McKay, R. J.: Textbook of Pediatrics, ed. 9. Philadelphia, W. B. Saunders Company, 1969.)

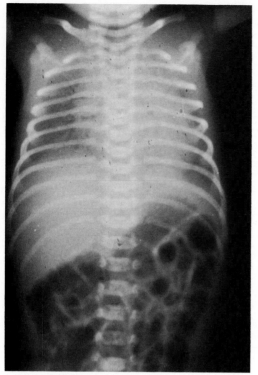

Figure 389 Anteroposterior x-ray view of a neonate with extensive hyaline membrane disease. Complete homogeneous density of the lung fields may be seen, but the typical diffuse granular pattern is shown here, representing areas of focal atelectasis.

noted. Atelectasis is also an integral part of the complete picture. It is usually attributed to obstruction of the smaller air spaces by the material forming the membranes. It may be related to diminished amounts of *surfactant* (see Chapter 6), the phospholipid present in healthy, mature lungs that is normally responsible for decreasing the surface tension within the alveolar spaces (Avery).

Treatment of infants with respiratory distress syndrome is largely supportive. Properly humidified oxygen should be administered as needed, with care being taken to avoid hyperoxygenation if possible. Warmth is essential because of the known adverse effects of hypothermia to which all sick neonates are particularly prone. Combined metabolic and respiratory acidosis is present in these infants and undoubtedly plays a major role in their death. Continuous monitoring of the acid-base balance and blood gases and correction of detected imbalances are, therefore, important aspects of therapy. Currently, antibiotics are administered to these infants because of the frequency of superimposed pneumonia.

INTRAVENTRICULAR HEMORRHAGE

Hemorrhage into the ventricles is responsible for about 10 per cent of all neonatal deaths and is seen especially in small premature infants who die. It is almost nonexistent in full-term infants. Although trauma may be contributory to its development, intraventricular hemorrhage is more often due to hypoxia and is not truly traumatic in origin. The role of prematurity in the development of subependymal and intraventricular hemorrhages probably depends on a number of factors, including softness of the skull and the brain, an increased incidence of anoxia, deficient development of elastic fibers in the vascular system and increased capillary fragility.

Clinical manifestations of intraventricular hemorrhage may be apparent at the time of delivery, with death usually occurring within 24 to 36 hours after birth. In some instances, however, clinical manifes-

few hours after delivery, but a distinct pattern may not become evident for 6 to 18 hours (Peterson and Pendleton). As the process progresses, the miliary densities coalesce so that ultimately both lungs are diffusely opacified. This pattern of diffuse, complete opacification is a very serious sign and is almost always fatal (Donald). Infants with less severe x-ray changes may survive, usually clearing their lungs by one week of age. Death usually occurs within one to two days after delivery in infants with fatal pulmonary hyaline membranes.

The pathogenesis of pulmonary hyaline membranes is not established, and various theories have been proposed. To date, the evidence indicates that the membranes are not formed from protein derived from the amniotic fluid, but are derived from fetal blood. Thus, they are probably related to the intense capillary pulmonary congestion (Duran-Jorda et al.) which is regularly tations may be delayed for several hours or even several days. During this latent period, there may be no unusual signs or symptoms. Clinically, the baby may become lethargic and unresponsive, with a weak cry, progressive pallor, dyspnea, vomiting and seizures. Rapid progression to apnea and death is usual. Survivors may have no residua or may demonstrate a wide range of neurologic abnormalities according to the location and degree of brain tissue destroyed (see below). There may be a fall in the hematocrit associated with extensive intraventricular hemorrhage. The cerebrospinal fluid is xanthochromic or frankly bloody.

With extensive intraventricular hemorrhage, there is usually considerable blood in the cisterna magna at autopsy, extending anteriorly in the subarachnoid space along the anterior surface of the pons into the interpeduncular cistern and sometimes into the Sylvian fissures (Fig. 390). Small, probably nonlethal, intraventricular hemorrhages may be confined to the posterior horn of one or both lateral ventricles,

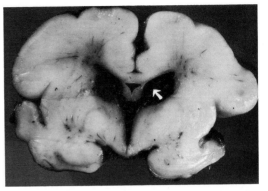

Figure 391 Cut section of the brain showing gross bilateral subependymal hemorrhages in the region of the linea terminalis, giving rise to extensive intraventricular hemorrhage. The hemorrhage in the lateral ventricles extends through the foramina of Monro into the third ventricle. The floor of the lateral ventricle is indicated by the arrow.

and then there usually is no associated hemorrhage in the subarachnoid space at the base of the brain.

The source of intraventricular hemorrhage is not always clear. Small hemorrhages confined to the occipital horns of the lateral ventricles and frequently overlying the choroid plexuses apparently arise from the engorged vessels of the choroid plexus. More extensive hemorrhages, however, usually arise as the result of a subependymal hemorrhage located about the terminal vein between the caudate nucleus and the thalamus (Fig. 391). Such subependymal hemorrhages probably account for the latent period between birth and the onset of manifestations.

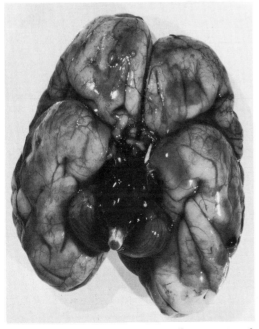

Figure 390 Gross appearance of extensive subarachnoid hemorrhage at the base of the brain in a premature infant dying as a result of an intraventricular hemorrhage. Note the blood in the region of the cisterna magna, on the anterior surface of the pons and in the vicinity of the optic chiasm.

SUBDURAL HEMORRHAGE

Intracranial hemorrhage in the newborn infant usually refers either to intraventricular hemorrhage or to subdural hemorrhage. The latter is a lesion associated with intracranial trauma. It is seen with less and less frequency as obstetric care improves, as excessively problematic labors are more often terminated by cesarean section and as the difficult, potentially injurious operative delivery procedures are eliminated from clinical practice. Nevertheless, whereas intraventricular hemorrhage is the most common variety of intracranial

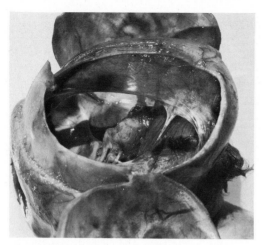

Figure 392 Interior of the skull of a newborn infant illustrating an unusual complete tear of the left leaf of the tentorium cerebelli, exposing the underlying cerebellar hemisphere. The falx cerebri is intact. The parietal bones are reflected laterally and the cerebral hemispheres have been removed.

bleeding seen in the premature infant, subarachnoid hemorrhage is most frequent at term (Haller et al.). Clinical manifestations are essentially the same as for intraventricular hemorrhage, except for the likelihood that traumatic hemorrhages tend to be more severe and, therefore, associated with more rapid progression.

Subdural hemorrhages arise from a variety of intracranial injuries, including tears involving (1) the superior cerebral veins where they enter from the superior sagittal sinus, (2) the great cerebral vein of Galen at its entrance into the straight venous sinus at the base of the brain and (3) the straight sinus itself or the transverse venous sinus. Damage to the falx cerebri or tentorium cerebelli (Fig. 392) or both is commonly coassociated with disruption of these vessels. Tears of the dural septums alone are not lethal lesions; it is the subdural and infratentorial hemorrhages which may accompany them that are usually responsible for death.

Such damage may result from excessive molding of the fetal head during labor or excessive instrumental compression, especially when the forces are misdirected, as in brow-mastoid applications. Precipitate vertex delivery, with its rapid alteration in the shape of the head, also tends to produce intracranial trauma. In a few in-

stances, lethal intracranial trauma may even occur after an apparently normal spontaneous delivery.

BRAIN DAMAGE

The clinical sequelae of intracranial hemorrhage vary with the site and degree of involvement. Motor, sensory, intellectual or personality defects and seizures may ensue, as well as syndromes of epilepsy, mental retardation and congenital blindness or deafness. Some survivors will manifest subtle damage in the form of specific reading disabilities and perceptual and cognitive disorders.

Cerebral palsy comprises a group of clinical syndromes characterized by chronic motor abnormalities, whether paralysis, weakness, incoordination, involuntary motion or any other motor aberration caused by involvement of the motor control centers of the brain. A child with cerebral palsy may have other associated disabilities. The disorder occurs about once in 2000 births.

Cerebral palsy is classified according to the motor defect as (1) spastic, (2) dyskinetic and (3) ataxic. The common spastic form shows exaggerated stretch reflex and increased tendon reflexes; the dyskinetic form has involuntary, uncoordinated movements, often with athetosis and tremors; the rare ataxic form is manifest by disturbed balance and dyssynergia. There is a close correlation between the type of motor defect and the etiology (Perlstein).

Cerebral palsy is more common in premature infants and in overly large neonates, in the firstborn and in those infants born to older women. It is more common in males than in females (5:4), and in whites than in blacks.

There is probably a constitutional factor which determines why some newborn infants with ostensibly severe degrees of anoxia or skull injury may recover without clinical sequelae, whereas others with relatively minor degrees of anoxia, jaundice or trauma may have extensive, permanent damage.

Severe hypoxia and cerebral contusion or hemorrhage are the most important causes of cerebral palsy. Brain cells are highly sensitive to lack of oxygen. If prolonged, anoxia causes irreparable damage because neural tissue, unlike most other tissues, does not have the property of regeneration.

In the fetus and newborn infant, the midbrain, the basal nuclei and their cortical connections seem to be more vulnerable to oxygen deprivation than the cortical cells and pyramidal tracts. Therefore, when anoxia interferes with normal metabolic functions, the clinical syndromes are usually those characterized by quadriplegic athetosis.

The most common primary cause of cerebral palsy is related to vascular injury or to direct brain trauma. Paradoxically, anoxic mechanisms are actually much more frequent in causing brain damage, but the lesions that result are more often lethal so that there are fewer surviving damaged babies. Most traumatic cerebral hemorrhages are asymmetrically located near the cortical motor areas or the internal capsule. Thus, they are likely to cause unilateral or asymmetric lesions and a clinical syndrome of spasticity with hemiplegic or asymmetric quadriplegic involvement.

Hemorrhages secondary to severe anoxia, by contrast, tend to be intraventricular and are more symmetrically distributed. Thus, primary anoxic damage to the brain is more likely to produce athetosis or related dyskinesias, whereas primary trauma or hemorrhage is more likely to cause spasticity.

Other known causes of brain damage include hyperbilirubinemia, rubella and other viremias, and maternal thyroid, adrenal and pancreatic dysfunction. The hazards to the fetus of untreated increases in circulating indirect bilirubin have been dealt with in Chapter 52, but it should be emphasized that the syndrome of kernicterus, with athetosis, extrapyramidal rigidity and hearing defects, is very serious. There may be coassociated discoloring and dysplasia of the enamel of the deciduous teeth as well. It is imperative that such permanent damage be averted by appropriate measures to combat excessive jaundice in the neonate. Prevention of the cerebral palsy syndromes due to this factor is now possible by means of exchange transfusion, when indicated.

FETAL TRAUMA

Skull Fracture

Traumatic fractures of the cranial bones during parturition are usually accompanied by an overlying cephalhematoma (Fig. 393). However, cephalhematoma is often

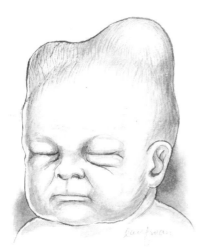
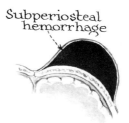

Subperiosteal hemorrhage

Figure 393 Drawing of a neonate with bilateral cephalhematomas. Inset at right shows location of the blood subperiosteally and limited to the region of the specific cranial bone underlying it by the periosteal attachment at the suture line.

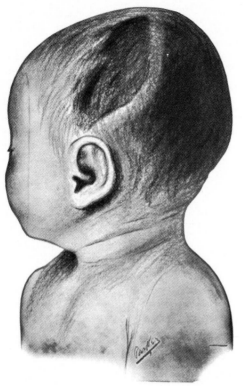

Figure 394   Depression of the parietal bone, erroneously called depression fracture, associated with forceps delivery.

Caput Succedaneum

Caput succedaneum is a commonly occurring swelling of the soft tissues of the presenting part (see Fig. 164). During labor, and especially after rupture of the membranes, that portion of the presenting part overlying the cervical os is subject to differential pressures resulting in venous engorgement and subsequent subcutaneous exudation of serous fluid and extravasation of blood.

The scalp is the usual site of a caput succedaneum. With prolonged labor, the caput overlying the vertex may be so extensive as to obtund palpatory recognition of cranial landmarks. Similar swellings, often associated with hemorrhage, are present over the face when this is the presenting part, and over the buttocks and scrotum or labia in infants presenting by the breech. The edematous swelling of the soft tissues rapidly disappears, usually by the end of the fourth day after birth. Complications of a caput succedaneum are almost nonexistent.

Cephalhematoma

Cephalhematoma, a subperiosteal accumulation of blood (Fig. 393), is less frequent than a caput succedaneum. The two conditions are similar in appearance, often coexist, and must be differentiated. Cephalhematoma usually represents a more severe injury than caput succedaneum. Since each bone of the calvarium is covered by its own independent periosteal membrane, the blood which accumulates within a cephalhematoma is of necessity confined to the surface of a single bone and does not cross the suture lines. However, multiple cephalhematomas may be present in 15 per cent of affected infants, and may make the diagnosis difficult. They are caused by tearing of some of the subperiosteal vessels.

Linear fractures of the underlying bone (see above) are sometimes found associated with cephalhematomas. Bleeding from the fractured cranial bone may contribute to their content of blood. Neither the fracture nor the cephalhematoma is ap-

seen without an accompanying fracture (see below); one in four cephalhematomas is related to an underlying skull fracture (Kendall and Woloshin). Short linear fractures are usually found in the lines of cleavage of the parietal bone at right angles to the sagittal suture.

Rarely, fractures of the base of the skull occur, located in the relatively weak suture line between the paired lateral exoccipital bones and the squamous portion of the occipital bone. They are encountered most often after breech deliveries. They may be associated with tearing of the occipital sinus or its tributaries.

Depressed fractures of the parietal bone (Fig. 394) or the frontal bone are not true fractures, but simply depressions of the bone where it is compressed against the maternal symphysis pubis or sacral promontory. Many of these will regain their normal contour spontaneously.

parently responsible for any symptoms unless underlying brain is concomitantly damaged.

Cephalhematomas may be present over one or both parietal bones or over the squamous portion of the occipital bone, the frontal bone or even the temporal bone. They are somewhat more common over the right parietal bone than elsewhere. The cephalhematoma may be obscured at the time of birth by a caput succedaneum and thus may not be apparent until the latter has receded.

It presents as an asymptomatic mass which initially is soft and fluctuant because of its content of fluid blood. Subsequently, it may be absorbed slowly and disappear or it may become organized and be converted into bone. Periosteal new bone is first laid down at the angle between the elevated periosteum and the underlying bone and, subsequently, as a thin shell of bone which completely encloses the hematoma. Rarely, hematomas persist for many years as roentgenographically demonstrable areas of cystic rarefaction. Treatment is generally not necessary. Because of possible secondary infection, it is best not to incise them.

Fractured Clavicle

The clavicle may be broken in its midportion in difficult shoulder deliveries, sometimes deliberately in order to resolve an impaction (see Chapter 60). Clinically, there may be diminished use of the arm on the affected side with absence of the Moro reflex unilaterally. Sometimes there is no apparent disability and the initial manifestation may be a palpable callus discovered one to two weeks after birth. The prognosis is excellent even without therapy.

Fracture of the Extremities

The arms and the legs are fractured much less often than the clavicle. The humerus and the femur are most frequently involved, the fractures usually being located in the midportion of the diaphysis, generally in association with breech presentations or delivery by ver-

sion and extraction. Spontaneous movement and the Moro reflex are usually absent in the involved extremity. The site of the fracture may or may not be palpable. Although the radial nerve is commonly injured with fractures of the humerus, permanent disability is rare.

Separation of the epiphysis of the upper end of the femur or the humerus or even dislocation of the humerus may result from trauma incurred during delivery, but such accidents are rare.

Vertebral Fractures

Fractures and dislocations of the spinal vertebras are rare and result from excessive force used in extraction of the aftercoming head in a breech presentation or, less frequently, of the shoulders in a cephalic presentation. Injuries are especially apt to occur when the spine is hyperextended or when lateral traction is exerted. The lower cervical and upper dorsal vertebras are most often involved.

The amount of injury to the spinal cord depends on the degree of displacement of the vertebral body and the extent of hemorrhage and tearing in the cord itself; severe damage to the cord may occur even without vertebral fracture. Damage is due to stretch injury or to compression of the cord and brain stem incurred mainly through excessive traction and flexion of the fetal vertebral column in cephalic as well as in breech delivery. In a recent revealing study, Abroms et al. found 21 per cent cervical cord injuries associated with hyperextension of the fetal head in breech presentations delivered vaginally and none in comparable fetuses delivered by cesarean section.

There usually is associated extensive hemorrhage into the spinal cord and canal and adjoining soft tissue. With severe injuries, especially those involving the cervical region, damage to the phrenic nerve or even to the medulla is apt to occur and be responsible for respiratory difficulty and early death of the infant.

The baby may survive with less severe injuries. In a very few instances, the initial paralysis may disappear, although total recovery is very unusual. The damage to the cord in these infants is presumably the result of edema and hemorrhage which subsequently subside. Paralysis below the level of the injury, associated with flexion deformities and urinary and fecal incontinence, is most often the outcome in those who survive.

Cord injuries in neonates who die soon after birth may not be diagnosed at autopsy unless the spinal cord is routinely removed and examined (Towbin). One should suspect cord injury in association with premature birth, breech and precipitate delivery, and in newborn infants with respiratory depression, shallow respirations, gasping or secondary apnea, who die in a few hours.

Peripheral Nerve Injuries *cranial nerve!*

Facial Palsy. The most common site of injury to a peripheral nerve during delivery is the facial nerve. Facial paralysis (Fig. 395) usually results from injury to the nerve near its exit from the stylomastoid foramen or as it crosses the ramus of the mandible. It is almost always unilateral and usually the result of forceps trauma.

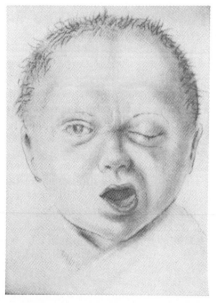

Figure 395 Neonate with right facial palsy, demonstrating absence of the nasolacrimal fold, open eye and lack of facial muscle activity during crying. (Courtesy of A. C. Posner.)

Rarely, the injury can be attributed to prolonged pressure by the maternal sacral promontory or symphysis pubis, or by the fetal shoulder. The eye on the affected side remains open as a result of paralysis of the orbicularis oculi muscle; this may be the only sign when the infant is not crying. When the infant cries, the affected side becomes obvious by lack of muscular response and the absence of a nasolabial fold. Since the damage to the nerve is generally produced by edema and hemorrhage in and about the facial nerve, the paralysis is usually temporary and disappears within a few weeks. Infrequently, there may be permanent paralysis if the nerve is severed.

Brachial Palsy. Injury to the brachial plexus may be caused by strong lateral traction on the neck during a difficult delivery, as during extraction of impacted shoulders or the delivery of the aftercoming head. Digital pressure against the axilla or hyperextension and abduction of the arm during delivery may also be responsible for injury to this plexus.

Unilateral *Duchenne-Erb's paralysis* (Fig. 396) is the most common form of brachial palsy. It is generally due to upper trunk injury at the junction of the fifth and sixth cervical nerves; tearing of the nerve roots and partial avulsion of their ganglions may also be responsible. The injury may consist only of edema and hemorrhage in and about the nerves, or there may be tearing of the nerve sheaths and fibers and hemorrhage into the soft tissue.

The triceps muscle is unaffected so that the arm is extended but, owing to loss of innervation of the biceps, it cannot be flexed. The ability to abduct and externally rotate the upper arm and to supinate the forearm is lost, so that the arm is adducted and internally rotated with pronation of the forearm; the palm of the hand is directed posteriorly or even posterolaterally. The Moro and biceps reflexes are absent on the affected side.

Prognosis depends on the degree of neural injury. If there is no improvement in a few months, it is probable that the nerve fibers have been torn. Neuroplastic procedures may then be beneficial.

Klumpke's paralysis is much less common, comprising only about two per cent of all brachial palsies. It is especially apt to

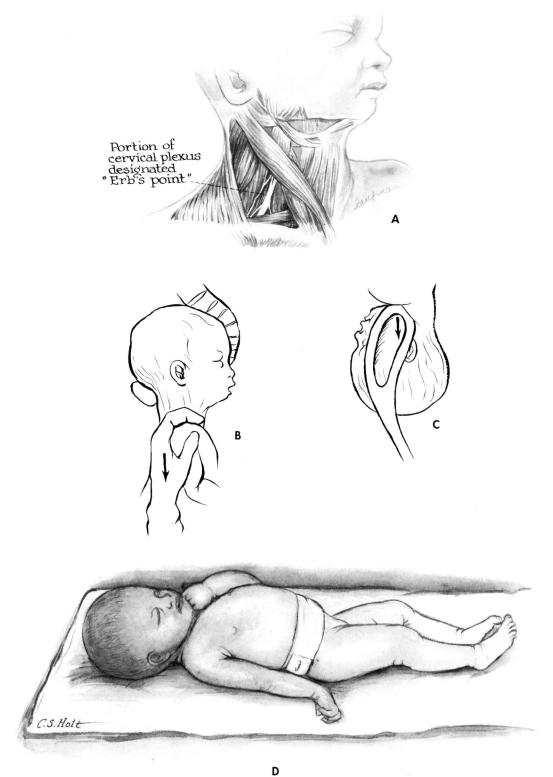

Figure 396 *A*, Neck dissection in the newborn showing anatomic relationships of Erb's point and the cervical plexus usually involved in Duchenne-Erb's paralysis. Mechanisms by which injury occurs include *B*, inappropriate traction on the aftercoming head or *C*, compression with forceps. *D*, Characteristic positioning of the arm in Duchenne-Erb's palsy on the right side.

result from forceful hyperextension and abduction of the arm during delivery, with resultant stretching and even tearing of the lower part of the brachial plexus. It is usually unilateral and is caused by damage to the lower part of the trunk, distal to the union of the eighth cervical and first thoracic nerves.

There is paralysis of the small muscles of the hand and of most of the long flexors of the fingers and wrist as a result of destruction of motor fibers which course in the ulnar and median nerves. The grasp reflex is absent and the hand is often swollen. Preganglionic sympathetic nerve damage affecting the first thoracic nerve will often produce a concomitant contraction of the pupil and drooping of the eyelid on the affected side (Horner's syndrome).

Paralysis of the whole arm results from damage to the entire brachial plexus, probably involving primarily the nerve roots themselves. All the muscles of the arm, forearm and hand are paralyzed. There is extensive loss of superficial and deep sensation. Such extensive damage is apt to be the result of tearing of the nerve fibers, making the prognosis for recovery of function poor.

Phrenic Nerve Paralysis. This is a result of injury sustained during delivery. It is usually unilateral and associated with Duchenne-Erb's paralysis. However, it may occur in the absence of other apparent injuries. The manifestations are dyspnea, cyanosis and a thoracic type of respiration with no bulging of the abdomen during inspiration. These signs usually appear within 24 hours after delivery, but may be delayed for several days. Fluoroscopic examination reveals elevation of the diaphragm on the affected side and parodoxical see-saw movements of the two sides of the diaphragm during respirations. Spontaneous recovery is likely, but is usually slow, and pulmonary infections are a serious complication.

Radial Nerve Palsies. In the newborn, radial nerve palsies have been attributed to pressure from a uterine constriction ring or injury by forceps (Feldman). The prognosis for recovery of function is good.

REFERENCES

Abroms, I. F., Bresnan, M. J., Zuckerman, J. E., Fischer, E. G., and Strand, R.: Cervical cord injuries secondary to hyperextension of the head in breech presentations. Obstet. Gynec., 41:369, 1973.

Avery, M. E.: The Lung and Its Disorders in the Newborn Infant, ed. 2. Philadelphia, W. B. Saunders Company, 1968.

Bruns, P. D., and Shields, L. V.: The pathogenesis and relationship of the hyaline-like pulmonary nembrane to premature neonatal mortality. Amer. J. Obstet. Gynec. 61:953, 1951.

Claireaux, A. E.: Hyaline membrane in the neonatal lung. Lancet 2:749, 1953.

Donald, I.: Neonatal respiration and hyaline membrane. Brit. J. Anaesth. 29:553, 1957.

Duran-Jorda, F., Holzel, A., and Patterson, W. H.: A histochemical study of pulmonary hyaline membrane. Arch. Dis. Child. 31:113, 1956.

Feldman, G. V.: Radial nerve palsies in the newborn. Arch. Dis. Child. 32:469, 1957.

Haller, E. S., Nesbitt, R. E. L., and Anderson, G. W.: Clinical and pathologic concepts of gross intracranial hemorrhage in perinatal mortality. Obstet. Gynec. Survey 11:179, 1956.

Himwich, H. E.: The Development of Enzyme Systems: The Maturation of the Respiratory Enzymes in the Central Nervous System of Experimental Animals, in Prematurity, Congenital Malformation and Birth Injury. Association for the Aid of Crippled Children, 1953.

Kendall, N., and Woloshin, H.: Cephalhematoma associated with fracture of the skull. J. Pediat. 41:125, 1952.

Landing, B. H.: Pathologic features of respiratory distress syndromes in newborn infants. Amer. J. Roentgen. 74:796, 1955.

Macgregor, A. R.: Some observations on aspiration of liquor amnii and the so-called "vernix membrane." In Delafresnaye, J. F., and Oppé, T. E., eds.: A Symposium on Anoxia of the New Born Infant. Springfield, Ill., Charles C Thomas, 1953.

Perlstein, M. A.: Perinatal brain injury with special reference to cerebral palsy. In Greenhill, J. P.: Obstetrics, ed. 13. Philadelphia, W. B. Saunders Company, 1965.

Peterson, H. G., Jr., and Pendleton, M. E.: Contrasting roentgenographic pulmonary patterns of the hyaline membrane and fetal aspiration syndromes. Amer. J. Roentgen. 74:800, 1955.

Smith, M. H. D.: Bacterial pathogens of the respiratory tract of the newborn infant. Pediat. Clin. N. Amer. 4:69, 1957.

Towbin, A.: Spinal cord and brain stem injury at birth. Arch. Path. 77:620, 1964.

Tran-Dinh-De and Anderson, G. W.: Hyaline-like membranes associated with diseases of the newborn lungs: A review of the literature. Obstet. Gynec. Survey 8:1, 1953.

Windle, W. F.: Asphyxial brain damage at birth with reference to the minimally affected child. In Greenhill, J. P., ed.: Year Book of Obstetrics and Gynecology, 1970. Chicago, Year Book Medical Publishers, Inc., 1970.

Chapter 69

Fetal Malformations

Fetal malformations account for 10 to 20 per cent of the deaths of fetuses and infants weighing more than 500 gm. They are also an important cause of intrauterine deaths during the first trimester of pregnancy and of many instances of crippling and death appearing months and years after birth. Probably less than half of the congenital malformations which will ultimately lead to permanent disability or death are apparent at birth (McIntosh et al.). The overall incidence is, therefore, not well defined, but it is estimated to be in excess of three per cent of all births. Lethal anomalies incompatible with life occur in about 0.5 per cent of infants born alive. If all minor malformations are included, the frequency of occurrence may be as high as 10 per cent.

Congenital malformations are not necessarily inherited genetic traits. They may result from abnormal environmental conditions acting on a genetically normal embryo or they may result from genetic abnormalities in the presence of apparently normal intrauterine environmental conditions. Often, moreover, they are probably dependent on an interaction between genetic and environmental factors. Among recognized environmental teratogens are radiation, certain infections of the mother, and drugs taken by her. Known causes account for only a very small proportion of all fetal anomalies.

Fetal malformations may be induced experimentally in animals by many different means. In spite of the advances in the knowledge of teratology accrued from such experimental work, little is known about the causes of congenital malformations in man Our inability to apply experimental information readily to humans is based large'y on species differences in response to given factors, differences in organ or tissue response at a given developmental stage during embryogenesis and on what is now recognized as individual differences in susceptibility. The latter relate both to the presence of and the interaction between environmental and genetic influences. The effect of a known teratogen, for example, may be nullified by optimizing the embryological environment or may be enhanced by an unfavorable environment so that a defect develops. Thus, in fetuses that are susceptible to developing a given anomaly (based on species, genetic make-up and the presence of an effective teratogen), the threshold of that susceptibility wi l be altered according to the prevailing environmental circumstances.

ETIOLOGY

Maternal rubella, especially during the first trimester of pregnancy, is a recognized cause of certain congenital malformations in infants (see Chapter 40), but the mechanism by which these malformations are produced is not clear. The neonate usually presents with heart malformations, cataracts, deafness and sometimes microcephaly. In addition, one may encounter thrombocytopenia, hepatitis, interstitial pneumonia, osteomyelitis and encephalitis (Monif). Transplacental fetal viremia is causative even though manifestations of rubella in the mother may be minimal or absent.

A number of other infectious diseases in the mother, such as Coxsackie B, influenza A, hepatitis and mumps virus infections, have been reported to be associated with

715

an increased incidence of congenital malformations, but evidence for a cause and effect relationship in most of them is not firmly established. Toxoplasmosis may cause severe intrauterine disease and destructive calcific brain lesions, but there is no conclusive evidence that it causes congenital malformations as a result of impaired early cerebral development. Cytomegalic inclusion disease may also be responsible for active intrauterine infection and lesions of the central nervous system, including microgyria, porencephaly and cerebral or cerebellar hypoplasia.

Exposure of a pregnant mother to ionizing irradiation may lead to malformations of the fetus (Fraser and Fainstat). Microcephaly with mental retardation was also observed in infants exposed *in utero* to atomic radiation, the incidence depending on dose and gestational age. There is little doubt that genetic damage, with a resultant effect on future generations, may be produced by such irradiation. The relative hazards of diagnostic radiation are balanced against its potential benefits in Chapter 12. Therapeutic levels of radiation are best avoided in pregnancy if the fetus is expected to be carried to viability.

Pharmacologic teratogens in humans include antimetabolites, such as folic acid antagonists (for example, Aminopterin), and the sedative thalidomide. The phocomelia which can result from ingestion of thalidomide during pregnancy is now well recognized (Fig. 397). In this syndrome the bones between the hands and shoulders are defective or absent, and the hands or rudimentary fingers derive directly from the ends of the affected bones. Both sides are affected, but usually not with equal severity. The legs may also be affected, but less severely. In extreme cases the arms and legs are absent. Most of these children are mentally normal. Of interest is the fact that thalidomide does not invariably cause this defect, but acts only at a specific interval in pregnancy and somewhat inconstantly even during that time span.

The fetus may develop massive enlargement of the thyroid gland from maternal administration of large doses of iodide-containing drugs over long periods of time. Thyroid suppressant agents that cross the placenta, such as propylthiouracil, and destructive radioisotopes that concentrate in fetal thyroid, such as radioactive iodine, may produce cretinism. Hypervitaminosis D may cause skeletal and aortic malformations in the fetus. Androgenic substances taken by the mother, including certain progestational agents, may be virilizing to some female fetuses, who show labial fusion and clitoral hypertrophy.

The teratogenic potentiality of most drugs has not been clearly determined. Animal studies are inapplicable to man, and investigation in humans is at best difficult and at worst unethical. Observations on the teratogenicity of specific agents consist of testimonials, with the result that an effect (such as that of thalidomide) must be common and catastrophic before it is recognized, and then only after perhaps

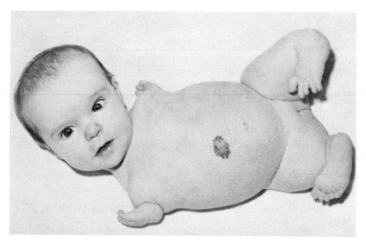

Figure 397 Baby born to a mother who had taken thalidomide in the early weeks of pregnancy. Note absence of humerus, radius and ulna, tibia and fibula, and foreshortened femur bilaterally. The infant is otherwise normal. (Courtesy of P. Ryan.)

tens of thousands of babies have been adversely affected. Moreover, any subtle effect goes unrecognized. To ensure against a fetal malformation from drugs not yet appreciated to be teratogenic, physicians should caution patients against taking any unnecessary medication during pregnancy, and they should not prescribe any agent that is not clearly indicated. Drugs which may be deleterious to pregnancy in other ways are discussed in Chapter 51.

Certain fetal defects are obviously hereditary, determined by factors transmitted through the germ cells. Some follow a simple mendelian pattern of transmission, including hydrocephalus, cataract, cleft palate, chondrodystrophy, polydactylism and brachydactylism. Some are inherited as dominant traits, such as osteogenesis imperfecta and achondroplasia; others are inherited as recessive, including cystic fibrosis and phenylketonuria.

However, it should not be inferred that all such defects are genetically determined, since clinically indistinguishable malformations (for example, hydrocephalus) may also result from adverse environmental factors *in utero*. In some instances, moreover, environmental factors may influence the manifestations of genetic defects as stated earlier. An example of this group is cleft palate.

Not all chromosomal defects are inherited. Some are newly created mutants. Chromosomal errors of this kind are likely to be lethal to the germ cell, interdicting fertilization, or lethal to the zygote, resulting in early spontaneous abortion. Thus, most conceptuses with chromosomal mutations do not survive to viability. Among those that do mature, there are recognizable clinical syndromes of malformations according to the type of chromosomal defect that exists (see below). A 45-chromosome anomaly with absence of the Y chromosome, for example, is manifest clinically by the picture of Turner's syndrome (XO) with webbed neck, cubitus valgus and lymphangiectatic edema of feet and hands. An extra chromosome forming a trisomy-21 is Down's syndrome (mongolism). Deletion of part of chromosome 5 yields a baby with *cri du chat* syndrome, characterized by moon facies, micrognathia, low-set ears, hypertelorism and a peculiar catlike cry.

Such well-defined entities are rare, however. Most of the genetic defects are manifested subtly. Although currently available techniques for studying chromosomal damage (see below) are much too coarse to detect any but the grossest of changes in chromosomal consistency, major genetic distortion may result from small losses or translocations of chromosomal fragments. Manifestations may not appear till later in life and may be indistinguishable from disorders due to other causes. Some individuals may be entirely normal (for example, translocation carriers) phenotypically, perhaps passing the defect on to the next generation.

DIAGNOSIS

In order to understand the diagnostic approaches to fetal malformations, particularly those due to chromosomal disturbances, it is necessary to review briefly some of the concepts of human cytogenetics. The nucleic acid and protein composition of the chromosomes is well recognized. They are the physical transmitters of hereditary data, containing the genetic complement. Genes are distributed in very precise geographic sites on the chromosomes.

Every body cell in man contains 22 pairs of autosomal chromosomes, numbered 1 through 22 in order of diminishing length, and one pair of sex chromosomes. The sex chromosomes are designated XX in females and XY in males; the Y is morphologically distinct. Chromosomes vary in size from 1.5 to 7.0 microns and can be grouped into seven categories, A–G, according to their size and the configuration of the pairs at metaphase. Characteristically, the location of the *centromere* (primary constriction of the paired *chromatids* where they appear to be joined) is useful in identifying autosomal groups; it may be centrally located (metacentric) along the long axis of the chromosome, off-center (submetacentric) or near the end of the chromosome (acrocentric). Chromosomes within groups cannot be identified morphologically, but techniques are now available for doing so autoradiographically by means of differen-

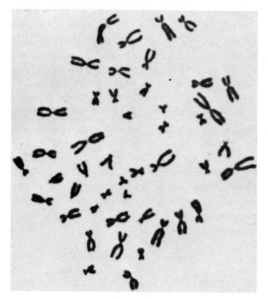

Figure 398 Cell division arrested in metaphase with chromosome pairs spread apart by exposure to hypotonic solution to show the 46 chromosomes of a normal male somatic cell.

tiating the rates of DNA synthesis through uptake of radioisotopically labeled DNA.

The systematic arrangement of chromosomes for purposes of detailed analysis is called the *karyotype*. The kinds of cells suitable for study are most often lymphocytes from the peripheral blood, but may also be marrow, skin, fascia or fetal cells obtained from amniotic fluid. Such cells in tissue culture are induced to divide by using phytohemagglutinin; they are then treated with colchicine to arrest division in the metaphase of mitosis and the cytoplasm is expanded by exposing the cells to a hypotonic solution so that the chromosomes are spread apart for study (Fig. 398). After fixation and staining, photomicrographs are obtained and the chromosome images on the printed photographs are cut up for karyotyping (Fig. 399).

The normal human karyotype consists of three large metacentric pairs of chromosomes comprising group A, two large submetacentric pairs (group B), eight or nine medium-sized submetacentric pairs (7 in group C and 1 or 2 X chromosomes that are morphologically identical), three medium acrocentrics (group D), three short submetacentrics (group E), three short metacentrics (group F) and two or three short acrocentrics (2 in group G and, in males, a Y chromosome).

The complement of chromosomes may be abnormal in several different ways and give rise to major malformations in development. Chromosome morphology may be distorted by means of *translocation* (exchange of genetic material between chromosomes), *inversion* (end-to-end reversal of a segment of a single chromosome that changes the gene order in a single chromosome) or *deletion* (loss of some genetic material from a chromosome); chromosome number may be affected *(aneuploidy)* with extra pairs (trisomy) or too few (monosomy). Aneuploidy results from *nondisjunction* (failure of diads or chromatids to separate) during either the first or second meiotic division in gametogenesis with unequal distribution of chromosome complement to the gamete.

Nondisjunction may also occur during mitotic division of the zygote after fertilization and yield a condition called *mosaicism* in which there are two or more cell lines of different chromosomal composition. This is to be distinguished from *chimerism* in which cell lines are derived from different zygotes. Anaphase lag also yields mosaicism by permitting unequal distribution of chromosome material during cell division, some being excluded as a consequence of failure to migrate from the metaphase plate.

Another important and more easily utilized diagnostic technique involves recognition of the *Barr body* or *sex chromatin*. In resting female somatic cells, one often sees a distinctive, basophilic chromatin mass lying against the nuclear membrane (Fig. 400); it is absent in males. It has been shown that the number of Barr bodies in a given cell is equal to one less than the number of X chromosomes present. Theoretically (Lyon), one X chromosome is heteropyknotic and genetically inactive. Inactivation occurs early in embryological development. Thus, normal males (XY) and females with Turner's syndrome (XO) have no Barr bodies; males with Klinefelter's syndrome (XXY) have one.

Demonstration of the Barr body can be done by the simple technique of scraping cells from the inner surface of the cheek, or by studying cells obtained from the

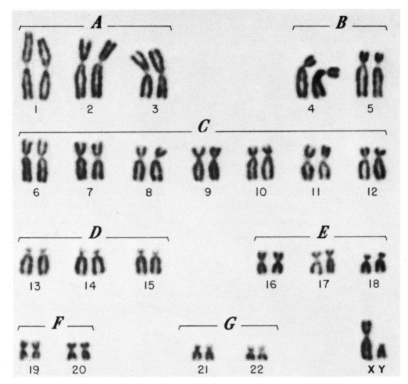

Figure 399 Karyotype of chromosome pairs in photomicrograph similar to that shown in Figure 398, cut up and arranged systematically to illustrate a normal male pattern of 22 pairs of autosomes and an XY sex chromosome complement.

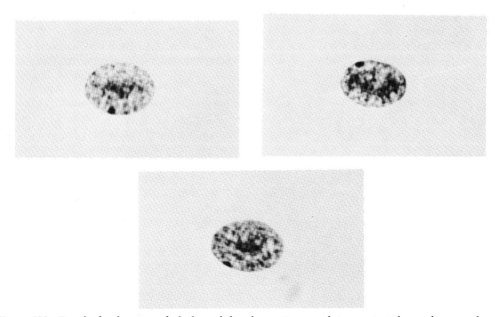

Figure 400 Barr body shown as dark, basophilic chromatin mass lying against the nuclear membrane in epithelial cells desquamated in a buccal smear obtained from a normal female. Sex chromatin-positive cells are found in at least 20 per cent of cells examined in females. (Carbol fuchsin stain, magnification × 1800.)

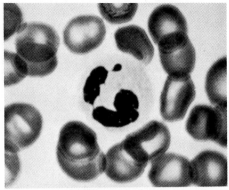

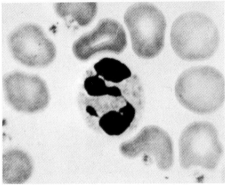

Figure 401 High-power photomicrograph of a blood smear, demonstrating polymorphonuclear neutrophilic leukocytes with drumstick lobulation of nuclear lobe characteristic of three per cent of female white cells. (Giemsa stain, magnification × 1800.)

vagina, bladder or amniotic fluid. Tissue culture techniques are seldom needed except for fetal cells derived from amniotic fluid. A thick smear is fixed, stained and examined microscopically. Normal females should have at least 20 per cent (usually 30 to 40 per cent) of cells chromatin positive, showing the characteristic Barr body.

A unique characteristic of some three per cent of neutrophilic polymorphonuclear leukocytes of females is the drumstick lobulation of a nuclear lobe (Fig. 401). Good quality blood smears can be used for the purpose of detecting drumstick neutrophils as a diagnostic tool.

CLINICAL SYNDROMES

It is impossible to review in detail the host of recognizable malformations. The interested reader is referred to extensive dissertations on this subject. Smith describes 135 clearly defined syndromes in his fine monograph. We will deal here only with those of special interest to obstetricians because of the prognostic implications of chromosomal disturbances.

Down's Syndrome (Mongolism)

The first and most common chromosomal aberration found to cause an autosomal abnormality was the trisomy 21 of Down's syndrome (Lejeune et al.). It occurs in 1 to 2 per 1000 births. About 20 per cent of affected babies are born to women over age 40, 50 per cent over age 35 (Lilienfeld). Collmann and Stoller estimated that the risk of a mother having a mongoloid child increases from 1:1000 at the beginning to 1:45 at the end of the reproductive period. The etiology of this disorder is unknown, but the finding of Australian antigen in 30 per cent of affected patients is highly suggestive epidemiologically. The genetic error (Fig. 402) results from nondisjunction of chromosome 21 during gametogenesis in a normal parent.

There is a small group of patients with Down's syndrome (about three per cent) in whom the extra chromosome 21 is translocated onto another chromosome. The chromosome count is 46. The standard trisomic and translocation trisomic mongols cannot at present be distinguished from each other except by chromosome analysis. Mosaicism is another unusual cytogenetic finding in Down's syndrome. The patient's tissues are then made up of two cell populations, one with trisomy 21 and the other normal.

The typical baby with Down's syndrome is hypotonic and has a tendency to keep its mouth open and protrude its tongue. There is hyperflexibility of the joints. Brachycephaly with flattened occiput and shortened neck is seen. There is an upward slant to the palpebral fissures with characteristic epicanthal folds. Speckling of the iris occurs. Dermatoglyphic patterns on the palms and soles are also unique, with a diagnostic Simian crease in 45 per cent. Hypoplasia of the middle phalanx of

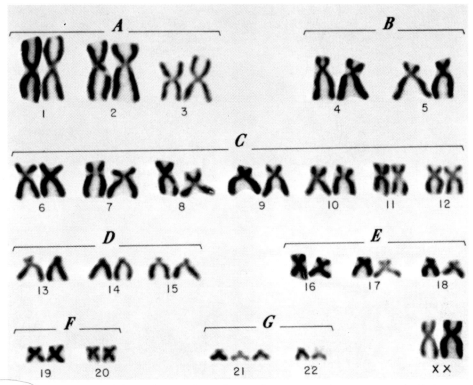

Figure 402 Karyotype of baby with Down's syndrome, showing typical trisomy 21 with 47 chromosomes in all. Other variants include translocation of the extra chromosome 21 onto another chromosome, retaining a total count of 46.

the fifth finger is found. The hair is fine, sparse and straight. The skin is dry and hyperkeratotic. The ears are consistently malformed, with the upper helix turned down (Fig. 403). The characteristic mental deficiency does not become apparent till later in life. Coassociated congenital heart disease is common and may be a major cause of early mortality. Additionally, these children are prone to develop serious respiratory infections.

D_1-Trisomy Syndrome (Trisomy 13)

Trisomy in the 13-15 (D) group causes multiple, severe congenital defects, and the infants almost always die during the first few weeks or months of life (Patau et al.). It is not known which of the three chromosomes in group 13-15 is trisomic in this syndrome. It has been called the D_1 syndrome (or 13 trisomy) because theoretically there could be three D syndromes,

two of them yet to be discovered, with differing defects depending on which member of the group is trisomic.

Characteristic of the syndrome are cleft palate, cleft lip (Fig. 404), microphthalmus, polydactyly and retroflexible thumb. Capillary hemangiomas of the forehead are seen. Microcephaly with sloping forehead is noted. The ears may be low set with an abnormal helix. A Simian palmar crease is common. Of diagnostic importance at birth is the finding of a single umbilical artery.

There is faulty development of the brain with mental retardation. Anomalies of the heart and gastrointestinal tract occur. Although most of these babies die in infancy, those that survive have severe mental deficiency and are subject to seizures. The D_1 syndrome is considerably less frequent than Down's syndrome. D-trisomy introduces a genetic error so severe that it is likely to be lethal in the early stages of embryogenesis.

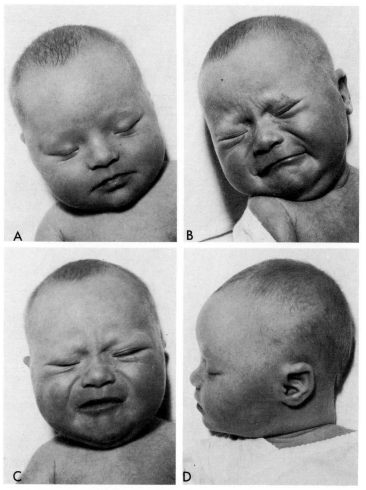

Figure 403 A 10-day-old neonate with Down's syndrome, showing upward slant of eyes and epicanthal folds (*A*); characteristic grimace (*B*); relative broadening of the face (*C*); brachycephaly, fat pad at back of neck and helical distortion of the ear (*D*). (From Potter, E. L.: Pathology of the Fetus and the Infant, ed. 2. Chicago, Year Book Medical Publishers, Inc., 1961.)

E-Trisomy Syndrome (Trisomy 18)

Another rare syndrome is caused by trisomy in the 16-18 (E) group of autosomes (Edwards et al.). It is second only to Down's syndrome in order of frequency of multiple malformation syndromes, occurring in about 3 per 10,000 neonates, mostly in females.

Infants with E syndrome are small at birth. They are feeble, have a weak cry, suck poorly and fail to thrive. Death in early infancy is the rule; others no doubt die *in utero*. The ears are set low and are usually malformed, the occiput is promi-

nent and the mandible is small (Fig. 405). The fingers are clenched and the index finger usually overlies the third finger; the fifth finger may also overlap the fourth. Prominence of the heels and convexity of the soles give the feet a "rocker-bottom" appearance. There may also be cardiac anomalies, such as ventricular septal defect or patent ductus arteriosus, renal anomalies and umbilical or inguinal hernias. At least 130 different abnormalities have been reported to be associated with E trisomy (Smith). Among the few survivors of infancy, there will be signs of defective maturation of the brain, including hypertonicity and mental retardation.

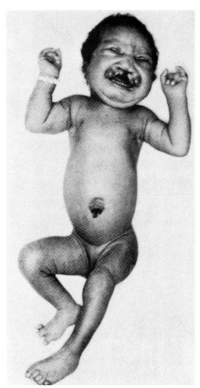

Figure 404 An infant with D₁-trisomy syndrome with cleft palate and lip and low-set ears. (Courtesy of P. E. Conen.)

Deletion Syndromes

Patterns of multiple malformations are recognized to result from deletion of the short arm of autosomes 4 or 5 (the latter called *cri du chat syndrome*) as well as the long arm of chromosome 18. The cri du chat syndrome takes its name from the characteristic catlike cry of the neonate. Affected infants tend to be small at birth and to grow slowly. Microcephaly with hypertelorism, downward sloping of the eyes, epicanthal folds and a Simian crease are common. Survivors manifest mental deficiency and may be troubled by congenital heart disease.

A somewhat different clinical pattern emerges with the rarer deletion of part of chromosome 4, which cannot be distinguished from the partial deletion of 5 except by autoradiography (German et al.). These severely retarded infants are small and feeble at birth, with a tendency to seizures. They grow slowly and have res-

piratory infections commonly. Cleft lip and palate are seen with short upper lip and downturned fishlike mouth. Strabismus, deformities of the iris and epicanthal folds are typical. Deletion of part of chromosome 18 yields mental deficiency with hypotonus, microcephaly and midfacial hypoplasia with deep-set eyes. Visual and hearing problems are frequent. There may be a prominent antihelix and antitragus deformity of the ear.

Sex Chromosome Abnormalities

The X chromosome bears many genes that have no direct concern with sex determination. McKusick catalogued X-borne mutations in man, listing 58 conditions for which X-linkage is considered proved or very likely. Many of the mutations are rare, but include those causing color blindness, hemophilia, agammaglobulinemia, the Duchenne type of muscular dystrophy, glucose-6-phosphate dehydrogenase deficiency and the recently discovered Xg blood group system.

The role of the X chromosome in embryonic differentiation of the ovaries is far from clear. Rudimentary "streak" ovaries are usually present when there is an XO error or when one of two X chromosomes is deficient because of partial deletion or other structural abnormality. This correlation suggests that sex-determining genes carried by two normal X chromosomes are required as a rule for normal development of the ovaries.

In a more general sense, however, the chromosome complement must contain female-determining genes in addition to those for ovarian differentiation on the X chromosome. Testes almost always develop when the sex chromosome complex includes a Y chromosome.

The main types of sex chromosome abnormalities are (1) an abnormal number of sex chromosomes, (2) a structural abnormality of sex chromosomes and (3) a mosaicism, consisting of two or more cell populations with different sex chromosome complexes. These errors introduce deviations from the normal genetic coding that are usually reflected in abnormal development. The numerical errors, which are the

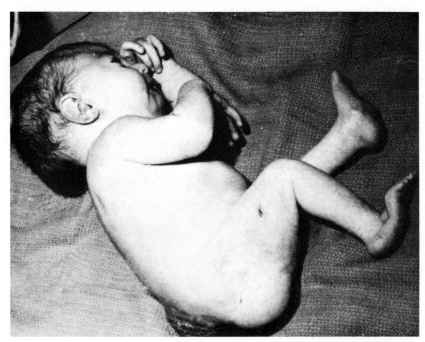

Figure 405 Lateral view of 10-day-old infant with E-trisomy syndrome, showing overlapping index finger and "rocker-bottom" convexity of the feet. Meningomyelocele, a less common coassociated defect, is also present.

most common and most straightforward, include omission of one X (Turner's syndrome, XO), triple-X or tetra-X females, XYY male phenotype and Klinefelter's syndromes (XXY, XXYY, XXXY, XXXYY and XXXXY). Various developmental defects result from structural errors, including partial deletion of X or Y, X-isochromosomes, ring-shaped X and others.

XO Errors. Turner's syndrome is the only known nonlethal instance in man of a chromosome occurring singly (monosomy). There are only 45 chromosomes in any somatic cell. The chromosome that should have been contributed by one of the parents is absent. If autosomal and YO monosomy occur in the zygote, it is probably lethal. Many XO monosomies probably do not survive early embryological life as indicated by studies of aborted specimens.

The XO abnormality (Fig. 406) (Ford et al.) occurs in 1:5000 neonates and is associated with a triad of sexual infantilism, webbing of the neck and cubitus valgus. The ovaries are represented by streaks of connective tissue (gonadal dysgenesis). The external genitals are female and the uterus and tubes are normal, although

often rather small. There is failure of breast development at puberty, unless induced by estrogen therapy.

Growth throughout childhood is usually retarded and these patients seldom attain a height in excess of 5 feet. Other abnormalities include widely spaced nipples, congenital heart defects (especially coarctation of the aorta) and renal anomalies (such as horseshoe kidney or double or cleft renal pelvis). The ears are usually prominent and the posterior hairline may come rather low down on the neck. Inner canthal folds are also sometimes seen.

One should be alerted to the possibility of the XO error in a female newborn if there are excessive looseness of the skin of the back of the neck and lymphedema of the lower extremities (Fig. 407). The looseness of the skin is gradually converted into lateral webbing of a short, thick neck, and the edema of the legs and feet subsides during the first year of life.

About one-fourth of patients with Turner's syndrome are sex chromatin-positive. Some of them have cellular mosaicism such as XO/XX or XO/XX/XXX; in others, only XX cells are demonstrable.

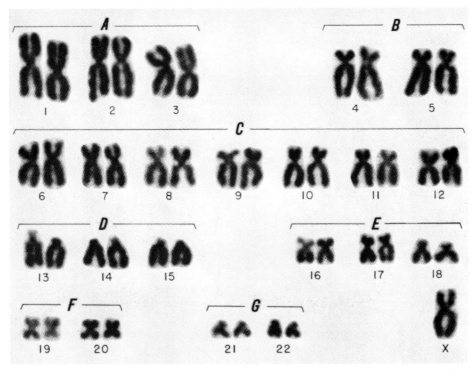

Figure 406 Karyotype of the X-monosomy, manifested by the clinical picture of Turner's syndrome. Note presence of only one X chromosome (XO).

The latter subjects may be hidden mosaics or they may be phenocopies of the XO abnormality, caused by mutant genes or nongenetic factors.

XXX Errors. Although more frequent than Turner's syndrome, XXX females are less frequently detected because the XXX error does not produce a well-defined clinical syndrome. Two of the three X chromosomes are heteropyknotic and visible as sex chromatin in many cells. They are probably relatively inert genetically. Some protection may thus be provided against trisomy of the large X chromosome, which might otherwise have a very deleterious effect on development.

Patients with X chromosome trisomy (Johnston et al.) often have normal menses and are fertile. They may have various defects, such as growth retardation, upward eye slant, patent ductus arteriosus, and be mentally retarded. Some appear to be without structural or developmental defects at all. Tetra-X and penta-X patterns occur very rarely and are associated with mental defectiveness and structural abnormalities of various kinds.

XXY Errors. The XXY abnormality is the most common of a group of complexes that are essentially intersexual because they include at least two X chromosomes and at least one Y chromosome. Klinefelter et al. first recognized the syndrome now known to be caused by the XXY sex chromosome abnormality (Jacobs and Strong) and characterized by tall stature, testicular atrophy with aspermatogenesis and gynecomastia. It results from meiotic nondisjunction.

Development during childhood is normal except that one in four of these children is mentally retarded to a varying degree. Cardinal findings in the Klinefelter syndrome include small testes, a chromatin-positive buccal smear and elevated urinary gonadotropins. The condition is one of the causes of male infertility.

A proportion of patients who satisfy the phenotypical requirements for inclusion in the Klinefelter's syndrome have chro-

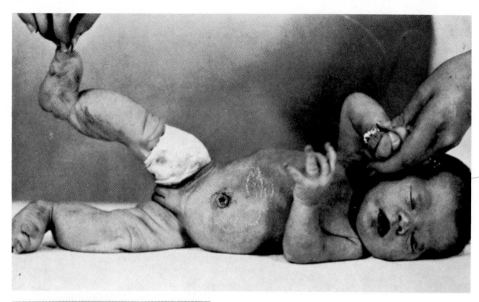

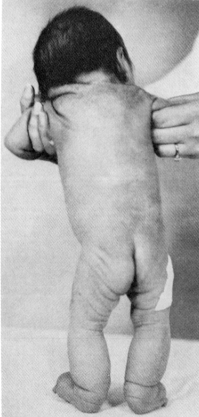

Figure 407 Neonate with Turner's syndrome, illustrating lymphedema of hands and legs, cubitus valgus, low-set hairline on back of neck, looseness of the skin in this area and the short thick neck. (From Grumbach, M. M., 1957).

matin-negative nuclei and XY sex chromosomes. Some may be concealed mosaics (for example, XY/XXY), but the etiologic factor in most of them is not known.

Structural Abnormalities. The X chromosome may show several kinds of structural abnormality, either in all cells or in one cell population of a mosaicism. The simplest abnormality involves an X chromosome with partial deletion. Phenotypic expression of the genetic defect is varied, but the patient often has features of Turner's syndrome (see above).

An X-isochromosome results from division of the centromere at the beginning of anaphase in a plane at right angles to the length of the chromosome. The daughter chromosomes then consist of homologous arms with an exactly median centromere, and one arm of the normal chromosome is missing. Several instances are on record in which patients with signs of Turner's syndrome had a normal X chromosome and an X-isochromosome consisting of duplicated long arms.

Very rarely, gonadal dysgenesis results from a complex consisting of a normal X chromosome and a ring X chromosome. The latter is produced when a break occurs near each end of the chromosome followed by union of the broken ends to form a ring. The Y chromosome varies in length in normal males, but instances of definite partial deletion of the Y chromosome are known. Partial Y deletion is likely to cause, in varying degree, defective development of the male reproductive system.

Mosaicism. Sex chromosome mosaicisms are not uncommon and should be borne in mind when the findings are atypical with respect to syndromes known to be caused by a sex chromosome abnormality. For example, typical and atypical Klinefelter subjects may show such mosaicisms as XY/XXY, XX/XXY, XY/XXXY and others that include a cell line with an intersexual sex chromosome complex.

PROGNOSIS

Prognostication after the delivery of a malformed infant is the very essence of genetic counseling. It involves applying the science of human genetics to practical problems. Some of the risk factors are summarized in Table 13 based on empirical data compiled by Anderson and Reed. The relative risks are enhanced by consanguineous marriages. Offspring of first cousins, for example, have twice the probability of having malformations as offspring of nonrelatives (Reed). Recessively inherited diseases, including phenylketonuria, alkaptonuria, Wilson's disease, xeroderma pigmentosum and familial cretinism, are more common in children of cousins (Motulsky).

Special consideration is given to diagnosis of the underlying defect in Down's syndrome. If it can be shown that the affected baby has merely a trisomy 21, the prognosis for future pregnancy is no different from that of any other woman. On the other hand, diagnosis of a translocation error carries a much more serious outlook. It implies that one of the parents is a translocation carrier, with a probability of having another infant with Down's syndrome rising to 25 to 33 per cent. For the concerned gravida over age 40 or one who has already delivered an affected baby, culture and karyotyping of desquamated fetal cells in amniotic fluid is feasible (see Chapter 13) and can give valuable information.

Since most trisomy 13 and 18 cases die *in utero* and are aborted, the recurrence risks are small. Spontaneous abortion does not carry the same sociologic or emotional hazards as delivery of a viable anomalous infant. However, it is also important to try to uncover translocation carriers among the parents because the risks of repeating in subsequent pregnancies are so much greater. Inherited translocations have also been reported in the *cri du chat* syndrome.

Knowledge concerning the genetic potentiality of a given malformation is essential, particularly as to whether it is heritable and, if inherited, whether as a recessive or a dominant trait. A detailed family history may be helpful in this regard, particularly when it is necessary to distinguish a known heritable disorder from one that is an acquired phenocopy (for example, hydrocephalus). With ever-increasing availability of intrauterine diag-

TABLE 13   INCIDENCE AND PROGNOSTIC RISK AFTER BIRTH OF A MALFORMED INFANT*

	Incidence in Population	Risk Figure in Later Siblings
All malformations	1 in 65	1 in 20
Central nervous system malformations (35%)		
Anencephaly	1 in 450 ⎫	1 in 50 ⎫
Spina bifida	1 in 375 ⎬ 1 in 200	1 in 25 ⎬ 1 in 22
Hydrocephalus	1 in 550 ⎭	1 in 60 ⎭
Mongolism	1 in 600	1 in 20
Muscular-skeletal malformations (25%)		
Harelip with or without cleft palate	1 in 1000	1 in 7
Cleft palate alone	1 in 2500	1 in 7
Polydactylia	1 in 1200	1 in 2
Syndactylia	1 in 2000	1 in 2
Clubfoot	1 in 1000	1 in 30
Malformed arms, hands	1 in 5000	
Achondroplasia	1 in 7000	
Congenital hip dislocation	1 in 1500	1 in 20
Cardiovascular malformations (20%)		
All congenital hearts	1 in 200	1 in 50
Patent ductus arteriosus	1 in 2500	1 in 50
Genitourinary malformations (6%)		
Hypospadias	1 in 1000	1 in 50 (?)
Polycystic kidney (infant)	1 in 15,000	1 in 4
Gastrointestinal malformations (3%)		
Exomphalos	1 in 4000	less than 1 in 100
Diaphragmatic hernia	1 in 10,000	
Tracheoesophageal fistula	1 in 6000	less than 1 in 100
Atresia ani	1 in 5000	less than 1 in 100
Multiple malformations (11%)		
Miscellaneous		
Pyloric stenosis	1 in 350	1 in 17

*From Anderson, R. C., and Reed, S. C., 1954.

nosis (see Chapter 13) and the wherewithal to terminate unwanted pregnancies bearing malformed fetuses (see Chapter 35), the issue is no longer academic, but is, instead, of considerable practical importance. Much valuable information for diagnosis and counseling can be obtained from regional centers equipped for these purposes.*

*Contact National Foundation, 800 Second Avenue, New York, New York 10017, to obtain information concerning relevant centers.

REFERENCES

Anderson, R. C., and Reed, S. C.: Likelihood of recurrence of congenital malformations. J. Lancet 74:175, 1954.

Collmann, R. D., and Stoller, A.: A survey of mongoloid births in Victoria. Amer. J. Public Health 52: 813, 1962.

Edwards, J. H., Harnden, D. G., Cameron, A. H., Crosse, V. M., and Wolff, O. H.: A new trisomic syndrome. Lancet 1:787, 1960.

Ford, C. E., Jones, K. W., Polani, P. E., de Almeida, J.

C., and Briggs, J. H.: A sex-chromosome anomaly in a case of gonadal dysgenesis (Turner's syndrome). Lancet 1:711, 1959.

Fraser, F. C., and Fainstat, T. D.: Causes of congenital defects: A review. Amer. J. Dis. Child. 82:593, 1951.

German, J., Lejeune, J., MacIntyre, M. N., and De Grouchy, J.: Chromosomal autoradiography in the cri-du-chat syndrome. Cytogenetics 3:347, 1964.

Jacobs, P., and Strong, D. A.: A case of human intersexuality having a possible XXY sex-determining mechanism. Nature *183*:302, 1959.

Johnston, A. W., Ferguson-Smith, M. A., Handmaker, S. D., Jones, H. W., and Jones, G. S.: The triple-X syndrome. Clinical, pathological and chromosomal studies in three mentally retarded cases. Brit. Med. J. *2*:1046, 1961.

Klinefelter, H. F., Jr., Reifenstein, E. C., Jr., and Albright, F.: Syndrome characterized by gynecomastia, aspermatogenesis with a-Leydigism, and increased excretion of follicle-stimulating hormone. J. Clin. Endocr. *2*:615, 1942.

LeJeune, J., Turpin, R., and Gautier, M.: Études des chromosomes somatiques de neuf enfants mongoliens. Compt. Rend. Acad. Sci. *248*:1721, 1959.

Lilienfeld, A. M.: Epidemiology of Mongolism. Baltimore, Johns Hopkins Press, 1969.

Lyon, M. F.: Sex-chromatin and gene action in the mammalian X-chromosome. Amer. J. Hum. Genet. *14*:135, 1962.

McIntosh, R., Merritt, K. K., Richards, M. R., Samuels, M. H., and Bellows, M. T.: The incidence of congenital malformations: A study of 5,964 pregnancies. Pediatrics *14*:505, 1954.

McKusick, V. A.: On the X chromosome of man. Quart. Rev. Biol. *37*:69, 1962.

Monif, G. R. G.: Viral Infections of the Human Fetus. London, Macmillan Company, 1969.

Motulsky, A. G.: Children of marriages between first cousins. J.A.M.A. *187*:244, 1964.

Patau, K., Smith, D. W., Therman, E., Inhorn, S. L., and Wagner, H. P.: Multiple congenital anomaly caused by an extra chromosome. Lancet *1*:790, 1960.

Smith, D. W.: Recognizable Patterns of Human Malformation: Genetic, Embryologic, and Clinical Aspects. Philadelphia, W. B. Saunders Company, 1970.

SECTION SIX

PATHOLOGY OF THE PUERPERIUM

Chapter 70

Puerperal Infection

The term *puerperal infection* includes all the inflammatory processes which arise from bacterial invasion of the genital organs during labor or the puerperium. Other terms for this condition are *puerperal sepsis, puerperal septicemia, puerperal fever* and *childbed fever.* The introduction of antibiotics has unfortunately made some physicians cavalier in their attitudes toward prevention and treatment of puerperal infection, once the most dreaded of parturitional complications. Resistant organisms develop; patients become sensitized to antibiotics or have adverse effects from them; puerperal infection becomes difficult to manage. Puerperal infection must still be considered to be potentially a most serious, even sometimes fatal, problem (Jewett et al.). It accounts for 20 per cent of maternal deaths.

Febrile morbidity has been defined uniformly on the basis of temperature elevations to 38° C. (100.4° F.) or more occurring on any two of the first ten days post partum, exclusive of the first 24 hours (that is, from day 2 through day 11 after delivery). The patient's temperature should be taken by mouth by a standard technique at least four times daily. British standards are somewhat more stringent (Browne), using 100° F. instead.

ETIOLOGY

The pathologic process in puerperal infection is the same acute suppurative inflammation seen in other surgical infections. Because of the special susceptibility of the recently gravid uterus and other genital organs and tissues, secondary to the anatomic and physiologic changes of pregnancy, labor and the puerperium, important variations exist which demand special consideration.

The bacteria most often found to cause puerperal infection are anaerobic streptococci and enterococci. In addition, beta-hemolytic streptococci (chiefly Lancefield Groups A, C and G), alpha-hemolytic streptococci and staphylococci may be the offenders. On rare occasions, other organisms may be causative, including Clostridia, Klebsiella, Pseudomonas and even Neisseria. Mixed flora are common.

The history of the quest to understand the modes of transmission of infection to the genital tract, dating from the times of Holmes and Semmelweis, is a saga which every person who cares for obstetric patients should read. Only in this way can we ensure that the tragic errors of the past will not be repeated. Of particular importance in this regard is the physician's own role in introducing infection.

Autoinfection

Autoinfection is the term applied to infection arising from endogenous pathogenic organisms already present in the generative tract or elsewhere in the patient. There are three sources of autoinfection: (1) from bacteria in the genital tract; (2) from a distant site of suppuration by hematogenous spread; and (3) from contiguous disease, for example, appendiceal abscess.

Conditions favoring autoinfection are excessive bruising of the tissues from prolonged labor, traumatic delivery manipulation and instrumentation and retention of pieces of placenta, membranes and blood clots in the uterus. Exhaustion and hemorrhage, when superimposed on trauma, are classically associated with the development of puerperal infection. Severe anemia, debilitation, malnutrition and some chronic illnesses enhance susceptibility. Autoinfections tend to be relatively mild. Fatalities are rare.

Heteroinfection

External or exogenous sources of infection are by far the most common and should always be considered first when fever develops in a puerpera. Infection may be introduced into the genital tract from the outside in many ways. It is essential that all who attend parturients and puerperas be keenly aware of these.

1. Most often it is the physician or other attendant medical or nursing personnel who infect the woman. Virulent bacteria from the physician's nasopharynx or fingers or from an instrument insufficiently sterilized or subsequently contaminated may be introduced into the genitals. These bacteria may have been brought from another patient who is infected. The physician himself or other hospital personnel may have an acute infection or harbor pathogens which are carried without overt manifestations. Of special concern here is the individual who is the unwary carrier of streptococci in his upper respiratory tract. He disseminates these potentially virulent organisms directly to the patient or into the air for further spread by coughing, sneezing or even just talking. The usual surgical face mask is not effective in preventing the spread of germ-laden droplets of saliva and mucus.

2. The environment has much to do with puerperal infection. Many puerperal infections are caused by the bacteria-laden dust in the air of hospitals and other places where births occur. Bacteria from puerperal women, from the dried pus of suppurations, from the autopsy room, the pathology laboratory and from the innumerable sources of infection of a general hospital gain access to air and dust, in droplets and droplet nuclei, and are carried by air currents in ventilating ducts or free to all parts of an institution, including the delivery rooms. The infectious material settles on sterilized tables, towels, hand solutions, bedclothes and the vulva. From these loci the bacteria are carried into the vagina by properly scrubbed and gloved fingers and by instruments, sponges and sutures.

3. The patient's marital partner may be a source of infection. He may infect her with gonorrhea or syphilis at the time of conception or during pregnancy. Intercourse near term is generally not considered to be an important factor (see Chapter 9), but it is interdicted once the membranes have ruptured.

4. The patient herself may carry infection on her fingers from a distant area to the genitals.

Intrapartum Infection

Uterine infection during labor may be carried over from pregnancy; it may result from prolonged labor, instrumental interference, a nearby focus of infection, such as appendicitis or pyelonephritis, or it may arise at a distance from the pelvic organs. Bacteria usually invade the uterus if the membranes have been ruptured a long time. Infections dormant or arising in labor are an important cause of puerperal infection.

During labor, the clinical manifestations of infection are the same as at any other time. Fever is the most common objective sign and is usually coassociated with tachycardia and leukocytosis. The fetus is endangered because it, too, may become infected. Fetal tachycardia may be an indicator of intrapartum infection, alerting the physician to its presence.

In advanced cases, the amniotic fluid is discolored and malodorous, depending on the kind of bacteria present, and the introitus and cervix may be covered with a grayish exudate. Pus may escape from the genitals. When fever begins, contractions are usually strengthened.

The differential diagnosis of the cause of the fever must be made to rule out dehydration and other focal or generalized infections. A stained smear of cervical discharge is sometimes helpful in pinpointing the infection to the uterus. One can be reasonably certain if the smear shows many bacteria and leukopedesis. If the membranes are intact, one may obtain a sample of amniotic fluid for study by transabdominal amniocentesis (see Chapter 52). Cultures are essential.

The prognosis for the mother and the fetus depends on the type of bacteria, the time when the infection began, the complicating conditions and the rapidity, ease and safety with which the labor can be terminated.

When infection develops in delayed labor, treatment will depend on the cause of the delay. In the absence of special indications, expectancy gives the best results. It is wiser to await spontaneous termination, at least until the head comes down onto the perineum, intervening only when absolutely necessary. One must exercise extreme care not to tear or bruise the parturient tract by overstimulation in labor or instrumentation at delivery. A chill with a sharp rise of temperature often follows operative intervention, but the fever usually subsides in several hours.

Cesarean section is indicated for the acute infection only if it is clear that vaginal delivery will not occur within a reasonable time, say 8 to 12 hours, or the infection is so fulminating that any delay in evacuating the uterus and establishing drainage is unthinkable. There no longer seems to be any rationale for use of extraperitoneal techniques of cesarean sections.

With the wide availability and use of effective antibiotics, the conduct of labor in the presence of fever is much less fearsome than it was formerly, but these drugs should not lull the physician into taking undue risks. The third stage requires as much consideration as the delivery. Manual exploration is essential. It must be ascertained that there are no perforating injuries in the genital tract; neglect of this can be fatal. A rupture demands hysterectomy, but lesser lacerations are left wide open for drainage after hemostasis is secured. Hemorrhage is stopped by suture ligation.

TYPES OF PUERPERAL INFECTION

At present, because of the early and even prophylactic use of antibiotics, the clinical picture of puerperal infection has changed considerably. Many patients are cured with medication before an accurate diagnosis is made. Nevertheless, whenever possible, an attempt should be made to determine the exact type of infection present by means of appropriate bacteriologic studies.

Vulvitis

The causes of vulvar infection are trauma and infection during labor. After operative deliveries, there is some contusion of the tissue, as well as small wounds and abrasions. These wounds may be covered with grayish or greenish exudate. Even superficial ulceration may occur. If the perineorrhaphy wound becomes infected, the tissues are swollen and have a brawny exudate. The edges are red and their line of apposition is separated by pus. Sloughing tissue with serum and pus oozes out of the suture holes until the wound opens spontaneously or is drained.

If drainage is free, there are no pronounced symptoms. The patient complains of some inability to urinate, pain and discomfort from the swelling and a sense of local heat. The temperature is seldom above 38.3° C. (101° F.). If sutures prevent the exit of the infected exudations or if the infective agent is a virulent streptococcus, chills and fever may usher in the disease. Treatment requires removal of the sutures to effect optimal drainage. Soaking the area by having the patient sit in a tub of hot water several times a day is also useful.

Vaginitis

Prolonged labor, frequent examinations, bruising from inept operating and laceration by obstetric forceps favor infection by producing conditions which cause the tissues to become less resistant to the bacteria normally present in the vagina. A gauze sponge inadvertently left in the vagina at delivery may be causative also.

The symptoms are more severe than those of vulvitis, especially if the bacteria are more virulent. If drainage is free, the general reaction is usually mild; if the discharges are retained, severe symptoms become manifest in the form of chills, high fever, pelvic pain, urinary retention and dysuria.

Endometritis

Few puerperal infections occur without involvement of the endometrium. The cervix and the endometrium are the ports of entry to the parametrium, the myometrium, the uterine tubes, the peritoneum and the blood.

The lochia may be retained if the uterus becomes acutely flexed on itself at the cervix or the cervix is obstructed by clots or retained placental or membrane fragments. This condition is called *lochiometra*. It usually causes a severe chill and fever which disappear quickly if the cause is removed by free drainage.

For the first two or three days the puerpera is fairly well, but careful observation will disclose nonspecific indications of trouble, such as slight malaise and prolonged afterpains or their recurrence after they had subsided. On the third, fourth or fifth day, the temperature climbs and all the usual febrile symptoms develop. The pulse is between 100 and 140 per minute and the temperature 38.3 to 40° C. (101 to 104° F.), depending on the severity of the infection. The abdomen is perhaps a trifle

distended; the uterus is usually larger than it should be and softer than normal. The lochial discharge at first is unaltered, but within 48 hours it becomes serous or seropurulent.

Unless the infection is virulent, the temperature subsides by lysis, the pulse slows down and in 6 to 10 days recovery is nearly complete.

Salpingitis and Oophoritis

Rarely, an infection spreads from the uterine cavity into the tubes to produce *salpingitis* and even beyond to the ovaries to produce *oophoritis*. Abscesses may form in the tubes or in the ovaries. A mild salpingitis after delivery may pass unnoticed and be responsible for one-child sterility.

Manifestations may be nonexistent clinically or there may be a full-blown picture of acute salpingo-oophoritis with abscess formation, exactly analogous to acute pelvic inflammatory disease as it occurs in the nongravid state. Unilateral or, more often, bilateral lower quadrant abdominal pain with signs of pelvic peritonitis is encountered, associated with high spiking fever (see below).

Pelvic Cellulitis

Pelvic cellulitis (often inappropriately called *parametritis*) is caused by bacteria which gain entrance to the connective tissue. Generally, the atrium of infection is a wound of the cervix or lower uterine segment, but the site of injury may have been in the vagina or even the perineum.

Symptoms usually begin on the third or fourth day, but may start as late as the ninth day. Nearly always the symptoms of endometritis precede those of pelvic cellulitis. They include chills, high fever, tachycardia and severe local pain. The fever is at first characteristically continuous; later, if pus has formed, it may be intermittent. Repeated chills then occur and sweats accompany the defervescence. The patient may die of exhaustion unless drainage is established and the pus is evacuated. The symptoms disappear rapidly after the abscesses are drained.

Early, the large, soft, sensitive uterus of infection and subinvolution will be found. At either side, deep in the flanks, there is pronounced tenderness on pressure. The whole pelvis is hot and soft, with one exquisitely sensitive spot, usually in the lateral fornix, and an ill-defined thickening may be present in this area.

If suppuration occurs in the mass, the numerous tiny abscesses fuse into a large one, palpable to the finger. It may begin to point. Vaginally, the soft abscess may be felt bulging down one of the fornices or it may be felt better through the rectum. Abdominally, the tumor causes a prominence above one or the other of Poupart's ligaments, the skin becomes slightly edematous and red, the tissues break down over the abscess and the pus escapes externally. If resorption occurs, the tumor hardens and shrinks, at first rapidly, later slowly. Three to twelve weeks are required for its resolution.

If symptoms of irregular fever, chills and emaciation suggest suppuration in the mass or if fluctuation is demonstrated, the abscess is to be opened. Abscesses of the broad ligament should be opened just above Poupart's ligament, extraperitoneally. If an abscess bulges in the posterior culdesac, it is opened there. If the abscess bulges into one of the lateral fornices, it should be opened as near the midline as possible to avoid injuring the ureter or uterine vessels. Prolonged expectancy is required, since pelvic cellulitis usually heals by absorption.

Peritonitis

Pelvic peritonitis accompanies many forms of local puerperal infections, such as cellulitis, endometritis and salpingitis. Both local and general signs and symptoms depend on the manner in which the infection reaches the peritoneum.

Rupture of an abscess is almost always attended by serious and stormy symptoms. They resemble the symptoms of ruptured ectopic pregnancy, including sharp, severe pain at the site of the abscess, tenderness and collapse, followed by fever and evidences of rapidly spreading peritonitis. Vomiting is almost always a constant occurrence, and paralytic ileus leads to immense abdominal distention. Later, foul diarrhea is observed. Thirst is excessive, restlessness is distressing, but usually the mind is clear until near the end when delirium or coma supervenes, or a paradoxical state of well-being begins. This is ominous.

The patient lies on her back, with her knees drawn up to relax the abdominal muscles and to support the weight of the bedclothes. Her expression is anxious and her coloring is at first reddened, later pale and gray or subicteric. The face at first presents a febrile aspect, but later this is replaced by one of collapse, with sunken eyes, a cold, pointed nose and a cool forehead covered with clammy sweat. In short, this is the typical *facies Hippocratica*. The tongue soon becomes dry and brown, and the breath is foul. The urinary output is sharply reduced in amount and contains albumin, casts, indican and often the causative bacteria. The temperature during and after the usual initial chill is often as high as 40.6° C. (105° F.); the pulse becomes rapid. Respiration is rapid and costal.

The abdomen is tympanitic over its lower part at first and, as the infection spreads, it may be immensely distended. The walls are usually rigid and exquisitely tender. If the infection is virulent, the symptoms become worse rapidly; the temperature remains high until shortly before death (when it drops); the pulse mounts in frequency (the two curves cross on the chart); collapse follows and pulmonary edema or exhaustion precedes death.

If the infection begins as an acute puerperal peritonitis, antibiotics must be administered without delay (see below). Of course, these drugs should be given when any infection is evident, and the earlier the better. The drug of choice is substituted after the results of the culture and sensitivity tests are available. The use of these drugs has so radically changed the treatment of puerperal infection that serious infections are seldom fatal any longer.

When there is localization, one must drain and culture the abscess that forms. The vagina is exposed with a short, broad speculum; the cervix is steadied, but not pulled down with a vulsellum; a needle is gently inserted into the culdesac to be sure that pus is present and to indicate the site

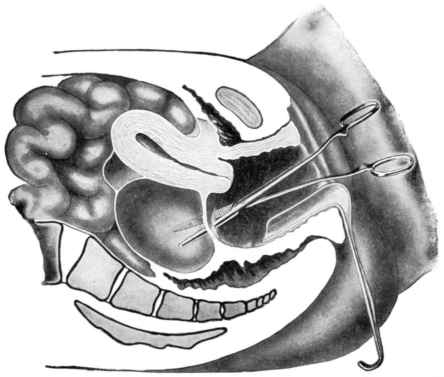

Figure 408 Draining the pelvic abscess vaginally. First, the culdesac is aspirated as in Figure 230, leaving the needle in place. Then, following alongside the needle with a scalpel or sharp-pointed scissors, the abscess cavity is perforated gently and the opening is enlarged by spreading the jaws of a clamp as shown here. Observe how easily the roof of the sac might be traumatized to discharge pus into the peritoneal cavity.

for drainage. After pus is aspirated, the posterior fornix and culdesac are cut gently with a sharp knife or sharp-pointed scissors. The opening is enlarged by stretching with an artery clamp (Fig. 408). The sac must not be punched into because delicate adhesions in the roof of the abscess may give way and pus will escape into the peritoneal cavity.

After the pus is cultured and evacuated, one finger may be passed into the cavity to find other loculations of abscesses. If any are found, they should be drained through the same opening. A rubber drainage tube should be left in place. Drainage usually persists for many weeks. Irrigations are unnecessary and may be harmful.

Bacteremia

This is an acute infectious disease resulting from the entrance into the blood of bacteria, usually streptococci, and their toxins which cause dissolution of the blood, degenerative changes in the organs and the symptoms of rapid intoxication. Most often the Group A beta-hemolytic streptococcus is the cause. Different clinical pictures are produced, depending on the mode of invasion.

The lymphatic form of bacteremia usually develops from an endometritis; the bacteria pass along the lymph spaces of the uterus and broad ligaments into the blood or out onto the surface of the peritoneum. The vascular form of bacteremia begins as a phlebitis, usually in uterine veins and venous sinuses at the placental site, with thrombus formation. From these infected thrombi, bacteria reach the blood and spread to distant organs, such as the lungs, the brain, the joints and the valves of the heart. Thus, a true bacteremia develops. *Metastatic abscesses* may also arise by embolization of bits of infected thrombi in foci of *septic thrombophlebitis* arising by contiguity in pelvic veins draining the infected uterus (see below).

An incubation period of one to three

days usually precedes the outbreak of the severe symptoms. Ordinarily, the prodromal stage is manifested by the signs and symptoms of the local process at the site where the bacteria gained access to the blood.

A severe chill ushers in the infection. The skin is pale and the lips and fingers are cyanotic. The temperature rises rapidly to 39.4 or 40° C. (103 or 104° F.) and the pulse increases rapidly to above 120 per minute. The patient is pallid and respiration is rapid.

Symptoms of peritonitis start early and if medication is not effective, the Hippocratic facies shows that the fatal termination is not distant. The lochial discharge is usually profuse, pungent and putrid. The puerperal wounds become necrotic. If the patient lives, the picture becomes one of virulent peritonitis.

The disease lasts from 2 to 10 days. It is especially virulent if it begins during labor and then its course is usually short and violent. A marbling of the skin, which shows the course of the superficial veins, is a bad omen because it indicates general hemolysis. Examination of the blood reveals the streptococcus or other organism, especially if the bacteremia is of vascular origin.

Thrombophlebitis

Acute inflammatory involvement of the veins of the pelvis and the legs is a very serious sequel of puerperal infection and a common route of spread. It demands astuteness for diagnosis, especially when one is dealing with a patient whose septic postpartum course is unresponsive to aggressive antibiotic therapy. The silence of the pelvic manifestations in terms of objective findings is well recognized.

The clinical picture and management of lower extremity thrombophlebitis occurring during pregnancy are discussed in Chapter 27. The principles are the same in the puerperium and will not be repeated. We will deal here only with the more serious problem of septic or suppurative thrombophlebitis as a special aspect of puerperal infection.

In *suppurative thrombophlebitis* the myometrial and parametrial venous plexuses are infected with pyogenic organisms. The infected thrombi may remain localized or extend by propagation through the uterine veins into the hypogastric and iliac veins or via the ovarian veins to the left renal vein or the vena cava. Liquefaction of the thrombus frequently takes place, and small mycotic emboli may be released. These may lodge in the lungs and cause infarctions, abscesses, pneumonia and pleurisy. They may also occasionally pass into the systemic circulation. Multiple pyemic abscesses may develop, especially in the lungs and the kidneys. Heart valves may be secondarily involved also, particularly if they are already damaged by a preexisting cardiopathy.

The clinical picture is one of severe general infection with localizing signs pointing to the pelvis as the source. Fever and chills may be severe. Positive blood cultures and, occasionally, roentgenographic evidence of widespread pulmonary involvement help to establish the diagnosis. Most patients respond to massive doses of appropriate antibiotics, anticoagulant therapy and general care. Ligation of the involved pelvic veins or even the inferior vena cava (Collins et al.) may be necessary in a small percentage of patients (see Chapter 27).

TREATMENT OF PUERPERAL INFECTION

Prevention plays the transcendentally important role in puerperal infection. Much can be done during pregnancy to get the woman into perfect condition for labor. Preexisting infection and anemia should receive appropriate treatment. The gravida should not expose herself to contagious diseases.

General resistance against infection is strengthened by good health and antepartum care. During labor, the physician must preserve the woman's forces by having her get sufficient sleep, rest and liquids. Infection may follow a protracted labor, particularly one in which exhaustion and acidosis combine to reduce resistance. Bleeding should be prevented during labor.

Puerperal wounds should be minimized or averted. It is good obstetrics to avoid trauma to tissues. Stringent attention to the details of sterile technique is essential at all times.

The third stage should be conducted as physiologically as possible. Intervention should be instituted only on strict indication. Manual removal of the placenta should be reserved primarily for occasions when bleeding occurs or there is a delay in expulsion. Great care is exerted to obtain the complete placenta and all the membranes. The uterus should not be bruised by Credé expression of the placenta or too forcible massage.

After every operative delivery, breech delivery and in all patients who have had rapid dilatation of the cervix, the whole uterovaginal tract should be examined for lacerations. All lacerations of the perineum should be repaired. Many infections originate in perineal wounds.

Everything that will improve the woman's general health will help her combat the disease. Sleep is a prime necessity. The sick woman should be isolated to prevent spread of infection and to ensure quiet for her. Visitors are excluded. Nursing the child is stopped.

If the patient vomits, food by mouth is withheld and appropriate fluid and electrolytes are given intravenously every day. Attention to details of fluid balance is important at all times. Blood transfusion may also be given, if needed, to combat anemia due to acute blood loss at delivery.

Specific treatment consists of antibiotics. They should be chosen for the offending organisms, if possible, and given in adequate amounts. They are not a panacea, however. Therefore, the utmost in maintaining the strictest possible aseptic techniques must be observed.

The great number of antibiotic and chemotherapeutic drugs available today offers the physician a remarkable choice in selecting a drug to combat a specific infection. The intelligent choice of an agent requires exact knowledge of the nature of the invading organisms. Bacteria vary widely in their response to these drugs and failure to effect a cure may be due to organism resistance or to improperly prescribed therapy. Specimens of blood, tissue, pus and discharges must be obtained for culture and sensitivity tests before therapy is begun, since isolation of bacteria is difficult once antibacterial treatment has been instituted. However, it is not advisable to await the results of these tests before starting treatment. A Gram stain may be most helpful in identifying the offending organism.

If, after several days of therapy, there is no improvement, results of the cultures and sensitivity tests will be available and the medication can then be changed to a drug specific for the isolated organism. In addition, sensitivity tests may be used as a guide to proper dosage of the drug used. Although clinical response and *in vitro* sensitivity tests are not always closely correlated, the results are sufficiently consistent to recommend use of these tests, thus avoiding dangerous trial and error methods.

As resistant strains of organisms arise and new antibiotics are introduced, recommendations for management change. This holds true especially for initial administration of drugs for an infection before the reports of the cultures are available. Combinations of penicillin and streptomycin or tetracycline have been used effectively for years to combat puerperal infection due to a wide range of the common causative organisms. If the patient is not responsive to this regimen, kanamycin or gentamicin may be substituted for the tetracycline. However, by this time the bacteriologic results of the sensitivity studies should be available so that the specific antibiotic to which the organism is known to be sensitive *in vitro* can be given.

The patient who is still unresponsive to specific antibiotic therapy given in suitable amounts must be considered to have septic thrombophlebitis or abscess formation or both. Intensive search for the pus collection should be initiated, using all laboratory and clinical measures possible. If none is found, although it is possible that an abscess has been overlooked, the diagnosis of pelvic thrombophlebitis must be entertained and anticoagulant therapy started. This diagnosis is often made by exclusion unless pulmonary embolization has occurred. Defervescence may occur within two to three days after treatment is begun.

There is general agreement regarding surgical drainage procedures for the treatment of localized suppurations, such as pelvic abscess, pyosalpinx, ovarian abscess, uterine abscess and necrotic leiomyomas. When the diagnosis is clear, drainage must be instituted.

Hysterectomy, on the other hand, is more difficult to justify. The main problem lies in assessing the indication for this operation. If the local lesion in the uterus is the predominant factor, hysterectomy is justified. Such local conditions include infection associated with (1) rupture of the uterus, (2) a degenerated leiomyoma, (3) coexistent cancer of the uterus, (4) hydatidiform mole, (5) placenta accreta, (6) myometrial abscess, (7) gangrene of the uterus and (8) an inverted or prolapsed uterus. In general it is best to avoid the added operative trauma and blood loss of such surgery unless it is clearly indicated and cannot be postponed.

REFERENCES

Browne, F. J.: Standards in obstetrics: A plea for uniform standards in maternity statistics and hospital reports. J. Obstet. Gynaec. Brit. Emp. 65:826, 1958.

Collins, C. G., Nelson, E. W., Ray, C. T., Weinstein, B. B., and Collins, J. H.: Ligation of the vena cava and ovarian vessels: A follow-up study of 59 cases. Amer. J. Obstet. Gynec. 58:1155, 1949.

Holmes, O. W.: Puerperal Fever as a Private Pestilence. Boston, Ticknor & Fields, 1855.

Jewett, J. F., Reid, D. E., Safon, L. E., and Easterday, C. L.: Childbed fever: A continuing entity. J.A.M.A. 206:344, 1968.

Semmelweis, I. P.: Die Aetiologie, der Begriff und die Prophylaxis des Kinderbettfiebers. Vienna, C. A. Hartleben, 1861.

Chapter 71

Diseases of the Breast

DISORDERS OF FUNCTION

Engorgement

Simple breast engorgement is common. It occurs on the third or fourth day after delivery. It is due to the venous and lymphatic distention that precedes lactation. It may occur also when acutely weaning the child because the usual relief produced by nursing is absent.

The breasts are very heavy, painful and hot, but there is no rise of body temperature. One should not ascribe a febrile reaction to the fictional entity "milk fever." Fever at such a time is usually the result of infection. Examination shows the breasts to be enlarged, tender, very warm to the touch, hard, bluish and mottled. The nipple is flattened and the secretion of milk may cease because tissue engorgement occludes the lactiferous ducts. When the part of the mammary gland coursing up into the axilla becomes congested, the patient cannot bring her arm to the side.

If left alone, the engorgement disappears gradually, the glands become soft and the milk flows readily when the child nurses. A tight breast binder is applied and supplemented by ice bags and mild analgesic agents for the pain.

Galactorrhea

The continuous flow of a milklike secretion from the breasts, irrespective of nursing and persisting after weaning, is called *galactorrhea*. A comparable disorder occurs in the nonpuerperal patient in association with amenorrhea. It is rare and in-

tractable. The cause is most likely a pituitary or hypothalamic dysfunction. Its true nature may soon be elucidated now that a reliable assay for prolactin is available. It is associated with low estrogen levels and diminished follicle-stimulating hormone.

In some patients persistent abnormal or erogenous stimulation of the breasts may be responsible. It may be unilateral or bilateral, stopping for a few days or weeks, to recur again; it may follow abortions or full-term labors. It may be slight or profuse. Primary therapy is compression of the breasts with a binder. Effective treatment with clomiphene has recently been described (Mass).

Abnormal Milk

Illness of the mother may affect the quality and quantity of the milk. Bacteria circulating in the maternal blood may be excreted in the milk. The infant may be infected from the bacteria thus swallowed or from the organisms contained in pus which escapes from a mammary abscess. However, women with septic infections have nursed their babies without apparent problems. Many drugs administered to the mother pass to the child by way of the milk. Nicotine is excreted in the milk, but lactation is little affected by moderate smoking.

Agalactia or Failing Lactation

A common complaint of nursing mothers is scarcity of milk. The causes are ill health, malformations or diseases of the nipples which render nursing impossible

739

or too painful, occlusion of the milk ducts, atrophy of the glandular tissue with aging, destruction of gland tissue from mastitis, insufficient stimulation of the breast by a child with poor sucking reflex, congenital insufficiency of gland tissue and febrile disorders. Emotional states, such as worry, fright, pain and anger, reduce or temporarily stop the flow; menstruation rarely reduces it. A pleasant, cheerful environment with much interpersonal encouragement, especially from nursing personnel, is particularly conducive to good milk production.

A large breast does not mean a good supply of milk; it may be made up mainly of fat with little gland tissue. Small breasts made up mostly of active mammary gland tissue usually yield sufficient milk. Principles of care of the puerperal breast are outlined in Chapter 26.

The symptoms of deficient milk supply are (1) distress and weight loss of the child and (2) absence of secretion. The child is dissatisfied with the nipple; he may suck for a short while but, finding nothing there, will refuse it and cry. Absence or insufficiency of milk is proved if the child's weight is the same before and after nursing or only slightly greater.

Caked Breast

So-called caked breast is a local engorgement affecting one or more lobules or lobes. It sometimes results from occlusion of the lactiferous ducts, but may be due to a simple congestion from an injury that may have antedated the gestation. A lump made up of hard, irregular masses of gland tissue may be present. The breast is sensitive to the touch, but there is no inflammation or any general reaction. Caked breast does not usually lead to mastitis (see below). The possibility of carcinoma, although remote, should be considered and in doubtful instances a biopsy should be obtained and examined microscopically. Mammography may be helpful in the differential diagnosis. The patient should be instructed to leave the breasts alone, and not to attempt to massage the lumps away.

NIPPLE FISSURES

Sore nipples are a frequent complication of the first weeks of nursing. They are exceedingly painful, may prevent lactation and may lead to infection of the breasts, resulting in an abscess. Primiparas suffer from sore nipples more often than multiparas; fair-skinned women, older women and those whose nipples are retracted or deformed are especially prone. If the nipple is flat or inverted, the child will be unable to take hold of it. If efforts at nursing are persisted in too long, cracks and fissures occur; infection may be introduced and an abscess result.

The conditions favoring sore nipples are erosions, blisters, cracks or fissures and ulcerations. Erosions are caused by maceration of the thin epithelium and the sucking of the infant. If the skin cracks, a little blood pours out; it hardens to a scab under which a droplet of pus sometimes is found. Cracks are either circular or vertical. Circular cracks are usually at the base of the nipple, at its junction with the areola, and if the ulceration is deep, the nipple may be partly amputated. Vertical cracks may split the nipple in two. Bacteria are always present on and in sore nipples and may cause illness in the baby. If the cracks bleed, the child may swallow blood, which reappears in the stools and thereby produces a false melena.

For the treatment of nipple pain and nipple damage, a nipple shield and topical ointments are useful. The child should not nurse from the affected breast if such measures are not promptly effective. Harsh soaps should be avoided to minimize local trauma and soreness. The nipple should be kept dry and exposed to the air to promote healing.

MASTITIS

Inflammation of the breast occurs almost exclusively in nursing women, and is seen especially in primiparas. The bacteria most often found in mastitis are coagulase-positive *Staphylococcus aureus*. Much less commonly, one encounters *Staphylo-*

coccus albus, Streptococcus pyogenes, Escherichia coli, pneumonococcus, gonococcus, *Candida albicans* and blastomyces. These microorganisms are brought to the breasts by the hands of the attendants or by the mother, in whom the usual source is the lochia. Special hand care with antiseptic soap is mandatory for all personnel who handle babies and puerperas (Plueckhahn and Banks). The child may also be the source of infection.

When the breast is injured, bacteria invade it. It is possible for organisms to gain access via the blood. This is probably the most common way for mastitis and mammary abscesses to arise. During epidemics of influenza, there is a definite increase of mammary infection. While cracks and fissures are usually emphasized as causes of mastitis, in actuality cracks of the nipples are infrequent with mastitis or mammary abscess.

The infection (Fig. 409) may be limited at first to the areola outside the lamina cribrosa, forming a *subareolar abscess*

around the nipple, in one of the tubercles of Montgomery or in the milk glands attached to them. Then it may involve the lactiferous tubules to form *parenchymatous* or *glandular mastitis* or *galactophoritis.* The bacteria may next gain access to the connective tissue through a crack or deep fissure, burrow into the fat around the lobes and lobules and cause *interstitial, intramammary* or *phlegmonous mastitis.* This cellulitis may be superficial or deep; occasionally, the latter two forms are combined. The infection may also pass directly through the gland to the areolar tissue under it and produce a *retromammary abscess. Subcutaneous abscesses* rarely form.

Symptoms. The parenchymatous form is the most common and seldom begins before the seventh postpartum day; most often it begins from the tenth to the twentieth day. Frequently, there is slight pain in one portion of the breast, exaggerated while nursing, and occasionally slight fever for a day or two preceding the outbreak, when there may be a severe chill

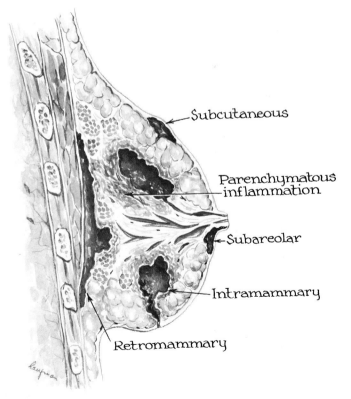

Figure 409 Lateral view of the breast in cross section to show schematically the several types of inflammatory processes which may occur in the puerperal breast and the possible loci of abscess formation.

Subcutaneous

Parenchymatous inflammation

Subareolar

Intramammary

Retromammary

and fever. The temperature may reach 41° C. (106° F.), but usually it does not rise above 39.4° C. (103° F.); the febrile symptoms are moderate.

Mammary pain is the rule and the affected lobe is red and sensitive. Any quadrant of the organ may be inflamed, though usually it is the outer half, and then one or more large lumps may be palpated.

Under appropriate treatment, the temperature and pain subside within 36 hours unless both breasts are affected. Suppuration usually appears if the fever continues for more than 48 hours. The temperature then becomes remittent, chills occur and the affected portion of the breast, containing a large hard mass, swells. At one spot this mass softens and redness of the skin, with a bluish tinge, indicates where the pus is pointing.

Unless properly treated, successive lobes are involved until the whole breast is riddled with abscesses. These must all be opened and drained. Healing often requires weeks or even months. Sometimes the acute symptoms subside and the physician believes the process is at an end, but a few weeks later fever again develops and the breast suppurates or pus is discharged through the nipple.

In the phlegmonous variety, the infection spreads into the gland from a fissure and along the connective tissue septums, and fan-shaped redness, spreading from the crack, may be seen around the nipple. If the deeper lymphatic glands are involved, the case resembles one of deep cellulitis with brawny swelling of the skin. Usually, the streptococcus is the incriminating organism. The fever, though at first less intense, persists longer. Suppuration is much more common in this form.

In the retromammary abscesses, the pus collects behind the gland and edema appears at the periphery. The general symptoms are most threatening; unless the abscesses are evacuated promptly, the pus may burrow deeply and the patient may die of bacteremia.

Treatment. The following has been found successful: (1) Remove the infant from the breast; there must be no massage or pumping of the breast. (2) Apply a tight breast binder. (3) Use cold or heat to allay the inflammation. Heat may take the form of hot-water bags or a heat lamp, and is preferable if suppuration is present. After the temperature has been normal for 24 hours, the child may be put back to the breasts to nurse. He should be observed carefully because he may be harboring the responsible organisms and either cause reinfection or develop overt manifestations of infection himself.

Acute puerperal mastitis may be treated according to the type of organism present and its sensitivity. Cultures should be taken of the milk before instituting treatment. Penicillin is generally quite effective. If the organism is penicillin-resistant, other agents should be substituted. Therapy should not be discontinued too quickly after defervescence because recrudescence is common.

If an abscess forms, it must be incised under general anesthesia as soon as it is diagnosed. To avoid ugly scars, the incision should be made at the edge of the nipple or at the rim of the areola. If the abscess is pointing, it may be drained at that spot. The abscess is evacuated and the septums between the pus pockets are punctured by inserting a finger so that all loculations are opened. Each involved lobe is treated separately. A drainage tube is inserted into the cavity. If all pus cavities are opened and drained, the condition will subside promptly and healing will occur. It is unwise to resume nursing after drainage of an abscess of the breast.

REFERENCES

Mass, J. M.: Amenorrhea-galactorrhea syndrome: Before, during and after pregnancy. Fertil. Steril. *18*:857, 1967.

Plueckhahn, V. D., and Banks, J.: Breast abscess and staphylococcal disease in a maternity hospital. Brit. Med. J. *2*:414, 1964.

OPERATIVE OBSTETRICS

Chapter 72

Principles of Operative Obstetrics

During labor, the physician's role is both prophylactic and remedial. First, he studies the physiologic processes of nature and tries to recognize and understand the pathologic deviations so as to determine when, where and how he may be of assistance. He must always bear in mind that he should never interfere unless something goes wrong during labor or the puerperium. Second, he studies what he must do and, third, when he should do it.

That which commands intervention or treatment is an *indication*. In each obstetric case are factors which determine or specify the nature of the procedure to be instituted. These are *conditions*. Therefore, a condition is a prerequisite to be fulfilled before the procedure demanded by the indication may be carried out.

The study of the case and the determination that a reason exists for adopting a particular line of treatment require delicate balancing of all the conditions. This principle applies to all therapeutic procedures and regimens in medicine; namely, one must always balance the risks of the untreated problem against the hazards of the treatment, the dangers of interference against those of inaction and the risks of one program of therapy against another.

All indications for intervention consist of aspects of immediate or prospective danger to the mother or the fetus. The conditions will be found in the state of the mother at the time of the intended treatment. Only when the conditions necessary for carrying out the procedure are present may one act, but the indication may be so strong that one has to force the condition, that is to say, one may have to modify what one ordinarily would consider to be optimal prerequisites for proceeding or else modify the procedure to fit the conditions. For example, a woman is bleeding. This is an indication to empty the uterus, but the cervix is tightly closed. A condition for rapid delivery is an open cervix; therefore, one must either open the cervix or choose an operation that does not require this condition. A condition that prohibits one from acting on an indication is called a *contraindication*.

Selection of an operation depends on the indications and conditions, but often there are other extenuating circumstances, particularly the skill of the physician and the availability of assistance, anesthesia, suitable operating facilities, blood bank and ancillary laboratory support.

DIAGNOSIS

Before every obstetric procedure, the physician must have made a careful general examination. He must know the blood pressure and the condition of the blood, kidneys, heart and lungs. Such knowledge is a *sine qua non* before giving any anesthesia or performing any operative procedure. Minimum laboratory evaluation includes hematocrit or hemoglobin and urine analysis. Other studies will depend on the prevailing problem, time constraints and sophistication of the obstetric unit or institution.

Just before an operative delivery, with the patient on the operating table and perhaps anesthetized, the examination of the local pelvic conditions, concentrating on fetal station, presentation, position, fetal heart, cervical dilatation and effacement and status of the membranes, must be repeated because the conditions may have changed in the time intervening or the first diagnosis may have been wrong. If the local findings are different from those expected, the original plan may have to be altered. Any other course taken that is less favorable to the patient endangers the mother and fetus. It may be best to put the woman back in bed and select an entirely different line of treatment. One must never feel irrevocably committed to a course of action merely because an operative procedure was decided upon at an earlier time. When the procedure is subsequently shown to be inappropriate, the honest physician will not let his false pride interfere with good judgment.

After the diagnosis is made, the physician should mentally rehearse the steps of the operation and take cognizance of the complications that may arise. If he will construct a mental picture of the conditions before him and then review the steps of the operation in his mind, he will facilitate the procedure considerably.

ASSISTANTS

For good obstetric operating, optimally at least three assistants are required: an anesthetist, an assistant physician and a nurse. Most surgeons demand more help than this, but most obstetricians usually have less and consider themselves fortunate when this minimum is available. In practice in most communities, it is sometimes impossible to obtain any assistants, even one to give the anesthetic. Local infiltration anesthesia helps a great deal to eliminate the need for an assistant, but this does not substitute for the expertise which the anesthetist can provide in acute cardiopulmonary care of the mother and resuscitation of the neonate (see Chapter 22 for the role of the anesthetist and principles of anesthesia administration). Good surgical care demands that a competent medical anesthetist be available for major procedures.

PREVENTION OF INJURIES

Obstetric operations require a clear head and a steady hand. Only too easily is the mother injured and the fetus harmed so seriously that its future is affected. Loss of sleep, the suffering of the patient, sympathy for her and the importunities of the family may wear down a physician. If he must then perform a complicated and delicate operation, he may, when suddenly confronted with an unexpected difficulty, lose his good judgment and operate with undue haste, harming the mother or the fetus, or both. To combat this tendency, obstetricians should be ever mindful of the old but still relevant mottos of our professional forebears: *Primum non nocere* (First of all do no damage) and *Non vi sed arte* (Not with force, but with skill).

PREPARATIONS

The technique for operative deliveries is identical to that of surgical operations, including all necessary operating theater accessories, instruments and equipment. In addition, one must make suitable preparation for the complications presented by the sudden accidents of delivery and the attention required by the baby. The obstetrician prepares himself with surgical cap and mask in fresh, clean, scrub clothes, having first divested himself of all street clothing; he appropriately scrubs his hands and forearms, and dons sterile gown and gloves.

When the woman is put on the operating table, the exposed area of mons, vulva and perineum is disinfected with antiseptic solution (Betadine is currently recommended for this purpose), a pair of sterile leggings is put on and a sterile towel is laid over the abdomen. Only the area immediately around the vulva, which has been disinfected, and the towel over the abdomen are to be considered sterile and may be touched by the physician.

An aseptic technique is not the final word in the prevention of infection. A good operative technique that handles tissues gently and avoids trauma, the preservation of the woman's own resistance by prevention of shock and hemorrhage and the proper selection of an operation all contribute much to success.

POSITIONING THE PATIENT

The patient for operative vaginal delivery should be so placed that the buttocks hang over the edge of the table about 3 inches. It is then easier to insert a hand for any manipulation since the perineum is not crowded inward and upward. Whenever a hand is inserted into the vagina, it is passed from above under the pubic arch (Fig. 410); the possibility of contamination from the rectum is always kept in mind and precautions are taken to prevent it.

POSTPARTUM EXAMINATION

It is a good rule to examine the parturient canal from the fundus to the vulva and the adjacent viscera and pelvis after every difficult, operative, vaginal delivery. With the patient under anesthesia, a hand is inserted into the uterus; the placental site is palpated; any adherent placental fragments, membranes and blood clots are removed; the lower uterine segment is carefully studied digitally to discover any laceration or injury; the vagina and finally the vulva are then examined. A careful search is made for tears. The pubic joint is palpated; the bladder is catheterized; lastly, after all repairs have been made, a

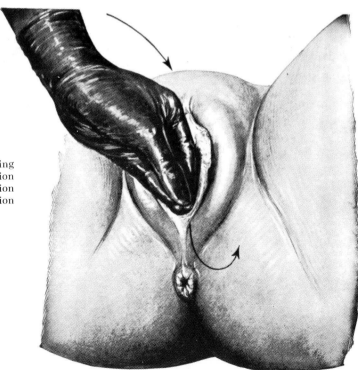

Figure 410 Method of introducing hand to avoid fecal contamination when undertaking manual exploration of uterus and vagina or manipulation of any sort.

finger is inserted into the rectum to determine if any stitches encroach on the lumen or if it is otherwise injured.

After operative delivery, the child also requires an especially careful examination by the obstetrician and by the pediatrician.

REFLECTION

After delivery, a most profitable procedure is a review of the details of the case and what was done. The physician should examine himself and his course of action to see if his judgment was good and his technique perfect; then he should decide what he would do the next time he is confronted by a similar patient or if the same woman became pregnant again. All these impressions should be written down in the patient's hospital record and the physician's own record; they will be invaluable for future reference, for self-instruction, for teaching others and for individual improvement.

Chapter 73

Cephalic Manipulations

MANUAL ROTATION

Faulty attitudes of the head occasionally require digital or manual correction because they give rise to dystocic problems. When arrest of descent is diagnosed (see Chapter 55) and cephalopelvic disproportion has been ruled out, the unfavorable position or deflexion may be considered to be contributory. Contractile forces can be improved with oxytocin infusion and then the attitude corrected by manual manipulation, if still necessary.

A simple and relatively safe method of bringing about anterior rotation of the occiput is the intravenous infusion of oxytocin. This procedure is most helpful with conduction anesthesia. With this type of anesthesia there is a high incidence of persistent occiput posterior and occiput transverse positions. The judicious use of oxytocin intravenously will considerably reduce the need for manual and forceps rotation of the occiput.

Occiput posterior positions only occasionally require correction because most occiputs rotate anteriorly spontaneously. The position may have to be corrected during the progress of labor or prior to delivery by forceps. In the former, after the correction is made, the woman is allowed to complete her labor by herself. Further interference to effect delivery may be indicated by circumstances which dictate more rapid termination for maternal or fetal problems. In the latter instance, having decided on forceps, one attempts manual rotation of the occiput to the front before the blades are applied. The type of manipulation depends on the station of the head.

There are certain prerequisite conditions for manual correction that must be fulfilled. (1) The pelvis must not be contracted; (2) the fetus must be living; (3) the cervix must be dilated to admit a hand; (4) the membranes must be ruptured or are to be ruptured; (5) the uterus must not be in tetanic contraction or on the point of rupture; and (6) there must be no placenta previa or prolapse of the cord.

When the occiput is deep down in the pelvis, a combined internal and external procedure can be done. Under sterile precautions, the head is grasped by obtaining a purchase on the skull behind the ear with two fingers of one hand, with the fingertips in or near the dependent lambdoidal suture. The occiput is pulled downward and forward to flex the head and rotate it; at the same time, the other hand placed suprapubically pushes the forehead toward the back of the pelvis (Fig. 411). In a large pelvis, one may use two hands in the vagina to apply added rotational pressure with two fingers on the malar bone from behind the pubis (Fig. 412).

For higher heads, the occiput is pulled anteriorly with the hand in the vagina. Here the fingers are behind the ear, and the forehead is pushed backward with the thumb (Fig. 413). At the same time, the anterior shoulder is pulled toward and beyond the midline with the hand outside. This is very important. Success in obtaining and maintaining an anterior position depends on getting the fetal back to the front; otherwise, the head will turn back as soon as pressure is released.

It may be necessary to rotate the body by the following special technique in order to ensure permanent anterior rotation of the occiput. With the patient under deep anes-

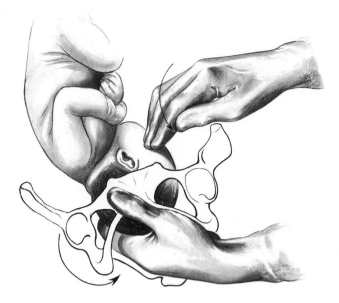

Figure 411 Rotating the occiput anteriorly by combined manual manipulation. The internal hand flexes and turns the head from the right occiput posterior position clockwise to the right occiput transverse and anterior, while the external hand presses the forehead posteriorly.

thesia, a hand is passed into the uterus and the fetal head is pushed up slightly. The head should not be displaced out of the pelvis, if possible. The fingertips seek the posterior shoulder, which is then swung around to the front. At the same time, the hand on the abdomen pulls the fetal back to the front or, better still, to the opposite side.

The head fits into the hollow of the in-

ternal hand and rotates with the trunk. As the head is led with the hand into its new position, pressure on the occiput with the hand outside forces it down so that the occiput enters under the pubic ramus. The malposition has thus been corrected. It is appropriate to allow the anesthesia to abate at this point and await further progress in descent unless there is some overriding indication for delivery. Be-

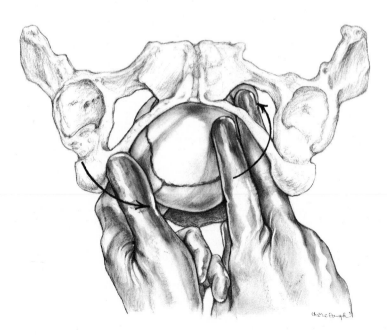

Figure 412 Rotating a head from the right occiput posterior position by flexion and synchronized clockwise rotary motion using two fingers of each hand inside the pelvis. The arrows indicate the flexion forces applied.

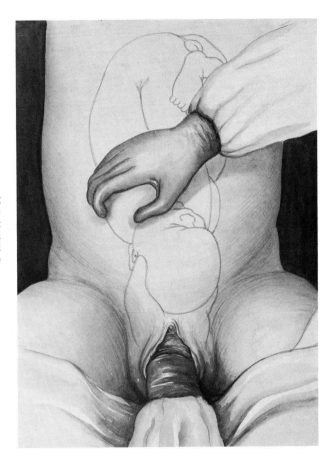

Figure 413 Combined manner of rotating a head that is not deeply engaged from the right occiput posterior position to occiput anterior. The head is rotated with the hand inside while the anterior shoulder is pulled toward and beyond the midline with the hand outside.

cause the head has been elevated and a loop of umbilical cord may have become occultly prolapsed, it is imperative that the fetal heart be listened to especially at the conclusion of this procedure. Bradycardia may be expected during manipulation on the basis of the vagal response to cranial compression.

It is not wise to attempt correction of an occiput posterior until the cervix is dilated fully because sometimes an unexpected indication for rapid delivery arises during the operation, such as prolapse of the cord or abruptio placentae. Furthermore, if one waits for the cervix to dilate completely, the occiput will usually rotate to the front spontaneously, making manual or instrumental rotation unnecessary. When manual correction fails, the fetus should preferably be delivered as an occiput sacral. This is far safer than resorting to a potentially traumatic forceps rotation (see Chapter 56).

FACE AND BROW CONVERSION

An indication for the operation to effect conversion of a face to a vertex presentation is the mentum posterior position (see Chapter 56), when the physician, from close observation of the course of labor, is convinced that the case is not likely to terminate with spontaneous anterior rotation of the chin. If the procedure is not successful, cesarean is indicated for mentum posterior position. Indeed, cesarean section is usually preferable. Another indication is the brow presentation which does not spontaneously convert itself to a face or a vertex presentation (see Chapter 56).

The conditions that must be met for conversion include the following: (1) The cervix must be fully dilated because the hand has to be introduced and it may become necessary to deliver at once. (2) The membranes must be ruptured. (3) The fetus

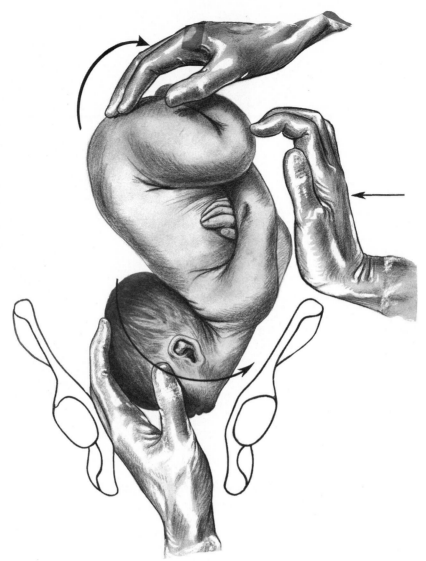

Figure 414 Combined technique for converting a face to a vertex presentation, showing the internal hand elevating the face and pulling the occiput down to flex the head, while two external hands try to convert the S curve of the trunk (shown here) to the flexed C of the normal intrauterine fetal attitude.

must not be too large nor the pelvis too small. (4) The uterus must not be too thin nor on the point of rupturing. (5) The head must not be deeply engaged in the pelvis. (6) Placenta previa must not be present. (7) The fetus must be living and viable.

Techniques in use to effect conversion involve a simultaneous combination of maneuvers to flex the head and to convert the S curvature of the fetal body (Fig. 414) to the normal, well-flexed configuration. Unless the latter is done at the same time, successful conversion will be unlikely. All

current methods are a modification of those of Thorn, who combined those originally described by Schatz and by Baudelocque. They involve placing the patient in the lithotomy position with the buttocks well over the edge of the table to allow the physician to sink his elbow. Deep anesthesia is indispensable.

With the usual stringent sterile precautions, the hand is introduced into the vagina and advanced to the lower uterine segment. In the right mentum posterior position, the left hand is used so that the

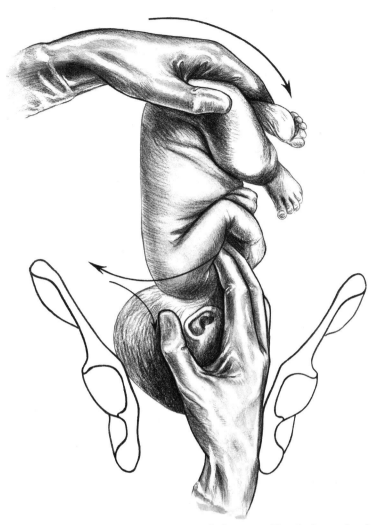

Figure 415 Continuation of maneuver in Figure 414 with the internal hand advanced to the anterior chest for purposes of aiding flexion of the thorax. Note the thumb of the vaginal hand pulling the occiput down, while the abdominal hand continues to exert pressure to flex the body.

palm will lie against the face. First the chin and then the face are pushed up to flex the head, while the occiput is pressed down with the hand outside. At the same time, the breech is being pulled forward and the chest impressed by the hands of an assistant applied externally as shown in Figure 414. The importance of this latter maneuver has been stressed above.

The hand inside is now passed further into the uterus until the chest and shoulder of the fetus are reached with the fingertips. Obtaining a hold on the shoulder, the fingers are flexed, throwing the chest first into a straight line and then into a concavity. Simultaneously, downward traction is made on the occiput with the thumb. The occiput is then brought into the palm of the hand. Meanwhile, the breech is pushed to the side on which the chin lies (Fig. 415).

Holding the flexed head, one gently leads the head into the pelvis, applying pressure on the uterine fundus. Pressure should be maintained over the course of several contractions to aid descent and prevent recurrence of the malpresentation. DeLee recommended use of forceps for this purpose, but it is generally unnecessary. Once engagement has taken place, recurrence of the face or brow presentation is no longer possible. One may then wait for natural delivery or apply forceps for delivery, depending on the circumstances then prevailing.

REFERENCES

Baudelocque, J. H.: L'Art des Accouchements. Paris, Méquignon, 1781.

DeLee, J. B.: The Principles and Practice of Obstetrics, ed. 7. Philadelphia, W. B. Saunders Company, 1938.

Schatz, F.: Die Umwandlung von Gesichtslage zu Hinterhauptslage durch alleinigen äusseren Handgriff. Arch. Gynäk. 5:306, 1873.

Thorn, W.: Zur manuellen Umwandlung der Gesichtslagen in Hinterhauptslagen. Z. Geburtsh. Gynäk. 13:186, 1886.

Chapter 74

Breech Procedures

Details of breech presentation and the mechanisms of labor associated with it are discussed in Chapter 57. The distinctions between spontaneous delivery, partial breech extraction (or assisted breech delivery) and breech extraction are also outlined. This material should be reviewed.

PARTIAL BREECH EXTRACTION

This term and its synonym, *assisted breech delivery,* are applied to extraction by the physician of the lower part of the body after the fetus has been extruded as far as the umbilicus by the uterine and abdominal forces. When the breech has been delivered, the woman is urged to bear down. If this does not elicit progress beyond delivery of the umbilicus, the indication for *partial breech extraction* is present.

An anesthetic should be used. These cases are ideal for pudendal block, but many obstetricians prefer inhalation anesthesia. In nulliparas, a deep mediolateral episiotomy should be routinely done just as the breech lateroflexes over the perineum, before the lower body is born. It is difficult to cut an episiotomy after the fetal body has partially delivered. The episiotomy facilitates all the manipulations of the delivery, preserves the fetus from injury, saves time (which lessens the danger of asphyxia), and safeguards the sphincter ani from laceration. If the fetus is astride the cord, the cord is loosened gently and slipped over one thigh. If this fails, the cord is cut between two clamps and the delivery is ended quickly. The bladder must be empty.

The maneuvers involved in partial breech extraction include: (1) engaging the shoulders by traction on the fetal pelvis to deliver the scapula and rotation of the body until the anterior shoulder stems under the symphysis; (2) delivering the shoulders by gently sweeping the anterior arm across the chest and rotating in the opposite direction to deliver the opposite shoulder; and (3) delivering the head by flexing it over the perineum with combined suprapubic and mandibular pressure. These steps are described in detail below in our discussion of total breech extraction.

TOTAL BREECH EXTRACTION

This term refers to delivery of the entire body of the fetus by the physician. It is a particularly hazardous procedure and should not be undertaken unless there are strong indications and no other alternatives are available. Because the risks of this procedure are so great, it is necessary that the hazards of *not* doing it must be substantial before one should entertain it seriously.

The criteria to be fulfilled before proceeding include: (1) a fully dilated cervix, (2) an adequate pelvis with no fetopelvic disproportion, (3) the bladder and the rectum empty, (4) the uterus intact and not excessively thinned so that rupture may be imminent, (5) the fetus alive and viable, and (6) the mother deeply anesthetized so that the uterus is relaxed. Breech extraction should always be done under optimally sterile conditions.

The procedure itself is divided into four

maneuvers: (1) bringing out the breech and legs; (2) delivery to the shoulders; (3) disengaging the shoulder girdle; and (4) delivery of the head. The last three are identical with the manipulations of partial breech extraction.

Deep anesthesia and the Trendelenburg position always enable one to reach the lower extremity, no matter how firmly the breech seems to be wedged in the pelvis. It is essential that one, or preferably both, legs be identified (see Fig. 324, Chapter 57) and grasped. The anterior limb is selected whenever possible, because doing so will bring the back to the pubis, but the posterior leg is grasped if too much trouble is experienced.

Delivery by inserting a finger into the groin may be used in some breech cases, but is not recommended because it may traumatize the hip joint or the femur. Cesarean section is far safer for the mother and fetus if there are overriding indications for effecting delivery quickly.

In a frank breech presentation, it will be necessary to flex the leg in order to grasp it for traction. Flexion is accomplished by the Pinard maneuver (Fig. 416) which insinuates a finger into the popliteal space, pressing the thigh and knee toward the fetal abdomen, causing the foreleg to flex and bringing the foot down so that it can be grasped. By splinting the long bones with the fingers, one may pull gently on the leg until the anterior hip is delivered (Fig. 417). Lateroflexion is followed in the delivery of the posterior hip as in a normal mechanism (Fig. 418) and the opposite leg is delivered either spontaneously or by the Pinard maneuver. At this point the umbilicus is born. The remaining maneuvers are the same for both partial and total breech extractions.

Grasping the fetal pelvis in two hands as shown in Figure 419, the physician makes gentle traction downward, perpendicular to the axis of the plane of the pelvic inlet, until the anterior scapula appears. If there has been no pressure applied to the uterus abdominally, the arms will usually be well flexed and crossed against the chest.

At this time the anterior arm can be delivered by gently sweeping it across the chest (Fig. 420). Once this is accomplished, the other arm can be similarly de-

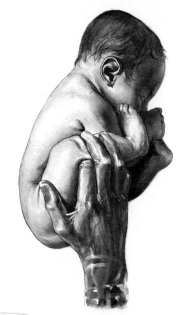

Figure 416 Bringing down a foot by Pinard's maneuver in breech extraction. A hand is passed up high into the uterus avoiding the cord. The index finger is pressed into the popliteal space, shortening the hamstring muscles and flexing the leg. The three fingers slip over the knee to the ankle. The foot is now slid along the other thigh posteriorly into the pelvis and out. No move is made during contractions.

livered; if this cannot be done, the body should be rotated so that the posterior shoulder is brought anteriorly. The rotation should be in the direction of the chest in order to keep the undelivered arm well flexed. It can best be done by merely grasping the delivered arm, as if shaking hands, and rotating the fetus by gently pulling the free arm across the chest. If either arm cannot be delivered, one should consider the probability that one is dealing with an extended arm or nuchal hitch (see below). Special procedures are needed to correct this serious problem.

The head is delivered by flexion. If all has gone well to this point, the back is up and the occiput anterior. The body of the fetus should be supported by the forearm, with its arms and legs straddling (Fig. 421). An airway can be established by inserting a finger into the baby's mouth posteriorly over the perineum. The perineal tissues can be retracted away and the oropharynx aspirated with a suction bulb. This accomplished, the fetus can breathe freely. Suprapubic pressure will cause

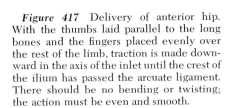

Figure 417 Delivery of anterior hip. With the thumbs laid parallel to the long bones and the fingers placed evenly over the rest of the limb, traction is made downward in the axis of the inlet until the crest of the ilium has passed the arcuate ligament. There should be no bending or twisting; the action must be even and smooth.

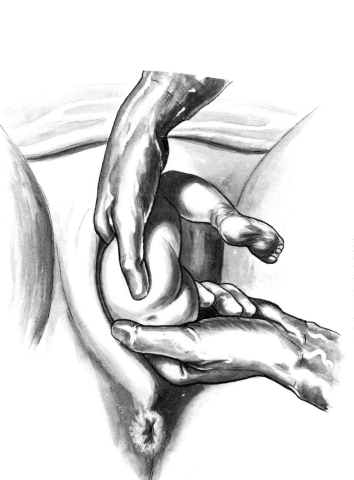

Figure 418 Delivery of posterior hip. The index finger of the other hand is passed over the back, along the crest of the ilium, into the posterior groin. With combined traction, the whole pelvis is brought out, following the usual lateroflexion mechanism. The second leg is allowed to drop out or is reduced by Pinard's maneuver.

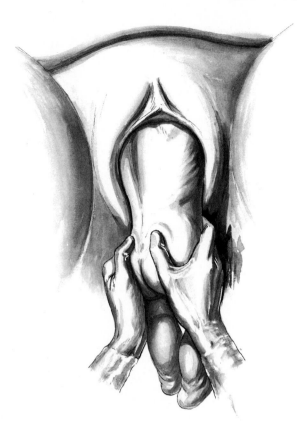

Figure 419 Delivery from umbilicus to shoulders in assisted breech delivery. The physician takes the breech in his two hands with the thumbs over the back of the sacrum; the index fingers rest on the anterior superior iliac spines. Gentle, even traction is made downward in the direction of the axis of the inlet, until the anterior shoulder blade comes well under the pubis.

Figure 420 Bringing down the anterior arm. Deliver the arms as they lie. Two fingers are slipped upward under the pubis over the fetal back and down to its elbow flexure. By flexing the two fingers and twisting his wrist, the physician sweeps the arm of the fetus over its chest and down and out.

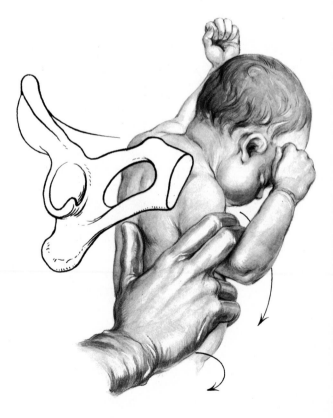

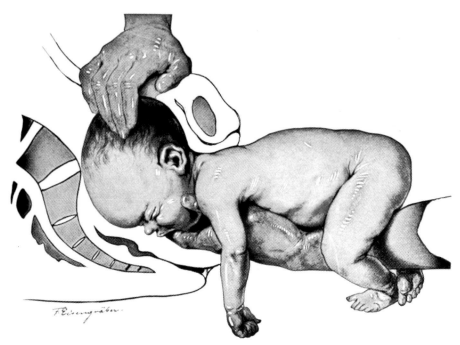

Figure 421 Wigand method of delivering the aftercoming head. With the fetal body straddling the forearm, the hand is inserted into the vagina and fingers are passed to the mouth. By gentle pressure from above, the head is brought down into the pelvis, rotated and delivered, following the natural mechanism. The chin is kept well flexed and, when the nape of the neck stems behind the pubis, the chin, face, forehead and vertex are brought slowly over the perineum.

flexion, especially when used in conjunction with occipital pressure from fingers inserted under the pubis.

As the head descends, the physician's elbow can be raised to effect delivery of the head. Traction must never be applied to the body. To do so is analogous to hanging the fetus by its neck. The chin is kept well flexed by the finger in or near the mouth, taking care to avoid traumatizing the jaw. The nape of the neck stems behind the symphysis and the chin, face, forehead and vertex are successively delivered over the perineum.

Complications

There are three major complications which may occur in breech deliveries: (1) constriction of the external os around the fetal neck, (2) arrest of the head in descent after delivery of the body, and (3) extension of one or both arms behind the fetal head. In addition, various hazards may affect the fetus or the mother.

If the posterior leg is brought down during total breech extraction, the anterior hip may impinge on the pubic ramus. During extraction this may be corrected by gently turning the fetal body so that the anterior leg moves away from behind the pubis. Occasionally, the foot drags the cord down with it and this demands rapid delivery if appropriate conditions are fulfilled, but not so rapid that the fetus is seriously injured.

A large fetus or a contracted pelvis may make delivery from the breech to the shoulders difficult. Care must be exercised in applying pressure on the fetus to avoid injury to the viscera. If more than ordinary resistance is encountered, the fingers are passed alongside the fetus to discover if a distended abdomen exists. With large fetuses it is wise to deliver the arms before the shoulders have become wedged into the pelvis. Therefore, it is best not to draw the trunk down until the scapula is palpable under the pubis but to begin sweeping the arms out sooner. Moderate pressure from above and slow traction from below will almost always succeed in bringing the shoulder girdle within reach.

Extended Arms

Normally, the arms lie crossed over the chest and, if nothing interferes, they are delivered in this position. The arms may be arrested and stripped up above the fetal head or actually come to rest behind the neck, a condition called *nuchal hitch* or *nuchal arms* (Fig. 422). This is most likely to occur if traction is made on the body too soon, if the pelvis is small, if Kristeller pressure is applied to the top of the uterus (especially when the uterus is relaxed), if a constriction ring is present and if the cervix is not sufficiently dilated.

For the arm that is merely extended upward, it is necessary to pass four fingers high into the pelvic inlet, leaving the thumb outside, and glide them over the fetal back, shoulders, humerus and elbow to the forearm; the forearm is pushed to the side of the pelvis, slid across the face and then down and out. The more accessible arm, usually the posterior, is delivered first. A deep episiotomy must be done in advance to provide space for manipulation.

It may be well to push the fetus back a little to loosen the arms from the wedge-like action of the head. If it is too difficult to deliver the posterior arm, the anterior arm should be brought down from behind the pubis. If this fails, the fetus may be rotated ventrally so as to bring the anterior arm to the hollow of the sacrum, and this arm is liberated first. The trunk is then rotated back for the other arm. During these maneuvers, there should be no pressure on the uterus except to assist the hand inside to reach the fetal arm.

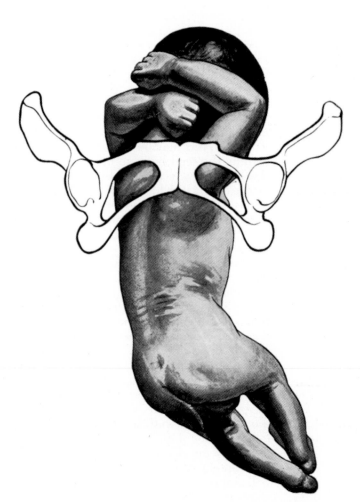

Figure 422 Nuchal hitch, bilateral, with the fetal arms at the nape of the neck. These arms can be made more accessible by manipulation from the outside or by rotating the body first 180° in one direction (here counterclockwise) to dislodge one arm and then 180° in the other direction to dislodge the other arm.

The more serious complication of nuchal arms is recognized only when the fingers are inserted to liberate the posterior arm. Without delay, the body of the fetus is pushed back a few inches to release the imprisoned arm and the hand is inserted directly up the fetal back to the forearm. The fetal elbow and forearm are then slid past the sacral promontory to the other half of the pelvis, down and out. The fetus should be pushed back a little farther if this maneuver does not succeed, and a second attempt made. If this fails, the anterior arm should be liberated, if possible, by the same sweeping motion.

It may be necessary to rotate the body 180° or more to release the nuchal arms. Rotation in one direction will generally release one arm, which can then be delivered as just described for the extended arm. It may also be necessary to rotate the body in the opposite direction to release the other arm and effect its delivery.

Gentle rotation of the trunk facilitates the release of the arm, but one must be particularly on guard against trauma, especially Erb's palsy. The arm must not be brought down over the back. Delivery of the head without previous liberation of the arms is dangerous and inexcusable.

Arrest of the Head

If the fetus is large or the pelvis is small, the head wedges into the inlet with the sagittal suture in the transverse diameter. Every effort should be made to anticipate such difficulties; cesarean section is appropriate for any breech presentation in association with fetopelvic disproportion. Extension occurs and the mouth is thrown up high. The head must be brought through the inlet in the transverse diameter or obliquely according to the best available pelvic diameters (Wigand). The head should not be strongly flexed or rotated to bring the occiput forward until it is deep in the midplane. Pressure suprapubically should be applied lightly and in a downward direction in the axis of the inlet. Traction on the neck from below is decried.

It is best to desist if the head cannot be brought into the pelvis with moderate force applied above because the end sought, a living uninjured child, will be defeated and the mother will also suffer unnecessary and irreparable injury. The fetus has almost always died by this time.

When the head is arrested in the midplane or, more rarely, at the outlet, a quick examination determines if the delay is caused by the cervix or by the bony pelvis. A tight cervix must be stripped back, stretched with two or three right-angle retractors inserted quickly, or cut; this is not a simple matter. Forceps should be applied inside the cervix if the head cannot be delivered with ease.

It is good practice to apply forceps to the aftercoming head if it does not quickly follow moderate traction (Fig. 423). In breech cases, the Piper forceps should be ready for immediate use at all times. They are especially useful for the aftercoming head because of the backward curving of the shanks, making it possible to apply them to the head from beneath the baby's body. The body and arms are cradled in a sling fashioned of a sterile towel as shown in Figure 423. The entire body is elevated slightly. The Piper forceps may then be readily applied. Gentle traction on the forceps in the proper axis and slow flexion of the head, combined with gradual elevation of the fetal body, soon bring the mouth and nose into view over the perineum. Leaving the legs and feet exposed by this method enables the physician to guard constantly against overextension of the fetal cervical spine, a particularly dangerous situation from the point of view of possible spinal cord injury.

A valuable maneuver, mentioned earlier but worth repeating, is the retraction of the perineum with the hands or with broad specula, wiping the vagina and oropharynx dry and allowing the fetus to breathe with its head still in the pelvis. A stiff rubber tube may also be inserted into the pharynx of the fetus.

BRACHT METHOD

The Bracht method of breech delivery, which simulates the natural mechanism of labor, is widely used abroad. The breech is

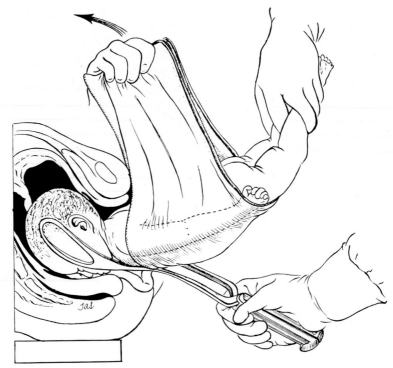

Figure 423   Forceps delivery of the aftercoming head, using Piper forceps. The body and arms are elevated slightly with a sling made of a towel. (From Savage, J. E.: Obstet. Gynec. 3:55, 1954.)

allowed to deliver spontaneously up to the umbilicus, and the body and extended legs are held together with both hands maintaining the upward and anterior rotation of the body (Fig. 424). When the anterior rotation is almost complete, the fetal body is held, not pressed, against the mother's symphysis. The force applied should be equivalent to the force of gravity, that is, just enough to support the weight of that portion of the fetus already delivered.

Maintenance of this position, added to the effects of uterine contractions and moderate suprapubic pressure during contractions by an assistant, suffices to complete the delivery by the spontaneous mechanisms just described. The arms are maintained in position against the chest and are delivered spontaneously during expulsive efforts as the fetus is supported against the symphysis progressively higher in the upward projection of the continuation of pelvic curve (Fig. 425). The head follows over the perineum by the same process (Fig. 426).

Under deep surgical anesthesia, the fetus lacks the tone necessary to play the passive role outlined and the mother's expulsive efforts are completely negated so that the maneuver is likely to fail. For the same reason, the Bracht maneuver cannot be used for delivery of a dead or macerated fetus. A reasonable degree of cooperation and minimal anesthesia are prerequisites. Short intermittent inhalation anesthesia alone or superimposed on local or pudendal block is ideal.

ABNORMAL ROTATION MECHANISM

Thus far, delivery has been considered when the mechanism of labor has been the usual one with the back anterior. Just as in vertex presentations, there are errors in the mechanism caused by abnormal rotation. In some breech deliveries, the fetal back turns to the mother's back and the abdomen lies anteriorly behind the pubis. This complication occurs more often in footling presentations when the posterior leg has come down or after version when

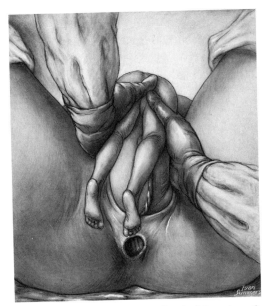

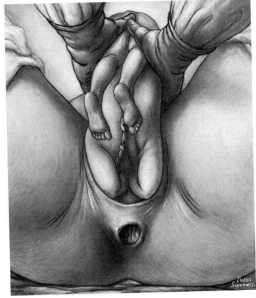

Figure 424 Bracht method of delivering the breech spontaneously to the umbilicus. The body and legs are held together with the hands merely supporting the breech against gravity and allowing it to move upward in the anteriorly curved projection of the pelvic curve. (Figures 424 to 426 from Plentl, A. A., and Stone, R. E.: Obstet. Gynec. Survey 8:313, 1953.)

Figure 425 Holding the baby against the mother's symphysis pubis leads to spontaneous and simultaneous delivery of the elbows as shown, followed by the arms and the shoulders in transverse position. No traction is made.

the physician has grasped the posterior leg. Rarely, it may occur during an otherwise natural breech labor when inadequate attempts at rotation have been made.

Nature almost always rectifies the abnormal start of the mechanism by turning the back three-fourths of a circle past the promontory and through the other half of the pelvis to the front. The back rotates in the direction opposite from that which one would expect. The physician may cause the back to remain posterior by not appreciating this point and resisting the natural mechanism.

The head may be arrested at the inlet with the chin caught over the pubic ramus or it may engage in the pelvis with the chin anterior. These cases may terminate either by flexion or by extension. In flexion, the body drops, the chin remains applied to the sternum, and the face, forehead and vertex roll out from behind the pubis with the nape of the neck resting on the perineum. By extension, the chin leaves the sternum and, if the fetus is lifted up onto the mother's abdomen, the occiput, the vertex and the face come successively

over the perineum with the neck resting behind the pubis.

The physician may attempt to turn the head so as to bring the occiput to the front and the chin to the rear. The chin should

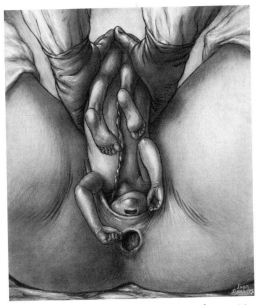

Figure 426 Maintaining the baby in this position leads to spontaneous delivery of the head, which passes through the outlet in its most favorable diameter. Delivery is accomplished by the mother's expulsive efforts alone.

be turned to the side if the pelvis is a flat contracted one. This rotation can be accomplished by obtaining a purchase on the malar bone with two fingers behind the pubis to push the chin posteriorly while using the abdominal hand to pull the occiput anteriorly.

If rotation of the head does not take place quickly, it may be better to try to deliver the head without turning the chin behind. Van Hoorn's (modified Prague) method is used if the occiput has not engaged in the pelvis. Gentle pressure is applied suprapubically on the forehead. This pressure should accomplish most of the work. The body is lifted up, with the chest applied to the pubis, and the occiput rolls past the promontory into the hollow of the sacrum. Too much force will fracture the fetal neck. Anterior rotation of the occiput is still possible at this time; if not, delivery by spontaneous mechanisms or by forceps should follow, usually by extension.

VERSION

Version is a maneuver with limited value and significant risk. It changes the polarity of the fetus with reference to the mother; the object is to change an abnormal relationship into a normal one. Thus, version may change a shoulder presentation to a longitudinal one or a breech presentation to a cephalic, or *vice versa*.

Version is a procedure unto itself. Although it is sometimes done in conjunction with breech extraction, they are two separate procedures with different indications. After completion of a version, a new indication must be present for extraction, which should not be performed unless there is an indication for it (see above).

Version is called *cephalic* when the head is brought down and *podalic* when the legs or breech are brought down into the pelvis. Version may be done by purely external manipulation or by combined internal and external manipulation. The latter is sometimes called *bipolar version.* Internal version alone is not done because the hand outside is always used to aid the one inside.

External Cephalic Version

External cephalic version has only limited use in a shoulder presentation. The lack of rationale for its use in breech presentations is discussed in Chapter 57. The indications for this procedure in transverse lie and the conditions that must be fulfilled are detailed in Chapter 58.

Dangers during the manipulation are (1) injury to the uterus, (2) partial or complete separation of the placenta and (3) kinking or prolapse of the cord, all of which jeopardize the fetus. External version should not be attempted under circumstances in which there is risk of abruptio placentae (for example, in gravidas with hypertensive states), placenta previa (with antepartum hemorrhage), placental dysfunction or rupture of the uterus from overdistention, excessive thinning or previous cesarean section.

Anesthesia must not be given in order to ensure the utmost in gentle manipulation limited by the patient's threshold of discomfort. For the patient with a shoulder presentation in active labor, one lowers the head of the table.

Wigand's technique of external version places the patient, with bladder and rectum empty, in a moderate Trendelenburg position. She is asked to relax the abdomen. The head-down tilt of the Trendelenburg position causes the fetus to drop away from the inlet and to become more movable. Talcum powder is liberally applied to the skin. The fetus is mobilized by gentle manipulation. One hand then draws the breech out of the inlet onto one iliac fossa, while the other hand presses the head down onto the opposite flank (Fig. 427). Movement is accomplished by alternate stroking and pushing movements. If the patient is having uterine contractions, one operates between them during uterine quiescence. One should never be hasty.

An attempt should be made to turn the fetus by flexion of the trunk, using synchronous action on its two poles. This short route is preferable. One should try to turn the fetus in the opposite direction if resistance is met. The fetus should be held in its new position for five minutes. The fetal heart should be listened to after each step. The fetus may be so adversely affected by a cord complication that the ef-

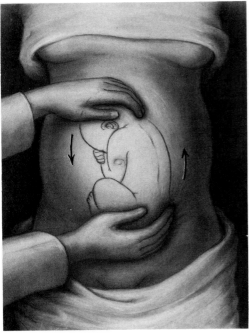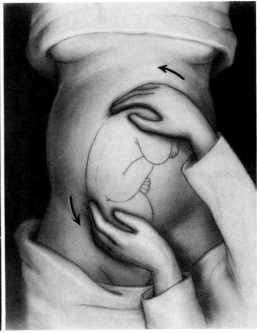

A   B

Figure 427 External version of breech to cephalic presentation. *A,* The first maneuver is an attempt to push the breech away from the pelvic inlet with one hand and at the same time to pull the head with the other hand in the direction in which the face lies. *B,* By continual pushing of the breech gently upward and away from the pelvic inlet while pulling the head downward toward the pelvis, the fetus is turned from a breech to a cephalic presentation. This must be done without force.

fort must be suspended and the fetus returned to its original position. One must never cause pain or use force if difficulties are encountered.

After external version, the foot of the table is lowered and the fetal head is gently forced down into the inlet, where it is held for five minutes or until the contractions fix it there. During this time, the fetal heart rate should be observed continuously to ascertain that the fetus has not been embarrassed by the procedure. If the cervix is dilated completely in active labor (provided the cord or the extremities have not prolapsed), the membranes may be ruptured while an assistant holds the head firmly in the inlet. The membranes should not be ruptured if the cervix is not fully dilated or if the cord lies over the os. Cesarean section is far better treatment for shoulder presentation than external version (see Chapter 58).

Podalic Version

When version is mentioned, it is usually the combined podalic version that is meant. Of historical interest only is the Hicks version, no longer done or condoned, in which two fingers are insinuated through the cervix and through the forelying placenta (in a previable pregnancy with placenta previa) to pull the fetal leg down to tamponade the placenta. The terrible hazards of this technique outweigh any possible benefits.

There are few indications still applicable to and acceptable for podalic version: (1) for transverse lie with intact membranes and (2) most commonly for the delivery of the second twin. Version in head presentations is often very dangerous. Although still occasionally done for prolapsed cord in the second stage with the cervix fully dilated or for face or brow presentations, the risks are so great to both fetus and mother that cesarean section is much more preferable.

No operation in obstetrics is more dangerous than bimanual podalic version, especially if performed without due consideration of the conditions that must be fulfilled. These include the following: (1) The cervix must be retracted and dilated fully. (2) The pelvis must be adequate for the delivery of the fetus. (3) The case must not be one of neglected transverse lie with the uterus on the point of rupture. (4) The fetus must be mobile within the uterus; this usually means that the membranes are intact or only recently ruptured. (5) The fetus must be alive unless it is small and the version promises to be exceptionally easy. In a shoulder presentation, if the uterus is not contracted around the fetus, it is permissible to perform a version on a dead fetus because it is less dangerous than a destructive operation. (6) The blad-

der and rectum must be empty. The indications, pros and cons are discussed in Chapter 58.

Deep narcosis and anesthesia are necessary for version because the uterus must be completely relaxed for the procedure. The dorsal lithotomy position is usually sufficient, but a moderate Trendelenburg position may be used. Very long, sterile gauntlet gloves are useful. Full surgical preparation is essential.

The hand the palm of which will lie against the breech should be the one in-

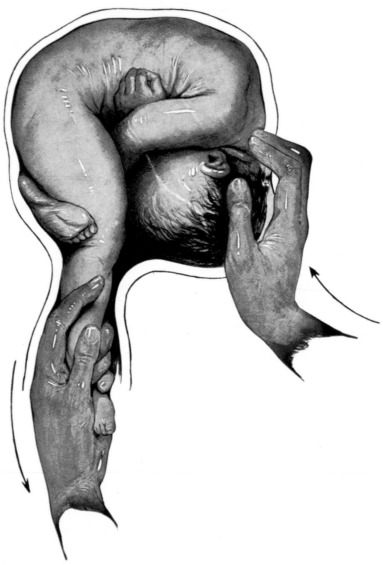

Figure 428   Bimanual podalic version grasps and draws a foot down in the axis of the inlet with the hand in the vagina, while at the same time the abdominal hand pushes the head of the fetus upward and inward toward its abdomen, thus shaping the body of the fetus into a ball which rotates better in the uterus.

troduced into the uterus; for example, when the breech is to the left, the right hand is passed through the cervix. The postured, if they are still intact, just as the hand is passed through the cervix. The possibility that the umbilical cord may slip down must be remembered.

In back-anterior presentations, the lower foot is brought down and in back-posterior presentations, the upper one is grasped. In either case, the back of the fetus will rotate anteriorly; this will be most favorable in the subsequent extraction. However, when it is at all difficult to reach the feet, the first foot identified is grasped.

If an arm prolapses, it is best to put a sling on it to ensure that it will not be withdrawn back into the uterus during the version, causing contamination. The end of the tape is placed on one groin. Later, during the extraction, an assistant maintains light traction on it to hold the arm alongside the trunk.

While the uterus is steadied with the outside hand, the foot is grasped and gently extracted toward the vagina as shown in Figure 428. The abdominal hand simultaneously elevates the head toward the uterine fundus. While elevating the head, one should maintain good flexion of the body to minimize the overall volume of the fetus within the uterus. No movement should be attempted during uterine contractions. Extreme care must be taken to avoid damage to the uterine wall or to the fetus.

In nearly all instances, the version is followed by immediate breech extraction of the fetus. However, this is not essential unless there is some indication for this additional procedure. In some cases, one may wait until the fetus is delivered spontaneously by the mother just as in an ordinary breech presentation.

The hazards of version must never be estimated lightly. Prognosis depends largely on the skill of the physician. Version may be fatal to the mother from rupture of the uterus or lethal to the fetus from placental or cord complications, or from direct trauma.

REFERENCES

DeLee, J. B.: The Principles and Practice of Obstetrics, ed. 7. Philadelphia, W. B. Saunders Company, 1938.

Hicks, J. B.: On Combined External and Internal Version. London, Longman, Green, Longman, Roberts & Green, 1864.

Pinard, A.: Cited by Farabeuf, L. H., and Varnier, H.: Introduction à l'étude clinique des accouchements. Paris, Steinheil, 1891.

Piper, E. B., and Bachman, C.: Prevention of fetal injuries in breech delivery. J.A.M.A. 92:217, 1929.

Plentl, A. A., and Stone, R. E.: The Bracht maneuver. Obstet. Gynec. Survey 8:313, 1953.

Savage, J. E.: Management of the fetal arms in breech extraction: A method to facilitate application of Piper forceps. Obstet. Gynec. 3:55, 1954.

van Hoorn, J.: Die zwo um ihrer Gottesfurcht und Treue willen von Gott wohlbelohnte Weh-Mütter Siphra un Pua, welche in Frag und Antwort treulich unterwiesen, ed. 3. Stockholm, G. Kiesewetter, 1737; 1743.

Wigand, J. H.: Von einigen äussern Handgriffen, wodurch man unter der Geburt die regelwidrigen Lagen der Frucht verbessern kann. Hamb. Mag. Geburtsh. 1:52, 1807.

Chapter 75

Forceps Operations

Forceps operations in obstetrics utilize an instrument designed to extract the fetus by its head from the maternal passages without injury to it or to the mother. Although of considerable benefit when well conceived and properly carried out, such procedures can cause much damage if undertaken under inappropriate circumstances and unskillfully conducted.

DESCRIPTION OF OBSTETRIC FORCEPS

The forceps consists of two articulating parts. They are designated right and left, respectively, according to the side of the mother's pelvis in which they lie when applied. The right blade is held in the right hand during insertion and is applied to the right side of the fetal head normally. Each part has a *handle*, a *shank*, a lock and a hooklike projection which grasps the head and is referred to as the *blade* of the forceps. The distal end of the blade is called the *toe* or *apex*; the part nearest the shank is the *heel* of the blade. The blades are curved on the flat to fit the head, producing the *cephalic curve*, and on the edge to fit the concavity of the pelvis, producing the *pelvic curve*. The cephalic and pelvic curves are perpendicular to each other in all forceps except the Barton forceps (see below). The two blades are fitted together by an articulating lock located on the shanks. The English type of sliding lock consists of opposing shoulders with a flange; the French lock, a screw or pin; and the German lock, a combination of both principles. Blades may be solid or fenestrated.

More than 600 kinds of forceps have been invented (Das). Most fall into the category of classic forceps; a few are considered special forceps. The special forceps, including the Kielland, Barton and Shute types, will be discussed at the end of this chapter; Piper forceps for delivery of the aftercoming head in breech presentation was described in Chapter 74.

There are two large categories of classic forceps, easily distinguished by the configuration of their shanks. *Simpson-type forceps* have separated shanks (Fig. 429); *Elliot-type forceps* have overlapping shanks. The significance of this difference lies in the cephalic curvature that results from the excursion of the blade out from its heel to the maximum point of separation: a broader, flatter arc results when the blade starts further out from the midline with separated shanks; a shorter, fuller arc is produced by overlapping shanks. Thus, the Simpson-type forceps yield a tapered cephalic curve; the Elliot type, a rounded cephalic curve.

In practice, the Simpson type is used for elongated, molded heads and the Elliot type for rounded, unmolded heads. The hundreds of variants of each of these basic types involve usually minor changes in lengths, curvatures and thickness of the blades, lengths of the shanks, the kinds of locking or articulating devices, design of the handles and mechanisms for axis traction (see below).

The history of obstetric forceps is steeped in mystery and intrigue. Although it is no credit to our professional forebears, there is considerable fascination in the conduct of the Chamberlen family who kept the secret for generations during the sixteenth and seventeenth centuries. The

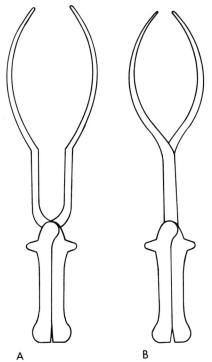

Figure 429 Comparison of Simpson type of forceps (*A*) and Elliot type (*B*). Note separated versus overlapping shanks which determine tapering or rounded cephalic curve.

interested reader is referred to the excellent monographs on the subject by Das and by Witkowski.

FUNCTIONS OF FORCEPS

As currently used, obstetric forceps provides a means for (1) traction, (2) rotation, (3) flexion or extension, (4) compression and (5) protection of the fetal head. It is not designed for use in shoulder or breech presentations.

Although not generally acknowledged or appreciated, compression of the head by forceps is inevitable, but it should be reduced to a minimum. The volume of the fetal head is reduced only slightly by extraneous force, but even this is attended by great danger. If one bears in mind that the widest dimension between the two blades when articulated is no greater than 7.5 cm. in all currently available obstetric forceps, one must accept the fact that some degree of compression will take place whenever forceps procedures are done on term babies whose biparietal diameters average 9.5 cm. Every effort must be made to avoid squeezing the handles of the articulated forceps together, thereby to prevent exerting maximal compressive force on the head.

Compression of the head has a harmful effect on the brain. Circulation may be hindered, causing asphyxia and hemorrhages in addition to direct injury to the cranial bones, tentorium, falx, vessels and brain (see Chapter 68). Fetuses vary much in their ability to withstand compression. Episiotomy helps to reduce compression.

Forceps may provide protection of the very small, delicately constructed head of a premature baby during delivery (see Chapter 67). Often however, abuse of this principle may counterbalance its theoretical benefits by applying the forceps too soon so that the head must be pulled and compressed excessively. Therefore, a generous episiotomy and spontaneous delivery are preferable.

While traction is the dominant function of forceps, a skillful physician can use the forceps also as a rotator to correct the position of the fetal head without injury to the mother or the fetus. Rotation with forceps must take into account the angle between the blades and the handle which forms the pelvic curve of the forceps. In order to make the head rotate around its own axis, it is necessary to sweep the handles through a large circle outside the pelvis (Fig. 435). Describing this large arc with the handles will impart the necessary rotary motion to the head. Use of forceps to effect conversion of a brow presentation by flexion to a vertex or by extension to a face presentation will be discussed later (see below).

How much traction may be applied safely is difficult to determine. It is rarely necessary to pull with more than the strength of the biceps. The objective of forceps traction is to mimic nature in the amount of force, the direction in which it is applied and its intermittent characteristic. To do otherwise is decried. To brace the feet against the table and pull with all one's strength is brutal. Only the greatest care and gentleness will preserve the fetus and the mother from injury.

INDICATIONS FOR FORCEPS

Most forceps operations are done without clear-cut indication, ostensibly as prophylactic measures. *Prophylactic forceps*, introduced by DeLee in 1920, is a popular concept in the United States based on the rationalization that it will (1) reduce the effort and discomfort of the second stage of labor, (2) save the pelvic floor and adjacent fascia from overstretching, (3) reduce blood loss and (4) preserve the fetal brain from prolonged compression. Whether or not these alleged benefits are true has never been verified or refuted. DeLee warned against the wide adoption of this procedure, believing that this would result in a high maternal and neonatal mortality, defeating the very purposes intended. Intelligent expectancy should still be the guide for the clinician and he should intervene only in the presence of an immediate or a prospective danger to the mother or the fetus.

Aside from prophylactic forceps, most indicated forceps operations are done to correct *arrest of progress* with the fetal head on the perineal floor. This is usually associated with (1) insufficient uterine and expulsive forces, (2) excessively resistant or inelastic perineal tissues, (3) a somewhat enlarged fetal head or (4) a malposition or a malpresentation. Combinations of these factors are common. Among malpositions, arrest of rotation, especially with persistent occiput posterior positions, is a frequent indication for use of forceps. Usually, spontaneous rotation is stopped in the transverse diameter of the pelvis to produce a *deep transverse arrest.*

Fetal distress warrants a forceps operation if conditions are appropriate for delivery. One must always weigh the relative risks of this procedure against those of other methods for delivery, such as cesarean section, or further delay to allow more optimal conditions to evolve for spontaneous delivery or a less hazardous forceps operation. Indeed, whenever a forceps procedure is undertaken, the fullest consideration must be given to the prevailing conditions (see below).

Complications which affect the mother or the fetus may serve as indications to justify use of forceps. Some of these are hypertensive states, pulmonary tuberculosis, heart disease, maternal exhaustion, abruptio placentae and prolapse of the cord.

CONDITIONS FOR FORCEPS DELIVERY

Certain conditions must always be fulfilled before forceps procedures are undertaken in order to minimize maternal and fetal hazards. (1) It is mandatory that forceps never be used by the uninitiated or unskilled; the requisite skills are acquired by manikin practice and closely supervised, extensive experience under very selective, optimal circumstances. This point bears emphasis. (2) The pelvis must be large enough to permit delivery of an undamaged fetus. A forceps procedure in which the instrument is applied when this fact is unknown or in doubt is considered a *trial forceps;* this exception will be considered separately later (see below). (3) The cervix must be completely effaced and dilated. (4) The patient's bladder and rectum must be empty. (5) Anesthesia is required. (6) The fetus must be in cephalic presentation. (7) The fetal presentation and position must be known precisely. (8) The head must be engaged with the biparietal diameter well below the inlet. (9) The membranes must be ruptured so that a good purchase can be obtained with the forceps on the head without risk of slippage. (10) The fetus must be alive.

TYPES OF FORCEPS OPERATIONS

Aside from forceps to the aftercoming head (see Chapter 74), forceps operations are divided into *outlet forceps, midforceps* and *high forceps.* They are defined on the basis of the station and the position of the head at the time the instrument is applied. The following are the current official definitions adopted by the American College of Obstetricians and Gynecologists (Hughes):

DEFINITIONS —

"A *low forceps operation* is the application of obstetric forceps to the fetal skull when the scalp is or has been visible at the introitus without separating the labia, the skull has reached the pelvic floor, and the sagittal suture is in the anteroposterior diameter of the outlet of the pelvis.

"A *midforceps operation* is the application of obstetric forceps to the fetal skull when the head is engaged, but the conditions for low forceps have not been met. In the context of this term, any forceps operation requiring artificial rotation, regardless of the station from which extraction is begun, shall be designated a 'midforceps operation.'

"A *high forceps operation* is the application of obstetric forceps at any time prior to the engagement of the fetal head." High forceps delivery carries such great risks to both mother and baby that it is never justified and is categorically condemned.

Greater scientific accuracy in describing the specific procedure may be obtained by designating the precise station (see Chapter 19) and position. According to this scheme, for example, the forceps application is at station +2 to a head in the right occiput posterior position. In this way, this operation can be separately designated

from a midforceps procedure done on a fetal head in the same position, but at station +4 or +5.

TECHNIQUE OF FORCEPS DELIVERY

When the sagittal suture of the fetal head lies in the anteroposterior diameter of the pelvis and the forceps is applied to the head so that the axis of the blades lies in the transverse, the head will be grasped in the most favorable manner and delivery will be attended with the least difficulty. This might be called the ideal or normal application (Fig. 430).

The ideal application of the forceps for any given fetal head is with the axis of the shanks perpendicular to the sagittal suture, with the toes or apices of the blades anchored around the zygomatous processes of the maxilla bilaterally. The anterior or front edge of each blade (that is, the side of the concavity on which the lock opens) should lie just in front of the fetal ear. The front of the forceps faces the occiput and is close to and equidistant from the lambdoidal sutures on either side; the

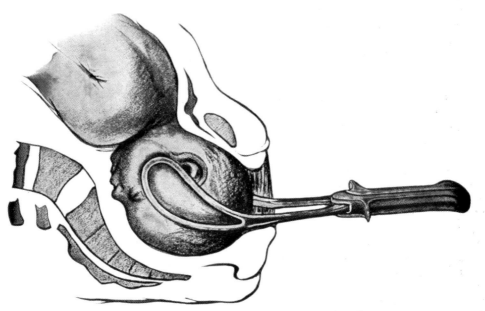

Figure 430   The forceps applied in its most favorable position to a head in a direct occiput anterior position over the perineum. Note location of blades in front of the fetus' ears, anchored below the zygoma.

heels of the blades overlie the parietal bones.

A forceps procedure consists of five separate maneuvers: (1) applying the blades, (2) checking the application, (3) adapting, adjusting and locking, (4) extracting the head and (5) removing the instrument.

Application to the Head

The bladder is catheterized with a soft rubber catheter. Two fingers are passed into the vagina to examine the region carefully. Special attention is directed to ascertaining that all conditions are met, especially with reference to the cervix, membranes, station and position. Anesthesia is given, either by inhalation or regional or local block.

Choice of the type of forceps to be used will depend on the degree of molding anticipated, the shape of the pelvis and any special problems encountered. Generally, for the well-molded head resulting from a long labor, especially in a nullipara, a Simpson type, such as the DeLee forceps or the like, can be used to advantage; for the relatively unmolded head in a multipara after a short labor, one of the Elliot type, such as the Tucker-McLane forceps or equivalent, is used.

The blade to be inserted first, right or left, depends on the position of the fetal head. For occiput anterior and left occiput anterior positions, the left blade is applied first; for right occiput anterior position, it is necessary to insert the right blade first. By applying the more posterior blade first, one prevents the head from rotating to the posterior during the wandering maneuver (see below) that must take place while the anterior blade is adjusted.

Sometimes, the occiput will rotate anteriorly during the insertion of the posterior blade. In fact, it is a common practice to make a deliberate effort to effect anterior rotation by applying slight internal pressure (clockwise in a right occiput anterior). When a single blade of a forceps is used alone in this manner, it is called a *vectis;* it is occasionally quite useful in this regard.

The preference for applying the left blade whenever there is equal option is based on the construction of all locks

which necessitate laying the right blade on top of the left, where the lock is located, to articulate properly. Otherwise, the handles would have to be recrossed outside the vulva after the application; this might subject the maternal tissues and the fetus to injury. Furthermore, this manipulation might allow the cord to fall into the grasp of the blades.

If the left blade is chosen, its handle is held lightly in the left hand, and the right hand is introduced into the vagina along the left side of the maternal pelvis. The toe of the forceps blade is introduced along the palm of the hand in the vagina as shown in Figure 431. The handle is poised at first vertically over the introitus so that the blade can be passed along the pelvic curvature with utmost gentleness and delicacy.

Nothing must lie between the forceps and the head; to be certain of this, the fingers should be passed up as high as possible, guarding the tip of the forceps blade until it passes beyond reach. As the blade is slipped along the fingers in the vagina, the toe is held close to the head. The thumb of the right hand is used to guide and press the blade into place. The handle is lowered progressively as the blade advances inside the pelvis. Pressure is never applied to the handle to advance the blade into the pelvis; to do so may cause great damage. Usually, the blades, if properly applied, fall into the right position by their own weight.

The right blade is then passed in like manner, four fingers of the left hand being inserted to act as a guide and to protect maternal tissues. If the fetal position is directly occiput anterior, the right blade will be introduced precisely as the left one had been and will seek its proper location opposite the left blade at the side of the pelvis. If the position is left occiput anterior, however, the left blade will lie in the left posterolateral aspect of the pelvis; the right blade must be *wandered* by the left hand in the vagina, using the gentlest pressure, in a clockwise direction until it is seated properly alongside the head in the right anterolateral pelvis.

The same technique is used if the position is right occiput anterior, except the right blade is introduced first into the right

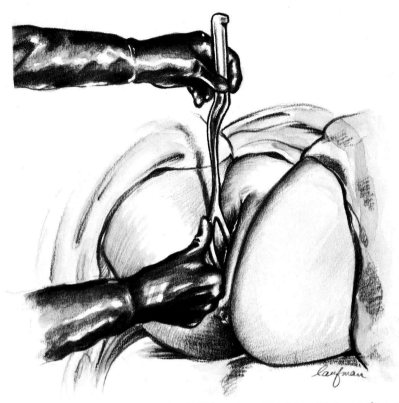

Figure 431 The left blade of the forceps, which is held loosely in the left hand, is inserted into the left side of the pelvis along the left side of the fetal head in an occiput anterior position.

posterolateral pelvis. Then the left blade is inserted and wandered to the left antero-lateral location. Subsequently, the blades are crossed and locked.

Checking the Application

After both blades are in place, they are articulated and the application is carefully checked for accuracy. The points to be remembered are: (1) the shanks are exactly perpendicular to the sagittal suture; (2) the lambdoidal sutures are each about 1 cm. anterior to the front edge of the forceps blades and equidistant; (3) no more than one fingertip can be insinuated under the heel of each blade over the parietal bones.

If the shanks are not perpendicular, the instrument is not aligned with the head and it will be necessary to unlock and adjust the blades so that both are moved clockwise or counterclockwise to fit the head more correctly. This error is con-

firmed by finding that the lambdoidal sutures are not equidistant from the front of the blades. If equidistant but greater than 1 cm., the position of the lambdoidal sutures demonstrates the application to a deflexed head; this, too, will have to be adjusted.

If there is more than one fingertip of space beneath the heels, it is likely either that the forceps chosen is too long or too tapered for the head or that the toes are anchored behind the zygomas; both possibilities are very serious errors because of the danger of trauma from slippage that is likely to result.

Adaptation, Adjustment and Locking

This movement will depend on the presentation and position of the head, since the blades must be applied to fit the head in the best way. If the head is low and the occiput has rotated to the front, the blades will fit naturally to the sides of the head. Often, however, they need a little adjusting before it is possible to fit the lock neatly. The easiest way to bring the blades into position is to press the unlocked handles gently downward onto the perineum. Forced locking always results in injury to the mother or the fetus.

Usually, the physician will find he has made a diagnostic error as to position if the blades will not lock easily. To correct this he must determine precisely the direction and the degree of the error in terms of the forceps application according to the guidelines just described. If the error is rotational (the fetal head is in left occiput anterior position, but the forceps is applied as if it were direct occiput anterior, for example), one must adjust the blades smoothly to the sides of the head by making one blade wander a little anteriorly and the other a little posteriorly. The wandering maneuver involves unlocking the blades and with the appropriate hand in the vagina (the right hand for the left blade) lifting or lowering the blade gently into place. The external hand applies no pressure whatsoever and merely supports the handle.

If the error is one of deflexion, this is correctable by disarticulating the blades, and raising them toward the occiput one at a time before rearticulating and locking them. The error of poor fit (toes anchored behind the zygomas, for example) connotes a poor choice of instrument or a badly misapplied forceps; in either instance, the forceps should be removed entirely.

After the blades are locked, the heart tones should be auscultated. If they suddenly become faint or slow, the cord may be in the grasp of the forceps. The blades should be unlocked at once. By pushing one or two fingers up along the back of the fetal neck, behind the pubis, it is possible to feel the cord if it encircles the neck. The instrument must be removed and reapplied if the cord is being compressed by the toe of the forceps.

Extraction of the Head

The principles of traction are the following: (1) Each traction is made to imitate uterine contractions. The pull is gradual at first, slowly reaches an acme, is held for a moment and then slowly relaxed. (2) As little force is used as possible, regulating the amount by the advance of the head. With the elbows at the sides and the arms flexed, the strength of the biceps alone should suffice. Time should be disregarded, but the fetal heart tones should be watched carefully. (3) If rotation is complete, the traction should be simple and direct in the proper pelvic axis. It should not be combined with pendulum, corkscrew or twisting motions. (4) Traction should not be straight out, but forward and downward, following the curve of the pelvic canal (Fig. 432). The proper direction can be obtained by combined outward traction on the handles and downward pressure on the shanks; the vector force that will result from this combined maneuver, called the *Saxtorph-Pajot maneuver,* will be more in the pelvic axis (see *Axis Traction,* below, and Fig. 437). (5) Avoid compressing the fetal head by insinuating a finger between the handles.

The handle is grasped by the left hand with the right hand on the shank (Fig. 432). Traction is applied as indicated above in terms of amount, timing and direction. The progress of the head is determined carefully and the head is allowed to recede very slowly; the heart tones are then auscultated. The forceps is loosened after each traction, but the handles are not separated too far. After a minute, another and slightly stronger traction is made, if necessary.

The descent and rotation of the head are determined by frequent examinations. Traction is made upward along the outward projection of the pelvic axis as the head bulges the perineum. To deliver the infant, the physician grasps the forceps at the shank with one hand and gently and slowly draws the head up and out over the perineum, mimicking the spontaneous mechanism.

To save the pelvic floor, one will often need an episiotomy, especially in nulliparas. If the physician wishes to deliver without an episiotomy, he must bring the head through the pelvic floor very slowly, allowing the perineum to stretch slowly and taking as much time as a natural delivery would require.

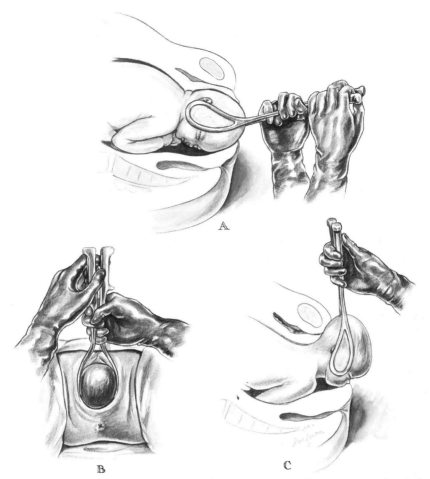

Figure 432 Low forceps delivery. *A*, The forceps are in place; the handles are separated with the left index finger and thumb; the pull is forward and downward with combined forces. *B*, Traction is continued, but with partial extension of the head; the handles are separated to avoid compression of the fetal head. *C*, The head is delivered by further extension over the perineum.

Removal of the Forceps

When the widest diameter of the fetal head is about to pass the vulvar ring, the forceps is removed. The slight lessening in circumference (by 5 to 8 mm.) from removing the instrument may be advantageous in averting tissue injury. Sometimes it is necessary to leave the forceps on until after the head is delivered; at other times, one may remove it earlier and proceed with the modified Ritgen maneuver (see Chapter 20) to effect a more natural delivery.

Removal of forceps is the reverse of application, taking care not to injure the fetal scalp or ear or maternal soft tissue. The blades are unlocked, disarticulated and removed one at a time, holding them by the handles and pulling gently in an upward direction toward the opposite side, maintaining the cephalic curve and toe closely applied to the head. As the blades come off the head, the handles come to lie over the mother's abdomen (the handle of the left blade goes to the right lower abdominal quadrant). The rest of the delivery is exactly the same as in a spontaneous delivery, with all appropriate measures taken to care for the fetus and the mother (see Chapter 20).

MORE COMPLEX FORCEPS PROCEDURES

Most forceps operations will involve the techniques described above. Only occasionally will other circumstances be encountered to warrant use of forceps. These include persistent occiput posterior positions, deep transverse arrests and face and brow presentations, all of which will be discussed here. We have already dealt with forceps to the aftercoming head in Chapter 74.

Forceps in Occiput Posterior Position

The pros and cons of manual and forceps rotations versus delivery as occipitosacral have been presented in Chapter 56, to which the reader is referred. If it were possible to rotate the head to occiput anterior without trauma, this would undoubtedly be preferable for delivery. However, because rotation may not be easy to accomplish, it may be necessary to deliver the head with the posterior fontanel over the perineum (Fig. 433) as an occipitosacral. This is particularly true in women with android and anthropoid pelves in which prominent ischial spines may prevent one from rotating the head past the transverse (see below).

The technique of forceps delivery as an occiput posterior is identical with that for occiput anterior, except that the forceps is applied to the head as if it actually were in the occiput anterior position; however, since it must fit the pelvis, the instrument

is applied in reverse fashion to the head so that the posterior fontanel is located toward the back of the blades rather than to the front. Moreover, since flexion tends to be rather poor in this position, attention must be directed at correcting it before applying traction for the delivery. In addition, since the presenting fetal diameters are larger and the actual plane in which the biparietal diameter lies tends to be higher, the axis of direction of the traction must be lower and the episiotomy larger.

For forceps deliveries in occiput posterior with rotation to occiput anterior, four objectives must be accomplished: flexion, synclitization, rotation and extraction. Disregard of the first two may render the others difficult or impossible. It is understood that the cervix must be retracted and completely dilated out of the way.

First, a correct diagnosis of the position, station, flexion and synclitism must be made; the cephalopelvic relationships should be reevaluated to ensure adequacy before proceeding. It would be traumatic to try to turn the head in a direction opposite to that which is optimal for the fetus according to how the body lies. If the back is to the right, for example, the occiput should be rotated around the right side of the pelvis; in back left positions, it is swung to the left side. If the caput succedaneum is large and obliterates the usual landmarks, an ear should be located

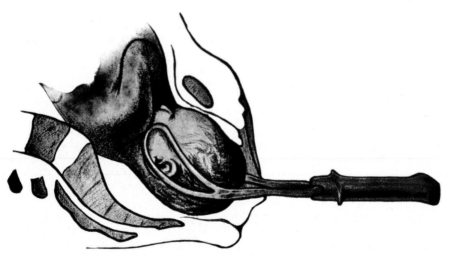

Figure 433 Forceps applied in the occipitosacral position on the pelvic floor. The larger presenting fetal diameters require more distention of the perineum and delivery by flexion of the head through the pelvic curve.

and its direction identified; the tragus points to the face.

An attempt should be made, under anesthesia, to effect *manual rotation*. The right hand is inserted in left occiput posterior positions and the left hand in right positions. The fingers are applied to the posterior parietal boss and the thumb is placed over the anterior malar bone to grasp the head. With a slow twist of the wrist, the occiput is turned part of the way around as described in Chapter 73. Supinating the hand before grasping the head will allow one to pronate through a longer arc, thereby sometimes bringing the occiput a full 180° anteriorly. If rotation past the transverse cannot be accomplished in either direction, the forceps may be applied to effect delivery as an occiput posterior or, alternatively, to attempt forceps rotation (see below).

As stated above, to deliver the head as an occiput posterior, the forceps application is made as for an occiput anterior position, but the front of the forceps points toward the forehead. Articulation and locking the blades are the same as usual. After they are locked, the handles are raised a little toward the pubis to increase flexion. Traction is made in the appropriate axis as described earlier for forceps traction in occiput anterior positions. The occiput is delivered first over the perineum with the forehead resting behind the pubis; the brow and face then come from under the pubis.

As a rule it is advisable to perform a deep episiotomy to avoid extensive lacerations of the pelvic floor and anal sphincter. Use of axis-traction forceps for this procedure, preferred by some obstetricians, will be discussed later in this chapter.

Forceps in Deep Transverse Arrest

With delay in the second stage manifest by arrest of descent for some time, examination may reveal the head well down in the pelvis, the sagittal suture in the transverse diameter and both fontanels on the same level. This condition is called *deep transverse arrest* and is troublesome. One must first be concerned over the possibility that cephalopelvic disproportion may

be the cause of this serious problem (see Chapter 63). This should be critically evaluated before proceeding. If disproportion is present, vaginal delivery should not be attempted. The principles of treatment for the remainder are similar to those of occiput posterior positions in general. If manual correction fails, reliance is to be placed on forceps.

It is obvious that, in transverse arrest, if the forceps were applied to the sides of the head, the blades would have to lie in the conjugate diameter of the pelvis. This is mechanically poor because there would be danger of injury, especially to the bladder by the anterior blade. If the instrument were placed transversely, on the other hand, the head would be grasped over the face and occiput, causing serious damage. Application of the classic forceps under these circumstances is very difficult to accomplish correctly without injuring the mother or fetus.

For transverse arrest with the fetal head in right occiput transverse, the forceps can sometimes be applied by the following maneuvers, recognizing its traumatic potentiality: The right blade is introduced directly posteriorly to seat itself across the right maxilla in front of the sacrum. By placing the right blade first, one prevents the head from rotating to an occiput posterior position during the next step which involves wandering the left blade over the face. The left blade is held in the left hand and introduced along the palm of the right hand which has been insinuated along the posterolateral aspect of the left side of the pelvis. As the left blade is being advanced, the fingers and thumb of the right hand exert slight counterclockwise pressure to cause the blade to wander over the face (Fig. 434), past the frontal bosses, until it is just beneath the symphysis pubis and in place alongside the left maxilla. At the same time, the handle is moved through an arc of nearly 180° from the vertical pointing up first during introduction and then to the vertical pointing down at completion.

Once in place, the two blades are articulated, the application checked and corrected, if necessary, and they are locked. When they are correctly in position and the head is properly flexed, the handles will point transversely to the right thigh.

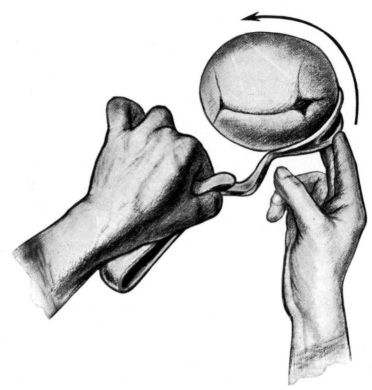

Figure 434 Schematic demonstration of the wandering maneuver in right occiput transverse position. The left blade has been introduced posterolaterally into the left side of the pelvis and wandered counterclockwise across the frontal bosses by gentle digital pressure applied with the right hand in the vagina.

For left occiput transverse, all maneuvers are opposite those just described, left substituting for right.

The difficulties inherent in this application are based on (1) the unphysiologic position of the forceps when in place, (2) the trauma to the bladder if traction should be applied, (3) the problem of wandering the blade across the face, and (4) the commonly coassociated prominent ischial spines and narrowed transverse diameter of the midplane. As to this last point, it is the very cause of the deep transverse arrest that makes it so difficult to effect good forceps applications using classic types of instruments; special varieties have been devised for this particular purpose (see below).

If the application has been attempted and is successful, it is imperative that no traction be made while the pelvic curve of the forceps is at right angles to the patient's own pelvic curve. To do so would cause great damage.

Forceps rotation should be done instead at this time to effect correction of the malposition to occiput anterior and then to mimic the natural mechanisms. Forceps rotation must be done with the greatest delicacy. A great deal of force can be exerted in rotations that may damage maternal and fetal tissues severely. Rotation is not accomplished by twisting the handles in their own axis; this would result in attempting to swing the toes through an arc within the pelvis (Fig. 435). Instead, the handles are carried gently through a wide arc in front of the perineum.

For the right occiput transverse application just described, the handles begin at 9 o'clock facing the right thigh and are rotated to 12 o'clock facing vertically up. In this way the occiput moves from the right transverse to directly anterior. The same principle applies to the forceps rotation from occiput posterior positions.

Forceps rotation may sometimes be done even when the application to the fetal head is imperfect, albeit considerably more hazardous. It is accomplished by the

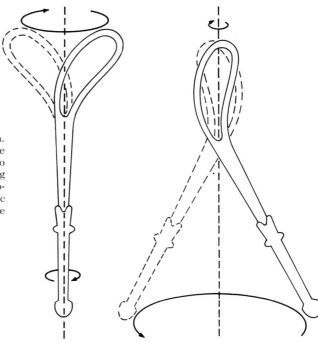

Figure 435 Principle of forceps rotation. *A*, If handles of the classic forceps were to be twisted as shown, the blades would tend to describe an arc in the pelvis, perhaps tearing the vagina and damaging the fetus. *B*, Rotating handles correctly through a wide arc imparts a smooth rotary movement to the blades in the pelvis.

A   B

so-called *key-in-lock maneuver.* Forceps are applied to the head in posterior or transverse position to fit the pelvic curve, essentially ignoring the fact of misapplication as a brow-mastoid or occipitomental application. Traction in such poor applications would almost surely damage the fetus, but gentle rotation should not. The forceps handles are carried through a short segment of its wide arc to rotate the occiput toward the anterior a few degrees; the blades are disarticulated, readjusted to fit the pelvis again and relocked. Then another partial rotation is carried out, and the performance repeated until rotation is complete and the head is in an occiput anterior position with the forceps properly applied to both the head and the pelvis.

After rotation is complete, the forceps may be removed and the birth left to nature if the heart tones are good. This may be desirable in nulliparas with slightly contracted outlets or large fetuses. In a few hours the contractions will have molded the head so as to permit spontaneous delivery after episiotomy or an easy outlet forceps application. The benefits may outweigh the objections to such a two-stage

procedure. More often, however, because of the anesthesia, the fetal condition or the mother's exhaustion, delivery is effected as previously described with appropriately directed, intermittent traction in the occiput anterior mechanism.

Scanzoni-Smellie Operation. This method of dealing with occiput posterior positions (often called *Scanzoni maneuver* or *Scanzoni rotation*) is fraught with great danger to the maternal soft tissues and to the fetus. It involves two forceps applications: the first to effect rotation, the second for delivery. Because this technique is still widely used, it is described here for completeness; but its hazards do not warrant its continued use.

The blades of a classic type of forceps are applied with the front pointing toward the forehead as described for delivery as occipitosacral (see above). By gently rotating the instrument through a wide arc of 180°, the occiput is brought anteriorly; this, of course, inverts the forceps so that the toes are pointing to the sacrum. Traction is impossible.

The instrument is removed and reapplied just as in an occiput anterior position. Usually, to prevent the head from rotating back to the occiput transverse or posterior position, one or both blades of the first instrument are left on and a different pair is used for the second application. After the second pair has been applied, the first is removed and delivery then effected.

Fenestrated forceps should not be used as the first instrument here because the blades of the second may be introduced inadvertently through the fenestration, interdicting any possibility of the first being removed afterwards. The procedure is completed as usual after rotation has occurred. Manual rotation is much safer than rotation with forceps.

Forceps in Face Presentation

Face presentation by itself is not an indication for forceps delivery, but labor may be delayed and help is frequently required with all the deflexion attitudes. In addition to all the conditions demanded for forceps in general, the chin must not be posterior to the transverse diameter of the pelvis. Anterior rotation of the chin, at least to the transverse diameter, must have occurred. Atraumatic delivery cannot be

note!

expected with a mentum posterior position unless rotation can be effected; such rotation to a mentum anterior can sometimes be done with Kielland forceps (see below).

Application of the blades of classic forceps after the chin has rotated is easy, although care is required not to injure the eyes of the fetus. Adaptation and locking are different from occiput cases. It is usually necessary to raise the handles before locking them. This sinks the toes of the blades toward the hollow of the sacrum and thus a firmer hold over the parietal bosses is obtained. The blades will slip anteriorly over the sinciput off the narrow brow if they are placed and locked in the usual manner. After locking, the handles are lowered to increase extension (Fig. 436) and reduce the presenting diameters.

Traction is first downward to increase deflexion further, then in the horizontal plane until the chin is well out from under the pubis and finally upward to follow the projection of the pelvic curve. Upward traction should not be as acute as in occiput presentations because the delicate fetal larynx may be injured if acutely flexed and pressed against the undersurface of the pubic bone. Episiotomy should be the rule with face presentation, especially in nulliparas.

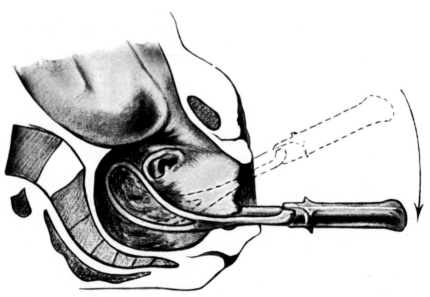

Figure 436 Forceps applied in face presentation to the mentum anterior position. Dotted lines show the forceps as it is first applied. After the handles are lowered to increase extension of the head, traction may be used to effect delivery of the face over the perineum by flexion through the pelvic curvature.

Forceps in Brow Presentation

What was said about face presentation applies here if it is the intention to deliver as a brow presentation with the bregma anterior. The brow, instead of the chin, must be brought to the pubis and appear in the vulva; the face is to remain behind the symphysis until the occiput can be brought over the perineum, after which the face comes down from behind the pubis. However, Kielland forceps (see below) can often be used successfully to flex a head to a vertex presentation by successive locking-flexing-disarticulating combinations of movements or to extend the head to a face presentation by comparable extension maneuvers.

Axis-Traction Procedures

Some obstetricians recommend the axis-traction forceps for deliveries begun when the head is not deeply engaged. Midforceps procedures which utilize this device permit force to be applied to the head parallel to the axis of the pelvis at all levels.

The head must traverse the pelvic curve. Because of the forward projection of the sacrum and the perineum, traction cannot be applied easily in the axis of the inlet. If applied in any other line, the force is misapplied and may cause serious injury to mother and fetus. If a deep episiotomy is performed, the lower pelvic curve is straightened out to a degree, but it is usually inadequate for purposes of effecting traction above station +3 or +4.

Figure 437 shows the effect of the ordinary forceps when applied on the head in midplane; if traction is made in the usual way, a large part of the force will be exerted against the symphysis. The Saxtorph-Pajot maneuver may accomplish a more appropriate pull in the proper axis by summating two vector forces: by pulling downward with one hand over the lock

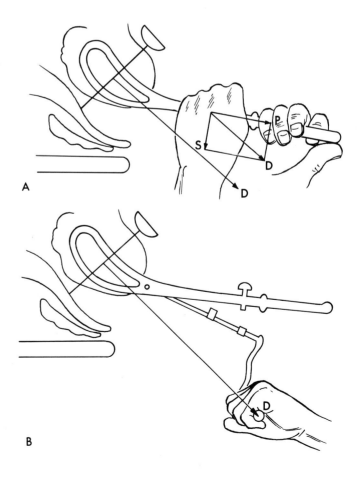

Figure 437 Axis-traction principle illustrating head with biparietal diameter at level of the inlet plane. *A*, Using classic forceps, traction on handles alone supplies force *P*; adding Saxtorph-Pajot downward pressure on the shanks *S* yields vector force *D* in the proper pelvic axis. *B*, Forceps equipped with axis-traction bar attached to the heels of the blades will provide the same directional force *D*.

and pulling straight out with the other hand, the net direction one achieves should approximate the correct axis of pull. By varying the amount of pressure applied either to the shank or to the handle, one can change the axis of pull without actually changing the position of the forceps relative to the head or the pelvis.

Axis-traction forceps, first conceived by Tarnier, is designed to provide a means for traction on the head in the exact axis of the pelvis. Moreover, the head has sufficient mobility while being pulled so that it can respond fairly easily to labor mechanisms. The hazards of its use, however, may outweigh its theoretical advantages. Axis-traction forceps allows the physician to begin traction before the head is well down in the pelvis, potentially causing trauma. Needless to say, this is not the fault of the instrument but rather of the physician who undertakes to do a difficult operation ill-advisedly. Moreover, the axis-traction handle does permit use of greater traction forces for delivery; such forces are decried because of the damage they inflict.

SPECIAL FORCEPS

Kielland Forceps

Kielland introduced a forceps especially designed for rotation of the fetal head from occiput posterior or transverse positions to the anterior in an anthropoid pelvis. He eliminated the pelvic curve so that the instrument could be applied directly and correctly to the fetal head whatever its position in the pelvis and almost without regard for the relationship of the forceps to the pelvis. Kielland forceps has overlap-

ping shanks and a sliding lock; it is light-weight and has a small knob on each handle to indicate the direction of the occiput (Fig. 438).

The blades adapt to the sides of the head when it lies with its long diameter in the transverse diameter. They may also be used as a simple rotator to deliver a transverse arrest or persistent occiput posterior with ease and safety, as well as for correction of a mentum posterior position or brow presentation. They can also correct asynclitism because of the special design of the sliding lock.

Kielland forceps has a definite place in the specialist's armamentarium. In occipitosacral position, the forceps is applied "upside down" (with the knobs on the shanks pointing down to the occiput). The rotation is then accomplished in the axis of the forceps handles rather than in the wide arc of classic forceps. After the rotation is completed, the occiput is in an anterior position, with the forceps still correctly applied.

Traction can be made in the usual manner, except that the handles cannot be raised over the horizontal because the blades are almost straight and to do so would cause the toes to dig into the vaginal sulci. To effect extension of the fetal head over the perineum, it is merely necessary to disarticulate the blades, lower them one at a time, rearticulate them and raise them again to the horizontal. This can be repeated again and as often as needed to accomplish the delivery without endangering the maternal tissues. This disadvantage aside, the Kielland forceps is much more effective and less traumatic than classic forceps for such rotations in anthropoid pelves.

In transverse arrest, there are two different ways in which Kielland forceps can

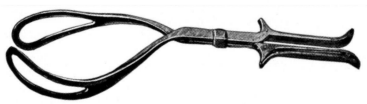

Figure 438 Kielland forceps showing almost total absence of a pelvic curve, sliding lock on overlapping shanks, lightweight construction and small knobs on the handles to designate direction of the occiput.

be applied. Kielland described an inversion method by which the anterior blade (the left blade in right occiput transverse) is inserted behind the symphysis pubis upside down (that is, with the cephalic curve facing up away from the head) and then gently rotated into position inside the lower uterine segment against the head. The toe is guided by the fingertips and inserted so that it hugs the anterior aspect of the head as it advances into the lower segment; the handle is progressively lowered and, as the narrow heel passes under the symphysis, slight rotational pressure on the handle will pull the blade over away from the occiput, turning it 180° over on itself to seat it in place. The left blade rotates clockwise in right occiput transverse applications, with the front curvature held against the left side of the fetal head.

This requires the utmost in delicacy and skill to avoid traumatizing the bladder or perforating the lower uterine segment. One should never persist against resistance. It should not be undertaken at all if there is pelvic narrowing or thinning of the lower segment. Use of Kielland forceps is contraindicated in flat pelves.

The alternative to the inversion method is the wandering technique previously described. Wandering the blade is less hazardous than direct insertion, but when wandering cannot be accomplished, as in a deep transverse arrest with prominent ischial spines, direct application is a useful maneuver.

After Kielland forceps has been applied to the transverse position of the head, asynclitism is recognized by the fact that, when articulated, the blades are not directly apposed to each other. By sliding one handle along the other by means of the sliding lock, one corrects the asynclitism automatically.

Barton Forceps

Barton forceps (Fig. 439) differs from classic forceps in having both pelvic and cephalic curves in the same plane instead of at right angles; in addition to a sliding lock and a hinged anterior blade, Barton forceps has axis-traction handles available. The hinge on the anterior blade allows this

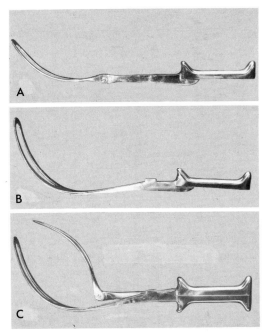

Figure 439 Barton forceps demonstrating (*A*) hinged anterior blade extended fully, (*B*) sharply angulated posterior blade and (*C*) articulated forceps with congruent pelvic and cephalic curves, overlapping shanks and sliding lock.

blade to be aligned with the shank for easier insertion.

This special forceps was constructed so that it could be applied correctly in a flat pelvis to the fetal head arrested in a transverse position, without disturbing its relationship to the pelvic axis. The blades join the shanks at an angle corresponding to the 135° angle made by the intersection of the axis of the pelvic brim and outlet. Both blades are fenestrated, flat on their inner surface.

The anterior blade is straightened (Fig. 440) in order for it to be introduced into the posterior pelvis. It is then wandered around the occiput (rarely around the brow) until it is in place beneath the symphysis. During the wandering maneuver, the anterior blade is "folded" at the hinge. The posterior blade is placed along the sacrum and is articulated with the anterior blade. The two blades are aligned along their sliding lock to correct asynclitism; traction is then applied in the correct pelvic axis utilizing combined downward pressure on the shank and slight pull on the handles. Alternatively, the axis-trac-

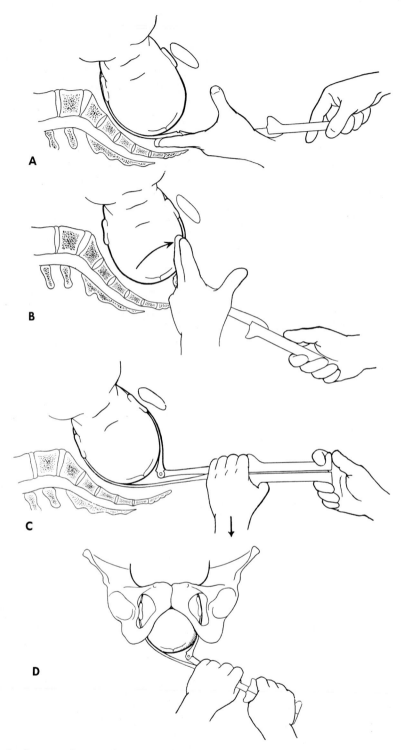

Figure 440 Application of Barton forceps to a head in right occiput transverse position at station +2 in a flat pelvis. *A*, The anterior blade is extended and introduced posteriorly along the sacrum. *B*, It is wandered 180° clockwise over the occiput to beneath the symphysis pubis; during the wandering maneuver, the blade is flexed at the hinge. *C*, The posterior blade is introduced posteriorly and the blades are articulated; traction is applied by pressure on the shanks (arrow) and slight pull on the handles. *D*, Rotation of the handles through widest arc brings the occiput to the anterior only after the head has reached the perineum.

tion handle may be used to good advantage.

After the head has advanced to the outlet in the transverse position, rotation may be effected by very gently rotating the handle through the widest arc so that the occiput comes to the front and the handle faces one thigh. Care must be taken not to lift the blades above the horizontal from this point on because of the damage that may occur to the vaginal sulci from the toes of the blades. The technique for extending the head described for Kielland forceps (see above) is equally applicable here, although it is generally easier to remove the Barton forceps and proceed with delivery using the modified Ritgen maneuver (see Chapter 20).

Parallel Forceps

Several varieties of special forceps have been devised as convenient instruments, using the principles of parallelism (Shute) and divergence (Laufe). Thierry used two spatulas as extensions of his hands, manipulating them individually. The parts do not cross or articulate and appear to be useful for gentle traction, rotation and flexion maneuvers without inflicting injury.

The advantages of the Shute forceps (Fig. 441) are the following: (1) The blades move easily in complete parallelism, thus fitting almost every head accurately regardless of size. (2) The blades are shorter and straighter than those of classic forceps so that they can rotate a head with a straight twisting motion, as with the Kielland forceps. (3) Since the cephalic curve is straight and the blades narrow, the parallel forceps can be applied more easily in almost any fetal position. (4) The mechanism of the lock is simple and will maintain perfect parallelism even though the handles or shanks are not completely apposed to each other. (5) The technique of using the parallel forceps is simple and effective.

Pearse and Kolbeck recently reported good experience with these forceps. They measured compressive forces and found them to be somewhat less than that of comparably applied Simpson-type forceps.

The Laufe forceps does not cross, but

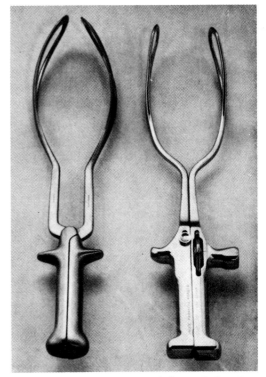

Figure 441 Comparison of classic DeLee-Simpson forceps (left) with Shute parallel forceps (right), illustrating differences in cephalic curves and scissors articulation versus parallel blades.

has a pivot lock at the distal end of the handles (Fig. 442). The lateral mobility that this provides allows the forceps to fit any size head, but without maintaining parallelism. A perineal curve is incorporated into the shank and handles to permit axis traction automatically when the finger grips are used. The instrument is useful for outlet forceps delivery. It appears to diminish compressive forces on the head somewhat.

Vacuum Extractor

Malmström developed a sophisticated instrument based on an ancient principle of scalp traction using a suction device for purchase. It has found wide acceptance abroad, where it has largely replaced forceps in some areas, but has not become popular in the United States. Malmström's vacuum extractor (Fig. 443) attaches a metal traction cup to the scalp by applying negative pressure to create a "chignon" of artificial caput succedaneum (Fig. 444). Traction is made on a chain passed through the suction tube. Cups of 30, 40 and 50 mm. diameters are available for use.

The site of application of the traction cup should, if possible, be the vertex area over the posterior fontanel. Negative pressure is built up slowly over at least a 10-minute interval to one atmosphere vacuum (−0.7 kilogram per square centimeter).

Vacuum extractor delivery is a series of tractions synchronized with the labor contractions and applied in the appropriate pelvic axis. To accomplish traction in the proper axis, one hand pulls on the chain and the other presses the head and the cup toward the sacrum to effect the necessary vector force. During descent, the head undergoes spontaneous rotation to accommodate itself optimally to the pelvic dimensions. The direction of traction is changed continuously along the pelvic axis.

The main indication for the vacuum ex-

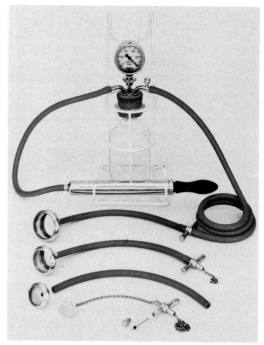

Figure 443   Constituent components of the Malmström vacuum extractor. From bottom up, traction chain; 30, 40 and 50 mm. scalp traction cups with suction tubing, chain and traction handle attached; hand pump (now almost entirely replaced by electrical suction equipment); glass vacuum trap and gauge.

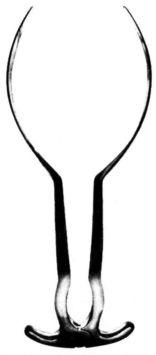

Figure 442   The Laufe divergent forceps showing pivot lock and finger grips at distal end of handles for use in effecting traction in low forceps operations. The perineal curve of the shank is not apparent in this view. (From Laufe, L. E.: Amer. J. Obstet. Gynec. 101:509, 1968.)

tractor is dysfunctional labor without cephalopelvic disproportion. Pathologic presentations and positions can be corrected by using the vacuum extractor, and it may even accelerate labor and delivery. The instrument is easy to use and effective.

Trauma to the scalp is common, however, especially if the vacuum is applied rapidly or maintained for excessively long periods of time (more than 30 minutes). Subgaleal hematomas, scalp lacerations and necrosis occur. Similarly, maternal soft tissues may be injured. Intracranial and intraocular hemorrhages have also been reported. However, in the hands of the novice, there is little doubt that less damage can be done with the vacuum extractor than with obstetric forceps (Chalmers).

Paradoxically, the ease with which this device can be used by the unskilled is perhaps its greatest disadvantage; forceful traction is too easily substituted for critical study, judgment and understanding of pathologic labor mechanisms. Thus, the

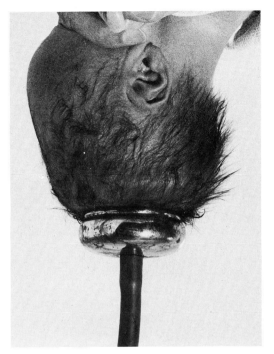

Figure 444 Malmström vacuum extractor attached to scalp of a recently delivered infant showing metal cup in place over the artificial caput succedaneum.

trauma reported to result occasionally from the use of the vacuum extractor may reflect its use under the most unfavorable circumstances, perhaps even when operative vaginal delivery is contraindicated and should not be undertaken.

TRIAL FORCEPS AND FAILED FORCEPS

By *trial forceps* is meant an attempt at delivery with forceps, knowing in advance that the operation may not succeed. One should not persist in such efforts lest the fetus and the mother be injured. When trial forceps are undertaken in the presence of possible disproportion, cesarean section should be done if firm, but gentle, tractions are ineffective in advancing descent.

Failed forceps, on the other hand, is an unsuccessful attempt at forceps delivery when one fully expects to deliver the fetus. These attempts are, unfortunately, usually forceful, and the fetus may be seriously injured. The forceps should be removed and the cause of the failure searched for by detailed investigation. Errors in position, insufficient preparation of the soft parts (for example, incompletely dilated cervix), constriction ring and significant disproportion will be found to be the usual causes.

Subsequent management will depend on the findings at this time. Cesarean section is indicated for disproportion; rest and time, for an incompletely dilated cervix; rotation, for malposition. Attention should be paid to hydration, electrolyte balance, analgesia, rest and moral support. The difference between trial forceps and failed forceps is a matter not only of intent but also of risk. Failed forceps procedures are especially hazardous.

DESTRUCTIVE OPERATIONS

Rarely, it will be necessary to undertake an operative procedure to effect vaginal delivery by reducing the size of the fetal head. This is indicated only if there is no possibility of salvaging a living, intact fetus. Cesarean section may be done instead, but is less preferable if it is possible that the uterus can be evacuated vaginally without traumatizing the mother.

The most commonly encountered situation in this category is the hydrocephalic fetus whose enlarged cranial diameters obstruct descent. *Ventricular tap* with a long needle or trocar will effectively reduce the head size to allow delivery to take place (see Chapter 60). This can be accomplished either transvaginally or transabdominally with relative ease.

Craniotomy involves perforation of the head of a fetus that is already dead by any one of several instruments available for this purpose so as to evacuate the intracranial contents. One may use any sharp device to do this, but Smellie scissors are specifically designed for this purpose. They are scissorlike instruments with the sharp edges on the outside for piercing. After the procedure, cranial contents will be discharged by the forces of labor, and descent and delivery will usually follow quickly.

The use of other special destructive instruments to diminish skull size by compression or to dismember the fetus is merely of historical interest. They are mentioned only to be condemned because they can cause irreparable maternal damage.

REFERENCES

Barton, L. G., Caldwell, W. E., and Studdiford, W. E.: New obstetric forceps. Amer. J. Obstet. Gynec. 15:16, 1928.

Chalmers, J. A.: The Ventouse: The Obstetric Vacuum Extractor. Chicago, Year Book Medical Publishers, 1971.

Das, K. N.: Obstetric Forceps (Its History and Evolution). Calcutta, Art Press, 1929; St. Louis, C. V. Mosby Company, 1929.

DeLee, J. B.: The prophylactic forceps operation. Amer. J. Obstet. Gynec. 1:34, 1920.

Hughes, E. C., ed.: Obstetric-Gynecologic Terminology. Philadelphia, F. A. Davis Company, 1972.

Kielland, C.: Ueber die Anlegung der Zange am nicht rotierten Kopf mit Beschreibung eines neuen Zangenmodelles und einer neuen Anlegungsmethode. Mschr. Geburtsh. Gynäk. 43:48, 1916.

Laufe, L. E.: A new divergent outlet forceps. Amer. J. Obstet. Gynec. 101:509, 1968.

Laufe, L. E.: Obstetric Forceps. New York, Harper & Row, 1968.

Malmström, T.: The vacuum extractor: An obstetrical instrument and the parturiometer, a tokographic device. Acta Obstet. Gynec. Scand. 36:Suppl. 3, 1957; 43:Suppl. 1, 1964.

Pajot, C.: Discussion relative au nouveau forceps de M. Tarnier. Ann. de gynéc. 7:241, 1877.

Pearse, W., and Kolbeck, T. J.: Compressive forces of the Shute forceps. Amer. J. Obstet. Gynec. 113:44, 1972.

Saxtorph, M.: De diverso partu ob diversam ad pelvim relationem mutuam. Hafniae, typ. viduae A. H. Godiche, 1771.

Shute, W. B.: An obstetrical forceps which uses a new principle of parallelism. Amer. J. Obstet. Gynec. 77:442, 1959.

Smellie, W.: A Treatise on the Theory and Practise of Midwifery, ed. 2. London, D. Wilson & T. Durham, 1752.

Thierry, E.: Les spatules: Manoeuvre du toboggan. Presse Méd. 68:317, 1960.

von Ritgen, F.: Uber ein Dammschutzverfahren. Mschr. Geburtsh. Frauenk. 6:321, 1855.

von Scanzoni, F. W.: Lehrbuch der Geburtshilfe, ed. 2. Vienna, L. W. Seidel, 1853.

Witkowski, G.-J.: Accoucheurs et Sages-Femmes Célèbres: Esquisses Biographiques. Paris, G. Steinheil, 1887.

Chapter 76

Cesarean Section

Cesarean section is the delivery of a fetus, the product of an intrauterine pregnancy, through an incision in the abdominal wall and the uterus. The term should not be applied to the removal of a fetus from the abdomen in an extrauterine abdominal pregnancy or after rupture of the uterus. Cesarean section is a major surgical procedure that should never be undertaken lightly and without serious consideration of the justifications, preparations and all essential ancillary support.

INDICATIONS

It is unfortunate that there are practitioners who inappropriately resort to cesarean section whenever they are confronted with a difficult obstetric situation or a medical or surgical problem in an obstetric patient. Although some of these operations are clearly justified, many are not. Clinicians are admonished to understand that delivery by cesarean section must be reserved only for those patients in whom vaginal delivery cannot be accomplished without seriously jeopardizing fetal or maternal life and health.

In balance, the risks of the surgical procedure must be outweighed by the hazards of either vaginal delivery or further delay until vaginal delivery is feasible. Appropriate indications include (1) previous cesarean section, (2) fetopelvic disproportion, (3) certain maternal disorders, such as hypertensive states and diabetes, but only under specific circumstances, (4) malpresentations, such as shoulder presentation, (5) tumor obstruction in the pelvis, (6) after certain uterine or vaginal surgical procedures like myomectomy, vaginal plasty,

cervical encirclage or fistula repair, and (7) documented fetal distress.

A previous cesarean section is undoubtedly the most common indication for cesarean section. If the indication for the first cesarean operation is still present, such as a contracted pelvis, all subsequent deliveries of normal-sized fetuses must be by cesarean section. If the indication for the first abdominal delivery is no longer present, such as placenta previa, and the patient has previously delivered *per vaginam*, one may consider vaginal delivery under certain special circumstances. These include optimal facilities for close observation and everything in readiness for immediate operation, especially anesthesia, blood bank, surgical team and support. Without these the risk of rupture of the uterine scar with intraperitoneal hemorrhage and fetal demise is too great to be acceptable.

Such patients, if allowed to labor, must be watched continuously with no conduction anesthesia and minimal analgesia to ensure that the earliest manifestations of rupture will be detected. Labor may be permitted to continue after cesarean section with constant watchfulness if a patient goes into labor spontaneously, the cervix dilates rapidly and the head descends.

Since these precautionary conditions are not feasible in most obstetric units, it is by far the most common practice to accept the dictum "once a cesarean, always a cesarean." The strongest argument in favor of this approach is the fact that maternal deaths from cesarean section are almost unknown, whereas the danger from uterine rupture is substantially greater, albeit still small when managed expeditiously (see Chapter 65).

When choosing the time for an elective

cesarean section, it must be known that the fetus is mature enough to survive. The methods for evaluating fetal size and maturity are detailed in Chapter 13. The best way to determine the proper time to perform a repeat elective cesarean section is to wait for the onset of labor or the spontaneous rupture of the membranes. Although premature infants may still be delivered by this approach, at least one is certain that the number is an irreducible minimum.

Disproportion between the fetal head and the pelvis warrants cesarean section, but this can seldom be determined definitely until after the patient has had a fair test of labor (see Chapter 64). X-ray pelvimetry is a useful guide (see Chapter 12), but only when adjudged in conjunction with the evolving dilatation and descent patterns. The clearest indication for cesarean section is disproportion, documented by pelvimetry, in the presence of secondary arrest of dilatation, prolonged deceleration phase or arrest of descent patterns. This concept holds equally for nulliparas and multiparas; just because a patient has delivered a term-size baby previously does not ensure her against fetopelvic disproportion in a subsequent pregnancy with a larger fetus. Objective evidence of fetopelvic disproportion in association with a breech presentation warrants section even without a test of labor (see Chapter 57).

Cesarean section should be done after myomectomy if the myomectomy incision extended into the uterine cavity. In general these patients are managed like those who have had a previous cesarean section because of the concern over the possibility of uterine rupture. The incidence of rupture following myomectomy is about the same as that after classic cesarean section (Pedowitz and Felmus). In threatened rupture of the uterus from any cause, cesarean section is indicated.

Tumors blocking the exit of the fetus, such as a cervical leiomyoma or an ovarian cyst in the culdesac, require abdominal delivery not only to effect evacuation of the uterus safely but also to determine the nature and extent of the tumor. In the event of an ovarian cystic tumor, it is important that its contents not be spilled into the peritoneal cavity in the course of parturition. If this should occur, neoplastic cells may be spread widely or serious chemical peritonitis may develop. Cesarean section will prevent this and allow extirpation as needed. Such obstructions are rare in labor.

The indications for cesarean section in hypertensive states are discussed in Chapter 36, where optimal timing is stressed. The relevant principles with regard to diabetes mellitus are dealt with in Chapter 49. Delivery by cesarean section is often indicated in placenta previa (see Chapter 37) and in abruptio placentae (see Chapter 38) when the circumstances demand it.

Shoulder presentation often warrants cesarean section (see Chapter 58), especially in nulliparas or in association with a contracted pelvis. Similarly, abdominal delivery should be done for cord prolapse if vaginal delivery cannot be effected quickly and atraumatically. This principle also applies in the presence of objective evidence of placental insufficiency or fetal distress (see Chapter 13).

Cesarean section for premature rupture of the membranes, when induction has failed, is practiced in some communities, based on the fear that amnionitis will develop. While there is no objection to performing a cesarean section for amnionitis if vaginal delivery cannot be quickly effected (Wynn), the rationale for section in all such cases to prevent amnionitis (which will occur only in a very small number of these cases) is not entirely defensible.

The safety of cesarean section should interdict such obsolete and potentially dangerous procedures as version with breech extraction (with rare exceptions as noted in Chapter 74), traumatic forceps operations and vaginal hysterotomy.

CONTRAINDICATIONS

Generally, cesarean section should not be done if the fetus is dead. Exceptions are frequent, however. In total placenta previa, for example, it will be necessary to empty the uterus abdominally in order to avoid serious maternal hemorrhage. Similarly, in some severe instances of abruptio placentae, cesarean section is needed when the mother's life is threatened by hemorrhage and coagulopathy. Insurmountable disproportion, neglected malpresentation, double monsters and obstruction by tumors all warrant cesarean section, even if the fetus is no longer alive.

Cesarean section may be contraindicated temporarily by the mother's general condition. If feasible, the procedure should be delayed until her status is more optimal to withstand the anesthesia and the operative strain. Examples include the eclamptic patient during and shortly following convulsions, the cardiac gravida in congestive failure (when section may be indicated for some relevant obstetric reason), the diabetic in ketoacidosis and the patient with a full stomach or an upper respiratory infection.

TYPES OF CESAREAN SECTIONS

There are four methods of abdominal delivery: (1) the *classic cesarean section,* for which a vertical incision is made in the upper uterine segment; (2) the *low segment* or *low cervical operation,* in which the incision is either transversely or vertically transperitoneal in the lower uterine segment; (3) the *extraperitoneal operation,* in which the lower uterine segment is reached extraperitoneally; and (4) *cesarean hysterectomy,* a combination of cesarean section (usually classic) followed by hysterectomy (preferably total).

The most commonly done technique is the transverse or Kerr incision low segment cesarean section. Both the classic incision and the vertical or Krönig incision in the lower segment are seldom used any longer, and extraperitoneal cesarean section is almost never done today. The advantages of the Kerr incision over the classic incision are (1) reduced hemorrhage because it traverses a thin fibrous area, (2) ease of repair, (3) less risk of subsequent rupture, (4) less opportunity for postoperative formation of adhesions and, therefore, less hazard of bowel obstruction and (5) the general impression that postoperative

morbidity is less. The only disadvantages are the additional time it takes to develop the peritoneal flap and advance the bladder (see below) and the possibility of lacerating the uterine vessels if the incision should extend laterally.

The speed and ease of the classic incision through the upper segment are its main advantages. It is especially useful when the lower pelvic anatomy is obscured by adhesions or leiomyomas. Some physicians consider the use of the classic incision to be preferable in placenta previa (see Chapter 37) and with a transverse lie (see Chapter 58). The counterbalancing disadvantage of the classic incision is the need to traverse the full thickness of myometrium, causing (1) hemorrhage, (2) hematoma formation, (3) febrile morbidity, (4) poorer healing and greater risk of rupture; in addition, (5) it is more difficult to repair and (6) postoperative bowel adhesions are more common and obstruction more likely to occur.

The Krönig incision has some of the disadvantages of both the Kerr and the classic incisions and essentially none of the advantages of either. It cuts through both the fibrous lower segment and the muscular upper segment so that the upper part heals poorly while presenting a greater risk of hemorrhage; it is time consuming to prepare the peritoneal flap; extension of the lower pole may injure the bladder. It is not a preferred technique.

Similarly, extraperitoneal section, once reserved for use in a grossly infected uterus, is no longer justified as a means of preventing peritonitis. The uterus is entered in the lower segment after dissection is carried down suprapubically in the space of Retzius between the bladder and its overlying peritoneum, attempting to keep the peritoneal cavity intact and unentered. The space of Retzius is actually just as vulnerable to infection and probably handles contamination less efficiently than the peritoneal cavity. The technical difficulty of this method and the risk of bladder and ureteral injury associated with it do not warrant its use in this era of effective antibiotics.

Cesarean hysterectomy may be indicated when leiomyomas are present, especially if they are large or block the pelvis.

Myomectomy may be performed instead in favorable cases if the woman desires to have more children. In rare cases of abruptio placentae, especially with a Couvelaire uterus, and in isolated instances of placenta previa when bleeding cannot be controlled, hysterectomy may be necessary. Placenta accreta, intractable postpartum bleeding and infection are other rare indications. Uterine rupture also usually requires hysterectomy.

Cesarean hysterectomy is also a method of sterilizing women (Brenner et al.) who have had several cesarean sections, especially if there are theological constraints regarding tubal ligation, a more preferable and less hazardous procedure. Although cervical cancer may be treated surgically, it is recommended that definitive therapy not be done at the time of delivery unless the obstetrician is a fully competent gynecological oncologist capable of executing radical surgical techniques.

SURGICAL TECHNIQUES

Low Segment Kerr Incision

Before proceeding, one should recall that it is essential that properly crossmatched whole blood or packed red cells be at hand, that a suitably skilled anesthetist be available and that someone capable of resuscitating the baby be present.

The bladder is catheterized and the abdomen is prepared as a sterile field. Under appropriate anesthesia with the patient in the Trendelenburg position, a median suprapubic, transverse muscle-cutting or Pfannenstiel incision is made. The abdomen is opened, taking care not to injure the bladder. The lower uterine segment is exposed with retractors. The loose peritoneum between the bladder and the uterus is incised near its attachment to the uterus, transversely and in a semilunar fashion, with the concavity upward, about 5 cm. on each side of the midline (Fig. 445). After the peritoneum is incised, it is stripped gently with a finger toward the pubis, undermining the bladder. A wide retractor (such as the anterior blade of the Balfour

retractor) is inserted to retract the bladder beneath the symphysis pubis and expose the lower uterine segment.

With a sharp knife, the uterus is incised in a transverse elliptical manner, scoring the myometrium along the entire proposed incision, and entering the uterus in the midline only. Usually, the membranes rupture at this point and suction of the amniotic fluid will be necessary to clear the field for visualization. With bandage scissors, the uterine wall is then incised, first to the right and then to the left, curving the incision upward at the ends (Fig. 446) so that it parallels the sides of the uterus; thus, if it should extend, it will not lacerate the uterine vessels. The incision should be large enough to permit delivery of the fetal head. Instead of scissors, the opening in the lower uterine segment can be made with two fingers, one index finger of each hand, inserted in the midline opening and pulled apart along the previously scored incision line. One must avoid incision or tearing of the uterine arteries.

After the incision is made, one inserts a hand between the symphysis pubis and the fetal head, with the palm facing the head. All abdominal retractors are removed as the occiput is rotated into the wound. The head is pressed gently upward while at the same time pressure is applied at the fundus by an assistant. In this combined manner, the head will be delivered by extension. Rarely will it be necessary to use instruments, such as a vectis or small Simpson forceps, or transvaginal pressure applied from below, to dislodge a head tightly wedged in the pelvis. Once the head is delivered, it is usually a simple matter to deliver the shoulders slowly one at a time, analogous to the manner of delivering the shoulders vaginally.

The cord is then doubly clamped and divided, and the baby is resuscitated by an assistant as required. Meanwhile, the placenta is manually dissected free of its attachments to the uterus. Oxytocin or ergotrate is given slowly intravenously to effect strong uterine contraction and to aid in hemostasis. The endometrial surface is carefully examined and wiped clean of any residual membranes. The internal os of the cervix is probed with a finger to ensure

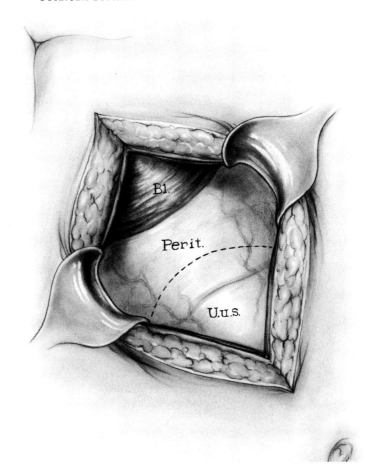

Figure 445 Low segment cesarean section. The abdomen has been opened by a longitudinal incision and the operative field is exposed. The dotted line shows the intended elliptical incision in the loose pubocervical peritoneum. *Bl.*, bladder; *Perit.*, peritoneum; *U.u.s.*, upper uterine segment. The patient is oriented here so that her head is down and to the right.

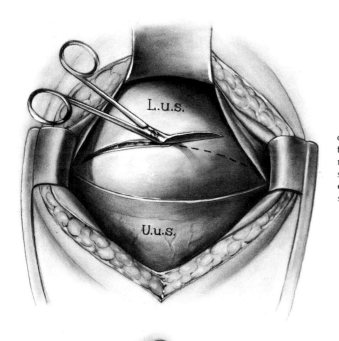

Figure 446 The peritoneal flap has been developed and the bladder is retracted under the symphysis pubis. An elliptical incision is made transversely across the lower uterine segment (*L.u.s.*) and curved upward at the ends to avoid the uterine vessels. Bandage scissors prevent injury to the fetus.

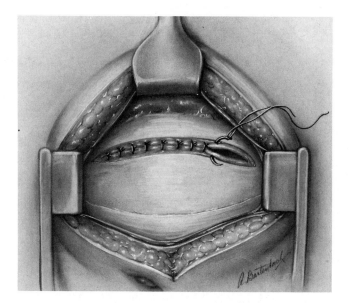

Figure 447 Suture of transverse incision in the lower uterine segment by interrupted chromic catgut sutures; continuous sutures may also be used. Two layers of sutures are inserted for good approximation and hemostasis.

there will be adequate lochial drainage postoperatively.

The wound is closed with two rows of continuous or interrupted size 0 chromic catgut sutures (Fig. 447), taking great pains to secure apposition of the myometrium and hemostasis, especially at the angles of the uterine incision. It does not seem to matter whether or not endometrium is included in the first layer of sutures, although some feel it is important to place the sutures in myometrium in such a way as to exclude the endometrium.

If there is considerable bleeding, temporary hemostasis may be obtained by placing Allis or T-clamps on the edges of the cut myometrium prior to and during the closure. Reperitonealization is done by apposing the edges of cut peritoneum (Fig. 448) with a fine continuous catgut suture. Some overlap the lower edge over the upper peritoneal surface, but there is no particular advantage to this technique. Before proceeding to close the abdominal wall in layers, the tubes and ovaries should be inspected and the peritoneal cavity should be explored thoroughly and cleaned of any accumulated blood and detritus.

Classic Cesarean Section

The bladder is catheterized and the abdomen is prepared as for the low segment cesarean section. A midline suprapubic abdominal wall incision is generally needed. The uterus is examined to detect sinistro- or dextrorotation and then rotated to the midline. A longitudinal incision about 11 cm. is made through the thickness of the uterine wall into the amniotic sac, being careful not to cut the fetus. Amniotic fluid gushes out and is suctioned.

Since the placenta is frequently implanted on the anterior surface of the uterine cavity, it is common to encounter the placenta when opening the uterus during a classic cesarean section. It is best to dissect quickly along the cleavage plane to the edge of the placenta, where the membranes are punctured and the amniotic sac entered. It is less preferable to cut through the placenta, although this is often done, because considerable fetal hemorrhage is possible. In either case the procedure should be carried out expeditiously to minimize fetal hypoxia.

Once the amniotic cavity has been entered, a hand is inserted to locate, identify and grasp one, or preferably both, feet. Gentle breech extraction is carried out to deliver the fetus through the uterine wound. The cord is divided between clamps; the placenta is delivered; the uterotonic agent is given; the endometrial lining is wiped clean, and the internal os is probed, all exactly the same as with the Kerr incision (see above).

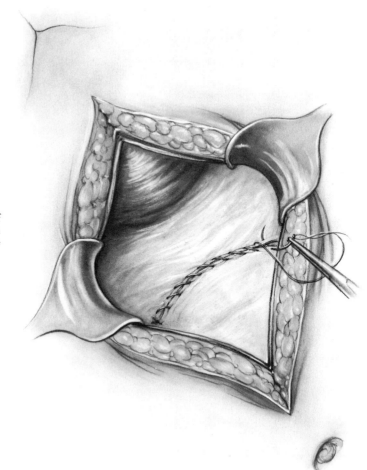

Figure 448 The bladder flap of peritoneum is reapproximated with a continuous chromic catgut suture to the upper edge of peritoneum.

The wound is closed in at least three layers of continuous or interrupted size 0 chromic catgut sutures, carefully apposing the myometrium and closing all dead space (Fig. 449). Hemostasis must be assured before the final peritoneal layer is placed. Abdominal exploration and peritoneal toilet are carried out before closing the abdominal wound.

Low Segment Krönig Incision

The Krönig technique differs from the Kerr-type section only insofar as the incision is concerned. Preparations and abdominal incision are the same. The peritoneal flap is created as for the Kerr incision except that the upper peritoneum requires considerably more dissection to ensure that the longitudinal uterine incision will later be covered by peritoneum. The uterine incision is made vertically in the lower segment and extended with bandage scissors down toward the bladder, while protecting the bladder from injury by a retractor and careful visualization, and up into the lower part of the upper uterine segment subperitoneally. If the patient has been in advanced labor for some time, the lower uterine segment can be expected to be stretched and elongated so that it is sometimes possible for the entire Krönig incision to be made in this segment.

Subsequent manipulations for delivery

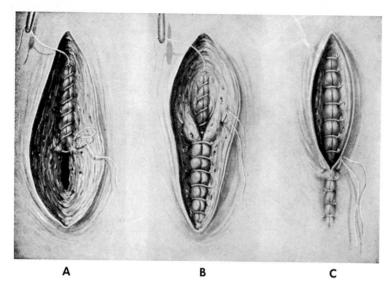

Figure 449 Closure of uterine incision in a classic cesarean section. *A*, First row approximates edge of myometrium with continuous or interrupted chromic catgut suture. *B*, Second row closes dead space and ensures hemostasis; additional rows may be needed. *C*, Peritoneal edges are apposed carefully.

    A   **B**   **C**

of the fetus and the placenta are carried out as usual. Closure requires two or more layers of continuous or interrupted size 0 chromic catgut sutures securing hemostasis. The peritoneal edges are apposed with a continuous size 00 chromic catgut suture. One should be careful not to advance the bladder too far up the uterine wall, as this will cause great difficulty in a subsequent cesarean section if it should ever be necessary. Some obstetricians suture the upper peritoneal edge down to the myometrium with fine sutures and then suture the lower edge to or over the upper edge; this has the effect of diminishing the dead space somewhat, but seems to be an unnecessary detail. The rest of the procedure is identical with both Kerr and classic cesarean sections.

Cesarean Hysterectomy

The term *Porro operation* is inappropriately applied when a cesarean section is performed and is followed by removal of the uterus; this is properly called *cesarean hysterectomy.* The first term should not be used because Porro was not the first to amputate the uterus after abdominal delivery, and the procedure he did involved hysterectomy with the fetus *in situ.* The first to amputate the uterus after cesarean section was Storer (Bixby).

The technique of cesarean hysterectomy is identical with that of hysterectomy in a nongravid patient. After the baby is delivered and the placenta removed, the uterine wound is oversewn for hemostasis. The round ligaments are divided between clamps (Fig. 450) and the broad ligaments are opened bluntly to expose the avascular spaces (Fig. 451). The uteroovarian ligaments and proximal ends of the uterine tubes are doubly clamped, divided and ligated (Figs. 452 and 453). If the tubes and ovaries are to be removed, the infundibulopelvic ligaments are divided at this step instead, taking care not to injure the underlying ureter. The peritoneum in the pubocervical fold above the bladder is incised transversely and the bladder freed of its loose areolar attachment to the cervix (Fig. 454), if it has not already been done in the course of preparation for the low segment cesarean section. The uterine vessels are skeletonized and divided between clamps (Fig. 455), placing the clamps close to the uterus to avoid ureteral damage. The uterine vascular pedicle should be doubly ligated with size 0 chromic catgut sutures (Fig. 456).

For supravaginal hysterectomy the cervix is incised above the level of the ligated uterine arteries, beveling the incision in an inverted cone fashion into the cervical canal (Figs. 457 and 458) to remove as much cervical glandular tissue as possible.

(*Text continued on page 799*)

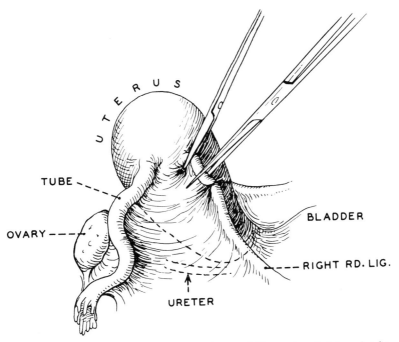

Figure 450 Hysterectomy (here shown in a nongravid uterus) illustrating division of right round ligament. (Figures 450 to 458 and 462 from Greenhill, J. P.: Surgical Gynecology, ed. 4. Chicago, Year Book Medical Publishers, Inc., 1969.)

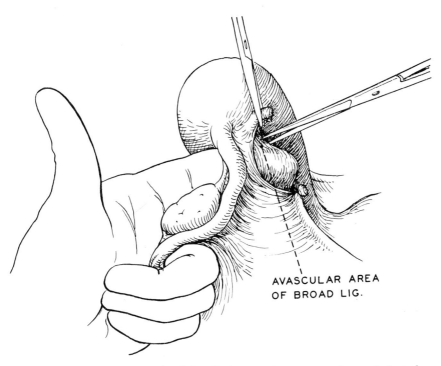

Figure 451 Round ligament has been divided and a finger is being inserted posteriorly to demonstrate the avascular area of the broad ligament.

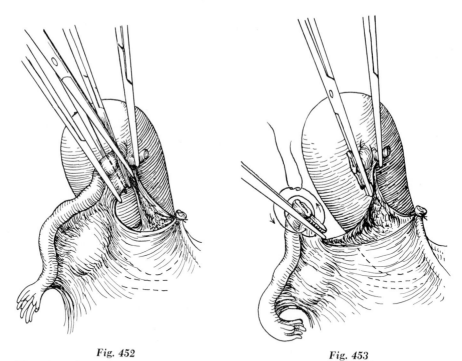

Fig. 452   Fig. 453

Figure 452   The right uteroovarian ligament and tube are doubly clamped and are about to be divided. If salpingo-oophorectomy were to be done, this step would involve resection across the infundibulopelvic ligament instead.

Figure 453   The uteroovarian ligament and tube have been divided and are being suture-ligated. Note the leaves of the broad ligament opening to permit access to the uterine vessels.

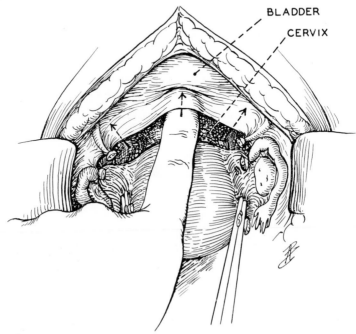

Figure 454   The pubocervical fold of peritoneum has been cut transversely and the bladder is being bluntly dissected free of its loose attachments to the cervix.

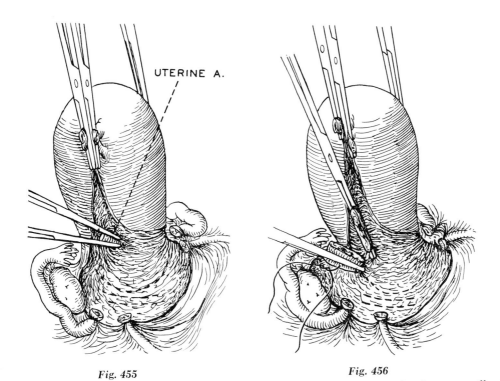

Fig. 455

Fig. 456

Figure 455 The uterine vessels are doubly clamped close to the uterus to ensure that the ureter will not be injured.

Figure 456 The uterine vasculature pedicle has been divided and ligated with a transfixing suture. A second suture of this stump is recommended.

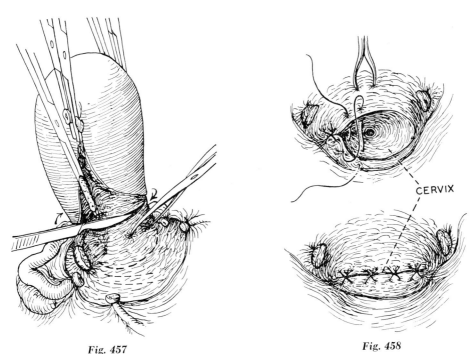

Fig. 457

Fig. 458

Figure 457 The uterus is amputated for a supravaginal hysterectomy by incising the cervix just above the uterine ligatures.

Figure 458 The cervical glands have been coned out during the uterine amputation. The cervix is closed with interrupted figure-eight chromic catgut sutures for approximation and hemostasis.

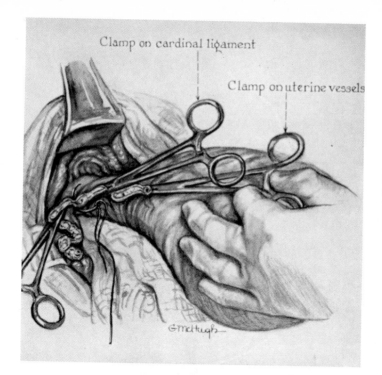

Clamp on cardinal ligament

Clamp on uterine vessels

Figure 459 Total hysterectomy showing technique for clamping and dividing the cardinal ligament adjacent to the cervix. The distal pedicle of the first bite of the cardinal ligament is here being suture-ligated after it was divided.

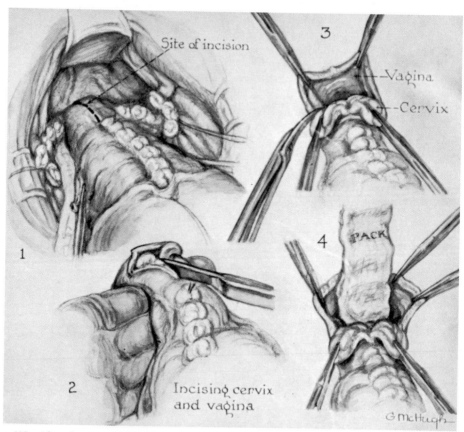

Site of incision

3

Vagina

Cervix

1

4 PACK

2 Incising cervix and vagina

Figure 460 After the parametrium has been completely resected (1), the cervix is incised longitudinally (2) to identify the cervicovaginal junction by inserting a finger down to the vagina or visualizing it directly. The cervix is identified and grasped (3) and the vagina transected at the fornices. A gauze pack may be inserted into the vagina through the incision (4) to prevent peritoneal contamination from collected vaginal contents; the pack is to be removed vaginally after the procedure is completed.

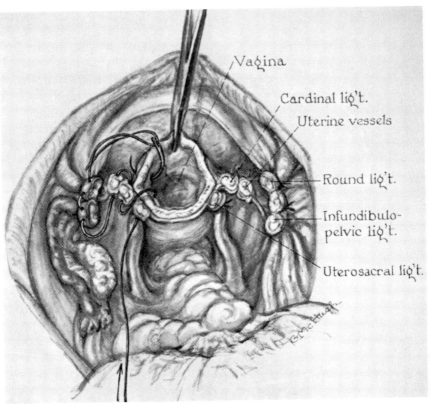

Figure 461 The vaginal vault is supported and made hemostatic by full-thickness sutures incorporating the stumps of cardinal and uteroovarian ligaments into the angles as shown here.

The cervical stump is sutured with figure-eight size 0 chromic catgut sutures in one or more layers. For total hysterectomy, which is preferred, the pubocervical fascia is transected transversely and the cuff of fascia pushed bluntly caudad. The cardinal ligaments are clamped and divided close to the cervix (Fig. 459). Several bites may be needed to completely separate the parametrium from the cervix over its entire length. The uterosacral ligaments should be divided posteriorly and ligated.

Identifying the cervicovaginal junction is an especially difficult task if the cervix has been effaced and dilated in the labor which preceded the hysterectomy. To accomplish this it may be necessary to incise the cervix longitudinally (Fig. 460) so as to insert a finger down into the vagina, or actually open into the vagina in order to visualize the junction. Then the vagina can be transected at the fornices and the cervix completely removed. The vaginal vault is supported and made hemostatically secure by interrupted chromic catgut sutures, incorporating the stumps of the cardinal and uteroovarian (or infundibulopelvic) ligaments into the lateral angles as shown in Figure 461. Whether or not the vault is actually closed with sutures appears to be unimportant.

Peritonealization is accomplished by reapposing the cut edges while imbricating and burying the pedicles of the round and the uteroovarian or infundibulopelvic ligaments (Fig. 462), thereby leaving a smooth peritoneal surface to minimize adhesion formation.

AGONAL CESAREAN SECTION

A fetus may live up to 20 minutes after the death of its mother, although one can-

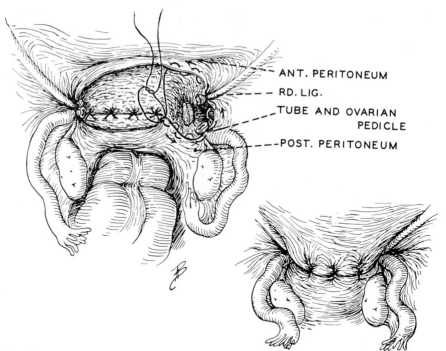

ANT. PERITONEUM

RD. LIG.

TUBE AND OVARIAN
PEDICLE

POST. PERITONEUM

Figure 462 Reperitonealization showing a method of bringing the peritoneal edges together while imbricating the cut pedicles of round and uteroovarian ligaments so that they are buried, using a purse-string suture.

not generally expect the infant to be undamaged if delivered after about five to eight minutes. The survival time depends on the suddenness of the mother's death. The more acute the death, the more likely the fetus to be alive for a finite interval. The physician has an ethical responsibility (and perhaps a legal obligation) to provide the viable near-term fetus with an opportunity to survive. In recent times postmortem or agonal cesarean section has been performed with encouraging results (Weber).

If the pregnancy has advanced beyond the twenty-eighth week, there should be no delay in opening the abdomen and uterus after the mother's life is definitely extinct. No time should be lost trying to hear the heart tones because several fetuses have been saved when the heart tones were inaudible. It is not necessary legally to obtain the consent of the husband or the family, although for his own protection the physician should secure permission in advance if possible (Bacon).

If death is anticipated in a gravida, one should have an emergency kit at hand at her bedside. Sterile precautions are unnecessary. A classic incision is made, the baby delivered, the cord clamped and aggressive resuscitation instituted rapidly. Artificial ventilation of the mother and cardiac massage may help increase the fetus' chances of survival if instituted immediately and maintained until the fetus is delivered (Weber). One should be sure to remove the placenta because there are reported cases in which the placenta was subsequently expelled vaginally after death.

REFERENCES

Bacon, C. S.: Legal aspects of postmortem cesarean section. Surg. Gynec. Obstet. *12*:168, 1911.

Bixby, G. H.: Extirpation of the puerperal uterus by abdominal section. J. Gynec. Soc. Bost. *1*:223, 1869.

Brenner, P., Sall, S., and Sonnenblick, B.: Evaluation

of cesarean section hysterectomy as a sterilization procedure. Amer. J. Obstet. Gynec. *108*:355, 1970.

Kerr, J. M. M.: The technique of cesarean section with special reference to the lower uterine segment incision. Amer. J. Obstet. Gynec. *12*:729, 1926.

Krönig, B.: Transperitonealer Cervikaler Kaiserschnitt. *In* Döderlein, A., and Krönig, B., eds.: Operative Gynäkologie, ed. 3. Leipzig, Georg Thieme, 1912.

Pedowitz, P., and Felmus, L. B.: Rupture of myomec-

tomy scars during subsequent pregnancies: A review. Obstet. Gynec. Survey 7:305, 1952.

Porro, E.: Della amputazione utero-ovarica come complemento di taglio cesareo. Milano, frat. Rechiedei, 1876.

Weber, C. E.: Postmortem cesarean section: Review of literature and case reports. Amer. J. Obstet. Gynec. *110*:158, 1971.

Wynn, R. M.: Premature rupture of the membranes. Chicago Med. 72:39, 1969.

Chapter 77

Conception Control

Family planning is an essential and integral part of total obstetric care. Most obstetric patients will seek out such care and express intimate concern over family spacing. For those who do not overtly voice their interest or needs, it is the obligation of the physician to make appropriate inquiries and to provide both information and counsel. Patients are most receptive immediately post partum during the hospital stay before returning home. This is an optimal time to pursue the matter, although most physicians routinely prescribe contraception at the time of the first return visit six weeks or so after delivery. For economic, sociologic and personal health reasons, it is important that the opportunity be seized during the hospitalization. This principle deserves emphasis because, unfortunately, those most in need of this advice may be uninformed, unaware, apathetic or fearful as a result of misinformation and may not reappear for their postpartum checkup, or they may return already pregnant again (admonitions to the contrary notwithstanding).

Scattered throughout this book in our discussions of various maternal disorders and pregnancy complications, including hypertensive states, heart and lung diseases, diabetes mellitus and sickle cell anemia, are recommendations for contraception or sterilization as indicated. These recommendations are made with the clear understanding that, although mentioned where applicable, they are not meant in any way to suggest coercion of the patient who cannot or will not accept any form of birth control on theological grounds. It should be pointed out, nonetheless, that most couples utilize some form of contraception control during much of their reproductive lives. This appears to be the case even for many Roman Catholic couples, despite the fact that the official papal stand is still adamantly against all forms except rhythm (see below).

There is today a rapidly growing awareness, especially on the part of young people who are entering their reproductive years, of the economic, sociologic and ecologic impact of childbearing on themselves and on the world about them. We are witnessing a dramatic attitudinal change from individual to collective responsibility, manifest especially in the zero-population-growth (ZPG) movement. The ZPG concept holds that if we are to prevent the inevitable overcrowding of this globe by a population explosion that will rapidly outgrow available limited supplies of consumables, we must voluntarily limit our own reproduction so that each couple replicates itself by having no more than two children.

Whether on this basis or as a result of other motivating forces, the birth rate in the United States and in some other developed areas of the world has dropped dramatically during the past two to three years. This is undoubtedly the direct result of greater utilization of easy-to-use and readily available contraceptive methods, such as oral contraceptive pills.

Currently known contraceptive measures are divisible into temporary or intermittent techniques and permanent forms of sterilization. The latter include vas ligation and tubal ligation or cauterization. Temporary measures include those that (1) prevent ovulation (the oral contraceptives), (2) use spermicidal agents (foams, gels, suppositories, creams), (3) occlude the cervix (diaphragm and jelly, cervical cap), (4) avert implantation (intrauterine devices, morning-after pill, perhaps prostaglandins), (5) shun the ovulatory interval (rhythm) and (6) preclude intravaginal ejaculation (condom, withdrawal, abstinence).

The value of the temporary contraceptive method in preventing pregnancy depends on its use-effectiveness as well as its acceptability. No method works if it has limited acceptability. Thus, there may be a wide discrepancy between the theoretical or optimal effectiveness of a technique and its actual efficacy in a population of users. Oral contraceptives are especially noteworthy in this regard. Ideally (Calderone), there should be less than one pregnancy per 100 women-years (100 women-years refers to the experience of 100 women using a technique for one year or 20 women for five years and so forth), but rates as high as 25 pregnancies per 100 women-years have been encountered in actual users (Tietze and Lewis).

Among sexually active individuals in the reproductive age one would expect about 80 pregnancies per 100 women-years if no contraception is practiced: ideally, rhythm results in 14; withdrawal, 16; foam, 3 or more; condom, 2 to 3; diaphragm, 2 to 3; intrauterine device, 1 to 3; and oral contraceptive, less than 1. Constant users, who are faithful and take all necessary and appropriate precautions, tend to have effectiveness data approaching these ideals; poorly motivated individuals, who are careless, casual and inconstant in usage or in their attention to the details of usage, fall far short of these figures.

WITHDRAWAL OR COITUS INTERRUPTUS

The ancient technique of withdrawal of the penis from the vagina before ejaculation is still widely practiced. Coitus is practiced without constraints, except that the male must maintain delicate control and awareness so that withdrawal will occur before emission. Moreover, it is necessary to ensure that ejaculation takes place away from the external genitalia.

Pregnancy results not only from semen deposited on the vulva, but also from the preejaculatory sperm-containing fluid which escapes from the penis prior to withdrawal. Although its use-effectiveness rate is relatively poor, it should be emphasized that its ready availability to all and lack of cost make it considerably better than nothing at all. Ungratified sexual needs are a major drawback second only to the high risk of pregnancy.

RHYTHM OR THE SAFE PERIOD

The most natural and the least harmful method of birth control is that commonly known as the rhythm method, the safe period, or the Ogino-Knaus method. It depends for its effectiveness on abstinence during that interval of the menstrual cycle when the patient is fertile, that is, when there is a recently expelled, viable ovum capable of being fertilized by a viable sperm present in the upper generative tract. While human oocytes appear to be capable of fertilization for only about 12 to 24 hours (and certainly no longer than 48 hours) following ovulation, the fertilizing capability of the spermatozoon is at least two days and possibly as long as four days. Thus, in order for the rhythm system to work, it is necessary for the couple to avoid intercourse for four days before the expected time of ovulation and two or three days afterwards. Ovulation is anticipated about 14 days prior to the onset of menstruation.

For example, women with cycles of 28 to 30 days' duration should ovulate between days 14 and 16. Subtracting four days for sperm viability at the beginning of this interval and adding three days after it, we can calculate that it is possible for such women to conceive between days 10 and 19. In general terms, one subtracts 18 days from the shortest cycle duration (14 days for ovulation plus four days for sperm viability) to obtain the beginning of the period requiring abstinence, and one subtracts 11 days from the longest interval (14 days for ovulation less three days for ovum viability) to date the end of this interval.

Obviously, this approach is valueless for patients who ovulate at irregular intervals and as a consequence have menstrual cycles that vary in length. This is especially problematic in adolescents, in women following childbirth and in premenopausal females when cyclic irregularity is common. Rhythm requires considerable motivation on the part of the couple and some degree of intelligence as well. There are no religious constraints to its use. Many women use it successfully, but it cannot be applied as universally as its proponents suggest. Only women who have fairly regular cycles and are strongly motivated are candidates for this method of birth control.

CONDOM

The use of the condom (variously called prophylactic, sheath, rubber, skin, safety or safe) is universal as an effective mechanical means of birth control. Sheaths made of latex rubber or processed lamb ceca are fitted over the erect penis to collect the ejaculated semen and prevent it from being deposited in the vagina.

Failures result from carelessness, especially during removal. The condom may slip off and spill its contents in or near the vagina if the rim is not held during withdrawal after ejaculation, or if detumescence is allowed to occur prior to withdrawal. Rarely does a well-made condom break unless it is reused, improperly stored in a warm place or lubricated with petroleum jelly so that it deteriorates.

The advantages of the condom are its convenience, ready availability, lack of any side effects and relative cheapness. Additionally, it does provide some protection against venereal disease. There are no clinical contraindications to its use, but some men find it diminishes sensation somewhat and some women report irritation of the vaginal walls or allergy to the rubber.

SPERMICIDAL AGENTS

Spermicides in the form of gel, cream, foam or suppository have as their purpose destruction of the spermatozoa which are deposited in the vagina during intercourse. The vehicle for the chemicals may also act as a mechanical barrier. The agent is placed deep in the vagina in the vicinity of the cervix just prior to intercourse; the effectiveness rarely exceeds an hour. Douching must be avoided for six to eight hours subsequent to coitus.

Parenthetically, douches are totally unsatisfactory means of contraception regardless of whether plain water is used or chemicals are added to the douche water. Spermatozoa appear in the cervical mucus within a matter of seconds (variously reported as early as 15 seconds) so that there is no way possible for douching to be effective.

Spermicides are available without prescription. They are obtainable cheaply and easy to use. They are especially valuable for women who are unable or unwilling to take the oral contraceptive pill or to use a diaphragm or an intrauterine device. They have the disadvantage of necessitating interruptions in sexual foreplay for the purpose of insertion. An occasional individual is allergic to the chemicals in one or another commercial preparation. Pregnancies are common, probably on the basis of forgetting to administer the agent prior to each intercourse or failure to insert enough in the right place (against the cervix) to be effective. They work best when used in combination with another method, such as the condom.

DIAPHRAGM AND JELLY

The combination of a vaginal diaphragm and a spermicidal jelly or cream provides satisfactory contraception when properly used. The diaphragm is a round rubber dome with a metal spring rim that is coated with a spermicidal agent and placed in the vagina prior to intercourse so that the dome covers the cervix and blocks the sperm from entering the uterus by means of both a mechanical and a chemical barrier.

The diaphragm must be fitted to the patient by a physician to be sure it is seated along the anterior vaginal wall between the posterior fornix and the vesicovaginal angle behind the symphysis covering the cervical os. If too small, the diaphragm may be incorrectly inserted into the anterior fornix and thus leave the cervix uncovered; if too large, it will be uncomfortable and may even occlude the urethra. Diaphragms are available with metal spring rims of various kinds, including coil spring, flat spring and arcing spring. The variety chosen depends on the comfort and fit.

After selecting the correct size (usually available in 5 mm. increments from 60 to 90 mm. diameter), the physician must carefully instruct the patient as to how to apply the jelly or cream to the inner aspect of the dome, squeeze the opposite rims together and insert the diaphragm deep into the vagina with the fingers or an inserter. Insertion is aided by squatting or elevating one leg or lying on the back. The diaphragm may have to be pressed up behind the pubic bone to be seated correctly. The cervix should always be checked to ensure that it is covered; the patient must be taught to recognize the cervix which can be likened to the nose in terms of its characteristic firmness.

The diaphragm is inserted no more than two hours before intercourse and must be left in place for at least eight hours afterwards to ensure that all spermatozoa are dead. More jelly or cream is needed if coitus is repeated beyond two hours; it is applied without disturbing the diaphragm by means of a special syringe-like applicator. To remove the diaphragm eight hours or more after the last intercourse, the patient inserts the index finger behind the front rim and pulls down and out. The diaphragm is then washed, dried, powdered and stored in a cool place. Cared for in this way a diaphragm should last at least a year, sometimes two years. Before and after each use, the diaphragm must be examined for defects.

Patients should be rechecked annually to ensure the proper fit. Refitting should also be done about three months after starting intercourse, after a term pregnancy or an abortion, after a rapid weight change of more than 10 pounds in either direction and after vaginal surgery.

Certain anatomic features make use of a diaphragm inappropriate or unacceptable, such as vaginal atresia, uterine prolapse or loss of levator ani muscle support. Some patients develop allergic sensitivity to the rubber or to the spermicidal agent. Some women find its use unaesthetic and even repugnant; but many are entirely satisfied with it as an effective technique, especially if they cannot use or object to taking oral contraceptives.

INTRAUTERINE CONTRACEPTIVE DEVICES

Use of intrauterine foreign bodies to prevent pregnancy in animals has long been known, as evidenced by the effectiveness of camel-stones used in North Africa. Graefenberg introduced a metal intrauterine ring which worked well, but was associated with bleeding, expulsion, infection and occasional pregnancy, leading to its almost universal condemnation. Renewed interest in recent years has led to improvement in design and composition.

Inert plastic and stainless steel intrauterine devices (called IUD, IUCD, coil or loop) are now widely used. Numerous varieties are available, including an assortment of loops, coils, bows, rings, shields, springs and M- and T-shaped devices. Most recently, devices containing progesterone or metallic copper are being studied for possible special effectiveness and added benefit. Most devices in current use are tailed so that a string or bead is left protruding through the cervix into the vagina; this is useful in enabling the patient and the physician to check that it has not been expelled. The tail aids in removal should this be desired.

Mechanisms of action are unknown; ovulation and fertilization are unimpeded, but implantation does not take place. The device is inserted under sterile conditions by means of a special applicator while the cervix is held with a tenaculum. Optimally, devices are inserted during menstruation or shortly thereafter and most easily post partum.

Intrauterine devices are contraindicated under certain circumstances, such as when pregnancy is suspected, in patients with the residua of pelvic inflammatory disease, in those with recent infected abortion or postpartum endometritis, in patients with leiomyomas or history of abnormal uterine bleeding and in those with acute cervicitis.

Patients may experience uterine cramping during insertion and for a variable period afterward. Pain subsides gradually and is generally easy to control with mild analgesics if the patient is well motivated. Subsequent periods may be heavy for several cycles. Up to 80 per cent of women have some menstrual changes after insertion, including most often shorter intervals as well as longer and heavier periods. If either pain or bleeding is excessive or unacceptable to the patient, the device will have to be removed merely by gently pulling on the tail or by using a crochet hook-like device for this purpose.

Expulsion is not uncommon, especially in the first month after insertion, occurring spontaneously in seven to nine per cent during the first year. The larger the device, the less the likelihood of expulsion; also, older patients and multiparas have fewer expulsions.

Perforation of the uterus occurs about once in 1500 to 2000 insertions, more often with certain devices such as the bow. Perforation is avoidable by taking great care in sounding the uterus for depth and direction before insertion; straightening the corpus so that it is aligned with the cervix by traction on the cervix with a tenaculum is very helpful in this regard.

If perforation is suspected, attempts should be made to remove the device transcervically. If this is not feasible, because the tail has broken off or vanished, hysterography with radiopaque dye injected into the uterus is of use. Although devices in the peritoneal cavity are usually removed surgically, only the closed rings or bows which could theoretically serve to incarcerate a loop of bowel must be dealt with in this aggressive manner. Despite the fact that instrumentation of the uterus may flare up a dormant subacute or chronic pelvic inflammatory disease, there is no clear evidence that a device will initiate such a process.

Ectopic pregnancies can develop, as might be expected, but the absolute incidence is not increased. Since fertilization takes place, it is possible for tubal implantation to occur if tubal transport is somehow impeded; the device does not influence this process.

Intrauterine pregnancies do occur with the device in place, although most of them result from expulsion that has gone unnoticed. Because expulsions may take place silently, it is recommended that women check digitally for the tail string or bead after each period and at weekly intervals. Spontaneous abortions may be increased with the device *in situ*, but usually the pregnancy is undisturbed and goes to term normally. The device may be found embedded in the membranes after delivery. Fetal malformations do not result if pregnancy occurs with a device in the uterus.

The major disadvantages of intrauterine devices are the high rates of expulsion and symptoms requiring them to be removed. For those remaining, the contraceptive effectiveness is very good and may be improved by additives currently being studied, such as progesterone and metallic copper. The overriding advantage is that, once inserted, its effectiveness does not depend on any special motivation or action or attention to detail by the patient herself.

ORAL CONTRACEPTIVES

By far the most popular and most extensively used method of birth control in the United States and other developed areas is the group of oral contraceptives, commonly called *the pill* or OC. They work by preventing ovulation through the action of estrogen and progesterone in combination or sequentially.

All mechanisms are not fully defined, but they appear to inhibit the release of pituitary gonadotropins that are needed for ovulation, perhaps by direct hormone effect on the hypothalamus. Additionally, the endometrial lining may be stimulated to undergo predecidual stromal and regressive glandular changes to make it unfavorable for implantation; the cervical mucus is made more viscid and hostile to sperm; tubal transport of the blastocyst is modified; sperm capacitation may also be inhibited. These latter effects are less likely to occur with sequential agents which mimic natural cyclic hormonal changes; this probably accounts for the higher failure rates with sequential regimens than with combined estrogen-progestogen preparations.

The many commercial products in use today contain varying kinds and dosages of synthetic estrogenic and progestational compounds. They vary pharmacologically in potency and side effects; there is also a wide variability in the way individual patients respond to them.

Commonly, women complain of nausea, edema, breast engorgement, dizziness, leg cramps, leukorrhea and chloasma. The gastrointestinal manifestations subside after a while if the patient persists with the agent; occasionally, it will be necessary to discontinue or change the agent because of these side effects. More serious side effects, such as thrombophlebitis, although rare occurrences, must nevertheless be watched for and guarded against.

Thus, oral contraceptives are contraindicated in a woman who has had thrombophlebitis or pulmonary embolism in the past. Along the same lines, because there are reported or theoretically relevant problems, they should not be given to women who have breast malignancy, undiagnosed vaginal bleeding, liver disease, diabetes or a strong family history of diabetes, migraine, epilepsy, multiple sclerosis, otosclerosis or porphyria.

Other side effects include breakthrough intermenstrual bleeding, usually with preparations containing small amounts of estrogen; menstrual flow tends to diminish and shorten; amenorrhea is rare, but may be associated with infertility; leiomyomas may enlarge, if present, both from edematous change and from proliferative stimulation; alopecia has been reported; hypertension has been shown to result in susceptible women; corneal edema may make it difficult for women to continue to wear contact lenses. Detailed review of these and other side effects is beyond our scope here, but the reader is referred to recent reports on this important subject (Advisory Committee; Tietze and Lewis; Cleary and Dajami; Calderone). Considerable controversy has arisen in this regard. Complications and side effects are gener-

ally considered to be far outweighed by the advantages offered in great effectiveness, ease of administration, acceptability and dissociation from the sex act.

The oral contraceptive agent is usually taken in pill form once daily beginning on the fifth day, counting from the first day of menstruation, for 20 or 21 days. Patients should be instructed to take the pill at the same time every day to establish the habit pattern. Some take it in the evening to diminish the nausea they experience.

If a day is missed, two pills should be taken the next day; if two days are missed, doubling up for two days will usually prevent breakthrough bleeding, but ovulation may occur and another concomitant form of contraceptive is advisable. Following the end of the 20 to 21 day treatment cycle, the patient will usually begin her next period within two to three days. She begins timing again from the first day of menstrual bleeding. If no period occurs, she begins taking the pills again after one week on the assumption that the amenorrhea is hormonally induced rather than due to a pregnancy. If there is no bleeding for two cycles, she should be checked for pregnancy, however.

To reduce or eliminate the confusion sometimes arising from the need to follow the timing precisely (three weeks on hormones, one week off), there has recently been introduced a 28-day package containing seven placebo pills. The patient merely takes a pill a day continuously without interruption for correct contraceptive control; active hormone is taken from day 5 through day 26 and inactive pills for days 27 to 28 and the first five days of the next cycle.

FEMALE STERILIZATION

Lest there be some possibility of misinterpretation, it should be stressed that male sterilization by *vas ligation* is a much simpler and safer operative procedure than any currently available technique for sterilizing the female. There is, fortunately, a growing trend toward vas ligation which has much to commend it; however, the subject is not validly a part of obstetrics for discussion here. Thus, although we recommend vas ligation as a preferable means for permanent contraception for a couple, we will deal here only with the techniques useful in the female.

For purposes of contrast and perspective, one should bear in mind that vas ligation is an office procedure done under local anesthesia; the vas deferens is isolated in the scrotum, divided and tied bilaterally; neither hospitalization nor long-term disability is involved; sexuality is unaffected, but sperm may still be present in the semen for many weeks.

Tubal ligation, on the other hand, requires major intraabdominal surgery with anesthesia in a hospital operating unit. Complications are those of comparable anesthesia and surgery. Hospitalization may be prolonged and postoperative recovery slow. This latter is acceptable when the sterilization procedure is being done at the same time as other indicated intraabdominal operations, such as cesarean section. Similarly, when done under an anesthesia that is being given for another reason, such as vaginal delivery, it is reasonable to operate; also when done during the first two to three days after a term delivery, it tends to be a relatively easy procedure because the puerperal uterus is enlarged and the tubes are held up out of the pelvis within easy reach through a small abdominal wall incision. At all other times and under other circumstances, tubal ligation must be considered a major undertaking with all the risks inherent in major abdominal surgery.

Tubal cauterization through a laparoscope is clearly preferable as an interval procedure. Although it does require general anesthesia for adequate pneumoperitoneum, the operation can be done quickly; hospitalization is short, lasting one or two days only; recovery is rapid; complications are few, but bleeding or bowel injury may occur and can be serious. Both Steptoe and Cohen report extensive experience with this technique, indicating its effectiveness, ease of performance and low morbidity.

Using carbon dioxide pneumoperitoneum (the gas administered by a transabdominal needle), one visualizes the pelvic organs by a fiber optic laparoscope inserted subumbilically; the midportion of one tube is grasped, cauterized and cut by a special instrument introduced through another opening in the lower abdomen; the other tube is then treated in the same way. The procedure cannot be done if the tubes are fixed by inflammatory or operative adhesions, hidden by bowel or involved in an inflammatory process.

There are several different techniques for tubal ligation, including Madlener, Pomeroy, and Irving operations in the order of their reported effectiveness. Garb found 1.44 per cent failure from Madlener procedures; 0.4 per cent after Pomeroy operations; and almost none after Irving sterilizations. The Madlener procedure is falling into disfavor because the other techniques are more certain of success.

The Madlener operation crushes and ligates a loop of the midportion of the tube using nonabsorbable suture; the Pomeroy sterilization merely resects a loop of the midportion and ligates the stump with absorbable catgut; the Irving procedure buries the proximal end of the divided tube in the myometrium. Nichols reviewed current practices and pointed out that, although the Irving technique is almost foolproof, it is technically more difficult and time consuming. He stressed the success of the *Uchida technique* which injects saline-epinephrine solution into the serosa of the tube to balloon the mesosalpinx for incision. The midportion of tube is delivered through the serosal incision and resected; 5 cm. is excised and ligated with chromic catgut; the proximal end is buried in the mesosalpinx and the distal end left protruding into the peritoneal cavity.

The *Pomeroy method* (Bishop and Nelms) of sterilization is simple, bloodless, requires only a few minutes and yields good results. The tube is grasped with an Allis forceps at about its midportion and elevated, thereby producing a loop (Fig. 463). A suture of plain No. 0 or 00 catgut is inserted through the mesosalpinx directly under this loop and both arms of the loop of tube are ligated. The segment of the tube above the ligature is excised. The same operation is performed on the opposite tube. When healing takes place, the two sealed ends of the cut tube separate for about 1 cm.

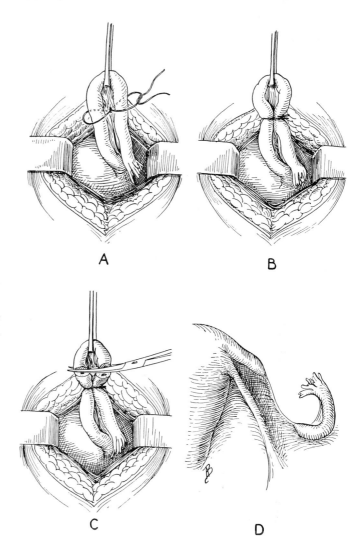

Figure 463 Pomeroy method of sterilization. *A*, One uterine tube is grasped at its midportion with an Allis clamp, and a ligature of plain catgut is placed around the loop. *B*, The catgut suture is tied. *C*, The loop of tube above the ligature is cut off. The same procedure is carried out on the other tube. *D*, The appearance of a tube some time after the Pomeroy operation has been carried out. The two ends of the cut have become sealed off and have separated widely.

The *Irving operation* is performed as follows (Fig. 464): In the bite of a clamp a tube is elevated 3 to 4 cm. from its cornual insertion. The mesosalpinx beneath this point is pierced by a hemostat in a bloodless area. The distal portion of the tube is ligated with No. 0 chromic catgut. Proximal to this, a double suture ligature of the same material, mounted on a half-curved, round-pointed needle and knotted about 7 to 8 cm. from its ends, is tied about the tube. The tube is divided between the two ligatures.

A stab wound is then made in the myometrium near the proximal end of the tube and spread open with a hemostat. A grooved director is inserted in this pit as far as it will go, and the half-curved needle on a needle holder is passed along the director to the extreme depth of the pit and brought out on the surface of the uterus. The director is removed. Traction on the suture ligature causes the tube to enter the pit. One strand of the double suture ligature is cut, a cross stitch is made in the superficial portion of the uterine wall and the free ends are tied, thus anchoring the tube deeply in the myometrium. The small wound at the point of entrance of the tube is closed with a figure-eight suture of chromic catgut, thus completing the operation. The distal portion of the divided tube is not treated in any way; it is not necessary to bury its cut end in the broad ligament.

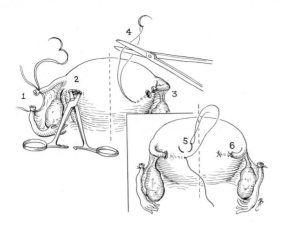

Figure 464   Technique of Irving sterilization operation. The tube is divided and ligated distally (1). The myometrium is tunnelled (2). The proximal end of the cut tube is pulled into the myometrial tunnel (3) and the traction suture cut (4). The tube is fixed in place by suturing to the serosa (5), and the myometrial opening is closed (6).

The other tube is treated in the same way

Sexuality is unaffected following tubal ligation or coagulation. It is important to stress this to the patient. Moreover, the procedure is immediately effective in preventing pregnancy. It is considered to be permanent; reanastomosis is possible, but requires another major surgical procedure and the results are poor at best. Hysterectomy as a means of sterilization may be justified when the uterus is diseased, but generally it carries so much more risk than tubal ligation that it cannot be rationalized on an elective basis.

REFERENCES

Advisory Committee on Obstetrics and Gynecology: Second Report on the Oral Contraceptives. Food and Drug Administration. Washington, Superintendent of Documents, U.S. Government Printing Office, 1969.

Bishop, E., and Nelms, W. F.: Simple method of tubal sterilization. New York J. Med. 30:214, 1930.

Calderone, M. S., ed.: Manual of Contraceptive Practice, ed. 2. Baltimore, Williams and Wilkins Company, 1969.

Cleary, R. E., and Dajami, R. M.: Current status of oral contraceptives. Med. Clin. N. Amer. 54:168, 1970.

Cohen, M. R.: Laparoscopy, Culdoscopy and Gynecography. Philadelphia, W. B. Saunders Company, 1970.

Garb, A. E.: A review of tubal sterilization failures. Obstet. Gynec. Survey 12:291, 1957.

Graefenberg, E.: Die Intrauterine Methode der Konzeptionsverhütung. In Haire, N., ed.: Proceedings of the Third Congress World League for Sexual Reform. London, Keegan, Paul, Trench, Trubner & Company, 1930.

Irving, F. C.: A new method of insuring sterility following cesarean section. Amer. J. Obstet. Gynec. 8:335, 1924.

Nichols, E. E.: Current practices in female sterilization in the United States: Incidence and methods. Amer. J. Obstet. Gynec. 101:345, 1968.

Steptoe, P. C.: Laparoscopy in Gynaecology. Edinburgh, E. & S. Livingstone Ltd., 1967.

Tietze, C., and Lewis, S.: The IUD and pill: Extended use-effectiveness. Fam. Plan. Prosp. 3:53, 1971.

INDEX

Note: Page numbers in *italic* indicate illustrations. Page numbers followed by t indicate tables.